TIMBY'S FUNDAMENTAL

Nursing Skills and Concepts

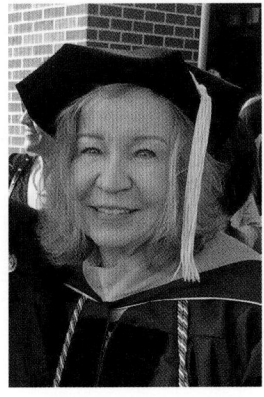

Loretta A. Donnelly-Moreno, DNP, RN, MSN

LVN/LPN Program Director
Nurse Faculty
Hallmark University
San Antonio, Texas

THIRTEENTH EDITION

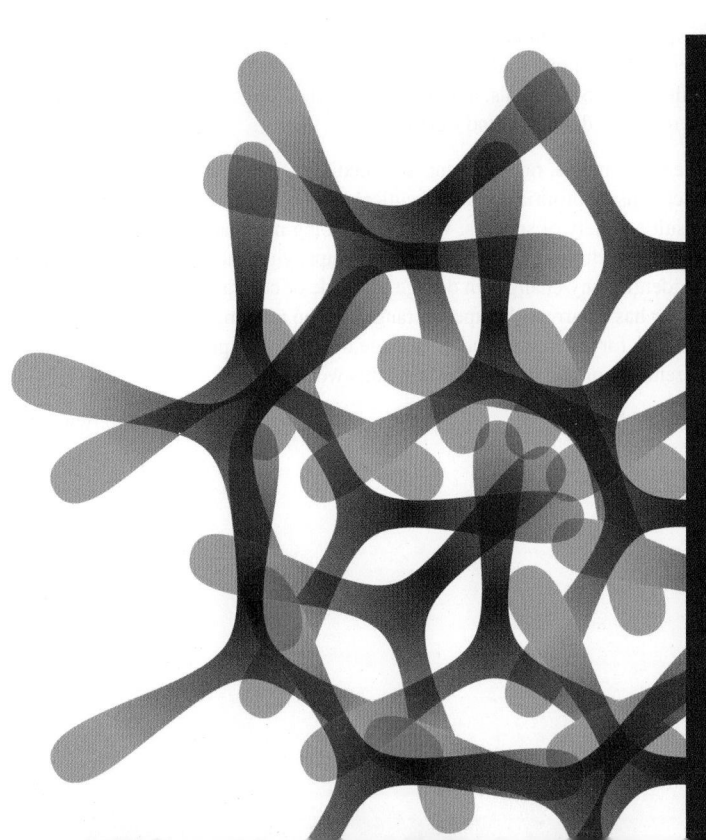

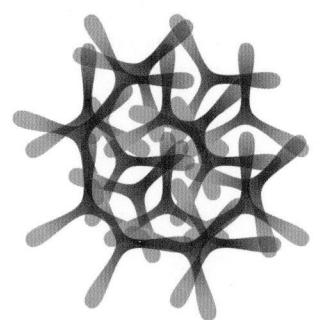
. Wolters Kluwer

Philadelphia • Baltimore • New York • London
Buenos Aires • Hong Kong • Sydney • Tokyo

Vice President and Publisher: Julie K. Stegman
Manager, Nursing Education and Practice Content: Jamie Blum
Senior Acquisitions Editor: Jonathan Joyce
Development Editor: Phoebe Jordan-Reilly
Editorial Coordinator: Erin E. Hernandez
Senior Production Project Manager: Catherine Ott
Marketing Manager: Wendy Mears
Manager, Graphic Arts & Design: Stephen Druding
Art Director, Illustration: Jennifer Clements
Prepress Vendor: S4Carlisle Publishing Services

Thirteenth Edition

9 8 7 6 5 4 3 2 1

Printed in Mexico

Library of Congress Cataloging-in-Publication Data available on request from publisher.

ISBN-13: 978-1-975220-77-8

Library of Congress Control Number: 2024913382

shop.lww.com

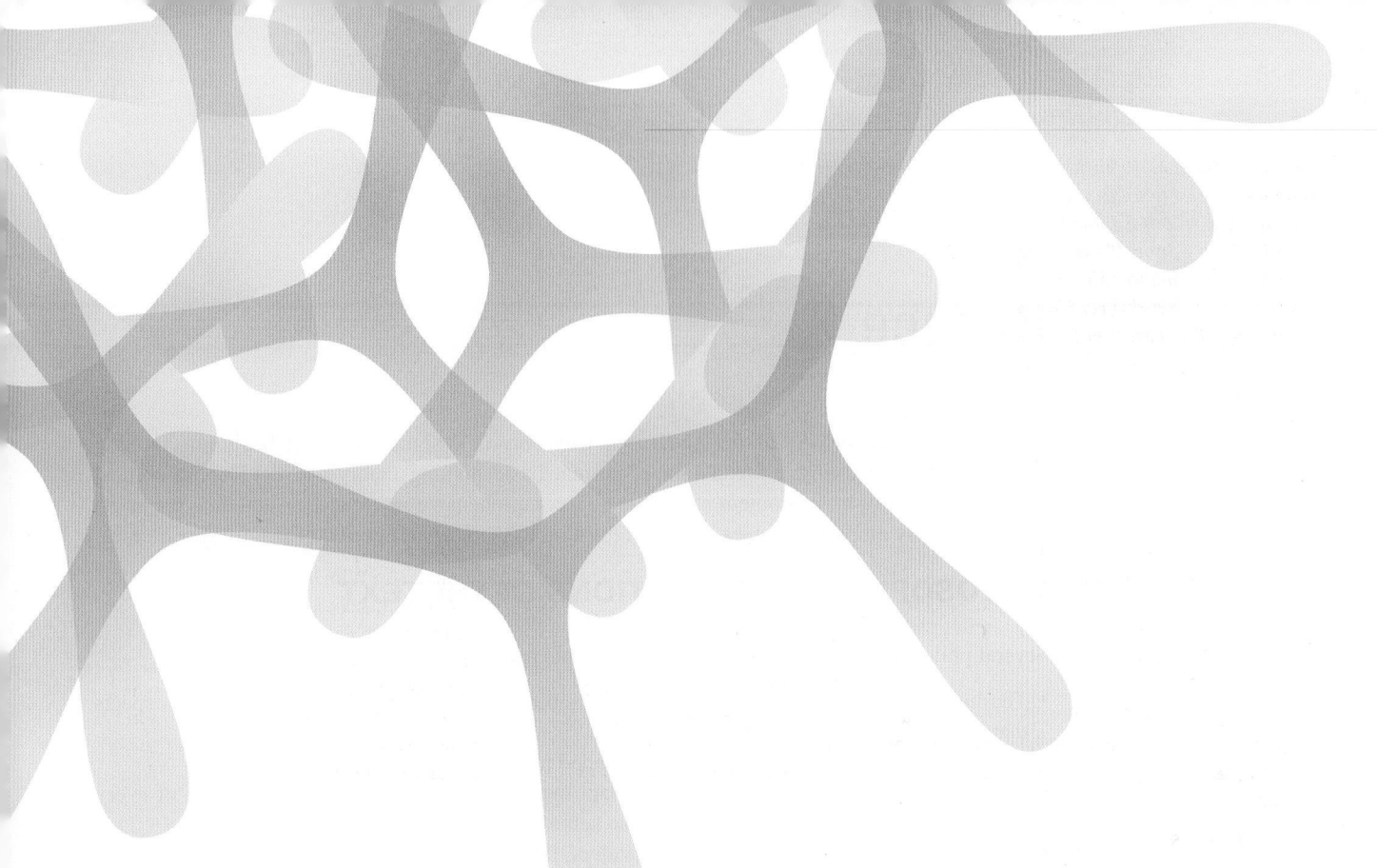

This edition of **Timby's Fundamental Nursing Skills and Concepts**
*is dedicated to all current and future nursing students. I hope this
fundamental nursing textbook supports and facilitates
students beginning their nursing careers.*

I am proud to be teaching in this wonderful and ever-changing profession.

*I also dedicate this book to my family, for all of their faithful support.
Thank you!*

—Loretta A. Donnelly-Moreno

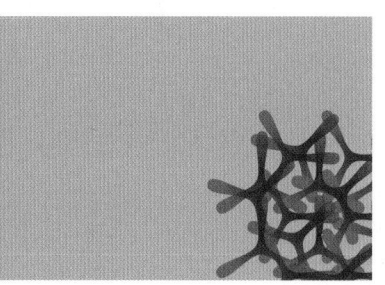

Preface

Timby's *Fundamental Nursing Skills and Concepts* is designed to assist beginning nursing students in acquiring a foundation of current basic nursing theory and developing clinical skills. In addition, its content can serve as a comprehensive reference for updating the skills of currently employed nurses or those returning to work after a period of inactive practice.

PHILOSOPHICAL FOUNDATIONS OF THE TEXT

Several philosophical concepts are the basis for this text:

- The human experience is a composite of physiologic, emotional, social, and spiritual aspects that affect health and healing.
- Caring is the essence of nursing and is extended to every client.
- Each client is unique, and nurses must adapt their care to meet the individual needs of every person without compromising safety or the achievement of desired outcomes.
- A supportive network of health care providers, family, and friends promotes health restoration and health promotion. Therefore, it is essential to include the client's significant others in teaching, formal discussions, and provision of services.
- Licensed and student nurses are accountable for their actions and clinical decisions; consequently, each must be aware of legislation as it affects nursing practice.

In today's changing health care environment, nurses face many challenges and opportunities. The 13th edition of *Fundamental Nursing Skills and Concepts* has been written to help nurses meet these challenges and take advantage of expanding opportunities.

NEW TO THIS EDITION

- **Current Lippincott Advisor nursing diagnoses and terminology.** The Lippincott Advisor diagnoses labels and definitions found in the Nursing Implications and accompanying Nursing Care Plans throughout the text have been updated according to the latest Lippincott Advisor Nursing Diagnoses, 2023.
- **Key Points.** At the end of each chapter, important information is included in outline format to assist the reader with studying key information from each chapter.
- **Gerontologic Considerations** have been moved to the beginning of each chapter. This reflects changes made to *Timby's Introductory Medical–Surgical Nursing* textbook.
- **NEXT-GENERATION NCLEX-STYLE REVIEW QUESTIONS** and clinical scenarios, with related questions, have been added to the chapters.
- **New Content.** The entire text has been revised and updated to reflect current medical and nursing practice. Additionally, several skills and sections contain pertinent content. The following are some highlights:
  - » Chapter 1, "Nursing Foundations," traces the origin and growth of nursing practice in the United States. It provides the current definition of nursing from the American Nurses Association and other theorists' explanations about the practice of nursing from Florence Nightingale to more contemporary nurses. This chapter introduces the term *evidence-based practice* and relates its significance to current nursing practice. Based on data provided by the U.S. Bureau of Labor Statistics, this chapter reinforces the projected increase in the demand for licensed practical nurses (LPNs) in a variety of health care settings. Because LPNs, as well as registered nurses (RNs), work with unlicensed assistive personnel (UAPs), Chapter 1 expands the

criteria for appropriate delegation. Updated statistics on enrollments and numbers of licensed nurses in various nursing programs demonstrate a continuing shortage of nurses as well as trends toward a demand for higher levels of nursing education, specialty certifications, and continuing education. The content describes the crises in health care and how efforts through federal legislation would somewhat help relieve the shortage of nurses in the United States. One example is the effort to continue designing ladder programs to advance the education of nurses from one level of practice to the next. In addition, it notes that the American Nurses Association and the National Council of State Boards of Nursing have endorsed the delegation of supportive nursing care to UAP, emphasizing that such delegation demands supervision and ultimate accountability on nurses who work with them.

» Chapter 2, "Nursing Process," defines and emphasizes the role of critical thinking in the nursing process. It continues to describe how creating nursing care plans promotes and refines the ability of students to think critically while gathering data that are significant and organizing the interventions for client care using evidence-based practice.

» Chapter 3, "Laws and Ethics," expands on the significance of the Health Insurance Portability and Accountability Act (HIPAA) in setting standards for ensuring the security of health information. It also reinforces that the National Practitioner Data Bank and Healthcare Integrity and Protection Data Bank track unfit health care practitioners within a database shared by licensing boards and health care facilities that hire nurses.

» Chapter 4, "Health and Illness," discusses various government-funded health programs. It provides statistics on enrollments in the Patient Protection and Affordable Care Act, a health reform law.

» Chapter 5, "Homeostasis, Adaptation, and Stress," relates to the body being in a stable state and how it reacts to stress using mechanisms of adaption. It describes the relationship between mind and body, and the physiologic and psychological stress responses.

» Chapter 6, "Culture and Ethnicity," updates the demographic information on the various ethnic groups that make up the population of the United States. This chapter also discusses various methods for communicating with deaf clients, clients who do not speak English, or those who speak English as a second language, including the use and certification of language interpreters. It introduces and defines integrative medicine, a new term for health care that combines conventional treatment with complementary and alternative medicine (CAM).

» Chapter 7, "The Nurse–Client Relationship," expands its discussion of special techniques to be used in communicating with older adults.

» Chapter 8, "Client Teaching," correlates the domains of client learning with the manner in which test questions on the National Council Licensure Examination (NCLEX) are classified according to their level of difficulty. It supports how questions in the Next-Generation NCLEX-Style Review Questions at the end of each chapter in the text are similarly classified. The chapter recommends using the "teach-back method" as a technique for confirming that a client has understood what has been taught by asking the client to repeat the information in their own words.

» Chapter 9, "Recording and Reporting," provides more information on electronic charting as well as its advantages and disadvantages.

» Chapter 10, "Asepsis," differentiates the rationales for broad- and narrow-spectrum antibiotic therapy. The mechanism of action for antiviral medications is explained. The World Health Organization's campaign identified as "Five Moments for Hand Hygiene" is provided to link hand hygiene with direct client care.

» Chapter 12, "Vital Signs," contains additional information on reasons why infants and older adults have difficulty maintaining normal body temperature. A more detailed discussion is provided on the correct use of infrared temporal thermometers, including circumstances when this type of thermometer is more advantageous than other types of thermometers. Assessing for postural hypotension is expanded with nursing measures for restoring or maintaining normotension.

» Chapter 13, "Physical Assessment," discusses cultural competence in physical assessments, including evaluating cultural biases in health care and the need to increase the diversity of languages used for health care resources.

» Chapter 14, "Special Examinations and Tests," includes the most revised guidelines from the American Cancer Society, the Association of Reproductive Health Professionals, and the American College of Obstetricians and Gynecologists (ACOG) regarding when women should be screened for cervical cancer and human papillomavirus infection.

» Chapter 15, "Nutrition," expands the information on trans fats, also known as partially hydrogenated oils (PHOs), to include the fact that the Food and Drug Administration (FDA) no longer considers PHOs safe in any human food and therefore mandates that food manufacturers remove them from their products. Values and significance for cardiac risk according to lipid laboratory test results established by the American Heart Association (AHA) have been updated.

» Chapter 16, "Fluid and Chemical Balance," contains more depth in explaining facilitated diffusion of glucose. The consequences of blood donation by individuals who have been actually or potentially exposed to Ebola are discussed.

» Chapter 17, "Hygiene," contains information on various types of assistive listening devices that amplify sounds, reduce the effect of distance between persons with hearing loss and the sound source, minimize background noise, and compensate for poor acoustics.

» Chapter 18, "Comfort, Rest, and Sleep," discusses how inadequate sleep is increasingly identified as a risk factor for obesity and is now considered an important lifestyle behavior linked to health. The stages of sleep and their characteristics have been revised and updated to correlate with the latest information on non–rapid eye movement (NREM) and REM sleep. Sleep requirements for various age groups have been revised to coincide with information from the National Sleep Foundation.

» Chapter 19, "Safety," reinforces the risk for latex allergy and measures that must be taken to prevent its occurrence. The pathophysiology of carbon monoxide poisoning is described as well as actions to take when victims succumb to its inhalation. Fall prevention is emphasized not only because falls are a leading cause of injury and death but also because the Centers for Medicare and Medicaid Services (CMS) will no longer cover the cost of care that was incurred by a fall. Private insurers are following a similar nonpayment policy.

» Chapter 20, "Pain Management," describes several pain theories that explain how pain is transmitted, perceived, and ameliorated. The list of common reactions of others who are in relationships with persons with chronic pain has been revised. The discussion of surgical approaches to pain relief has been updated in light of more recent less invasive techniques. The latest information on the "opioid crisis," with suggestions for alternative pain relief methods, is provided.

» Chapter 21, "Oxygenation," adds a discussion of the tripod position to improve breathing and the use of a BiPaP mask.

» Chapter 22, "Infection Control," elaborates on various classifications of infectious diseases with an emphasis on health care–associated infections. It refers readers to the Centers for Disease Control and Prevention (CDC) guidelines for infection control practices for Ebola, COVID-19, and other illnesses when caring for exposed or infected clients and health care workers returning to the United States. It also clarifies the sequence for removing personal protection equipment.

» Chapter 23, "Body Mechanics, Positioning, and Moving," added an algorithm for the safe transfer of clients to and from bed and integrated actions within related skills.

» Chapter 24, "Fitness and Therapeutic Exercise," has been retitled to reflect the current discussion on maintaining and improving general health and stamina. A table has been included for assessing fitness using a pedometer, and a discussion has been added on isokinetic exercise. The objectives of the health initiative *Healthy People 2030* are included.

» Chapter 27, "Perioperative Care," updates the Universal Protocol for Preventing Wrong Site, Wrong Procedure, Wrong Person Surgery, developed by The Joint Commission.

» Chapter 28, "Wound Care," adds to the discussion on wound healing. It includes additional information on types of dressings; describes maggot therapy and negative pressure wound therapy (vacuum-assisted closure); and notes that wet-to-dry dressings are now considered a substandard practice.

» Chapter 29, "Gastrointestinal Intubation," revises the information on determining tube location and the reasons why former assessment methods are no longer recommended. It revises information about gastric residual measurements and recommended actions and provides new information on methods for clearing an obstruction within a tube.

» Chapter 30, "Urinary Elimination," discusses the rationale for using soap and water versus antiseptic swabs when a clean-catch urine specimen is required. It eliminates the need to test the balloon before inserting a retention catheter because this is no longer necessary.

» Chapter 31, "Bowel Elimination," adds a discussion about fecal immunologic and stool DNA tests to detect colorectal cancer. It identifies current guidelines for endoscopic screenings for colorectal cancer.

» Chapter 32, "Oral Medications," includes a discussion about The Joint Commission's *Medication Management Standards* that requires hospitals to develop a list of look-alike/sound-alike medications they store, dispense, or administer to promote the safe administration of medications. It includes a reference to The Institute for Safe Medication Practices for a List of Confused Drug Names as well as error-prone abbreviations, symbols, and dose designations. It elaborates on the circumstances in which verbal and telephone orders are justified and on precautions the nurse must take in regard to these types of medication orders.

» Chapter 34, "Parenteral Medications," adds to the discussion about insulin pumps, and provides new information and guidelines regarding the glucose monitoring systems.

» Chapter 36, "Airway Management," elaborates on the parts of a tracheostomy tube. It adds information on how to obtain a sputum specimen using a suction catheter and mucous trap.

» Chapter 37, "Resuscitation," reflects the most recent changes in the AHA's chain of survival and the International Cardiopulmonary Resuscitation (CPR) and Emergency Cardiovascular Care (ECC) guidelines for performing basic life support techniques.

» Chapter 38, "End-of-Life Care," provides the most recent information regarding life expectancies in the United States, according to the CDC's National Center for Health Statistics. It describes the difference between a medical examiner and a coroner; identifies what types of deaths are reported to a medical examiner or coroner; explains the difference between a clinical autopsy and forensic autopsy; and includes the variations in preparing a body during postmortem care when a forensic autopsy will be performed. Updated information on "Living Wills" and "Advance Directives" is included.

• **Art and Photography Program.** Contemporary nursing practice is illustrated by the many full-color photos and line drawings. These illustrations assist visual learners to become familiar with the latest equipment, techniques, and practices in today's health care environment.

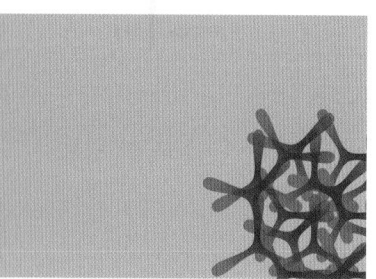

Features and Learning Tools

Table of Contents. Based on market feedback, Units 1 to 3 include chapters related to fundamental nursing concepts. Units 4 to 11 focus on fundamental nursing skills, beginning with Chapter 10, "Asepsis," to underscore the importance of hand hygiene and other aseptic practices when providing nursing care.

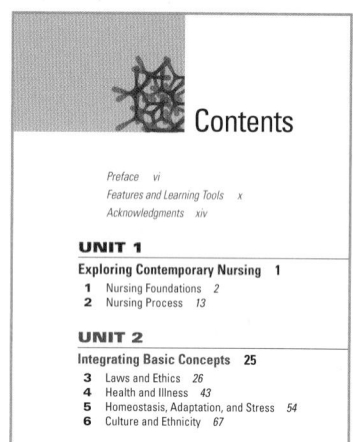

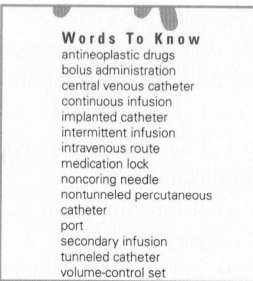

Words To Know. These key terms are listed at the beginning of each chapter and set in boldface type within the text where they appear with or near their definition. Additional technical terms are italicized throughout the text. Words To Know and their definitions can also be found in the glossary in alphabetical order.

Words To Know
antineoplastic drugs
bolus administration
central venous catheter
continuous infusion
implanted catheter
intermittent infusion
intravenous route
medication lock
noncoring needle
nontunneled percutaneous
catheter
port
secondary infusion
tunneled catheter
volume-control set

Learning Objectives

On completion of this chapter, the reader should be able to:

1. Name the types of veins into which intravenous (IV) medications are administered.
2. Describe appropriate situations for administering IV medications.
3. Describe one method for giving bolus administrations of IV medications.
4. Name ways by which IV medications are administered.
5. Describe methods for administering medicated solutions intermittently.
6. Explain the technique for administering a secondary piggyback infusion.
7. Discuss purposes for using a volume-control set.
8. Describe a central venous catheter (CVC).
9. Name types of CVCs.
10. Discuss techniques for protecting oneself when administering

Learning Objectives. These student-oriented objectives appear at the beginning of each chapter to serve as guidelines for acquiring specific information. They are numbered so that the corresponding student and instructor resources can be easily matched.

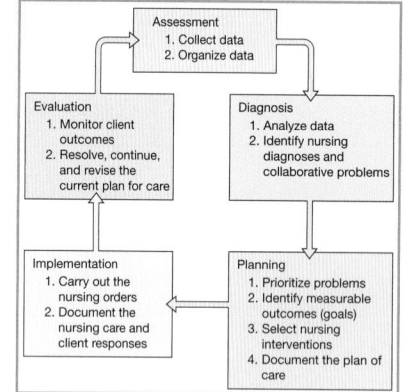

Nursing Process Focus. The focus on the nursing process continues to be strong. The concepts and paradigm for the nursing process appear in Chapter 2. The premise is that early familiarity with its components will reinforce its use in the Skills and sample Nursing Care Plans throughout the text. Each skills chapter has the most recent applicable nursing diagnoses that correlate with the types of problems recipients of the respective skills may have.

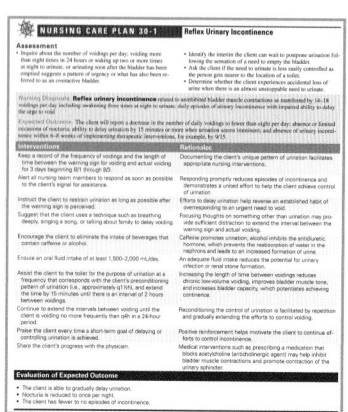

Nursing Care Plans. Nursing Care Plans are accompanied by a representative photo of a client and a description of a clinical scenario. This feature helps students identify with a "real person" and their subsequent individualized care. The diagnostic statements contain three parts for actual diagnoses and two parts for potential diagnoses. A double-column format lists interventions on one side and corresponding rationales on the other. The evaluation step is reinforced by evidence indicating expected outcome achievement.

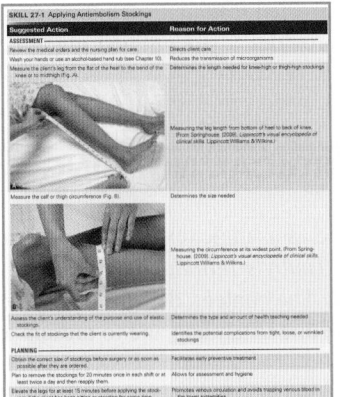

Skills. The Skills break down clinical skills that nurses use on a daily basis step by step. In addition, each illustration within the Skills has been closely reviewed to ensure that it complies with Standard Precautions and infection control guidelines from the Centers for Disease Control and Prevention.

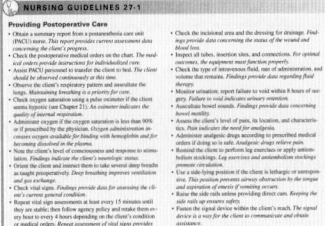

Nursing Guidelines. These mini-procedures provide directions for performing various kinds of nursing care, or suggestions for managing client care problems. Illustrations are included to facilitate visual learning.

Client and Family Teaching 27-1
Performing Forced Coughing

The nurse teaches the client and the family as follows:
- Sit upright.
- Take a slow, deep breath through the nose.
- Make the lower abdomen rise as much as possible.
- Lean slightly forward.
- Exhale slowly through the mouth.
- Pull the abdomen inward.
- Repeat, but this time cough three times in a row while exhaling.

Client and Family Teaching Boxes. These specially numbered boxes found throughout the chapters highlight essential education points for nurses to communicate to clients and their families.

CRITICAL THINKING EXERCISES

1. The following data are reviewed by a nurse preparing a client for surgery: The client is 60 years old; weighs 205 lb; has a history of chronic pulmonary disease; quit smoking 10 years ago; vital signs are BP 140/88 mm Hg, temperature 101.8°F, pulse rate 92, and respiratory rate 28 breaths/minute. Which finding is most important to report to the surgeon?
2. A client reports having taken only one shower with chlorhexidine gluconate rather than two the night before surgery. What actions could the nurse take?

Critical Thinking Exercises. Critical thinking questions appear at the end of each chapter to facilitate application of the material, using clinical situations or rhetorical questions.

NEXT-GENERATION NCLEX-STYLE REVIEW QUESTIONS

1. Assuming a client is admitted the evening before surgery, when is it best for the nurse to perform preoperative skin antisepsis and hair removal, if the latter is necessary, on a client who is scheduled for a procedure at 1300?
   a. The night before surgery
   b. After the morning shower
   c. Before transport to the receiving area
   d. When in the operating room
   Test-Taking Strategy: Note the key word, "best." Select the option that is better than any of the others for reducing the risk of a surgical infection.
2. What information is essential to verify during a presurgical time-out? Select all that apply.
   a. The client's room number
   b. The client's identity
   c. The name of the surgeon
   d. The name of the procedure
   e. The type of anesthesia
   f. The site of the procedure

NEXT-GENERATION NCLEX-STYLE REVIEW QUESTIONS. NCLEX-Style Review Questions help students apply their acquired knowledge by answering items that reflect the formats within the NCLEX-PN test plan. An effort has been made to include many alternate format items to assist students with the types of questions they will eventually encounter on their licensing examination, including using clinical scenarios with related questions, to reflect the next-generation NCLEX format.

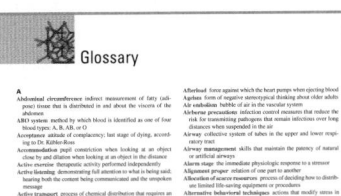

Glossary. Found at the back of the book, this is a quick reference of definitions for Words To Know that are used throughout the text. The glossary provides the key terms in alphabetical order.

Bibliography. This is a comprehensive listing of references and suggested readings, including general recommendations as well as unit-specific citations, which provides a streamlined guide to current literature about topics discussed in the text.

USE WITH INTRODUCTORY MEDICAL–SURGICAL NURSING

Timby's Fundamental Nursing Skills and Concepts may be adopted as a single text for students in a nursing program. Additionally, the book may be adopted with *Timby's Introductory Medical–Surgical Nursing* as well as *Lippincott's NCLEX-PN Review Book*. The content, designs, features, and styles of these texts have been coordinated closely to facilitate understanding and to present a consistent approach to learning.

TEACHING–LEARNING PACKAGE

The 13th edition of *Timby's Fundamental Nursing Skills and Concepts* features a compelling and comprehensive complement of additional resources to help students learn and instructors teach.

RESOURCES FOR STUDENTS

Valuable learning tools for students are available on thePoint®:

- **Concepts in Action** animations and **Watch and Learn** video clips demonstrate important concepts related to various topics explored in the accompanying text.
- Journal articles about relevant topics enable students to stay aware of the latest research and information available in the current literature.

RESOURCES FOR INSTRUCTORS

The above student-oriented materials are available for instructors on thePoint®. Additionally, instructors have access to the following tools to assist with teaching:

- An extensive collection of materials is provided for each chapter:

  » **PowerPoint presentations** provide an easy way to integrate the textbook with students' classroom experience, via either computerized slide shows or handouts.
  » **Guided Lecture Notes** walk instructors through the chapters, objective by objective, and provide corresponding PowerPoint slide numbers.
  » An **Image Bank** provides the photographs and illustrations from this textbook to be used in a way that best suits instructor needs, including in PowerPoint slides.

- A **sample syllabus** provides guidance for structuring a licensed practical nurse (LPN)/licensed vocational nurse (LVN) course.
- The **Test Generator** lets teachers assemble exclusive new tests from a bank containing more than 900 questions to help assess students' understanding of the material. These questions are formatted to match the NCLEX, so students can practice preparing for this important examination.
- Answer Keys for the Stop, Think, and Respond boxes, Next-Generation NCLEX-Style Review Questions, and Critical Thinking Exercises can be shared with students to check their comprehension of textbook presentations as desired.

LIPPINCOTT® COURSEPOINT

Lippincott® CoursePoint is an integrated, digital curriculum solution for nursing education that provides a completely interactive and adaptive experience geared to help students understand, retain, and apply their course knowledge and be prepared for practice. The time-tested, easy-to-use, and trusted solution includes engaging learning tools, evidence-based practice, case studies, and in-depth reporting to meet students where they are in their learning, combined with the most trusted nursing education content on the market to help prepare students for practice. This easy-to-use digital learning solution of Lippincott® CoursePoint, combined with unmatched support, gives instructors and students everything they need for course and curriculum success!

Lippincott® CoursePoint includes:

- Engaging course content with a variety of learning tools to engage students of all learning styles
- Adaptive and personalized learning to help students learn the critical thinking and clinical judgment skills needed to help them become practice-ready nurses
- Immediate, evidence-based, online nursing clinical-decision support with Lippincott® Advisor
- Unparalleled reporting that provides in-depth dashboards with several data points to track student progress and help identify strengths and weaknesses
- Unmatched support that includes training coaches, product trainers, and nursing education consultants to help educators and students implement Lippincott® CoursePoint with ease

BUILDING CLINICAL JUDGMENT SKILLS

Nursing students are required to obtain nursing knowledge and apply foundational nursing processes to practice effective clinical judgment. Being able to apply clinical judgment in practice is critical for patient safety and optimizing outcomes. The content provided in this text includes features such as Critical Thinking Exercises, Nursing Care Plans, and Next-Generation NCLEX-Style Review Questions that strengthen students' clinical judgment skills by giving them opportunities to apply knowledge and practice critical thinking. Additionally, accompanying products CoursePoint and Lippincott NCLEX-PN PassPoint provide an adaptive experience that allows students to build confidence by answering questions like those found on the Next-Generation NCLEX (NGN) examination.

A NOTE ABOUT THE LANGUAGE USED IN THIS BOOK

Wolters Kluwer recognizes that people have a diverse range of identities, and we are committed to using inclusive and nonbiased language in our content. In line with the principles of nursing, we strive not to define people by their diagnoses, but to recognize their personhood first and foremost, using as much as possible the language diverse groups use to define themselves, and including only information that is relevant to nursing care.

We strive to better address the unique perspectives, complex challenges, and lived experiences of diverse populations traditionally underrepresented in health literature. When describing or referencing populations discussed in research studies, we will adhere to the identities presented in those studies to maintain fidelity to the evidence presented by the study investigators. We follow best practices of language set forth by the *Publication Manual of the American Psychological Association*, 7th edition, but acknowledge that language evolves rapidly, and we will update the language used in future editions of this book as necessary.

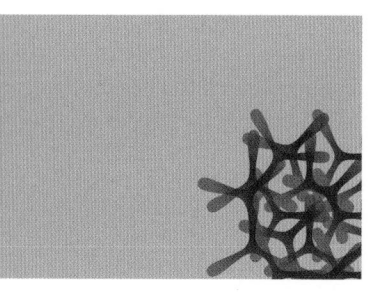

Acknowledgments

t is my belief that this text and its ancillary package will facilitate learning and produce safe, effective practitioners, capable of providing quality care for diverse clients in a variety of settings. Thanks go to the people at Wolters Kluwer for their help in preparing this book and for supporting the revision and new ideas and organization of the text material.

—Loretta A. Donnelly-Moreno

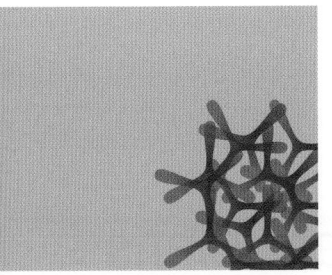

Contents

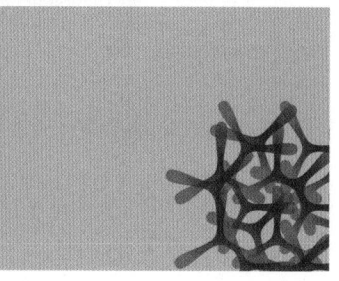

Quick Reference to Nursing Care Plans

UNIT 1 | Exploring Contemporary Nursing

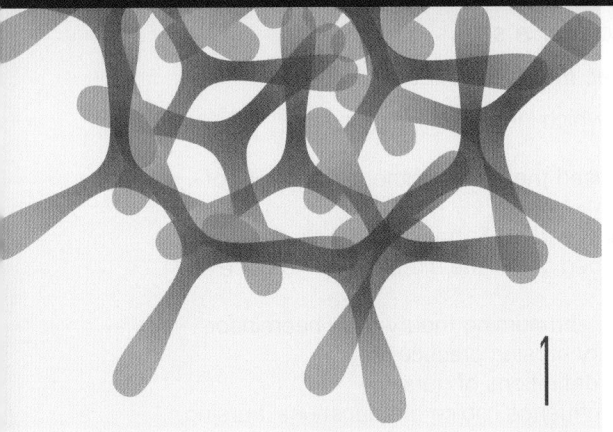

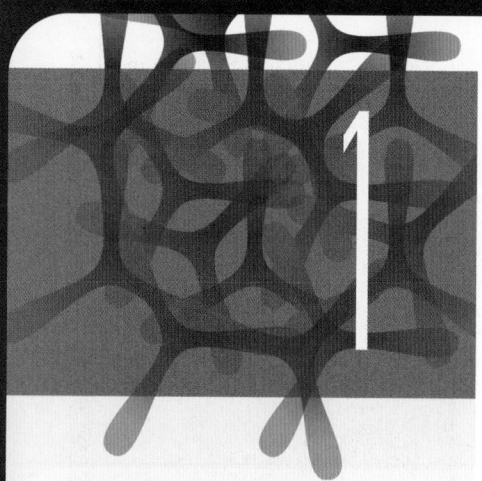

1

Nursing Foundations

Learning Objectives

On completion of this chapter, the reader should be able to:

1. Identify the reforms for which Florence Nightingale is responsible.
2. Name the ways nurses used their skills in the early history of U.S. nursing.
3. Describe the way in which early U.S. training schools deviated from those established under the direction of Florence Nightingale.
4. Explain how art, science, and nursing theory have been incorporated into contemporary nursing practice.
5. Discuss the evolution of definitions of nursing.
6. Identify the factors that influence choice of educational nursing program.
7. List types of educational programs that prepare students for beginning levels of nursing practice.
8. Explain the importance of continuing education in nursing.
9. List examples of current trends affecting nursing and health care.
10. Discuss the shortage of nurses and methods to reduce the crisis.
11. Describe four skills that all nurses use in clinical practice.

INTRODUCTION

This chapter traces the historical development of nursing from its simple beginning to its current sophisticated practice. Nurses in the 21st century owe a debt of gratitude to their pioneering counterparts who served clients in their homes, on battlefields, and in urban settlement houses. Ironically, nursing is returning to its original community-based practice model.

ORIGINS OF NURSING

Nursing is one of the youngest professions but one of the oldest arts. It evolved from the familial roles of nurturing and caretaking. Early responsibilities included assisting pregnant people during childbirth, suckling healthy newborns, and ministering to people with illnesses, older adults, and those with functional needs within households and surrounding communities. Its hallmark was caring more than curing.

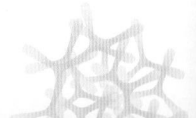

THE NIGHTINGALE REFORMATION

In the midst of deplorable health care conditions, Florence Nightingale, an English woman born of wealthy parents, announced that God had called her to become a nurse. Despite her family's protests, she worked with nursing deaconesses, a Protestant order of women who cared for the sick in Kaiserswerth, Germany. After becoming suitably prepared through her nursing apprenticeship, Nightingale embarked on the next phase of her career.

The Crimean War

While Nightingale was providing nursing care for residents at the Institution for the Care of Sick Gentlewomen in Distressed Circumstances, England found itself allied with Turkey, France, and Sardinia in defending the Crimea, a peninsula on the north shore of the Black Sea (1854 to 1856). Reports of high death rates and complications among the war casualties caused outrage among the British people. As a result, the government became the object of national criticism.

It was then that Nightingale offered a strategic plan: she proposed that the sick and injured British soldiers in Turkey would fare better if a team of women trained in nursing skills could care for them. Nightingale selected women who would accept the discipline and hard work necessary for this looming task.

The arrival of this group of women intimated to the soldiers that the men were incapable of providing adequate care. Jealousy and rivalry caused them initially to refuse any help from Nightingale and her 38 volunteers. When it became clear that the daily death rate, averaging about 60%, was not subsiding, the medical staff allowed Nightingale's nurses to work. Under Nightingale's supervision, the women cleaned the filth, eliminated the vermin, and improved ventilation, nutrition, and sanitation. In sharp contrast with the military orderlies, Nightingale made rounds at night with illumination from an oil lamp, comforting and caring for the war casualties and infirm. The practice led to her public persona as "the lady with the lamp."

Nightingale and her collective recruits helped lower the death rate to 1%. To show appreciation, donated funds were given to sustain her great work. Nightingale used this money to start the first training school for nurses at St. Thomas Hospital in England (Fig. 1-1). This school became the model for others in Europe and the United States.

Nightingale's Contributions

Nightingale changed the negative image of nursing to a positive one. She is credited with:

- Training women for future work
- Selecting only those with upstanding characters as potential nurses
- Improving sanitary conditions for the sick and injured
- Significantly reducing the death rate of British soldiers
- Providing classroom education and clinical teaching
- Advocating that nursing education should be lifelong

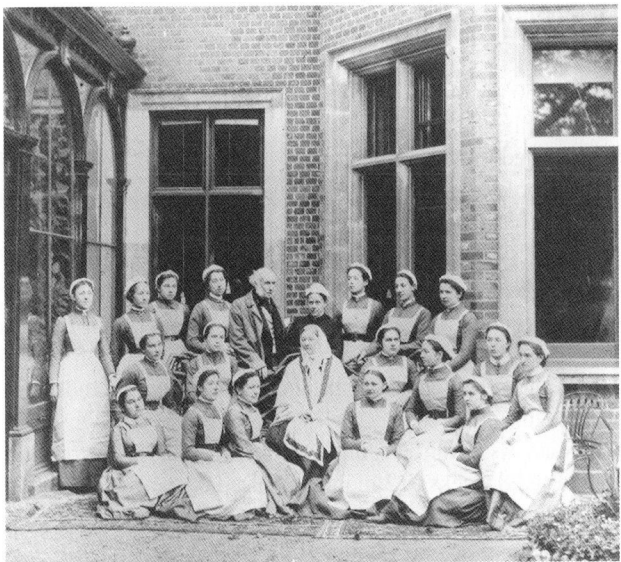

FIGURE 1-1 Florence Nightingale (center), her brother-in-law, Sir Harry Verney, and Miss Crossland, the nurse in charge of the Nightingale Training School at St. Thomas Hospital, with a class of student nurses. (Courtesy of The Florence Nightingale Museum Trust, London, England.)

>> *Stop, Think, and Respond 1-1*
How did Florence Nightingale convince the English and others that formal education of people who cared for the sick and injured was essential?

NURSING IN THE UNITED STATES

Colonial Period

In colonial times, there were no hospitals. By the late 1700s, a few were located in larger, more populous cities like Philadelphia and New York. For the most part, itinerant physicians practiced in isolated rural settings. The initial and extended care for people with illnesses and injuries, older adults, and pregnant people during childbirth often fell to female family members or kind neighbors in the community. With little more than experiential knowledge and a desire to relieve suffering, local women provided nursing care and temporarily carried out tasks such as housekeeping, laundry, and meal preparation for those entrusted to their care.

Civil War Nursing

The American Civil War occurred around the same time as the Nightingale reformation. Like England, the United States found itself involved in a war without any organized trained nursing staff to care for the sick and wounded. The military had to rely on untrained corpsmen and civilian volunteers, who were often the mothers, wives, and sisters of soldiers. They traveled with the troops from battlefield to battlefield giving supportive but inexperienced care.

Out of necessity, the Union government appointed Dorothea Lynde Dix, a social worker who had proven her worth by reforming health conditions for people with mental illnesses, to select and organize female volunteers to care for the troops.

In 1862, Dix followed Nightingale's advice and established the following selection criteria. Applicants were to be:

- 35 to 50 years old
- Matronly and plain looking
- Educated
- Neat, orderly, sober, and industrious with a serious disposition

Post–Civil War Nursing

Because women had demonstrated their commitment and value during the Civil War, there was some support for training women to meet peacetime health care needs. In 1890, one of the first courses for training "attendants for the sick" was begun in New York by the Brooklyn Young Women's Christian Association (Johnston, 1966). The brief training that lasted 8 weeks to 3 months focused on caring for people with chronic illnesses, adults, and children. It did not include any hospital experience. Later, the condensed training was extended to include home nursing skills such as household duties, hygiene, bowel regulation, bed changing, reading a thermometer, counting the pulse, and care of pressure injuries (Johnston, 1966).

Attendants for the sick were now referred to as practical nurse attendants. Later this title changed from "attendant nurses" to "practical nurses."

Nursing Schools in the United States

With the growing acceptance that work as a nurse was as respectable as teaching, sewing, and domestic service, more training schools for nurses began to be established. Unfortunately, however, the standards of these schools deviated substantially from those of the Nightingale paradigm. While planned and consistent formal education was the priority in Nightingale's schools, the training of nurses in the United States was like an unsubsidized apprenticeship. Eventually, the curricula and content of the U.S. training schools became more organized and uniform. Training periods lengthened from 6 months to 3 full years. Graduate nurses received a diploma attesting to their successful completion of training.

Expanding Horizons of Practice

Diplomas in hand, nurses trained in the United States began the 20th century by distinguishing themselves in caring for sick and disadvantaged people outside of hospitals (Fig. 1-2). Some nurses moved into communities and established "settlement houses" where they lived and worked among immigrants experiencing poverty. Others provided midwifery services, especially in rural Appalachia. The success of their public health efforts in administering prenatal and obstetric care, teaching child care, and immunizing children is well documented.

Like their previous counterparts, nurses continued to volunteer during wars. They helped fight yellow fever, typhoid, malaria, and dysentery during the Spanish–American War. During World Wars I and II, community hospitals needed more staff to assist nurses caring for civilians. Consequently, greater numbers of practical nurses and Red Cross–trained

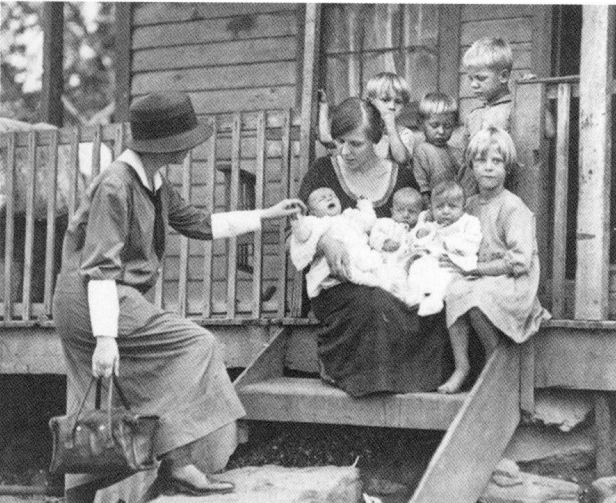

FIGURE 1-2 A nurse makes a home visit as did others during the late 1800s to early 1900s. (Courtesy of Visiting Nurse Association, Inc., Detroit, MI.)

aides were hired. They helped replenish the deficit caused by nurses pursuing careers.

During wartime, nurses worked alongside physicians in Mobile Army Surgical Hospitals (MASH). During the Korean War, nurses acquired knowledge about trauma care that later would help reduce the mortality rate of the U.S. soldiers in Vietnam. More recently, nurses again answered the call during the conflicts in Iraq and Afghanistan. Whenever and wherever there has been a need, nurses have put their own lives on the line.

CONTEMPORARY NURSING

Nursing is both an art and a science. During the 20th century, the nursing theories and nursing organizations developed to qualify, quantify, and codify what is now the profession of nursing.

Combining Nursing Art with Science

At first, the training of nurses consisted of learning the **art** (ability to perform an act skillfully) of nursing. Students learned this art by watching and imitating the techniques performed by other more experienced nurses. In this way, mentors informally passed skills on to students.

Contemporary nursing practice has added another dimension: science. The English word "science" comes from the Latin word *scio*, which means "to know." A **science** (body of knowledge unique to a particular subject) develops from observing and studying the relationship of one phenomenon to another. By developing an accumulating body of unique scientific knowledge, it is now possible to predict which nursing interventions are most likely to produce desired outcomes, a process referred to as **evidence-based practice**.

Integrating Nursing Theory

The word **theory** (opinion, belief, or view) comes from a Greek word meaning vision. For example, a scientist may study the relation between sunlight and plants and derive a theory of photosynthesis that explains how plants grow. Others who believe in the theorist's view may then apply the theory for their own practical use.

Nursing has undergone a similar scientific review. Florence Nightingale and others have examined the relationships among humans, health, the environment, and nursing. The outcome of such analysis becomes the basis for **nursing theory** (proposed ideas about what is involved in the process called nursing). Nursing programs then adopt a theory to serve as the conceptual framework or model for their philosophy, curriculum, and, most importantly, approach to clients. Similarly, psychologists have adopted and used Freud's psychoanalytic theory or Skinner's behavioral theory, for example, as a model for diagnostic and therapeutic interventions with clients.

Table 1-1 summarizes some nursing theories and how each has been applied to nursing practice. These are only a few of many; additional information can be found in current nursing literature and academic courses in nursing theory.

TABLE 1-1 Nursing Theories and Applications

THEORIST	THEORY	EXPLANATION
Florence Nightingale 1820–1910	**Environmental Theory**	
	Synopsis of theory	External conditions such as ventilation, light, odor, and cleanliness can prevent, suppress, or contribute to disease or death.
	Application to nursing practice	Nurses modify unhealthy aspects of the environment to put the client in the best condition for nature to act.
	Person	An individual whose natural defenses are influenced by a healthy or unhealthy environment
	Health	A state in which the environment is optimal for the natural body processes to achieve reparative outcomes
	Environment	All the external conditions capable of preventing, suppressing, or contributing to disease or death
	Nursing	Putting the client in the best condition for nature to act
Virginia Henderson 1897–1996	**Basic Needs Theory**	
	Synopsis of theory	People have basic needs that are the components of health. The significance and value of these needs are unique to each person.
	Application to nursing practice	Nurses assist in performing those activities that the client would perform if the client had the strength, will, and knowledge.
	Person	An individual with human needs that have unique meaning and value
	Health	The ability to independently satisfy human needs composed of 14 basic physical, psychological, and social elements
	Environment	The setting in which a person learns unique patterns for living
	Nursing	Temporarily assisting a person who lacks the necessary strength, will, and knowledge to satisfy one or more of 14 basic needs
Dorothea Orem 1914–2007	**Self-Care Theory**	
	Synopsis of theory	People learn about behaviors that they perform on their own behalf to maintain life, health, and well-being.
	Application to nursing practice	Nurses assist clients with self-care to improve or to maintain health.
	Person	An individual who uses self-care to sustain life and health, to recover from disease or injury, or to cope with its effects
	Health	The result of practices that people have learned to carry out on their own behalf to maintain life and well-being
	Environment	External elements with which people interact in the struggle to maintain self-care
	Nursing	A human service that assists people in progressively maximizing their self-care potential
Sister Callista Roy 1939–	**Adaptation Theory**	
	Synopsis of theory	Humans are biopsychosocial beings; a change in one component results in adaptive changes in the others.
	Application to nursing practice	Nurses assess biologic, psychological, and social factors interfering with health; alter the stimuli causing the maladaptation; and evaluate the effectiveness of the action taken.
	Person	A social, mental, spiritual, and physical being affected by stimuli in the internal and external environments
	Health	A person's ability to adapt to changes in the environment
	Environment	Internal and external forces in a continuous state of change
	Nursing	A humanitarian art and expanding science that manipulates and modifies stimuli to promote and to facilitate humans' ability to adapt

Defining Nursing

To clarify what nursing encompasses, for the public and nurses themselves, various working definitions have been proposed. Nightingale is credited with the earliest modern definition: "putting individuals in the best possible condition for nature to restore and preserve health."

Other definitions have been offered by nurses who are recognized as authorities, and therefore qualified spokespersons, on the practice of nursing. One such authority was Virginia Henderson (1897 to 1996). Her definition, adopted by the International Council of Nurses, broadened the description of nursing to include health promotion, not just illness care. As Henderson stated in 1966, "the unique function of the nurse is to assist the individual, sick or well, in the performance of those activities contributing to health or its recovery (or to a peaceful death) that he would perform unaided if he had the necessary strength, will or knowledge and to do this in such a way as to help him gain independence as rapidly as possible."

Henderson proposed that nursing is more than carrying out medical orders. It involves a special relationship and service between the nurse and the client (and the client's family). According to Henderson, the nurse acts as a temporary proxy, meeting the client's health needs with knowledge and skills that neither the client nor family members can provide.

In *Nursing's Social Policy Statement*, 3rd edition (2010), the American Nurses Association (ANA) defines nursing as:

- Protection, promotion, and optimization of health and abilities
- Prevention of illness and injury
- Alleviation of suffering through the diagnosis and treatment of human response
- Advocacy in the care of individuals, families, communities, and populations

The ANA (2010) further attests that six essential features characterize nursing: (1) provision of a caring relationship that facilitates health and healing; (2) attention to the range of human experiences and responses to health and illness within the physical and social environments; (3) integration of objective data with knowledge gained from an appreciation of the client's or group's subjective experience; (4) application of scientific knowledge to the processes of diagnosis and treatment through the use of judgment and critical thinking; (5) advancement of professional nursing knowledge through scholarly inquiry; and (6) influence on social and public policy to promote social justice.

These statements from the ANA demonstrate that nursing has an independent area of practice in addition to traditional dependent and interdependent functions involving physicians. As the role of the nurse evolves, the definition of nursing and the scope of nursing practice will undergo further revisions.

THE EDUCATIONAL LADDER

Two basic educational options are available to those interested in a nursing career: practical (vocational) nursing and registered nursing. Several types of programs prepare graduates in registered nursing. Each educational track provides the knowledge and skills for a particular entry level of practice. The following factors influence the choice of a nursing program:

- Career goals
- Geographic location of schools
- Costs involved
- Length of programs
- Reputation and success of graduates
- Flexibility in course scheduling
- Opportunity for part-time versus full-time enrollment
- Ease of movement into the next level of education

Practical/Vocational Nursing

During World War II, when many registered nurses (RNs) enlisted in the military, civilian hospitals, clinics, schools, and other health care agencies faced an acute shortage of nurses. To fill the void expeditiously, abbreviated programs in practical nursing were developed across the country to teach essential nursing skills. The goal was to prepare graduates to care for the health needs of infants, children, and adults who were mildly or chronically ill or convalescing so that RNs who remained stateside could be used effectively to care for acutely ill clients.

After the war, many RNs opted for part-time employment or resigned to become full-time homemakers. Thus, the need for practical nurses persisted. It became obvious that the role of practical nurses would not be temporary. Consequently, leaders in practical nursing programs organized to form the National Association for Practical Nurse Education and Service, Inc. This group worked to standardize practical nurse education and to facilitate the licensure of graduates. There are currently over 1,000 state-approved schools, in addition to many programs offered online and hybrid (combining in classroom and online education). To become licensed, graduates must successfully pass the National Council Licensing Examination for Practical Nurses (NCLEX-PN).

Career centers, vocational schools, hospitals, independent agencies, and community colleges generally offer practical nursing programs and arrange clinical experiences at local community hospitals, clinics, and nursing homes. The length of a practical nursing program averages from 12 to 18 months, after which graduates are qualified to take the licensing examination. Because this nursing preparatory program is the shortest, many consider it the most economic. Practical nursing programs are also considered as a stepping stone to associate and baccalaureate nursing degrees.

Enrollments in practical and vocational schools continued to attract candidates (Fig. 1-3). In 2022, a total of 47,635 U.S.-educated candidates passed the NCLEX-PN on the first attempt (National Council of State Boards of Nursing, 2018). Licensed practical nurses (LPNs)/licensed vocational nurses (LVNs) have a projected job growth of 12% from 2016 through 2026 (NCSBN, 2018). However, hospitals are not likely to be the primary employers. LPNs will in all probability secure positions in skilled nursing homes,

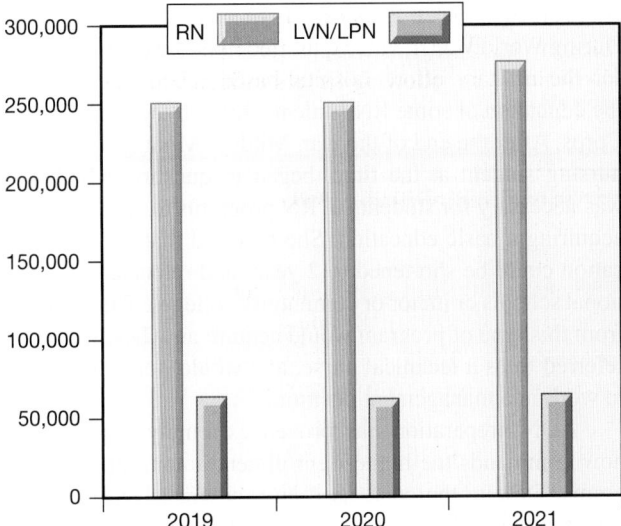

FIGURE 1-3 Trends in enrollments from 2019 to 2021 based on pass rates among LPN/LVNs and RNs who were candidates taking the NCLEX for the first time. LPN/LVNs, licensed practical nurses/licensed vocational nurses; RNs, registered nurses. (From National Council of State Boards of Nursing. [2021]. *2021 fact sheet*. https://www.ncsbn.org/publications/2021-nclex-fact-sheet)

physicians' offices, home health care agencies, outclient centers, residential care facilities, correctional institutions, and government agencies.

LPNs are a vital link between the RN and the **unlicensed assistive personnel** (UAP). They work under the supervision of an RN, physician assistant, physician, or dentist, but their role may be expanded to include supervision of UAPs in circumstances like long-term care (National Council of State Boards of Nursing). LPNs or LVNs in California and Texas provide nursing care to clients with common health needs that have predictable outcomes. The scope of practice is described in the nurse practice act in the state in which the nurse is licensed. Each state interprets the limits of practice differently. For example, in one state, an LPN may monitor and hang intravenous solutions, discontinue the infusion, and dress the site. The same may not be true in another state. An LPN also may delegate tasks to UAPs, who may or may not have acquired state certification. The LPN, therefore, must know the extent to which nursing assistants can function and the outcomes of their actions (see guidelines for delegation under "Registered Nursing"). Because of the geographic disparities in LPN practice, educational programs, and state regulations, the National Council of State Boards of Nursing (NCSBN) is researching and pursuing strategies to promote more consistency. Additional information on nursing practice standards for the LPN/LVN can be obtained from the National Federation of Licensed Practical Nurses (NFLPN) website. The ANA and the NCSBN have jointly endorsed delegating supportive nursing care to UAP. The role of UAPs is to assist licensed nurses with client care activities. UAPs must be trained and demonstrate competence for tasks carried out in a clinical setting. Client care provided by a UAP must be supervised by the delegating nurse who is ultimately accountable for the UAP's actions.

Opportunities for postlicensure certifications in pharmacology and long-term care are available through the National Association for Practical Nurse Education and Services, Inc. (NAPNES). Achieving certification via testing demonstrates knowledge above minimum standards. To provide career mobility, many schools of practical nursing have developed "articulation agreements" to help graduates enroll in another school or another program within the same school that offers a path to registered nursing through associate or baccalaureate degrees.

Registered Nursing

RNs work under the direction of a physician or dentist in various health care settings ranging from preventive to acute care. They provide and coordinate client care, educate clients and the public about various health conditions, and provide advice and emotional support to clients and their families. RNs care for clients who are stable but have complex health needs or those who are unstable with unpredictable outcomes. RNs delegate client care to LPNs and UAPs when appropriate.

Regardless of whether it is an RN delegating to an LPN or UAP or an LPN delegating to the UAP, delegation requires adhering to the following five guidelines:

- Right task: matching the client's needs with the caregiver's skills
- Right circumstance: ensuring that the situation is appropriate
- Right person: knowing the unique competencies of the caregiver
- Right directions and communication: providing sufficient information
- Right supervision and evaluation: being available for assistance; validating that the task was completed, obtaining the results, and analyzing if further actions are necessary (Barrow & Sharma, 2023)

Students can choose one of the three paths to become an RN: a hospital-based diploma program; a program that awards an associate degree in nursing (ADN); or a baccalaureate nursing program. All three meet the requirements for taking the national licensing examination (NCLEX-RN). A person licensed as an RN may work directly at the bedside or supervise others in managing the care of groups of clients.

Hospital-Based Diploma Programs

Diploma programs were the traditional route for nurses through the middle of the 20th century. Their decline became obvious in the 1970s, and the number of diploma programs continues to be lowest among other basic nursing educational programs (Fig. 1-4). The reasons for their decline are twofold. First, there has been a movement to increase professionalism in nursing by encouraging education in colleges and universities. Second, hospitals can no longer financially subsidize schools of nursing.

Diploma nurses were and are well trained. Because of their vast clinical experience (compared with students from other types of programs), they are often characterized as more self-confident and more easily socialized into the role requirements of a graduate nurse.

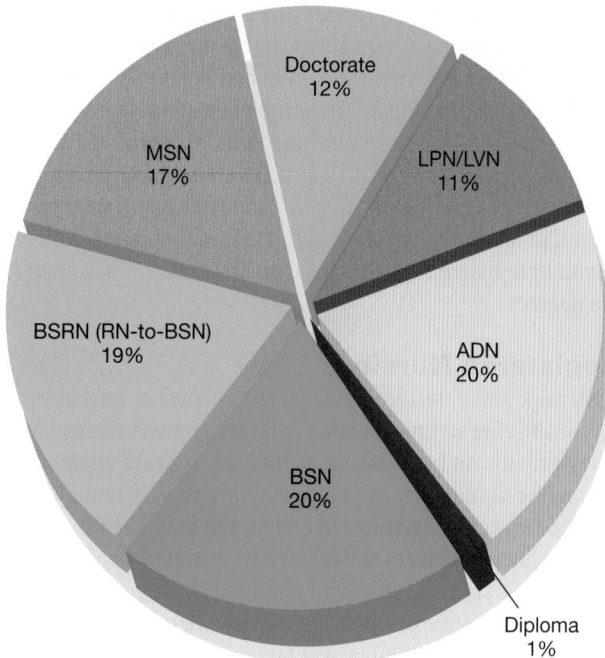

FIGURE 1-4 Enrollments in nursing programs by program type, 2021. ADN, associate degree in nursing; BSN, baccalaureate degree nursing; BSRN, bachelor of science registered nurse; LPN/LVN, licensed practical nurse/licensed vocational nurse; MSN, master of science in nursing. (From National League for Nursing. [2021]. *NLN faculty census survey 2020–2021.* https://www.nln.org/nlnNews/newsroom/nursing-education-statistics)

A hospital-based diploma program generally lasts 3 years. Many hospital schools of nursing collaborate with nearby colleges to provide basic science and humanities courses; graduates can transfer these credits if they choose to pursue associate or baccalaureate degrees later.

Associate Degree Programs

During World War II, when qualified nurses were being used for the military effort, hospital-based schools accelerated the education of some RN students through the Cadet Nurse Corps. After the end of the war, Mildred Montag, a doctoral nursing student at the time, began to question whether it was necessary for students in RN programs to spend 3 years acquiring a basic education. She believed that nursing education could be shortened to 2 years and relocated to vocational schools or junior or community colleges. The graduate from this type of program would acquire an ADN, would be referred to as a technical nurse, and would not be expected to work in a management position.

ADN preparation has proven extremely popular and now commands the highest enrollment among all RN programs. Despite the condensed curriculum, ADN graduates have demonstrated a high level of competence in passing the NCLEX-RN. Furthermore, ADN graduates are using this level of entry into practice as a springboard to higher programs of learning.

Application to nursing programs has been difficult for some because of the problems in transferring credits for courses they took during their diploma or associate degree programs. To increase enrollment, some collegiate programs are offering nurses an opportunity to obtain credit by passing "challenge exam initiations." Additionally, many colleges and universities provide satellite or outreach programs to accommodate nurses who cannot go to school full-time or travel long distances. Despite a renewed interest in acquiring a nursing education, approximately 25% of qualified LPN/LVN applicants for admission were rejected in 2021 (National League for Nursing, 14; Fig. 1-5). Qualified applicants are being rejected or waitlisted because (1) there

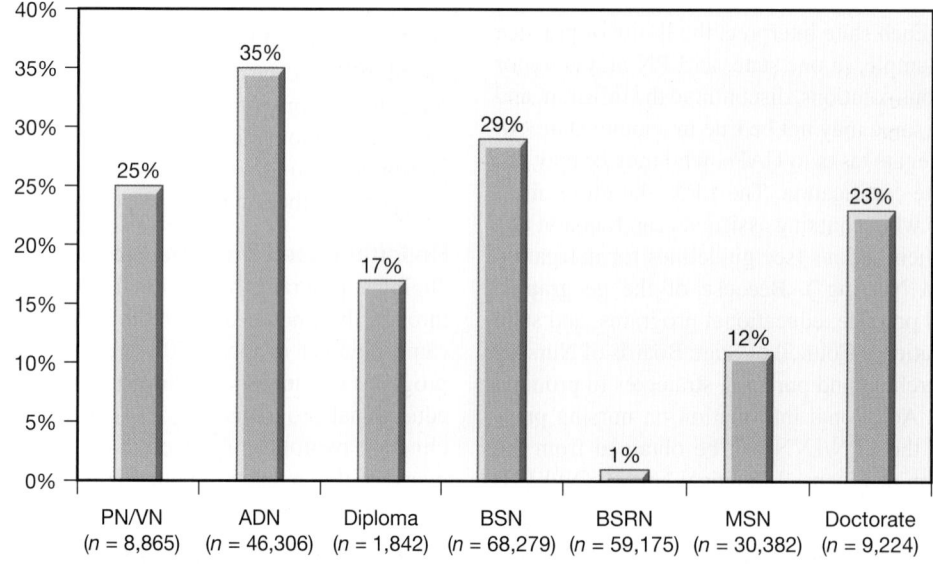

FIGURE 1-5 Percentages of qualified applicants turned away by program type in 2020 academic year. ADN, associate degree in nursing; BSN, baccalaureate degree nursing; BSRN, bachelor of science registered nurse; MSN, master of science in nursing; PN/VN, practical nurse/vocational nurse. (National League of Nursing. [2020]. *NLN biennial survey of schools of nursing 2020.* https://www.nln.org/docs/default-source/uploadedfiles/research-statistics/percentage-of-qualified-applications-turned-away-by-program-type-2020.pdf?sfvrsn=4a41a10d_0)

is a shortage of master's and doctoral-prepared nursing faculty who are available to teach required courses; (2) there is a lack of placements for clinical experiences; (3) there is a lack of space in educational institutions; (4) there are budget cuts among institutions that provide nursing programs; and (5) there is intense competition for selective admissions (American Association of Colleges of Nursing [AACN], 2022).

Baccalaureate Programs

Although collegiate nursing programs were established at the beginning of the 20th century, until recently they did not attract many students. Their popularity has been increasing at a progressive rate, perhaps because of proposals by the ANA, the National League for Nursing (NLN), and the Institute of Medicine (IOM) to establish baccalaureate education as the entry level into nursing practice. The deadline for implementation of this goal, once set for 1985, was delayed for three reasons:

- The date coincided with a national shortage of nurses.
- There was tremendous opposition from nurses without degrees, who believed that their titles and positions would be jeopardized.
- Employers feared that paying higher salaries to personnel with degrees would escalate budgets beyond their financial limits.

Although a baccalaureate preparatory program is the longest and most expensive, graduate nurses have the greatest flexibility in qualifying for nursing positions, both staff and managerial. Nurses with baccalaureate degrees are usually preferred in areas requiring substantial independent decision-making. They are more likely to be employed in hospital administrative positions, outclient care centers, public health, and home health nursing.

Graduate Nursing Programs

Graduate nursing programs are available at both the master's and the doctoral levels. These **advanced practice** nurses fill roles as clinical specialists, nurse practitioners, certified nurse anesthetists, certified midwives, administrators, and collegiate educators. Unfortunately, too few are pursuing advanced degrees in sufficient numbers to fill the positions vacated by retiring faculty. Although a graduate degree in nursing is preferred, some nurses pursue advanced degrees in fields outside of nursing, such as business, leadership, and education, to enhance their nursing careers.

Continuing Education

Continuing education in nursing is any planned learning experience beyond the basic nursing program. Nightingale is credited with having said, "to stand still is to move backwards." The principle that learning is a lifelong process still applies. Box 1-1 lists reasons why nurses in particular pursue continuing education. Many states now require nurses to show a prescribed number of hours as proof of continuing education to renew their nursing licenses.

BOX 1-1 **Rationales for Acquiring Continuing Education**

- No basic program provides all the knowledge and skills needed for a lifetime career.
- Current advances in technology make previous methods of practice obsolete.
- Assuming responsibility for self-learning demonstrates personal accountability.
- To ensure the public's confidence, nurses must demonstrate evidence of current competence.
- Practicing according to current nursing standards helps ensure care is legally safe.
- Renewal of state licensure is often contingent on evidence of continuing education.

TRENDS IN NURSING

"The federal government projects that more than 203,000 new registered nurse positions will be created each year from 2021 to 2031" (AACN, 2022). Two major issues dominate nursing today. The first concerns methods of eliminating the shortage of nurses. The second involves strategies for responding to a growing aging population with chronic health problems.

Health care officials hope that enrollment in all nursing programs and continuing education will reduce the current and projected critical shortage of nurses. However, the near future looks alarming.

Some factors contributing to the nursing shortage include:

- Increased aging population requiring health care
- Disappointing salaries for nurses with longevity employment
- Job dissatisfaction as a result of stress and the unrelenting rigor of working in health care
- Heavier workloads and sicker clients
- Policies regarding mandatory overtime
- Downsizing nursing staff from dwindling revenues and managed care policies
- Negative stereotypes about nursing as a traditionally female occupation
- More lucrative opportunities in nonnursing fields

Governmental Responses

The federal government has addressed the shortage of nurses by approving the American Recovery and Reinvestment Act in 2009. This legislation authorized:

- Loan repayment programs and scholarships for nursing students
- Funding for public service announcements to encourage more people to enter nursing
- Career ladder programs to facilitate advancement to higher levels of nursing practice
- Establishment of nurse retention and client safety enhancement grants
- Grants to incorporate gerontology into nursing curricula
- Loan repayment programs for nursing students who agree to teach after graduation (AACN, 2020)

Another governmental response was to implement the Affordable Care Act. With this act, the government funded innovative models of community-based care for older adults with chronic illnesses and created many new roles for nurses.

Proactive Strategies

Rather than taking a "wait-and-see" position about the nursing shortage and the ramifications of the Recovery and Reinvestment Act, many nurses have been and are proactively responding to the trends affecting their role in health care (Box 1-2).

BOX 1-2   Trends in Health Care and Nursing

Health Care
- The most underserved health care populations include older adults, ethnic minorities, and the poor, who delay seeking early treatment because they cannot afford it.
- Medicare and Medicaid benefits are being modified and reduced.
- Chronic illness is a primary health problem.
- Disease and injury prevention and health promotion are priorities.
- Medicine tends to focus on high technology, which improves outcomes for a select few.
- Hospitals are downsizing and hiring unlicensed personnel to perform procedures once in the exclusive domain of licensed nurses for cost containment.
- There are fewer primary care physicians in rural areas.
- Changes in reimbursement practices have created a shift in decision-making from hospitals, nurses, and physicians to insurance companies.
- Health care costs continue to increase despite **managed care practices** (cost-containment strategies used to plan and coordinate a client's care to avoid delays, unnecessary services, or overuse of expensive resources).
- **Capitation** (strategy for controlling health care costs by paying a fixed amount per member) encourages health providers to limit tests and services to increase profits.
- Hospitals, health care providers, and health insurance companies are required to measure, monitor, and manage quality of care.

Nursing
- Enrollments and numbers of graduates from LPN/LVN and RN educational programs are not keeping pace with projected shortages.
- More licensed nurses are earning baccalaureate, master's, and doctoral degrees.
- There continues to be a shortage of nurses in various health care settings because of decreased enrollments, retirement, attrition, and cost-containment measures.
- Hospital employment is decreasing.
- Client-to-nurse ratios in employment settings are higher.
- More high-acuity clients are in previously nonacute settings such as long-term and intermediate health care facilities.
- Job opportunities have expanded to outclient services, home health care, hospice programs, community health, and mental health agencies.

Nurses are dealing with the unique challenges of the 21st century by:

- Switching from part-time to full-time positions
- Delaying retirement
- Pursuing postlicensure education
- Training for advanced practice roles to provide cost-effective health care in areas in which numbers of primary care physicians are inadequate
- Becoming **cross-trained** (able to assume nonnursing jobs, depending on the census or levels of client acuity on any given day). For example, nurses may be trained to provide respiratory treatments and to obtain electrocardiograms, duties that nonnursing health care workers previously performed.
- Learning more about **multicultural diversity** (unique characteristics of diverse cultural groups) as it affects health beliefs and values, food preferences, language, communication, roles, and relationships
- Supporting legislative efforts toward national health insurance and other health care reforms that involve nurses in primary care (the first health care worker to assess a person with a health need)
- Promoting wellness through home health and community-based programs
- Helping clients with chronic diseases learn techniques for living healthier and consequently longer lives
- Referring clients with health problems for early treatment, a practice that requires the fewest resources and thus minimizes expenses
- Coordinating nursing services across health care settings—that is, **discharge planning** (managing transitional needs and ensuring continuity)
- Providing older adults with a variety of nursing services such as physical assessment during periods of illness, teaching, and managing medications, in assisted living facilities at less cost than care in nursing homes
- Developing and implementing **clinical pathways**, standardized multidisciplinary plans for a specific diagnoses, or procedures that identify aspects of care to be performed during a designated length of stay
- Participating in **quality assurance** (process of identifying and evaluating outcomes)
- Concentrating on the knowledge and skills to manage the health needs of older Americans over age 65 whose numbers will reach 95 million by 2060 (Population Reference Bureau, 2019)

UNIQUE NURSING SKILLS

Although employment locations and how they carry out **nursing skills** (activities unique to the practice of nursing) differ according to educational preparation, all nurses share the same philosophy. In keeping with Nightingale's traditions, contemporary nursing practice continues to include assessment skills, caring skills, counseling skills, and comforting skills.

Assessment Skills

Before being able to determine what care a person requires, the nurse must determine the client's needs and problems.

This requires the use of **assessment skills** (acts that involve collecting data), which include interviewing, observing, and examining the client and, in some cases, the client's family ("family" is used loosely to refer to the people with whom the client lives and associates). Although the client and family are the primary sources of information, the nurse also reviews the client's medical record and talks with other health care providers to obtain facts. Assessment skills are discussed in more detail in Unit 4.

Caring Skills

Caring skills (nursing interventions that restore or maintain a person's health) may involve actions as simple as assisting with **activities of daily living** (ADLs), the acts people normally do every day, for example, bathing, grooming, dressing, toileting, and eating. Increasingly, however, the nurse's role is expanding to include the safe care of clients who require invasive or highly technical equipment. This textbook introduces beginning nurses to the concepts and skills needed to provide care for clients whose disorders have fairly predictable outcomes. After this foundation has been established, students may add to their knowledge base.

Traditionally, nurses have always been providers of physical care for people unable to meet their own health needs independently. But caring also involves the concern and attachment that result from the close relationship of one human being with another. Nevertheless, the nurse ultimately wants clients to become self-reliant. Like a parent who continues to tie a child's shoes long after the child is capable of doing it themselves, the nurse who assumes too much care for clients often delays their independence.

Counseling Skills

A counselor is one who listens to a client's needs, responds with information based on the counselor's area of expertise, and facilitates the outcome that a client desires. Nurses implement **counseling skills** (interventions that include communicating with clients, actively listening during exchanges of information, offering pertinent health teaching, and providing emotional support) in relationships with clients.

To understand the client's perspective, the nurse uses therapeutic communication techniques to encourage verbal expression (see Chapter 7). The use of **active listening** (demonstrating full attention to what is being said, hearing both the content being communicated and the unspoken message) facilitates therapeutic interactions. Giving clients the opportunity to be heard helps them organize their thoughts and evaluate their situations more realistically.

When the client's perspective is clear, the nurse provides pertinent health information without offering specific advice. By reserving personal opinions, nurses promote the right of every person to make their own decisions and choices on matters affecting health and illness care. The role of the nurse is to share information about potential alternatives, to allow clients the freedom to choose, and to support the final decision.

While providing care, the nurse finds many opportunities to teach clients how to promote healing processes, stay well, prevent illness, and carry out ADLs in the best possible way. People know much more about health and health care today than ever before, and they expect nurses to share accurate information with them.

Because clients do not always communicate their feelings to strangers, nurses use **empathy** (intuitive awareness of what the client is experiencing) to perceive the client's emotional state and need for support. This skill differs from **sympathy** (feeling as emotionally distraught as the client). Empathy helps the nurse become effective at providing for the client's needs while remaining compassionately detached.

 Concept Mastery Alert

Health Promotion and Illness Prevention

Promoting health and preventing illness go hand in hand and are two major areas often addressed in client education. But there are subtle differences. Activities for promoting health focus on increasing a client's control over behaviors to maintain health. It is broad and nonspecific in scope. An example would be a heart-healthy diet. Preventing illness, however, is more specific, focusing on reducing risk factors as well as measures to slow or stop the progression of the illness and minimize its effects. Smoking cessation is an example of preventing illness.

Comforting Skills

Nightingale's presence and the light from her lamp communicated comfort to the frightened British soldiers in the 19th century. As a result of that heritage, contemporary nurses understand that illness often causes feelings of insecurity that may threaten the client's or family's ability to cope; they may feel vulnerable. At this point, the nurse uses **comforting skills** (interventions that provide stability and security during a health-related crisis). The nurse becomes the client's guide, companion, and interpreter. This supportive relationship generally increases trust and reduces fear and worry.

As a result of one woman's efforts, modern nursing was born. It has continued to mature and flourish ever since. The skills Nightingale performed on a grand scale are repeated today during each and every nurse–client interaction.

》》 Stop, Think, and Respond 1-2

Identify the following nursing actions as assessment skills, caring skills, counseling skills, or comforting skills: (a) the nurse discusses with a family the progress of a client undergoing surgery; (b) the nurse provides information on advance directives, which allows a client to identify end-of-life decisions; (c) the nurse asks a client to identify their current health problems; (d) the nurse provides medication for a client in pain.

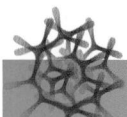

- Florence Nightingale helped reform nursing by changing the negative image of nursing to a positive one, recommending basic care of improved ventilation, nutrition, and sanitation.
- Contemporary nursing combined the art of nursing with science, creating evidence-based nursing.
- Nursing is defined by:
  - Protection, promotion, and optimization of health and abilities
  - Prevention of illness and injury
  - Alleviation of suffering through the diagnosis and treatment of human response
  - Advocacy in the care of individuals, families, communities, and populations

- Licensed nursing can be achieved through four different educational programs:
  - LPN/LVN
  - Associate degree RN (ADN)
  - Hospital-based diploma nursing RN
  - Baccalaureate degree nursing RN (BSN)
- Future trends in nursing focus on the nursing shortage and the increase in the aging population.
- The unique skills the nurses learn in nursing school are:
  - Assessment skills
  - Caring skills
  - Counseling skills
  - Comforting skills

CRITICAL THINKING EXERCISES

1. Describe some outcomes that may result if the nursing shortage is not reduced or resolved.
2. There are four major categories of questions on the NCLEX-PN: safe and effective care environment; health promotion and maintenance; psychosocial integrity; and physiologic integrity (refer to NCSBN, 2022; 2023 NCLEX-PN Detailed Test Plan). Based on your personal experiences during wellness or illness care, identify nursing skills (other than those in Stop, Think, and Respond Box 1-2) that would be examples of each of the four NCLEX-PN categories.
3. How might the shortage of RNs affect LPNs both positively and negatively?
4. If Florence Nightingale were alive today, how might she view the current education and practice of nursing?

NEXT-GENERATION NCLEX-STYLE REVIEW QUESTIONS

1. Before delegating the task of assessing a client's blood glucose to a UAP, what should the LPN do first?
   a. Review the client's trends in blood glucose measurements.
   b. Check the diabetic medications prescribed for the client.
   c. Determine whether the UAP is qualified to check the blood glucose.
   d. Assess what the client knows about controlling blood glucose.
   Test-Taking Strategy: Note the key word, "first." Apply principles concerning delegation to select an answer.
2. After receiving an assignment from the RN in charge, list in order of priority (a-d), which client the LPN would assess first.
   a. Client A, who will be discharged in the morning
   b. Client B, who returned from surgery an hour ago

   c. Client C, who received recent pain medication
   d. Client D, who has not urinated in 4 hours
   Test-Taking Strategy: Note the key word, "first."
3. Number the first to fourth options by priority. What information is most important for an LPN to obtain during a report on an assigned postoperative client?
   a. The client's age
   b. The client's occupation
   c. The client's last consumption of food
   d. The client's most recent blood pressure
   Test-Taking Strategy: Note the key word and modifier, "most important." Select the option that reflects the most pertinent data about the client's current condition.
4. After an LPN delegates the assessment of a client's blood pressure to a UAP, what is the most important action to take next?
   a. Check the results of the delegated task.
   b. Recheck the client's blood pressure.
   c. Teach the client about controlling blood pressure.
   d. Assess the client's family history for heart disease.
   Test-Taking Strategy: Note the key word and modifier, "most important." Recall that the person who delegates a task is still ultimately responsible for it.
5. When an RN determines an LPN's assignment, which client assignment is most reasonable for the LPN to question?
   a. Client A, who has unrelieved chest pain
   b. Client B, whose fractured leg is in traction
   c. Client C, who is recovering after an appendectomy
   d. Client D, whose white blood cell count is elevated
   Test-Taking Strategy: Note the key word and modifier, "most reasonable." Use the process of elimination to select the client whose outcome is least predictable.

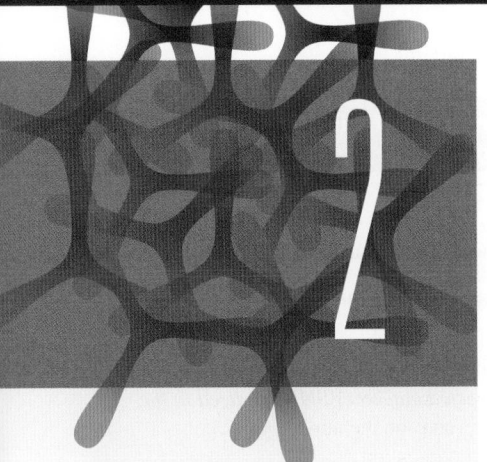

Nursing Process

Words To Know

assessment
collaborative problems
critical thinking
database assessment
diagnosis
evaluation
focus assessment
functional assessment
goals
health promotion diagnosis
implementation
long-term goals
nursing care plans
nursing diagnosis
nursing orders
nursing process
objective data
outcome criteria
planning
problem-focused diagnosis
risk diagnosis
short-term goals
signs
standards for care
subjective data
symptoms
syndrome diagnosis
The Joint Commission

Learning Objectives

On completion of this chapter, the reader should be able to:

1. Define the term "nursing process."
2. Describe the characteristics of the nursing process.
3. List the steps of the nursing process.
4. Identify sources of assessment data.
5. Differentiate among database, focus, and functional assessments.
6. List the parts of a nursing diagnostic statement.
7. Distinguish between a nursing diagnosis and a collaborative problem.
8. Describe the rationale for setting priorities.
9. Discuss appropriate circumstances for short- and long-term goals.
10. Identify ways to document a plan of care.
11. Describe the information that is documented in a plan of care.
12. Discuss the outcomes that result from an evaluation.
13. Identify learning strategies used by educators to help students implement the nursing process.

INTRODUCTION

In the past, nursing practice consisted of actions based mostly on common sense and the examples set by older, more experienced nurses. The actual care of clients tended to be limited to the physician's medical orders. Although nurses today continue to work interdependently with physicians and other health care providers, they now plan and implement client care more independently. Nurses are held responsible and accountable for providing client care that is safe and appropriate and reflects currently accepted standards for nursing practice.

 Gerontologic Considerations

■ All Medicare- and Medicaid-funded nursing homes and home care agencies must periodically complete the Minimum Data Set (MDS) for Resident Assessment and Care Screening to document a client's functional assessment. The MDS is widely recognized as a standardized tool for improving care based on ongoing assessments.

DEFINITION OF THE NURSING PROCESS

A process is a set of actions leading to a particular goal. The **nursing process** is an organized sequence of problem-solving steps used to identify and manage the health problems of clients (Fig. 2-1). Although the sequence appears to progress from one step to the next in a circular fashion, in actual practice, it is a dynamic process of interacting feedback loops among the various components.

The nursing process is the infrastructure of nursing practice in all health care settings. When nursing practice follows the nursing process, clients receive quality care in minimal time with maximal efficiency. Nurse practice acts hold nurses accountable for demonstrating all the steps in the nursing process when caring for clients. To do less implies negligence. Its importance is further evidenced by the fact that the nursing process is the foundation for the national licensing examinations and other nursing testing services such as those of the National League for Nursing. It serves as the basis for the standards of the American Nurses Association (Box 2-1). In addition, the nursing process serves as a framework for nursing documentation in medical records, and when medical records are subpoenaed for court cases.

CHARACTERISTICS OF THE NURSING PROCESS

The nursing process has seven distinct characteristics:

- *Within the legal scope of nursing.* Most state nurse practice acts define nursing as an independent problem-solving role that involves the diagnosis and treatment of human responses to actual or potential health problems.
- *Based on knowledge.* The ability to identify and resolve client problems requires **critical thinking**, which is a process of objective reasoning or analyzing facts to reach a

| BOX 2-1 | Standards of Clinical Nursing Practice |

Standard I—Assessment
The nurse collects patient health data.

Standard II—Diagnosis
The nurse analyzes the assessment data to determine diagnoses.

Standard III—Outcome Identification
The nurse identifies expected outcomes individualized to the patient.

Standard IV—Planning
The nurse develops a plan of care that prescribes interventions to attain expected outcomes.

Standard V—Implementation
The nurse implements the interventions identified in the plan of care.

Standard VI—Evaluation
The nurse evaluates the patient's progress toward attainment of outcomes.

American Nurses Association. (2021). *Nursing: Scope and standards of practice* (4th ed.).

valid conclusion. Critical thinking enables nurses to determine which problems necessitate collaboration with the physician and which fall within the independent domain of nursing. Critical thinking helps nurses select appropriate evidence-based nursing interventions for achieving predictable outcomes.

- *Planned.* The steps of the nursing process are organized and systematic. One step leads to the next in an orderly and interrelated fashion.
- *Client-centered.* The nursing process makes it easier to formulate a comprehensive and unique plan of care for each client. Clients are expected, whenever possible, to be actively included in participating in their care.
- *Goal-directed.* The nursing process involves a united effort between the client and the nursing team to achieve desired outcomes.
- *Prioritized.* The nursing process provides a focused way to resolve the problems that represent the greatest threat to the client's health.
- *Dynamic.* Because the health status of any client is constantly changing, the nursing process acts like a continuous loop. Evaluation, the last step in the nursing process, involves data collection, beginning the process again.

STEPS OF THE NURSING PROCESS

The steps of the nursing process, each of which is discussed in detail throughout this chapter, are as follows:

1. Assessment
2. Diagnosis
3. Planning
4. Implementation
5. Evaluation

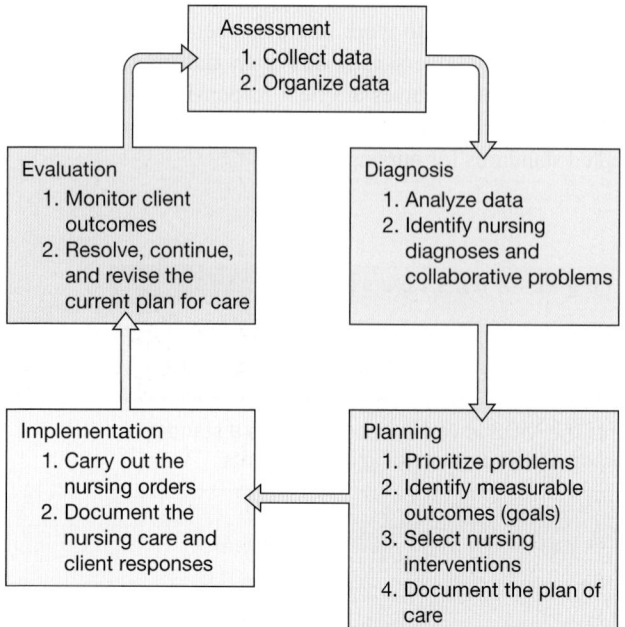

FIGURE 2-1 The steps in the nursing process.

TABLE 2-1 Levels of Responsibilities for the Nursing Process

	PRACTICAL/VOCATIONAL NURSE	ASSOCIATE DEGREE NURSE	BACCALAUREATE NURSE
Assessing	Gathers data by interviewing, observing, and performing a basic physical examination of people with common health problems with predictable outcomes	Collects data from people with complex health problems with unpredictable outcomes, their families, medical records, and other health team members	Identifies the information needed from individuals or groups to provide an appropriate nursing database
Diagnosing	Contributes to the development of nursing diagnoses by reporting abnormal assessment data	Uses a classification list to write a nursing diagnostic statement, including the problem, its etiology, and signs and symptoms Identifies problems that require collaboration with the physician	Conducts clinical testing of approved nursing diagnoses Proposes new diagnostic categories for consideration and approval
Planning	Assists in setting realistic and measurable goals Suggests nursing actions that can prevent, reduce, or eliminate health problems with predictable outcomes Assists in developing a written plan of care	Sets realistic, measurable goals Develops a written individualized plan of care with specific nursing orders that reflect the standards for nursing practice	Develops written standards for nursing practice Plans care for healthy or sick individuals or groups in structured health care agencies or the community
Implementing	Performs basic nursing care under the direction of an RN	Identifies priorities Directs others to carry out nursing orders	Applies nursing theory to the approaches used for resolving actual and potential health problems of individuals or groups
Evaluating	Shares observations on the progress of the client in reaching established goals Contributes to the revision of the plan of care	Evaluates the outcomes of nursing care routinely Revises the plan of care	Conducts research on nursing activities that may be improved with further study

Note that each more advanced practitioner can perform the responsibilities of those identified previously.

RN, registered nurse.

Licensed practical nurses (LPNs) and registered nurses (RNs) have different responsibilities related to the nursing process (Table 2-1). For example, RNs may delegate some parts of an initial assessment to an LPN, but the RN is still responsible for ensuring that data collection is complete. After obtaining the assessment data, the RN develops the initial plan of care. Differences exist in various locales as to whether the LPN makes changes to the plan of care independently or collaboratively with the RN (National Council of State Boards of Nursing, 2022).

Assessment

Assessment, the first step in the nursing process, is the systematic collection of facts or data. Assessment begins with the nurse's first contact with a client and continues as long as a need for health care exists. During assessment, the nurse collects information to determine areas of abnormal function, risk factors that contribute to health problems, and client strengths.

Types of Data

Data are either objective or subjective (Box 2-2). **Objective data** are observable and measurable facts and are referred to as **signs** of a disorder. An example is a client's blood pressure measurement. **Subjective data** are information that only the client feels and can describe, and these are called **symptoms**. An example is pain.

>> *Stop, Think, and Respond 2-1*

Which of the following represents objective data?

- *A client rates his pain as 8 on a scale of 0 to 10, with 10 being the most pain he has ever experienced.*
- *A client has an incisional scar in the right lower quadrant of the abdomen.*
- *A client says she slept well and feels rested.*
- *A client's blood pressure is 165/86 mm Hg.*
- *A client's heart rate is irregular.*

BOX 2-2 | **Examples of Objective and Subjective Data**

Objective Data	Subjective Data
Weight	Pain
Temperature	Nausea
Skin color	Depression
Blood cell count	Fatigue
Vomiting	Anxiety
Bleeding	Loneliness

Sources of Data

The primary source of information is the client. Secondary sources include the client's family, reports, test results, information in current and past medical records, and discussions with other health care providers.

Types of Assessments

There are three types of assessments: database assessment, focus assessment, and functional assessment (Table 2-2).

Database Assessment

A **database assessment** (initial information about the client's physical, emotional, social, and spiritual health) is lengthy and comprehensive. The nurse obtains database information during the admission interview and physical examination (see Chapter 13). Health care facilities generally provide a form that is printed or available on a computer for use as a guide (Fig. 2-2). Information obtained during a database assessment serves as a reference for comparing all future data and provides the evidence used to identify the client's initial problems. Comparisons of ongoing assessments with baseline data help determine whether the client's health is improving, deteriorating, or remaining unchanged.

Focus Assessment

A **focus assessment** is information that provides more details about specific problems and expands the original database. For instance, if during the initial interview the client tells the nurse that they are constipated more often than not, more questions follow. The nurse obtains data about the client's dietary habits, level of activity, fluid intake, current medications, frequency of bowel elimination, and stool characteristics. The nurse may ask the client to save a stool for inspection.

Focus assessments are generally repeated frequently or on a scheduled basis to determine trends in a client's condition and responses to therapeutic interventions. Examples include conducting postoperative surgical assessments (see Chapter 27), monitoring the client's level of pain before and after administering medications, and checking the neurologic status of a client with a head injury.

Functional Assessment

A **functional assessment** is a comprehensive evaluation of a client's physical strengths and weaknesses in areas such as (1) the performance of activities of daily living (see Box 2-3 for an example that relates to bathing); (2) cognitive abilities; and (3) social functioning. The results of the functional assessment help formulate an individualized plan for care that identifies specific interventions for achieving the maximum possible functioning to ensure a better quality of life.

Organization of Data

Interpreting data is easier if information is organized. Organization involves grouping related information. For example, consider the following list of words: apple, wheels, orchard, pedals, tree, and handlebars. At first glance, they appear to be a jumble of terms. If asked to cluster the related terms, however, most people would correctly group apple, tree, and orchard together, and wheels, pedals, and handlebars together.

>>> *Stop, Think, and Respond 2-2*
Organize the following data into two related clusters: cough, dry skin, infrequent urination, fever, nasal congestion, and thirst.

TABLE 2-2 Comparison of Database, Focus, and Functional Assessments

DATABASE ASSESSMENT	FOCUS ASSESSMENT	FUNCTIONAL ASSESSMENT
Obtained on admission	Compiled throughout subsequent care	Completed within the first 14 days of admission
Consists of predetermined questions and systematic head-to-toe examination	Consists of unstructured questions and a collection of physical assessments	Can follow various assessment tools, one of which is standardized MDS
Performed once	Repeated each shift or more often	Repeated at least every 12 months or immediately after a significant change in physical or mental status; reviewed every 3 months
Suggests possible problems	Rules out or confirms problems	Identifies physical, psychological, and social factors that affect self-care
Findings documented on an admission assessment form	Findings documented on a checklist or in progress notes	Findings documented on various assessment tools, one of which is standardized MDS
Time-consuming, may take 1 hour or more	Completed in a brief amount of time (about 15 minutes)	Labor-intensive, may involve a multidisciplinary team with final completion by an RN
Supplies a broad, comprehensive volume of data	Collects limited data	Comprehensive evaluation of current strengths and the potential for avoidable decline
Provides breadth for future comparisons	Adds depth to the initial database	Provides comparative data
Reflects the client's condition upon entering the health care system	Provides comparative trends for evaluating the client's response to treatment	Data may also be used as a facility's quality indicator.

MDS, Minimum Data Set; RN, registered nurse.

ADMISSION ASSESSMENT RECORD

RESPIRATION

[ ] PROBLEM	HISTORY OF	[ ] CHEST PAIN [ ] PNEUMONIA [ ] BRONCHITIS [ ] ASTHMA [ ] EMPHYSEMA

SHORTNESS OF BREATH
[ ] YES   [ ] WITH EXERCISE   [ ] WITHOUT EXERCISE
[ ] NO

[ ] POTENTIAL FOR REFERRAL

COUGH
[ ] YES   [ ] PRODUCTIVE   [ ] NON-PRODUCTIVE   [ ] SPUTUM COLOR
[ ] NO

BREATH SOUNDS (DESCRIBE)

RATE	RHYTHM	QUALITY [ ] LABORED [ ] SHALLOW	SKIN COLOR [ ] PINK [ ] PALE [ ] CYANOTIC

ACCESSORY MUSCLES

COMMENTS

CIRCULATION

[ ] PROBLEM	HISTORY OF	[ ] BLOOD CLOTS [ ] EDEMA [ ] ABNORMAL EKG [ ] NUMBNESS [ ] TINGLING [ ] POOR CIRCULATION [ ] FATIGUE [ ] HYPERTENSION

APICAL RATE	APICAL RATE [ ] REGULAR [ ] IRREGULAR	RHYTHM

[ ] POTENTIAL FOR REFERRAL

NECK VEIN DISTENSION [ ] PRESENT [ ] ABSENT	NAIL BEDS [ ] PINK [ ] PALE [ ] CYANOTIC

PEDAL EDEMA   [ ] PRESENT   [ ] ABSENT

PEDAL PULSES   LEFT [ ] PRESENT [ ] WEAK [ ] ABSENT   RIGHT [ ] PRESENT [ ] WEAK [ ] ABSENT

COMMENTS

NUTRITIONAL/METABOLIC

[ ] PROBLEM	HISTORY OF	[ ] DIABETES [ ] HYPOGLYCEMIA [ ] THYROID PROBLEMS	NUTRITIONAL STATUS [ ] WELL NOURISHED [ ] EMACIATED [ ] OBESE

MEALS PER DAY	DIET AT HOME	DIET PREFERENCE	LAST MEAL [ ] A.M. [ ] P.M.	RECENT WEIGHT CHANGES

[ ] POTENTIAL FOR REFERRAL

NUTRITIONAL DISTURBANCES
[ ] VOMITING   [ ] NAUSEA   [ ] ANOREXIA   [ ] CHEWING PROBLEMS   [ ] OTHER (DESCRIBE)

JAUNDICE PRESENT [ ] YES [ ] NO	DENTAL HYGIENE (DESCRIBE)	TEETH [ ] OWN [ ] DENTURES	TONGUE CONDITION [ ] DRY [ ] COATED [ ] MOIST [ ] SWOLLEN	ORAL MUCOSA [ ] DRY [ ] MOIST	COLOR

COMMENTS

ELIMINATION

[ ] PROBLEM	BOWEL HABITS COLOR [ ] SOFT FORMED [ ] CONSTIPATED LAST BOWEL MOVEMENT STOOLS PER DAY _____ [ ] DIARRHEA [ ] USE LAXATIVE

BLADDER [ ] DYSURIA	[ ] URGENCY [ ] NOCTURIA	[ ] CALCULI [ ] FREQUENCY	[ ] HEMATURIA [ ] PROSTATE PROBLEM	BOWEL SOUNDS [ ] PRESENT [ ] ABSENT OSTOMIES OR TUBES (DESCRIBE)

[ ] POTENTIAL FOR REFERRAL

ABDOMEN [ ] TENDER [ ] SOFT [ ] FIRM [ ] DISTENDED [ ] NOT DISTENDED	URINARY DEVICES (DESCRIBE)

COMMENTS

COGNITIVE/PERCEPTUAL

[ ] PROBLEM	HISTORY OF	[ ] SEIZURES [ ] FREQUENT [ ] INFREQUENT [ ] HEADACHES [ ] FREQUENT [ ] INFREQUENT	LIMITATION OR RESTRICTION RELATED TO [ ] HEARING - IMPAIRED [ ] YES [ ] NO [ ] VISION - IMPAIRED [ ] YES [ ] NO

LEVEL OF CONSCIOUSNESS
[ ] ALERT   [ ] LETHARGIC   [ ] CONFUSED   [ ] LISTLESS   [ ] RESPONDS TO PAIN   [ ] UNRESPONSIVE

[ ] POTENTIAL FOR REFERRAL

ORIENTED TO [ ] TIME [ ] PLACE [ ] PERSON	AFFECT [ ] CALM	[ ] WITHDRAWN [ ] APPREHENSIVE	[ ] OTHER (DESCRIBE)

BEHAVIOR [ ] COOPERATIVE [ ] UNCOOPERATIVE	PUPILS [ ] EQUAL [ ] REACTIVE	[ ] OTHER (DESCRIBE)

COMMUNICATION
[ ] SPEAKS ENGLISH   [ ] ABLE TO READ   [ ] ABLE TO WRITE   [ ] COMMUNICATES ADEQUATELY

AWARENESS
[ ] NO PROBLEM WITH MEMORY   [ ] PROBLEM WITH MEMORY

DISCOMFORT/PAIN [ ] YES [ ] NO	WHERE	TYPE	PAIN MANAGEMENT	POTENTIAL RISK OF FALLS [ ] YES [ ] NO

COMMENTS

FIGURE 2-2 One page of a multipage admission assessment form is shown.

Nurses organize assessment data similarly. Using knowledge and past experiences, they cluster related data (Box 2-4). Data organized into small groups are easier to analyze, and they take on more significance than when the nurse considers each fact separately or examines the entire group at once.

Diagnosis

Diagnosis, the second step in the nursing process, is the identification of health-related problems. Diagnosis results from analyzing the collected data and determining whether they suggest normal or abnormal findings.

BOX 2-3 **Functional Assessment as Applied to Bathing**

5: Unable to assist in any way
4: Able to cooperate, but cannot assist
3: Able to wash hands, face, and chest with supervision; needs help with completing the bath
2: Able to wash face, chest, arms, and upper legs; needs help with completing the bath
1: Bathes self but requires devices (e.g., long-handled sponge)
0: Bathes self independently

BOX 2-4 **Organization of Data**

Assessment Findings
Lassitude; distended abdomen; dry, hard stool passed with difficulty; fever; weak cough; thick sputum

Related Clusters
Lassitude, fever
Weak cough, thick sputum
Distended abdomen; dry, hard stool passed with difficulty

Nursing Diagnoses

Nurses analyze data to identify one or more nursing diagnoses. A **nursing diagnosis** is a health issue that can be prevented, reduced, resolved, or enhanced through independent nursing measures. It is an exclusive nursing responsibility. Nursing diagnoses are categorized into four groups: problem-focused (formerly called actual); risk diagnosis; syndrome diagnosis; and health promotion (Table 2-3).

Collaborative Problems

Collaborative problems are those potential complications from a disorder, test, or treatment that the nurse cannot treat independently, for example, hemorrhage. They represent an

---

⟫⟫ *Stop, Think, and Respond 2-3*

Data: The client eats only bites of the food served. She has lost 15 lb in the last 3 weeks and currently weighs 130 lb, which is more than 10% underweight for her height. She has been experiencing chronic vomiting after eating for the last 3 weeks and is physically weak.

Which nursing diagnostic statements is written correctly based on the data and the information in this chapter?

1. Risk for imbalanced nutrition: Less than body requirements related to vomiting
2. Imbalanced nutrition: Less than body requirements related to inadequate intake of food secondary to vomiting as manifested by caloric intake below daily requirements, recent weight loss of 15 lb, and current weakness
3. Weight loss related to vomiting as evidenced by reduced intake of food
4. Possible malnutrition due to inadequate consumption of nutrients

---

TABLE 2-3 Categories of Nursing Diagnoses

TYPE	EXPLANATION AND EXAMPLE
Problem-focused diagnosis	A problem that currently exists *Impaired gas exchange related to abnormal blood gases and respiratory diagnosis*
Risk diagnosis	A problem the client is uniquely at risk for developing *Infection risk for potential infection from injury or surgery*
Syndrome diagnosis	Cluster of problems related to an event or situation that can be managed together *Deconditioning, bathing/hygiene ADL deficit*
Health promotion diagnosis	A concern with which a healthy person desires nursing assistance to maintain or achieve a higher level of wellness *Altered health maintenance*

ADL, activities of daily living.

---

interdependent domain of nursing practice (Fig. 2-3). The role of the nurse is to monitor to detect the complication(s) and, if detected, manage the complication(s) cooperatively with nurse- and physician-prescribed interventions.

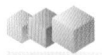 Concept Mastery Alert

Collaborative Problems

For collaborative problems, always think of "monitoring for complications." When caring for clients with collaborative problems, nurses play a key role in monitoring clients for trends or changes that might indicate the client is developing a complication.

The diagnosis of a specific condition or illness, whether it is based in clinical, biochemical, and radiologic criteria, was traditionally seen as the domain of medicine; it is now considered much more of a collaborative activity (Table 2-4).

The nurse is specifically responsible and accountable for:

- Correlating medical diagnoses or medical treatment measures with the risk for unique complications
- Documenting the complications for which clients are at risk
- Making pertinent assessments to detect complications
- Reporting trends that suggest development of complications
- Managing the emerging problem with nurse- and physician-prescribed measures
- Evaluating the outcomes

BOX 2-5 **Parts of a Nursing Diagnostic Statement (PES)**

1. Disturbed sleep pattern = Problem
2. Related to excessive intake of coffee = Etiology
3. As evidenced by difficulty in falling asleep, feeling tired during the day, and irritability with others = Signs and symptoms

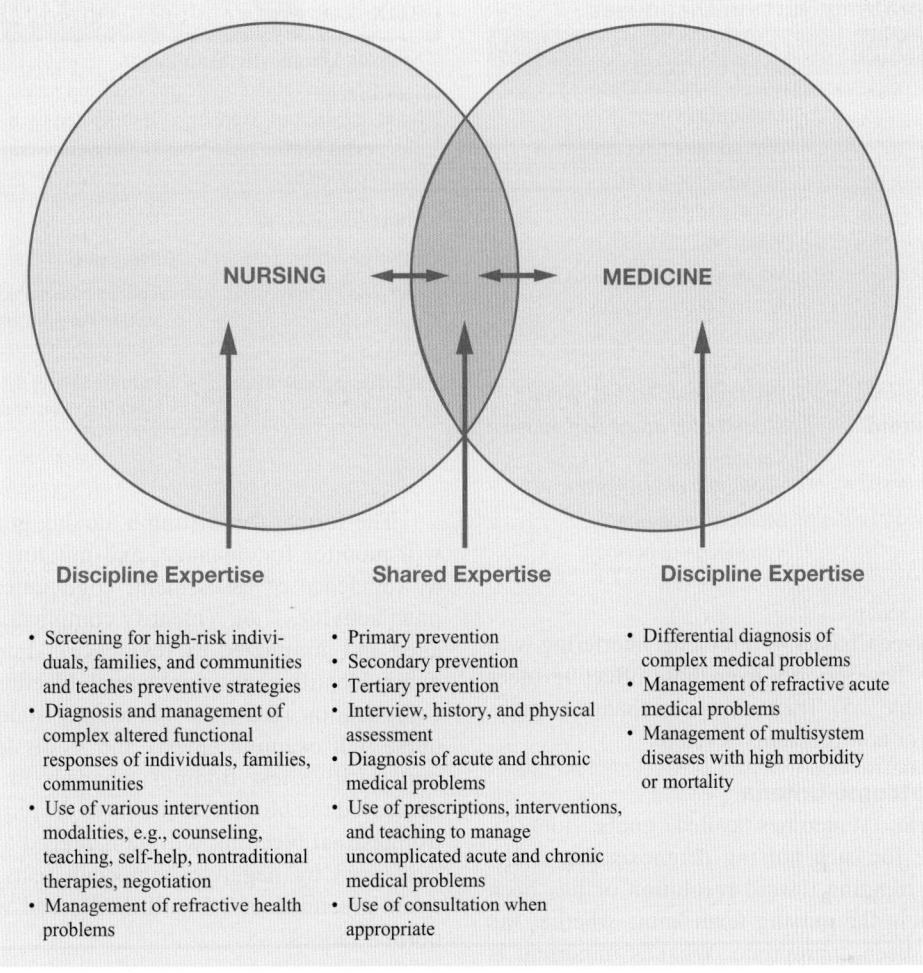

FIGURE 2-3 These two overlapping circles illustrate that the nurse independently treats nursing diagnoses. Doctors, other health providers, and nurses work together on collaborative problems.

Planning

The third step in the nursing process is **planning**, or the process of prioritizing nursing diagnoses and collaborative problems, identifying measurable expected outcomes, selecting appropriate interventions, and documenting the plan of care. Whenever possible, the nurse consults the client while developing and revising the plan.

Setting Priorities

Since many clients' problems take time to resolve, it is important to determine which problems require the most immediate attention. This is done by setting priorities. Prioritization involves ranking those that are most serious or immediate to those of lesser importance.

There is more than one way to determine priorities. One method nurses frequently use is Maslow's Hierarchy

TABLE 2-4 Correlation of Collaborative Problems		
MEDICAL DIAGNOSIS OR MEDICAL TREATMENT	**POSSIBLE CONSEQUENCE**	**COLLABORATIVE PROBLEM**
Myocardial infarction (heart attack)	Abnormal heart rhythm	RC: Dysrhythmias
Heart failure	Fluid in the lungs	RC: Pulmonary edema
Severe burns	Serum moves into tissue, depleting blood volume	RC: Hypovolemic shock
HIV positive	Decreased blood cells that fight infection	RC: Immunodeficiency
Gastric decompression (suctioning stomach fluid)	Removes acid and electrolytes	RC: Alkalosis
		RC: Electrolyte imbalance
Cardiac catheterization (inserting a catheter into the heart)	Arterial bleeding	RC: Hemorrhage

RC, risk for complication.

TABLE 2-5 Prioritizing Nursing Diagnoses

HUMAN NEED	EXAMPLES OF NURSING DIAGNOSES
Physiologic	Malnutrition risk
	Altered breathing pattern
	Acute/Chronic pain
	Urinary retention
Safety and security	Injury risk
	Visual impairment
	Acute/Chronic anxiety
	Fear
Love and belonging	Social isolation
	Psychosocial/Spiritual needs
Esteem and self-esteem	Altered body image perception
	Caregiver fatigue
	Ineffective breastfeeding
Self-actualization	Memory impairment
	Knowledge deficiency

BOX 2-6 **Components of Short-Term Goals**

Nursing Diagnostic Statements
Constipation related to decreased fluid intake, lack of dietary fiber, and lack of exercise as manifested by no normal bowel movement for the past 3 days, abdominal cramping, and straining to pass stool

Short-Term Goal

The client will	Client-centered
have a bowel movement	Identifies measurable criteria that reflect the problem portion of the diagnostic statement
in 2 days (specify date)	Identifies a target date for achievement within a realistic time frame

of Human Needs (see Chapter 4). Problems interfering with physiologic needs have priority over those affecting other levels of needs (Table 2-5). The ranking can change as problems are resolved or new problems develop.

Establishing Outcome Criteria

Outcome criteria, sometimes called **goals**, identify specific evidence for each nursing diagnosis that a client's problem is trending toward resolution or has been resolved. They help the nursing team know whether the nursing care has been appropriate. What is important is that the statement contains objective evidence for verifying that the client has improved. Depending on the agency, client-centered goals may identify short-term criteria, long-term criteria, or both.

Short-Term Goals

Nurses use **short-term goals** (outcomes achievable in a few days to 1 week) more often in acute care settings because most hospital stays are only a few days or no longer than 1 week. Short-term goals (Box 2-6) have the following characteristics:

- Developed from the problem portion of the diagnostic statement
- Client-centered, reflecting what the client will accomplish, not what the nurse will accomplish
- Measurable, identifying specific criteria that provide evidence of goal achievement
- Realistic, to avoid setting unattainable goals, which can be self-defeating and frustrating
- Accompanied by a target date for accomplishment (the predicted time when the goal will be met), which establishes a timeline for evaluation

Long-Term Goals

Nurses generally identify **long-term goals** (outcomes that take weeks or months) that report, record, evaluate, and promote early detection and treatment.

The format for writing a nursing goal is, "The nurse will monitor for, manage, and minimize (complication) by (evidence of assessment, communication, and treatment activities)" or "(identify complication) will be managed and minimized by (evidence)." For example, if the nurse identifies gastrointestinal bleeding as a risk for complication (RC), the nurse may state the goal, "The nurse will examine emesis and stools for blood and report positive test findings, changes in vital signs, and decreased red blood cell counts to the physician," or "Gastrointestinal bleeding will be managed and minimized as evidenced by negative hemoccult tests, red blood cell count greater than 2.5 million/dL, and vital signs within normal ranges."

Selecting Nursing Interventions

Planning the measures that the client and nurse will use to accomplish outcome criteria involves critical thinking. Critical thinking is a process by which a person reaches a goal based on objectively analyzing, interpreting, and evaluating observations, experiences, and information. In nursing, critical thinking leads to selecting nursing interventions that are directed at eliminating the etiologies. The nurse selects strategies based on evidence-based knowledge that certain nursing actions produce desired effects. Whatever interventions are planned, they must be safe, within the legal scope of nursing practice, and compatible with medical orders. Initial interventions are generally limited to selected measures with the potential for success. Nurses should reserve some interventions in case a client does not accomplish the goal.

Documenting the Plan of Care

The Joint Commission and similar entities are not-for-profit organizations that accredit health care organizations in the United States. They require that every client's medical record provides evidence of the planned interventions for meeting the individualized client's needs, but not necessarily a nursing plan of care. Plans of care can be written by hand (Fig. 2-4), standardized on printed forms, computer-generated, or based on an agency's written standards or clinical pathways.

Name: Mrs Rita Willard   Age: 68   Date of Admission: 11/10

Diagnosis on admission: DVA left-sided weakness

Nursing diagnosis: Fall Risk, Injury Risk, Situational Low Self-Esteem

Long-term goals: Independent mobility using walker or quad cane, record of personal safety, positive self-regard

DATE	PROBLEM	GOAL	TARGET DATE	NURSING ORDERS
11/10	#1 Fall Risk related to left sided weakness as manifested by decreased muscle strength in left leg and arm, slowed gait, dragging foot.	The client will stand and pivot from bed to wheelchair or commode.	11/24	1) Passive ROM t.i.d. to left arm and leg 2) Physical therapy b.i.d. for practice at parallel bars 3) Apply left leg brace and sling to left arm when up 4) Assist to balance on right leg at bedside before and after physical therapy daily C. Meyer, RN
11/10	#2 Injury Risk related to motor deficit	The client will transfer from bed to wheelchair without injury.	12/1	1) Keep side rails and trapeze over bed 2) Use shoe & nonskid sold on right foot (leg brace on left) before transfer 3) Dangle for 5 minutes before attempting to stand 4) Lock wheels on wheelchair before transfer 5) Obtain help of second assistant 6) Block left foot to avoid slipping during pivot 7) Place signal light on right side within reach at all times C. Meyer, RN
12/2	#3 Situational Low Self-Esteem related to dependence on others as manifested by statements. "I need as much help as a baby; I feel so useless; How embarrassing to be so dependent."	The client will identify one or more positive feelings regarding improved mobility and self-care.	12/18	1) Allow to express feelings without disagreeing or interrupting 2) Reinforce concept that the right side of body is unaffected. 3) Help to set and accomplish one realistic goal daily. S. Moore, RN

FIGURE 2-4 Sample written nursing care plan.

Standardized care plans are preprinted. Both computer-generated and standardized plans provide general suggestions for managing the nursing care of clients with a particular problem. It is up to the nurse to transform the generalized interventions into specific nursing orders and to eliminate whatever is inappropriate or unnecessary.

Agency-specific **standards for care** (policies that indicate which activities will be provided to ensure quality client care) and clinical pathways (see Chapter 1) relieve the nurse from writing time-consuming plans. Both tools help nurses use their time efficiently and ensure consistent client care.

Writing Nursing Orders

Nursing orders (directions for a client's care) within a nursing care plan identify the what, when, where, and how for performing nursing interventions (see Fig. 2-4). They provide specific instructions so all nursing team members know exactly what to do for the client (Box 2-7). Nursing orders are also signed to indicate accountability.

BOX 2-7	Nursing Orders

Nursing Order
Encourage fluids

Weaknesses
Lacks specificity

Likely to Be Interpreted Differently
May result in inconsistent or less than adequate care

Improvement
Provide 100 mL of oral fluid every hour while awake

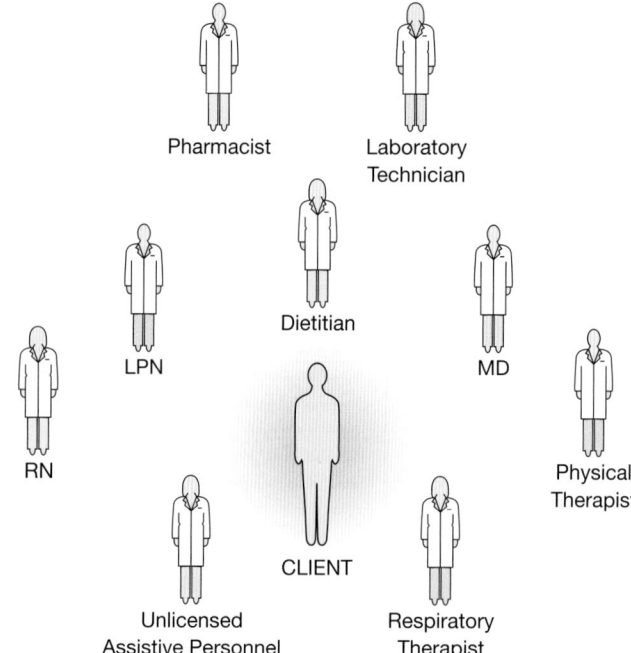

FIGURE 2-5 Members of the health care team. LPN, Licensed practical nurse; MD, medical doctor; RN, registered nurse.

Communicating the Plan of Care

Clients need consistency and continuity of care to achieve goals. Therefore, the nurse shares the plan of care with nursing team members, the client, and the client's family. In some agencies, the client signs the plan of care.

The plan of care is a permanent part of the client's medical record. It is placed in the client's chart, kept separately at the client's bedside, or located in a temporary folder at the nurses' station for easy access. Wherever it is located, each nurse assigned to the client refers to it daily, reviews it for appropriateness, and revises it according to changes in the client's condition.

Implementation

Implementation, the fourth step in the nursing process, means carrying out the plan of care. The nurse implements medical orders as well as nursing orders, which should complement each other. Implementing the plan involves the client and one or more members of the health care team. A wide circle of care providers with assorted roles may be called on to participate, either directly or indirectly, in carrying out one client's plan of care (Fig. 2-5).

The medical record (chart) is legal evidence that the plan of care has been more than just a paper trail. The information in the chart shows a correlation between the plan and the care that has been provided. In other words, the nurse's charting (see Chapter 9) reflects the written plan. Nurses are just as accountable for carrying out nursing orders as they are for carrying out physician's orders.

In addition to identifying the nursing interventions that have been provided, the record also describes the quantity and quality of the client's response. Quoting the client helps identify the client's point of view and safeguards against incorrect assumptions. In short, appropriate documentation maintains open lines of communication among members of the health care team, ensures the client's continuing progress, complies with accreditation standards, and helps ensure reimbursement from government or private insurance companies.

Evaluation

Evaluation, the fifth and final step in the nursing process, is the way by which nurses determine whether a client has reached a goal. Although this is considered the last step, the entire process is ongoing. By analyzing the client's response, evaluation helps determine the effectiveness of nursing care (Table 2-6).

Before revising a plan of care, it is important to discuss any lack of progress with the client. In this way, both the nurse and the client can speculate on what activities need to be discontinued, added, or changed. Other health team members who are familiar with a particular client or problems similar to those of the client may offer their expertise as well. The evaluation of a client's progress may be the subject of a nursing team conference. Some units even invite the client and family to participate.

USE OF THE NURSING PROCESS

Use of the nursing process is the standard for clinical nursing practice. More detailed discussions of the nursing process can be found in specialty texts and in some of the suggested readings at the end of this book. Nursing Guidelines 2-1 reiterates the sequence of the nursing process.

Nursing educational programs use learning strategies to develop nursing care plans that incorporate the steps in the nursing process. This learning strategy may serve as a bridge between theory and practice by allowing students to organize knowledge, prioritize care, link relationships, and promote critical thinking (Garwood et al., 2018). Typically, students are required to create **nursing care plans,** written assignments on standardized worksheets that contain a column for nursing diagnoses, outcome criteria, nursing interventions, and the rationales for each intervention for each assigned client. The activity often requires multiple pages and hours to complete.

TABLE 2-6 Outcomes from Evaluation

ANALYSIS	REASON	ACTION
The client has reached the goals.	Plan was effective and implemented consistently.	Discontinue the nursing orders.
The client has made some progress.	Care has been inconsistent.	Check that nursing orders are clear and specific.
	Target date was too ambitious.	Continue care as planned; readjust target date.
	Client's response has been less than expected.	Revise the plan by adding nursing interventions or more frequent implementation.
The client has made no progress.	The initial diagnosis was inaccurate.	Revise problem list; write new goals and nursing orders.
	New problems have occurred.	Add new problems, goals, and nursing orders.
	The target date was unrealistic.	Revise expected date for achievement.
	Nursing interventions were ineffective.	Add new nursing orders; discontinue ineffective measures; and readjust target date.

NURSING GUIDELINES 2-1

Using the Nursing Process

- Collect information about the client. *Data collection is the basis for identifying problems.*
- Organize the data. *Organizing related data simplifies the process of analysis.*
- Analyze the data for what is normal and abnormal. *Abnormalities provide clues to the client's problems.*
- Identify problem-focused, risk, syndrome, and health promotion nursing diagnoses and collaborative problems. *Problem identification directs the nurse to select methods for maintaining or restoring the client's health.*
- Prioritize the problem list. *Setting priorities targets problems that require the most immediate attention.*
- Establish specific criteria for evaluating whether the problems have been prevented, reduced, or resolved. *Goals predict the expected outcomes from nursing care.*
- Select a limited number of appropriate nursing interventions. *The nurse uses evidence-based knowledge to determine which measures will be most effective in accomplishing the goals of care.*
- Give specific directions for nursing care. *Specific directions promote consistency and continuity among caregivers.*
- Document the plan of care using whatever format is acceptable. *A documented plan provides a means of communication and reference for the nursing team to follow.*

- Discuss the plan with nursing team members, the client, and the family. *Verbally sharing the plan ensures that everyone is informed and goal-directed.*
- Put the plan into action. *Work produces results.*
- Observe the client's responses. *Evaluating outcomes is the basis for determining the effectiveness of the plan of care.*
- Chart all nursing activities and the client's responses. *Documentation demonstrates that planned care has been implemented and provides information about the client's progress.*
- Compare the client's responses with the outcome criteria. *If the planned care is appropriate, there should be some measure of progress toward accomplishing goals.*
- Discuss the progress, or lack of it, with the client, family, and other nursing team members. *Pooling resources may provide better alternatives when revising the plan of care.*
- Change the plan in areas that are no longer appropriate. *The nursing care plan changes according to the needs of the client.*
- Continue to implement and evaluate the revised plan of care. *The nursing process is continuous; it is repeated until the goals have been met.*

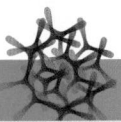

KEY POINTS

- The nursing process consists of five steps:
  - Assessment
  - Diagnosis
  - Planning
  - Implementation
  - Evaluation
- The assessment portion of the nursing process consists of:
  - Database assessment
  - Focus assessment
  - Functional assessment

- The outcome criterion or goal may be a short-term goal, long-term goal, or both depending on the health care setting or agency.
- Nursing students are educated in the nursing care process using nursing care plan. This educational strategy encourages students to apply the nursing process by collecting, interpreting, analyzing, synthesizing, and evaluating data.

CRITICAL THINKING EXERCISES

If an unconscious client is brought to the nursing unit, how can a nurse gather data?

1. Three nursing diagnoses are on a client's plan of care: ineffective breathing pattern; social isolation; and anxiety. Which diagnosis has the highest priority and why?

2. While reviewing a client's plan of care, a nurse notices that the client has made no progress in accomplishing a goal by its projected target date. What actions are appropriate at this time?

3. A nurse plans a 1,800-calorie diet for a client with the nursing diagnosis of obesity, but the client rejects that intervention, instead choosing to exercise 30 minutes each day. What nursing action is appropriate in this situation?

NEXT-GENERATION NCLEX-STYLE REVIEW QUESTIONS

1. When managing the care of a client, arrange the list in order from a to d according to client priority needs.
   a. Develop a plan of care.
   b. Determine the client's needs.
   c. Assess the client physically.
   d. Collaborate on goals for care.
   Test-Taking Strategy: Note the key words and modifier, "most appropriate" and "first." Use the steps in the nursing process to guide the selection of the answer.

2. According to most nurse practice acts, if a charge nurse assigns an LPN to admit a new client, what is the practical nurse's primary role?
   a. Create an initial nursing care plan.
   b. Gather basic information from the client.
   c. Develop a list of the client's nursing diagnoses.
   d. Report assessment data to the client's physician.
   Test-Taking Strategy: Apply the responsibilities of the practical nurse to help select the answer.

3. When staff members discuss a client's nursing diagnoses at a team meeting, which nursing diagnosis is of the highest priority?
   a. Ineffective airway clearance
   b. Ineffective coping
   c. Deficient diversional activity
   d. Interrupted family processes
   Test-Taking Strategy: Note the key words and modifier, which in this case is "highest priority." Apply Maslow's Hierarchy of Needs to select the answer.

4. The LPN notes that an expected outcome of bathing independently has not been reached by the target date. What action is most appropriate to take at this time?
   a. Urge the client to try harder to bathe independently.
   b. Limit bathing until the client can bathe independently.
   c. Suggest that the staff reduce their assistance with bathing.
   d. Revise the interventions or target date for achieving the goal.
   Test-Taking Strategy: Note the key word and modifier, "most appropriate." Select an answer for revising the plan of care when progress has not been made.

5. When gathering nursing data on a newly admitted client, which is the most appropriate source to consult for additional information?
   a. The client's visitors
   b. The client's family
   c. The client's clergy
   d. The client's employer
   Test-Taking Strategy: Note the key word and modifier, "most appropriate." Consider the next best source for data other than the client.

UNIT 2 | Integrating Basic Concepts

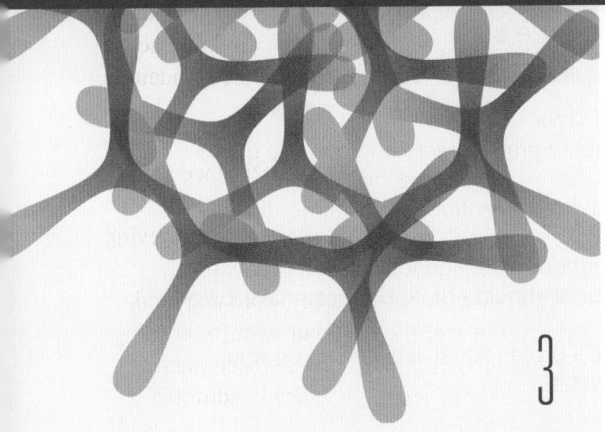

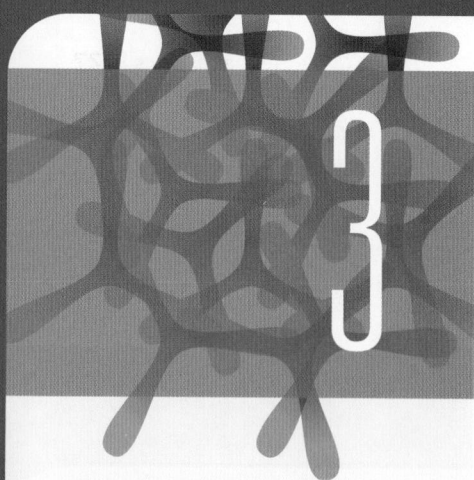

3

Laws and Ethics

Words To Know

administrative laws
advance directive
allocation of scarce resources
anecdotal record
assault
assumption of risk
autonomy
battery
beneficence
board of nursing
civil laws
code of ethics
code status
common law
confidentiality
criminal laws
defamation
defendant
deontology
documentation
durable power of attorney for
health care
duty
ethical dilemma
ethics
false imprisonment
felony
fidelity
Good Samaritan laws
gross negligence
Health Insurance Portability and
Accountability Act
incident report
intentional tort
invasion of privacy
justice
laws
liability insurance
libel
living will
malpractice
misdemeanor
National Practitioner Data Bank
negligence
nonmaleficence
nurse licensure compacts

Learning Objectives

On completion of this chapter, the reader should be able to:

1. Identify different types of laws.
2. Discuss the purpose of nurse practice acts and the role of the state board of nursing.
3. Explain the difference between intentional and unintentional torts.
4. Describe the difference between negligence and malpractice.
5. Identify reasons why a nurse should obtain professional liability insurance.
6. List the ways that a nurse's professional liability can be mitigated in the case of a lawsuit.
7. Define the term "ethics."
8. Explain the purpose of a code of ethics.
9. Describe two types of ethical theories.
10. Name and explain the ethical principles that apply to health care.
11. List ethical issues common in nursing practice.

INTRODUCTION

Laws, ethics, client rights, and nursing duties affect nurses regularly throughout their careers. This chapter introduces basic legal and ethical concepts and issues that affect the practice of nursing.

 Gerontologic Considerations

■ **Telehealth services,** technology that facilitates the transmission of health assessment and monitoring data with audio, video, and internet-based devices, contribute to the welfare of homebound older adults or those who live in rural, remote, or underserved areas for health care.

■ Nurses providing Medicare-reimbursed skilled home care services are increasingly incorporating telehealth monitoring to improve health outcomes in patients with chronic conditions, such as diabetes and heart failure.

LAWS

Laws (rules of conduct established and enforced by government) are intended to protect both the general public and each person. The six categories of laws are constitutional, statutory, administrative, common, criminal, and civil (Table 3-1).

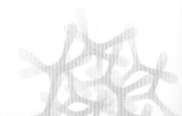

Words To Know *(continued)*
nurse practice act
Nursing Home Reform Act
plaintiff
reciprocity
restraints
risk management
slander
statute of limitations
statutory laws
telehealth services
telenursing
teleology
tort
truth telling
unintentional tort
values
veracity
whistle-blowing

TABLE 3-1 Types of Laws

CATEGORY	PURPOSE	EXAMPLES
Constitutional law	Protects fundamental rights and freedoms of U.S. citizens Defines the duties and limitations of the executive, legislative, and judicial branches of government	Bill of Rights, freedom of speech
Statutory law	Identifies local, state, or federal rules necessary for the public's welfare	Public health ordinances, tax laws, nurse practice acts
Administrative law	Develops regulations by which to carry out the mission of a public agency	State boards of nursing, which enact and enforce rules as they relate to nurse practice acts
Common law	Interprets legal issues based on previous court decisions in similar cases (legal precedents)	Tarasoff v. Board of Regents of University of California (1976), which justifies breaching a client's confidentiality if they reveal the identity of a potential victim of crime
Criminal law	Determines the nature of criminal acts that endanger all of society	Identifies the differences in first- and second-degree murder, manslaughter, etc.
Civil law	Determines the circumstances and manner in which a person may be compensated for being the victim of another person's action or omission of an action	Derelict of duty, negligence

Constitutional Law

The founders of the United States wrote the country's first formal laws within the Constitution. This document, which has endured with amendments, divides power among three branches of government and establishes checks and balances that protect the entire nation from any one entity gaining too much power. It also identifies the rights and privileges to which all U.S. citizens are entitled. Two examples of rights protected by constitutional law are free speech and privacy.

Statutory Laws

Statutory laws (laws enacted by federal, state, or local legislatures) are sometimes identified as public acts, codes, or ordinances. For example, state legislatures are responsible for enacting statutes that ensure the competence of health care providers. A **nurse practice act** (statute that legally defines the unique role of the nurse and differentiates it from that of

other health care providers, such as physicians) is one example of a statutory law (Box 3-1). Although each state's nurse practice act is unique, all generally contain common elements:

- They define the scope of nursing practice.
- They establish the limits to that practice.
- They identify titles that nurses may use, such as licensed practical nurse (LPN), licensed vocational nurse (LVN), or registered nurse (RN).
- They authorize a board of nursing to oversee nursing practice.
- They determine what constitutes grounds for disciplinary action.

Administrative Laws

Administrative laws (legal provisions through which federal, state, and local agencies maintain self-regulation) affect the power to manage governmental agencies. Some

Vocational/Practical nursing means a directed scope of nursing practice, including the performance of an act that requires specialized judgment and skill, the proper performance of which is based on knowledge and application of the principles of biological, physical, and social science as acquired by a completed course in an approved school of vocational/practical nursing. The term does not include acts of medical diagnosis or the prescription of therapeutic or corrective measures. Vocational/Practical nursing involves: (A) collecting data and performing focused nursing assessments of the health status of an individual; (B) participating in the planning of the nursing care needs of an individual; (C) participating in the development and modification of the nursing care plan; (D) participating in health teaching and counseling to promote, attain, and maintain the optimum health level of an individual; (E) assisting in the evaluation of an individual's response to a nursing intervention and the identification of an individual's needs; and (F) engaging in other acts that require education and training, as prescribed by board rules and policies, commensurate with the nurse's experience, continuing education, and demonstrated competency.

Nursing Practice Act, Nursing Peer Review, & Nurse Licensure Compact Texas Occupations code. From https://www.bon.texas.gov/pdfs/law_rules_pdfs/nursing_practice_act_pdfs/NPA2023.pdf

administrative laws authorize federal and state governments to ensure citizen health and safety.

State Boards of Nursing

The state board of nursing is an example of an administrative agency that enforces administrative law. Each state's **board of nursing** (regulatory agency for managing the provisions of a state's nurse practice act) has a primary responsibility to protect the public receiving nursing care within the state. Some activities of the state's board of nursing include (1) reviewing and approving nursing education programs in the state; (2) establishing criteria for licensing nurses; (3) overseeing procedures for nurse licensing examinations; (4) issuing and transferring nursing licenses; (5) investigating allegations against nurses licensed in that state; and (6) disciplining nurses who violate legal and ethical standards. The state's board of nursing is responsible for suspending and revoking licenses and reviewing applications asking for **reciprocity** (licensure based on evidence of having met licensing criteria in another state). A license in one state does not give a person a right to automatic licensure in another.

Nurse Licensure Compacts

Several states have enacted **nurse licensure compacts**, agreements between states in which a nurse licensed in one state can practice in another without obtaining an additional license (Fig. 3-1). Under this agreement, the nurse acknowledges that they are subject to each state's nurse practice act and discipline. Advantages include:

- Simplifies the licensing process and removes barriers, thus increasing employability and access to nursing care

- Is more cost-effective than multiple licensing fees
- Decreases barriers for nurses who live in one state and want to work in another nearby
- Reduces the need for duplicate listings of nurses working in more than one state for disaster planning and preparedness or during other times of need for qualified nursing services
- Facilitates a cost-effective alternative when a nurse is employed to provide **telenursing**, health triage, or information from their state through electronic or telephonic access to residents in another state
- Responds to the health care delivery trend in which nurses are employed in small hospitals or satellite agencies that have merged with multistate health care systems

The traditional method of separate licenses for each state of practice provides a legal loophole when one state revokes a nurse's license as a disciplinary measure. Some nurses move to the state where their licenses are still active and continue to work. Legislation has been enacted, however, to track incompetent health care practitioners. The **National Practitioner Data Bank** (NPDB) merged with the Healthcare Integrity and Protection Data Bank (HIPDB) in 2013; it serves as a tracking system designed to protect the public from unfit health care practitioners. Included in the database are the names of licensed health care providers who have been disciplined by hospitals, courts, licensing boards, professional associations, insurers, and peer review committees. State Boards of Nursing report individuals whose licenses have been revoked or suspended and those who have been subject to reprimands, censure, or probation (National Council of State Boards of Nursing, 2020a, 2020b). The information is made available nationwide to licensing boards and health care facilities that hire nurses, should they choose to check it, but it is unavailable to the general public. Under the nurse licensure compact, the state of licensure and the state where the client was located during an incident may take disciplinary action against a nurse working under a multistate agreement. Some employers are also requiring potential and current employees to undergo state or federal background checks and drug screens.

Common Law

Common law (decisions based on prior similar cases) is also known as *judicial law*. It is based on the principle of *stare decisis* ("let the decision stand"), in which prior outcomes guide decisions in other jurisdictions dealing with comparable circumstances. Common law refers to litigation that falls outside the realm of constitutional, statutory, and administrative laws.

Criminal Laws

Criminal laws (penal codes that protect all citizens from people who pose a threat to the public good) are used to prosecute those who commit crimes. The state represents "the people" when prosecuting those accused of crimes. Crimes are either misdemeanors or felonies. A **misdemeanor** is a minor criminal offense (e.g., shoplifting). If a person is convicted of a misdemeanor, a small fine, a short period of

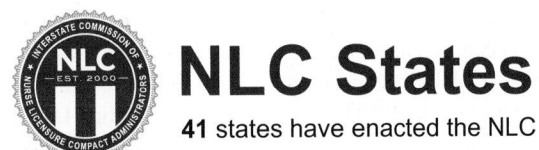

NLC States

41 states have enacted the NLC

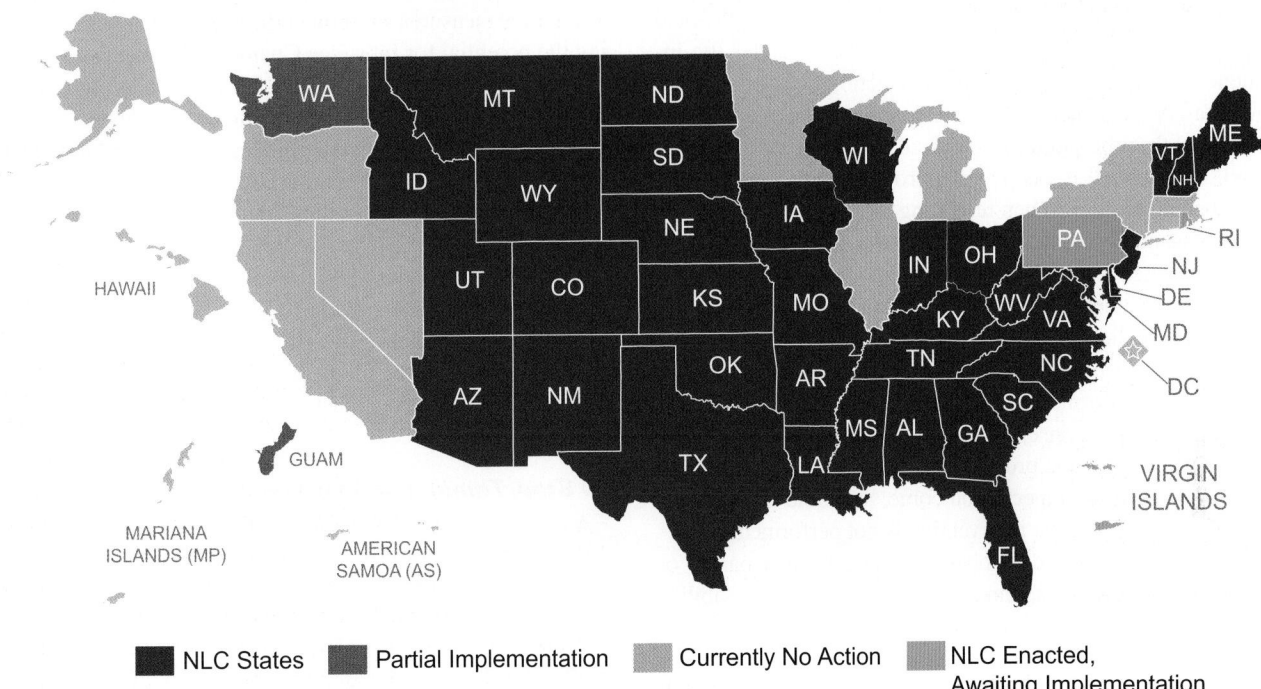

■ NLC States   ■ Partial Implementation   ■ Currently No Action   ■ NLC Enacted, Awaiting Implementation

FIGURE 3-1 States participating in the nurse licensure compact (NLC) and those in which their status is pending as of December 2022. **Guam:** Pending implementation in 2022, tentatively. Nurses holding a multistate license in other NLC states may practice in Guam. Guam residents cannot obtain a multistate license until implementation is complete. **Pennsylvania (PA):** NLC enacted July 1, 2021. Implementation date is to be determined. Criminal background checks must also be implemented. PA residents cannot obtain a multistate license until implementation is completed. Nurses in other NLC states with a multistate license may not practice in PA until implementation is complete. **Virgin Islands (VI):** NLC enacted December 6, 2021. Implementation date is to be determined. Criminal background checks must also be implemented. VI residents cannot obtain a multistate license until implementation is completed. Nurses in other NLC states with a multistate license may not practice in VI until implementation is complete. (National Council of State Boards of Nursing. [2023]. *Nurse licensure compact administrators*. Map of NLC States. https://www.ncsbn.org/public-files/NLC_Map.pdf)

incarceration, or both may be levied. The fine is paid to the state. A **felony** is a serious criminal offense, such as murder, falsifying medical records, insurance fraud, and stealing narcotics. Conviction is punishable by a lengthy prison term or even execution. The state generally prohibits felons from obtaining occupational licenses, and the state will revoke such a license if its holder is convicted of a felony.

Civil Laws

Civil laws (statutes that protect personal freedoms and rights) apply to disputes between individual citizens. Some examples include laws that protect the right to be let alone, freedom from threats of injury, freedom from offensive contact, and freedom from character attacks. In civil cases, the **plaintiff** (person claiming injury) brings charges against the **defendant** (person charged with violating the law). The case is referred to as a **tort** (litigation in which one person asserts that a physical, emotional, or financial injury was a consequence of another person's actions or failure to act). A tort implies that a person breached their duty to another

person. A **duty** is an expected action based on moral or legal obligations.

It does not take the same quality or quantity of evidence to be convicted in a civil lawsuit as in a criminal case. If a defendant is found guilty of a tort, they are required to pay the plaintiff restitution for damages. Torts are classified as intentional or unintentional.

Intentional Torts

Intentional torts are lawsuits in which a plaintiff charges that a defendant committed a deliberately aggressive act. Examples include assault, battery, false imprisonment, invasion of privacy, and defamation.

Assault

Assault is an act in which bodily harm is threatened or attempted. Such harm may be physical intimidation, remarks, or gestures. The plaintiff interprets the threat to mean that force may be forthcoming. A nurse may be accused of assault if they verbally threaten to restrain a client unnecessarily (e.g., to curtail the use of the signal light).

Battery

Battery (unauthorized physical contact) can include touching a person's body, clothing, chair, or bed. A plaintiff can claim battery even if contact causes no actual physical harm. The criterion is that contact happened without the plaintiff's consent.

Sometimes, nonconsensual physical contact can be justified. For example, health care providers can use physical force to subdue clients with mental illness or under the influence of alcohol or drugs if their actions endanger their own safety or that of others. Documentation must show, however, that the situation required the degree of restraint used. Excessive force is never appropriate when less would have been effective. When recording information about such situations, nurses must describe the behavior and the client's response when lesser forms of restraint were used first.

To protect health care providers from being charged with battery, adult clients are asked to sign a general permission for care and treatment during admission (Fig. 3-2) and additional written consent forms for tests, procedures, or surgery. When seeking a client's consent for specific treatments, the physician must describe the proposed intervention, potential benefits, risks involved, expected outcome, available alternatives, and consequences if the intervention is not performed.

Health care providers obtain consent from a parent or guardian if the client is a minor, has a developmental disability, or is mentally incompetent. In an emergency, consent can be implied. In other words, it is assumed that in life-threatening circumstances, a client would give consent for treatment if they were able to understand the risks. In most cases, another physician must concur that the emergency procedure is essential.

False Imprisonment

A plaintiff can allege **false imprisonment** (interference with a person's freedom to move about at will without legal authority to do so) if a nurse detains a competent client from leaving the hospital or other health care agency. If a client wants to leave without being medically discharged, it is customary for them to sign a form indicating personal responsibility for leaving against medical advice (AMA) (Fig. 3-3). If the client refuses to sign the paper, however, health care providers cannot bar them from leaving. The signed form or the client's refusal is documented in the medical record.

Forced confinement is legal under two conditions: if there is a judicial restraining order (e.g., a prisoner admitted for medical care) or if there is a court-ordered commitment (e.g., a client with mental illness who is dangerous to self or others).

Restraints are devices or chemicals that restrict movement. They are used with the intention to subdue a client's activity. Types include cloth limb restraints, bedrails, chairs with locking lap trays, and sedative drugs. Unnecessary or unprescribed restraints can lead to charges of false imprisonment, battery, or both.

The **Nursing Home Reform Act** of the Omnibus Budget Reconciliation Act (OBRA), federal legislation that sets standards of care and establishes certain rights for older adults, states that residents in nursing homes have "the right to be free of, and the facility must ensure freedom from, any restraints imposed or psychoactive drug administered for purposes of discipline or convenience, and not required to treat the residents' medical symptoms." This is not to say that restraints cannot be used, rather, they should be used as a last resort. Use must be justified and accompanied by informed consent from the client or a responsible relative.

Before using restraints, the best legal advice is to try alternative measures for protecting wandering clients, reducing the potential for falls (see Chapter 19), and ensuring that clients do not jeopardize medical treatment by pulling out feeding tubes or other therapeutic devices. If less restrictive alternatives are unsuccessful, nurses must obtain a medical order before each and every instance in which they use restraints. In acute care hospitals, medical orders for restraints are renewed every 24 hours. When restraints are applied, charting must indicate regular client assessment; provisions for fluids, nourishment, and bowel and bladder elimination; and attempts to release the client from the restraints for a trial period. When the client is no longer a danger to themselves or others, nurses must remove the restraints.

>>> **Stop, Think, and Respond 3-1**
A nurse warns a weak and debilitated older adult that if she continues to get out of bed during the night without calling for assistance, it will be necessary to apply wrist restraints. Can the nurse legally restrain the client who may be harmed if the behavior does not change?

Invasion of Privacy

Civil and federal laws protect citizens from **invasion of privacy** (failure to leave people and their property alone). Nonmedical civil examples of offenses include trespassing, illegal search and seizure, wiretapping, and revealing personal information about someone, even if true. Examples of privacy violations in health care include photographing a client without consent, revealing a client's name in a public report, and allowing an unauthorized person to observe the client's care. Privacy curtains are used during care; permission is obtained if a nursing or medical student will observe a procedure.

The **Health Insurance Portability and Accountability Act** (HIPAA), legislation that sets national standards for the security of health information, ensures that an individual's electronic, paper, or oral health information is protected (see Chapter 9). Therefore, to protect clients' rights to privacy, medical records and information are kept confidential. Personal names and identities are concealed or obliterated in case studies or research.

Defamation

Defamation (an act in which untrue information harms a person's reputation) is unlawful. Examples include **slander** (character attack uttered orally in the presence of others) and **libel** (damaging statements written and read by others). Injury is considered to occur because the derogatory remarks attack a person's character and good name.

If a client accuses a nurse of defamation of character, the client must prove that there was malice, misuse of

Example Memorial Hospital
AUTHORIZATION FOR HOSPITAL TREATMENT

* C O N S E N T *

Patient's Name: _____

1. **CONSENT FOR TREATMENT:** I, the undersigned, request and authorize the Hospital and all its physicians, surgeons, technicians, nurses, and other qualified personnel, whether employed directly by the Hospital or brought in on a consulting basis, to provide any medical/surgical treatment, diagnostic tests and hospital care which the attending physician or designee(s) may deem necessary or beneficial for my health.

   I understand that the results of any treatments, tests or care cannot be guaranteed. I also understand that I have the right to refuse any drugs, treatment, or procedures to the extent permitted by law.

   I understand that medical, nursing, and other health care personnel in training may be observing and participating actively in my care under the supervision of authorized personnel. I hereby give my consent to such observations and/or participation.

2. **RELEASE OF RESPONSIBILITY FOR PERSONAL VALUABLES:** I have been made aware that the Hospital provides special facilities for the safekeeping of valuables. I release the Hospital from any responsibility for the loss or damage to any valuable possession (including valuables brought in to me by other persons) that I choose to keep in my personal possession and do not deposit with the Hospital for safekeeping.

3. **RELEASE OF INFORMATION:** To obtain payment for services, I authorize the Hospital to furnish and release to my insurance carrier(s) or their representatives insuring the patient named, any or all portions of my medical record which may be necessary for completion of my patient care insurance claims. I understand that billing agencies for specialized services such as radiology, emergency services, and anesthesia will also receive information necessary for billing.

   I authorize the release of copies or summaries of my medical record to any health care facility or home care provider to which I may be transferred or referred. I further authorize release of my medical information to any physician involved in providing my care. I hereby release the Hospital from all legal liability that may arise from the release of the information requested and provided. A photocopy of this authorization shall be as binding as the original.

4. **ASSIGNMENT OF BENEFITS/FINANCIAL RESPONSIBILITY:** I request that payment of authorized benefits be made on my behalf and do hereby authorize payment directly to Example Memorial Hospital and/or its physician of any benefits that otherwise would be payable directly to me for this period of hospitalization or treatment. I understand that I am financially responsible to the hospital and/or physician for charges not covered by this authorization.

I have read this consent form, I have had it explained to me and understand its contents. I hereby agree to all terms and conditions set forth above.

Patient Rights & Responsibilities Brochure _____ Received _____ Denied.

_____
Date and/Time of Signing

_____
Patient's Signature

_____
Witness to Signature

_____
Authorized Representative's Signature & Relationship (if patient is unable to sign)

AFFIX PATIENT LABEL

FIGURE 3-2 Example of consent for treatment form. (From Donnelly-Moreno, L., Moseley, B., & Timby, B. K. [2021]. *Introductory medical-surgical nursing.* Lippincott Williams & Wilkins.)

THREE RIVERS HOSPITAL
THREE RIVERS, MICHIGAN 49093

Release from Responsibility for Discharge

Date: _____ Time: _____ A.M.
                                                                  P.M.

CLIENT: _____

This is to certify that I _____, a client in
the _____ Hospital, am being discharged
against the advice of the attending physician and the hospital administration. I acknowledge that I have
been informed of the risk involved and hereby release the attending physician and the hospital from all
responsibility for any ill effects that may result from such discharge.

Witnesses:

_____

_____

(Signature of Client)

(To be signed by the legal
representative in case of a
minor or of a client who
is not mentally competent,
otherwise by the client.)

FIGURE 3-3 Example of a release form for discharging oneself against medical advice.

privileged information, and spoken or written untruths. Nurses are at risk for defamation of character suits if they make negative comments in public areas (e.g., elevators, lunch rooms, and agency cafeterias) or assert opinions regarding a client's character in the medical record. To avoid accusations of defamation, nurses must avoid making or writing negative comments about clients, physicians, or other coworkers.

Unintentional Torts

Unintentional torts result in an injury, though the person responsible did not mean to cause harm. The two types of unintentional torts involve allegations of negligence and malpractice.

Negligence

Negligence (harm that results because a person did not act *reasonably*) implies that a person acted carelessly. In cases of negligence, a jury decides whether any other prudent person would have acted differently than the defendant, given the same circumstances. For example, a car breaks down on the highway. The driver moves to the side of the road, raises the hood, and activates the emergency flashing lights. If another vehicle strikes the disabled car and the driver of the second car sues, the guilt or innocence of the driver of the disabled car depends on whether the jury believes their action was reasonable. *Reasonableness is based on the jury's opinion of what constitutes good common sense.*

Malpractice

Malpractice is professional negligence, which differs from simple negligence. It holds professionals to a higher standard of accountability. Rather than being held accountable for acting as an ordinary, reasonable layperson, in a malpractice case, the court determines whether a health care provider acted in a manner comparable to that of their peers. The plaintiff must prove four elements to win a malpractice lawsuit: duty, breach of duty, causation, and injury (Box 3-2).

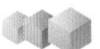 Concept Mastery Alert

Laws and Safety Laws and regulations, regardless of where and by whom they were established, go hand in hand with public safety.

BOX 3-2	Elements in a Malpractice Case

Duty—An obligation existed to provide care for the person who claims to have been injured or harmed.
Breach of duty—The caregiver failed to provide appropriate care, or the care provided was given negligently, that is, in a way that conflicts with how others with similar education would have acted given the same set of circumstances.
Causation—The caregiver's action, or lack of it, caused the plaintiff harm.
Injury—Physical, psychological, or financial harm occurred.

Because the jury may be unfamiliar with the scope of nursing practice, the plaintiff may present other resources in court to prove breach of duty. Some examples include the employing agency's standards for care, written policies and procedures, care plans or clinical pathways, and the testimony of expert witnesses (Fig. 3-4).

The best protection against malpractice lawsuits is competent nursing. Nurses demonstrate competency by participating in continuing education programs, taking nursing courses at colleges or universities, and becoming certified. Defensive nursing practice also involves thorough and objective documentation (see Chapter 19).

One of the best methods for avoiding lawsuits is to administer compassionate care. The "golden rule" of doing unto others as you would have them do unto you is a good principle to follow. Clients who perceive the nurse as caring and concerned tend to be satisfied with their care. The following techniques communicate a caring and compassionate attitude:

- Smiling
- Introducing yourself
- Calling the client by the name they prefer
- Touching the client appropriately to demonstrate concern
- Responding quickly to the call light
- Telling the client how long you will be gone if you need to leave the unit; informing the client who will provide care in your absence; alerting the client when you return
- Spending time with the client other than while performing required care
- Being a good listener
- Explaining everything so that the client can understand it
- Being a good host or hostess—offering visitors extra chairs, letting them know where they can obtain snacks and beverages, and directing them to the restrooms and parking areas
- Accepting justifiable criticism without becoming defensive
- Saying "I'm sorry"

Clients can sense when a nurse wants to do a good job, rather than just get a job done. The relationship that develops is apt to reduce the potential for a lawsuit, even if harm occurs.

PROFESSIONAL LIABILITY

All professionals, including nurses, are held responsible and accountable for providing safe and appropriate care. Because nurses have specialized knowledge and proximity to clients, they have a primary role in protecting clients from preventable or reversible complications.

The number of lawsuits involving nurses is increasing. It is to every nurse's advantage to obtain liability insurance

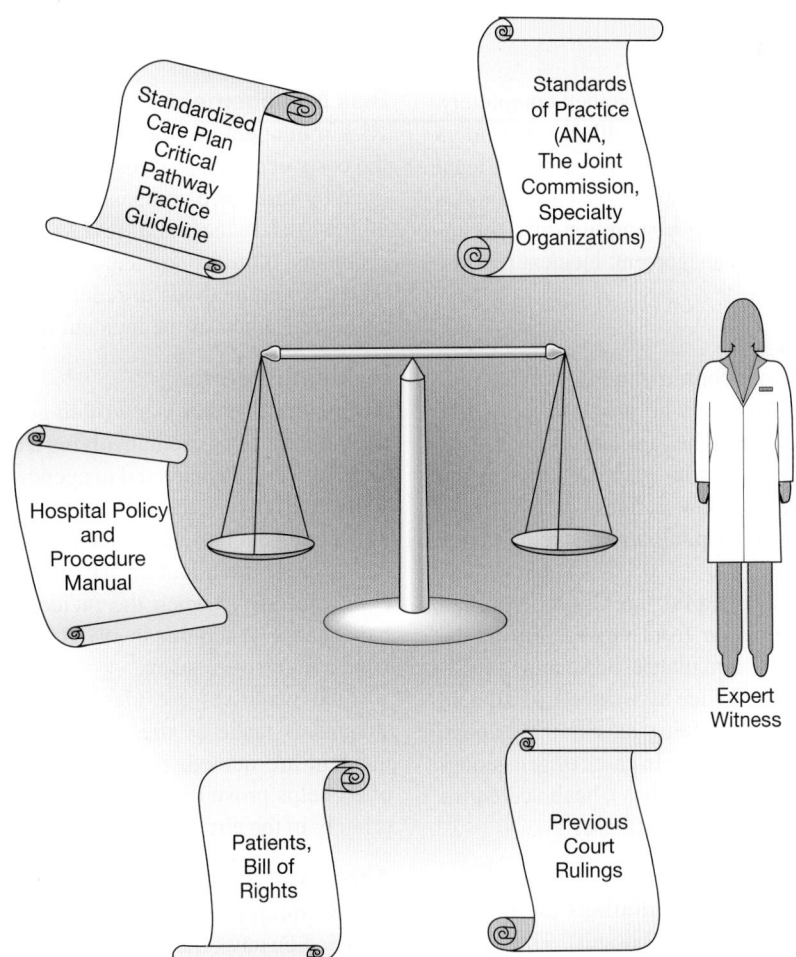

FIGURE 3-4 Data that establish standards of care. ANA, American Nurses Association.

and to become familiar with legal mechanisms, such as Good Samaritan laws and statutes of limitations, that may prevent or relieve culpability, as well as with strategies for providing a sound legal defense, such as written incident reports and anecdotal records.

Liability Insurance

Liability insurance (a contract between a person or corporation and a company willing to provide legal services and financial assistance when the policy holder is involved in a malpractice lawsuit) is necessary for all nurses. Although many agencies have liability insurance with an umbrella clause that includes its employees, nurses should obtain their own personal liability insurance. The advantage of personal liability insurance is that a nurse involved in a lawsuit will have a separate attorney working on their sole behalf. Because the damages sought in malpractice lawsuits are so costly, attorneys hired by health care facilities sometimes are more committed to defending the facility against liability and negative publicity rather than defending an individual nurse whom they also are being paid to represent.

Student nurses are held accountable for their actions during clinical practice and should also carry liability insurance. Liability insurance is available through the National Federation for Licensed Practical Nurses (NFLPN), the National Student Nurses' Association, the American Nurses Association (ANA), and other private insurance companies.

Reducing Liability

It is unrealistic to think lawsuits can be avoided completely. Some avenues protect nurses and other health care providers from being sued or provide a foundation for a sound legal defense. Examples include Good Samaritan laws, statutes of limitations, principles regarding assumption of risk, appropriate documentation, risk management, incident reports, and anecdotal records.

Good Samaritan Laws

Most states have enacted **Good Samaritan laws**, which provide legal immunity to passersby who provide emergency first aid to victims of accidents. The legislation is based on the biblical story of the person who gave aid to a beaten stranger along a roadside. The law defines an emergency as one occurring outside of a hospital, not in an emergency department.

Although these laws are helpful, no Good Samaritan law provides absolute exemption from prosecution in the event of injury. Paramedics, ambulance personnel, physicians, and nurses who stop to provide assistance are still held to a higher standard of care because they have training above and beyond that of average laypeople. In cases of **gross negligence** (total disregard for another's safety), health care providers may be charged with a criminal offense.

Statute of Limitations

Each state establishes a **statute of limitations** (designated time within which a person can file a lawsuit). The length varies among states and is generally calculated from when the incident occurred. When the injured party is a minor, however, the statute of limitations sometimes does not commence until the victim reaches adulthood. When the time expires, an injured party can no longer sue, even if their claim is legitimate.

Assumption of Risk

An **assumption of risk** is determined by whether a client is forewarned of a potential safety hazard and chooses to ignore the warning. If that occurs, the court may hold the client responsible. For example, if a hospitalized client objects to having the side rails up or lowers the rails independently, the nurse or health care facility may not be held fully accountable for an injury. It is essential that the nurse document that they warned the client and that the client disregarded the warning. The same recommendation applies when nurses caution clients about ambulating only with assistance.

Documentation

A major component to limiting liability is accurate, thorough **documentation** (record keeping). Nurses are held responsible or liable for information that they either include or exclude in reports and charting. Each health care setting requires accurate and complete documentation. The medical record is a legal document and is used as evidence in court. Records must be timely, objective, accurate, complete, and legible (see Chapter 9). The quality of the documentation, including neatness and spelling, can influence a jury's decision.

Risk Management

Risk management (the process of identifying and reducing the costs of anticipated losses) is a concept originally developed by insurance companies. Health care institutions now employ risk managers to review all the actual and potential problems in the workplace, identify common elements, and then develop methods to reduce the risk. A primary tool of risk management is the incident report.

Incident Reports

An **incident report** is a written account of an unusual, potentially injurious event involving a client, employee, or visitor (Fig. 3-5). It is directed to agency administrators and kept separate from the medical record. Incident reports determine how to prevent hazardous situations and serve as a reference in case of future litigation. They must include five important components: (1) when the incident occurred; (2) where it happened; (3) who was involved; (4) what happened; and (5) what actions were taken.

All witnesses are identified by name. Any pertinent statements made by the injured person before or after the incident are quoted. Accurate and detailed documentation often helps prove that the nurse acted reasonably or appropriately in the circumstances.

Anecdotal Records

An **anecdotal record** (personal account of an incident) is not recorded on any official form, nor is it filed with administrative records. The nurse personally retains the information,

THREE RIVERS AREA HOSPITAL INCIDENT REPORT
CONFIDENTIAL—DO NOT DUPLICATE
Forward to Risk Management within 48 hours

Identification	Sex	Age	Incident Date	Time	Shift	Department	Addressograph
__ Inpatient	__ M		__ / __ / __	__ : __	__ 1st ___		
__ Outpatient	__ F				__ 2nd ___		
__ Visitor					__ 3rd ___		

Reason for hospitalization/presence on premises: _____

I. Location of Incident:
　__ Patient room # ___
　__ Patient bathroom
　__ Corridor
　__ Other _____

II. Type of Incident:
　__ Fall
　__ Medication
　__ Infusion
　__ Lost/found
　__ Burn
　__ Treatment/procedure
　__ Equipment
　__ Needle/sponge count
　__ Other _____

III. Description of Incident: _____

IV. Nature of Incident:
　A. FALLS:

Activity Order:	Pt. Condition Prior to:	Fall Involved:	Patient/Visitor was:
__ Restraints	__ Weak, unsteady	__ Chair, W/C	__ Lying
__ Bed rest	__ Alert, oriented	__ Stretcher	__ Standing
__ BRP	__ Disoriented/confused	__ Tub/shower	__ Getting on/off
__ Up w/asst.	__ Senile	__ Toilet	__ Sitting
__ Up AD LIB	__ Unconscious	__ Floor condition (below)	__ Ambulating
	__ Medicated/sedated	__ Bed	__ Other _____
	Med. name ___	__ Side rails up	
	Last dose ___	__ Side fails down	

　B. MEDICATIONS:
　Incident Involved:

		Factors:	
__ Wrong Med, Tx, procedure	__ Adverse reaction	__ Patient ID not checked	__ Charting
__ Wrong patient	__ Infiltration	__ Transcription	__ Wrong med from pharmacy
__ Wrong time	__ Other _____	__ Labeling	__ Defective equipment
__ Omission		__ Physician orders not clear	__ Communications
__ Incorrect dose		__ Physician orders not checked	__ Other _____
__ Incorrect method of administration		__ Misread label/dose	

　C. OTHER:
　__ Loss of property
　__ Struck by object, equipment
　__ Equipment malfunction
　__ Anesthesia
　__ Patient I.D.
　__ Other

V. Nature of Injury (Injury sustained as a result of incident):
　__ Asphyxia, strangulation, inhalation
　__ Head injury
　__ Contagious or infectious disease exposure
　__ Fracture or dislocation
　__ Viscera injury
　__ Sprain or strain
　__ Contusion, cut, laceration
　__ Burn or scald
　__ Chemical burn
　__ No injury
　__ No apparent injury
　__ Other _____

VI. Actions Taken:

Physician notified:	Pt./visitor seen by MD/T&EC:	MD Name	Time
__ Yes __ No	__ Yes __ No	_____	__ : __

Physician's findings: _____

Follow-up: __ No __ Yes–Specify _____

Name of Person Reporting	__ / __ / __ Date	Department Director	__ / __ / __ Date
Supervisor	__ / __ / __ Date	Risk Management	__ / __ / __ Date

FIGURE 3-5 Example of an incident report form.

which is safeguarded and may be used later to refresh the nurse's memory if a lawsuit develops. Anecdotal notes can be used in court on advice of an attorney.

Malpractice Litigation

Malpractice is a claim that a professional person's actions failed to meet a standard of care or conduct of similar professionals, resulting in injury to a client. A successful outcome in a malpractice lawsuit depends on many variables, such as physical evidence and attorney expertise. The appearance, demeanor, and conduct of a nurse charged with malpractice inside and outside of the courtroom can help or damage the case. Suggestions in Box 3-3 may help if a nurse becomes involved in malpractice litigation.

BOX 3-3　　**Legal Advice**

1. Notify the claims agent of your professional liability insurance company.
2. Contact the National Nurses Claims Database through the ANA. This confidential service provides information that supports nurses involved in litigation.
3. Discuss the particulars of the case only with your attorney.
4. Tell your attorney everything.
5. Avoid giving public statements.
6. Reread the client's record, incident sheet, and your anecdotal notes before testifying.
7. Ask to reread information in court if it will help to refresh your memory.
8. Dress conservatively, in a business-like manner. Avoid excesses in makeup, hairstyle, or jewelry.
9. Look directly at the person asking a question.
10. Speak in a modulated but audible voice that the jury and others in the court can hear easily.
11. Tell the truth.
12. Use language with which you are comfortable. Do not try to impress the court with legal or medical terms.
13. Say as little as possible in court under cross-examination.
14. Answer the prosecuting lawyer's questions with "yes" or "no;" limit answers to only the questions asked.
15. If you do not know or cannot remember information, say so.
16. Wait to expand on information if asked by your defense attorney.
17. Remain calm, objective, and cooperative.

ETHICS

The word "ethics" comes from the Greek word *ethos*, meaning customs or modes of conduct. **Ethics** (moral or philosophical principles) helps classify actions as either right or wrong. Various organizations, such as those representing nurses, have identified standards for ethical practice, known as a code of ethics, for members within their discipline.

Codes of Ethics

A **code of ethics** (a list of written statements describing ideal behavior) serves as a model for personal conduct. The National Association for Practical Nurse Education and Services, the NFLPN, and the International Council of Nurses all have composed codes of ethics. The ANA released the latest revision of *Code of Ethics with Interpretive Statements* in 2015. Because of rapidly changing technology, no code is ever specific enough to provide guidelines for every dilemma that nurses may face.

Ethical Dilemmas

An **ethical dilemma** (choice between two undesirable alternatives) occurs when individual values and laws conflict. This is especially true in relation to health care. Occasionally, nurses find themselves in situations that are legal but are personally unethical, or are ethical but illegal. For instance, abortion is legal, but some believe it is unethical. Assisted suicide is illegal except in California, Colorado, Hawaii,

Oregon, Vermont, Montana, New Jersey, Washington, and Washington, D.C., which has legalized physician-assisted suicide (State by State Guide to Assisted Suicide, 2018), but some believe it is ethical.

Ethical Theories

Nurses generally use one of two ethical problem-solving theories to guide them in solving ethical dilemmas. These are teleology and deontology.

Teleologic Theory

Teleology is ethical decision-making based on final outcomes. It is also known as utilitarianism because the ultimate ethical test for any decision is based on what is best for the most people. Stated from a different perspective, teleologists believe "the end justifies the means." Thus, the choice that benefits many people justifies the harm that may come to a few. A teleologist would argue that selective abortion (destroying some embryos in a multiple pregnancy) is ethical because it is done to ensure the full-term birth of those that remain. In other words, termination can be justified in some situations but may not be justified in all cases.

Teleologists analyze ethical dilemmas on a case-by-case basis. They propose that an action is not good or bad in and of itself. Instead, the consequences determine whether the action is good or bad. The primary consideration is a desirable outcome for those most affected.

Deontologic Theory

Deontology is ethical decision-making based on duty or moral obligations. It proposes that the outcome is not the primary issue; rather, decisions must be based on the morality of the act itself. In other words, certain actions are always right or wrong regardless of circumstances. Deontologists would argue that destroying any fetus is wrong, whether done to save others or not, because killing is immoral. Deontology proposes that health care providers have a moral duty to maintain and preserve life. Thus, deontologists would consider it immoral for a nurse to assist with abortion, suicide for the terminally ill, or execution of a convicted prisoner.

Deontology also proposes that moral duty to others is equally as important as consequences. A duty is an obligation to perform or to avoid an action to which others are entitled. For example, deontologists believe that lying is never acceptable because it violates the duty to tell the truth to those entitled to honest information. Nurses ultimately have a professional duty to their clients, and clients have rights to which they are entitled (Box 3-4).

Ethical Principles

It is sometimes impossible or impractical to analyze ethical issues from solely a teleologic or deontologic point of view. In lieu of using one ethical theory exclusively, nurses can base ethical decisions on six principles that form a foundation for ethical practice: (1) beneficence, (2) nonmaleficence, (3) autonomy, (4) veracity, (5) fidelity, and (6) justice. These principles may at times conflict with each other.

1. Patients have the right to information necessary to make decisions about their health care that is provided in their primary language in ways they can understand.
2. Patients have the right and responsibility to choose health care providers they trust and who they believe are best able to treat them successfully.
3. Individuals deserve immediate access to emergency medical care when needed.
4. Patients have the right to know options and the responsibility to participate in decisions regarding their health care, or to authorize a representative to make decisions for them.
5. Patients have the right to respect and consideration and should never suffer from discrimination based on differences by health care professionals or health care plan representatives.
6. Patients have the right to consult privately with their health care providers, to see and discuss their personal medical records, and to request changes to those records as specifically listed in HIPAA.
7. Patients must have access to procedures that guarantee a timely, confidential, and fair review of any complaints they may have concerning care, facilities and personnel, or their health care insurer.

HIPAA, Health Insurance Portability and Accountability Act.
A compilation of standard practices based on the HIPAA of 1966, The Consumer Bill of Rights and Responsibilities of 1998, and the Patient Safety Act of 2005; Reynolds, L. (n.d.). *What is the patient bill of rights?* Retrieved March 4, 2015, from http://www.ehow.com/facts_4868817_what-patient-bill-rights.html?ref=Tract2utm_source=ask

>> *Stop, Think, and Respond 3-2*
How might a teleologist and a deontologist approach an ethical dilemma such as managing the care of an infant with microcephaly (small brain and severe cognitive impairment) who develops a high fever as a result of an infection?

Beneficence and Nonmaleficence

Beneficence means "doing good" or acting for another's benefit. To do good, an ethical person prevents or removes any potentially harmful factor. For example, if a client has cancer, the beneficent act is to eliminate the cancer with surgery, drugs, or radiation. The difficulty, for example, is that a health care provider's approach to doing good may not be what the client feels is best. The client may prefer no treatment of the cancer.

Nonmaleficence means "doing no harm" or avoiding an action that deliberately harms a person. Sometimes, however, "harm" is necessary to promote "good." In the previous example of cancer, available treatments can cause pain, nausea, vomiting, hair loss, and susceptibility to infection. Yet, the ultimate benefit is eradicating the cancer. This is an example of the *principle of double effect*. The following criteria can help to resolve cases involving double effect:

- The action itself must not be intrinsically wrong; it must be good or neutral.
- Only the good effect must be intended even though the harmful effect is foreseen.
- The harmful effect must not be the means of the good effect.
- The good effect must outweigh the harmful effect.

Autonomy

Autonomy refers to a competent person's right to make their own choices without intimidation or influence. For a person to make a decision, they must have all relevant information, including treatment options in a language they understand. The client always has the option of obtaining a second opinion from another health care provider. One outcome may be that the client declines all possible options for treatment, a decision that must be respected.

Conflict can arise if the client's choice poses more risk than potential benefit; is illegal (e.g., requesting assistance with suicide), morally objectionable, or medically inappropriate; or interferes with the needs of another person whose case merits higher priority. An example is a young woman who seeks the removal of both breasts because she fears breast cancer though there is no evidence she is at a high risk for it. In such a case, the duty to respect the client's wishes may be nullified. One option may be to refer the client to another health care provider.

Veracity

Veracity means the duty to be honest and avoid deceiving or misleading a client. This principle causes conflict when the truth may harm the client by interfering with recovery or worsening the present condition.

Fidelity

Fidelity means being faithful to work-related commitments and obligations. Its application relates to the caregiver's obligation to clients. For example, nurses are obligated to be competent in performing skills and services required for safe and appropriate care. This implies that nurses pursue continuing education and maintain current certification for cardiopulmonary resuscitation (CPR). It also requires that nurses respect clients, provide compassionate care, protect confidentiality, honor promises, and follow their employer's policies.

Justice

Justice mandates that clients be treated impartially without discrimination according to age, gender, race, religion, socioeconomic status, weight, marital status, or sexual orientation. In other words, everyone should have equal distribution of goods and services. In reality, circumstances may force nurses to devote more attention to an unstable client. For example, a person arrives in the emergency department with fever and vomiting. Shortly thereafter, another person presents with chest pain. The nurse decides to attend to the client with chest pain first. Another example of inequality is when more than one client needs a scarce resource, such as an organ for transplantation. Although several clients may qualify for the organ, only one can receive it.

When goods and services cannot be allocated equally, decisions are based on need, merit, or potential for contribution. In the example of the transplant organ, based on need, the most critically ill person would receive it. Based on merit, the organ would be given to the person who worked hardest or made the greatest effort at this point in their life.

Values and Ethical Decision-Making

When a nurse has not taken a course in ethics, their ethical decisions are often the result of values. **Values** are a person's most meaningful beliefs and the basis on which they make most decisions about what is right or wrong. Values are commonly (1) acquired from parental models, life experiences, and religious tenets; (2) reinforced by a person's world view; (3) modeled in personal behavior; (4) consistent over time; and (5) defended when challenged.

The following serve as guidelines to ethical decision-making:

- Make sure that whatever is done is in the client's best interest.
- Preserve and support the rights of clients (see Box 3-4).
- Work cooperatively with the client and other health care providers.
- Follow written policies, codes of ethics, and laws.
- Follow your conscience.

Ethics Committees

Ethical decisions are complex, especially when they affect the lives of clients. Because making a judgment for another is a weighty responsibility, many health care agencies have established ethics committees. These committees consist of a broad cross-section of professionals and nonprofessionals within the community with varying viewpoints. Most ethics committees will include a board member of the institution, a lay person, an administrator, and a member of the clergy. Their diversity encourages healthy debate about ethical issues. Ethics committees are best used in a policy-making capacity before any specific dilemma. They are also called upon to offer advice, to protect clients' best interests, and to avoid legal conflicts.

Common Ethical Issues

Several ethical issues recur in nursing practice. Examples include telling the truth, maintaining confidentiality, withholding or withdrawing treatment, advocating for ethical allocation of scarce resources, and protecting vulnerable people from unsafe practices or practitioners.

Truth Telling

Truth telling proposes that all clients have the right to complete and accurate information. It implies that physicians and nurses have a duty to tell clients the truth about matters concerning their health. Personnel demonstrate respect for this right by explaining to the client the status of their health problem, the benefits and risks of treatment, alternative forms of treatment, and consequences if the treatment is not administered.

It is the physician's duty to inform clients. Conflict occurs when the client has not been given full information, when facts have been misrepresented, or when a client misunderstands information. In some cases, physicians are reluctant to talk honestly with clients or present the proposed treatment in a biased manner. Often, the nurse is forced to choose between remaining silent in allegiance to the physician and providing the client with the truth. Either action may have frustrating consequences.

Confidentiality

Confidentiality, or safeguarding a person's health information from public disclosure, is the foundation for trust. Nurses must not divulge health information to unauthorized people without the client's written permission. Even giving medical information to a client's health insurance company requires a signed release. Consequently, nurses must use discretion when sharing verbal information so that others do not hear it indiscriminately. Now that vast information about clients is stored on computers, the duty to protect confidentiality extends to safeguarding both written and electronic data (refer to the discussion of the HIPAA).

Withholding and Withdrawing Treatment

Technology is often used to prolong life at all costs, beyond justifying its benefits. Decisions involving life and death may sometimes continue to circumvent clients, a clear violation of ethical principles. Completing advance directives and determining a client's code status ensure that a person's health care is in accordance with their wishes.

Advance Directives

Legislation now mandates the discussion of terminal care with clients. Since Congress approved the Patient Self-Determination Act in 1990, health care agencies reimbursed through Medicare must ask clients whether they have executed an **advance directive** (written statement identifying a competent person's wishes concerning terminal care). The two types of advance directives are a living will and a durable power of attorney for health care. A **living will** is an instructive form of an advance directive; that is, it is a written document that identifies a person's preferences regarding medical interventions to use—or not use—in a terminal condition, irreversible coma, or persistent vegetative state with no hope of recovery (Fig. 3-6). Clients must share advance directives with health care providers to ensure that they are implemented.

A **durable power of attorney for health care** (Fig. 3-7) designates a proxy for making medical decisions when the client becomes so incompetent or incapacitated that they cannot make decisions independently. The designee can give or withhold permission for treatments on the client's behalf in end-of-life circumstances or when the client is temporarily unconscious.

Living wills and durable powers of attorney for health care are not just measures reserved for older adults; any competent adult can initiate them. They are best composed before a health crisis develops to assist care providers and significant others to comply with the client's wishes. A living will and health care proxy can avoid legal expenses, delays in obtaining guardianship, or unwanted decisions made by an ethics committee or court. Thus, nurses should inform all clients about their right to self-determination, encourage them to compose advance directives, and support their decisions (see Client and Family Teaching 3-1).

LIVING WILL

A living will allows a principal to select end-of-life treatment options in the chance of incapacitation with no viable cure.

I choose to: (check one)

_____ ☐ - Have a living will.
_____ ☐ - Not have a living will. Part II of this form is intentionally left blank.

A. PRINCIPAL. I, _____, with a mailing address of _____,
City of _____, County of _____, State of _____, with the
last four (4) digits of my social security number (SSN) being XXX - XX - _____ ("Principal") desire to advise my doctors and medical
providers of my wishes for my health care in the event I am not able to communicate my wishes.

B. LIFE SUPPORT.

I desire that my doctor make a concerted effort to return me to an acceptable quality of life using then available treatments and therapies.
However, if my quality of life becomes unacceptable as I have defined below, and my doctors have determined that my condition will not
improve (is irreversible), I direct that all treatments that extend my life be withdrawn.

An unacceptable quality of life means (initial and check all that apply):

_____ ☐ - Chronic coma or persistent vegetative state
_____ ☐ - No longer able to communicate my needs
_____ ☐ - No longer able to recognize family or friends
_____ ☐ - Total dependence on others for daily care
_____ ☐ - Other: _____.

Initial and check one (1) only:

_____ ☐ - Even if I have the quality of life described above, I still wish to be treated with food and water by tube or intravenously (IV).
_____ ☐ - If I have the quality of life described above, I do NOT wish to be treated with food and water by tube or intravenously (IV).

C. CERTAIN LIFE-SUSTAINING TREATMENT. (initial and check all that apply)

Some people do not wish to have certain life-sustaining treatments under any circumstance, even if recovery is a possibility. Check the treatments
below, if any, that you do not wish to have under any circumstances:

_____ ☐ - Cardiopulmonary Resuscitation (CPR)
_____ ☐ - Ventilation (breathing machine)
_____ ☐ - Feeding tube
_____ ☐ - Dialysis
_____ ☐ - Other: _____.

D. END OF LIFE WISHES. (hospice care, funeral arrangements, etc.):

When I am near death, it is important to me that:
_____
_____
_____

I have signed this document on this ____ day of _____, 20____.

Principal's Signature: _____

Print Name: _____

Depending on your State's laws, you either two (2) witnesses and/or notary public may be required for signing this form.

FIGURE 3-6 Example of a living will.

MEDICAL POWER OF ATTORNEY

A medical power of attorney allows you the right to name someone else to make health care decisions on your behalf.

I choose to: (check one)

_____ ☐ - Have a medical power of attorney.

_____ ☐ - Not have a medical power of attorney. Part I of this form is intentionally left blank.

A. PRINCIPAL. I, _____, with a mailing address of _____,
City of _____, State of _____, Zip Code: _____ ("Principal") hereby designate:

B. AGENT. _____, with a mailing address of _____, City of _____,
State of _____, Zip Code: _____ ("Agent").

AGENT'S TELEPHONE (CELL): (____) ____-_____

I select the above-named person as my Agent to act in all matters relating to my health care (including my mental health care) and including, without limitation, the power to give or refuse consent to all medical and surgical treatments, hospitalizations, and all related health care. This power of attorney is effective at the point when I am no longer able to communicate my health care wishes. My Agent's decisions under this power of attorney, during any period when I am unable to make and/or communicate my health care decisions or when there is uncertainty as to whether I am dead or alive, are binding on my heirs, devisees, and personal representatives.

C. ALTERNATE AGENT. If my Agent is unable or unwilling to serve or make a decision in a timely manner,
I select _____, with a mailing address of _____, City of _____,
State of _____, to act as my alternate agent ("Alternate Agent"):

ALTERNATE AGENT'S TELEPHONE (CELL): (____) ____-_____

I intend for my Agent to receive any and all of my health records and information as if I were the one requesting such information. This release authority applies to any information governed by the Health Insurance Portability and Accountability Act of 1996 (aka HIPAA), 42 USC 1420D, and 45 CFR 160-164.

FIGURE 3-7 Example of a medical power of attorney form.

Client and Family Teaching 3-1
Advance Directives

The nurse teaches the following points:

- An advance directive is not required, but it is encouraged.
- A lawyer is not needed to create an advance directive; printed forms are available from health care agencies, organizations such as the American Association of Retired Persons, and various internet sites such as Legal Zoom and Legal Nature (http://www.aarp.org/relationships/care-giving/info-03-2012/free-printable-advance-directives.html).
- When filling out the form, indicate specific wishes for the initiation or withdrawal of life-sustaining medical treatments such as cardiopulmonary resuscitation, kidney dialysis, mechanical ventilation, use of a tube for administering food and water, obtaining comfort measures such as pain medication, and donation of organs.
- Write additional instructions if something is not addressed in the form; for example, your instructions may be different if you are pregnant.
- Obtain the signatures of two witnesses, other than your physician or spouse.
- Give a copy to your physician for your medical file.
- Tell family members or your lawyer that you have an advance directive and its location.
- Keep the original advance directive in a place where it can be found easily.
- Bring a copy of your advance directive whenever you are hospitalized or admitted to a health care facility (e.g., nursing home, extended care facility).
- Change your advance directive by revoking or adding instructions at any time; share the revised copy with those who will carry out your instructions.
- A separate or different advance directive is not needed for each state; they are generally recognized universally within the United States.

Code Status

A **code status** refers to how health care providers are required to manage care in the case of cardiac or respiratory arrest. Without a written order from the physician to the contrary, the client is designated as a full code. A full code means that all measures to resuscitate the client are used.

After a discussion with the physician, some clients indicate that they want no resuscitative efforts, that is, "no code" or "do not resuscitate (DNR)." Alternately, they may select a combination of interventions that constitute less than a full code. Some clients specify using drugs, but refuse cardiac defibrillation or endotracheal intubation for mechanical ventilation. For anything less than a full code, the physician must write an order to that effect in the client's medical record.

Allocation of Scarce Resources

Allocation of scarce resources is the process of deciding how to distribute limited life-saving equipment or procedures among several who could benefit. Such decisions are difficult. In effect, those who receive the resources have a greater chance to live, while those who do not may die prematurely. One strategy is "first come, first served." Another is to project what would produce the most good for the most people.

Whistle-Blowing

Whistle-blowing (reporting incompetent or unethical practices), as the name implies, calls attention to unsafe or potentially harmful situations. Usually, it occurs in the institution where the reporting person is employed. For instance, a nurse may report another nurse or physician who cares for clients while under the influence of alcohol or a controlled substance.

Whenever a problem is identified, the first step is to report the situation to an immediate supervisor. If the supervisor takes no action, the nurse faces an ethical dilemma about any further steps. Going beyond the administrative hierarchy and making public revelations may be necessary.

The decision to "blow the whistle" involves personal risks and may result in grave consequences such as character assassination, retribution in the form of crimes against one's person or property, negative evaluations, demotions, or shunning. Nevertheless, the ethical priority is protecting clients in general and the community at large.

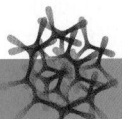

KEY POINTS

- There are six categories of laws that we must abide by:
- Constitutional law
- Statutory law (includes nurse practice acts)
- Administrative law
  - State Boards of Nursing
  - Nurse licensure compacts
- Common law
- Criminal laws
- Civil laws
- The nurse practice act defines the scope of practice specific to an RN, LPN, advanced nurse practitioner, and nurse anesthetist. It represents all laws that regulate a nurse's scope of practice in the state or states of America in which the nurse is licensed to work. These laws protect patients from harm as well as lay the rules and regulations for the specific level of a nurse's educational and licensure requirements.
- Negligence versus malpractice
  - Negligence: harm that results because a person did not act *reasonably*
  - Malpractice: professional negligence; the health care provider did not act in a manner comparable to that of their peers.
- Ethics (moral or philosophical principles) classifies actions as either right or wrong. A code of ethics is a list of written statements describing ideal behavior and serves as a model for personal conduct.
- Beneficence versus nonmaleficence
  - Beneficence: "Doing good" or acting for another's benefit

- Nonmaleficence: "Doing no harm" or avoiding an action that deliberately harms a person
- Guidelines to ethical decision-making:
  - Make sure that whatever is done is in the client's best interest.
  - Preserve and support the rights of clients.
  - Work cooperatively with the client and other health care providers.
  - Follow written policies, codes of ethics, and laws.
  - Follow your conscience.
- Advance directives
  - Living will: An instructive form of an advance directive; identifies a person's preferences regarding medical interventions to use—or not use—in a terminal condition, irreversible coma, or persistent vegetative state with no hope of recovery; must be provided to the health care provider.
  - Durable power of attorney for health care: Designates a proxy for making medical decisions when the client becomes so incompetent or incapacitated that they cannot make decisions independently; the designee can give or withhold permission for treatments on the client's behalf in end-of-life circumstances or when the client is temporarily unconscious.
- Code status: Unless there is written order from a physician or designated in advance directives, a client is designated as a "full code," meaning all measures to resuscitate the client are used; "no code" or "DNR" means no measures are to be used; clients may also indicate which measures are acceptable and which are not.

CRITICAL THINKING EXERCISES

1. What actions might protect a nurse from being sued when a client assigned to their care falls out of bed?
2. A client who fell while ambulating to the bathroom sues the assigned nurse. Based on the elements necessary in a malpractice lawsuit, what must the client's lawyer prove? What defense may the nurse's lawyer offer?
3. Which criteria justify assisted suicide?
4. Two people need a liver transplant; only one liver is available. What information might a teleologist and a deontologist use to determine who should receive the organ?

NEXT-GENERATION NCLEX-STYLE REVIEW QUESTIONS

1. What is the first action the nurse should take if there is a suspicion that a colleague is stealing narcotics and recording their administration to assigned clients?
   a. Refer the nurse to the ethics committee.
   b. Notify the local police department.
   c. Share concerns with nursing peers.
   d. Report suspicions to a supervisor.
   Test-Taking Strategy: Note the key words, "first action." Select the option that represents the most immediate line of authority, communication, and responsibility within the organization.
2. What information is most important for the nurse to obtain in a preoperative assessment?
   a. Birth certificate
   b. Social security number
   c. Advance directive
   d. Proof of insurance
   Test-Taking Strategy: Note the key word and modifier, "most important." Use the process of elimination to select the data that have the highest priority for nursing care.

3. What nursing action is most appropriate after caring for a client who has fallen out of bed? List in order of priority.
   a. Institute fall precautions.
   b. Complete an incident report.
   c. Call the nursing supervisor.
   d. Notify the client's family.
   Test-Taking Strategy: Note the key word and modifier, "most appropriate." Use the process of elimination to select the action that provides a written account regarding an injury or potential injury. All of the answers are correct. List them in order of priority for fall precautions.
4. What nursing action is most appropriate when an unresponsive client with terminal cancer and no advance directive or "do not resuscitate order" stops breathing and has no pulse?
   a. Note the time of death.
   b. Notify the physician.
   c. Perform postmortem care.
   d. Begin resuscitative efforts.
   Test-Taking Strategy: Note the key word and modifier, "most appropriate," and additional information in the stem that states, "no advance directive." Use the process of elimination to select the option that corresponds with a nurse's responsibility in the absence of any written order to withhold emergency care.
5. What nursing action is best when a client has never created an advance directive?
   a. Recommend contacting a lawyer.
   b. Ask the client about terminal care.
   c. Consult with the client's family.
   d. Provide an advance directive form.
   Test-Taking Strategy: Note the key word, "best." Use the process of elimination to select the option that allows the client to document information regarding their end-of-life wishes.

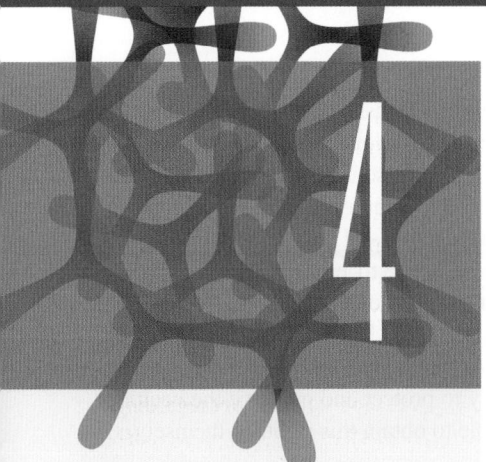

4

Health and Illness

Learning Objectives

On completion of this chapter, the reader should be able to:

1. Describe how the World Health Organization (WHO) defines health.
2. Discuss the difference between values and beliefs, and list health beliefs common among Americans.
3. Explain the concept of holism.
4. Identify the five levels of human needs.
5. Define illness and terms used to describe illness.
6. Differentiate primary, secondary, tertiary, and extended care.
7. Name programs that help finance health care for older, disabled, and low-income populations.
8. List methods for controlling escalating health care costs.
9. Identify national health goals targeted for the year 2030.
10. Discuss methods that nurses use to administer client care.

INTRODUCTION

Neither health nor illness is an absolute state; rather, there are fluctuations along a continuum throughout life (Fig. 4-1). Because it is impossible to be (or get) well and stay well forever, nurses are committed to helping people prevent illness and restore or improve their health.

Nurses accomplish these goals by:

- Helping people live healthy lives
- Encouraging early diagnosis of disease
- Implementing measures to prevent complications of disorders

 Gerontologic Considerations

■ Shorter lengths of hospital stays along with increasing prevalence of chronic conditions in older adults have led to the development of a broad range of extended care services for the growing population of older adults.

■ Despite the major contribution of health insurance programs in paying for health care services, out-of-pocket expenses have been increasing steadily for older adults.

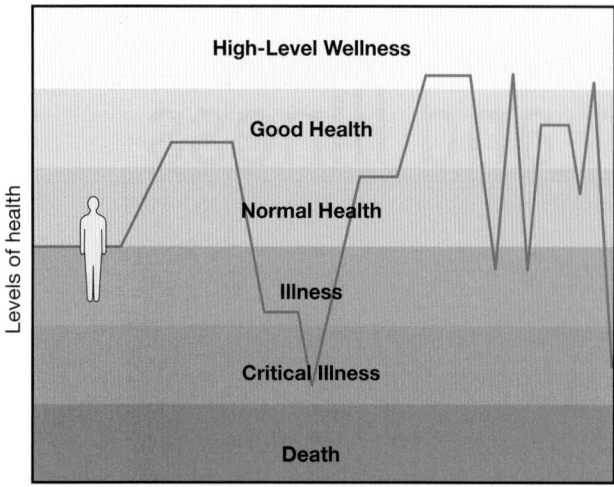

FIGURE 4-1 The health–illness continuum shows the different levels of health a person experiences over a lifetime.

HEALTH

The World Health Organization (WHO) is globally committed to "health for all." In the preamble to its constitution, the WHO defines **health** as a state of complete physical, mental, and social well-being, not merely the absence of disease or infirmity. Each person perceives and defines health differently. Nurses must recognize the importance of respecting such differences rather than imposing standards that may be unrealistic for a given person.

A person's behaviors are the outcomes of their values and belief systems. **Values** are ideals that a person feels are important (e.g., knowledge, wealth, financial security, marital fidelity, health). **Beliefs** are concepts that a person holds to be true (e.g., how people see themselves and the world). Beliefs and values guide a person's actions. Both health values and beliefs demonstrate or affirm what is personally significant. When a person values health, they take actions to preserve it.

Many Americans believe that health is a limited resource, health is a right, and/or health is a personal responsibility.

Health: A Limited Resource

A resource is a possession that is valuable because its supply is limited and there is no substitute. Given that definition, health is considered quite precious. People often say, "as long as you have your health, you have everything" and "health is wealth." Personal health depends in some measure on the active and passive signs people observe and adopt about their own health. These include a person's individual actions for preventing or minimizing the effects of a disease.

Health: A Right

The United States Declaration of Independence proclaims that "all men are created equal" and are entitled to life, liberty, and the pursuit of happiness. Based on this premise, the U.S. laws aim to ensure that everyone, regardless of age, gender, level of education, religion, sexual orientation, ethnic origin, social position, or wealth, receives equal services for sustaining

health. However, as will be discussed later, health disparities exist among various groups within the United States. These groups include people of lower socioeconomic (SES) status, members of racial and ethnic minorities, those affected by gender differences, older adults, and people with disabilities. Efforts are underway, however, to eliminate health barriers and to promote equal access to health care (see discussion of *Healthy People 2030* later in this chapter). If all are equally entitled to health, it follows that the nation in general and nurses in particular have a duty to protect and preserve the health of those who may be unable to obtain this right for themselves.

Health: A Personal Responsibility

Health requires continuous personal effort. There is as much potential for illness as there is for health. Each person is instrumental in their own health outcomes. Nurses stand ready to provide assistance and to advocate on behalf of others.

Wellness

Wellness refers to a full and balanced integration of all aspects of health. It involves physical, emotional, social, and spiritual health. **Physical health** exists when body organs function normally. **Emotional health** results when one feels safe and copes effectively with the stressors of life. **Social health** is an outcome of feeling accepted and useful. **Spiritual health** is characterized as believing that one's life has purpose. The four components are collectively referred to as the concept of holism.

Holism

Holism (the sum of physical, emotional, social, and spiritual health) determines how "whole" or well a person feels (Fig. 4-2). Any change in one component, positive or negative, automatically creates repercussions in the others. Take,

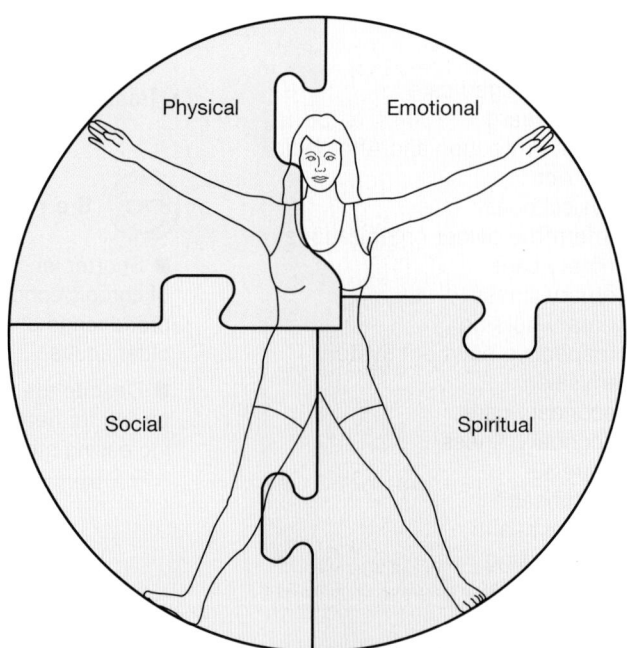

FIGURE 4-2 Holism is a concept that considers all aspects of a person.

for example, the person who has a heart attack. Their physical health is immediately impaired. In addition, heart attack affects the emotional, social, and spiritual aspects of health. For example, the client may experience psychological anxiety over this health change. Their social roles may temporarily or permanently change. The client may explore philosophical and spiritual issues as they consider the potential of death.

Nurses are often considered "holistic practitioners" because they are committed to restoring balance in each of the four aspects of wellness. They base their strategies for doing so on a hierarchy of human needs.

Hierarchy of Human Needs

In 1954, Abraham Maslow, a psychologist, identified five levels of **human needs** (factors that motivate behavior) in his book, *Motivation and Personality*. He grouped the needs in tiers, or a sequential hierarchy (Fig. 4-3), according to their significance: physiologic (first level), safety and security (second level), love and belonging (third level), esteem and self-esteem (fourth level), and self-actualization (fifth level).

The first-level physiologic needs are the most important to survival. They are the activities necessary to sustain life, such as breathing and eating. Each level is less important to survival than the one(s) below it. Maslow believed that until a human satisfies their physiologic needs, that person cannot or will not seek to fulfill other needs. By progressively satisfying needs at each level, however, the person will realize their maximum potential for health and well-being.

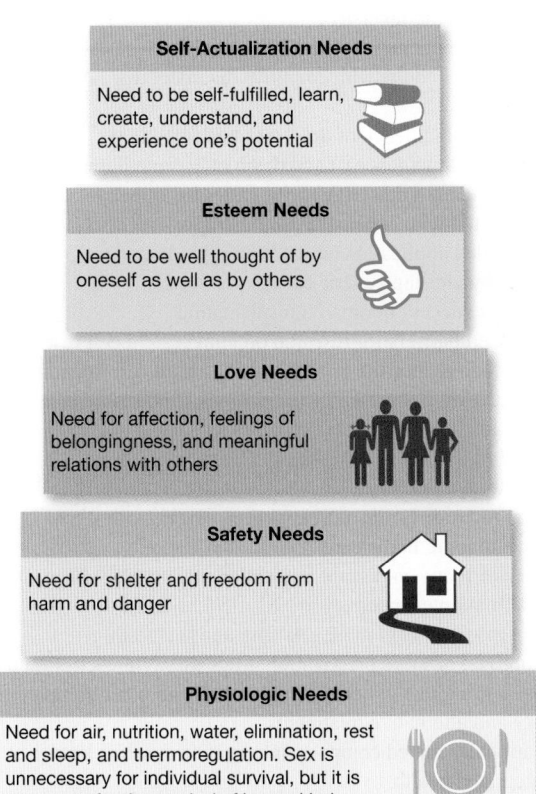

FIGURE 4-3 Maslow's hierarchy of human needs. (From Craven, R. F., & Himle, C. J. [2021]. *Fundamentals of nursing* [9th ed.]. Lippincott Williams & Wilkins.)

Nurses have adopted Maslow's hierarchy as a tool for setting priorities for client care. For example, in the case of the client who has had a heart attack, the nurse considers the client's physical needs, such as managing pain, as a priority. The nurse addresses other needs, such as assisting the client with a possible change in role performance or spiritual distress, after the client's health condition stabilizes.

ILLNESS

Illness is a state of being unhealthy when disease, deterioration, or injury impairs a person's well-being. Several terms are used commonly when referring to illnesses: morbidity and mortality; acute, chronic, and terminal; primary and secondary; remission and exacerbation; and hereditary, congenital, and idiopathic.

Morbidity and Mortality

Morbidity (incidence of a specific disease, disorder, or injury) refers to the rate or the numbers of people affected. Federal statistics are compiled on the basis of age, gender and/or biologic sex, or per 1,000 people within the population. **Mortality** (incidence of deaths) denotes the number of people who died from a particular disease or condition. Table 4-1 lists the 10 leading causes of death among all Americans of all ages in 2020.

Acute, Chronic, and Terminal Illnesses

Describing an illness as an **acute illness** (one that comes on suddenly and lasts a short time) is one method for classifying a change in health. Influenza is an example of an acute illness. Many acute illnesses are curable. Some lead to long-term problems because of their **sequelae** (singular: sequela; ill effects that result from permanent or progressive organ damage caused by a disease or its treatment). The risk for **chronic illness** (one that comes on slowly and lasts a long time) increases as people age. A **terminal illness** (one for which there is no potential for cure) is one that eventually is fatal. The terminal stage of an illness is one in which a person is approaching death.

TABLE 4-1 Leading Causes of Death in the United States in 2020

RANK	CAUSE OF DEATH	NUMBER
1	Heart disease	696,962
2	Cancer	602,350
3	COVID-19	350,831
4	Accidental (unintentional injuries)	200,955
5	Stroke	160,264
6	Chronic lower respiratory diseases	152,657
7	Alzheimer disease	134,242
8	Diabetes	102,188
9	Influenza and pneumonia	53,544
10	Kidney disease	52,547

Data from Murphy, S. L., Kochanek, K. D., Jiaquan, X., & Arias, E. (2021). Mortality in the United States, 2020. *NCHS Data Brief No. 427.* National Center for Health Statistics. https://doi.org/10.15620/cdc:112079

Primary and Secondary Illnesses

A **primary illness** (one that develops independently of any other disease) differs from a **secondary illness** (disorder that develops from a preexisting condition). For example, pulmonary disease acquired from smoking is a primary illness. If pneumonia or heart failure occurs as a consequence of smoke-damaged lung tissue, it is considered a secondary problem. In essence, the primary condition predisposes a person to the secondary condition.

Remission and Exacerbation

Remission is the disappearance of signs and symptoms associated with a particular disease. Although remission resembles a cured state, the relief may be only temporary. The duration of remission is unpredictable. An **exacerbation** (reactivation of a disorder, or one that reverts from a chronic to an acute state) can occur periodically in clients with long-standing diseases. Often, remissions and exacerbations are related to how well or how poorly the immune system is functioning, the stressors the client is facing, and the client's overall health status (e.g., nutrition, sleep, hydration).

Hereditary, Congenital, and Idiopathic Illnesses

A **hereditary condition** (disorder acquired from the genetic codes of one or both parents) may or may not produce symptoms immediately after birth. Cystic fibrosis, a lung disease, and Huntington chorea, a neurologic disorder, are examples of inherited illnesses. The first is diagnosed soon after birth; the second does not manifest until adulthood.

Congenital disorders (those present at birth but which are the result of faulty embryonic development) cannot be genetically predicted. Maternal illness, such as rubella (German measles), infection with the Zika virus, or exposure to toxic chemicals or drugs, especially during the first 3 months of pregnancy, often predisposes the fetus to congenital disorders. Several decades ago, many pregnant people took the drug thalidomide and subsequently gave birth to infants with missing arms and legs. There is a great deal of concern about the role of alcohol in producing fetal alcohol spectrum disorders, permanent but preventable forms of cognitive impairment, and the effects of exposure to other environmental toxins. Although the etiologies for some congenital disorders are well established, they can occur randomly.

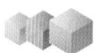 Concept Mastery Alert

Hereditary and Congenital Illnesses

Hereditary and congenital illnesses are often confused. To avoid this confusion, think "genes" for hereditary and "embryonic" for congenital.

An **idiopathic illness** is an illness of unknown cause. Treatment focuses on relieving the signs and symptoms because the etiology is unknown. Examples of idiopathic conditions include hypertension for which there is no known cause or a fever of undetermined origin.

HEALTH CARE SYSTEM

The **health care system** (the network of available health services) involves agencies and institutions where people seek treatment for health problems or assistance with maintaining or promoting their health. The health care system, clients, and their diseases have drastically changed during the past 25 years (Box 4-1). Advances in technology and discoveries in science have created more elaborate methods of diagnosing and treating diseases, creating a need for more specialized care. What was once a system in which people sought medical advice and treatment from one physician, clinic, or hospital has now developed into a complex system involving primary, secondary, tertiary, and extended care.

Primary, Secondary, and Tertiary Care

Primary care (health services provided by the first health care provider or agency a person contacts) is usually provided by a family practice physician, nurse practitioner, or physician assistant in an office or clinic. Cost-conscious health care reforms advocate the provision of primary care by advanced practice nurses.

An example of **secondary care** (health services to which primary caregivers refer clients for consultation and additional testing) is the referral of a client to a cardiac

BOX 4-1	Trends in Health and Health Care

- Increase in the older adult population
- Greater ethnic diversity
- More chronic but preventable illnesses
- More older adults with cognitive disorders (e.g., Alzheimer disease)
- Increased incidence of drug-resistant infections
- Decreased incidence of and death rates from human immunodeficiency virus (HIV) with increased life expectancy associated with expensive drug therapy
- Expanded application of genetic engineering (treating diseases by altering genetic codes)
- Greater success in organ transplantation
- Reduced barriers for research on human stem cell research
- Efforts to reduce the growth in U.S. health care spending
- Potential for increased health care via health insurance under the Affordable Care Act
- More outpatient or ambulatory (1-day stay) care
- Shorter hospital stays
- Less invasive forms of treatment
- Shift to more home care
- Greater focus on disease prevention, health promotion, and health maintenance
- Movement toward more self-care and self-testing
- Approval of more prescription drugs for nonprescription use
- Greater interest in herbal supplements and other complementary and alternative treatments
- Nationally linked computer information systems known as integrated health
- Computerized medical record systems
- Shift to criterion-based treatment (clients must meet established criteria to justify treatment measures)
- Increased litigation against health care providers

catheterization laboratory. **Tertiary care** includes health services provided at hospitals or medical centers where complex technology and specialists are available. The growing trend is to provide as many secondary and tertiary care services as possible on an outpatient basis or to require no more than 24 hours of inpatient care.

>>> *Stop, Think, and Respond 4-1*

A friend reports having frequent bouts of indigestion. Explain how primary, secondary, and tertiary care might be involved in this friend's care.

Extended Care

Extended care (services that meet the health needs of clients who no longer require acute hospital care) includes rehabilitation, skilled nursing care in a person's home or a nursing home, and hospice care for dying clients. Extended care is an important component of the health care system because it allows earlier discharge from secondary and tertiary care agencies and reduces the overall expense of health care.

Health Care Services

As a whole, health care services include those that offer health prevention, diagnosis, treatment, or rehabilitation. As the types of health services expand, the health care delivery system becomes more complex, costly, and in many cases less accessible. Children, older adults, members of underrepresented groups, and people of lower socioeconomic status (SES) are likely to be underserved. Many people delay seeking early treatment for their health problems because they cannot afford to pay for services. When an illness becomes so severe that the only choice is to seek medical attention, many turn to their local hospital emergency departments for care. Inappropriate use of emergency departments is expensive and involves long waits and often no follow-up care.

Government-Funded Health Care

"The nation's uninsured rate declined significantly in 2021 and early 2022, reaching an all-time low of 8.0 percent for U.S. residents of all ages in the first quarter (January–March) of 2022, based on new data from the National Health Interview Survey, compared to the prior low of 9.0 percent in 2016" (U.S. Department of Health and Human Services, 2022). The increased number of insured clients is thought to be due to increased health care access and lower costs through the American Rescue Plan's enhanced Marketplace subsidies and state Medicaid expansions. Still, many uninsured people live below the federal poverty threshold due to unemployment; consequently, their access to health care is affected by the economic burden seeking care poses.

As the number of people covered by an employer's group health insurance has declined, reliance on government plans such as Medicare, Medicaid, and military health care known as Tricare has increased. Americans who are uninsured, those without health insurance through their employers, or those who are purchasing health insurance privately can now receive cost-assisted health insurance through health insurance marketplaces that will be discussed later.

As a result of the **Patient Protection and Affordable Care Act (ACA)**, a health reform law passed in 2010, more people have acquired health insurance. Due in part to each state's Children's Health Insurance Program (CHIP) and the fact that children up to the age of 26 were able to stay on their parents' plan, the number of insured clients has risen across the United States. Many more people were covered through employers who expanded coverage under the ACA and on private plans.

Medicare

Medicare (a federal program that finances health care costs of persons aged 65 years and older, permanently disabled workers of any age and their dependents, and those with end-stage renal disease) is funded primarily through withholdings from an employed person's income. Medicare is divided into Parts A, B, C, and D (the latter three are optional):

- Part A covers acute hospital care, rehabilitative care, hospice, and home care services.
- Part B is purchased for an additional fee and covers physician services, outpatient hospital care, laboratory tests, durable medical equipment, and other selected services. Although Medicare is primarily used by older Americans, it does not cover long-term care and limits coverage for health promotion and illness prevention.
- Part C (Medicare Advantage) is a Medicare-approved private health insurance plan that provides all of Parts A and B of Medicare plus additional benefits such as vision, dental, and hearing; many such plans include prescription drug coverage. Medicare Advantage can potentially save a person money because out-of-pocket expenses may be lower than with Medicare Parts A and B.
- Part D includes prescription drug coverage.

Medicare Part D became available in 2006. It provides a means of relieving the financial burden on older Americans and people with low incomes and disabilities who require prescription drugs. Everyone eligible for Medicare can receive prescription drug coverage regardless of income, resources, health status, or current prescription expenses. Nevertheless, a coverage gap, sometimes referred to as the "donut hole," remains (Fig. 4-4). People are being advised to compare Medicare benefits with Medicare Advantage plans offered by private companies. Some may choose to purchase an additional "Medigap" insurance plan to assist with the cost of deductibles and copayments and to cover the "gap" to supplement their Medicare coverage.

Medicaid

Medicaid is a federally funded, state-administered health care program for low-income families, people receiving Supplemental Security Income (SSI), pregnant women and children who qualify, and other qualifying groups (Centers for Medicare and Medicaid Services, n.d.). There is no required payment of premiums or deductibles for people who qualify for Medicaid based on personal income and assets. Health care providers who accept Medicaid cannot bill for any additional charges. Each state determines how the funds will be spent.

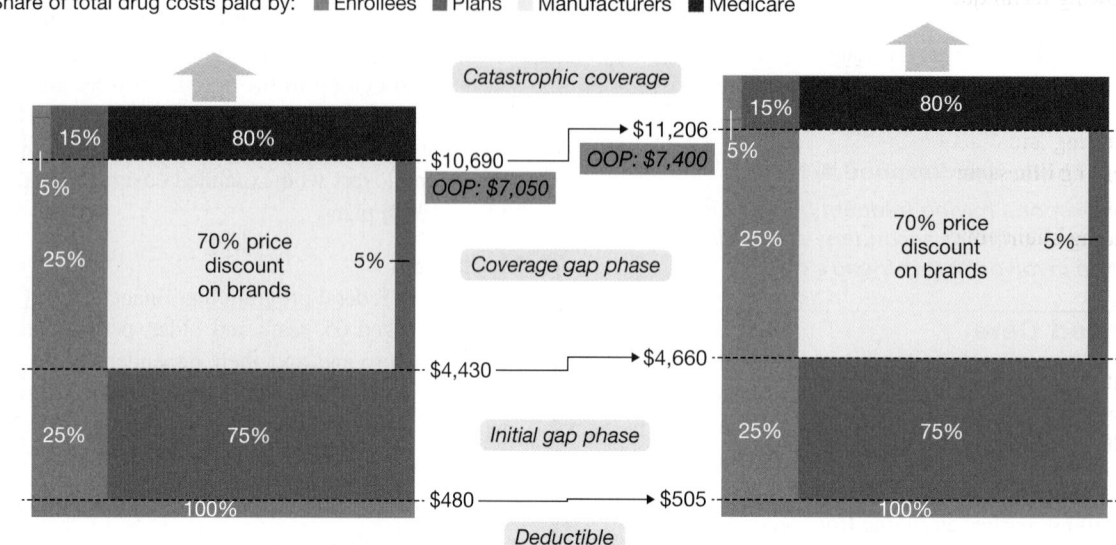

Medicare Part D Standard Benefit Parameters Will Increase in 2023

Share of total drug costs paid by: ■ Enrollees ■ Plans □ Manufacturers ■ Medicare

NOTE: Some amounts rounded to nearest dollar. OOP is out of pocket.
SOURCE: KFF, based on 2022 and 2023 Part D benefit parameters.

FIGURE 4-4 Standard Medicare prescription drug benefit, 2023. (From Medicare. [2023]. *An overview of the Medicare Part D prescription drug benefit.* https://www.kff.org/medicare/fact-sheet/an-overview-of-the-medicare-part-d-prescription-drug-benefit/)

In general, Medicaid programs cover prescription drugs, eyeglasses, preventive care, hospitalization, diagnostic tests, physician visits, rehabilitation, and outpatient care. However, coverage for health care services varies among states.

CHIP is also a national insurance program. It is designed to cover expenses of uninsured children who are not eligible for Medicaid.

Health Insurance Marketplaces

Health insurance marketplaces are state organizations that provide a means for individual people or employers with small numbers of employees to purchase affordable private health insurance under the provisions identified in the ACA. For states that have not established a marketplace, people can purchase a plan administered by the federal government.

Financing Health Care

Historically, private insurance, self-insurance systems, and Medicare paid for health care. Hospitals and approved providers received payment for what they charged; more charges increased income and profits. These plans offered no incentives to control costs. Disparities in access to health care and the high costs prompted evaluation of the entire health care system. Subsequently, this led to innovative cost-cutting approaches in government payment systems and those financed by private insurers and corporate health plans.

Prospective Payment Systems

In response to escalating health care costs, the federal government implemented a system of prospective payment in 1983 for people enrolled in Medicare. A **prospective payment system** uses financial incentives to decrease total health care charges by reimbursing hospitals on a fixed rate basis. Reimbursement is based on the **diagnostic-related group** (DRG; a classification system used to group clients with similar diagnoses). For example, all clients receiving a hip, knee, or shoulder replacement fall into DRG 209, total joint replacement, and the surgeries are reimbursed at basically the same rate. If actual costs are less than the reimbursed amount, the hospital keeps the difference. If costs exceed the reimbursed amount, the hospital is left with the deficit. Hospitals that are inefficient in managing clients' recoveries and early discharges can potentially lose vast revenue, possibly leading to closure of the facility.

Since its inception, the DRG system has been largely responsible for marked decreases in hospital lengths of stay. Subsequently, three major criticisms have surfaced: (1) some older clients are discharged prematurely so as not to exceed the fixed reimbursement; (2) families have had to assume responsibility for the care of clients who cannot function independently after discharge; and (3) increased hospital care costs have been charged to clients with private insurance to make up for the lost Medicare revenues. In response to cost-shifting and other economic forces, private insurance companies have countered by aggressively challenging hospital charges, refusing payment for unjustified billings, and developing their own cost-containment reimbursement system known as managed care.

Managed Care

Managed care organizations (MCOs; private insurers who carefully plan and closely supervise the distribution of their clients' health care services) control costs of health care and focus on prevention as the best way to manage costs using the following techniques:

- Using health care resources efficiently
- Bargaining with providers for quality care at reasonable costs
- Monitoring and managing fiscal and client outcomes
- Preventing illness through screening and health promotion activities
- Providing client education to decrease the risk for disease
- Minimizing the number of hospitalizations of clients with chronic illness

The two most common types of managed care systems are health maintenance organizations (HMOs) and preferred provider organizations (PPOs). Capitation is the third emerging MCO financial strategy.

Health Maintenance Organizations

Health maintenance organizations (HMOs) are corporations that charge preset, fixed, or yearly fees in exchange for providing health care for their members. The fee remains the same regardless of the type of health service required or the frequency of care. These organizations are able to remain fiscally sound because they offer preventive services, periodic screenings, and health education to keep their members healthy and out of the hospital.

HMOs provide ambulatory, hospitalization, and home care services. Some HMOs have their own health care facilities; others use facilities within the community. A member of an HMO must receive permission for seeking additional care, such as second opinions from specialists or unauthorized diagnostic tests. Those members who fail to do so are responsible for the entire bill. In this way, HMOs serve as gatekeepers for health care services.

Preferred Provider Organizations

Preferred provider organizations (PPOs) are agents for health insurance companies that control health care costs on the basis of competition. PPOs create a network of a community's physicians who are willing to discount their fees for service in exchange for a steady supply of referred clients. The subscriber's clients can lower their health care costs by receiving care from any of the preferred providers. If they select providers outside the network, they pay a higher percentage of the costs.

Capitation

An approach that is fundamentally different from HMOs and PPOs is **capitation**, a payment system in which a preset fee per member is paid to a health care provider (usually a hospital or hospital system) regardless of whether the member requires services. Capitation provides an incentive to providers to control tests and services as a means of making a profit. If members do not receive costly care, the provider makes money.

Outcomes of Structured Reimbursement

In many cases, the changes in reimbursements have shifted economic and decision-making power from hospitals and physicians to insurance companies. One criticism is that it is

---

| BOX 4-2 | **Integrated Delivery Systems' Services** |

Integrated delivery systems provide:
- Wellness programs
- Preventive care
- Ambulatory care
- Outpatient diagnostic and laboratory services
- Emergency care
- Secondary and tertiary services
- Rehabilitation
- Long-term care
- Assisted living facilities
- Psychiatric care
- Home health care services
- Hospice care
- Outpatient pharmacies

---

difficult to obtain and provide health care without the economic pressure of insurers. Patient advocates claim that the profits of insurance companies come at the expense of quality care. For example, hospitals are using unlicensed assistive personnel to perform some duties that practical/vocational and registered nurses once provided. Current evidence shows that deaths in health care agencies increase as the number of licensed nurses decreases (American Hospital Association, 2022).

Cost-driven changes have had positive effects as well. As concern for cost meets concern for quality, health care institutions, nursing personnel, and other providers search for ways to ensure that all care, teaching, and preparation before the discharge date occur without overusing expensive resources.

In an attempt to reduce duplication of health care services and to increase revenue, hospitals and other health care facilities are forming networks known as integrated delivery systems. **Integrated delivery systems** (networks that provide a full range of health care services in a highly coordinated, cost-effective manner) offer diverse options to clients (Box 4-2) and result in shorter hospital stays, fewer complications such as hospital-acquired infections, and quicker returns to self-care.

NATIONAL HEALTH GOALS: *HEALTHY PEOPLE 2030*

An ongoing national health promotion effort referred to as *Healthy People* is a continuation of the 1979 Surgeon General's Report, *Healthy People*, and later, *Healthy People 2000: National Health Promotion and Disease Prevention, Healthy People 2010, Healthy People 2020,* and *Healthy People 2030*. The mission of *Healthy People* and its main goals for promoting the nation's health involve helping people achieve healthy, thriving lives; eliminating health disparities; creating health-promoting environments; promoting health across the lifespan; and engaging leaders and the public in designing health-promoting policies (Box 4-3).

Healthy People 2030's main goals are subdivided into multiple topic areas, each of which has identified

---

BOX 4-3   *Healthy People 2030* **Foundational Principles, Goals, and Plan of Action**

Foundational Principles

Foundational principles explain the thinking that guides decisions about *Healthy People 2030*.

- The health and well-being of all people and communities is essential to a thriving, equitable society.
- Promoting health and well-being and preventing disease are linked efforts that encompass physical, mental, and social health dimensions.
- Investing to achieve the full potential for health and well-being for all provides valuable benefits to society.
- Achieving health and well-being requires eliminating health disparities, achieving health equity, and attaining health literacy.
- Healthy physical, social, and economic environments strengthen the potential to achieve health and well-being.
- Promoting and achieving health and well-being nationwide is a shared responsibility that is distributed across the national, state, tribal, and community levels, including the public, private, and not-for-profit sectors.
- Working to attain the full potential for health and well-being of the population is a component of decision-making and policy formulation across all sectors.

Overarching Goals

- Attain healthy, thriving lives and well-being free of preventable disease, disability, injury, and premature death.
- Eliminate health disparities, achieve health equity, and attain health literacy to improve the health and well-being of all.
- Create social, physical, and economic environments that promote attaining the full potential for health and well-being for all.
- Promote healthy development, healthy behaviors, and well-being across all life stages.
- Engage leadership, key constituents, and the public across multiple sectors to take action and design policies that improve the health and well-being of all.

Plan of Action

- Set national goals and measurable objectives to guide evidence-based policies, programs, and other actions to improve health and well-being.
- Provide accurate, timely, and accessible data that can drive targeted actions to address regions and populations that have poor health or are at high risk for poor health.
- Foster impact through public and private efforts to improve health and well-being for people of all ages and the communities in which they live.
- Provide tools for the public, programs, policymakers, and others to evaluate progress toward improving health and well-being.
- Share and support the implementation of evidence-based programs and policies that are replicable, scalable, and sustainable.
- Report biennially on progress throughout the decade from 2020 to 2030.
- Stimulate research and innovation toward meeting *Healthy People 2030* goals and highlight critical research, data, and evaluation needs.
- Facilitate development and availability of affordable means of health promotion, disease prevention, and treatment.

HealthyPeople.gov. (n.d.). *Healthy People 2030 framework.* https://health.gov/healthypeople/about/healthy-people-2030-framework

---

interventions that consist of programs, policies, and information; *determinants* that identify social, economic, environmental factors and individual traits; and *outcomes*, such as behaviors, specific risk factors, diseases, mental disorders, disabilities, injuries, and qualities of life (Fig. 4-5). Examples of targeted health goals for achievement are:

- Increase the proportion of people with health insurance.
- In the health professions, allied and associated health professions, and nursing, increase the proportion of all degrees awarded to members of underrepresented racial and ethnic groups.
- Increase the proportion of health and wellness and treatment programs and facilities that provide full access for people with disabilities.
- Reduce the number of new cases of cancer as well as the illness, disability, and death caused by cancer.
- Reduce infections caused by key foodborne pathogens.
- Improve visual and hearing health nationally through prevention, early detection, treatment, and rehabilitation (HealthyPeople.gov, n.d.).

Healthy People 2030 was launched in 2020. The vision of *Healthy People 2030* is "a society in which all people can achieve their full potential for health and well-being across the lifespan." The mission is "to promote, strengthen, and evaluate the nation's efforts to improve the health and well-being of all" (HealthyPeople.gov, n.d.).

THE NURSING TEAM

The **nursing team** (Fig. 4-6) primarily includes the client and nursing personnel, but it may also include several types of professionals as well as allied health care providers with special training such as respiratory therapists, physical therapists, and technicians.

In particular, nurses use their unique skills in the hospital as well as other employment areas. Because they have skills that assist people who are healthy, people who are dying, and all others in between, nurses work in various settings such as HMOs, physical fitness centers, weight loss clinics, public health departments, home health agencies, and hospices. Wherever nursing personnel work together, they use

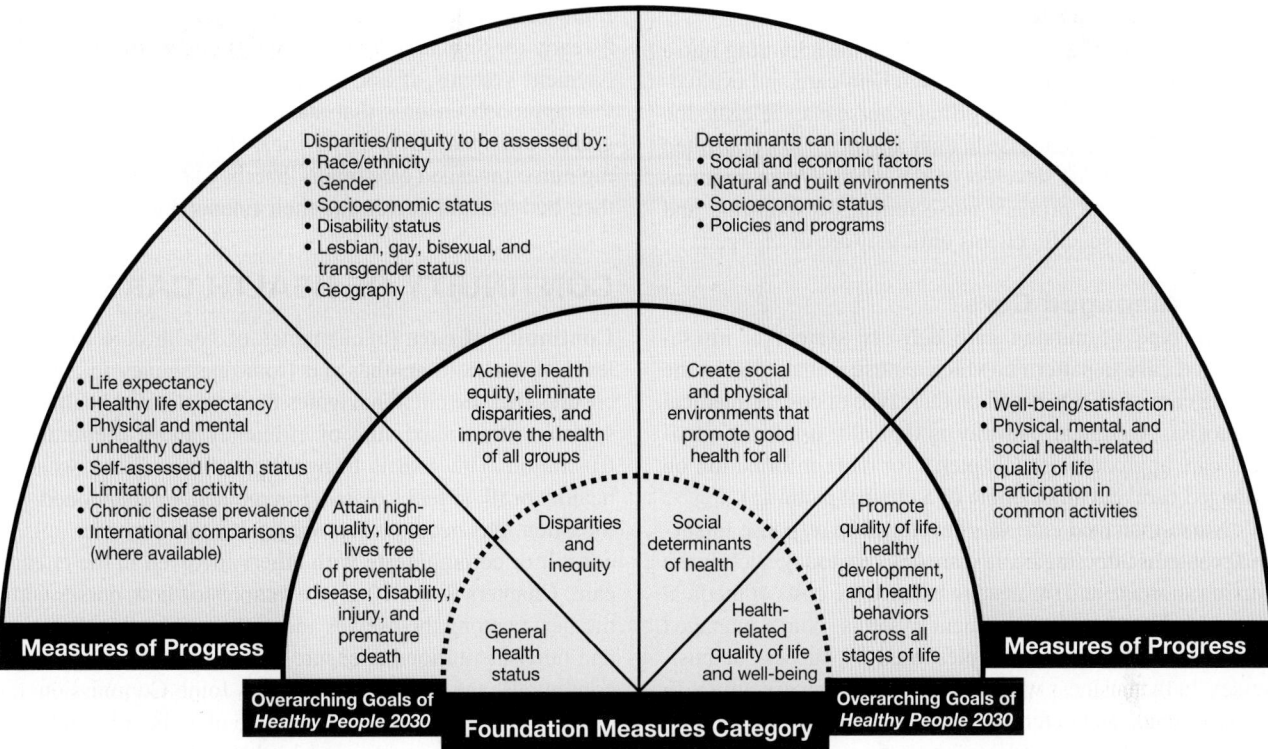

FIGURE 4-5 Components of *Healthy People 2030*.

one of several patterns for managing client care. The five common management patterns are functional nursing, case method, team nursing, primary nursing, and nurse-managed care. Each has advantages and disadvantages. Nursing students are likely to encounter several or all of these methods in their clinical experience.

Functional Nursing

One method used when providing client care is **functional nursing** (a pattern in which each nurse is assigned specific tasks). For example, one nurse is assigned to give all

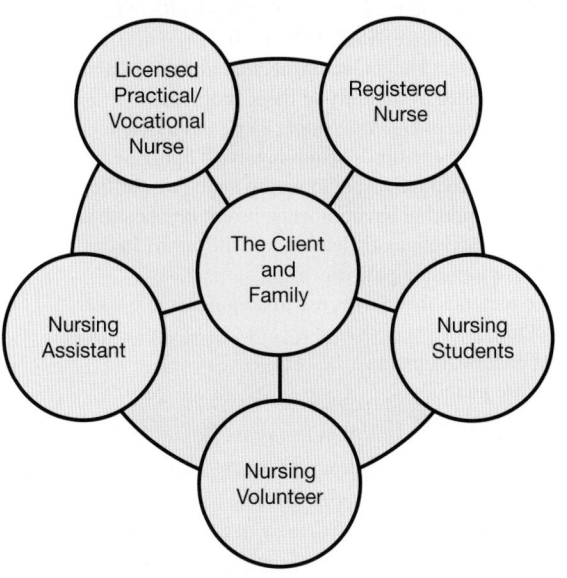

FIGURE 4-6 The nursing team.

the medications, another performs all the treatments (such as dressing changes), and another works at the desk transcribing physicians' orders and communicating with other nursing departments about client care issues. This pattern is being used less often because its focus tends to be more on completing the task rather than caring for individual clients.

Case Method

The **case method** (a pattern in which one nurse manages all the care a client or group of clients needs for a designated period of time) should not be confused with managed care, which is discussed later. The case method is most often used in home health, public health, and community mental health nursing. Nurses who deliver this type of care are referred to as case managers.

Team Nursing

Team nursing (a pattern in which nursing personnel divide the clients into groups and complete their care together) is organized and directed by a nurse called the team leader. The leader may assist with care but usually assigns and supervises the care that other team members provide. All team members report the outcomes of their care to the team leader. The team leader is responsible for evaluating whether the goals of client care are met.

Conferences are an important part of team nursing. They may cover a variety of subjects but are planned with certain goals in mind such as determining the best approaches to each client's health problems, increasing the team members' knowledge, and promoting a cooperative spirit among nursing personnel.

Primary Nursing

In **primary nursing** (a pattern in which the admitting nurse assumes responsibility for planning client care and evaluating the client's progress), the primary nurse may delegate the client's care to someone else in their absence but is consulted when new problems develop or the plan of care requires modifications. The primary nurse remains responsible and accountable for specific clients until they are discharged.

Nurse-Managed Care

Another type of nursing care delivery system is **nurse-managed care** (a pattern in which a nurse manager plans the nursing care of clients based on their type of case or medical diagnosis). A clinical pathway is typically used in a managed care approach (see Chapter 1 for more information on managed care and an example of a clinical pathway).

Nurse-managed care was developed in response to several problems affecting health care delivery today, such as the nursing shortage and the need to balance the costs of medical care with limited reimbursement systems. Nurse-managed care is similar to the principles used by successful businesses. In the business world, corporations pay executives to forecast trends and determine the best strategies for making profits. In nurse-managed care, a professional nurse evaluates whether predictable outcomes are met on a daily basis.

If the team meets the outcomes in a timely manner, the client is ready for discharge by the time designated by prospective payment systems, if not before. Pilot studies indicate that this approach ensures that standards of care are met with greater efficiency and cost savings. Hospitals that are adopting nurse-managed care report that they are operating within their budgets and decreasing their financial losses.

CONTINUITY OF HEALTH CARE

Continuity of care (maintenance of health care from one level of health to another and from one agency to another) ensures that the client navigates the complicated health care system with a maximum of efficiency and a minimum of frustration. The goal is to avoid causing a client, whether healthy or ill, to feel isolated, fragmented, or abandoned. All too often, this occurs when one health care provider fails to consult or communicate with others involved in the client's care. Chapters 9 and 10 give examples of how nurses communicate among themselves and with personnel in their own and other institutions to ensure that the client's care is both continuous and goal-directed. The Joint Commission requires discharge planning at the time of a client's admission to ensure that any additional health care services are preplanned when the client transitions to another level of care.

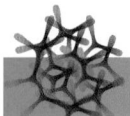

KEY POINTS

- Wellness: Full and balanced integration of all aspects of health, involving physical, emotional, social, and spiritual health
- Holism: Sum of physical, emotional, social, and spiritual health determines how "whole" or well a person feels
- Maslow's five levels of human needs include:
  - Physiologic
  - Safety and security
  - Love and belonging
  - Esteem and self-esteem
  - Self-actualization
- Illnesses may be categorized as:
  - Acute illness, one that comes on suddenly and lasts a short time
  - Chronic illness, one that comes on slowly and lasts a long time
  - Terminal illness, one for which there is no potential for a cure
  - Primary illness, one that develops independently of any other disease
  - Secondary illness, disorder that develops from a preexisting condition
  - Hereditary, a disorder acquired from the genetic codes of one or both parents
  - Congenital, a disorder present at birth that is the result of faulty embryonic development
  - Idiopathic, an illness of unknown cause
- Health care can be categorized as:
  - Primary care: Usually given by a family practice physician, nurse practitioner, or physician assistant in an office or clinic
- Secondary care: Given per referral from primary caregivers for consultation and additional testing
- Tertiary care: Health services provided at hospitals or medical centers where complex technology and specialists are available
- Extended care: Services that meet the health needs of clients who no longer require acute hospital care; includes rehabilitation, skilled nursing care in a person's home or a nursing home, and hospice care
- Government-funded health care in the United States includes Medicare, Medicaid, and state-run health insurance marketplaces. The Patient Protection and Affordable Care Act expanded availability of these programs.
- The mission of *Healthy People 2030* and its main goals for promoting the nation's health involve helping people achieve healthy, thriving lives; eliminating health disparities; creating health-promoting environments; promoting health across the lifespan; and engaging leaders and the public in designing health-promoting policies.
- Five methods that nurses use to administer client care include:
- Functional nursing
- Case method
- Team nursing
- Primary nursing
- Nurse-managed care

CRITICAL THINKING EXERCISES

1. If you were asked to participate in planning the goals and strategies for *Healthy People 2030*, what suggestions would you make to promote health and to reduce chronic illness?

2. Which pattern for managing client care seems most advantageous for nurses? Which pattern might clients prefer? Give reasons for your selections.

3. What arguments would you offer to persuade others that health care reform such as that provided by the ACA is beneficial for promoting wellness among people living in the United States?

4. Why might people who manage their diabetes effectively profess that they are "healthy?"

NEXT-GENERATION NCLEX-STYLE REVIEW QUESTIONS

1. Which client problem is of highest priority for nursing management?
   a. Low self-esteem
   b. Labored breathing
   c. Feeling powerless
   d. Lack of family support
   Test-Taking Strategy: Note the key word and modifier, "highest priority." Apply Maslow's hierarchy of needs to select an answer.

2. What is the most appropriate initial nursing referral for a person who is experiencing frequent headaches?
   a. Refer the client to a drug company seeking clinical trial volunteers for a headache medication.
   b. Refer the client to a neurologic institute conducting investigational research on headaches.
   c. Refer the client to a hospital's emergency department for immediate medical treatment.
   d. Refer the client to a family practice physician for a baseline physical examination.
   Test-Taking Strategy: Identify the key word in the stem of the question, "initial." Consider the action that should be performed before all others.

3. A hospital nurse's referral to which type of organization is best for promoting continuity of care for a client with terminal cancer?
   a. PPO
   b. Home health nursing organization
   c. HMO
   d. MCO
   Test-Taking Strategy: Identify the key word in the stem of the question, "best." Use the process of elimination to exclude strategies for controlling health care costs rather than caring for a client.

4. Place the components of Maslow's hierarchy of human needs in progressive sequence, beginning with that which is most basic.
   a. Love and belonging
   b. Physiologic care
   c. Self-actualization
   d. Esteem and self-esteem
   e. Safety and security
   Test-Taking Strategy: Analyze the stem to determine what the question asks. In this case, it asks for a sequential listing of Maslow's hierarchy of needs from the lowest to highest levels.

5. Which client problem is a nurse correct in identifying as one that compromises the human need for safety and security?
   a. Chronic anxiety
   b. Labored breathing
   c. Severe loneliness
   d. Sleep deprivation
   Test-Taking Strategy: Use Maslow's hierarchy to eliminate options affecting lower level needs.

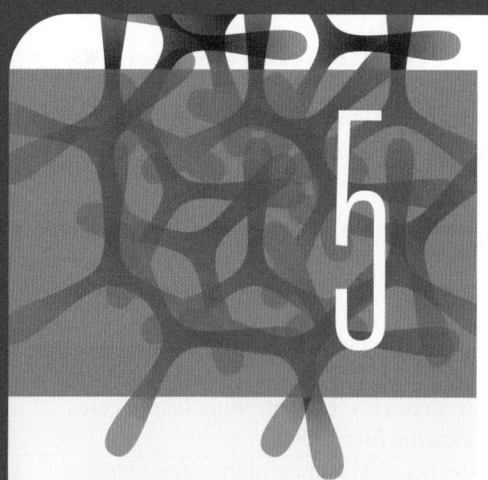

5

Homeostasis, Adaptation, and Stress

Words To Know

adaptation
alarm stage
alternative behavior techniques
alternative lifestyle techniques
alternative thinking techniques
catastrophize
coping mechanisms
coping strategies
cortisol
endocrine system
endorphins
feedback loop
fight-or-flight response
general adaptation syndrome
homeostasis
hypothalamus–pituitary–adrenal
  axis
neuropeptides
neurotransmitters
primary prevention
reframing
reticular activating system
secondary prevention
sensory manipulation
stage of exhaustion
stage of resistance
stress
stress management techniques
stress reduction techniques
stressors
stress-related disorders
tertiary prevention

Learning Objectives

On completion of this chapter, the reader should be able to:

1. Explain homeostasis and list categories of stressors that affect homeostasis.
2. Identify beliefs about the body and mind based on the concept of holism.
3. Identify the purpose of adaptation and possible outcomes of unsuccessful adaptation.
4. Trace the structures through which adaptive responses take place.
5. Differentiate sympathetic and parasympathetic adaptive responses.
6. Define stress and list factors that affect the stress response.
7. Discuss the stages and consequences of general adaptation syndrome.
8. Explain psychological adaptation and possible outcomes.
9. Name three levels of prevention that apply to reducing or managing stress-related disorders.
10. Describe nursing activities helpful in the care of clients prone to stress and approaches for preventing, reducing, or eliminating a stress response.

INTRODUCTION

Health is a tenuous state. To sustain it, the body continuously adapts to **stressors** (changes with the potential to disturb equilibrium). As long as stressors are minor, the body's responses are negligible and generally unnoticed. When stressors are intense or numerous, efforts to restore balance may cause uncomfortable signs and symptoms. With prolonged stress, related disorders and even death may occur.

 Gerontologic Considerations

■ With advanced age, networks of social support tend to dwindle or disintegrate, diminishing older adults' ability to cope. Social losses may provoke the onset of physical or emotional disorders.

■ Older adults' coping strategies are likely to focus on accepting limitations, adjusting expectations, and maintaining quality of life.

■ When caring for older adults, it is imperative to strengthen their social support resources as an intervention for reducing stress. It is also important to teach caregivers about stress reduction techniques.

TABLE 5-1 Common Stressors

PHYSIOLOGIC	PSYCHOLOGICAL	SOCIAL	SPIRITUAL
Prematurity	Fear	Gender, racial, age discrimination	Guilt
Aging	Powerlessness	Isolation	Doubt
Injury	Jealousy	Abandonment	Hopelessness
Infection	Rivalry	Poverty	Conflict in values
Malnutrition	Bitterness	Conflict in relationships	Pressure to join, abandon, or change
Obesity	Hatred	Political instability	religions
Surgery	Insecurity	Denial of human rights	Religious discrimination
Pain		Threats to safety	
Fever		Illiteracy	
Fatigue		Infertility	
Pollution			

HOMEOSTASIS

Homeostasis is a relatively stable state of physiologic equilibrium; it means "staying the same." Although it sounds contradictory, staying the same requires constant physiologic activity. The body maintains constancy by adjusting and readjusting in response to changes in the internal and external environments that foster disequilibrium.

Holism

Homeostasis is associated primarily with a person's physical status; however, emotional, social, and spiritual components also affect it. As discussed in Chapter 4, holism implies that factors in all these areas contribute to the whole of a person. Based on the principles of holism, stressors may be physiologic, psychological, social, or spiritual (Table 5-1).

Holism is the foundation of two commonly held beliefs: (1) Both the mind and the body directly influence humans, and (2) the relationship between the mind and the body can potentially sustain health as well as cause illness. Consequently, it is helpful to understand how the mind perceives information and makes adaptive responses. Both physical and psychological mechanisms of perception and adaptation are discussed later in this chapter.

>> *Stop, Think, and Respond 5-1*

List physiologic, psychological, social, and spiritual stressors that can affect homeostasis for a nursing student.

Adaptation

The purpose of **adaptation** (the response of an organism to change) is to maintain homeostasis. Adaptation requires the use of self-protective properties and mechanisms for regulating homeostasis. Neurotransmitters mediate homeostatic adaptive responses by coordinating functions of the central nervous system (CNS), autonomic nervous system, and endocrine system.

Neurotransmitters and Neuropeptides

Neurotransmitters (chemical messengers synthesized in the neurons) allow communication across the synaptic cleft

between neurons, subsequently affecting thinking, behavior, and bodily functions. When released, neurotransmitters temporarily bind to receptor sites on the postsynaptic neuron and transmit their information. After this is accomplished, the neurotransmitter is broken down, recaptured for later use, or weakened (Fig. 5-1).

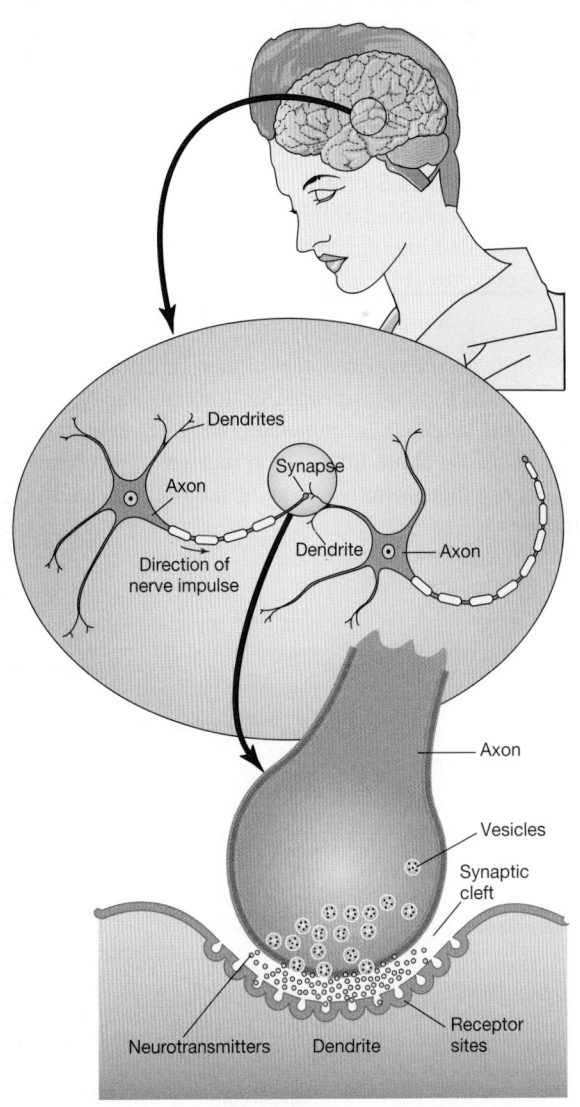

FIGURE 5-1 Neurotransmitter activity. (From Donnelly-Moreno, L., & Moseley, B. [2021]. *Introductory medical-surgical nursing* [13th ed.]. Lippincott Williams & Wilkins.)

Examples of neurotransmitters include serotonin, dopamine, epinephrine, norepinephrine (also called adrenaline and noradrenaline), acetylcholine, gamma-aminobutyric acid (GABA), and glutamate. **Neuropeptides** are types of neuromodulators; they help neurons communicate with each other. Numerous neuropeptides are located in the brain, where they have many effects on neuronal function (Jankovic, 2022). Neuropeptides include substance P, endorphins, enkephalins, and other neurohormones.

Neurotransmitters and neuropeptides exert different effects. Serotonin stabilizes mood, induces sleep, and regulates temperature. Epinephrine and norepinephrine heighten arousal and increase energy. Acetylcholine and dopamine promote coordinated movement. GABA inhibits the excitatory neurotransmitters, such as epinephrine, norepinephrine, and dopamine, which are classified as catecholamines. Substance P transmits the pain sensation, while endorphins and enkephalins interrupt the transmission of substance P and promote a sense of well-being.

Different brain areas contain different neurons that contain specific neurotransmitters. Receptors for these chemical messengers are found throughout the central nervous, endocrine, and immune systems, suggesting a highly integrated communication system sometimes referred to as the **hypothalamus–pituitary–adrenal (HPA) axis**.

Central Nervous System

The CNS is composed of the brain and the spinal cord. The brain is divided into the cortex and the structures that make up the subcortex (Fig. 5-2).

Cortex

The cortex is considered the higher functioning portion of the brain. It enables people to think abstractly, use and understand language, accumulate and store memories, and make decisions about information received. The cortex also influences other primitive areas of the brain located in the subcortex.

Subcortex

The subcortex consists of the structures in the midbrain and brain stem. The midbrain, which lies between the cortex and the brain stem, includes the basal ganglia, thalamus, and hypothalamus. The brain stem, so named because it resembles a stalk, contains the cerebellum, medulla, and pons. The subcortical structures are primarily responsible for regulating and maintaining physiologic activities that promote survival. Examples include regulation of breathing, heart contraction, blood pressure (BP), body temperature, sleep, appetite, and stimulation and inhibition of hormone production.

Reticular Activating System

The **reticular activating system** (RAS), an area of the brain through which a network of nerves pass, is the communication link between the body and the mind. Information about a person's internal and external environment is funneled through the RAS to the cortex on both conscious and unconscious levels (Fig. 5-3). The cortex processes the information and generates behavioral and physiologic responses through activation by the hypothalamus. The hypothalamus, in turn, influences the autonomic nervous system and endocrine functions (Fig. 5-4).

Activity in the RAS is affected by inhibitory neurotransmitters, such as GABA, and excitatory neurotransmitters, such as norepinephrine. Drugs such as alcohol, narcotic analgesics, and tranquilizers decrease brain activity and induce sleep by simulating or increasing GABA. Drugs such as caffeine, medications for attention-deficit/hyperactivity disorder, and psychostimulants like methamphetamine increase RAS activity, alertness, and the "thinking activity" of the cortex by stimulating receptors for norepinephrine.

Self-medication with alcohol and other sedative drugs that are frequently misused, such as narcotic analgesics and

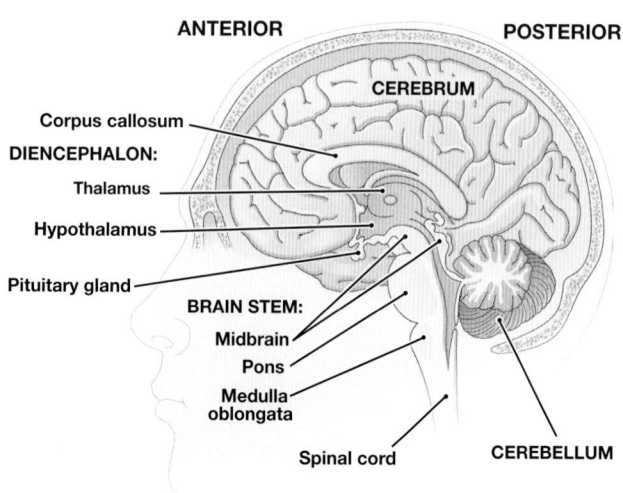

FIGURE 5-2 Central nervous system structures.

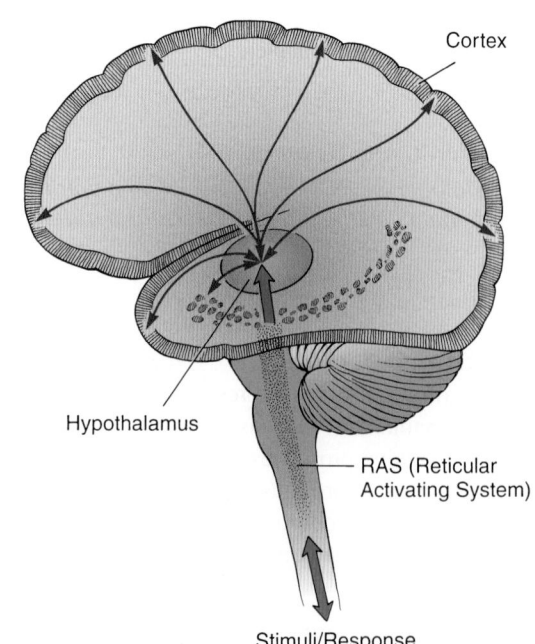

FIGURE 5-3 The reticular activating system is the communication link in the mind–body connection.

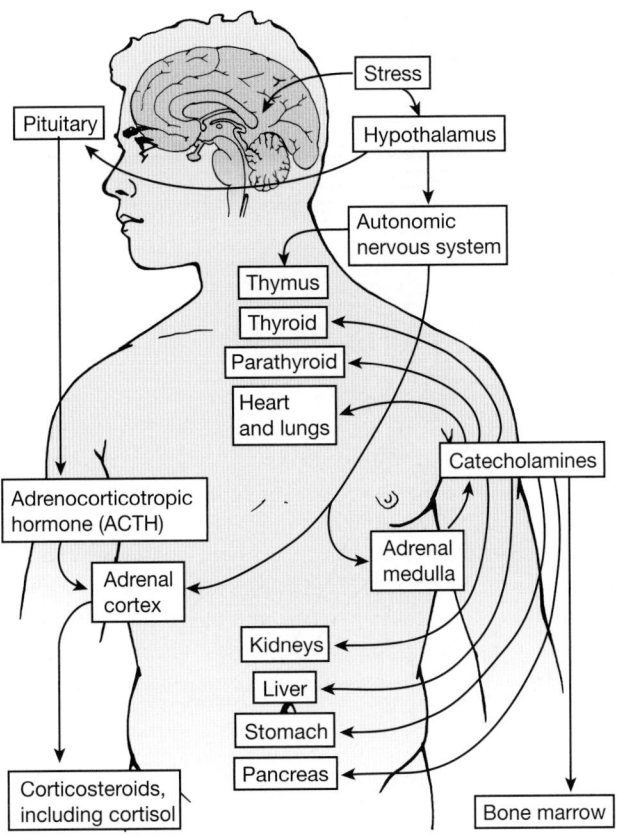

FIGURE 5-4 Homeostatic adaptive pathways.

 Pharmacologic Considerations

Self-medication to reduce stress by combining alcohol with drugs is increasing at a dramatic rate for all ages.

Autonomic Nervous System

The autonomic nervous system is composed of peripheral nerves affecting physiologic functions that are largely automatic and beyond voluntary control. It is subdivided into the sympathetic and parasympathetic nervous systems.

Both the sympathetic and parasympathetic divisions supply organs throughout the body with nerve pathways. Each division takes a turn being functionally dominant, depending on the appropriate physiologic response. For example, when increased heart rate is needed, the sympathetic division dominates; when heart rate needs to be slowed, the parasympathetic division takes over.

Sympathetic Nervous System

When a situation occurs that the mind perceives as dangerous, the sympathetic nervous system prepares the body for a **fight-or-flight response**. It accelerates the physiologic functions that ensure survival through enhanced strength or rapid escape. The person becomes active, aroused, and emotionally charged.

Parasympathetic Nervous System

The parasympathetic nervous system restores equilibrium after danger is no longer apparent. It does so by inhibiting the physiologic stimulation created by its counterpart, the sympathetic nervous system. The parasympathetic nervous system, however, does not produce an opposite reaction for every sympathetic effect (Table 5-2). For this reason, many neurologic researchers believe that the parasympathetic nervous system offers an alternate but equally effective mechanism for responding to threats from the internal or external environment. For example, physiologic deceleration, produced by the parasympathetic nervous system, has been linked to the manner in which opossums and other animals

tranquilizers, may decrease arousal and produce temporary relaxation. However, excessive or chronic substance abuse can lead to physical impairment, drug dependence, and legal problems, creating more stressors than those they were originally intended to relieve.

Because an unrelieved stress response is generally accompanied by anxiety and depression, short-term prescription drug therapy with antianxiety medication such as alprazolam (Xanax) or antidepressant drugs like fluoxetine (Prozac) may help a person to more realistically assess and address stressors.

TABLE 5-2 Sympathetic and Parasympathetic Effects

TARGET STRUCTURE	SYMPATHETIC EFFECT	PARASYMPATHETIC EFFECT
Irises of the eyes	Dilated pupils	Constricted pupils
Sweat glands	Increased perspiration	None
Salivary glands	Inhibited salivation	Increased salivation
Digestive glands	Inhibited secretions	Stimulated secretions
Heart	Increased rate and force of contraction	Decreased rate and force of contraction
Blood vessels in the skin	Constricted, causing pale appearance	Dilated, causing blush or flushed appearance
Skeletal muscles	Increased tone	Decreased tone
Bronchial muscles	Relaxed (bronchodilation)	Contracted (bronchoconstriction)
Digestive motility (peristalsis)	Decreased	Increased
Kidney	Decreased filtration	None
Bladder muscle (detrusor)	Inhibited (suppressed urination)	Stimulated (urge to urinate)
Liver	Release of glucose	None
Adrenal medulla	Stimulated	None

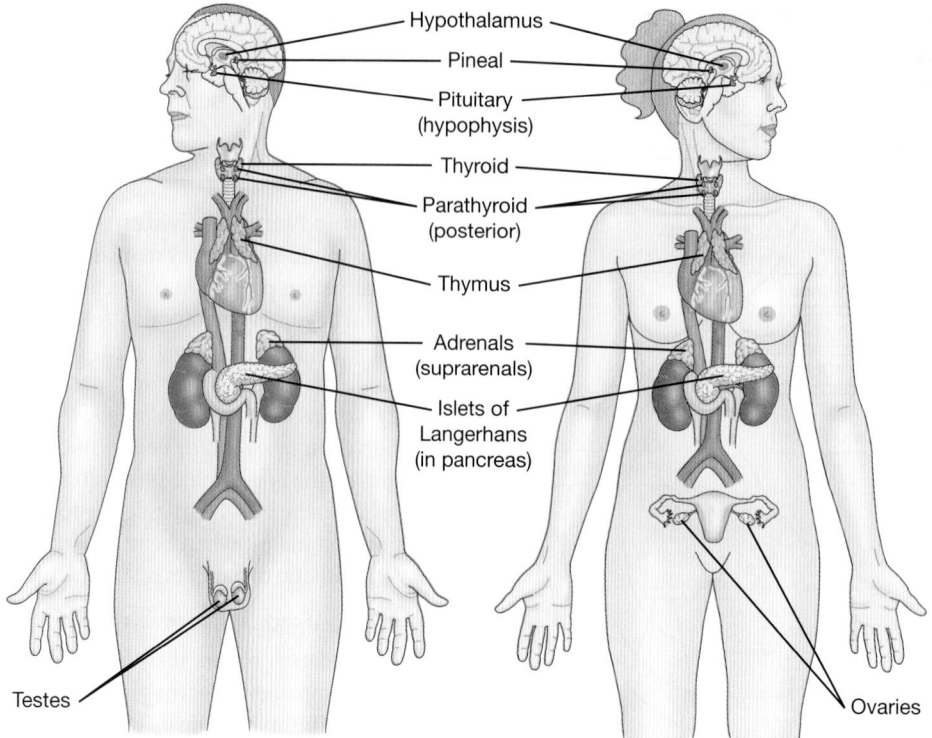

FIGURE 5-5 Endocrine glands.

"play dead" when they sense that predators are stalking them. This simulated appearance of death often prompts the predator to leave the animal alone, thus saving its life. It has been proposed that humans may also respond to stimuli not only by speeding physiologic responses, but also by slowing them down.

Endocrine System

The autonomic nervous system provides the initial and immediate response to a perceived threat through either sympathetic or parasympathetic pathways. The **endocrine system**, a group of glands found throughout the body that produce hormones, sustains the response (Fig. 5-5). Hormones are chemicals produced in one part of the body; their actions have physiologic effects on target cells elsewhere.

Neuroendocrine Control

The pituitary gland, located in the brain, is considered the master gland, producing hormones that influence other endocrine glands. The pituitary gland is connected to the hypothalamus, a subcortical structure, through both vascular connections and nerve endings. For pituitary function to occur, the cortex stimulates the hypothalamus, which then activates the pituitary gland.

Feedback Loop

A **feedback loop** is the mechanism for controlling hormone production (Fig. 5-6). Feedback can be negative or positive. Most hormones are secreted in response to negative feedback; when a hormone level decreases, the releasing gland is stimulated. In positive feedback, the opposite occurs, keeping concentrations of hormones within a stable range

at all times. Homeostasis is maintained when hormones are released as needed or inhibited when adequate.

STRESS

As long as demands on the central nervous, autonomic nervous, and endocrine systems are within adaptive capacity, the body maintains homeostasis. When internal or external changes overwhelm homeostatic adaptation, stress results. **Stress** is the physiologic and behavioral responses to disequilibrium. It has physical, emotional, and cognitive effects (Box 5-1).

Although all humans have the capacity to adapt to stress, not everyone responds to similar stressors in the same way. Differences vary according to the intensity of the stressor, the number of stressors, the duration of the stressor,

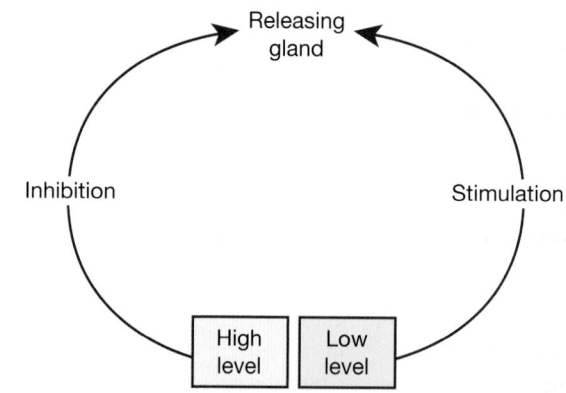

FIGURE 5-6 A feedback loop regulates hormone levels.

Physical
Rapid heart rate
Rapid breathing
Increased blood pressure
Difficulty falling asleep or excessive sleep
Loss of appetite or excessive eating
Stiff muscles
Hyperactivity or inactivity
Dry mouth
Constipation or diarrhea
Lack of interest in sex

Emotional
Irritability
Angry outbursts
Hypercriticism
Verbal abuse
Withdrawal
Depression

Cognitive
Impaired attention and concentration
Forgetfulness
Preoccupation
Poor judgment

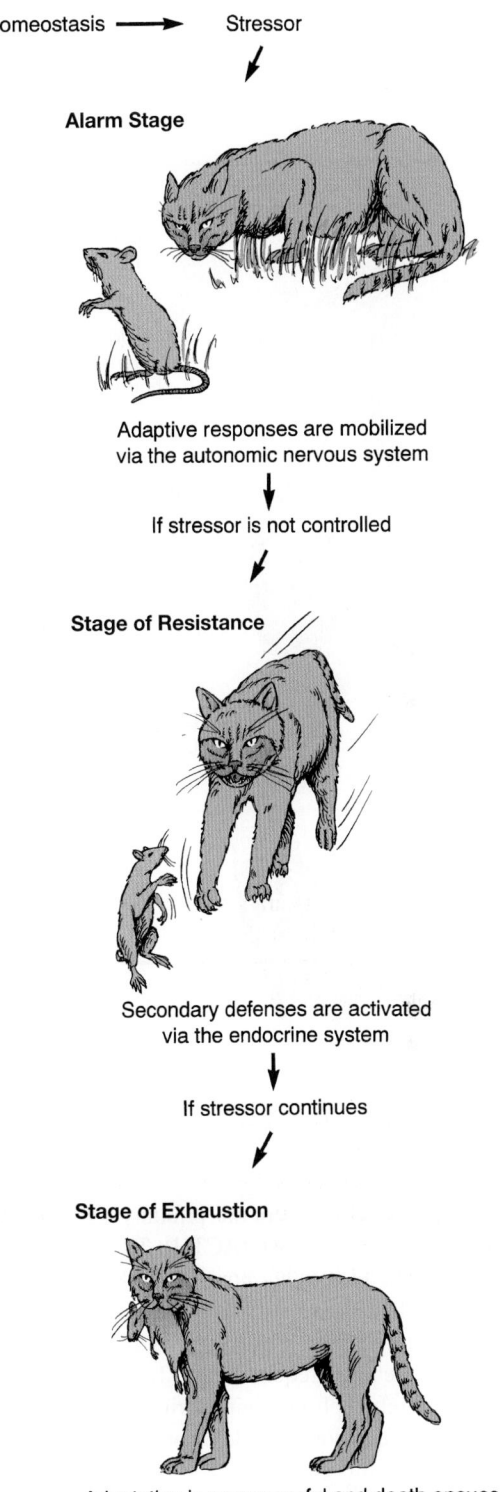

FIGURE 5-7 Stages of general adaptation syndrome.

physical health status, life experiences, coping strategies, social support, personal beliefs, attitudes, and values. Because of unique differences, outcomes may be adaptive or maladaptive, depending on each person's response. Some stress-prone people have a tendency to **catastrophize**, choosing to focus on all the potentially negative outcomes that may result from stressors, thus perpetuating and intensifying their responses to stress.

Physiologic Stress Response

Hans Selye, a Canadian physician who lived in the early 1900s, devoted much of his life to researching the collective physiologic processes of the stress response, which he called **general adaptation syndrome.** Selye observed that this syndrome occurs repeatedly and consistently regardless of the nature of the stressor. He maintained that (1) the body's physical response is always the same and (2) it follows a one-, two-, or three-stage pattern: alarm stage, stage of resistance, and in some cases, stage of exhaustion (Fig. 5-7). The first two stages parallel the adaptation processes of maintaining homeostasis (discussed earlier). Brief stress responses generally have adaptive outcomes, with restoration of equilibrium. If the stage of resistance is prolonged, however, the process can become maladaptive and pathologic. It can lead to stress-related disorders and in some cases, death.

Alarm Stage

The **alarm stage** is the immediate physiologic response to a stressor. At its onset, storage vesicles within sympathetic nervous system neurons rapidly release norepinephrine. Shortly thereafter, the adrenal glands secrete additional norepinephrine and epinephrine. These stimulating neurotransmitters and neurohormones prepare the person for a "fight-or-flight" response; that is, the person will either try to overcome the danger the stressor represents or flee to escape its threat. Almost simultaneously, there is a hypothalamic–pituitary–adrenal cascade of hormones (Fig. 5-8). The hypothalamus releases corticotropin-releasing

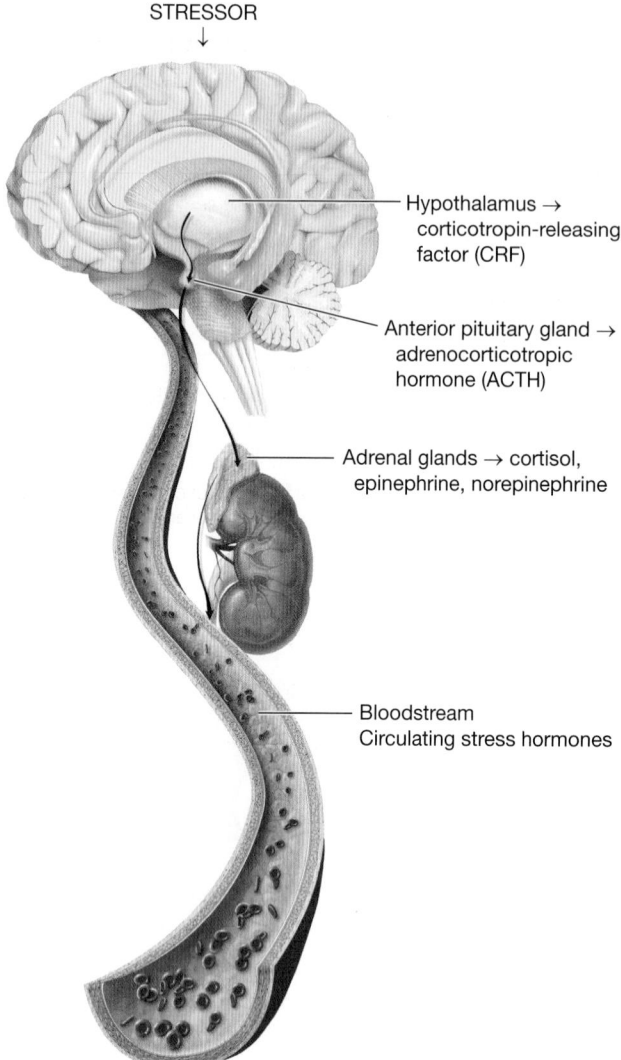

STRESSOR
↓

Hypothalamus →
corticotropin-releasing
factor (CRF)

Anterior pituitary gland →
adrenocorticotropic
hormone (ACTH)

Adrenal glands → cortisol,
epinephrine, norepinephrine

Bloodstream
Circulating stress hormones

FIGURE 5-8 The hypothalamus–pituitary–adrenal (HPA) axis carries out interactions and feedback in response to stress.

TABLE 5-3 Actions of Cortisol

MAJOR INFLUENCE	EFFECT ON BODY
Glucose metabolism	Stimulates gluconeogenesis (synthesis of glucose from amino acids and sources other than carbohydrates)
	Decreases glucose use by the tissues
Protein metabolism	Increases breakdown of proteins
	Increases plasma protein levels
Fat metabolism	Increases mobilization and use of fatty acids
Antiinflammatory action	Stabilizes membranes of inflamed cells, preventing release of proinflammatory mediators
	Decreases capillary permeability to prevent swelling of tissues
	Depresses phagocytosis by white blood cells
	Suppresses the immune response
	Causes atrophy of lymphoid tissue
	Reduces eosinophils (white blood cells active during infectious and allergic reactions)
	Decreases cell-mediated immunity
	Reduces fever
	Inhibits fibroblasts (connective tissue cells that promote wound healing)
Psychic effect	May contribute to emotional instability
Adaptive effect	Facilitates the response of tissues to physiologic changes, such as increased norepinephrine, during trauma and extreme stress

Porth, C. (2019). *Essentials of pathophysiology: Concepts of altered health states* (5th ed.). Lippincott Williams & Wilkins.

factor (CRF), which triggers the pituitary gland to secrete adrenocorticotropic hormone (ACTH). The result is the release of **cortisol**, a stress hormone, from the adrenal cortex. In responding to a stressor, cortisol plays various important roles, such as raising blood glucose and inhibiting insulin to meet increased energy requirements (Table 5-3). Prolonged elevation of norepinephrine, epinephrine, and cortisol levels, however, can predispose people to stress-related disorders discussed later in this chapter.

 N u t r i t i o n   N o t e s

The relationship between stress and eating is complex. Studies suggest that short-term physical stress (e.g., illness) leads to a decreased intake; conversely, people may eat more as a coping strategy for chronic psychological stress. Also, a prolonged increase in circulating cortisol due to chronic psychological stress may enhance appetite and visceral fat accumulation independent of dietary intake.

Stage of Resistance

The **stage of resistance**, the second phase in general adaptation syndrome, is characterized by physiologic changes that work to restore homeostasis. Neuroendocrine hormones, though temporarily excessive, endeavor to compensate for the physiologic changes of the alarm stage. If stress is protracted, however, resistance efforts remain activated. Consequently, one or more organs or physiologic processes may eventually lead to increased vulnerability for stress-related disorders or progression to the stage of exhaustion.

Stage of Exhaustion

The **stage of exhaustion** is the last phase of general adaptation syndrome. It occurs when one or more adaptive or resistive mechanisms are no longer able to protect the person experiencing a stressor. Once beneficial mechanisms now become destructive. For example, a prolonged high level of cortisol leads to higher-than-normal blood glucose levels and a lowered immune response. As a result, there are reduced natural killer cells, which attack viruses and cancer cells, and decreased secretory immunoglobulin A, an antibody involved in immune defense. These changes put the person at risk for frequent or severe infections or cancer (Randall, 2011). As resistance dwindles, there is risk of physical and mental deterioration, illness, and death.

>>> *Stop, Think, and Respond 5-2*

List the following stress-related responses in sequential order:
1. *The adrenal cortex releases cortisol.*
2. *The pituitary gland secretes ACTH.*
3. *The body prepares for fight or flight.*
4. *The blood glucose level rises.*
5. *The adrenal glands release norepinephrine and epinephrine.*
6. *The hypothalamus secretes CRF.*
7. *The immune system becomes suppressed.*
8. *Sympathetic neurons release norepinephrine.*

Psychological Stress Responses

Just as stress requires adaptation on the part of the body, stress also affects the psyche (mind). The mind, in turn, mounts additional defenses.

Coping Mechanisms

Sigmund Freud (1856 to 1939) posited that humans use **coping mechanisms** (unconscious tactics to defend the psyche) to prevent their ego, or reality base, from feeling inadequate (Table 5-4). These manipulations of reality act as psychological first aid, allowing people to temporarily avoid the emotional effects of stress. When appropriate and moderate, coping mechanisms enable people to maintain their mental equilibrium. Coping mechanisms that are overused or over-extended may have maladaptive effects, distorting reality to such an extent that the person fails to recognize and correct their weaknesses. Consequently, the person may avoid taking responsibility for solving personal problems.

Coping Strategies

Coping strategies (stress reduction activities consciously selected) help people deal with stress-provoking events or situations. They can be therapeutic and nontherapeutic. Therapeutic coping strategies usually help the person acquire insight, gain confidence in confronting reality, and develop emotional maturity. Examples include seeking professional assistance in a crisis, using problem-solving techniques, demonstrating assertive behavior, practicing progressive relaxation, and turning to a comforting person or higher power.

Maladaptation results when people use nontherapeutic coping strategies such as mind- and mood-altering substances, hostility and aggression, excessive sleep, avoidance of conflict, and abandonment of social activities. Negative coping strategies may provide immediate temporary relief from a stressor, but they eventually cause problems when used long-term.

 Concept Mastery Alert

Therapeutic Coping Strategies

Therapeutic coping strategies focus on helping the client gain insight and confidence to deal with stressors. They are not synonymous with a client going into therapy.

Stress-Related Disorders

Stress-related disorders are diseases that result from prolonged stimulation of the autonomic nervous and endocrine systems (Box 5-2). Many stress-related diseases involve allergic, inflammatory, or altered immune responses. The effect of prolonged stress can include both physical and mental health

TABLE 5-4 Coping Mechanisms

MECHANISM	EXPLANATION	EXAMPLE
Repression	Forgetting about the stressor	Removing from conscious memory the experience of being sexually abused
Suppression	Purposely avoiding thinking about a stressor	Resolving to "sleep on" a problem or turn the problem over to a higher power, such as God
Denial	Rejecting information	Refusing to believe a life-threatening diagnosis
Rationalization	Relieving oneself of personal accountability by attributing responsibility to someone or something else	Blaming failure on a test to the manner in which the test was constructed
Displacement	Taking anger out on something or someone who is less likely or unable to retaliate	Kicking the wastebasket after being reprimanded by one's boss
Regression	Behaving in a manner that is characteristic of a much younger age	Wanting to be bottle-fed like an infant sibling
Projection	Attributing that which is unacceptable in oneself onto another	Accusing a person of another race of being prejudiced
Somatization	Manifesting emotional stress through a physical disorder	Developing diarrhea that excuses one from dealing with stressful work tasks
Compensation	Excelling at something to make up for a weakness of another kind	A person feels bad about not being a good cook and overcompensates by having an extremely tidy, organized kitchen
Sublimation	Channeling one's energies into an acceptable alternative	Turning to sportscasting when an athletic career is not realistic
Reaction formation	Acting in a way that is in opposition to one's feelings	Being extremely nice to someone who one intensely dislikes
Identification	Taking on the characteristics of another person	Imitating the style of dress, speech, or behavior of another person

BOX 5-2 Stress-Related Disorders

- Hypertension
- Headaches
- Gastritis
- Asthma
- Rheumatoid arthritis
- Skin disorders
- Hyperinsulinism/hypoinsulinism
- Hyperthyroidism/hypothyroidism
- Bruxism (teeth grinding)
- Depressive disorders
- Cancer
- Low back pain
- Irritable bowel syndrome
- Allergies
- Anxiety disorders
- Infertility
- Erectile dysfunction

TABLE 5-5 The Social Readjustment Rating Scale

RANK	LIFE EVENT	LCU VALUE
1	Death of spouse	100
2	Divorce	73
3	Marital separation	65
4	Jail term	63
5	Death of close family member	63
6	Personal injury or illness	53
7	Marriage	50
8	Fired at work	47
9	Marital reconciliation	45
10	Retirement	45
11	Change in health of family member	44
12	Pregnancy	40
13	Sex difficulties	39
14	Gain of new family member	39
15	Business readjustment	39
16	Change in financial state	38
17	Death of close friend	37
18	Change to different line of work	36
19	Change in number of arguments with spouse	35
20	Mortgage over $10,000 annually	31
21	Foreclosure of mortgage or loan	30
22	Change in responsibilities at work	29
23	Child leaving home	29
24	Trouble with in-laws	29
25	Outstanding personal achievement	28
26	Spouse begins or stops work	26
27	Begin or end school	26
28	Change in living conditions	25
29	Revision of personal habits	24
30	Trouble with boss	23
31	Change in work hours or conditions	20
32	Change in residence	20
33	Change in schools	20
34	Change in recreation	19
35	Change in organized religious activities	19
36	Change in social activities	18
37	Mortgage or loan less than $10,000	17
38	Change in sleeping habits	16
39	Change in number of family get-togethers	15
40	Change in eating habits	15
41	Vacation	13
42	Christmas	12
43	Minor violations of the law	11

LCU, life change unit.
Social events are ranked from most stressful to least stressful. Each event is assigned an LCU that correlates with the severity of the stressor. The sum of LCUs over the past 6 months is calculated. A score of less than 150 LCUs is considered low risk, a score between 150 and 199 is an indication of mild risk, moderate risk is associated with a score between 200 and 299, and a score over 300 places the person at major risk; From Holmes, T. H., & Rahe, R. H. (1967). The social readjustment rating scale. *Journal of Psychosomatic Research, 11*(2), 216.

conditions (Cherry, 2021). They are characterized by physical conditions that cycle through asymptomatic periods (absence of the disorder) to episodes that usually develop when the person is under stress. The brain–immune connection suggests that changes in body chemistry during periods of stress may trigger the following: (1) an autoimmune (self-attacking) response like those associated with rheumatoid arthritis and other connective tissue disorders; (2) failure to respond, as in immunosuppression; or (3) a weakened immune response, which may contribute to infections and cancer.

NURSING IMPLICATIONS

Nurses must be aware of potential stressors affecting clients because they add to the cumulative effect of other stressful life events. When a person is experiencing a stressor, nurses may do one or several of the following:

- Identify the stressors.
- Assess the client's response to stress.
- Eliminate or reduce the stressors.
- Prevent additional stressors.
- Promote the client's physiologic adaptive responses.
- Support the client's psychological coping strategies.
- Assist in maintaining a network of social support.
- Implement stress reduction and stress management techniques.

Assessment of Stressors

Holmes and Rahe (1967) developed the social readjustment rating scale, a tool used to predict a person's potential for developing a stress-related disorder. The rating scale is based on the number and significance of social stressors a person has experienced within the previous 6 months (Table 5-5). The risk for a stress-related disorder increases as the person's score rises. Although the dollar amount in the mortgage-related item of the scale is outdated (with inflation, the $10,000 of the 60s is about $92,000 in today's money), being in debt is still a major stressor. With minor modifications, the assessment tool continues to have diagnostic value.

One research study ranked hospital stressors clients experience in a list modeled after the social readjustment rating scale (Box 5-3). By being aware of how an illness or interactions with health care providers and facilities can affect

BOX 5-3	Client-Related Stressors

- Thinking you might lose your sight
- Thinking you might have cancer
- Thinking you might lose an organ
- Knowing you have a serious illness
- Thinking you might lose your hearing
- Not being told what your diagnosis is
- Not knowing for sure what illness you have
- Not getting pain medication when you need it
- Not knowing the results or reasons for your treatments
- Not getting relief from pain medications
- Being fed through tubes
- Missing your spouse
- Not having your questions answered by the staff
- Not having enough insurance to pay for your hospitalization
- Not having your call light answered
- Having a sudden hospitalization you were not planning to have
- Being hospitalized far from home
- Knowing you have to have an operation
- Not having family visit you
- Feeling you are getting dependent on medications
- Having nurses or doctors talk too fast or use words you cannot understand
- Having medications that cause you discomfort
- Thinking about losing income because of your illness
- Having the staff be in too much of a hurry
- Not knowing when to expect things will be done to you
- Being put in the hospital because of an accident
- Being cared for by an unfamiliar doctor
- Not being able to call family or friends on the phone
- Having to eat cold or tasteless food
- Worrying about your spouse being away from you
- Thinking you might have pain because of surgery or test procedures
- Being in the hospital during holidays or special family occasions
- Thinking your appearance might be changed after your hospitalization
- Being in a room that is too cold or too hot
- Not having friends visit you
- Having a roommate who is unfriendly
- Having to be assisted with a bedpan
- Having a roommate who is seriously ill or cannot talk with you
- Being aware of unusual smells around you
- Having to stay in bed or the same room all day
- Having a roommate who has too many visitors
- Not being able to get access to media when you want them
- Having to be assisted with bathing
- Being awakened in the night by the nurse
- Having strange machines around
- Having to wear a hospital gown
- Having to sleep in a strange bed
- Having to eat at different times than you usually do
- Having strangers sleep in the same room with you

The events in this list are arranged in order of their perceived significance as a stressor. The first event is the most stressful, and the rest follow in descending order.

Reproduced with permission from Volicer, B. J., & Bohannon, M. W. (1975). A hospital stress rating scale. *Nursing Research, 24*(5), 352–359.

clients, nurses can be instrumental in supporting those who are especially vulnerable.

Prevention of Stressors

By offering appropriate interventions to people with severe or accumulated stressors, nurses can help prevent or minimize stress-related illness. Prevention takes place at three levels:

- **Primary prevention** involves eliminating the potential for illness before it occurs. An example is teaching adolescents principles of nutrition and methods to maintain normal weight and BP.
- **Secondary prevention** includes screening for risk factors and providing a means for early diagnosis of disease. An example is regularly measuring the BP of a client with a family history of hypertension.
- **Tertiary prevention** minimizes the consequences of a disorder through aggressive rehabilitation or appropriate management of the disease. An example is frequently turning, positioning, and exercising a client who has had a stroke to help restore functional ability.

Stress Reduction Techniques

Stress reduction techniques are methods that promote physiologic comfort and emotional well-being. Some general interventions appropriate during the care of any client include providing adequate explanations in understandable language, keeping the client and family informed, demonstrating confidence and expertise when providing nursing care, remaining calm during crises, being available to the client, responding promptly to the client's signal for assistance, encouraging family interaction, advocating on behalf of the client, and referring the client and family to organizations or people who provide postdischarge assistance.

Stress Management Techniques

People susceptible to intense stressors or those likely to experience stressors over a long period may benefit from additional stress management approaches. **Stress management techniques** are therapeutic activities used to reestablish balance between the sympathetic and the parasympathetic nervous systems (Table 5-6). Techniques that counter sympathetic stimulation have a calming effect; stimulating tactics counterbalance parasympathetic dominance. Interventions that cause the release of endorphins, manipulation of sensory stimuli, and adaptive activities also mediate physical and emotional responses to stress. Nurses help clients manage stress, for example, by teaching principles of time management and assertiveness techniques.

Endorphins

Endorphins are natural body chemicals that produce effects similar to those of opioid drugs such as morphine. In addition to decreasing pain, these chemicals promote a sense of pleasantness, tranquility, and well-being.

"Endorphins are created in your pituitary gland and hypothalamus, both located in the brain. Endorphins are a type

TABLE 5-6 Interventions for Stress Management

INTERVENTION	EXPLANATION
Modeling	Promotes the ability to learn an adaptive response by exposing a person to someone who demonstrates a positive attitude or behavior
Progressive relaxation	Eases tense muscles by clearing the mind of stressful thoughts and focusing on consciously relaxing specific muscle groups
Imagery	Uses the mind to visualize calming, pleasurable, and positive experiences
Biofeedback	Alters autonomic nervous system functions by responding to electronically displayed physiologic data
Yoga	Reduces physical and emotional tension through postural changes, muscular stretching, and focused concentration
Meditation and prayer	Have been found to create an even more significant decrease in anxiety by focusing on thankfulness and concern for others
Placebo effect	Alters a negative physiologic response through the power of suggestion

TABLE 5-7 Healthy Ways to Cope with Stress

METHODS	STRATEGIES
Taking breaks from news and social media	It's good to be informed, but consider limiting reading or listening to news to just a couple times a day. Disconnect from the phone, TV, and computer screens for a while.
Taking care of one's body	Eat plenty of fruits and vegetables, lean protein, whole grains, and fat-free or low-fat milk and milk products. Go to bed at the same time each night and get up at the same time each morning. Move more and sit less—every little bit of physical activity helps. Take deep breaths, stretch, or meditate. Limit alcohol intake. Avoid using prescription drugs in ways other than prescribed. Avoid smoking and the use of other tobacco products. Continue with regular health appointments.
Making time to unwind	Try to set aside time devoted to activities you enjoy.
Connecting with others	Talk with people you trust about your concerns and how you are feeling.
Connecting with community- or faith-based organizations	Gather with members of community-based and/or religious organizations.

Adapted from Centers for Disease Control and Prevention. (n.d.). *Coping with stress.* https://www.cdc.gov/mentalhealth/stress-coping/cope-with-stress/index.html

of neurotransmitter, or messenger in your body" (Cleveland Clinic, 2024). Some health care providers believe that certain activities, such as massage, sustained aerobic exercise, and laughter, trigger the release of endorphins. Once released, endorphins attach themselves to receptor sites in the brain—perhaps in the limbic system, the center where emotions are experienced.

Sensory Manipulation

Sensory manipulation involves altering moods, feelings, and physiologic responses by stimulating pleasure centers in the brain using sensory stimuli. Research is being conducted on the stress-reducing effects of certain colors; full-spectrum lighting in the home and workplace; music; and specific aromas that conjure pleasant associations, such as the smell of baking bread.

Adaptive Activities

To enhance adaptation, people experiencing stress may adopt alternative thinking, alternative behavior, and alternative lifestyle techniques.

Alternative Thinking Techniques

Alternative thinking techniques are those that facilitate a change in a person's perceptions from negative to positive. **Reframing** helps a person analyze a stressful situation from various perspectives and ultimately conclude that the situation is not as bad as it once seemed. For instance, instead of dwelling on the negative consequences of a minor car crash, such as the expense and inconvenience of repairs, the person can choose to focus on the positive aspect of being physically unharmed in the accident.

Alternative Behavior Techniques

Alternative behavior techniques are those actions that modify stress in order for the person to take control rather

than become immobilized. Making choices and pursuing actions promote self-confidence over feeling victimized. Procrastination only prolongs and intensifies the original stressor. In addition, sharing frustrations with others who are both objective and supportive is usually more therapeutic than brooding in isolation. Other behavioral approaches to reduce stress include prioritizing what needs to be accomplished and initially attending to that which is most important or difficult. Less important activities may be postponed or delegated to others. Although other positive behaviors can be cultivated, it is also important sometimes to say "no" to avoid becoming overwhelmed and more stressed.

Alternative Lifestyle Techniques

Alternative lifestyle techniques are those activities in which people who are prone to stress make a conscious effort to change their patterns of living. Some examples include improving diet; becoming more physically active; cultivating humor; and taking scheduled breaks throughout the day for leisure, power naps, or listening to uplifting music. Although pet ownership is not possible for everyone, those who do have pets often find it soothing and relaxing to stroke and touch an animal that responds affectionately regardless of a person's age, physical characteristics, or accomplishments. Pets tend to improve a person's feelings of self-worth in a way that extends to human relationships as well (Table 5-7).

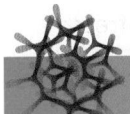

KEY POINTS

- Homeostasis: The body maintains constancy by adjusting and readjusting in response to changes in the internal and external environment that foster disequilibrium. The body does this by using adaptation and neurotransmitters.
- Autonomic nervous system: Peripheral nerves affecting physiologic functions that are largely automatic and beyond voluntary control
  - Sympathetic nervous system: Prepares the body for a fight-or-flight response
  - Parasympathetic nervous system: Restores equilibrium after danger is no longer apparent
- Stress is the physiologic and behavioral responses to disequilibrium. The physiologic responses to stress make up general adaptation syndrome, which consists of the following:
  - The alarm stage: The immediate physiologic response to a stressor (sympathetic nervous system)
  - The stage of resistance: Characterized by physiologic changes that work to restore homeostasis
  - The stage of exhaustion: Occurs when one or more adaptive or resistive mechanisms are no longer able to protect the person experiencing a stressor
- Coping mechanisms enable people to maintain their mental equilibrium.
- The three stages of stress prevention are:
  - Primary: Eliminating the potential for illness before it occurs

- Secondary: Screening for risk factors and providing a means for early diagnosis of disease
- Tertiary: Minimizing the consequences of a disorder through aggressive rehabilitation or appropriate management of the disease
- Stress reduction techniques the nurse can implement include the following:
  - Providing adequate explanations in understandable language
  - Keeping the client and family informed
  - Demonstrating confidence and expertise when providing nursing care
  - Remaining calm during crises
  - Being available to the client
  - Responding promptly to the client's signal for assistance
  - Encouraging family interaction
  - Advocating on behalf of the client
  - Referring the client and family to organizations or people who provide postdischarge assistance
- Stress management may include the following:
  - Endorphins: Natural body chemicals that can help decrease pain and promote a sense of pleasantness, tranquility, and well-being
  - Sensory manipulation: Altering moods, feelings, and physiologic responses by stimulating pleasure centers in the brain using sensory stimuli

CRITICAL THINKING EXERCISES

1. Identify at least five interventions that are both realistic and helpful in reducing the stressors associated with being a student.
2. What stressors are more unique to older adults than to people in other age groups?
3. Explain how the coping mechanism of denial can initially protect the self-image of a client with alcohol use disorder but can eventually cause harm.
4. Choose a coping mechanism from Table 5-3. How can it be positive or negative?

NEXT-GENERATION NCLEX-STYLE REVIEW QUESTIONS

1. When the nurse assesses a client, which make up a cluster of signs and symptoms suggesting the client is experiencing a stress response? Select all that apply.
   a. Rapid heart rate
   b. Nervousness
   c. Excessive thirst
   d. Impaired concentration
   e. Elevated BP

Test-Taking Strategy: Use the process of elimination to select manifestations of a stress response. Recall that during a stress response, the body is initially flooded with stimulating hormones, epinephrine, and norepinephrine and later with cortisol.

2. Which nursing intervention is initially most appropriate when providing information to a stress-prone client?
   a. Advise obtaining monthly BP assessments.
   b. Provide information about antihypertensive medications.
   c. Explore various stress management techniques.
   d. Teach the client the health hazards of hypertension.

Test-Taking Strategy: Identify the key word in the stem of the question, which is "initial." Recall that prevention has a higher priority than treatment.

3. When the nurse cares for an older adult, which recent event likely represents the greatest stressor?
   a. Death of a spouse
   b. Change in living conditions
   c. Planned retirement
   d. Change in financial state

Test-Taking Strategy: Use the process of elimination to select the situational event that has the most severe impact on a client's equilibrium.

4. When the nurse interacts with a client, which coping mechanism is being demonstrated when the client refuses treatment because they believe their breast biopsy indicating cancer is incorrect?
   a. Somatization
   b. Regression
   c. Displacement
   d. Denial

   Test-Taking Strategy: Analyze the information this question asks, which requires selecting a coping mechanism from among four options that correlates with one in which the client's belief contradicts factual evidence.

5. Which nursing activity would have the most benefit toward promoting health and wellness?
   a. Encouraging teenagers to never smoke cigarettes
   b. Offering suggestions for smoking cessation
   c. Explaining how to apply nicotine patches to the skin
   d. Advising smokers with a chronic cough to consult a physician

   Test-Taking Strategy: Identify the key word and modifier in the stem of the question, which in this case is "most benefit." Select the answer from among the four options that can prevent, rather than manage, the consequences of smoking.

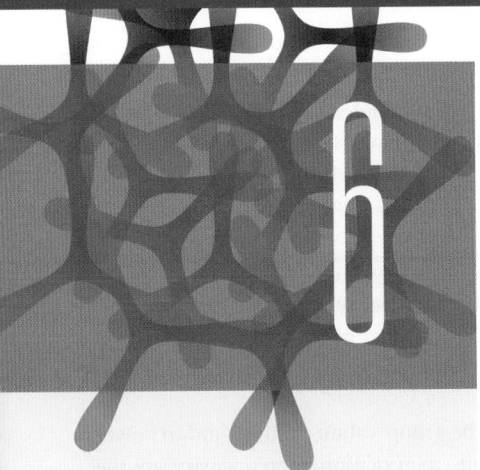

6

Culture and Ethnicity

Words To Know

African American
ageism
Asian Americans
bilingual
certified interpreter
cultural shock
culturally sensitive care
culture
diversity
ethnicity
ethnocentrism
folk medicine
generalization
Latino
limited English proficiency (LEP)
minority
Native American
race
stereotypes
telephonic interpreting
transcultural nursing
European American

Learning Objectives

On completion of this chapter, the reader should be able to:

1. Differentiate culture, race, and ethnicity.
2. Discuss factors that interfere with perceiving people as individuals.
3. Explain why U.S. culture is described as anglicized.
4. List the predominant cultures present in the United States.
5. List the diversities among people informed by their cultures.
6. Describe characteristics of culturally sensitive care.
7. List ways to demonstrate cultural sensitivity.

INTRODUCTION

Clients vary by age, sex, gender, race, health status, education, religion, occupation, and economic level, among other characteristics. Culture, the focus of this chapter, is another characteristic that contributes to client **diversity** (differences among groups of people).

Nurses have always cared for clients with differences of many sorts. Despite there being cultural differences among clients, the traditional tendency has been to treat clients as though those differences do not exist. However, ignoring differences can contradict the best interests of clients. Instead, nurses can practice **culturally sensitive care** (Table 6-1): "Culturally sensitive nursing care recognizes the need for respect and acknowledgement of the wholeness of all human beings, regardless of culture, race, ethnicity, heritage, religion – everyone has a unique background" (Culturally Sensitive Nursing Care, n.d.).

This chapter provides information about cultural concepts, cultural aspects of different ethnic and racial groups, and intercultural communication. Although components of culture are specific to a particular group of people, individual clients within a given cultural group may deviate from others within that group. Therefore, nurses are advised to always consider cultural needs from each individual client's perspective.

 Gerontologic Considerations

■ There were 54.1 million people aged 65 years and older living in the United States in 2019. By 2040, the population of older adults is projected to reach 80.8 million; by 2060, 94.7 million (ACL, 2024).

■ Some older adults may prefer their own culture's traditional healing practices with which they have been familiar since childhood. They may implement these practices instead of or along with care recommended by providers of Western-based health care.

Ageism, a form of negative stereotypical thinking, promotes false beliefs about older adults being physically and cognitively impaired, lacking interest in sex, and being burdensome to families and society. According to an article published in 2020, ageism may affect the quality of care shown to older clients, by nurses (Van Wicklin, 2020). Ageism was associated with shorter, less effective, and more superficial communication from nurses.

CONCEPTS RELATED TO CULTURE

Culture

Culture is "the ways in which people live and express themselves, and it is a central concern of sociology" (New Cultural Frontiers, 2022). It includes, but is not limited to, language, communication style, traditions, religion, art, music, dress, health beliefs, and health practices.

A group's culture is passed from one generation to the next. According to Hinkle and Cheever (2021), culture is learned from birth; shared by members of a group; influenced by environment, technology, and the availability of resources; and dynamic and ever-changing.

The United States has been described as a "melting pot" in which culturally diverse groups have become assimilated. However, people from various cultural groups have settled, lived, and worked in the United States while continuing to maintain unique identities.

Race

Race refers to physical differences that groups and cultures consider socially significant. For example, people might identify their race as Aboriginal, African American or Black, Asian, European American or White, Native American,

TABLE 6-1 Components of Culturally Sensitive Care

COMPONENT	DESCRIPTION
Awareness	Nurses can pay close attention to their own biases and how they react to people whose backgrounds and cultural experiences differ from their own.
Attitude	Once nurses tap into awareness, they can actively analyze their increased awareness and internal belief systems. They can examine the factors that lead to their cultural biases.
Knowledge	Nurses can work to acknowledge that a disconnect can exist between beliefs and behaviors and view knowledge as an important element of developing culturally sensitive care.
Skills	Nurses put their awareness, attitude, and knowledge into practice by integrating culturally sensitive behaviors into their daily interactions. These behaviors include effective and respectful communication and body language. For example, nonverbal communication methods, such as gestures, can mean very different things to people within different cultural groups.

Adapted from Deering, M. (2022). *Cultural Competence in Nursing.* https://nursejournal.org/resources/cultural-competence-in-nursing/

Native Hawaiian or Pacific Islander, Māori, or some other race (American Psychological Association, 2024). Race is not the same thing as ethnicity or culture.

Minority

A **minority** group is a culturally, ethnically, or racially distinct group that coexists with but has less political or economic power compared to another group. By itself, minority status does not necessarily correlate to population (Britannica, 2024).

Rather, it refers to the group's status with regard to power and control. For example, men of European ancestry are the current majority in the United States. Slightly more women than men make up the population of the United States, but women are considered the minority group. According to the U.S. Census Bureau (2022b), the most prevalent racial group in the United States was the non-Hispanic White population at 57.8%; this represents a decrease from 63.7% in 2010. The projected American Indian and Alaska Native population either alone or in combination with other race groups on July 1, 2060, will be about 2.5% of the projected total U.S. population (U.S. Census Bureau, 2022a). Racial minority groups will make up 57% of the population by 2060. Despite making up the majority of the population at that time, until these groups acquire more political and economic power in society, they will continue to be classified as minorities (Fig. 6-1).

Ethnicity

Ethnicity refers to shared cultural characteristics. These characteristics include, but are not limited to, ancestry, beliefs, languages, and cultural practices. A person's identification with their ethnicity may exist regardless of whether they have ever lived in the country of their family's heritage. People may express a connection to their ethnicity by giving children names that reflect their heritage, wearing unique items of clothing, appreciating folk music and dance, and eating dishes from the region of their family's heritage.

Often, cultural characteristics represent what may be considered the majority in a homogeneous group; therefore, those characteristics are seen as expected or "normal." When cultural groups mix, however, as through the process of immigration, differences become more obvious. People within the groups may experience **cultural shock** (bewilderment over behavior that is culturally unfamiliar).

FACTORS THAT AFFECT PERCEPTION OF INDIVIDUAL PEOPLE

Stereotyping

Stereotypes are preconceived, fixed ideas that attribute particular characteristics to groups of people. Stereotypes are used to classify people according to age, gender, skin color, sexual orientation, ethnicity, and so on. These overgeneralized beliefs contribute to "mental shortcuts" the human brain uses to respond rapidly to situations. Those shortcuts rarely lead to accurate assessment of an individual person or a group. Stereotypes interfere with one's ability to see other people as unique individuals.

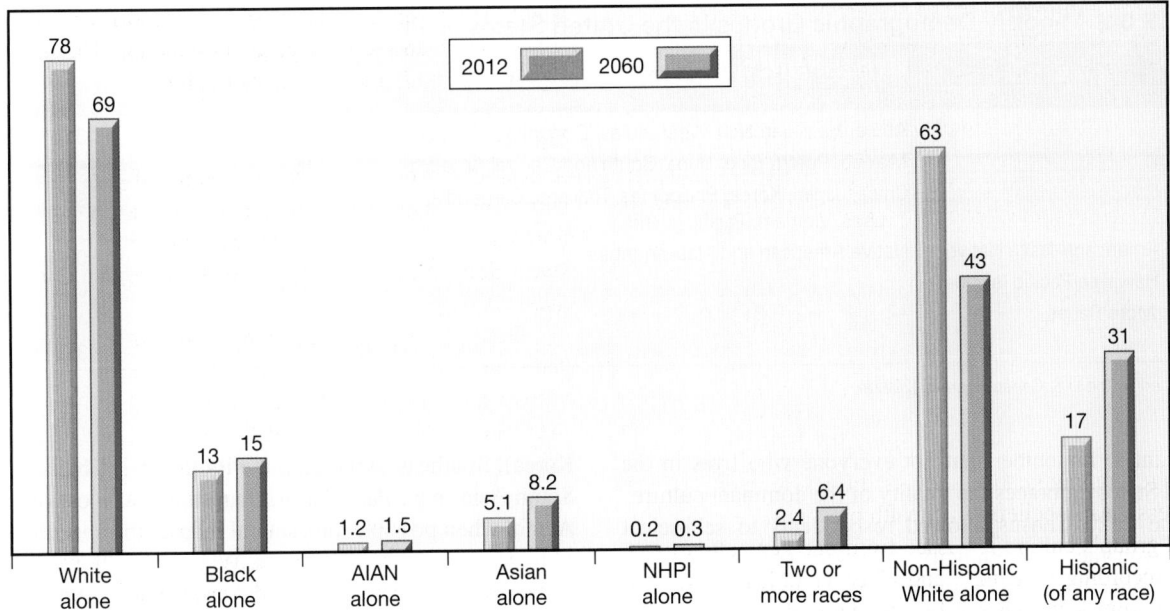

FIGURE 6-1 Percent of total population by race and Hispanic origin: 2012 and 2060. AIAN, American Indian and Alaska Native; NHPI, Native Hawaiian and Other Pacific Islander.

Generalization

Generalization (the supposition that a person shares cultural characteristics with others of a similar background) is different from stereotyping. Stereotyping is to develop a predetermined idea about a person or group (AFS USA .org). Assuming that all people who affiliate themselves with a particular group behave alike or hold the same beliefs is always incorrect. Despite what may appear to be a homogeneous group, diversity always exists among individuals in any group.

A generalization is by its nature flexible. It provides a springboard from which to explore a person's individuality. For example, when a nurse is assigned to care for a terminally ill client who immigrated to the United States from Venezuela, the nurse may assume that the client is Roman Catholic because Catholicism is common in many Latin American countries. However, before contacting a priest to assist with the client's spiritual needs, the culturally sensitive nurse understands that this generalization concerning religion may not be accurate. The nurse must seek information that confirms or contradicts the original generalization.

Ethnocentrism

Ethnocentrism (the belief that one's own ethnicity is superior to all others) has no place in intercultural relationships. Ethnocentrism provides rationalization for treating people outside one's ethnic group as deviant and undesirable.

CULTURES IN THE UNITED STATES

The United States can be described as anglicized, or English-based, because it evolved primarily from the culture and legal system of its early English settlers. Box 6-1 provides an overview of some common characteristics of U.S. culture. While these characteristics are common, it is

BOX 6-1 Examples of Common Cultural Characteristics in the United States

- English is the language of communication.
- The pronunciation or meaning of some words varies according to regions within the United States.
- The customary greeting is a handshake.
- A distance of 4 to 12 ft is customary when interacting with strangers or doing business (Giger, 2013).
- In casual situations, it is acceptable for people of all genders to wear pants; blue jeans are common apparel.
- The majority of Americans are Christians.
- Sunday is recognized as the Sabbath for Christians.
- Government is expected to remain separate from religion.
- Guilt or innocence for alleged crimes is decided by a jury of one's peers.
- Selection of a marriage partner is an individual person's choice.
- Legally, men and women are equals.
- Marriage is monogamous (only one spouse); fidelity is expected.
- Divorce and subsequent remarriages are common.
- Parents are responsible for their minor children.
- Aging adults live separately from their children.
- Status is related to occupation, wealth, and education.
- Common beliefs are that everyone has the potential for success and that hard work leads to prosperity.
- Daily bathing and use of a deodorant are standard hygiene practices.
- Many women shave the hair from their legs and underarms; men without beards shave their faces daily.
- Licensed practitioners provide health care.
- Drugs and surgery are expected forms of medical treatment.
- Americans tend to value technology and equate it with quality.
- Generally, Americans are time-oriented and, therefore, rigidly schedule their activities according to clock hours.
- Forks, knives, and spoons are used, except when eating "fast foods," for which the fingers are appropriate.

TABLE 6-2 Minority Demographic Groups in the United States as Projected for 2022 and 2060

GROUP	REPRESENTATIVE COUNTRIES	U.S. POPULATION ESTIMATE 2022 (%)	U.S. POPULATION PROJECTION FOR 2060 (%)
Black	Africa, Haiti, Jamaica, West Indies, Dominican Republic	10	13.0
Hispanic	Mexico, Puerto Rico, Cuba, South and Central America	15.6	28.6
Asian	China, Japan, Korea, Philippines, Thailand, Cambodia, Laos, Vietnam, Pacific Islands	5	9.1
Native American/Alaska Native	Native American and Alaskan tribes	0.9	0.6
Native Hawaiian/Pacific Islander		0.2	0.2
Two or More Races		8.5	4.9
White		52	43.6

As reported by the U.S. Census Bureau (2022a).

important to remember that not everyone who lives in the United States embraces the totality of the dominant culture.

The 2020 Census allowed respondents to self-select from seven race and ethnicity categories (Table 6-2). The reports generated from the census data included estimations of the distribution of the U.S. population among those categories in 2022 and 2060 (Table 6-3).

The term **African Americans** is used to identify people whose ancestral origin is Africa. People of African descent may be from Latin America, countries in Africa, Caribbean islands, regions of the United States, or other places. Some American people of African descent prefer "Black," while others prefer "African American." **Latino**, a shortened term for *Latino Americano*, refers to people originating from Latin American countries, including Brazil. Some people use the word *Hispanics* to refer to people who speak Spanish. Not all people in Latin America speak Spanish, however, so this cannot be used to universally refer to people of Latin American origin. The word Latino is gendered ("Latina" is the feminine form); nongendered forms include Latin@ and Latinx. In general, using the name of the nation of origin (e.g., referring to someone as Mexican American) is preferred to using the general labels Latino or Hispanic. The nurse should use the term the patient uses to refer to themself. **Asian Americans** are people of Asian ancestry who are from the United States. Discussion of Asian ancestry can be divided regionally, for example: East Asia (e.g., China, Japan, South Korea, and North

Korea), Southeast Asia (e.g., the Philippines, Thailand), and South Asia (e.g., Pakistan, Afghanistan, and most of India). Again, when possible, one should refer to the specific region or nation of the person's origin. While the U.S. Census uses the term "American Indian," the term **Native American** is typically preferred when referring to descendants of the Indigenous peoples of the United States. Native Americans belong to 574 federally recognized tribes in the United States (National Congress of American Indians, 2022). Specify the person's nation when possible.

Although **European American** culture predominates in the United States, people of African, Asian, Latino/Hispanic, Native American, and Hawaiian/Pacific Islander ancestry will soon outnumber people who trace their ancestry to the United Kingdom and Western Europe. This increased diversity in the U.S. population illustrates the continued importance of cultural sensitivity in nursing.

TRANSCULTURAL NURSING

Madeleine Leininger (1925 to 2012) coined the term **transcultural nursing** (providing nursing care within the context of the client's culture) in the 1970s. Aspects of transcultural nursing include:

- Assessments of a cultural nature
- Acceptance of each client as an individual

TABLE 6-3 Categories of Race and Ethnicity for Federal Statistics

CATEGORY	DESCRIPTION
White	A person having origins in any of the original peoples of Europe, the Middle East, or North Africa
Hispanic, Latino, or Spanish	Origins in Cuba, Mexico, Puerto Rico, South or Central America, or other Spanish culture, regardless of race
Asian	A person having origins in any of the original peoples of East Asia, Southeast Asia, or the Indian subcontinent
Black or African American	A person having origins in any of the Black racial groups of Africa or people who report responses such as African American, Jamaican, or Haitian
American Indian and Alaska Native	A person having origins in any of the original peoples of North and South America (including Central America) and who maintains tribal affiliation or community attachment
Native Hawaiian and Other Pacific Islander	A person having origins in any of the original peoples of Hawaii, Guam, Samoa, or other Pacific Islands
Two or more races	A person who identifies as a combination of more than one race category

U.S. Census Bureau. (2022). *2020 census redistricting data* (Public Law 94-171) summary file.

- Knowledge of health problems that affect particular racial or ethnic groups
- Planning of care within the client's health belief system to achieve the best health outcomes

To provide culturally sensitive care, nurses must become skilled at managing language differences, understanding biologic and physiologic variations, promoting health education that will reduce prevalent diseases, and respecting alternative health beliefs or practices.

Cultural Assessment

To provide culturally sensitive care, the nurse strives to gather data by asking clients to describe unique characteristics informed by their culture. Pertinent data include:

- Language and communication style
- Hygiene practices, including feelings about modesty and accepting help from others
- Special clothing or ornamentation
- Religion and religious practices
- Rituals surrounding birth, passage from adolescence to adulthood, illness, and death
- Family and gender roles, including child-rearing practices and kinship with older adults
- Proper forms of greeting and showing respect
- Food habits and dietary restrictions
- Methods for making decisions
- Health beliefs and medical practices

Assessment of these areas is likely to reveal many differences. Examples of variations include those in language and communication, eye contact, space and distance, touch, emotional expressions, dietary customs and restrictions, time, and beliefs about the cause of illness.

Language and Communication

Because language is the primary way to share and gather information, difficulty in communication is one of the biggest obstacles to providing culturally sensitive care. The nurse may encounter travelers from other countries or people living in the United States who speak English as their second language or do not speak it at all. It is estimated that 67.3 million people who live in the United States speak a language other than English at home; Spanish is the most often spoken language other than English in the United States (Fig. 6-2; Acutrans, 2022). People who can communicate in English may still prefer to use their primary languages, especially under stress.

Equal Access

Federal law, specifically Title IV of the Civil Rights Act of 1994, states that people with **limited English proficiency (LEP)**—an inability to speak, read, write, or understand English at a level that permits interacting effectively—are entitled to the same health care and social services as those who speak English fluently. In other words, all clients have the right to unencumbered communication with a health provider. Using children as interpreters or requiring clients to provide their own interpreters is a civil rights violation. The Joint Commission (TJC) requires that hospitals provide effective communication for each client.

The use of untrained interpreters, volunteers, or family to interpret information for a client undermines confidentiality and privacy. It also violates family roles and boundaries. It increases the potential of the interpreter to modify, condense, omit, or add information, or to project their own values during communication between the client and the health care provider.

The best form of communication with a client who has LEP is through a **certified interpreter**. A certified interpreter

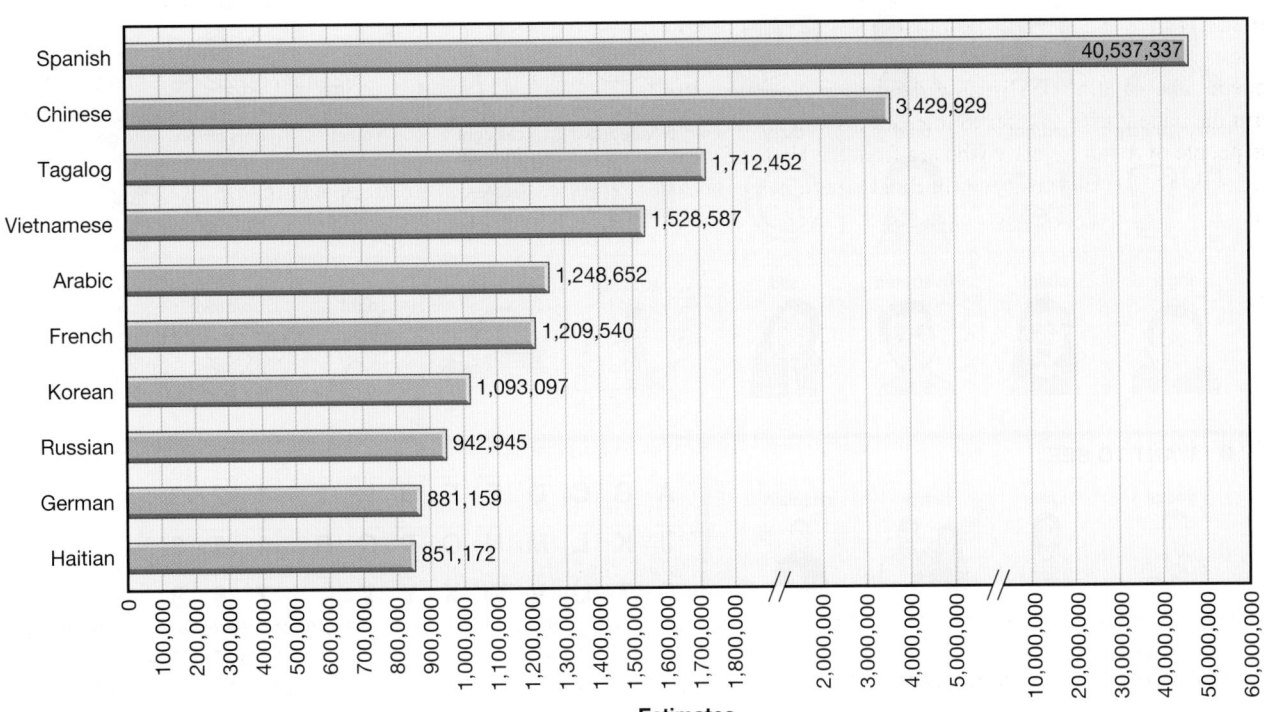

FIGURE 6-2 Top 10 languages other than English spoken at home in the United States. (Acutrans. [2022]. *Top 10 most spoken languages*. https://acutrans.com/top-10-most-spoken-languages/)

is a translator who is certified by a professional organization through rigorous testing based on appropriate and consistent criteria. However, interpreters who meet these qualifications are few and far between. To comply with the laws and accreditation requirements, health care agencies are strongly encouraged to train professional interpreters. A competently trained interpreter demonstrates the skills listed in Box 6-2.

When a trained or certified interpreter is not available in person or by video, there are a variety of other options. In descending order of preference, the following may be used: agency-employed interpreters, **bilingual** (able to speak a second language fluently) staff, volunteers, and least desirable, family or friends. TJC requires the use of qualified, professional interpreters to achieve compliance.

Qualifications and competencies can be met in various ways. Of utmost importance is that the interpreter is language-proficient, trained in the practice of interpreting, and qualified to translate health care information. For example, when an on-site interpreter is not available, use of a video or **telephonic interpreting** (over-the-phone translation) can be used as an alternative. Voice-to-text apps also exist, whereby one person speaks into their mobile device in one language and the other person does the same in their preferred language. Each message is translated into the other person's language in real time. In addition, though it does not meet all the needs of an LEP client, a picture or dual-language communication board may be useful for immediate bedside interactions between the client and the nursing staff (Fig. 6-3).

Culturally Sensitive Nurse–Client Communication

If the nurse is not bilingual (able to speak a second language fluently) and a trained interpreter is not available, the nurse must use an alternative method for communicating (see Nursing Guidelines 6-1 for more information).

Understanding some unique cultural characteristics involving aspects of communication may assist the nurse in practicing culturally sensitive care. It is helpful to be aware of general communication patterns among major cultural

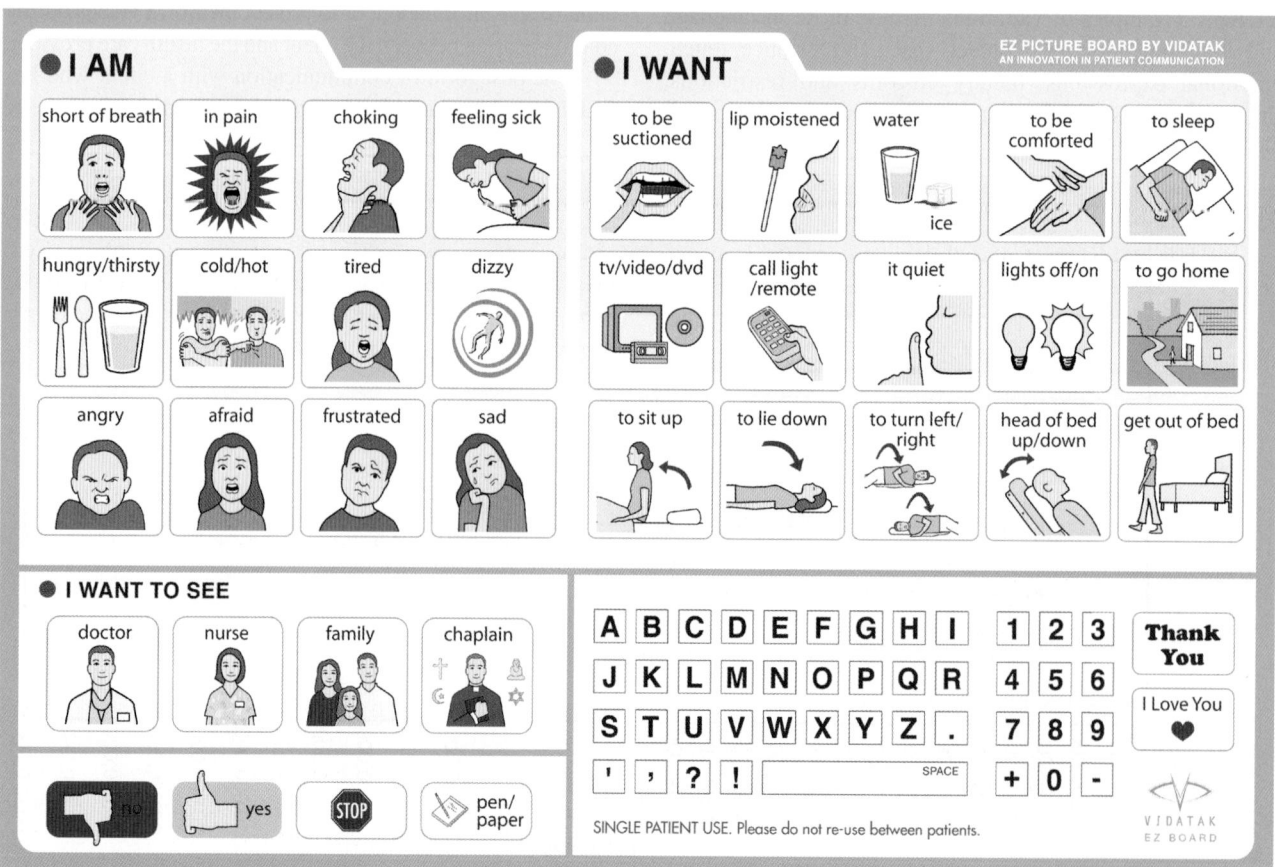

FIGURE 6-3 A picture communication board allows clients to point at appropriate images or use a wet-erase marker. (Courtesy of Vidatak, LLC. Los Angeles, CA 90069.)

NURSING GUIDELINES 6-1

Communicating with Clients Who Do Not Speak English

- Greet or say words and phrases in the client's language, even if carrying on a conversation is impossible. *Using familiar words indicates a desire to communicate with the client even if the nurse lacks the expertise to do so extensively.*
- With the client, use websites that translate English to several foreign languages and vice versa. Examples include Google and www.babelfish.com. *A computer with internet access provides sites with easy-to-use, rapid, free translations of up to 5,000 characters at a time.*
- Refer to an English/foreign language dictionary or use appendices in references such as *Taber's Cyclopedic Medical Dictionary. Some dictionaries provide medical words and phrases that may provide pertinent information.*
- Compile a loose-leaf folder or file cards of medical words in one or more languages spoken by clients in the community. Place it with other reference books in the nursing unit. *A homemade reference provides a readily available language resource for communicating with others in the local area.*
- Request a trained interpreter. If that option is impossible, call community organizations or church offices to obtain a list of people who speak the client's language and may be willing to act as emergency translators. *Someone proficient at speaking the language is more effective at obtaining necessary information and explaining proposed treatments than someone relying on a rough translation.*
- When several interpreters are available, select one who is of the same gender and approximately the same age as the client. *Some clients are embarrassed relating personal information to people with whom they have little in common.*
- Look at the client, not the interpreter, when asking questions and listening for responses. *Eye contact indicates that the client is the primary focus of the interaction and helps the nurse interpret nonverbal clues.*

- If the client speaks some English, speak slowly, not loudly, using simple words and short sentences. *Lengthy or complex sentences are barriers when communicating with someone not skilled in a second language.*
- Avoid using technical terms, slang, or phrases with a double or colloquial meaning. *The client may not understand the spoken vernacular, especially if they learned English from a textbook rather than conversationally.*
- Ask questions that can be answered with yes or no. *Direct questions avoid the need to provide elaborate responses in English.*
- If the client appears confused by a question, repeat it without changing the words. *Rephrasing tends to compound confusion because it forces the client to translate yet another group of unfamiliar words.*
- Give the client sufficient time to respond. *The process of interpreting what has been said in English and then converting the response from the client's language back to English requires extra time.*
- Use nonverbal communication or pantomime. *Pointing and pantomiming actions tend to be communicated and interpreted quite accurately.*
- Be patient. *Anxiety is communicated interpersonally and tends to heighten frustration.*
- Show the client written English words. *Some non–English-speaking people can read English better than they can understand spoken English.*
- Work with the health agency's records committee to obtain consent forms, authorization for health insurance benefits, and copies of client's rights written in languages other than English. *Legally, clients must understand that to which they are consenting.*
- Develop or obtain foreign translations describing common procedures, routine care, and health promotion. *All clients are entitled to explanations and educational services.*

groups in the United States. However, keep in mind that these are generalizations; awareness of the individual client's preferences is critical in providing culturally sensitive care.

Native Americans

Native American people have traditionally been fearful of the U.S. health care establishment (Satter et al., 2014). Consequently, Native American people may hesitate to share personal information with health care providers they do not know. They may interpret questioning as prying or meddling. The nurse should be patient when awaiting an answer and listen carefully because impatience may be considered disrespectful (Lipson & Dibble, 2012). Navajo people, members of the largest tribe of Native Americans, traditionally believe that no person has the right to speak for another. Therefore, they may refrain from commenting on a family member's health.

Because Native Americans traditionally preserved heritage through oral rather than written history, they may be wary of nurses who write down what they say. If possible, the nurse should write notes after, rather than during, the interview.

African Americans

African American people may be mistrustful of the medical establishment, in part because of unethical practices

employed in past research projects such as the U.S. Public Health Service Tuskegee Study of Untreated Syphilis (Centers for Disease Control and Prevention, 2013), during which health care providers told African American men they were receiving free health care. In reality, for 40 years, those providers withheld diagnosis and treatment from nearly 40 men with syphilis. The nurse must demonstrate professionalism by addressing all clients by their titles and last names and introducing themselves. The nurse should follow up thoroughly with requests, respect the client's privacy, and ask open-ended rather than direct questions until trust has been established.

Latino People

In general, Latino people are often comfortable sitting close to interviewers and letting interactions unfold slowly. Many Latino people speak English but, like native English speakers, have difficulty with medical terminology. They may be embarrassed to ask the interviewer to speak slowly, so the nurse must provide information and ask questions carefully. Latino men are traditionally protective and may be authoritarian regarding women and children. They may expect to be consulted in decisions concerning family members (Larson et al., 2017).

Asian Americans

Asian American people tend to respond with brief or more factual answers and little elaboration, perhaps because traditionally, many Asian cultures value simplicity, meditation, and introspection. Asian Americans may not openly disagree with authority figures, such as physicians and nurses, because of their respect for harmony. The appearance of agreement can conceal disagreement or potential nonadherence to a particular therapeutic regimen that is unacceptable from the client's perspective (Ruiz et al., 2022).

Eye Contact

Expectations and meanings associated with eye contact traditionally vary among cultural groups. European Americans generally value making and maintaining eye contact throughout communication. Direct eye contact may offend people from some Asian American or Native American cultures, who are more likely to believe that lingering eye contact is an invasion of privacy or a sign of disrespect. In Arab culture, strong eye contact can indicate honesty. Some Arab American women may avoid continued eye contact with men because in Arab culture, this may be interpreted as flirtation (Helal, 2017; Evanson, 2024).

Space and Distance

Providing personal care and performing nursing procedures often require entering a client's personal space, which can cause discomfort for members of some cultural groups. For example, Asian American clients may feel more comfortable with the nurse at more than an arm's length away. The physical closeness of a nurse who intends to provide comfort and support may be perceived as threatening to clients from various cultures. Therefore, it is always best to provide explanations when close contact during procedures and personal care is necessary.

Touch

Many people from Southeast Asia traditionally consider the head to be a sacred body part that only close relatives can touch. Nurses and other health care providers should ask permission before touching this area. Southeast Asian people also traditionally believe that the area between a female's waist and knees is particularly private and should not be touched by any male other than the woman's husband. For all clients, a nurse can relieve the client's anxiety by offering an explanation, requesting permission, and allowing the client's spouse or family members to stay in the room if desired.

Emotional Expression

In general, people from European American and African American backgrounds tend to freely express both positive and negative feelings. In contrast, people from East Asian backgrounds do not tend to rely as much as other cultures to express facial features of pain expressions and may not vary their expressions as much as pain intensities (Saumure et al., 2023). Stoicism should not be interpreted as a lack of feeling or caring (Eliopoulos, 2013). Similarly, Latino men may not demonstrate their feelings or readily discuss their symptoms because they may interpret doing so as less masculine. This response can be attributed to *machismo*, a traditional belief common to Latin American cultures that virile men are physically strong and must deal with emotions privately. Awareness

of such cultural expectations can assist the nurse in working to learn the emotional and physical needs of the individual client.

Dietary Customs and Restrictions

Food is necessary for survival: it relieves hunger, promotes health, and prevents disease. Eating also has social meanings that relate to communal togetherness, celebration, reward and punishment, and relief of stress. Culture may inform the types of food and how frequently a person eats, the types of utensils used, and the status of individual people, such as who eats first and who gets larger servings.

Religious practices within some cultures impose certain rules and restrictions such as times for fasting and foods that can and cannot be consumed (Table 6-4). Nurses should incorporate cultural and religious food preferences into dietary teaching to promote the client's adherence to a therapeutic diet for a medical disorder.

 Nutrition Notes

■ Dietary acculturation occurs when people change their eating behaviors after moving to a new area. The person will reject some traditional foods and add new foods or substitute them for traditional foods. Availability and cost influence dietary acculturation.

■ Acculturation can have a positive or negative effect on eating habits. Generally, when people immigrate to the United States and adopt the "typical American diet," their intake of fat, sugar, and calories increases, and their intake of fruit, vegetables, fiber, and protein decreases. Clients should be encouraged to retain any healthy eating practices.

■ Mexican Americans may drink *atole*, a heated mixture of masa harina (corn meal), *piloncillo* (Mexican brown sugar), cinnamon, vanilla, and, sometimes, chocolate or fruit, as a traditional celebration and comfort food. *Atole* is also consumed during *la cuarentena*, a 40-day period following the delivery of an infant, in the belief that it will help the new mother recover and increase the volume of breast milk.

■ The diet of some African Americans may include greens, grits, cornbread, and beans cooked with a generous amount of fat or fatty meats, reflecting Southern American roots.

■ The diets from different regions in the Asian culture show diets from Southeast and South Asia often lack fresh fruit and get unhealthy fat from cooking oils, such as coconut oil, while Southeast and Northeast diets get high levels of sodium from condiments, such as soy sauce, although regional favorites differ (Merschel, 2023).

■ Native Americans may consume what is grown locally like fry bread made from corn; meat that is hunted on land or fished from nearby rivers; and chicken, pigs, and cattle that are raised within the community.

■ Many Muslims buy *halal* meat (how the animal is slaughtered) from Muslim shopkeepers. Islam also includes rules about avoiding consumption of alcohol, including not eating at a table where alcohol is served (Islamic-laws.com, n.d.).

■ Jewish people have *kosher* rules for food, which must be certified as such by a rabbi. For example, utensils (including pots and pans and other cooking surfaces) that have come into contact with meat may not be used with dairy and vice versa. Utensils that have come into contact with nonkosher food may not be used with kosher food.

TABLE 6-4 Examples of Religious Beliefs and Practices That Affect Health Care

RELIGION	EXAMPLES	NURSING IMPLICATIONS
Orthodox Judaism and some nonorthodox Jewish sects (i.e., Conservative, Reform, and Reconstructionist)	Circumcision is a sacred ritual performed on the eighth day of life.	Provide information on care following circumcision before discharge.
	Kosher dietary laws allow consumption of animals that chew their cud and have cloven hoofs (e.g., cattle, sheep, goats, deer, and bison). Animals are slaughtered according to defined procedures; dairy products and meat are not eaten together. Seafood with fins and scales is permitted (i.e., no shellfish, like crabs and shrimp).	Notify the dietary department of the client's food preferences. Packaged food labeled *kosher* indicates it was prepared and preserved according to dietary laws. *Pareve* means "made without meat or milk."
	Sabbath begins on Friday at sundown and ends on Saturday at sundown.	Avoid scheduling nonemergency tests or procedures during this time.
	Autopsies are not allowed unless required by law.	All organs that are removed and examined during an autopsy must be returned to the body so that the body may remain intact for burial.
	Burial is preferred within 24 hours of death; Judaic law requires that the body not be left alone.	Contact the family to stay with the dying client. Orthodox family members may ask a son or other relative to close the mouth and eyes of the deceased.
Catholicism	Statues and medals of religious figures provide spiritual comfort.	Leave such items on or near the client; keep items safe and return promptly if removed.
	Artificial birth control and abortion are forbidden.	Explain how to decrease chances of pregnancy through methods such as checking basal body temperature and characteristics of cervical mucus.
	Baptism is necessary for salvation.	In an emergency, any baptized Christian may perform baptism by pouring water over the person's head three times and saying, "I baptize you in the name of the Father, and of the Son, and of the Holy Spirit."
Jehovah's Witnesses	Blood transfusions are refused even in life-threatening situations because they believe blood is the source of the soul.	Refer to physicians who practice blood conservation strategies such as autotransfusions and intravenous volume expanders (e.g., dextran).
Seventh Day Adventist	Strict dietary laws are followed based on the Old Testament of the Christian bible.	Request a consult with the dietitian to facilitate a vegetarian diet without caffeine.
	Saturday is the Sabbath.	Avoid scheduling medical appointments or procedures at this time.
Christian Scientist	Prayer is the antidote for any illness.	Expect that Christian Scientist clients will contact lay practitioners to assist with healing. Legal procedures may be an option when the well-being of minor children is threatened by parental refusal for medical care.
Church of Jesus Christ of Latter-Day Saints (Mormonism)	Coffee, tea, alcohol, tobacco, illegal drugs, and overuse of prescription drugs are prohibited.	Notify the dietary department to provide noncaffeinated beverages.
	Male members may anoint the sick with consecrated olive oil.	Facilitate anointing rituals before surgery or at the client's request.
Amish	Members may be reluctant to spend money on health care unnecessarily.	Assess home remedies and folk healing being used. Home deliveries are preferred; expect brief overnight stays following hospital births.
	Illness must be endured with faith and patience.	Offer comfort measures and analgesic medications rather than waiting for clients to request them.
	Members are formally educated up to the eighth grade.	Provide written health educational materials at the client's level of understanding.
	Photographs are not permitted.	Avoid photographing newborns.
Hinduism	Modesty and hygiene are valued.	Provide a daily bath, with the client's modesty in mind, but not following a meal; add hot water to cold, but not the reverse.
	The application of a *pundra*, a distinctive mark on the forehead, is religiously symbolic.	Avoid removing the *pundra*, or replace it as soon as possible.
	Hindus value self-control.	Offer comfort measures and analgesic medications rather than waiting for Hindu clients to request them.
	Men do not participate during labor and delivery.	Keep men informed of the birthing progress.
	Cleansing of the body after death symbolizes cleansing of the soul.	Inquire if the family wishes to wash a deceased client's body.
	Most Hindu people are vegetarians; beef is forbidden, and some do not consume eggs.	Request a consult with the dietitian. Clients may refuse medication in gelatin capsules because gelatin is made from animal byproducts.

(continued)

TABLE 6-4 Examples of Religious Beliefs and Practices That Affect Health Care (*continued*)

RELIGION	EXAMPLES	NURSING IMPLICATIONS
Islam (Muslims)	Prayer and washing are required five times a day.	Plan care around prayer and washing rituals, which occur at sunrise, midmorning, noon, afternoon, and sunset. Help clients face Mecca for prayer.
	Pork and alcohol are forbidden.	Clients may refuse medication in capsules and pork insulin. Request that the pharmacist omit alcohol in liquid medications, which usually contain this ingredient.
	Members prefer to die at home.	Expect that the client and their family will view life support as unacceptable if there is no hope for a reasonable recovery.
	Only relatives may touch or wash the body of a deceased Muslim	Consult the family before performing postmortem care.

Adapted from Andrews, J. D. (2021). *Cultural, ethnic and religious reference manual* (5th ed.). JAMARDA Resources.

Time

Throughout the world, people view clock time and social time differently (Clockify, 2021). Calendars and clocks define clock time, dividing it into years, months, weeks, days, hours, minutes, and seconds. Social time reflects attitudes concerning punctuality that vary among cultures. Punctuality is less important in some cultures than it is in others. Tolerating and accommodating cultural differences related to time facilitate culturally sensitive care.

Beliefs Concerning Illness

Generally, people embrace one of three cultural views (or some combination of these views) to explain illness or disease. The *biomedical* or *scientific perspective* is often shared by those from industrialized countries in which people base their beliefs about health and disease on research findings. An example of a scientific perspective is that microorganisms cause infectious diseases, and frequent hand hygiene reduces the potential for infection.

The *naturalistic* or *holistic perspective* espouses that humans and nature must be in balance or harmony to remain healthy; illness is an outcome of disharmony. Some Native Americans believe that positive outcomes result from living in congruence with Mother Earth (Native Hope, 2023). Another example is the traditional Chinese *yin/yang* theory, which refers to the belief that balanced forces promote health. Latin American and Caribbean traditional health systems apply the *hot/cold* theory, which implies that illness is caused by imbalance between components ascribed as having hot or cold attributes. Adding or subtracting heat or cold to restore balance can also restore health. This is also a consideration in Ayurveda, which has its origins in India.

Finally, there is the *magico–religious* perspective in which there is a cultural belief that supernatural forces contribute to disease or health. Some examples of the magico–religious perspective include faith healing or practice forms of the African Diaspora religions Hatian Vodou and Lousiana Voodoo (Vidal, 2023). Native Americans have a strong reverence for the Great Spirit's influence on health and illness. Traditional health care uses herbs and spiritual rituals performed by tribal leaders or medicine people to relieve illness (Learn Religions, 2022). Although the nurse may not understand or may disagree with a client's beliefs concerning causes of health or illness, the nurse's respect for the individual client helps achieve health care goals. As long as a culturally held health belief or practice is not harmful, the nurse should incorporate it into the client's care.

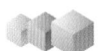 Concept Mastery Alert

Client Health Beliefs

Always incorporate a client's health beliefs in their care. For example, a Native American client with a strong belief in the Great Spirit's influence on health and illness will likely expect a tribal medicine person to play a major role in the care of their illness.

⟩⟩ *Stop, Think, and Respond 6-1*

How might a culturally competent nurse respond to a Vietnamese client who practices coining, which involves applying heated oil to a symptomatic area of the skin and then rubbing it with a smooth-edged hard object to draw negative energies out of the body? Coining is not painful, but it produces redness of the skin and superficial ecchymosis (bruising), and the oils used may be toxic.

Biologic and Physiologic Variations

The biologic characteristics of primary importance to nurses are those that involve the skin, hair, and certain physiologic enzymes.

Skin Characteristics

Skin assessment techniques that are commonly taught are biased toward White clients. To provide culturally sensitive care, nurses must modify their techniques to obtain accurate data on People of Color.

The best technique for observing baseline skin color in a person with dark skin is to use natural or bright artificial light. Because the palms of the hands, the feet, and the abdomen contain the least pigmentation and are less likely to have been tanned, they are often the best areas to inspect.

All skin, regardless of a person's skin color, contains an underlying red tone. Its absence or a lighter appearance indicates pallor, a characteristic of anemia or inadequate oxygenation. The color of the lips and nail beds, common sites for assessing cyanosis in White clients, may be highly pigmented in other groups, and nurses may misinterpret normal findings. The conjunctiva and oral mucous membranes are likely to provide more accurate data. The sclera or the hard palate, rather than the skin, is a better location for assessing jaundice. In some people of color, however, the sclera may have a yellow cast from carotene and fatty deposits; nurses should not misconstrue this finding as jaundice (Andrews & Boyle, 2019).

Rashes, bruising, and inflammation may be less obvious in people with dark skin. Palpating for variations in texture, warmth, and tenderness is a better assessment technique than inspection. Keloids (irregular, elevated thick scars) are more common among dark-skinned clients (Fig. 6-4). Keloids are thought to form from a genetic tendency to produce excessive transforming growth factor-beta (TGF-β), a substance that promotes fibroblast proliferation during tissue repair.

Some nurses, when bathing a client with dark skin, may misinterpret the brown discoloration on a washcloth as a sign of poor hygiene. However, this is due to the normal shedding of dead skin cells, which retain their pigmentation.

Hypopigmentation and hyperpigmentation are conditions in which the skin is not of a uniform color. Hypopigmentation may result when the skin becomes damaged. Regardless of a person's skin color, damaged skin characteristically manifests temporary redness, which then fades to a lighter hue; in clients with dark skin, the effect may be more obvious. Vitiligo, a disease that can affect clients of any skin color, produces irregular white patches on the skin as a result of an absence of melanin (Fig. 6-5). Other than hypopigmentation, there are no physical symptoms, but the cosmetic effects may create emotional distress. Clients concerned about uneven skin tone may use a pigmented cream to disguise noticeable areas.

Congenital dermal melanocytosis (CDM), an example of hyperpigmentation, are dark blue areas on the lower back and sometimes on the abdomen, thighs, shoulders, or arms of infants and children with dark skin (Fig. 6-6). Nurses may hear this condition referred to as "Mongolian spots." However, this term is considered to be marginalizing and outdated (Yale et al., 2021). CDM is due to the migration of melanocytes into the fetal epidermis. CDM is rare among

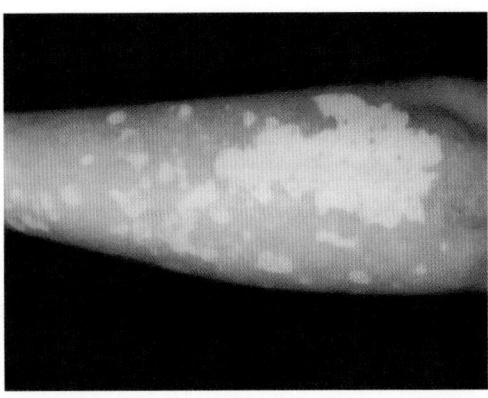

FIGURE 6-5 Vitiligo of the forearm in an African American client. (Courtesy of Neutrogena Care Institute.)

children with light skin and tends to fade by the time a child is 5 years old. Nurses unfamiliar with differences in skin color can mistake CDM as a sign of physical abuse or injury. They can differentiate the two by pressing the pigmented area: CDM will not produce pain when pressure is applied.

Hair Characteristics

Hair color and texture are also biologic variants. People with dark skin usually have dark brown or black hair. Hair texture results from the amount of protein molecules within the hair. Variations range from straight to very curly. The curlier the hair, the more difficult it may be to comb. In general, using a wide-toothed comb or pick, wetting the hair with water before combing, or applying a moisturizing cream makes grooming more manageable.

Enzymatic Variations

Three inherited enzymatic variations are prevalent among members of various U.S. demographic groups. They involve an absence or insufficiency of the enzymes lactase, glucose-6-phosphate dehydrogenase (G-6-PD), and alcohol dehydrogenase (ADH).

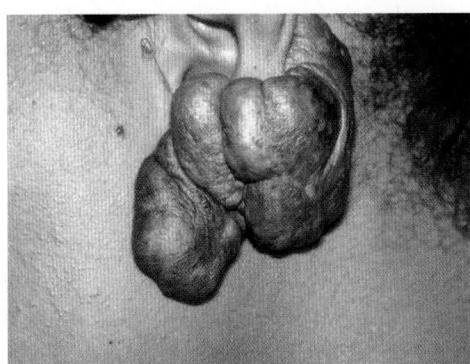

FIGURE 6-4 Keloids are raised, thick scars, as seen in this client's ear lobe, which was originally punctured to accommodate pierced earrings. (Photo by B. Proud.)

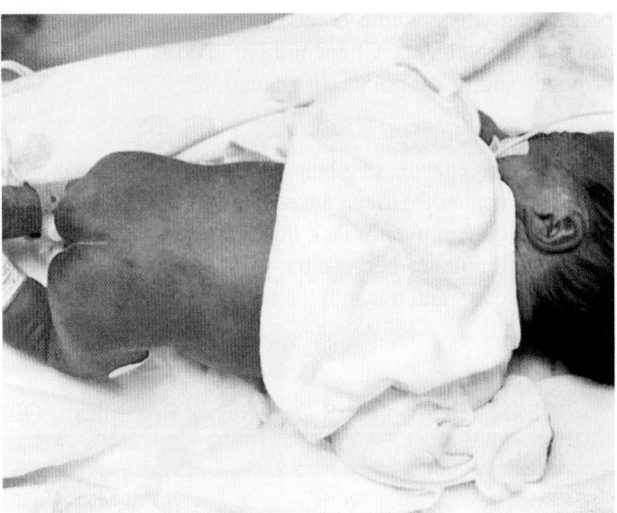

FIGURE 6-6 Congenital dermal melanocytosis. These bluish-pigmented areas are common in infants with dark skin. (Photo by K. Timby.)

Client and Family Teaching 6-1
Reducing or Eliminating Lactose

In order to reduce or eliminate lactose, the nurse teaches the client or the family to do the following:

- Avoid milk, dairy products, and packaged foods that list dry milk solids or whey among their ingredients (e.g., some breads, cereals, puddings, gravy mixes, caramels, chocolate).
- Use nondairy creamers, which are lactose-free, instead of cream or milk.
- Consume only small amounts of milk or dairy products at a time.
- Substitute milk that has been cultured with the *Acidophilus* organism, which converts lactose into lactic acid.
- Drink Lactaid, a commercial product in which the lactose has been converted into other absorbable sugars.
- Use kosher foods, which are prepared without milk; they can be identified with the word *pareve* on the label.

Lactase Deficiency

Lactase is a digestive enzyme that converts lactose, the sugar in milk, into simpler sugars, glucose and galactose. A lactase deficiency, common among people of African ancestry, Latino people, and Chinese people, causes intolerance to dairy products. Without lactase, people have cramps, intestinal gas, and diarrhea approximately 30 minutes after ingesting milk or foods that contain it. Symptoms may continue for 2 hours (Dudek, 2021). Eliminating or reducing sources of lactose in the diet may prevent the discomfort. Liquid tube-feeding formulas and those used for bottle-fed infants can be prepared using milk substitutes. Because milk is a good source of calcium necessary for health, nurses should teach affected clients to obtain calcium from other sources, such as green leafy vegetables, dates, prunes, canned sardines and salmon with bones, egg yolks, whole grains, dried peas and beans, and calcium supplements. Client and Family Teaching Box 6-1 provides additional points for education.

G-6-PD Deficiency

G-6-PD is an enzyme that helps red blood cells metabolize glucose. People of African ancestry and people of Mediterranean origin commonly lack this enzyme. The disorder is manifested in males because the gene is sex-linked, but females can carry and transmit the faulty gene.

A G-6-PD deficiency makes red blood cells vulnerable during stress, which increases metabolic needs. When this happens, red blood cells are destroyed at a much greater rate than in unaffected people. If the production of new red blood cells cannot match the rate of destruction, anemia develops.

Because several drugs can precipitate the anemic process (Table 6-5), it is important for the nurse to intervene if these drugs or those that depress red blood cell production are prescribed for clients who are at greatest risk. The nurse must monitor susceptible clients and advocate for laboratory tests, such as red blood cell count and hemoglobin levels, which will indicate any adverse effects.

Alcohol Dehydrogenase Deficiency

When a person consumes alcohol, a process of chemical reactions involving enzymes, one of which is ADH, eventually breaks down the alcohol into acetic acid and carbon dioxide. Some research suggests that people of Asian descent and Native Americans often metabolize alcohol at a different rate than other groups because of environmental differences and physiologic variations in their enzyme system (Olafuyi et al., 2021). The result is that affected clients experience dramatic vascular effects, such as flushing and rapid heart rate, soon after consuming alcohol. In addition, the middle metabolites of alcohol (those formed before acetic acid) remain unchanged for a prolonged period. Many scientists believe that the middle metabolites, such as acetaldehyde, are extremely toxic and subsequently play a primary role in causing organ damage.

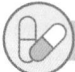

Pharmacologic Considerations

Pharmaceutical studies demonstrate that genetic variations can influence medication outcomes (Cleveland Clinic, 2023). For example, certain drug classes used for psychological illnesses such as those for depression or schizophrenia reduce symptoms more effectively in people of African and Asian descent than other classes of drugs. Protein variations in the genetic code are thought to influence these differences.

Disease Prevalence

Several diseases, including sickle cell anemia, hypertension, diabetes, and stroke, occur with much greater frequency among particular ethnic minority groups in the United States. The incidence of chronic illness affects morbidity differently as well (Table 6-6).

The incidence of some chronic diseases and their complications are related partly to variations in social factors,

---

TABLE 6-5 Examples of Drugs That Precipitate Glucose 6-Phosphate Dehydrogenase Anemia

DRUG CATEGORY	EXAMPLE	USE
Aspirin	Acetylsalicylic acid (Aspirin)	Treatment of pain, inflammation, and fever
Nonsteroidal antiinflammatory drugs (NSAIDs)	Ibuprofen (Advil) Naproxen (Aleve)	Treatment of pain, inflammation, and fever
Sulfonamides	Trimethoprim/sulfamethoxazole (Bactrim)	Treatment of urinary infections

TABLE 6-6 Leading Causes of Death Among U.S. Racial Groups 2019

RANK	ALL AMERICANS	BLACK OR AFRICAN AMERICAN	HISPANIC OR LATINO	NATIVE AMERICAN OR ALASKA NATIVE	ASIAN OR PACIFIC ISLANDER
1	Heart disease	Heart disease	Heart disease	Heart disease	Cancer
2	Cancer	Cancer	Cancer	Cancer	Heart disease
3	Chronic lower respiratory disease	Unintentional injuries	Unintentional injuries	Unintentional injuries	Cerebrovascular diseases
4	Unintentional injuries	Cerebrovascular diseases	Chronic lower respiratory disease	Chronic liver disease and cirrhosis	Unintentional injuries
5	Cerebrovascular diseases	Diabetes	Cerebrovascular diseases	Diabetes	Diabetes
6	Alzheimer disease	Chronic lower respiratory disease	Alzheimer disease	Chronic lower respiratory diseases	Alzheimer disease
7	Diabetes	Homicide	Diabetes	Cerebrovascular diseases	Chronic lower respiratory diseases
8	Influenza and pneumonia	Nephritis, nephrotic syndrome, and nephrosis	Nephritis, nephrotic syndrome, and nephrosis	Suicide	Influenza and pneumonia
9	Suicide	Alzheimer disease	Influenza and pneumonia	Nephritis, nephrotic syndrome, and nephrosis	Nephritis, nephrotic syndrome, and nephrosis
10	Nephritis, nephrotic syndrome, and nephrosis	Essential hypertension, hypertensive renal disease	Suicide	Influenza and pneumonia	Suicide

Leading causes of death and number of deaths, by culture in the United States, 2019 https://www.cdc.gov/nchs/data/hus/2020-2021/LCODRace.pdf

such as poverty. Underserved community members tend to be less affluent; consequently, their access to expensive health care is often limited (Ndugga & Artiga, 2023). The lack of preventive health care, early detection, and treatment contributes to higher death rates. The U.S. government, therefore, has committed itself to reducing disparities in health care among all Americans (see Chapter 4).

With the knowledge that underserved community members are at increased risk for chronic diseases, culturally sensitive nurses focus heavily on health education, participate in community health screenings, and campaign for equitable health services.

Health Beliefs and Practices

Many differences in health beliefs exist among U.S. demographic groups. These beliefs are informed by cultural and ethnic influences. Health beliefs affect health practices.

Folk medicine (health practices based on tradition rather than modern scientific practice) typically refers to methods of disease prevention or treatment outside mainstream conventional practice. Generally, folk medicine is not given by formally educated and licensed medical practitioners. In addition to culturally specific health practices, such as those sought from a *curandero* (traditional practitioner in Hispanic cultures who is thought to have spiritual and medicinal powers), a medicine person, or an herbalist, many people in the United States also turn to complementary and alternative medicine (CAM). CAM refers to therapies that are used in addition to or instead of conventional medical treatment for which there is some scientific evidence of safety and effectiveness. CAM is

often referred to as *integrative therapy* (Weil, 2012; Fig. 6-7, Box 6-3).

CAM attracts people for various reasons. Mainstream medical care is expensive, there may be dissatisfaction with prior treatment or progress, family or acquaintances may provide testimonials about their efficacy, or people may feel intimidated by the health care establishment.

Just because a health belief or practice is different from what the nurse generally practices does not make it wrong. Culturally sensitive nurses respect the client's belief system and help integrate folk and complementary practices into scientifically based treatment.

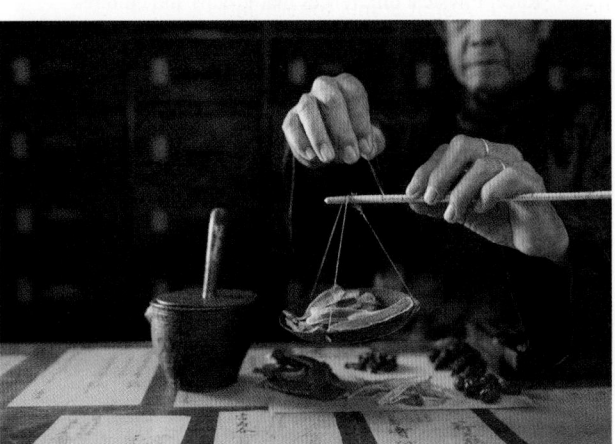

FIGURE 6-7 Treatment with herbal remedies may be more common among Asian American and Pacific Islander clients. (Dragon Images/Shutterstock.)

BOX 6-3	Examples of Complementary and Alternative Medicine

- Homeopathy is based on the principle of similarity; it uses diluted herbal and medicinal substances that cause symptoms similar to a particular illness in healthy people. For example, quinine is used to treat malaria because it causes chills, fever, and weakness (symptoms of malaria) when administered to healthy people.
- Naturopathy uses botanicals, nutrition, homeopathy, acupuncture, hydrotherapy, and manipulation to treat illness and restore a person to optimum balance.
- Chiropractic medicine is based on the belief that illnesses and pain result from spinal misalignment; it uses manipulation and readjustments of joint articulations, massage, and physiotherapy to correct dysfunction.
- Environmental medicine proposes that allergies to environmental substances in the home and workplace affect health, particularly for highly sensitive people. It advocates reduced exposure to chemicals to control conditions that adherents believe mainstream physicians have failed to diagnose or have underdiagnosed.
- Acupuncture is a key component of traditional Chinese medicine and is most commonly used to treat pain; increasingly, it is being used for overall wellness, including stress management.

CULTURALLY SENSITIVE NURSING

Accepting that the United States is multicultural is the first step toward culturally sensitive nursing care. The following recommendations are ways to demonstrate culturally sensitive nursing care:

- To improve interactions, use culturally sensitive techniques such as sitting in the client's comfort zone and making appropriate eye contact.
- Become familiar with physical differences among racial groups.
- Perform physical assessments, especially of the skin, using techniques that provide accurate data.
- Learn or ask clients about cultural beliefs concerning health, illness, and techniques for healing.
- Consult the client on ways to solve health problems.
- Never verbally or nonverbally ridicule a cultural belief or practice.
- Integrate helpful or harmless cultural practices within the plan of care.
- Guide the client in modifying or gradually changing culturally unsafe health practices.
- Avoid removing religious items or clothes that hold symbolic meaning for the client. If they must be removed, keep them safe and replace them as soon as possible.
- If the client has cultural food preferences, provide those foods.
- Advocate for routine screening for diseases to which clients are genetically or culturally prone.
- Facilitate rituals by the person the client identifies as a healer within their belief system.
- Apologize if you violate a client's cultural traditions or beliefs.
- Learn to speak a second language.

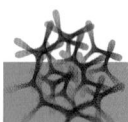

KEY POINTS

- Culturally sensitive nursing care: Care that respects and is compatible with each client's culture
  - Culture: The values, beliefs, and practices of a particular group
  - Race: Physical differences that groups and cultures consider socially significant
  - Ethnicity: Shared cultural characteristics (e.g., ancestry, beliefs, languages, and cultural practices)
- Factors that interfere with achieving culturally sensitive nursing:
  - Stereotypes: Preconceived, fixed ideas that attribute particular characteristics to groups of people
  - Generalization: Supposition that a person shares cultural characteristics with others of a similar background
- Ethnocentrism: Belief that one's own ethnicity is superior to all others
- Transcultural nursing: Providing nursing care within the context of another's culture
  - Assessments of a cultural nature
  - Acceptance of each client as an individual
  - Knowledge of health problems that affect particular racial or ethnic groups
  - Planning of care within the client's health belief system to achieve the best health outcomes
- Accepting that the United States is multicultural and that health care disparities exist is the first step toward culturally sensitive nursing care

CRITICAL THINKING EXERCISES

1. A nurse working for a home health agency is assigned to care for a non–English-speaking client from Pakistan. How would a culturally sensitive nurse prepare for this client's care?

2. A pregnant Nigerian client explains to a nurse that she is wearing a safety pin on her clothing to protect her unborn child from evil spirits and to help ensure a safe delivery. Discuss how it would be best to respond to this client from a culturally sensitive perspective.

3. Identify common characteristics of a cultural group in your community; include family patterns, dietary preferences or restrictions, health beliefs, and cultural practices.

4. Explore approaches used to meet the health needs of a particular ethnic group within the community in which you live; include methods for communicating with clients who may not speak English.

NEXT-GENERATION NCLEX-STYLE REVIEW QUESTIONS

1. In order of priority, list the steps a nurse should take when preparing to teach a Latino client about dietary measures to control diabetes mellitus.
   a. Review, with the client, a diabetic meal plan.
   b. Evaluate the client's ability to read a food label.
   c. Obtain a copy of a calorie-controlled exchange list.
   d. Determine the client's food likes and dislikes.
   Test-Taking Strategy: Put in order of importance for teaching about changes in diet for diabetes mellitus.

2. When conducting a cultural assessment during admission to a health care institution, what is the best technique for a culturally sensitive nurse to use when asking questions?
   a. Position themselves directly next to the client.
   b. Position themselves just beyond an arm's length away.
   c. Position themselves within the doorway to the room.
   d. Position themselves to facilitate occasional touching.
   Test-Taking Strategy: Use the process of elimination and knowledge of common cultural patterns to select an option that is better than any of the others.

3. While assessing an African American infant during a home visit, the nurse observes a bluish area on the baby's buttocks. What is the action that is best for the nurse to take?
   a. Document the information; it is a normal assessment finding.
   b. Report suspicion of physical abuse to Child Protective Services.
   c. Notify the physician in charge of the infant's care about the finding.
   d. Examine any and all children in the home for additional signs of abuse.
   Test-Taking Strategy: Use the process of elimination and knowledge of variations in skin color to select an option that is better than any of the others.

4. An Ojibwa community client reports that a tribal elder used "smudging," a ritual in which a substance like sweet grass is burned and the smoke is fanned about the body with an eagle feather, to cleanse negative energy during a recent illness. Which response by the nurse is most appropriate?
   a. Explain that smudging will not help restore the client's health.
   b. Suggest that the client include the physician's treatment regimen.
   c. Report the tribal elder for practicing medicine without a license.
   d. Advise the client to avoid treatment prescribed by the tribal elder.
   Test-Taking Strategy: Note the key words, "most appropriate," which indicates one choice is better than any of the others. Determine if the practice of smudging is harmful or harmless to the client's physical health.

5. Which of the following hospital menu suggestions would be appropriate for a person who practices Orthodox Judaism? Select all that apply.
   a. Breaded pork chop
   b. Crab salad
   c. Tuna filet
   d. Baked chicken
   e. Bacon, lettuce, and tomato sandwich
   Test-Taking Strategy: Use the process of elimination to exclude options that are not compatible with the dietary practices of Orthodox Jewish people.

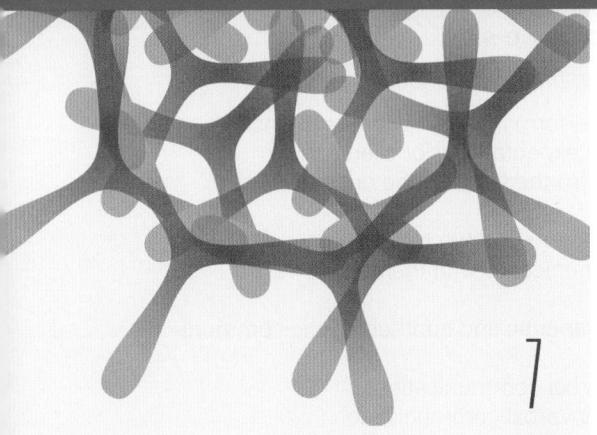

UNIT 3 | Fostering Communication

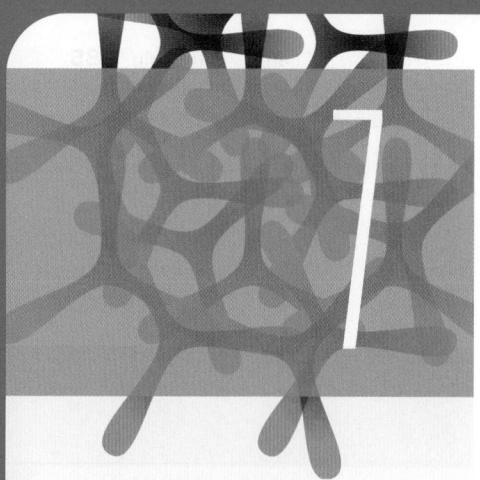

The Nurse–Client Relationship

Words To Know

active listening
affective touch
American Sign Language (ASL)
caregiver
collaborator
communication
Deaf
delegator
educator
empathy
expressive aphasia
hard of hearing
intimate space
introductory phase
kinesics
nonverbal communication
paralanguage
personal space
proxemics
public space
relationship
silence
social space
task-oriented touch
terminating phase
therapeutic relationship
therapeutic verbal communication
touch
verbal communication
working phase

Learning Objectives

On completion of this chapter, the reader should be able to:

1. Name the roles nurses perform in nurse–client relationships.
2. Describe the current role expectations for clients.
3. List the principles that form the basis of the nurse–client relationship.
4. Identify the phases of the nurse–client relationship.
5. Differentiate social communication and therapeutic verbal communication.
6. Provide examples of therapeutic and nontherapeutic communication techniques.
7. List factors that affect verbal communication.
8. Describe the forms of nonverbal communication.
9. Differentiate task-related touch from affective touch.
10. List situations in which affective touch may be appropriate.

INTRODUCTION

The client's confidence in the nurse's ability to care for them in a fair, unbiased manner is the basis for a nurse–client relationship. One of the primary keys to establishing and maintaining positive nurse–client relationships is the manner and style of the nurse's communication. This chapter offers information about techniques for communicating therapeutically, listening empathetically, sharing information, and providing client education, all of which are among the most basic processes within the context of nurse–client relationships.

 Gerontologic Considerations

■ Greet the client by giving your name and title and ask how the client prefers to be addressed. Use titles of respect such as "Mr" or "Mrs" Avoid using familiar or patronizing terms such as "dear," "sweetie," or "honey," no matter what age the client is.

■ Promote an older adult's control over decisions as much as possible by including them in discussions.

■ Avoid the "invisible client syndrome." Talking with someone else in the room as if the client is not there is disrespectful.

■ Never treat older adults as if they are children or are uneducated. Avoid using terms that are demeaning or that connote childlike or

infantile behavior (e.g., referring to incontinence products as "diapers").

■ In the event that it is difficult for an older adult to read the name tag or recall the nurse's name from a previous introduction, the client may appreciate if the nurse identifies themself by name and title before each interaction or posts this on a dry erase board in the room.

■ For older clients with diminished hearing, it may be helpful to reduce noise in the immediate environment. Identify which ear has the best hearing and take a position on that side. Speak at a normal volume without distorting words.

■ Maintain a face-to-face position and avoid covering your mouth.

■ Encourage reminiscing. Ask about past events and relationships associated with positive experiences and feelings. Giving older adults an opportunity to talk about earlier times in their lives reinforces their value and unique identity and promotes recall of situations in which they have demonstrated coping or adaptation.

■ Older adults may have difficulty perceiving nonverbal forms of communication due to visual impairments.

■ Avoid standing in front of bright lights when communicating with older adults because the glare may interfere with their ability to perceive what the nurse is communicating.

■ Although physical touch is an important form of nonverbal communication, use it purposefully as a primary method to reinforce verbal messages.

■ Recognize that touch as a form of communication is usually more important to older adults than to those who are younger.

■ Gender and age differences and cultural norms of the client and care provider may influence the acceptability of touch. Appropriate use of touch, as with eye contact, requires cultural competence.

NURSING ROLES WITHIN THE NURSE–CLIENT RELATIONSHIP

A **relationship** (an association between two or more people that develops over time) is established between the nurse and the client when nursing services are provided. Nurses provide services or skills that assist people (in this relationship, called clients or patients) in promoting or restoring health, coping with disorders that will not improve, and dying with dignity.

The nurse–client relationship requires the nurse to respond to the client's needs. The National Council of State Boards of Nursing, which develops the National Council Examination-Practical Nurse (NCLEX-PN), designates four categories of client needs as the structure for the test plan: (1) safe and effective care environment, (2) health promotion and maintenance, (3) psychosocial integrity, and (4) physiologic integrity. These four categories apply to all areas of nursing practice regardless of the stage in the client's life or the setting for health care delivery. To meet these client needs, nurses perform four basic roles: caregiver, educator, collaborator, and delegator.

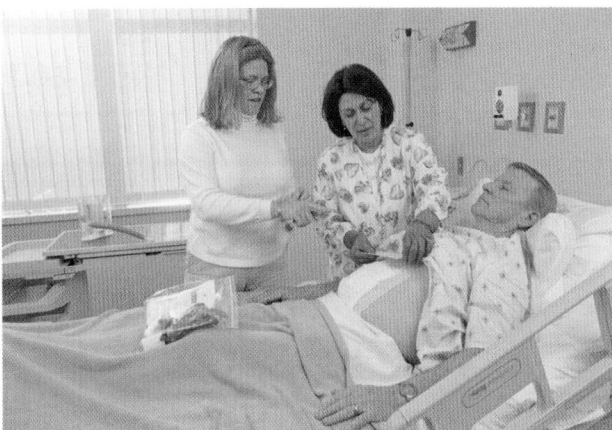

FIGURE 7-1 The nurse cares for a client's wound as the client's caregiver watches.

The Nurse as Caregiver

A **caregiver** is a person who performs health-related activities that a sick person cannot perform independently (Fig. 7-1). Caregivers provide physical and emotional services to restore or maintain functional independence. Table 7-1 highlights the many differences between the services that nurses provide and those that other caring people provide.

Although the traditional nursing role is associated with physical care, it also involves developing close emotional relationships. The contemporary caregiving role incorporates an understanding that illness and injury cause feelings of insecurity that may threaten a person's ability to cope. Nurses use **empathy** (an intuitive awareness of what a client is experiencing) to perceive the client's emotional state and need for support (Fig. 7-2). Empathy helps nurses become effective at providing for the client's needs while remaining compassionately detached.

TABLE 7-1 Differentiating Caring Acts from Nursing Acts

CARING ACTS	NURSING ACTS
Prompted by observing a person in distress	Prompted by a concern for the well-being of everyone
Motivated by sympathy	Motivated by altruism
Spontaneous	Planned
Goal is to relieve crisis	Goal is to promote self-reliance
Outcomes are short-term	Outcomes are long-term
Assume major responsibility for resolving the person's problem	Expect mutual cooperation in resolving health problems
Experience-based	Knowledge-based
Modeled on a personal moral code	Modeled on a formal code of ethics
Guided by common sense	Legally defined
Accountability based on acting reasonably prudent	Accountability based on meeting professional standards

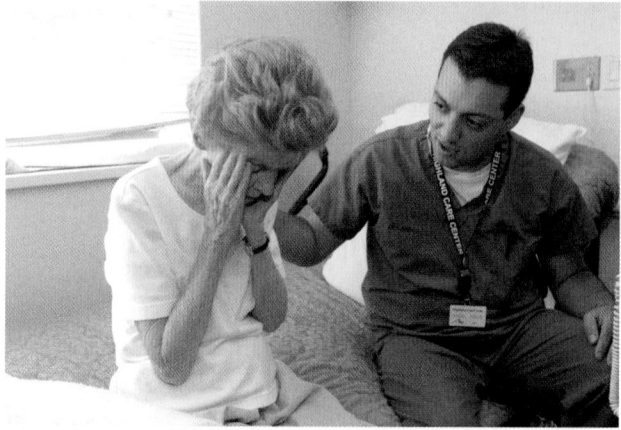

FIGURE 7-2 The nurse demonstrates empathy with a distraught client.

The Nurse as Educator

Being an **educator** (one who provides instruction) is a necessity in today's complex health care arena. Nurses provide health teaching pertinent to each client's needs and knowledge base (see Chapter 8). Some examples include explanations about diagnostic test procedures, self-administration of medications after discharge, techniques for managing wound care, restorative exercises like those performed after a mastectomy, and preventive measures to avoid complications (Fig. 7-3).

When it comes to treatment decisions, the nurse avoids giving advice, reserving the right of each person to make their own choices on matters affecting health and illness care. The nurse shares information on potential alternatives, promotes the client's freedom to choose, and supports the client's ultimate decision.

Nursing is considered a practice "without walls" because it extends beyond the original treatment facility. Consequently, nurses are resources for information about health services available in the community. This type of information empowers clients to become involved with self-help groups or those that offer rehabilitation, financial assistance, or emotional support.

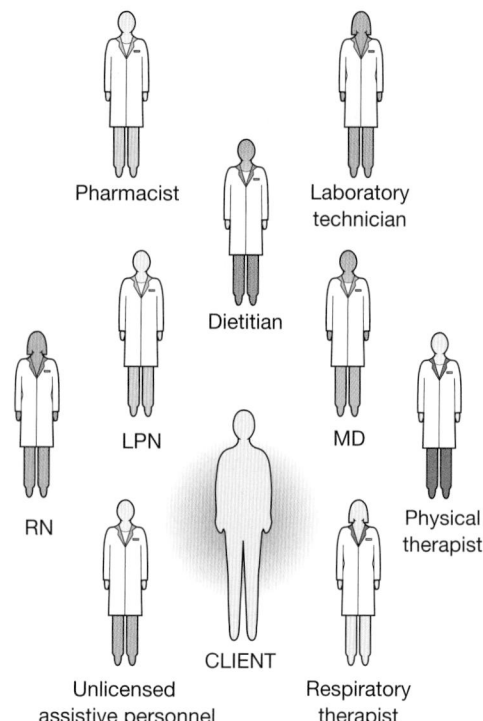

FIGURE 7-4 Collaboration may involve many members of the health care team. LPN, licensed practical nurses, MD, Medical Doctor; RN, registered nurse

The Nurse as Collaborator

The nurse also acts as a **collaborator** (one who works with others to achieve a common goal) (Fig. 7-4). The most obvious example of collaboration occurs between the nurse responsible for managing care and those to whom they delegate care (Fig. 7-5). Collaboration also occurs when the nurse and the physician share information and exchange findings with other health care providers.

>>> *Stop, Think, and Respond 7-1*
With whom would the nurse collaborate when caring for an older adult with a fractured hip?

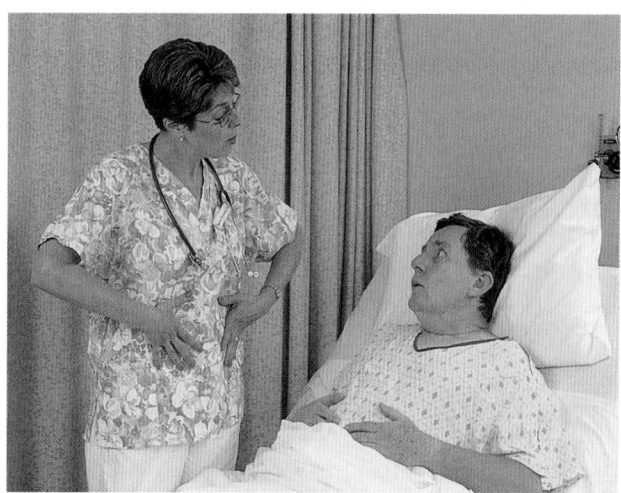

FIGURE 7-3 The nurse demonstrates breathing exercises when teaching a preoperative client.

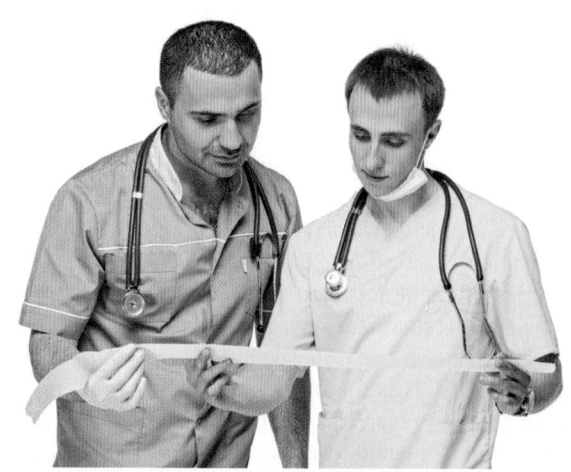

FIGURE 7-5 Two critical care nurses collaborate concerning current data during client care.

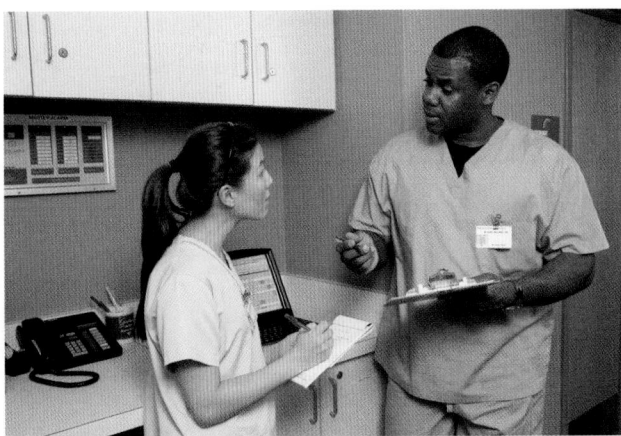

FIGURE 7-6 A nurse delegates tasks to a coworker.

The Nurse as Delegator

Before the nurse performs the role of **delegator** (one who assigns a task to someone), they must know what tasks are legal and appropriate for particular health care providers to perform (Fig. 7-6). A nurse may potentially be sued when delegating a task to someone who does not have the knowledge or expertise to perform it correctly. Once a task is assigned, it is still the delegator's responsibility to check that the task has been completed and determine the resulting outcome. For example, if a nurse asks a nursing assistant to change a client's position, the nurse verifies that the assistant carried out the nurse's request and obtains additional pertinent information such as the condition of the client's skin. If the delegated task is not performed or is performed incorrectly, the nurse is accountable for the inadequate care.

»» *Stop, Think, and Respond 7-2*

Before delegating the task of taking a client's vital signs (temperature, pulse, respiratory rate, and blood pressure) to a student nurse, how might the nurse determine whether the task is appropriate for the student? If appropriate, how might the nurse then confirm that it has been performed?

THE THERAPEUTIC NURSE–CLIENT RELATIONSHIP

The nurse–client relationship can be called a **therapeutic relationship** because the desired outcome of the association is almost always moving toward improving health. A therapeutic relationship differs from a social relationship. A therapeutic relationship is client-centered, with a focus on goal achievement. It is also time-limited; the relationship ends when goals are achieved.

The relationship between nurses and clients has changed. In the past, the role of a sick person was passive; others made decisions and the client was submitted to treatments without question or protest by the client or their family. Nurses now encourage and expect people for whom they care to become actively involved, communicate, question, assist in planning their care, and retain as much independence as possible (Box 7-1).

BOX 7-1	Responsibilities within the Nurse–Client Relationship

Nursing Responsibilities
- Possess current knowledge.
- Be aware of unique age-related differences.
- Perform technical skills safely.
- Be committed to client care.
- Be available and courteous.
- Facilitate participation of client and family in decisions.
- Remain objective.
- Advocate on the client's behalf.
- Provide explanations in easily understood language.
- Promote the client's independence.

Client Responsibilities
- Identify the current problem.
- Describe desired outcomes.
- Answer questions honestly.
- Provide accurate historical and subjective data.
- Participate to the fullest extent possible.
- Be open and flexible to alternatives.
- Adhere to the plan for care.
- Keep appointments for follow-up care.

Underlying Principles

A therapeutic nurse–client relationship is more likely to develop when the nurse treats each client as a unique person and respects the client's feelings. The nurse strives to promote the client's physical, emotional, social, and spiritual well-being and encourages the client to participate in problem-solving and decision-making. The nurse believes that a client has the potential for growth and change and communicates using terms and language the client understands. The nurse uses the nursing process to individualize the client's care; involves people to whom the client turns for support, such as family and friends, when providing care; and implements health care techniques compatible with the client's value system and culture.

Phases of the Nurse–Client Relationship

Nurse–client relationships are ordinarily brief. They begin when a person seeks services that will maintain or restore health or prevent disease. They end when the client can achieve their health-related goals independently. This type of relationship is generally described as having three phases: introductory, working, and terminating.

Introductory Phase

The relationship between client and nurse begins with the **introductory phase** (the period of getting acquainted). Each person usually brings preconceived ideas about the other to the initial interaction. These assumptions are eventually confirmed or dismissed.

Many experts agree that most people form their initial opinions within just a few seconds of meeting. Some techniques for facilitating a positive first impression include:

- Dressing appropriately
- Being well-groomed
- Smiling

- Making eye contact
- Greeting with a handshake
- Projecting confidence
- Avoiding offensive personal odors, such as the smell of cigarette smoke or strong scents of perfume or cologne

After the initial formalities, the client initiates the relationship by identifying one or more health problems for which they are seeking help. It is important for the nurse to demonstrate courtesy, active listening, empathy, competency, and appropriate communication skills to ensure that the relationship begins on a positive note.

Working Phase

The **working phase** (period during which tasks are performed) involves mutually planning the client's care and implementing the plan. Both the nurse and the client participate. Each shares in performing those tasks that lead to the desired outcomes mutually identified by the client and the nurse. During the working phase, the nurse tries to avoid impeding the client's independence; doing too much for the client can be as harmful as doing too little.

Terminating Phase

The nurse–client relationship is self-limiting. The **terminating phase** (the period when the relationship comes to an end) occurs when the nurse and client agree that the client's immediate health problems have improved. A caring attitude and compassion help facilitate the client's transition of care to other health care services or to independent living.

Barriers to a Therapeutic Relationship

The nurse likely will not develop a positive relationship with every client. Box 7-2 lists examples of behaviors that are

---

BOX 7-2 Barriers to a Nurse–Client Relationship

- Appearing unkempt: long hair that dangles on or over the client during care, offensive body or breath odor, wrinkled or soiled uniform, dirty shoes
- Failing to identify oneself verbally and with a name tag
- Mispronouncing or avoiding the client's name
- Using the client's first name without permission
- Showing disinterest in the client's personal history and life experiences
- Sharing personal or work-related problems with the client or with staff in the client's presence
- Using crude language or language the client may find distasteful
- Revealing confidential information or gossip about other clients, staff, or people commonly known
- Focusing on nursing tasks rather than the client's responses
- Being inattentive to the client's requests (e.g., food, pain relief, assistance with toileting, bathing)
- Abandoning the client at stressful or emotional times
- Failing to keep promises such as consulting with the physician about a current need or request
- Going on a break or to lunch without keeping the client informed and identifying who has been delegated for the client's care during the temporary absence

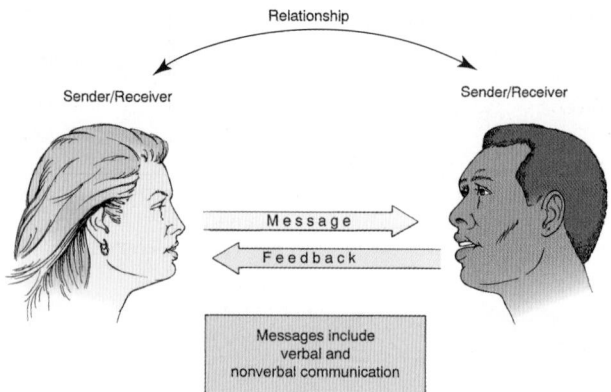

FIGURE 7-7 Communication is a two-way process between a sender and a receiver.

likely to interfere with developing a therapeutic relationship. The best approach is to treat all clients with the same level of respect.

COMMUNICATION

Communication (an exchange of information) involves both sending and receiving messages between two or more people followed by feedback indicating that the information was understood or requires further clarification (Fig. 7-7). Communication takes place simultaneously on verbal and nonverbal levels with the nonverbal level representing the stronger component in any interaction. Because no relationship can exist without both verbal and nonverbal communication, nurses develop skills that enhance their therapeutic interactions with clients.

Verbal Communication

Verbal communication (communication that uses words) includes speaking, reading, and writing. Both the nurse and the client use verbal communication to gather facts. They also use it to instruct, clarify, and exchange ideas.

Many factors affect the ability to communicate by speech or in writing. Examples include (1) attention and concentration; (2) language compatibility; (3) verbal skills; (4) hearing and visual acuity; (5) motor functions involving the throat, tongue, and teeth; (6) sensory distractions; (7) interpersonal attitudes; (8) literacy; and (9) cultural similarities. The nurse promotes the factors that enhance the communication of verbal content and controls or eliminates those that interfere with the accurate perception of expressed ideas.

Therapeutic Verbal Communication

Communication can take place on a social or therapeutic level. Social communication involves the ability to use language in social contexts, such as greeting someone, or requesting information. **Therapeutic verbal communication** (using words and gestures to accomplish a particular objective) is extremely important, especially when the nurse is exploring problems with the client or encouraging expression of feelings. Techniques that the nurse may find helpful are described in Table 7-2.

TABLE 7-2 Therapeutic Verbal Communication Techniques

TECHNIQUE	USE	EXAMPLE
Broad opening	Relieves tension before getting to the purpose of the interaction	"We are having some wonderful weather."
Giving information	Provides facts	"Your surgery is scheduled at noon."
Direct questioning	Acquires specific information	"Do you have any allergies?"
Open-ended questioning	Encourages the client to elaborate	"How are you feeling?"
Reflecting	Confirms that the nurse is following the conversation	Client: "I haven't been sleeping well." Nurse: "You haven't been sleeping well."
Paraphrasing	Restates what the client has said to demonstrate listening	Client: "After every meal, I feel like I will throw up." Nurse: "Eating makes you nauseous, but you don't actually vomit."
Verbalizing what has been implied	Shares how the nurse has interpreted a statement	Client: "All the nurses are so busy." Nurse: "You're feeling that you shouldn't ask for help."
Structuring	Defines a purpose and sets limits	"I can speak with you now. If your pain is relieved, we can discuss when your procedure will begin."
Giving general leads	Encourages the client to continue	"Tell me more," or "Go on."
Sharing perceptions	Shows empathy for the client's feelings	"You seem depressed."
Clarifying	Avoids misinterpretation	"Is this what you're saying?"
Confronting	Calls attention to manipulation, inconsistencies, or lack of responsibility	"You're concerned about your weight loss, but you didn't eat any breakfast."
Summarizing	Reviews information that has been discussed	"You've asked me to check on increasing your pain medication and getting your diet changed."
Silence	Allows time for considering how to proceed or arouses the client's anxiety to the point that it stimulates more verbalization	

The nurse must never assume that a quiet, uncommunicative client is problem-free or understands everything. However, it is never appropriate to probe and pry; rather, it may be advantageous to wait and be patient. It is not unusual for reticent clients to share their feelings and concerns after they conclude that the nurse is sincere and trustworthy.

Nurses must approach vocal and/or emotional clients delicately. For instance, when clients are angry or crying, the best nursing response is to remain nonjudgmental, allow the client to express emotions, and return later with a follow-up regarding legitimate complaints. Allowing clients to display their feelings without fear of retaliation or censure contributes to a therapeutic relationship.

Although nurses often have the best intentions of interacting therapeutically with clients, some techniques block or hinder verbal communication. Table 7-3 lists common examples of nontherapeutic communication techniques.

TABLE 7-3 Nontherapeutic Verbal Communication Techniques

TECHNIQUE AND CONSEQUENCE	EXAMPLE	IMPROVEMENT
Giving False Reassurance Trivializes the client's unique feelings and discourages further discussion	"You've got nothing to worry about. Everything will work out fine."	"Tell me your specific concerns."
Using Clichés Provides generalized, often unhelpful advice and curtails exploring alternatives	"Keep a stiff upper lip."	"It must be difficult for you right now."
Giving Approval or Disapproval Holds the client to a rigid standard; implies that future deviation may lead to subsequent rejection or disfavor	"I'm glad you're exercising so regularly." "You should be testing your blood glucose each morning."	"Are you having any difficulty fitting regular exercise into your schedule?" "Let's explore some ways that will help you remember to test your blood glucose each morning."
Agreeing Does not allow the client flexibility to change their mind	"You're right about needing surgery immediately."	"Having surgery immediately is one possibility. What others have you considered?"

(continued)

TABLE 7-3 Nontherapeutic Verbal Communication Techniques (*continued*)

TECHNIQUE AND CONSEQUENCE	EXAMPLE	IMPROVEMENT
Disagreeing		
Intimidates the client; may make them feel foolish or inadequate	"That's not true! Where did you get that idea?"	"Maybe I can help clarify that for you."
Demanding an Explanation		
Puts the client on the defensive; they may be tempted to make up an excuse rather than risk disapproval for an honest answer	"Why didn't you keep your appointment last week?"	"I see you could not keep your appointment last week."
Giving Advice		
Discourages independent problem-solving and decision-making; provides a biased view that may prejudice the client's choice	"If I were you, I'd try drug therapy before having surgery."	"Share with me the advantages and disadvantages of your options as you see them."
Defending		
Indicates such a strong allegiance that any disagreement is unacceptable	"Ms Johnson is my best nursing assistant. She would not have let your light go unanswered that long."	"I'm sorry you had to wait so long."
Belittling		
Disregards how the client is responding as an individual	"Lots of people learn to give themselves insulin."	"You're finding it difficult to inject yourself with a needle."
Patronizing		
Treats the client condescendingly, as if they are not capable of making an independent decision	"Are we ready for our bath yet?"	"Would you like your bath now, or should I check with you later?"
Changing the Subject		
Alters the direction of the discussion to a topic less likely to cause discomfort	Client: "I'm so scared that a mammogram will show I have cancer." Nurse: "Tell me more about your family."	Client: "I'm so scared that a mammogram will show I have cancer." Nurse: "It is a serious disease. What concerns you the most?"

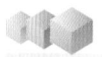 Concept Mastery Alert

Therapeutic and Nontherapeutic Communication

Communication in the nurse–client relationship is classified as either therapeutic or nontherapeutic. Therapeutic communication is interpersonal and purposeful, geared to achieve a specific goal.

Listening

Listening is as important during communication as speaking. In contrast with hearing, which involves perceiving sounds, **active listening** is an activity that includes attending to and becoming fully involved in what the client says. To facilitate active listening, other issues in one's personal agenda must be temporarily blocked in order to focus on the content of the present interaction.

Giving attention to what clients say provides a stimulus for meaningful interaction. It is important to avoid behaviors that indicate boredom, impatience, or the pretense of listening. For example, looking out a window or interrupting is a sign of disinterest. When communicating with most clients, it is best to position oneself at the client's level and make frequent eye contact (Fig. 7-8). Refer to Chapter 6

for cultural considerations in communication. Nodding and making comments, such as "Yes, I see," encourages clients to continue and shows full involvement in what is being said.

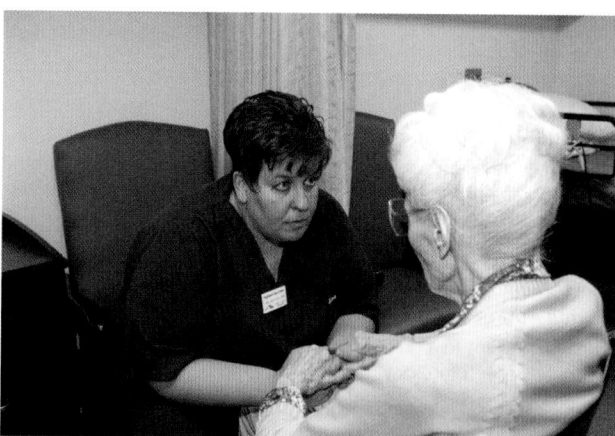

FIGURE 7-8 The nurse takes a position on the same level as the client when demonstrating concern for the client's emotional situation. (From Carter, P. J. [2019]. *Lippincott's textbook for long-term care nursing assistants.* Lippincott Williams & Wilkins.)

Silence

Silence (intentionally withholding verbal commentary) plays an important role in communication. It may seem contradictory to include silence as a form of verbal communication. Nevertheless, one of its uses is to encourage the client to participate in verbal discussions. Other therapeutic uses for silence include relieving a client's anxiety by providing a personal presence and offering a brief period during which the client can process information or respond to questions.

Clients may use silence to camouflage fears or to express contentment. They also use silence for introspection when they need to explore feelings or pray. Interrupting someone deep in concentration disturbs their thought process. A common obstacle to effective communication is ignoring the importance of silence and talking excessively.

Nonverbal Communication

Nonverbal communication (an exchange of information without using spoken or written words) involves what is not said. The manner in which a person conveys verbal information affects its meaning. Research suggests that 55% of what is communicated comes from body language, 38% from the tone of voice, and only 7% from spoken words (The University of Texas Permian Basin, 2022).

A person has less control over nonverbal than verbal communication. Words can be chosen with care, but facial expression and other forms of body language are harder to control. As a result, people often communicate messages more accurately through nonverbal communication. People communicate nonverbally through the following techniques: kinesics, paralanguage, proxemics, and touch.

Kinesics

Kinesics (body language) includes nonverbal techniques such as facial expressions, posture, gestures, and body movements. Clothing style and accessories such as jewelry may also affect the context of communication. Table 7-4 describes various examples of nonverbal behaviors and their meanings.

Knowledge of kinesics is important for the nurse being evaluated by their clients and vice versa. To create a positive impression during a client interaction, the nurse should:

- Assume a position at eye level with the client; stand or sit tall.
- Relax arms, legs, and feet; do not cross any body part.
- Maintain eye contact approximately 60% to 70% of the time or whatever is appropriate in consideration of the client's culture (see Chapter 6); in a group, focus on the last person who spoke.
- Keep the head level, both horizontally and vertically.
- Lean forward to demonstrate interest and attention.
- Keep the arms where they can be seen.
- Strike a balance in arm movements—neither too demonstrative nor reserved.
- Keep the legs as still as possible.

Paralanguage

Paralanguage (vocal sounds that are not actually words) also communicates a message. Some examples include facial expressions and gestures. Vocal inflections, volume, pitch, and rate of speech add another dimension to communication. Crying, laughing, and moaning are additional forms of paralanguage.

Proxemics

Proxemics (the use and relationship of space to communication) varies among people from different cultural backgrounds. Anthropologist Edward T. Hall (1914 to 2009) was the first to identify four zones of communication among Americans. The four zones that have remained the standard include **intimate space** (within 6 in), **personal space** (6 in to 4 ft), **social space** (4 to 12 ft), and **public space** (more than 12 ft; Fig. 7-9).

Most people in and from Western countries comfortably tolerate strangers in a 2- to 3-ft area. Venturing closer may cause some to feel anxious. Understanding the client's comfort zone helps the nurse know how spatial relations affect nonverbal communication. Closeness is common

---

TABLE 7-4 Examples of Body Language

POSITIVE	INTERPRETATION	NEGATIVE	INTERPRETATION
Tilt of head	Interested	Arms crossed	Blocking; oppositional
Open hands	Sincere	Clenched jaw	Angry; antagonistic
Brisk, erect walk	Confident	Downcast eyes	Remorseful; bored
Hand to cheek	Contemplative	Rubbing nose	Doubtful; deceitful
Rubbing hands	Anticipatory	Drumming fingers	Impatient
Steepled fingers	Authoritative	Fondling hair	Insecure
Nod	Agreement	Frown	Disagreement
		Stroking chin	Stalling for time
		Shifting from foot to foot	Desire to get away
		Looking at watch	Bored

healthline. *A beginner's guide to reading body language.* (2020). https://www.healthline.com/health/body-language#eyes

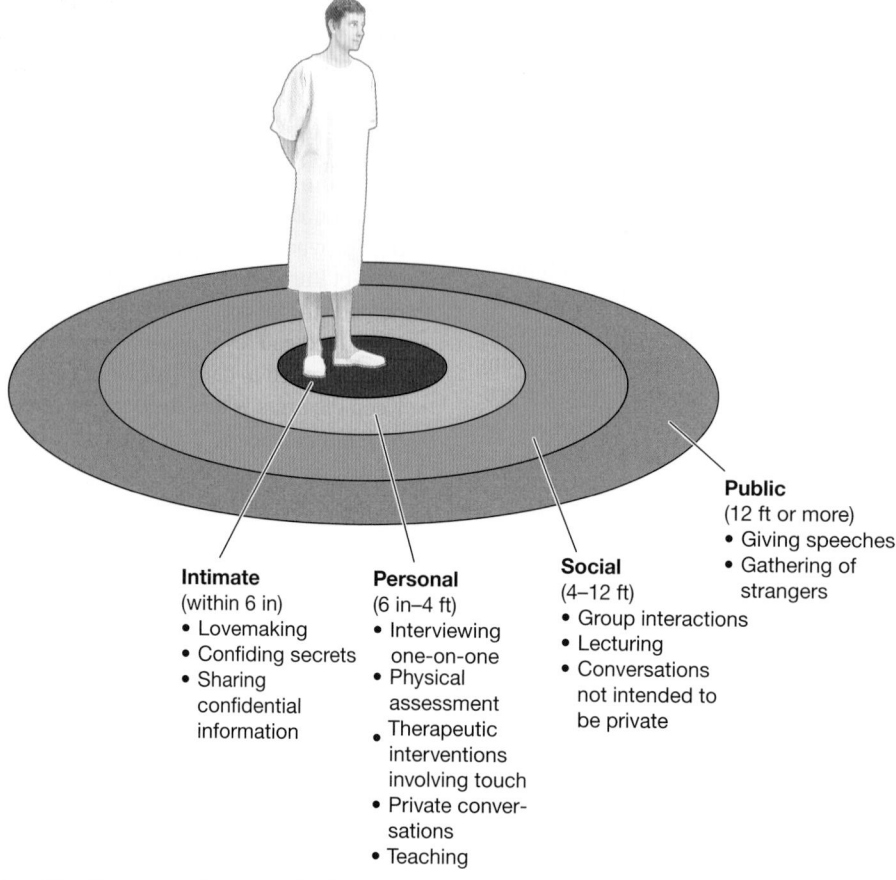

FIGURE 7-9 Activities within the zones of communication.

Intimate
(within 6 in)
• Lovemaking
• Confiding secrets
• Sharing
confidential
information

Personal
(6 in–4 ft)
• Interviewing
one-on-one
• Physical
assessment
• Therapeutic
interventions
involving touch
• Private conver-
sations
• Teaching

Social
(4–12 ft)
• Group interactions
• Lecturing
• Conversations
not intended to
be private

Public
(12 ft or more)
• Giving speeches
• Gathering of
strangers

in nursing because nurses and clients are often in direct physical contact within the client's intimate and personal spaces.

Touch

Touch (a tactile stimulus produced by making personal contact with another person or object) occurs frequently in nurse–client relationships. While caring for clients, touch can be task-oriented, affective, or both. **Task-oriented touch** involves the personal contact required when performing

nursing procedures (Fig. 7-10). **Affective touch** is used to demonstrate concern or affection (Fig. 7-11).

Affective touch has different meanings to different people depending on how they were raised and their culture. Because nursing care involves a high degree of touching, the nurse is sensitive to how clients may perceive it. Some people respond positively to touch, but some may prefer not to be touched. Therefore, nurses use affective touch cautiously even though its intention is to communicate caring and support. In general, affective touch is therapeutic when a client is:

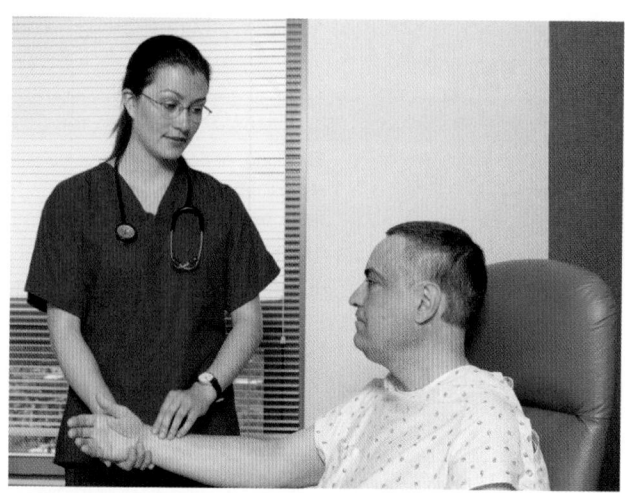

FIGURE 7-10 Examining a client involves task-oriented touch. (Photo by B. Proud.)

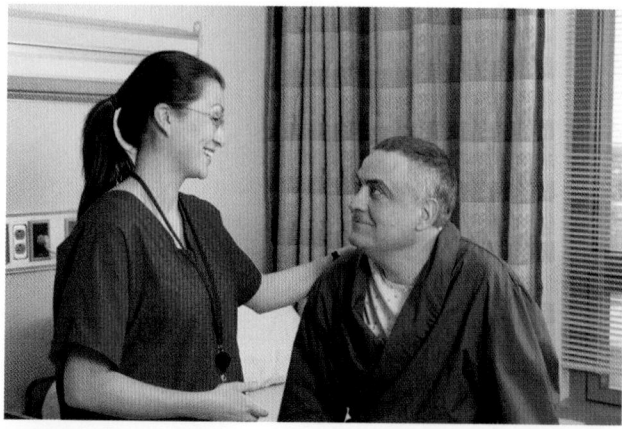

FIGURE 7-11 This nurse uses affective touch while talking with a client. (Photo by B. Proud.)

- Lonely
- Uncomfortable
- Near death
- Anxious, insecure, or frightened
- Disoriented
- Disfigured
- Semiconscious or comatose
- Visually impaired
- Sensory-deprived

Some clients can misinterpret physical nearness and touching in personal and intimate zones as having sexual connotations. Approaches that may prevent such misunderstanding include explaining beforehand how a nursing procedure will be performed, ensuring that a client is properly draped or covered, and asking that another staff person of the client's gender be present during a potentially sensitive examination or procedure.

Communicating with Members of Special Populations

The nurse will encounter clients who have challenges in communicating. These may include people who are verbally impaired, Deaf people, or people who have cognitive impairments due to conditions such as Alzheimer disease. Nurses and other health care providers must find ways to effectively communicate with these clients about their health problems and needs, so they can give informed consent, and so they understand health practices that will have an impact on their recovery or health maintenance. All clients have a right to quality care, and health care regulating agencies are adamant that health care providers facilitate communication in order to provide that care.

Communicating with Clients Who Are Verbally Impaired

There are instances when nurses and clients cannot communicate verbally despite the fact that both are proficient in English. For example, clients who have had a stroke sometimes experience **expressive aphasia**, an inability to use verbal language skills. Clients who have artificial airways (e.g., an endotracheal or tracheostomy tube) or who have their jaws wired following facial trauma cannot speak. Communication is a nursing priority as mandated by The Joint Commission's National Patient Safety Goals (see Chapter 19); therefore, the nurse must take steps to facilitate communication with these clients. The nurse may provide the verbally impaired client with a paper tablet and pencil or "magic slate," though this approach can be time-consuming. In some cases, the client may not have the use of their hands or the fine motor skills necessary to use a writing device. Other communication tools such as those discussed in Chapter 6 or visual communication boards may be used to communicate with verbally impaired clients; they may point to common phrases, spell with the alphabet, and identify relevant numbers. In addition, smart phones and other tablets can help clients with communication, allowing them to keep in touch with family and friends via email and texting. Text-to-speech features are also available on smart phones and can assist clients with reading comprehension. Word prediction software can facilitate writing, while some apps let users click on a picture or word to hear an audio description or pronunciation. Clients can also use mapping apps for audio navigation (American Stroke Association, 2024; Fig. 7-12).

Communicating with Deaf Clients

A **Deaf** person is unable to hear well enough to process spoken information, while a person who is **hard of hearing** has impaired hearing but is still able to perceive what is being said verbally when spoken at a louder level. If a Deaf client can read and write, writing can facilitate communication. However, written communication may not be useful for all clients. Many Deaf clients, especially those who were born Deaf or lost their hearing at an early age, have learned to lip read and use **American Sign Language (ASL)**, which uses signs made by hand movements and finger spelling, an alphabetical substitute for words that have no sign (Fig. 7-13). However, not all health care agencies have someone available who is proficient in ASL. Some hospitals therefore use a webcam. The webcam facilitates video interpreting, in which a person skilled in ASL communicates with the Deaf client in the presence of the nurse.

Communicating with Clients with Alzheimer Disease

Alzheimer disease is a progressive, deteriorating brain disorder. Its onset is insidious, with symptoms that may develop slowly over years. Memory loss is the classic symptom. Other symptoms include disturbances in behavior; diminished ability to care for oneself; and, eventually, compromised communication skills. Problems with speaking, reading, and writing affect communication. Clients with this disease have difficulty expressing themselves verbally, such as finding correct words, organizing words into logical sentences, finishing sentences, and understanding words. Eventually, they may become mute.

Techniques that may facilitate communicating with a client who has Alzheimer disease include the following:

- Gain the client's attention by approaching from the front and using the client's name.
- Smile to convey friendliness.
- Maintain eye contact to evaluate the client's attention and comprehension.
- Assume a relaxed posture to avoid agitating the client.
- Speak naturally at a normal rate and volume; avoid long sentences and difficult words.
- Wait for a response while the client processes the information.
- Rephrase information if the client does not seem to understand what has been said.
- Show patience when the client tries to put thoughts into words.
- Use visual cues like gestures that may clarify verbal meanings.
- Avoid correcting or arguing with the client.

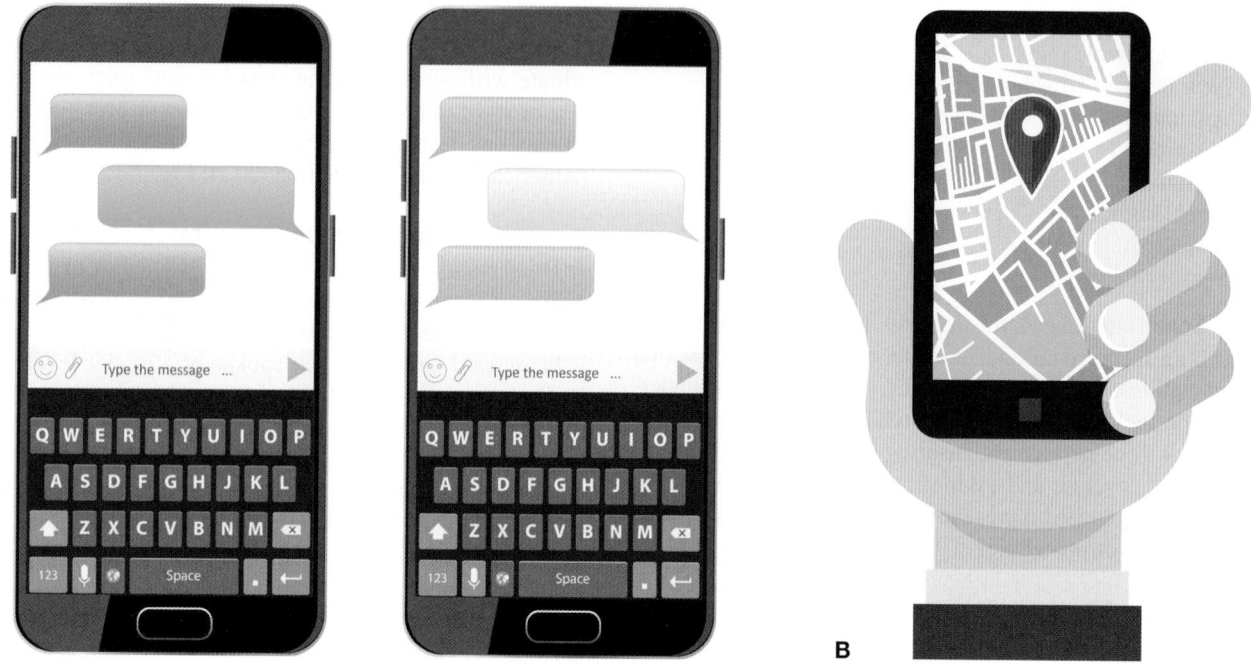

FIGURE 7-12 **A.** Smart phone with texting (Nice Vector Wow/Shutterstock). **B.** Smart phone with map application (Pretty Vectors/Shutterstock).

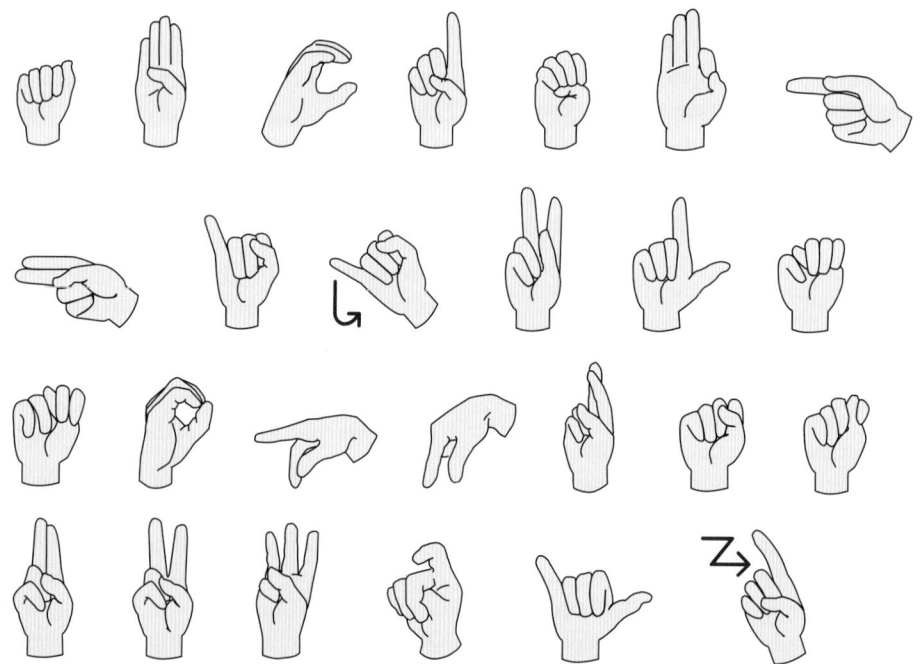

FIGURE 7-13 The alphabet in sign language.

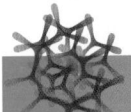

KEY POINTS

- Roles of the nurse in communication:
  - Caregiver: One who performs health-related activities that a sick person cannot perform independently
  - Educator: One who provides instruction
  - Collaborator: One who works with others to achieve a common goal
  - Delegator: One who assigns a task to someone
- Types of communication:
  - Verbal communication: Uses words; includes speaking, reading, and writing
  - Therapeutic verbal communication: Uses words and gestures to accomplish a particular objective, for example, exploring problems and expressing feelings
  - Active listening: Attending to and becoming fully involved in what the client says
  - Silence: Intentionally withholding verbal commentary; can relieve a client's anxiety with a personal presence and offer a brief period during which the client can process information or respond to questions
- Nonverbal communication: An exchange of information without using spoken or written words
- Kinesics: Body language
- Paralanguage: Vocal sounds that are not actually words
- Proxemics: The use and relationship of space to communication; personal space versus public space
- Touch: A tactile stimulus produced by making personal contact with another person or object
- Nontherapeutic verbal communication: Review Table 7-3 for examples and improvements in communication skills
- Communication with members of special populations requires alternate types and methods of communication skills.

CRITICAL THINKING EXERCISES

1. What specific services might a person expect within a nurse–client relationship that differ from those within a physician–client relationship?
2. Studies have shown that older adults are not touched with the same frequency as clients in other age groups. Discuss possible reasons for this.
3. What are possible explanations when a client does not respond as expected during nurse–client interactions?
4. How might a nurse relieve anxiety experienced by a client who requires health care in an emergency situation?

NEXT-GENERATION NCLEX-STYLE REVIEW QUESTIONS

1. A discouraged client says, "I'm sure this surgery won't help any more than the others." What is the best initial nursing response?
   a. "You're saying that you doubt you will improve."
   b. "Do you want to talk to the surgeon again?"
   c. "I'd recommend a more positive attitude."
   d. "Of course it will, you'll be up and around in no time."
   Test-Taking Strategy: Note the key words and modifier, "best initial response." Select the statement that should occur first and eliminate options that should be avoided or postponed until later.

2. When a terminally ill client does not respond to medical treatment, which nursing action is most helpful in assisting the client in dealing with their impending death?
   a. Providing literature on death and dying
   b. Allowing the client privacy to think alone
   c. Listening to the client talk about their feelings
   d. Encouraging the client to get a second opinion
   Test-Taking Strategy: Note the key word and modifier, "most helpful." Select the option that promotes nurse–client communication by eliminating options that hamper or avoid dealing with the client's emotionally charged situation.

3. An alarm caused by a loose cardiac monitor lead startles a client with chest pain. In order of priority, list the nursing interventions.
   a. Reassure the client regarding their health.
   b. Identify the client's current heart rhythm.
   c. Explain the reason the alarm sounded.
   d. Review with the client the need for the monitor.
   Test-Taking Strategy: All of the answers are correct, so list them in order of nursing priority. Think about what would help alleviate the client's medical concerns first, and then prioritize the answers.

4. A 2-year-old child has a high fever of unknown origin. Which task is appropriate for the nurse to delegate to a nursing assistant?
   a. Administer an aspirin suppository to reduce the child's fever.

b. Give the toddler a popsicle or other fluid every 30 minutes.
c. Call the laboratory for the results of diagnostic tests.
d. Listen to the child's lungs for sounds of congestion.

Test-Taking Strategy: Select an option that is compatible with a task that an unlicensed caregiver can perform. Eliminate tasks that correlate with those that a licensed nurse can perform.

5. What is the best nursing response when an 82-year-old client with Alzheimer disease says they are looking forward to a visit from their mother later today?
a. "Your mother has been deceased for years."
b. "Tell me more about your mother."
c. "Let me call and check on your mother."
d. "When did you last see your mother?"

Test-Taking Strategy: Note the key word, "best." Select an option that restores reality for the client. Eliminate options that may be emotionally upsetting or cognitively unrealistic, or that sustain the client's false expectation.

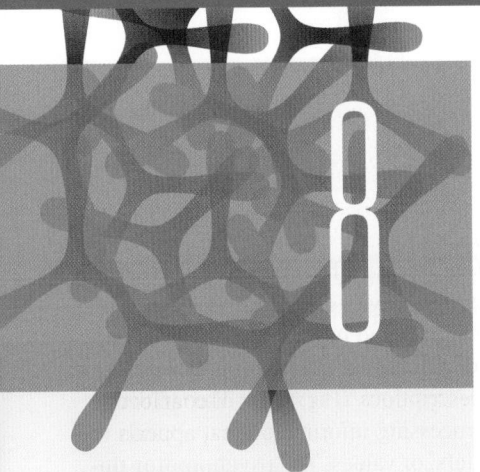

Client Teaching

Words To Know

adapting
affective domain
analyzing
andragogy
applying
capacity to learn
characterization
cognitive domain
creating
developmental level
discharge instructions
evaluating
formal teaching
functional illiteracy
geragogy
health literacy
illiterate
imitating
informal teaching
learning need
learning readiness
learning style
literacy
motivation
observing
organization
pedagogy
practicing
psychomotor domain
receiving
remembering
responding
teach-back method
telehomecare
understanding
valuing

Learning Objectives

On completion of this chapter, the reader should be able to:

1. Identify the authoritative bases that mandate client teaching.
2. List examples of client teaching provided by nurses.
3. List five benefits of client teaching.
4. Identify factors that nurses assess before teaching clients.
5. Describe the three domains of learning.
6. Discuss age-related categories of learners.
7. Discuss characteristics unique to older adult learners.

INTRODUCTION

Teaching is one of the most important uses of communication for nurses. Health teaching promotes the client's independent ability to meet their health needs. An old proverb that reinforces how education promotes self-care says, "Give a man a fish and he will eat for a day; teach a man to fish and he will eat for a lifetime."

Teaching is an essential nursing responsibility when caring for clients in a health care agency, at home, or in community settings. This chapter offers information on principles of teaching and learning.

 Gerontologic Considerations

■ During an assessment, older clients may interact in a socially appropriate manner and may indicate that they understand the material being taught. Asking a client to recall what has been discussed after approximately 15 minutes can help the nurse determine what information has actually been retained. A mental status examination may be indicated (see Chapter 13). If the client is cognitively impaired, a support person or caregiver should be present for the teaching sessions.

■ A calm demeanor and a quiet environment can decrease anxiety or distractions that interfere with learning. Peer teaching or reinforcement in support group settings may be helpful.

■ Many people are "creatures of habit" and are reluctant to make changes, especially without understanding the benefit of a change. Clients are more likely to incorporate changes in health behavior if the teaching session makes the purpose or anticipated benefit clear.

■ Stating a belief that the older adult can make the recommended health behavioral changes and providing encouragement may increase the client's self-confidence and result in increased learning.

■ Begin the teaching session by connecting the new information to the older person's lived experience.

■ When working with older adults, the following teaching strategies are particularly effective: presenting small amounts of information at a time, allowing enough time for the client to process information, expressing confidence in the older adult's ability to change health-related behaviors, and using positive feedback.

IMPORTANCE OF CLIENT TEACHING

Health teaching is a mandated nursing activity. State nurse practice acts require health teaching, and the Joint Commission (2010) has made it a criterion for accreditation. "Patient teaching is part of the LPN's (LVN's) duties—they are entrusted with discussing with the patient's guardians regarding their plan of care" (LPN scope of practice, 2023). Limited hospitalization time demands that nurses begin teaching as soon as possible after admission. Early attention to the client's learning needs is essential because learning takes place in four progressive stages:

1. Recognition of what has been taught
2. Recollection or description of information to others
3. Explanation or application of information
4. Independent use of new learning

SCOPE AND CONSEQUENCES OF CLIENT TEACHING

Client teaching generally focuses on combinations of the following subject areas:

- The plan of care, treatment, and services
- Safe self-administration of medications
- The pain assessment process and methods for pain management
- Directions and practice in using equipment for self-care
- Nutrition and dietary instructions
- Rehabilitation programs
- Available community resources
- Plan for medical follow-ups
- Signs of complications and actions to take

Some of the benefits of client teaching include reduced length of stay, cost-effectiveness of health care, better allocation of resources, increased client satisfaction, and decreased readmission rates.

A delay in teaching in turn delays optimum learning outcomes. If teaching standards are not met and a discharged client is readmitted or harmed because they were uninformed or failed to understand information the nurse taught, the nurse is at risk for being sued.

The best evidence of adherence to teaching standards is to document in the client's medical record the individual taught by the nurse other than the client (e.g., the client's spouse or caregiver); what the nurse taught; the teaching method; and the evidence of learning. Hospitals are asking clients to sign a copy of their **discharge instructions**, the information that is essential for promoting safety during the initial posthospitalization period.

ASSESSING THE LEARNER

To implement effective teaching, the nurse must determine the client's:

- Preferred learning style
- Age and developmental level
- Capacity to learn
- Motivation
- Learning readiness
- Learning needs

Learning Styles

A client's **learning style** refers to how a person prefers to acquire knowledge. Learning styles fall within three general domains: cognitive, affective, and psychomotor. The **cognitive domain** is a style of processing information by listening or reading facts and descriptions (Fig. 8-1). The **affective domain** is a style of processing information that appeals to a person's feelings, beliefs, or values. The **psychomotor domain** is a style of processing information that focuses on learning by doing.

One way to determine the client's preferred learning style is to ask a question such as, "When you learned to add fractions, what helped you most—hearing the teacher's explanation or reading about it in a mathematics book (cognitive domain), recognizing the value of the exercise (affective domain), or actually working out sample problems (psychomotor domain)?" Although most clients favor one domain, nurses can optimize learning by presenting information through a combination of teaching approaches. The bottom line is that learning improves when there is more active involvement.

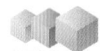 Concept Mastery Alert

Domains of Learning

To help differentiate the different domains of learning, remember the following: for cognitive, think "thinking"; for affective, think "feeling"; for psychomotor, think "doing."

Cognitive Domain

The cognitive domain addresses intellectual skills involved in learning. It is the foundation for learning because the remaining domains are integrated with a cognitive component. There are various levels of intellectual skills within the cognitive domain progressing from the basic level of thinking to the more advanced. Benjamin Bloom and his colleagues identified the cognitive levels in 1956. Although the original

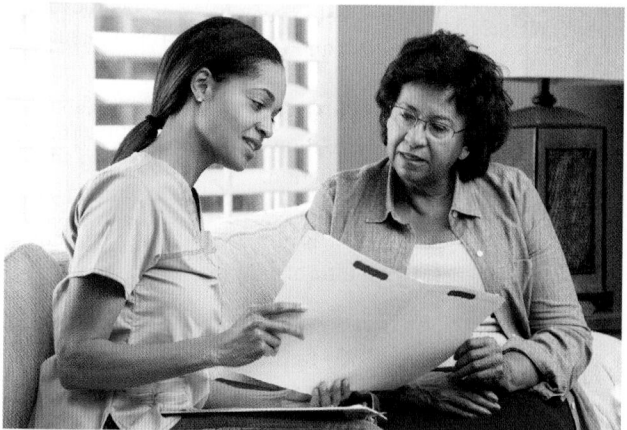

FIGURE 8-1 The nurse reviews medications with a client. (Monkey Business Images/Shutterstock.)

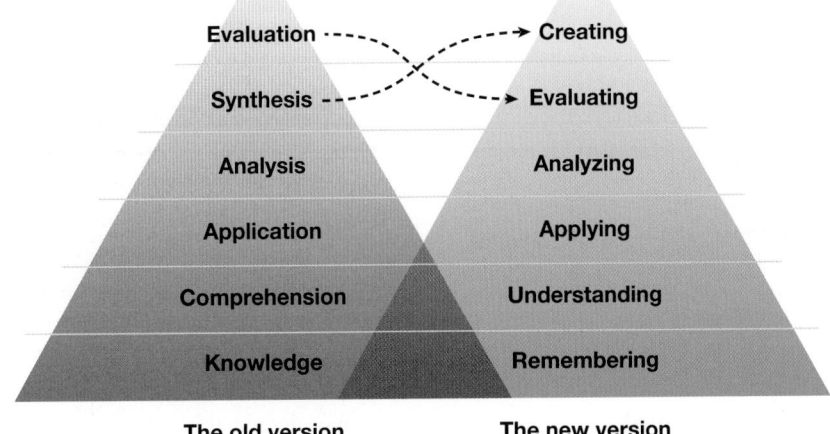

FIGURE 8-2 The older and newer versions of Bloom's taxonomy in the cognitive domain.

was a collaborative effort, the levels are typically referred to as Bloom's taxonomy (classification). In 2001, Anderson, one of Bloom's former students, and Krathwohl, one of Bloom's original coauthors, revised and rearranged the original taxonomy, changing nouns to verbs (Fig. 8-2).

Application of the Cognitive Domain to the National Licensing Examination

Each test question on the National Licensing Examination (NCLEX) is classified according to its level of difficulty, which coincides with a level of Bloom's taxonomy. Passing the examination depends on both the number of correctly answered questions and their levels of cognitive difficulty.

- **Remembering**, the lowest level of cognition, requires recalling information from prior memorization.
- **Understanding**, the next level, requires explaining ideas or concepts.
- **Applying**, the cognitive level at which the majority of NCLEX-PN items are written, requires using principles to solve or interpret information related to a client's health or its deviations.
- **Analyzing**, a cognitive level of further difficulty, requires using abstract and logical thought processes that form the basis for a nursing action. This level of thinking necessitates, for example, that a person compare or contrast information, distinguish cause and effect, identify differences, or question actions.
- **Evaluating**, the next-to-highest cognitive level, involves an ability to appraise a situation or information and to defend or support a selected action.
- **Creating**, the highest and most challenging degree of thinking, requires activities such as inventing, modifying, substituting, and reorganizing information to fashion new ideas.

Affective Domain

Krathwohl and others (1973) further expanded learning into affective levels based on the way people deal with feelings and emotions. The levels within the affective domain are similarly arranged from simple to complex. The focus in this domain includes motivation to learn, valuing what is learned,

and incorporating learning into one's life. Learners are characterized as (1) willing to listen (**receiving**), (2) willing to participate (**responding**), (3) accepting or committing to new information (**valuing**), (4) integrating the new information by changing behavior (**organization**), and (5) continuing to practice and act upon acquired information (**characterization**).

Psychomotor Domain

Psychomotor learning is the development of structured patterns of muscular activities guided by environmental signals (*Psychomotor learning*, 2022). The psychomotor domain is described as how a physical skill develops. For the purposes of simplicity, a summary of levels was developed within the psychomotor domain. **Observing** involves watching an experienced person perform a physical skill; **imitating** describes the learner's attempt to duplicate the observed skill; **practicing** is the act of performing a skill repeatedly; and **adapting** involves making minor changes in the performance of the skill when necessary adjustments are required (LUCIDWAY, 2022). This tier of actions describes how nursing students and others progress from novice to skilled practitioners. Table 8-1 outlines the model for the psychomotor domain established by R.H. Dave.

>> **Stop, Think, and Respond 8-1**

Identify the learning domain that relates to each of the following teaching methods:

1. *The nurse watches as a client with diabetes practices administering an injection.*
2. *The nurse asks a client who had a mastectomy to speak to clients attending a health seminar about the importance of monthly breast self-examinations.*
3. *The nurse explains the technique for performing leg exercises to a client scheduled for surgery.*
4. *The nurse helps a client self-administer nutritional formula through a gastrostomy tube.*
5. *The nurse gives a client with back strain a pamphlet on using good posture and body mechanics.*

TABLE 8-1 The Psychomotor Domain

LEVEL	DESCRIPTION	EXAMPLE
Imitation	Observing and patterning behavior after someone else Performance may be of low quality	Copying a work of art
Manipulation	Being able to perform certain actions by following instructions and practicing	Creating work on one's own, after taking lessons or reading about the process
Precision	Refining, becoming more exact Few errors are apparent.	Doing and redoing something, so it will be "just right"
Articulation	Coordinating a series of actions, achieving harmony and internal consistency	Producing a video that involves music, drama, color, sound, etc.
Naturalization	Having high-level performance become natural, without needing to think much about it	Michael Jordan playing basketball, Nancy Lopez hitting a golf ball, etc.

LUCIDWAY. (2022). *The psychomotor domain—Get Physical*. https://www.lucidway.com/the-psychomotor-domain-get-physical/

Age and Developmental Level

Learning takes place differently depending on a person's age and developmental level. **Developmental level** refers to physical, cognitive, social/emotional, and language characteristics that are norms at particular stages in life from infancy through adulthood. Teaching tends to be more effective when it is designed to accommodate unique age-related differences.

Recently, a distinction has been made between learners at the early and later ends of the aging spectrum. Currently, there are three major categories of teaching with age in mind:

- **Pedagogy** involves teaching children or adults with cognitive abilities comparable to those of children.
- **Andragogy** encompasses the principles of teaching adult learners.
- **Geragogy** includes the techniques that enhance learning among older adults.

Nurses and all those who provide health teaching must be aware of the typical learning characteristics of children, adults, and older adults (Table 8-2). Each learner is unique and may demonstrate characteristics associated with other age groups.

Although most clients with health problems are in their later years, nurse educators are advised to prepare themselves to teach adults who belong to Generation X, Generation Y, Generation Z, and Generation Alpha as they age. Generation X refers to those born between 1961 and 1981; Generation Y, also called millennials, refers to people who were born after 1981 through 1994; those born between 1995 and 2009 belong to the Net generation or Generation Z; and Generation Alpha refers to people born between 2010 and 2024. In general, individuals in these generations may share many learning characteristics:

- They are or will be technologically literate, having used or grown up with computers, smart phones, and tablet devices.
- They expect stimulation and quick responses.
- They expect immediate answers and feedback.
- They become bored with memorizing information and doing repetitive tasks.

TABLE 8-2 Typical Age-Related Differences among Learners

PEDAGOGIC LEARNERS	ANDRAGOGIC LEARNERS	GERAGOGIC LEARNERS
Physically immature	Physically mature	Undergoing degenerative changes
Lack experience	Building experience	Have vast experience
Compulsory learners	Voluntary learners	Crisis learners
Passive	Active	Passive/active
Need direction and supervision	Self-directed and independent	Need structure and encouragement
Motivated to learn by potential rewards or punishment	Seek knowledge for their own sake or for personal interest	Motivated by a personal need or goal
Learning is subject-centered	Learning is problem-centered	Learning is self-centered
Short attention span	Longer attention span	Attention may be affected by low energy level, fatigue, and anxiety
Convergent thinkers (unidirectional, e.g., see one application for new information)	Divergent thinkers (process multiple applications for new information)	Practical thinkers (process new information as it applies to a unique personal problem)
Need immediate feedback	Can postpone feedback	Respond to frequent feedback
Rote learning	Analytical learning	Experiential learning
Short-term retention	Long-term retention	Short-term retention unless reinforced by immediate use
Task-oriented	Goal-oriented	Outcome-oriented
Think concretely	Think abstractly	Think both concretely and abstractly
Respond to competition	Respond to collaboration	Respond to encouragement from significant others or caregivers

- They prefer a variety of instructional methods from which they can choose.
- They respond best when information is relevant.
- They appreciate visualizations, simulations, and other methods of participatory learning.

>> **Stop, Think, and Respond 8-2**

Identify the client age group for whom the following teaching techniques are most appropriate. Explain the basis for your analysis.

1. *The nurse plans for the teaching session to be no more than 20 minutes.*
2. *The nurse emphasizes knowledge or techniques that the client is interested in learning.*
3. *The nurse reinforces that the client's discharge from the health agency correlates with becoming competent in self-administering insulin injections.*
4. *The nurse indicates that the client can play a video game for 30 minutes when they can name the number of recommended servings in each category within the food pyramid.*
5. *The nurse challenges the client to devise a plan for managing their colostomy upon their return to work following discharge.*

Capacity to Learn

For a person to receive, remember, analyze, and apply new information, they must have a **capacity to learn**, that is, a certain amount of intellectual ability. Illiteracy, sensory deficits, cultural differences, shortened attention spans, and lack of motivation and readiness require special adaptations when implementing health teaching.

Literacy

It is essential to determine a client's level of **literacy** (ability to read and write) before developing a teaching plan. The Organization for Economic Cooperation and Development found that 50% of U.S. adults can't read a book written at an eighth-grade level (Wylie Communications, 2021). **Functional illiteracy** may be the consequence of a learning disability or lack of access to quality education, not below-average intellectual capacity.

Health Literacy

Personal **health literacy**, "the degree to which individuals have the ability to find, understand, and use information and services to inform health-related decisions and actions for themselves and others" (Centers for Disease Control and Prevention, 2023), is a factor in client teaching. It affects a client's ability to do the following:

- Locate health information
- Access health care services
- Share personal health information with professionals
- Analyze relative health risks and benefits
- Calculate drug dosages
- Evaluate information for credibility and quality
- Interpret test results

Detecting Health Illiteracy

Because many people who are **illiterate** or functionally illiterate are not always willing or able to volunteer information about their reading problems, literacy may be difficult to assess. Some indications that clients have low health literacy are missed appointments, incomplete health forms, nonadherence to medication regimen, inability to provide a coherent health history, and lack of follow-up on tests and referrals.

People who are illiterate or functionally illiterate may develop elaborate mechanisms to disguise or compensate for their learning deficits. To protect the client's self-esteem, the nurse can ask, "How do you learn best?" and plan accordingly.

Strategies for Promoting Health Literacy

Studies have shown that clients immediately forget 40% to 80% of medical information they receive and that nearly half of the information they retain is incorrect (Centre for Disease Control and Prevention, 2022).

Some useful approaches for promoting health literacy include the following:

- Using verbal and visual modes for instruction
- Avoiding technical language
- Limiting information to three to five key points
- Being specific rather than general
- Repeating directions several times in the same sequence so that the client can memorize the information
- Providing pictures, diagrams, audio recordings, and videos for future review

One method to determine if teaching has been effective is the **teach-back method**, a technique for confirming that a client has understood what has been taught. The nurse asks the client to repeat the information in their own words. It can be considered a form of "feedback." For example, the nurse can say, "I want to be sure that I explained your medication correctly. Can you tell me how you are going to take this medicine?" (The Teach-Back Method, Tool 5).

Sensory Deficits

Older adults tend to have visual and auditory deficits, though such deficits are not exclusive to this population. Deficits in the ability to see or hear can impact the client's learning. Nursing Guidelines 8-1 presents some techniques for teaching clients with sensory impairment. Figure 8-3 shows samples of printing that can be used as visual aids.

Cultural Competence in Client Teaching

Because teaching and learning involve language, the nurse must modify approaches if the client cannot speak English or if they speak English as a second language (see Chapter 6, Nursing Guidelines 6-1). Language differences between the nurse and client do not justify omitting health teaching. In most cases, if neither the nurse nor the client speaks a mutually understood language, a translator or acceptable alternative is needed.

NURSING GUIDELINES 8-1

Teaching Clients with Sensory Impairments

Ensure that the client with a visual impairment is wearing prescription eyeglasses or that the client with a hearing impairment is wearing a hearing aid, if available. *Visual and auditory aids improve the client's ability to perceive sensory stimuli.*

For clients with visual impairment:

- Speak in a normal tone of voice. *Clients with visual impairment do not necessarily also have hearing impairment. Increased volume does not compensate for reduced vision.*
- Use at least a 75- to 100-watt light source, preferably in a lamp that shines over the client's shoulder. *Ceiling lights tend to diffuse light rather than concentrate it on a small area where the client needs to focus.*
- Avoid standing in front of a window through which bright sunlight is shining. *It is difficult to look into bright light.*
- Provide a magnifying glass for reading. *Magnification enlarges standard or small print to a comfortable size.*
- Obtain pamphlets in large (12- to 16-point) print with serif lettering, which has horizontal lines at the bottom and top of each letter (see Fig. 8-3). *Letters and words are usually more distinct when set in large print with a style that promotes visual discrimination.*

- Avoid using materials printed on glossy paper. *Glossy paper reflects light, causing a glare that makes reading uncomfortable.*
- Select black print on white paper. *This combination provides maximum contrast and makes letters more legible.*

For clients with hearing impairment:

- Use a magic slate, chalkboard, flash cards, or writing pads to communicate. *Writing can substitute for verbal instructions.*
- Lower the voice pitch. *Hearing loss is generally in the higher pitch ranges.*
- Try to select words that do not begin with "f," "s," "k," and "sh." *These letters are formed with high-pitched sounds and therefore can be difficult for clients with hearing impairment to discriminate.*
- Rephrase rather than repeat when the client does not understand. *Rephrasing may provide additional visual or auditory clues to facilitate the client's understanding.*
- Insert a stethoscope into the client's ears and speak into the bell with a low voice. *The stethoscope acts as a basic hearing aid. It projects sounds directly to the ears and reduces background noise.*

Attention and Concentration

The client's attention and concentration affect the duration, delivery, and teaching methods employed. Some helpful approaches include the following:

- Observe the client and implement health teaching when they are most alert and comfortable.
- Keep the teaching session short.
- Use the client's name frequently throughout the instructional period; this refocuses their attention.
- Show enthusiasm, which may inspire enthusiasm for learning in the client.

- Use colorful materials, gestures, and variety to stimulate the client.
- Involve the client in an active way.
- Vary the tone and pitch of your voice to stimulate the client aurally.

Motivation

Learning is optimal when a person has **motivation**, or a purpose for acquiring new information. Relevance of learning depends on individual variables. The desire for learning may be to satisfy intellectual curiosity, restore independence, prevent complications, or facilitate discharge and return to the comfort of home. Less desirable reasons for individuals to learn may be to please others and to avoid criticism.

Learning Readiness

When both capacity and motivation for learning exist, the nurse can determine the final component—learning readiness. **Learning readiness** refers to the client's current physical and psychological well-being. For example, a person who is in pain, is too warm or cold, is having difficulty breathing, or is depressed or fearful is not in the best condition to learn. In these situations, it is best to restore comfort first and attend to teaching afterward.

Learning Needs

A **learning need** is the gap between what a client knows and what they have yet to learn. The best teaching and learning take place when teaching is individualized. For teaching to be most efficient and personalized, the nurse must gather pertinent information from the client. Guessing or assuming

---

12 pt. Times

Aa Bb Cc Dd Ee Ff Gg Hh Ii Jj Kk Ll
Oo Pp Qq Rr Ss Tt Uu Vv Ww Xx Yy

14 pt. Times

Aa Bb Cc Dd Ee Ff Gg Hh Ii Jj Kk
Oo Pp Qq Rr Ss Tt Uu Vv Ww Xx

16 pt. Times

Aa Bb Cc Dd Ee Ff
Oo Pp Qq Rr Ss Tt

FIGURE 8-3 Selecting printed materials with 12- to 16-point type, black print on white paper, and serif lettering help improve visual clarity.

what the client wants and needs to know often leads to wasted time and effort.

The following are questions a nurse can ask to assess the client's learning needs:

- What does being healthy mean to you?
- What factors in your life interfere with being healthy?
- What do you not understand as fully as you would like?
- With what activities do you need help?
- What do you hope to accomplish before being discharged?
- How can I help you at this time?

INFORMAL AND FORMAL TEACHING

Informal teaching is unplanned and occurs spontaneously when interacting with a client. **Formal teaching** requires a plan. Without a plan, teaching becomes haphazard. Furthermore, a lack of organization of time and content jeopardizes the potential for reaching goals, providing adequate information, and ensuring comprehension. Potential teaching needs are generally identified at the client's admission, but they may be amended as care and treatment progress. If ongoing teaching is necessary, furnishing clients with technology for **telehomecare** (visiting clients electronically in their home for the purpose of seeing and communicating in real time) may be beneficial, especially for clients located in rural areas.

A student nurse may work with a staff nurse or instructor in developing a teaching plan. Usually, one or more nurses carry out certain specific parts of a teaching plan (Fig. 8-4). This approach is the most desirable, as it helps

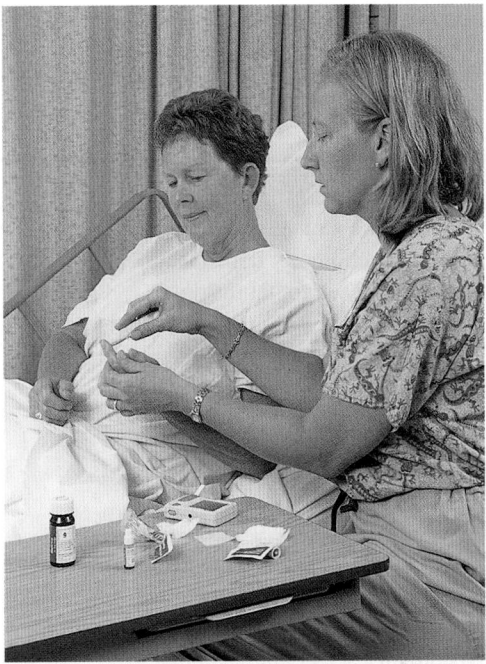

FIGURE 8-4 The nurse teaches about diabetes at the bedside. Multisensory stimulation is promoted by giving the client explanations and encouraging them to watch the technique for testing blood glucose as it is being performed. (Photo by B. Proud.)

keep the client from being overwhelmed with processing volumes of new information or learning skills that are difficult for novices to perform. Skill 8-1 serves as a model when an adult client needs teaching.

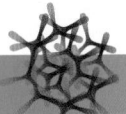

KEY POINTS

- Benefits of client teaching include:
  - Reduced lengths of hospitalizations
  - Cost-effectiveness of health care
  - Better allocation of resources
  - Increased client satisfaction
  - Decreased readmission rates
- Learning styles include:
  - Cognitive domain: A style of processing information by listening or reading facts and descriptions
  - Affective domain: A style of processing information that appeals to a person's feelings, beliefs, or values
  - Psychomotor domain: A style of processing information that focuses on learning by doing
- Teaching related to age and developmental level:
  - Pedagogy: Teaching children or adults with cognitive abilities comparable to those of children

- Andragogy: The principles of teaching adult learners
- Geragogy: Includes techniques that enhance learning among older adults
- Ways to approach clients to promote increasing health literacy include:
  - Using verbal and visual modes for instruction
  - Avoiding technical language
  - Limiting information to three to five key points
  - Being specific rather than general
  - Repeating directions several times in the same sequence so that the client can memorize the information
  - Providing pictures, diagrams, audio recordings, and videos for future review

CRITICAL THINKING EXERCISES

1. Identify reasons why health literacy is especially important in the 21st century.
2. How would a nurse teach techniques for toothbrushing differently to a child? To a person from the X, Y, Z, or Alpha generations?
3. What teaching strategies within the cognitive, affective, and psychomotor domains of learning could the nurse use to teach toothbrushing?
4. Give two examples of how a nurse could determine whether a client actually learned information that was taught, such as toothbrushing.

NEXT-GENERATION NCLEX-STYLE REVIEW QUESTIONS

1. When a nurse evaluates the outcomes of health teaching, which activities are compatible with a client who indicates their preferred learning style is in the cognitive domain? Select all that apply.
   a. Assembling equipment
   b. Listing needed equipment
   c. Identifying pieces of equipment
   d. Defending the choice of equipment
   e. Summarizing the use of equipment
   Test-Taking Strategy: Eliminate options that describe physical skills or skills that involve feelings or emotions.

2. Arrange the following steps in the order in which they should occur when a nurse performs health teaching.
   a. Encourage feedback from the client.
   b. Divide information into manageable amounts.
   c. Find out what the client wants to know.
   d. Document the client's evidence of learning.
   e. Determine the client's recall of information.
   Test-Taking Strategy: Apply the steps in the nursing process to arrange the options.

3. Which of the following is most important before the nurse teaches the parent of a 6-year-old child about nutrition?
   a. Assess the child's height and weight.
   b. Obtain a nutrition guidelines pamphlet.
   c. Develop a plan for 1 week of menus.
   d. Collect various nutritional recipes.
   Test-Taking Strategy: Note the key word and modifier, "most important." Use the nursing process to select an option that is necessary before other nursing actions.

4. After teaching a client how to perform breathing exercises, what is the best method the nurse can use for evaluating the effectiveness of the teaching?
   a. Request that the client explain the importance of breathing exercises.
   b. Have the client perform the breathing exercises as they were taught.
   c. Ask the client if they are performing the breathing exercises as required.
   d. Monitor the client's respiratory rate several times a day.
   Test-Taking Strategy: Select the option that provides the best evidence of learning.

5. Which teaching aid is developmentally appropriate when the nurse plans to prepare a preschool child for a diagnostic test such as a bone marrow puncture?
   a. Dolls or puppets
   b. Pamphlets or booklets
   c. Colored diagrams
   d. Commercial videotapes
   Test-Taking Strategy: Use the process of elimination to select the most age-appropriate method for teaching.

SKILL 8-1 Teaching Adult Clients

Suggested Action	Reason for Action
ASSESSMENT	
Find out what the client wants to know.	Personal interest facilitates learning.
Establish what the client should know to remain healthy.	Clients are not always aware of what information is vital to maintain their health and safety.
Determine the client's learning style.	Teaching is more effective when techniques support the client's preferred learning method.
PLANNING	
Collaborate with the client on content, goals, and realistic time frames.	Adult learners tend to prefer collaboration and active involvement in the learning process.
Develop a written plan that builds from simple to complex, familiar to unfamiliar, and expected to unexpected.	Adult learners learn best by applying information from present knowledge or past experiences.
Divide information into manageable amounts.	Too much information at once tends to overwhelm learners.
Select teaching strategies and resources that are compatible with the client's preferred style for learning.	Adult learners generally prefer one learning style, but multiple approaches enhance learning.
Use a variety of instructional methods from the cognitive, affective, and psychomotor domains.	Adults tend to retain more knowledge when a variety of instructional techniques are used.
Review the content that will be used during teaching.	Preparation and knowledge evoke self-confidence.
IMPLEMENTATION	
Teach when the client appears interested and physically and emotionally ready to learn, if possible.	Learning takes place more easily when the client can focus on the task at hand.
Provide an environment that promotes learning.	Learning occurs best in a well-lit room with a comfortable temperature. Distractions and interruptions interfere with concentration.
Identify how long the teaching session will last.	Clarifying the length of time prepares the client for the demands on their time and attention.
Begin with basic concepts.	Learning that builds from simple to complex is best.
Review previously taught information.	Repetition increases retention of information.
Use vocabulary within the client's personal level of understanding.	Teaching at the learner's level preserves dignity. The nurse is accountable for ensuring the client's comprehension.
Explain any and all new terms.	Clients are sometimes embarrassed to admit they do not understand.
Involve the client actively by encouraging feedback and handling of equipment.	Adult learners prefer active rather than passive learning situations.
Stimulate as many senses as possible.	Involvement of more than one sense enhances learning.
Invent songs, rhymes, or a series of key terms that correspond with the teaching content.	Creativity is stimulated by the right hemisphere of the brain where information is retrieved more easily.
Use equipment as similar as possible to what the client will use at home.	Becoming familiar with equipment is the best preparation for self-care at home.
Allow time for questions and answers.	Providing this opportunity helps the client clarify information and prevents misunderstandings.
Summarize the key points covered during the current teaching.	Reviewing reinforces important concepts.
Determine the client's level of learning.	The ability to recall or apply information and to demonstrate skills is proof of short-term learning.
Identify the time, place, and content for the next teaching session.	Planning the next meeting provides a time frame during which the client may review and practice what they have learned.
Arrange an opportunity for the client to use or apply the new information as soon as possible after it was taught.	Immediate application reinforces learning and promotes long-term retention.
Document the information taught and evidence demonstrating the client's understanding.	Documentation provides a written record of the client's progress and avoids omissions or duplications during future teaching sessions.
Review with the client the progress made toward goals.	Collaboration keeps the client focused on expected outcomes.
Evaluate the need for further teaching.	Evaluation is the basis for revising the teaching plan.

(continued)

SKILL 8-1 Teaching Adult Clients (*continued*)

Suggested Action	Reason for Action

EVALUATION

- The planned teaching content was covered.
- The client participated in the teaching process.
- The client recalled at least 50% of the concepts with accuracy.

DOCUMENT

- Date and time
- Content taught
- Evidence of the client's learning

SAMPLE DOCUMENTATION[a]

Date and Time Explained the times for taking two drugs that require self-administration after discharge. States, "I take the yellow pill once in the morning before breakfast and I take one blue pill three times a day when I eat breakfast, lunch, and supper."
_____ J. Doe, LPN

[a]In an electronic/computerized charting, the name and title of the person doing the documentation is automatically identified when the person logs on to the computer, so a signature and title are not necessary.

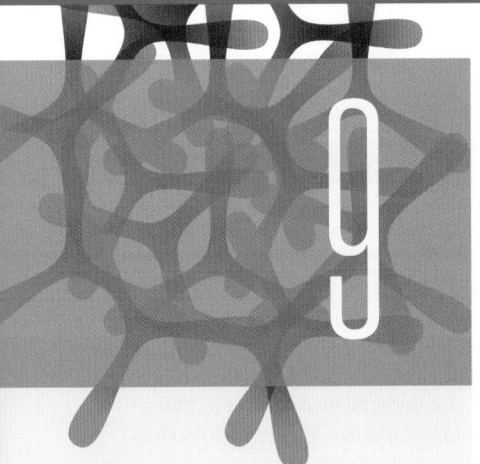

9

Recording and Reporting

Learning Objectives

On completion of this chapter, the reader should be able to:

1. Identify uses for medical records.
2. List components generally found in any client's medical record.
3. List legally defensible characteristics of written charting.
4. Differentiate between source and problem-oriented records.
5. Identify methods of charting.
6. List advantages and disadvantages of an electronic medical record.
7. Explain the purpose and applications associated with the Health Insurance Portability and Accountability Act (HIPAA).
8. List aspects of documentation required in the medical records of all clients cared for in acute settings.
9. Discuss why it is important to use only approved abbreviations when charting.
10. Explain how to convert traditional time to military time.
11. Identify written forms used to communicate information about clients.
12. List ways that health care providers exchange client information other than by reading the medical record.

INTRODUCTION

Nurses must communicate information clearly, concisely, and accurately when speaking and recording information. This chapter describes various written and spoken forms of communication and nursing responsibilities for record keeping and reporting.

 Gerontologic Considerations

■ State laws related to mandatory reporting of elder abuse and neglect, including self-neglect, take precedence over HIPAA regulations.

MEDICAL RECORD

A **medical record** is a collection of information about a person's health, the care provided by health care providers, and the client's progress. It is also referred to as a *health record* or *client record*. The medical record may consist of various agency-approved paper forms (Table 9-1), or the

TABLE 9-1 Common Agency Chart Forms

NAME OF FORM	CONTENT
Fact sheet	Provides information such as the client's name, date of birth, address, phone number, religion, insurer, admitting physician, admitting diagnosis, person to contact in case of emergency, and emergency phone number
Advance directive	Provides instructions about the client's choices for care should they be unable to make decisions later
History and physical examination	Contains the physician's review of the client's current and past health problems, results of a body system examination, medical diagnosis, and tentative plan for treatment
Physician's orders	Identifies laboratory and diagnostic tests, diet, activity, medications, intravenous fluids, and clinical procedures (instructions for changing a dressing, inserting tubes, and so forth) on a day-by-day basis
Physician's or multidisciplinary progress notes	Describes the client's ongoing status and response to the current plan of care and potential modifications in the plan
Nursing admission database	Documents information concerning the client's health patterns and initial physical assessment findings
Nursing or multidisciplinary plan of care	Identifies client problems, goals, and directions for care based on an analysis of collected data
Graphic sheet	Displays trends in the client's vital signs, weight, and daily summary of fluid intake and output
Daily nursing assessment and flow sheet	Indicates focused physical assessment findings by individual nurses during each 24-hour period and the routine care that was provided
Nursing notes	Provides narrative details of subjective and objective data, nursing actions, response of the client, outcomes of communication with other health care providers, or the client's family
Medication administration record	Identifies the drug name, date, time, route, and frequency of drug administration as well as the name of the nurse who administered each medication
Laboratory and diagnostic reports	Contains the results of tests in a sequential order
Discharge plan	Indicates the information, skills, and referral services that the client may need before being released from the agency's care
Teaching summary	Identifies content that was taught, evidence of the client's learning, and need for repetition or reinforcement

forms may be stored on the hard drive of a computerized electronic medical record (EMR). The American Recovery and Reinvestment Act informed physicians, who provided care to Medicare and Medicaid clients, that in order for them to continue to receive the payments, they must change to exclusively computerized health records and electronic information technology (IT). According to the Centers for Disease Control and Prevention (CDC), as of 2019, almost 90% of physicians have adopted electronic health records (EHRs).

Hard copy paper forms are placed in a **chart** (a binder or folder that promotes the orderly collection, storage, and safekeeping of a person's medical record). The paper forms in the chart are color-coded or separated by tabbed sheets. Most paper charts are being replaced by the EHRs. An EHR stored on a computer is accessed by using a password and selecting the desired form from a menu. EHRs can be printed if a hard copy is desired. All personnel involved in a client's health care contribute to the medical record by **charting**, **recording**, or **documenting** (the process of entering information).

Uses for Medical Records

Besides serving as a permanent health record, the collective information about a client provides a means to share information among health care providers, thus ensuring client safety and continuity of care. Occasionally, medical records also are used to investigate quality of care in a health agency, demonstrate compliance with national accreditation standards, promote reimbursement from insurance companies, facilitate health education and research, and provide evidence during malpractice lawsuits.

Permanent Account

The client's medical record is a written, chronologic account of a person's illness or injury and the care provided from the onset of the problem through discharge or death. The record is filed and maintained for future reference. Previous health records are often requested during subsequent admissions so that the client's health history can be reviewed.

Sharing Information

Because it is impossible for all health care providers to meet and exchange information on a personal basis at the same time, the medical record becomes central to communication (i.e., sharing information among personnel). The documentation serves as a way to inform others about the client's status and plan for care.

Sharing information prevents duplication of care and helps reduce the chance of error or omission. For example, if a client requests medication for pain, the nurse checks the client's current record to determine when the last pain-relieving drug was administered. Accurate and timely documentation prevents medication from being administered too frequently or withheld unnecessarily. Maintaining immunization records is another example of how documentation promotes continuity; the record ensures the administration of subsequent immunizations according to an appropriate schedule.

Quality Assurance

To maintain a high level of care, hospitals and other health care agencies use medical records to promote **quality assurance** (*QA*), **continuous quality improvement** (*CQI*), or **total quality improvement** (*TQI*) (an agency's internal process for self-improvement to ensure that the level of care reflects or exceeds established standards). One QA method involves investigating the documentation in a sample of medical records. If the analyzed data indicate less-than-acceptable compliance with standards of care, the committee recommends corrective measures and reevaluates the outcomes later.

Accreditation

The Joint Commission (TJC) is a private association that has established criteria reflecting high standards for client safety and institutional health care. Representatives of TJC or other accreditation agencies periodically inspect health care agencies to determine whether they demonstrate evidence of quality care.

The documentation in randomly selected medical records is just one component examined during an accreditation visit. To support a health care agency's accreditation, nursing documentation should include:

- Initial assessment and reassessments of physical, psychological, social, environmental, and self-care status; education; and discharge planning
- Identification of nursing diagnoses or client needs
- Planned nursing interventions or nursing standards of care for meeting the client's nursing care needs including the education and training provided to the client and fall precaution strategies
- Nursing care provided
- Client's response to interventions and outcomes of care, including pain management, discharge planning activities, and the client's or caregiver's ability to manage continuing care needs

If documentation is substandard, accreditation may be withheld or withdrawn.

Reimbursement

The costs of most clients' hospital and home care are billed to third-party payers such as Medicare, Medicaid, and private insurance companies. **Auditors** (inspectors who examine client records) survey medical records to determine whether the care provided meets the established criteria for reimbursement. Undocumented, incomplete, or inconsistent documentation of care may result in a denial of payment.

Education and Research

Published references are primary resources for health education. Examining the medical records of clients with specific disorders, however, provides a valuable supplement that enhances learning and future problem-solving. Client records also facilitate research. For example, some types of clinical investigations are difficult to conduct because few participants are in a particular locale or test facilities are limited. Consequently, stored, microfilmed, or EHR documents serve as an alternative resource for scientific data.

Nevertheless, to protect confidentiality, only authorized persons are allowed access to client records (see discussion on protecting health information). Formal permission must be obtained from the client, the health agency's administrator, or other authority whenever a client's record is used for a purpose other than treatment and record keeping.

Legal Evidence

The medical record is considered a legal document. Therefore, entries in medical records must follow legally defensible criteria (Box 9-1). Portions of the medical record can be subpoenaed as evidence by the defense or prosecuting attorney to prove or disprove allegations of malpractice. It is especially important to document safety precautions taken to protect the client, individuals who were notified about concerns and issues, and outcomes of the communication.

BOX 9-1 **Criteria for Legally Defensible Charting**

When making an entry in a client's medical record, the nurse should:

- Ensure that the client's name appears on each page.
- Never chart for someone else.
- Use the specified color of ink and ballpoint pen, or enter data on a computer.
- Date and time stamp each entry as it is made.
- Chart promptly after providing care.
- Make entries in chronologic order.
- Identify documentation that is out of chronologic sequence with the words "late entry."
- Write or print legibly.
- Use correct grammar and spelling.
- Reflect the plan of care.
- Describe the outcomes of care.
- Record relevant details.
- Use only approved abbreviations.
- Never scribble over entries or use correction fluid to obliterate what has been written.
- Draw a single line through erroneous information so that it remains readable, add the date, initial, and then document the correct information.
- Record facts, not subjective interpretations.
- Quote the client's verbal comments.
- Write "duplicate" or "recopied" on documentation that is not original; include the date, time, initials, and reason for the duplication.
- Never imply criticism of another's care.
- Document the circumstances for notifying a physician, the specific data reported, and the physician's recommendations.
- Identify specific information provided when teaching a client and the evidence that indicates the client has understood the instructions.
- Leave no empty spaces between entries and signature.
- Sign each entry by name and title.

Each person who makes entries in the client's medical record is responsible for the information they record and can be summoned as a witness to testify concerning what has been documented. Any written documentation that cannot be clearly read or that is vague, scribbled through, whited out, written over, or erased makes for a poor legal defense.

>>> *Stop, Think, and Respond 9-1*

Discuss how the nurse could improve each of the following documentation samples:
1. *01/11 0800 Ate well.*
2. *1400 Hygiene provided and ambulated.*
3. *1500 Depressed all day. S. Rogers.*

Client Access to Records

Historically, clients were not allowed to see their medical records. Since the passing of federal legislation regarding client confidentiality in 1996 known as the **Health Insurance Portability and Accountability Act** (HIPAA), with the latest revision or update in 2022, clients have the right to see their own medical and billing records, request changes to anything they feel is inaccurate, they must also be informed about who has seen their medical records (U.S. Department of Health and Human Services, 2022). Some highlights of the 2022 HIPAA update include potential changes to:

- Patient acknowledgment of notice of privacy practices
- The minimum necessary standard for protected health information (PHI) protection
- Allowable disclosures related to care coordination and case management
- Disclosures of PHI for health emergencies
- Citizens' rights to access their PHI
- Fees that organizations may charge individuals to access PHI

The latest version also includes updates and revisions to previous definitions of what constitutes a data breach (HIPAA Journal, 2022) and HIPAA rules for cloud computing (HHS.gov, 2017). Consequently, many institutions have written policies that describe the guidelines by which clients can access their own medical records. Policies range from complete, unrestricted access within 30 days of the client's written request to arranging access in the presence of the client's physician or hospital administrator. Nurses must follow the established agency policy.

Types of Client Records

Client records in most agencies contain similar information. They are generally organized in either a source-oriented or a problem-oriented format.

Source-Oriented Records

The traditional type of client record is a **source-oriented record** (records organized according to the source of documented information). This type of record contains separate forms on which physicians, nurses, dietitians, physical therapists, and other health care providers make entries about their own specific activities in relation to the client's care.

One of the criticisms of source-oriented records is that it is difficult to demonstrate a unified, cooperative approach for resolving the client's problems among caregivers. Frequently, the fragmented documentation gives the impression that each health care provider is working independently of the others.

Problem-Oriented Records

A second type of client record is the **problem-oriented record** (records organized according to the client's health problems). In contrast to source-oriented records that contain numerous locations for information, problem-oriented records contain four major components: the database, the problem list, the plan of care, and the progress notes. The information is compiled and arranged to emphasize goal-directed care to promote the recording of pertinent information and to facilitate communication among health care providers.

METHODS OF CHARTING

Nurses use various styles to record information within the client's record. Examples include narrative charting, SOAP charting, focus charting, PIE charting, charting by exception, and electronic computerized charting.

 Concept Mastery Alert

"If it wasn't documented it wasn't done"

- Good documentation is a clear, concise, and accurate description of the care that you have given.
- Poor documentation leaves the record open to questions, with no clear direction to follow.

(Texas Health and Human Services Department, n.d.)

Narrative Charting

Narrative charting (the style of documentation generally used in source-oriented records) involves writing information about the client and client care in chronologic order. There is no established format for narrative notations; the content resembles a log or journal (Fig. 9-1).

Narrative charting is time-consuming to write and read. The health care provider must sort through the lengthy notation for specific information about care and progress that correlates with the client's problems. Depending on the skill of the person writing a narrative entry, they may omit pertinent documentation or include insignificant information.

SOAP Charting

SOAP charting (the documentation style more likely to be used in a problem-oriented record) acquired its name from four essential components included in a progress note:

1. S = subjective data
2. O = objective data
3. A = analysis of the data
4. P = plan for care

Anytown General Hospital
214 Main Street
Anytown, USA 11001

DATE/TIME	NURSING NOTES
01/06/25, 1345	Pt. c/o nausea denies vomiting but states he feels like he may be sick, requests medication to ease stomach discomfort. VS: BP 100/64, P 70, R 18, T 98.4. O2 Sat 98% on room air. Abdomen is soft, BS active x4 quads. Pt reports some abdominal tenderness when palpated. Continent of bowel; reports last BM 01/05/22, normal consistency, and denies any history of diarrhea or constipation.
1350	Promethazine 25 mg. (one) given po, as per prn order for N&V.
1415	Reassessed pt. for c/o nausea and vomiting. Pt. reports nausea has subsided since taking medication at 1345. Denies vomiting or other complaints currently. Bed in low position, SR up x2, call light within reach.
1430	Continent of bladder with 18 Fr. indwelling foley catheter with leg band attached to right thigh, catheter is patent to gravity with approx. 200 cc pale yellow urine in foley bag. Skin is warm and dry to touch, turgor fair. Peripheral pulses present x2 upper and lower extremities with good capillary refill. Skin is warm and dry to touch, turgor fair, no edema noted. No skin tears or lacerations noted, no integumentary compromise noted on visual assessment. PERRLA. Lungs CTAB. Mucous membranes are pink and moist. _____ T. Jones, LVN@1430.

FIGURE 9-1 Sample of narrative charting.

Some agencies have expanded the SOAP format to SOAPIE or SOAPIER (I = interventions, E = evaluation, R = revision to the plan of care; Table 9-2).

Any variations in the SOAP format tend to focus the documentation on pertinent information that is required by a hospital accreditation agency. SOAP charting also helps demonstrate interdisciplinary cooperation because everyone involved in the care of a client makes entries in the same location in the chart.

Focus Charting

Focus charting (a modified form of SOAP charting) uses the word *focus* rather than *problem* because some believe that the word *problem* carries negative connotations. A focus can be the client's current or changed behavior, significant events in the client's care, or even a North American Nursing

Diagnosis Association International (NANDA-I) nursing diagnosis. Instead of using the SOAP format to make entries, focus charting follows a DAR model (D = data, A = action, R = response; Fig. 9-2). DAR notations tend to reflect the steps in the nursing process.

PIE Charting

PIE charting (a method of recording the client's progress under the headings of problem, intervention, and evaluation) is similar to the SOAPIE format. The PIE style prompts the nurse to address specific content in a charted progress note.

When nurses use the PIE method, they document assessments on a separate form and give the client's problems corresponding numbers. They use the numbers subsequently in the progress notes when referring to interventions and the client's responses.

TABLE 9-2 SOAPIER Charting Format

LETTER	EXPLANATION	EXAMPLE OF RECORDING
S = Subjective information	Information reported by the client	S—"I don't feel well"
O = Objective information	Observations made by the nurse	O—Temperature 102.4°F
A = Analysis	Problem identification	A—Fever
P = Plan	Proposed treatment	P—Offer extra fluids and monitor body temperature
I = Intervention	Care provided	I—750 mL of fluid intake in 8 hours; temperature assessed every 4 hours
E = Evaluation	Outcome of treatment	E—Temperature reduced to 101°F
R = Revision	Changes in treatment	R—Increase fluid intake to 1,000 mL per shift until temperature is ≤100°F

6/30/2024	D(ata)	Bladder distended 2 fingers above pubis.
1015		Has not urinated in 8 hrs. since
		catheter was removed.
	A(ction)	Assisted to toilet. Water turned on at
		faucet. Instructed to press over bladder
		with hands.
	R(esponse)	Voided 525 mL of clear urine. L. Cass, SN

FIGURE 9-2 Example of DAR charting.

Charting by Exception

Charting by exception is a documentation method in which nurses chart only abnormal assessment findings or care that deviate from a standard norm. Proponents of this method say that charting by exception is more efficient. It provides quick access to abnormal findings because it does not describe normal and routine information.

Electronic Charting

Electronic charting (documenting client information via computer) is a component of informatics. **Informatics** refers to the collection, storage, retrieval, and sharing of recorded data. Nursing informatics involves a combination of computer skills, knowledge of informatics, and information literacy.

Electronic charting is most efficient for nurses when documentation is done at the point of care (POC) on a bedside computer (Fig. 9-3) or on a computer on wheels. Having a terminal at the nursing station is a less desirable option because this removes the nurse from the source of the data; however, this may be the only alternative when there are limited computers for charting available. Centralized terminals generally are connected to large information systems (e.g., local area networks or LANs) that link departments in the institution (e.g., pharmacy, laboratory, admissions office, accounting); therefore, they are less specific for nursing use.

Although each computer system varies, electronic charting is generally done by using a computer and keyboard or touching the monitor screen with a finger or device such as a light pen to select from a list of menu options. Some systems allow a combination of keyboarding and touch-screen technology. Data entry by voice activation is also available. A

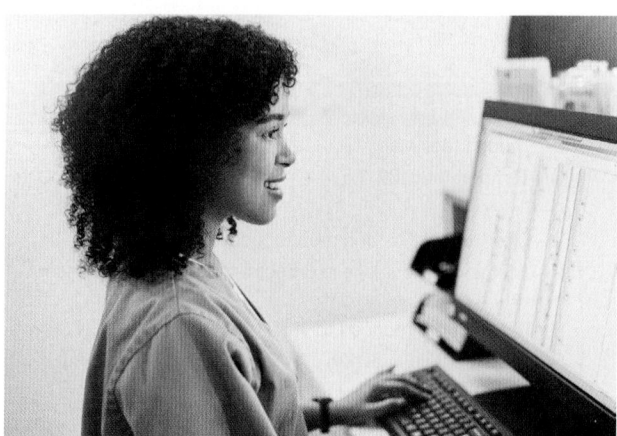

FIGURE 9-3 Portable computers allow for point-of-care documentation. (PeopleImages.com—Yuri A/Shutterstock.)

single keystroke saves the information displayed on the monitor to the client's record. Computerized electronic charting (Fig. 9-4) from a nursing point of view has many advantages:

- The information is always legible.
- It automatically records the date and time of the documentation.
- The abbreviations and terms are consistent with agency-approved lists.
- It eliminates trivia.
- Omissions are fewer because the computer prompts the nurse to enter specific information.
- It saves time because it eliminates delays in obtaining a physical chart.
- It reduces overtime costs for incomplete end-of-shift charting.
- Multiple health care providers can use the medical records simultaneously from many different work stations.
- Documentation formats prompt the nurse to enter data required by accreditation agencies such as pain and fall assessments.
- Entries are automatically credited to the user.
- Legibility and spelling are no longer issues.
- Reduces medication errors because the system alerts and prompts the physician regarding miscalculations of drug doses, medication interactions, or the client's allergies
- Allows obtaining test results quickly so that interventions can be implemented in a more timely manner
- Frees nurses from transcribing physicians' orders and making phone calls for the purpose of clarification
- Firewalls and passwords prevent breaches in confidentiality by protecting unauthorized access to confidential information.
- Electronic records are periodically backed up on systems outside of the agency of origin and are therefore protected from destruction should there be a fire or other type of disaster.

There are other nursing benefits from computer applications. Computers are being used to generate nursing care plans, develop staffing patterns that meet the current unit census and client acuity levels, analyze assessment data from monitoring equipment, and reduce medication errors by calling attention to drugs that have been newly ordered or not administered and by alerting the nurse to incompatibilities or contraindications to prescribed drugs.

Computerized documentation and EMRs have additional advantages for institutions, but there are also disadvantages, such as:

- Systems are expensive to purchase.
- Systems vary with institutions necessitating extensive training of new hires.
- Competency in using the system requires significant time.
- IT support staff are required.
- Passwords must be changed regularly.
- Downtime during system upgrades and power or electronic failures can interrupt and delay documentation and access to the full record.
- Temporary paper charting must be substituted when the system is down.

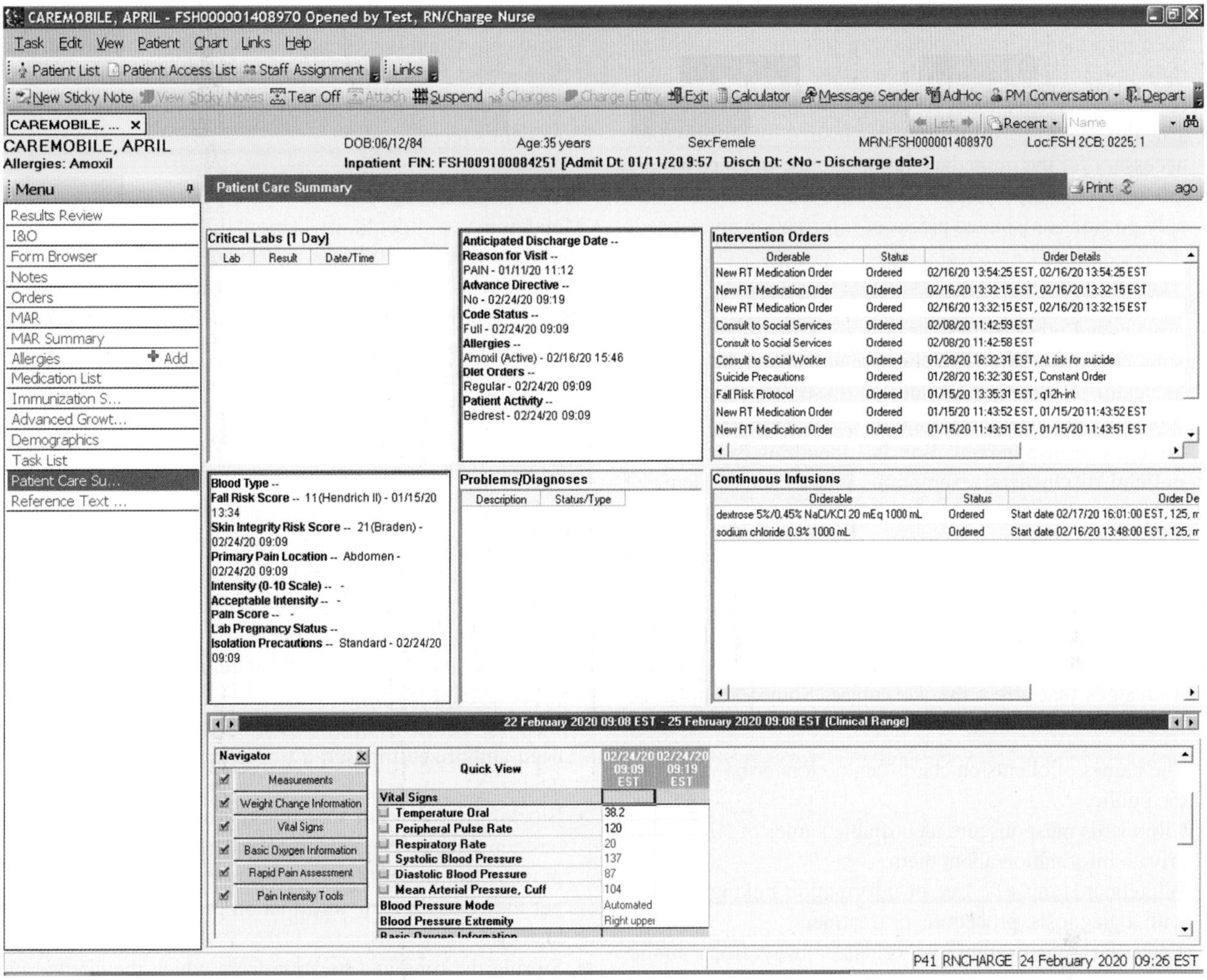

Sample of computerized charting figure (FIGURE 9-4).

FIGURE 9-4 Sample of computerized charting.

- There are fewer narrative entries due to structured options that are limited to multiple lists.
- Information is scattered among various files.
- They can promote **double charting** (repetitive entry of same information).

Confidentiality of information may be compromised if computer screens are left unattended, viewed by others at the bedside, accessed by unauthorized users, or if printouts are not secured or destroyed at the end of a shift.

Pharmacologic Considerations

■ Built-in safeguards are a feature of electronic medication administration records (MARs).
■ Screen pop-ups require the entry of data before the MAR screen can be viewed. This is designed to ensure that vital assessments such as blood pressure, pulse, or blood glucose levels are done before administering select medications, alerting the nurse and reducing the chance of serious consequences of incorrect medication administration.

PROTECTING HEALTH INFORMATION

Congress enacted the first HIPAA legislation to protect the rights of U.S. citizens to retain their health insurance when changing employment. To do so required transmitting health records from one insurance company to another. Transmission of the information resulted in the disclosure of personal health information to nonclinical individuals, a process that essentially jeopardized the individual's confidentiality and right to privacy. Subsequently, the original HIPAA legislation was expanded in 2022 to enact further measures to protect the privacy of health records and the security of that data. All health care agencies have been mandated to comply with the newest HIPAA regulations.

Privacy Standards

HIPAA regulations require health care agencies to safeguard written, spoken, and electronic health information in the following ways:

- Submit a written notice to all clients identifying the uses and disclosures of their health information such as to third parties for use in treatment or for payment for services.

- Obtain the client's signature indicating that the client has been informed of the disclosure of information and their right to learn who has seen the records. The law also indicates that agencies must limit released information from a health record to **minimum disclosure**, or information necessary for the immediate purpose only. In other words, it is inappropriate to release the entire health record when only portions or isolated pieces of information are needed.

Health care agencies must obtain specific authorization from the client to release information to family or friends, attorneys, and other parties for uses such as research, fundraising, and marketing. The client retains the right to withhold health information for any of these. There are some exceptions when health information can be revealed without the client's prior approval. Box 9-2 identifies examples of **beneficial disclosures** (exemptions when agencies can release private health information without the client's prior authorization).

Workplace Applications

In an effort to limit casual access to the identity of clients and health information, HIPAA legislation has created several changes that affect the workplace. Some examples of these regulations include:

- The names of clients on charts can no longer be visible to the public.
- Clipboards must obscure identifiable names of clients and private information about them.
- Whiteboards must be free of information linking a client with a diagnosis, procedure, or treatment.
- Computer screens must be oriented away from public view. Flat screen monitors are more difficult to read at obtuse angles.
- Conversations regarding clients must take place in private places where they cannot be overheard. This has led to a trend of providing private rooms for all hospitalized clients so that personal health information cannot be overheard by someone else sharing the room.
- Facsimile (fax) machines, filing cabinets, and medical records must be located in areas off-limits to the public.
- A cover sheet and a statement indicating that faxed data contain confidential information must accompany electronically transmitted information.

BOX 9-2   **Exemptions for Beneficial Disclosures**

- Reporting vital statistics (births and deaths)
- Informing the U.S. Food and Drug Administration of adverse reactions to drugs or medical devices
- Disclosing information for organ or tissue donation
- Notifying the public health department about communicable diseases
- Notifying an identified person of a credible threat for imminent harm

---

- Light boxes for examining X-rays or other diagnostic scans on which the client's name appears must be in private areas.
- Documentation must be kept of those who have accessed a client's record.

Data Security

Maintaining confidentiality is more difficult with computerized data keeping. Because multiple people who enter and retrieve information from computer files can access electronically stored data, it has been difficult to monitor use or to limit access to only authorized people within and outside a health care institution.

As a result of HIPAA legislation, health agencies are adopting the following methods to ensure the protection of electronic data:

- Assigning an access number and password to authorized personnel who use a computer for health records. These are kept secret and changed regularly.
- Using automatic save, use of a screensaver, or return to a menu if data have been displayed for a specific period
- Issuing a plastic card or key that authorized personnel use to retrieve information
- Locking out client information except to those who have been authorized through a fingerprint or voice activation device
- Blocking the type of information that personnel in various departments can retrieve. For example, laboratory employees can obtain information from the medical orders, but they cannot view information in the client's personal history.
- Storing the time and location from which the client's record is accessed in case there is an allegation concerning a breach in confidentiality
- Encrypting any client information transmitted through the internet

DOCUMENTING INFORMATION

Each agency sets its own documentation policies. In addition to identifying the method for charting, such policies generally indicate the type of information recorded on each chart form, the people responsible for charting, and the frequency for making entries on the record. Box 9-3 lists the general content of nursing documentation. Current standards of accreditation agencies require that the medical records of clients cared for in acute care agencies (e.g., hospitals) must identify the steps of the nursing process (assessment, diagnosis, planning, implementation, and evaluation of outcomes).

Because consistency in charting is important for legal purposes, nurses must follow the agency's documentation policy. Deviating from the charting policy reduces a nurse's legal protection if the record is subpoenaed (see Chapter 3).

Using Abbreviations

Abbreviations shorten the length of documentation and the time required for this task. Brevity, however, must never take

<table>
<tr><td>BOX 9-3</td><td>Content of Nursing Documentation</td></tr>
</table>

Nurses or those to whom they delegate client care are responsible for documenting:

- Assessment data[a]
- Client care needs
- Routine care such as hygiene measures
- Safety precautions that have been used
- Nursing interventions described in the care plan
- Medical treatments prescribed by the physician
- Outcomes of treatment and nursing interventions
- Client activity
- Medication administration
- Percentage of food consumed at each meal
- Visits or consults by physicians or other health professionals
- Reasons for contacting the physician and the outcome of the communication
- Transportation to other departments, like the radiography department, for specialized care or diagnostic tests, and time of return
- Client teaching and discharge instructions
- Referrals to other health care agencies

[a]In acute care settings, TJC requires a registered nurse to document the admission nursing assessment findings and develop the initial plan of care. The registered nurse may delegate some aspects of the initial data collection to the practical or vocational nurse.

priority over completeness and accuracy. It is better to write at length than to omit information or make vague entries.

Many abbreviations have common meanings; however, nurses cannot assume that all abbreviations are interpreted the same universally. Some may have one meaning in one locale or agency but may mean something different or be unfamiliar in another. To avoid confusion among caregivers and misinterpretation if the chart is subpoenaed as legal evidence, each agency provides a list of approved abbreviations and their meanings. *When documenting, nurses must use only those abbreviations on the agency's approved list.*

TJC has identified specific abbreviations that should not be used in order to protect the safety of clients (available via TJC's website; see the resources on thePoint' or by searching the term *"National Patient Safety Goals 02.02.01" in a search engine*). There may be future deletions of dangerous abbreviations, acronyms, symbols, and dose designations as accreditation agencies monitor and evaluate compliance. Currently, the ban on using unapproved abbreviations does not apply to health IT systems such as EMRs, but accreditation agencies recommend that they be eliminated from newly appropriated or upgraded systems. Some common abbreviations are listed in Table 9-3; more can be found in the Appendix.

Indicating Documentation Time

The nurse identifies the date and time of each entry in the record; this happens automatically with electronic documentation. Some hospitals use **traditional time** (time based on two 12-hour revolutions on a clock), which is identified with

TABLE 9-3 Commonly Used Abbreviations

ABBREVIATION	MEANING
abd.	abdomen
a.c.	before meals
ad lib	as desired
AMA	against medical advice
amt.	amount
approx.	approximately
b.i.d.	twice a day
BM	bowel movement
BP	blood pressure
bpm	beats per minute
BRP	bathroom privileges
c̄	with
C	Centigrade
CCU	coronary care unit
c/o	complains of
dc	discontinue
ED	emergency department
et	and
H_2O	water
I & O	intake and output
IM	intramuscular
IV	intravenous
kg	kilogram
L	liter
L and Lt	left
lb	pound
NKA	no known allergies
NPO	nothing by mouth
NSS	normal saline solution
O_2	oxygen
OB	obstetrics
OOB	out of bed
OR	operating room
per	by or through
P	pulse
p.c.	after meals
p.o.	by mouth
postop.	postoperative
preop.	preoperative
pt.	patient
PT	physical therapy
q	every
q.i.d.	four times a day
q.s.	quantity sufficient
R	respirations
R and Rt	right
s̄	without
SS	soap suds
stat	immediately
t.i.d.	three times a day
TPR	temperature, pulse, respirations
UA	urinalysis
via	by way of
WC	wheelchair
WNL	within normal limits
Wt.	weight

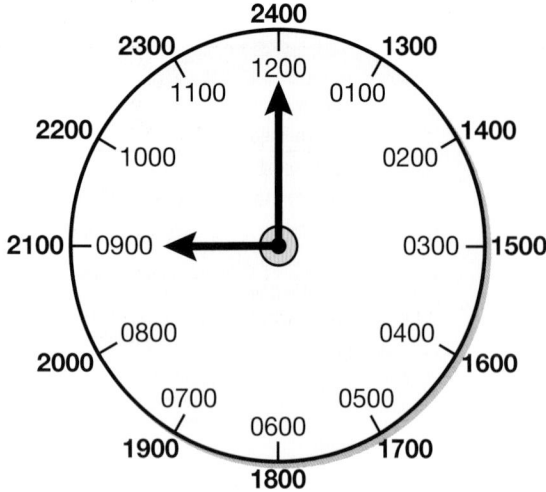

FIGURE 9-5 The military clock uses one 24-hour time cycle instead of two 12-hour cycles (e.g., 9:00 AM is 0900 and 9:00 PM is 2100).

the hour and minute, followed by AM or PM. Other agencies prefer **military time** (time based on a 24-hour clock), which uses a different four-digit number for each hour and minute of the day (Fig. 9-5 and Table 9-4). The first two digits indicate the hour within the 24-hour period, and the last two digits indicate the minutes.

The use of military time avoids confusion because no number is ever duplicated, and the labels AM, PM, midnight, and noon are not needed. Military time begins at midnight (2400 or 0000). One minute after midnight is 0001. A zero is placed before the hours of one through nine in the morning; for example, 0700 refers to 7 AM and is stated as "oh seven hundred." After noon, 12 is added to each hour; therefore, 1 PM is 1300. Minutes are given as 1 to 59. See Skill 9-1.

⟫ *Stop, Think, and Respond 9-2*

Convert the following from traditional time to military time:

1. *6:30 PM*
2. *Midnight*
3. *8:45 AM*
4. *9:05 PM*
5. *4:15 AM*

TABLE 9-4 Examples of Military Time Conversions

TRADITIONAL TIME	MILITARY TIME
Midnight	0000 or 2400
12:01 AM	0001
1:30 AM	0130
Noon	1200
1:00 PM	1300
3:15 PM	1515
7:59 PM	1959
10:47 PM	2247

COMMUNICATION FOR CONTINUITY AND COLLABORATION

Although the medical record serves as an ongoing source of information about the client's status, nurses use other methods of communication to promote continuity of care and collaboration among the health care providers involved in the client's care. These methods are in written or verbal forms.

Written Forms of Communication

Examples of written forms of communication include the nursing care plan, the nursing Kardex, checklists, and flow sheets.

Nursing Care Plans

A **nursing care plan** is a written or printed list of the client's problems, goals, and nursing orders for client care. It promotes the prevention, reduction, or resolution of health problems. The principles and style for writing a diagnostic statement, goals, and nursing orders are described in Chapter 2.

Presently, accreditation agencies' standards require that the record show evidence of plan of care. Many agencies require a separate nursing care plan as a means of demonstrating compliance. Nurses revise the plan of care as the client's condition changes.

Most agencies use preprinted care plans, computer-generated care plans, standards of care, clinical pathways, or cite the plan of care within progress notes.

Because the nursing care plan is part of the permanent record and thus is a legal document, it is compiled and maintained following documentation principles. All entries and revisions are dated. The written components are clear, concise, and legible. The information is never obliterated; only approved abbreviations are used. Each addition or revision to the plan is signed.

Nursing Kardex

The nursing **Kardex** is a quick reference for current information about the client and the client's care (Fig. 9-6). The Kardex forms for all clients are centrally located in a folder at the nursing station to allow caregivers to flip from one client's data to another. The Kardex has the following uses:

- Locate clients by name and room number.
- Identify each client's physician and medical diagnosis.
- Serve as a reference for a change-of-shift report.
- Serve as a guide for making nursing assignments.
- Provide a rapid resource for current medical orders on each client.
- Specify the client's code or do-not-resuscitate (DNR) status.
- Check quickly on a client's diet.
- Alert nursing personnel to a client's scheduled tests or test preparations.
- Inform staff of a client's current level of activity.
- Identify comfort or assistive measures a client may require.
- Provide a tool for estimating the personnel-to-client ratio for a nursing unit.

```
3/10/24        539                        Page 001      3/10/24        539                        Page 002

Stevens, James                          M 65            Stevens, James                          M 65
MR #: 00310593          Acct #: 9400037290             MR #: 00310593          Acct #: 9400037290
DR: J. Carrio                      2/W 204-01           DR: J. Carrio                      2/W 204-01
DX: Unstable angina          Date: 3/10/24             DX: Unstable angina          Date: 3/10/24

SUMMARY : 3/10        0701 to 1501                     SUMMARY: 3/10        0701 to 1501

PATIENT INFORMATION                                    SCHEDULED MEDICATIONS:
    3/10      ADVANCE DIRECTIVE : No.                      3/10      Nitroglycerin oint 2%, 1-1/2 in, apply to chest wall
              Advance directive does not exist                      q 8 h, starting on 3/10, 1800 hrs.
    3/10      ORGAN DONOR:  Yes                            3/10      Diltiazem tab 90 mg, #1, P.O., q 6 h 0800, 1400, 2000, 0200
    3/10      ADMIT DX:  Unstable angina                   3/10      Furosemide tab 40 mg, #1, P.O., daily 0900
    3/10      MED ALLERGY:  None known                     3/10      Potassium chloride tab 10 mEq, #1, P.O., daily 0900
    3/10      ISOLATION:  Standard precautions             3/10      Labetalol tab 100 mg, #1/2, P.O. bid 0900, 1800

MISC. PATIENT DATA                                     STAT/NOW MEDICATIONS:
                                                       3/10      Furosemide tab 40 mg, #1, P.O. now
NURSING CARE PLAN PROBLEMS                             3/10      Potassium chloride tab 10 mEq, #1, P.O., now
3/10      Acute pain  R/T: anginal pain
                                                       PRN MEDICATIONS:
ALL CURRENT MEDICAL ORDERS                                 3/10      Procardia nifedipine cap 10 mg, #1, subling. q 6 n, prn
                                                                    SBP > 170 or DSBP > 105
NURSING ORDERS:                                            3/10      Acetaminophen tab 325 mg, #2, P.O., q 4 h, prn for pain
3/10          Activity, OOB, up as tol.                    3/10      Temazepam cap 15 mg, #1, P.O. 1 HS, prn
3/10          Routine V/S q & h                            3/10      Alprazolam tabl 0.25 mg, #1/2, P.O., q 8 h, prn
              Telemetry
3/10          If 1800 PTT < 50, increase heparin drip   LABORATORY:
              to 1200 units/hr. If 50 to 100, maintain     3/10      CK & MB 1800 today
              1000 units/hr. If > 100, reduce to 900       3/10      CK & MB 0200 tomorrow
              units/hr.                                    3/10      Urinalysis floor to collect
DIET:                                                      3/10      PTT 1800 today
    3/10      Diabetic: 1600 cal., start with lunch today
I.V.s.:                                                LABORATORY:
    3/10      Peripheral line #1. . . . Start D2W 250 ml   3/10      Stress test persantine, perp H1, Patient handling:
              with heprin 25,000 units: rate, 1000                  Wheelchair, Schedule: tomorrow
              units/hr.

                                        (continued)                                 Last page
```

FIGURE 9-6 A computer-generated Kardex. (Holmes, H. N. [2006]. *Documentation in action* [pp. 231–232]. Lippincott Williams & Wilkins, used with permission.)

The information in the Kardex changes frequently, sometimes several times a day. The Kardex is not a part of the permanent record. Therefore, nurses can write information in pencil and erase it.

Checklists

A **checklist** is a form of documentation in which the nurse indicates the performance of routine care with a check mark or initials. It is an alternative to writing a narrative note. Nurses use paper checklists or a designated file on a computer primarily to avoid documenting types of care that are regularly repeated such as bathing and mouth care. This charting technique is especially helpful when the care is similar each day and the client's condition does not differ much for extended periods.

Flow Sheets

A **flow sheet** is a form of documentation with sections for recording frequently repeated assessment data. It enables nurses to evaluate trends because similar information is located on one form. Some flow sheets provide room for recording numbers or brief descriptions.

Interpersonal Communication

In addition to using written resources (e.g., the medical record) to exchange information, communication also takes place during personal interactions among health providers. Some examples include:

• Change-of-shift reports
• Client assignments
• Team conferences
• Rounds
• Telephone calls

Change-of-Shift Report

A **change-of-shift report** is a discussion between a nursing spokesperson from the shift that is ending and the arriving personnel (Fig. 9-7). It includes a summary of each client's condition and current status of care (Box 9-4).

To maximize the efficiency of change-of-shift reports, nurses should:

• Be prompt so that the report can start and end on time.
• Come prepared with a pen and paper or clipboard.
• Avoid socializing during reporting sessions.
• Take notes.
• Clarify unclear information.
• Ask questions about pertinent information that may have been omitted.

Some agencies scan and record the report, which saves time because there are no interruptions or digressions. In

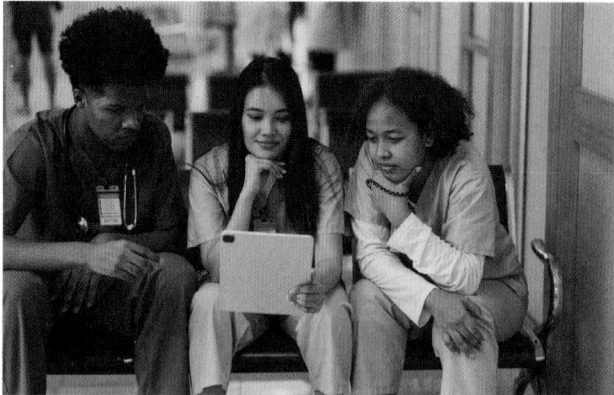

FIGURE 9-7 Nurses begin their shifts by receiving reports on their clients. (Party people studio/Shutterstock.)

addition, nurses can replay portions of the digital recording if information needs to be repeated. A recorded report, however, does not allow direct questions, elaboration, or clarification with the person who recorded the report.

Client Care Assignments

Client care assignments are made at the beginning of each shift. Assignments are posted, discussed with team members, or written on a worksheet (Fig. 9-8). Each assignment identifies the clients for whom the staff person is responsible and describes their care. Meals and break times may also be scheduled, as well as special tasks such as checking and restocking supplies.

Team Conferences

Conferences are commonly used to exchange information. Topics generally include client care problems, personnel conflicts, new equipment or treatment methods, and changes

BOX 9-4 Change-of-Shift Report

A change-of-shift report usually includes the following:

- Name of client, age, and room number
- Name of physician
- Medical diagnosis or surgical procedure and date
- Range in vital signs
- Abnormal assessment data
- Characteristics of pain, medication, amount, time last administered, and outcome achieved
- Type of diet and percentage consumed at each meal
- Special body position and level of activity, if applicable
- Scheduled diagnostic tests
- Test results, including those performed by the nurse, such as blood glucose levels
- Changes in medical orders, including newly prescribed drugs
- Intake and output totals
- Type and rate of infusing intravenous fluid
- Amount of intravenous fluid that remains
- Settings on electronic equipment such as amount of suction
- Condition of incision and dressing, if applicable
- Color and amount of wound or suction drainage

in policies or procedures. Team conferences often include the nursing staff, staff from other departments involved in client care, physicians, social workers, personnel from community agencies, and, in some cases, clients and their significant others (Fig. 9-9). Usually, one person organizes and directs the conference. Responsibilities for certain outcomes that result from the team conference may be delegated to various staff members who attend the meeting.

Client Rounds

Rounds (visits to the bedside of clients on an individual basis or as a group) are used as a means of learning firsthand about clients (Fig. 9-10). When done as a group, the client is a witness to and often an active participant in the interaction. Observing and conversing in the client's presence provides an opportunity to survey the client's condition and determine the status of equipment used in their care. It also tends to boost client confidence and security in their care. Since the passage of HIPAA regulations, however, agencies avoid this type of communication if another client shares the room or if the client has not authorized family members or friends who may be visiting to have access to their health information.

Telephone

Nurses use the telephone to exchange information when it is difficult for people to get together or when they must communicate information quickly. When using the telephone, the nurse:

- Answers as promptly as possible
- Speaks in a normal tone of voice
- Identifies themselves by name, title, and nursing unit
- Obtains or states the reason for the call
- Discreetly identifies the client being discussed to avoid being publicly overheard
- Spells the client's name if there is any chance of confusion
- Converses in a courteous and business-like manner
- Repeats information to ensure it has been heard accurately

When notifying a physician about a change in a client's condition, the nurse documents in the client's record the information reported and the instructions received. In an effort to support TJC's National Patient Safety Goals regarding the improvement of staff communication and identifying patient safety risks, the **SBAR format** (Table 9-5) has been recommended as a model for effective communication.

SBAR refers to:

- S (Situation): What is the situation about which you are calling?
- B (Background): Pertinent background information related to the situation
- A (Assessment): What is your assessment of the situation?
- R (Recommendation): Explain what is needed or wanted.

If the nurse believes that the physician has not responded in a safe manner to the information given, they notify the nursing supervisor or the head of the medical department.

NURSING ASSIGNMENT SHEET

TEAM MEMBER _Jane Doe L.P.N._
TEAM LEADER _Mary Black R.N._

BREAK _9:15 A.M._ CONFERENCE _10:30 A.M._ LUNCH _12:00 N._ DATE: _____

ASSIGNMENT _Filling and distributing water carafes on the Northwing_

ROOM	PATIENT	BATH	ACTIVITY	DIET	FLUIDS	TO BE CHECKED	TREATMENTS	SPECIMEN	COMMENTS
296¹	Flora Brown — Duodenal Ulcer	BED / SELF * / SHOWER / (TUB) / SITZ	BED / DANGLE / BRP / AMB·HELP / WALKER / CRUTCHES / WC	REGULAR / SOFT / SURG LIQ / FULL LIQ / (SPECIAL) Sippy / FASTING / TUBE FEEDING	FORCE / NPO / LIMIT / SIPS WATER / ICE CHIPS / IV / DIST WATER	(BLOOD PRESSURE) qd / TPR / TEST URINE A.C. & HS / SLIDING SCALE / I&O / LEVIN TUBE / CHEST TUBE / FOLEY / OXYGEN	ENEMA / DOUCHE / PERI CARE·LIGHT / WEIGH / ORAL HYGIENE / SPECIAL BACK CARE / PREPARE FOR SURG / PREPARE FOR X·RAY / OT·PT·ECT	(STOOL) qd / URINE / SPUTUM / BLOOD / CULTURE / TISSUE	
296²	Mary Green — Coronary	(BED) / SELF * / SHOWER / TUB / SITZ	(BED) / DANGLE / BRP·HELP / AMB·HELP / WALKER / CRUTCHES / WC	REGULAR / SOFT / SURG LIQ / (FULL LIQ) low / (SPECIAL) Na / FASTING / TUBE FEEDING	FORCE / NPO / LIMIT / SIPS WATER / ICE CHIPS / IV / DIST WATER	(BLOOD PRESSURE) 8-12 / TPR q4h / TEST URINE A.C. & HS / SLIDING SCALE / I&O / LEVIN TUBE / CHEST TUBE / FOLEY q4h·1 hr·q / (OXYGEN) q4h·1 hr·q	ENEMA / DOUCHE / (PERI CARE)·LIGHT / (WEIGH) / ORAL HYGIENE / SPECIAL BACK CARE / PREPARE FOR SURG / PREPARE FOR X·RAY / OT·PT·ECT	STOOL / URINE / SPUTUM / BLOOD / CULTURE / TISSUE	
298¹	John Snapp — C.O.P.D.	BED / (SELF *) / SHOWER / TUB / SITZ	BED / DANGLE / (BRP) / (AMB) č O₂ / WALKER / CRUTCHES / WC	REGULAR / (SOFT) / SURG LIQ / FULL LIQ / SPECIAL / FASTING / TUBE FEEDING	(FORCE) / NPO / LIMIT / SIPS WATER / ICE CHIPS / IV / DIST WATER	BLOOD PRESSURE / TPR / TEST URINE A.C. & HS / SLIDING SCALE / (I&O) / LEVIN TUBE / CHEST TUBE / FOLEY / (OXYGEN) 1-4/M cont.	(ENEMA) Fleets / DOUCHE / PERI CARE·LIGHT / WEIGH / ORAL HYGIENE / SPECIAL BACK CARE / PREPARE FOR SURG / PREPARE FOR X·RAY / OT·PT·ECT	STOOL / URINE / (SPUTUM) / BLOOD / CULTURE / TISSUE	1000 ml 5% D/W č 500 mg Aminophylline @ 900 ml/sec cont.
298²	Tom Henry — C.H.F.	(BED) / SELF * / SHOWER / TUB / SITZ	BED / (DANGLE) / BRP·HELP / AMB·HELP / WALKER / CRUTCHES / WC	REGULAR / SOFT / SURG LIQ / (FULL LIQ) 1200 / (SPECIAL) Na / FASTING / TUBE FEEDING	FORCE / NPO / (LIMIT) 300/sh / SIPS WATER / ICE CHIPS / IV / DIST WATER	(BLOOD PRESSURE) 8-12 / TPR / TEST URINE A.C. & HS / SLIDING SCALE / (I&O) / LEVIN TUBE / CHEST TUBE / (FOLEY) / OXYGEN 4 L/M cont.	ENEMA / DOUCHE / (PERI CARE)·LIGHT / WEIGH / (ORAL HYGIENE) 8-12 / (SPECIAL BACK CARE) / PREPARE FOR SURG / PREPARE FOR X·RAY / OT·PT·ECT	STOOL / URINE / SPUTUM / BLOOD / CULTURE / TISSUE	Change position q 2hr.
299	Jim Smith — Diabetes Mellitus	BED / (SELF *) / (SHOWER) / TUB / SITZ	BED / DANGLE / BRP / (AMB) / WALKER / CRUTCHES / WC	REGULAR / SOFT / SURG LIQ / (FULL LIQ) 1200 / (SPECIAL) Diabetic / FASTING / TUBE FEEDING	FORCE / NPO / LIMIT / SIPS WATER / ICE CHIPS / IV / DIST WATER	BLOOD PRESSURE / TPR / (TEST URINE A.C. & HS) / (SLIDING SCALE) / I&O / LEVIN TUBE / CHEST TUBE / FOLEY / OXYGEN	ENEMA / DOUCHE / PERI CARE·LIGHT / WEIGH / ORAL HYGIENE / SPECIAL BACK CARE / PREPARE FOR SURG / PREPARE FOR X·RAY / OT·PT·ECT	STOOL / URINE / SPUTUM / BLOOD / CULTURE / TISSUE	
		BED / SELF * / SHOWER / TUB / SITZ	BED / DANGLE / BRP / AMB·HELP / WALKER / CRUTCHES / WC	REGULAR / SOFT / SURG LIQ / FULL LIQ / SPECIAL / FASTING / TUBE FEEDING	FORCE / NPO / LIMIT / SIPS WATER / ICE CHIPS / IV / DIST WATER	BLOOD PRESSURE / TPR / TEST URINE A.C. & HS / SLIDING SCALE / I&O / LEVIN TUBE / CHEST TUBE / FOLEY / OXYGEN	ENEMA / DOUCHE / PERI CARE·LIGHT / WEIGH / ORAL HYGIENE / SPECIAL BACK CARE / PREPARE FOR SURG / PREPARE FOR X·RAY / OT·PT·ECT	STOOL / URINE / SPUTUM / BLOOD / CULTURE / TISSUE	
		BED / SELF * / SHOWER / TUB / SITZ	BED / DANGLE / BRP / AMB·HELP / WALKER / CRUTCHES / WC	REGULAR / SOFT / SURG LIQ / FULL LIQ / SPECIAL / FASTING / TUBE FEEDING	FORCE / NPO / LIMIT / SIPS WATER / ICE CHIPS / IV / DIST WATER	BLOOD PRESSURE / TPR / TEST URINE A.C. & HS / SLIDING SCALE / I&O / LEVIN TUBE / CHEST TUBE / FOLEY / OXYGEN	ENEMA / DOUCHE / PERI CARE·LIGHT / WEIGH / ORAL HYGIENE / SPECIAL BACK CARE / PREPARE FOR SURG / PREPARE FOR X·RAY / OT·PT·ECT	STOOL / URINE / SPUTUM / BLOOD / CULTURE / TISSUE	

CODE
* : YOU WASH BACK AND LEGS
BRP : BATHROOM PRIVILEGES
AMB : AMBULATORY
I&O : INTAKE AND OUTPUT

WC : WHEELCHAIR
BP : BLOOD PRESSURE
NPO : NOTHING BY MOUTH
DIST : DISTILLED WATER

ECT : ELECTRICAL CONVULSIVE THERAPY
OT : OCCUPATIONAL THERAPY
PT : PHYSICAL THERAPY

FIGURE 9-8 Sample of a nursing assignment sheet.

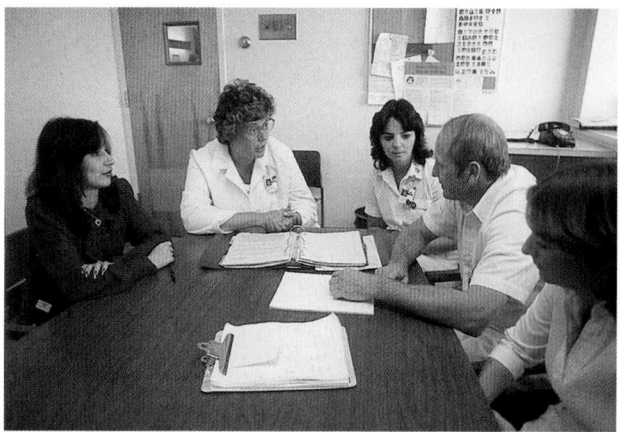

FIGURE 9-9 A team of personnel hold a conference to discuss the care of a client. (Rosdahl, C. B., & Kowalski, M. T. [2021]. *Textbook of basic nursing* [12th ed.]. Lippincott Williams & Wilkins.)

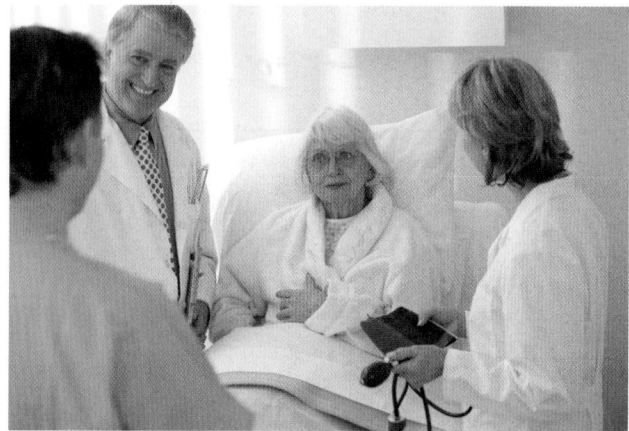

FIGURE 9-10 Rounds help acquaint oncoming staff with the client.

TABLE 9-5 SBAR Format

S	**Situation:** What is the situation you are calling about? Identify yourself, unit, patient, and room number. Briefly state the problem, what it is, when it happened or started, and how severe.
B	**Background:** Pertinent background information related to the situation could include: The admitting diagnosis and date of admission List of current medications, allergies, IV fluids, and labs Most recent vital signs Lab results: The date and time test was done and results of previous tests for comparison Code status Other clinical information
A	**Assessment:** What is your assessment of the situation?
R	**Recommendation:** What is your recommendation about what should happen next? For example, there may need to be notification that a patient has been admitted, that a patient needs to be seen immediately, or that an order must be changed.

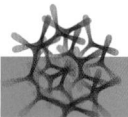

KEY POINTS

- Reasons for client charts and medical records:
  - Permanent account
  - Sharing information
  - QA
  - Accreditation
  - Reimbursement
  - Education and research
  - Legal evidence
- Methods of charting:
  - Narrative
  - SOAP
  - Focus
  - PIE
  - Charting by exception
  - Electronic
- HIPAA: Regulations that require health care agencies to safeguard written, spoken, and electronic health information

- Review abbreviations list for approved medical abbreviations and "do not use" lists.
- Review and understand the conversion of traditional time to military time: The military clock uses one 24-hour time cycle instead of two 12-hour cycles (e.g., 9:00 AM is 0900 and 9:00 PM is 2100, adding 12 hours to the 12-hour cycle time).
- Written forms of communication:
  - Nursing care plans
  - Nursing Kardex
  - Checklists
  - Flow sheets
- Interpersonal communication:
  - Change-of-shift report
  - Client care assignments
  - Team conferences
  - Client rounds
  - Telephone

CRITICAL THINKING EXERCISES

1. What are some reasons for protecting the information within a client's health record?
2. In your opinion, what is the most important reason for compiling and maintaining a client's health record?
3. When initially employed, how can the nurse ensure they are documenting information appropriately?
4. Explain the possible consequences if a nurse's documentation contains illegible writing, unapproved abbreviations, and misspelled words. How would you help the nurse improve their documentation?

NEXT-GENERATION NCLEX-STYLE REVIEW QUESTIONS

1. Which nursing action violates the HIPAA?
   a. The nurse assigns five clients equally to each person on the team.
   b. The nurse writes the names of clients on a dry erase board in a public area.
   c. The nurse posts the names of the assigned staff in the client's room.
   d. The nurse reviews the Kardex of each client during a shift report.
   Test-Taking Strategy: Use the process of elimination to exclude situations that do not apply to the HIPAA legislation. Recall that this law protects the confidentiality of clients from others who are not involved in the client's care.

2. When a nurse reviews the documentation of a nursing team member who has just been hired, which practice is most important to correct?
   a. The newly hired person documents in a partially filled space.
   b. The newly hired person charts information at 2-hour intervals.
   c. The newly hired person uses abbreviations in the documentation.
   d. The newly hired person signs an entry with first and last name and title.
   Test-Taking Strategy: Note the key word and modifier, "most important." Review the choices and select the option that contradicts the principles of legally defensible charting.

3. When electronically documenting at the bedside of a client, which nursing actions are most appropriate? Select all that apply.
   a. Logging on and off when entering data
   b. Returning the screen to the main menu
   c. Making entries in other client records
   d. Asking others to leave while making an entry
   e. Turning the computer off before leaving
   Test-Taking Strategy: Note the key word and modifier, "most appropriate." Select options that describe actions for documenting data electronically, saving the documentation, and restoring the status of the computer allowing its use by others.

4. When a client voices concern with a nurse about keeping his medical information confidential, which situation is the nurse correct in identifying as one exception to maintaining confidentiality?
   a. Confidentiality can be breached when a client has attempted suicide.
   b. Confidentiality can be breached when a client has a substance use problem.
   c. Confidentiality can be breached when a client wishes to terminate further treatment.
   d. Confidentiality can be breached when a client has a highly contagious disease.
   Test-Taking Strategy: Use the process of elimination to select an option that allows information about a client to be shared without the client's consent.

5. When a nurse recognizes they have made a mistake in documenting written information, what actions are appropriate? Select all that apply.
   a. Obliterate the incorrect information with a black marker.
   b. Draw a single line through the incorrect information.
   c. Erase the misinformation so it is no longer readable.
   d. Specify the nature of the incorrect information.
   e. Discard the page and rewrite the entire documentation.
   f. Initial and date the error; rewrite the correction.
   Test-Taking Strategy: Read all the options carefully. Apply principles of legally defensible charting that apply to correcting written documentation.

SKILL 9-1 Making Entries in a Client's Record

Suggested Action	Reason for Action
ASSESSMENT	
Review the agency's policy for the charting format it uses.	Some agencies require personnel to use a specific style (e.g., SOAP charting, narrative charting, PIE charting) for documentation.
Locate the agency's list of approved abbreviations.	Abbreviations must be compatible with those that have been approved for legally defensible reasons.
Determine the paper form that is appropriate to use for documenting the information or locate the file within an electronic record used for nursing documentation via a computer.	Data obtained initially from the client are entered on the admission form; periodic additions about the client's condition and care are entered on a form commonly called "nurses' notes" or on a progress sheet. A graphic sheet or *flow sheet* is used to document numbers or trends in assessment data.
Check that the client's name is identified on the chart form or computer file.	If a sheet of paper becomes separated from the chart, proper identification ensures that it is reinserted into the appropriate record. Electronic records are opened and stored using the client's name.
PLANNING	
Resolve to document information as soon as it is obtained or at least every 1–2 hours.	The potential for inaccuracies or omissions increases when documentation is delayed.
Use a pen or keyboard to make entries; use the color of ink indicated by the agency's policy.	Ink is permanent. Black ink photocopies better than other colors.
IMPLEMENTATION	
Record the date and time.	Information is recorded in chronologic order. The time of documentation is when the notation is written. Legal issues often involve the timing of events.
Write, print, or type information so that it can be read easily. Take care that keyboarding is accurate when a computer is used.	The entry loses its value for exchanging information if it is unreadable. Illegible entries become questionable in a court of law.
Use accurate spelling and grammar.	Literacy skills reflect a person's knowledge and education.
Be brief but complete; delete articles ("a," "an," "the").	Extra words add length to the entry.
Do not state the client's name; do not use *pt.* as an abbreviation for "patient."	It is understood that all the entries refer to the person identified on the chart form.
Use only agency-approved abbreviations and symbols.	Using approved abbreviations promotes consistent interpretation.
Document information clearly and accurately without any subjective interpretation. Quote the client if a statement is pertinent.	The chart is a record of facts, not opinions.
Avoid phrases such as "appears to be" or "seems to be."	Phrases implying uncertainty suggest that the nurse lacks reasonable knowledge.
Never use "ditto" marks.	Even if information is repetitious, it must be documented separately.
Identify actual or approximate sizes when describing assessment data rather than using relative descriptions such as large, moderate, or small.	Nonspecific measurements are subject to wide interpretation and are therefore less accurate and informative.
Record adverse reactions; include the measures used to manage them.	Documentation may be necessary to demonstrate that the nurse acted reasonably and that the care was not substandard.
Identify the specific information that is taught and the evidence of the client's learning.	Ensures continuity in preparing the client for discharge.
Fill all the space on each line of the form; draw a line through any blank space on an unfilled line.	Filling space reduces the possibility that someone else will add information to the current documentation.
Never chart nursing activities before they have been performed.	Making early entries can cause legal problems, especially if the client's condition suddenly changes.
Follow agency policy for the interval between entries.	Frequent charting indicates that the client has been observed and attended to at reasonable periods.
Indicate the current time when charting a late entry (documentation of information that occurred earlier but was unintentionally omitted); write "late entry for . . .," identifying the date and time to which the documentation refers.	Correlating time with actual events promotes logic and order when evaluating the client's progress.

SKILL 9-1 Making Entries in a Client's Record (*continued*)

Suggested Action	Reason for Action
Draw a line through a mistake rather than scribbling through or in any other way obscuring the original words.	Corrections are done in such a way that all words are readable. Obliterated words can cast suspicion that the record was tampered with to conceal damaging information.
Put the word "*error*" followed by a date and initials next to the entry and immediately enter the corrected information. Some agencies specify that the nurse must indicate the nature of the error (e.g., "wrong medical record").	A jury seeing the word "*error*" without any explanation might assume that the nurse made an error in care rather than in documentation.
Sign each entry with a first initial, last name, and title.	The signature demonstrates accountability for what has been written.
Log off the computer after documenting in an electronic client record.	Logging off returns the computer to a home or menu page, which prevents anyone else from entering information under the name of the person who originally logged in. Exiting to a home or menu page prevents those who are unauthorized from viewing anything confidential on the computer screen.

EVALUATION

The writer's entries are:
- Dated and timed
- Accurate, comprehensive, and up to date
- Legibly written according to the agency's format
- Spelled correctly without grammatical errors
- Objectively written
- Free of unapproved abbreviations
- Identified with the writer's name and title

SAMPLE DOCUMENTATION

Date and Time   Dressing changed. Abdominal incision and sutures are intact. No evidence of redness, swelling, or drainage.
_____ J. Doe, LPN

UNIT 4

Performing Basic Client Care

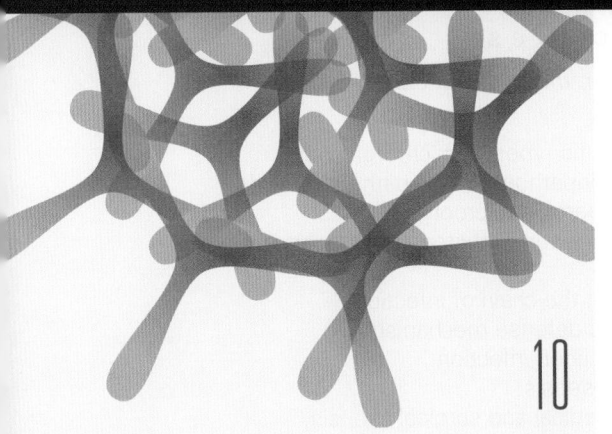

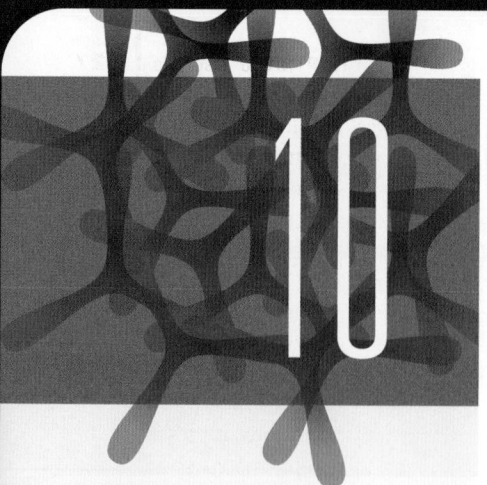

Asepsis

Words To Know

Learning Objectives

On completion of this chapter, the reader should be able to:

1. Describe microorganisms.
2. Name and describe specific types of microorganisms.
3. Differentiate between nonpathogens and pathogens and between aerobic and anaerobic microorganisms.
4. Give examples of the ways some microorganisms have adapted for survival.
5. Name the components in the chain of infection.
6. Cite examples of biologic defense mechanisms.
7. Define health care–associated infection.
8. Discuss the concept of asepsis.
9. Differentiate between medical and surgical asepsis.
10. Identify principles of medical asepsis.
11. List examples of medical aseptic practices.
12. Name techniques for sterilizing equipment.
13. Identify principles of surgical asepsis.
14. List nursing activities that require application of the principles of surgical asepsis.

INTRODUCTION

Preventing infections is one of the most important priorities in nursing. The most effective method is hand hygiene, an essential nursing activity that must be performed repeatedly when caring for clients. This chapter discusses how microorganisms survive and how to use **aseptic techniques**, measures that reduce or eliminate microorganisms.

 Gerontologic Considerations

■ Pneumonia, influenza, urinary tract and skin infections, and tuberculosis (TB) are common in older adults. Most cases of TB occur in people ages 65 or older living in long-term care facilities (QIAGEN, 2022). Adults 65 years of age or older had the highest TB incidence rate in 2020 (3.4 per 100,000 persons) and experienced the largest percentage decrease (24.3%) compared with 2019 (4.5 per 100,000 persons) (Centers for Disease Control and Prevention [CDC], 2020).

■ Pathogens may find a portal of entry into vulnerable older adults through devices such as indwelling urinary catheters, humidifiers, oxygen administration devices, and tissues compromised by equipment used for administering intravenous fluids, parenteral nutrition, tube feedings, and reprocessed endoscopy equipment that has not been thoroughly disinfected.

■ Many long-term care residents, older hospitalized clients, and health care providers are colonized with antibiotic-resistant bacteria, possibly with few or no symptoms.

■ Hospitals are now obtaining nasal cultures of clients to identify any that have been colonized with methicillin-resistant *Staphylococcus aureus* (MRSA).

■ In postmenopausal patients, thinning, drying, and decreased vascular supply to the skin and mucous membranes within the urinary tract due to a decline in circulating estrogen predispose the client to urinary tract infections.

■ An enlarged prostate, common in aging males, traps urine in the bladder, leading to urinary tract infections that are often overtreated with antibiotics leading to resistant pathogens.

■ Older adults often have comorbidities such as diabetes, which increases the risk for infections.

■ Visitors with respiratory infections need to wear masks or avoid contact with older adults in their homes or long-term care settings until their symptoms have subsided. In addition to the mask, frequent and thorough hand washing can help prevent the transfer of organisms.

■ Older adults, family members in close contact with older people, and all personnel in health care settings should obtain annual immunizations against influenza, a virus spread via respiratory secretions. People 65 years and older should receive an initial dose of the pneumococcal vaccine.

MICROORGANISMS

Microorganisms, living animals or plants visible only through a microscope, are commonly called "microbes" or "germs." What they lack in size, they make up for in numbers. Microorganisms are present everywhere—in the air, soil, and water and on and within virtually everything and everyone.

Once microorganisms invade, one of three events occurs: the body's immune defense mechanisms eliminate them, they reside within the body without causing disease, or they cause an infection or an infectious disease. Factors that influence whether an infection develops include the type and number of microorganisms, the characteristics of the microorganism (such as its **virulence**, the ability to overcome the immune system), and the person's state of health.

Types of Microorganisms

Microorganisms are divided into two main groups: **nonpathogens** or **normal flora** (harmless, beneficial microorganisms), and **pathogens** (microorganisms that cause illness).

Nonpathogens

Nonpathogens live abundantly and perpetually on and within the human body, which is their host. They are found in areas of the body exposed to the external environment, as well as internal areas such as the skin, nose, mouth, throat, lower urethra, and intestines. They have adapted to human defense mechanisms like acidic sweat and oil secretions on the skin. Most exist in the large intestine, having been introduced from food or substances on fingers, pencils, tableware, and other items placed in the mouth. Nonpathogens assume one of two relationships with the human host—mutually

beneficial or neither harming nor helping the host. They inhibit pathogenic growth and reproduction by competing for nutrients, vying for space, or producing substances that interfere with pathogens. They thus ensure a hospitable habitat for themselves.

Pathogens

Pathogens have a high potential for causing infectious **communicable diseases** (diseases that can be transmitted to other people), also called **contagious diseases** and **community-acquired infections**. Some examples of communicable diseases are measles, streptococcal sore throat, sexually transmitted infections, and TB. Although pathogenic infections can result in death, most of them lead only to temporary illness. They may cause illness in various ways. They may become established, grow, and proliferate when numbers of nonpathogens are reduced such as when **broad-spectrum antibiotics** (those prescribed to eliminate a wide range of bacteria) are prescribed. Pathogens may also cause infections when the host is immunosuppressed from acquired immunodeficiency syndrome (AIDS), cancer chemotherapy, or steroid drug therapy.

In addition, their structures and functions may promote virulence (the extent of dangerousness) of pathogens. Some have *fimbriae*, tiny hairs used to attach themselves to the host's tissue to avoid expulsion. Fimbriae prevent pathogens that reach the bladder from being eliminated during urination. Some pathogens use *flagella*, long tails that promote motility to reach a site less hostile to survival. Others release *toxins* (harmful chemicals). Many enter the host's cells and use their content to support their life cycles.

 Pharmacologic Considerations

Broad- and narrow-spectrum antibiotics each have unique benefits. Broad-spectrum antibiotics are active against a wide range of bacteria and preferred for use when:

■ Antiinfective therapy needs to start before the pathogen is identified.

■ Multiple pathogenic organisms are involved.

■ Resistance to narrow-spectrum drugs is identified.

Narrow-spectrum antibiotics target specific bacteria and are less likely to kill nonpathogenic bacteria or result in resistance when the bacterial pathogen is identified.

Nonpathogens and pathogens include bacteria, viruses, fungi, rickettsiae, protozoans, mycoplasmas, helminths, and prions.

Bacteria

Bacteria are single-celled microorganisms. They appear in various shapes: round (cocci), rod shaped (bacilli), and spiral (spirochetes) (Fig. 10-1). **Aerobic bacteria** require oxygen to live, while **anaerobic bacteria** exist without oxygen; this difference demonstrates how varied these life forms have become.

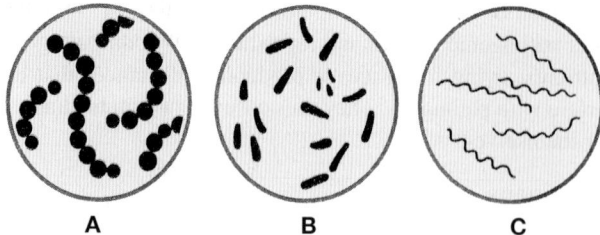

FIGURE 10-1 Classification of bacteria according to shape: cocci (**A**), bacilli (**B**), and spirochetes (**C**).

Viruses

Viruses, the smallest microorganisms known to cause infectious diseases, are visible only through an electron microscope. They are filterable, which means that they can pass through very small barriers. Viruses are unique because they do not possess all the genetic information necessary to reproduce; they require metabolic and reproductive materials from other living species. Some can remain dormant in a human and reactivate sporadically, causing recurrence of an infectious disorder. An example is the herpes simplex virus (HSV), which can cause cold sores (fever blisters) to repeatedly flare up after an initial infection.

Some viral infections, such as the common cold, are minor and self-limiting, that is, they terminate with or without medical treatment. Others, such as rabies, poliomyelitis, hepatitis, coronavirus, and AIDS, are more serious or fatal.

Fungi

Fungi include yeasts and molds. Only a few types of fungi produce infectious diseases in humans. The three types of fungal (mycotic) infections are superficial, intermediate, and systemic. Superficial fungal infections affect the skin, mucous membranes, hair, and nails. Examples include tinea corporis (ringworm), tinea pedis (athlete's foot), and candidiasis (a yeast infection that infects mucous membranes in the mouth and the vagina). Intermediate fungal infections affect subcutaneous tissues such as fungal granuloma (an inflammatory lesion under the skin). Systemic fungi infect deep tissues and organs, such as histoplasmosis in the lungs.

Rickettsiae

Rickettsiae resemble bacteria; like viruses, however, they cannot survive outside another living species. Consequently, an intermediate life form, such as fleas, ticks, lice, or mites, transmits rickettsial diseases to humans. For example, tiny deer ticks transmit Lyme disease, a problem found where people live, work, or enjoy activities in wooded areas.

Protozoans

Protozoans are single-celled animals classified according to their ability to move. Some use amoeboid motion, by which they extend their cell walls and their intracellular contents flow forward. Others move by cilia (hairlike projections) or flagella (whiplike appendages). Some cannot move independently at all.

Mycoplasmas

Mycoplasmas lack cell walls. They are referred to as *pleomorphic* because they assume various shapes. Mycoplasmas are similar but not related to bacteria. Primarily, they infect the surface linings of the respiratory, genitourinary, and gastrointestinal tracts.

Helminths

Helminths are infectious worms, some of which are microscopic. They are classified into three major groups: nematodes (roundworms), cestodes (tapeworms), and trematodes (flukes). Some helminths enter the body in the egg stage, while others spend the larval stage in an intermediate life form before finding their way into humans. Helminths mate and reproduce after they invade a species. They are then excreted, and the cycle begins again.

Prions

At one time, it was believed that all infectious agents contain nucleic acid, either deoxyribonucleic acid (DNA) or ribonucleic acid (RNA), compounds that control cellular functions and heredity. The idea of an atypical infectious agent (initially referred to as a rogue protein) was proposed in 1967. Dr Stanley Prusiner won a Nobel Prize in 1997 for his discovery of *prions*.

A prion is a protein containing no nucleic acid. Research suggests that a normal prion, which is present in brain cells, protects against dementia (diminished mental function). When a prion mutates, however, it can become an infectious agent that alters other normal prion proteins into similar mutant copies. The mutants, which can result from either genetic predisposition or transmission between same or similar infected animal species, cause transmissible spongiform encephalopathies. These are so named because they cause the brain to become spongy (i.e., full of holes). As a result, brain tissue withers, leading to uncoordinated movements. Examples of transmissible spongiform encephalopathies include bovine spongiform encephalopathy (mad cow disease), scrapie in sheep, and Creutzfeldt–Jakob disease in humans. Researchers are currently trying to determine whether prions are the cause of neurologic disorders such as Alzheimer disease, Parkinson disease, and Huntington disease; whether people with these disorders lack prions; and whether prions in people with these disorders are ineffective.

Survival of Microorganisms

Each species of microorganism is unique, but all microorganisms share one characteristic, that is, although infinitesimally small, they are powerful enough to cause disease. All they need is a favorable environment in which to survive. Conditions that promote survival include warmth, darkness, oxygen, water, and nourishment. Humans offer all these, and so they are optimal hosts for supporting the growth and reproduction of microorganisms.

Many pathogens have mutated to adapt to hostile environments and unfavorable living conditions. Such adaptability has ensured that they continue to pose a threat to humans. One example of biologic adaptation is the ability of some

- Prescribing antibiotics for minor or self-limiting bacterial infections
- Administering antibiotics prophylactically (for prevention) in the absence of an infection
- Failing to take the full course of antibiotic therapy
- Taking someone else's prescribed antibiotic without knowing whether it is effective for one's illness or symptoms
- Prescribing antibiotics for viral infections (antibiotics are ineffective for treating infections caused by viruses)
- Dispersing antibiotic solutions into the environment
- Depositing partially empty intravenous (IV) bags containing antibiotic drugs in waste containers
- Releasing droplets while purging IV tubing attached to secondary bags of antibiotic solution
- Expelling air from syringes before injecting antibiotics
- Administering antibiotics to livestock, leaving traces of drug residue that humans consume after their slaughter
- Spreading pathogens via unwashed or poorly washed hands

microorganisms to form spores. A **spore** is a temporarily inactive microbial life form that can resist heat and destructive chemicals and can survive without moisture. Consequently, spores are more difficult to destroy than their more biologically active counterparts. When conditions are favorable, spores can reactivate and reproduce.

Another example of adaptation is the development of antibiotic-resistant bacterial strains of *Staphylococcus aureus*, *Enterococcus faecalis* and *E. faecium*, and *Streptococcus pneumoniae*. Such strains no longer respond to drugs that once were effective against them (Box 10-1). Next-generation technologies are developing new and cost-effective treatments using genetic information for emerging antimicrobial resistance. Additionally, researchers speculate that resistant species can transmit their resistant genes to totally different microbial species (National Institute of Allergy and Infectious Diseases, 2018).

CHAIN OF INFECTION

By interfering with the conditions that perpetuate the transmission of microorganisms, humans can avoid acquiring infectious diseases. The six essential components in the **chain of infection** (the sequence that enables the spread of disease-producing microorganisms) must be in place if pathogens are to be transmitted from one location or person to another:

1. An infectious agent
2. A reservoir for growth and reproduction
3. An exit route from the reservoir
4. A means of transmission
5. A portal of entry
6. A susceptible host (Fig. 10-2)

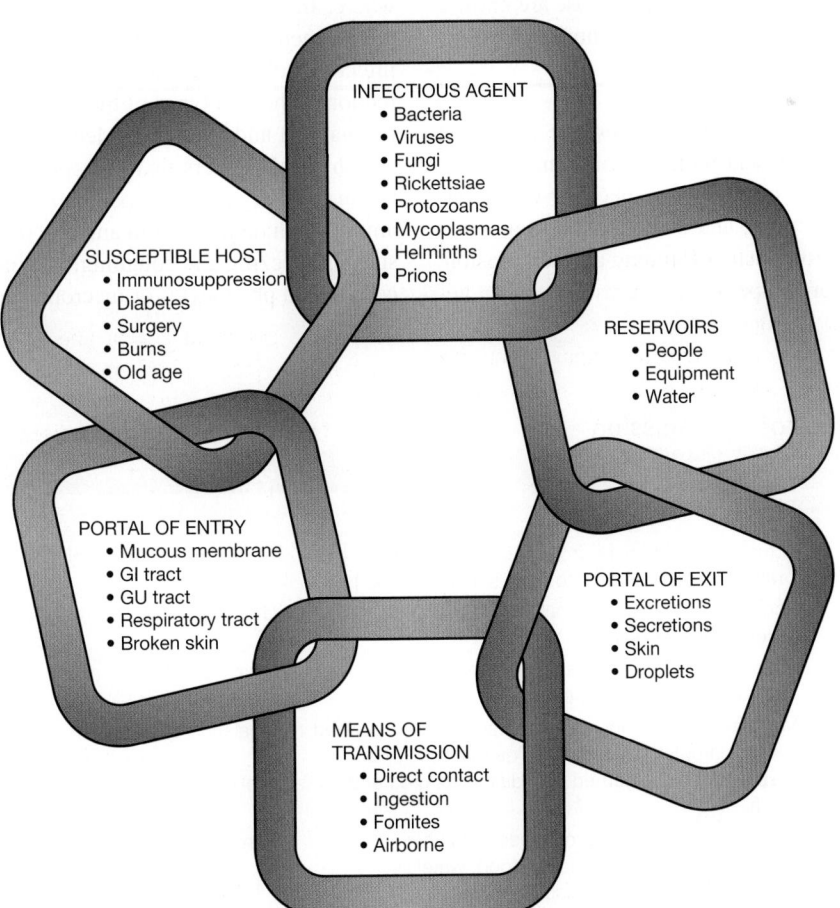

FIGURE 10-2 The chain of infection. GI, gastrointestinal; GU, genitourinary.

Infectious Agents

Some microorganisms are less dangerous than others. Just as some animal species coexist *symbiotically* (for mutual benefit), some normal flora help maintain healthy functioning. For example, intestinal bacteria help produce vitamin K that helps control bleeding. Vaginal bacteria create an acidic environment hostile to the growth of pathogens.

Unless the supporting host becomes weakened, normal flora remain controlled. If the host's defenses are weakened, however, even benign microorganisms can cause **opportunistic infections** (infectious disorders among people with compromised health). More commonly, however, infections result from pathogens that inherently produce illness after invading body tissues and organs.

Reservoirs

A **reservoir** is a place where microbes grow and reproduce, providing a haven for their survival. Microorganisms thrive in reservoirs such as tissues within the superficial crevices of the skin, on shafts of hair, in open wounds, in the blood, inside the lower digestive tract, and in nasal passages. Some grow abundantly in stagnant water, in uncooked and unrefrigerated food, and on used utensils or equipment. They are present in intestinal excreta and the earth's organic matter.

Asymptomatic clients or animals that harbor pathogens but do not show evidence of an infectious disease are known as **carriers**. Nonliving reservoirs are called **fomites**.

Exit Routes

The **exit route** is how microorganisms escape from the original reservoir. When present within or on humans, they are displaced by handling or touching objects or whenever blood, body fluids, secretions, and excretions are released. In the environment, factors such as flooding and soil erosion provide mechanisms for escape.

 Concept Mastery Alert

Common Exit Routes

Major key exit routes for organisms include the respiratory tract through coughing, sneezing, and possibly talking and the gastrointestinal tracts through vomiting and stool. Breaking the chain of infection at the link of the exit route can significantly reduce the risk for infectious diseases.

Means of Transmission

The **means of transmission** is how infectious microorganisms move to other locations. This component is important to the microorganism's survival because most microorganisms cannot travel independently. Microorganisms are transmitted by one of five routes: contact, droplet, airborne, vehicle, and vector (Table 10-1).

Portal of Entry

The **portal of entry** is where microorganisms find their way onto or into a new host, thus facilitating relocation. One of the most common ports of entry is an opening in the skin or mucous membranes. Microorganisms also can be inhaled, swallowed, introduced into the blood, or transferred into body tissues or cavities through unclean hands or contaminated medical equipment.

Although microorganisms exist in reservoirs everywhere, **biologic defense mechanisms** (anatomic or physiologic methods that stop microorganisms from causing an infectious disorder) often prevent them from producing infections. The two types of biologic defense mechanisms are mechanical and chemical. Mechanical defense mechanisms are physical barriers that prevent microorganisms from entering the body or that expel them before they multiply. Examples include intact skin and mucous membranes, reflexes such as sneezing and coughing, and infection-fighting blood cells called phagocytes or macrophages.

TABLE 10-1 Methods of Transmission

ROUTE	DESCRIPTION	EXAMPLE
Contact transmission		
Direct contact	Actual physical transfer from one infected person to another (body surface to body surface contact)	Sexual intercourse with an infected person
Indirect contact	Contact between a susceptible person and a contaminated object	Use of a contaminated surgical instrument
Droplet transmission	Transfer of moist particles from an infected person who is within a radius of 3 ft	Inhalation of droplets released during sneezing, coughing, or talking
Airborne transmission	Movement of microorganisms attached to evaporated water droplets or dust particles that have been suspended and carried over distances greater than 3 ft	Inhalation of spores
Vehicle transmission	Transfer of microorganisms present on or in contaminated items such as food, water, medications, devices, and equipment	Consumption of water contaminated with microorganisms
Vector transmission	Transfer of microorganisms from an infected animal carrier	Diseases spread by mosquitoes, fleas, ticks, or rats

Chemical defense mechanisms destroy or incapacitate microorganisms through natural biologic substances. For example, lysozyme, an enzyme found in tears and other secretions, can dissolve the cell wall of some microorganisms. Gastric acid creates an inhospitable microbial environment. Antibodies, complex proteins also called immunoglobulins, form when macrophages consume microorganisms and display their distinct cellular markers.

Susceptible Host

Humans become susceptible to infections when their defense mechanisms are diminished or impaired. A **susceptible host**, the last link in the chain of infection, is one whose biologic defense mechanisms are weakened in some way (Box 10-2). Ill clients are prime targets for infectious microorganisms because their health is already compromised. Health care providers who are sick should stay at home rather than exposing already ill clients to infectious microorganisms.

Particularly susceptible clients include those who:

- Are older adults or premature infants
- Are burn victims
- Have experienced major trauma
- Require invasive procedures such as endoscopy (see Chapter 14)
- Need indwelling equipment such as a urinary catheter
- Receive implantable devices such as intravenous catheters
- Are given antibiotics inappropriately, promoting microbial resistance
- Are receiving anticancer drugs and antiinflammatory drugs such as corticosteroids that suppress the immune system
- Are infected with human immunodeficiency virus (HIV)

⟩⟩ *Stop, Think, and Respond 10-1*

Use the chain of infection to trace the transmission of the common cold from one person to another.

ASEPSIS

Health care institutions are teeming reservoirs of microorganisms because of the sheer numbers of confined sick people. Add to this the number of caregivers, equipment, and treatment devices in constant use, and it is easy to understand why infection control is so important. Nurses must understand and practice methods to prevent **health care–associated infections** (infections acquired while a person is receiving care in a health care agency).

Asepsis refers to those practices that decrease or eliminate infectious agents, their reservoirs, and vehicles for transmission. It is the major method for preventing and controlling infection. Health care providers use medical and surgical asepsis to accomplish this goal.

Medical Asepsis

Medical asepsis means those practices that confine or reduce the numbers of microorganisms. Also called *clean technique*, it involves measures that interfere with the chain of infection in various ways. The following principles underlie medical asepsis:

- Microorganisms exist everywhere except on sterilized equipment.
- Frequent hand hygiene and maintaining intact skin are the best methods for reducing the transmission of microorganisms.
- Blood, body fluids, cells, and tissues are considered major reservoirs of microorganisms.
- Personal protective equipment such as gloves, gowns, masks, goggles, and hair and shoe covers serve as barriers to microbial transmission.
- A clean environment reduces microorganisms.
- Certain areas like the floor, toilets, and the insides of sinks are more contaminated than others.
- Cleaning should be done in order from cleaner to dirtier areas rather than vice versa.

Examples of medical aseptic practices include using antimicrobial agents, performing hand hygiene, wearing protective garments, confining and containing soiled materials appropriately, and keeping the environment as clean as possible. Measures used to control the transmission of infectious microorganisms are discussed in more detail in Chapter 22.

Using Antimicrobial Agents

Antimicrobial agents are chemicals that destroy or suppress the growth of infectious microorganisms (Table 10-2). Some antimicrobial agents are used to clean equipment, surfaces, and inanimate objects. Others are applied directly to the skin or administered internally. Examples are antiseptics, disinfectants, and antiinfective drugs.

Antiseptics

Antiseptics, also known as *bacteriostatic agents*, inhibit the growth of but do not kill microorganisms. An example is alcohol. Antiseptics generally are applied to the skin or mucous membranes. Some are also used as cleansing agents.

Disinfectants

Disinfectants, also called *germicides* and *bactericides*, destroy active microorganisms but not spores. Phenol, household bleach, and formaldehyde are examples. Disinfectants are rarely applied to the skin because they are very strong; rather, they are used to kill and remove microorganisms from equipment, walls, and floors.

BOX 10-2	Factors Affecting Susceptibility to Infections

- Inadequate nutrition
- Poor hygiene practices
- Suppressed immune system
- Chronic illness
- Insufficient white blood cells
- Prematurity
- Advanced age
- Compromised skin integrity
- Weakened cough reflex
- Diminished blood circulation

TABLE 10-2 Antimicrobial Agents

TYPE	MECHANISM	EXAMPLE	USE
Soap	Lowers the surface tension of oil on the skin, which holds microorganisms; facilitates removal during rinsing	Dial, Safeguard	Hygiene
Detergent	Acts as soap, except detergents do not form a precipitate when mixed with water	Dreft, Tide	Sanitizing eating utensils, laundry
Alcohol	Injures the protein and lipid structures in the cellular membrane of some microorganisms (70% concentration)	Isopropyl ethanol	Cleansing skin, instruments
Iodine	Damages the cell membrane of microorganisms and disrupts their enzyme functions; not effective against *Pseudomonas*, a common wound pathogen	Betadine	Cleansing skin
Chlorine	Interferes with microbial enzyme systems	Bleach, Clorox	Disinfecting water, utensils, blood spills
Chlorhexidine	Damages the cell membrane of microorganisms, but is ineffective against spores and most viruses	Hibiclens	Cleansing skin and equipment
Glutaraldehyde	Inactivates cellular proteins of bacteria, viruses, and microbes that form spores	Cidex	Sterilizing equipment

Antiinfective Drugs

The two groups of drugs used most often to combat infections are antibacterials and antivirals.

The chemical actions of antibacterials, which consist of antibiotics and sulfonamides, alter the metabolic processes of bacteria but not viruses. They damage or destroy bacterial cell walls or the mechanisms that bacteria need to reproduce. When used, the intent is to kill or control pathogens; however, these drugs have the capacity to similarly affect normal nonpathogenic bacteria. Before the advent of antibacterial therapy, wound infections, dysentery, and many contagious diseases shortened life expectancy. Some believe that humans will return to the days of epidemics, plagues, and pestilence when antibacterial agents can no longer control microorganisms. A current example of this phenomenon is the emergence of MRSA and vancomycin-resistant *Enterococcus* (VRE).

Antiviral agents were developed more recently, most likely in response to the rising incidence of influenza and blood-borne viral diseases such as hepatitis and AIDS. Most antivirals do not destroy infecting viruses; rather, they control **viral replication**, or the release of copies from the infected cells, to limit the **viral load** (the number of viral copies), or stimulate the immune system to interfere with the infectious process. Viruses such as HSV-1 and HSV-2 that cause cold sores and genital infections as well as varicella-zoster virus (HZV), another type of herpes virus that causes shingles, remain dormant and can potentially reactivate from time to time. In a similar fashion, when a person with AIDS becomes drug-resistant or discontinues drug therapy, the HIV replicates again.

 Pharmacologic Considerations

The discovery and use of antiviral medications has turned once-deadly viral infections (such as HIV and hepatitis C) into chronic diseases.

Hand Hygiene

Hand hygiene refers to removing surface contaminants on the skin by either hand washing or hand antisepsis. **Hand washing** is a medical aseptic practice that involves cleaning the hands with soap, water, and friction to mechanically remove dirt and organic substances. It is the preferred method of hand hygiene when the hands are visibly dirty, when the hands are soiled with blood or other body fluids, after using the toilet, or when exposure to potential spore-forming pathogens is strongly suspected or proven (CDC, 2022b). Hand washing removes **resident microorganisms** (generally, nonpathogens constantly present on the skin) and **transient microorganisms** (pathogens picked up during brief contact with contaminated reservoirs).

Although transient microorganisms are more pathogenic, hand washing removes them more easily. They tend to cling to grooves and gems in rings, the margins of chipped nail polish and broken or separated artificial nails, and long fingernails. Thus, these items are contraindicated when caring for clients. Without conscientious hand washing, transient microorganisms become residents, thereby increasing the potential for transmission of infection. One possible explanation for the increase of antimicrobial-resistant pathogens is that health care–acquired pathogens are replacing the normal flora of clients when health care providers fail to wash their hands at appropriate times for a minimum of 20 seconds (CDC, 2022b). Considering how often health care providers use their hands when touching or using equipment in their care, it is no surprise that *hand hygiene is the single most effective way to prevent infections*. Skill 10-1 describes the steps of hand washing. Certain situations require hand washing; in others, nurses may substitute hand antisepsis (Box 10-3).

In 2009, the World Health Organization (WHO) introduced a simplified campaign identifying "Your 5 Moments for Hand Hygiene" (Fig. 10-3) (WHO, 2022) to help health care providers link hand hygiene with direct client care. Health care agencies and their personnel have since adopted the process worldwide.

BOX 10-3	Hand Washing and Hand Antisepsis Guidelines

Soap and Water	Alcohol-Based Hand Sanitizer
• Before, during, and after preparing food • Before eating food • Before and after caring for someone who is sick • Before and after treating a cut or wound • After using the bathroom, changing diapers, or cleaning up a child who has used the bathroom • After blowing your nose, coughing, or sneezing • After touching an animal, animal food or treats, animal cages, or animal waste • After touching garbage • If your hands are visibly dirty or greasy	• Before and after visiting a friend or a loved one in a hospital or nursing home, unless the person is sick with *Clostridium difficile* (if so, use soap and water to wash hands). • If soap and water are not available, use an alcohol-based hand sanitizer that contains at least 60% alcohol, and wash with soap and water as soon as you can. NOTE: Do NOT use hand sanitizer if your hands are visibly dirty or greasy: for example, after gardening, playing outdoors, or fishing or camping (unless a hand washing station is not available). Wash your hands with soap and water instead.

Centers for Disease Control and Prevention. (2021). *Hand sanitizer use out and about.* https://www.cdc.gov/handwashing/hand-sanitizer-use.html#:~:text=DO%20NOT%20use%20hand%20sanitizer,with%20soap%20and%20water%20instead

>> *Stop, Think, and Respond 10-2*

Discuss actions for ensuring appropriate hand washing before and after caring for a client in their home. Use a scenario in which the client has a bar soap that rests on the bathroom sink and terrycloth hand towels shared among an entire family.

Performing Hand Antisepsis

Research has shown that health care workers comply with the minimum requirements for hand washing less than 50% of the time (Institute for Healthcare Improvement, 2014). To improve compliance with hand hygiene, guidelines for hand antisepsis with alcohol-based hand rubs have been developed. **Hand antisepsis** means the removal and destruction of transient microorganisms without soap and water (Skill 10-2). It involves products such as alcohol-based liquids, thick gels, and foams. Alcohol-based hand rubs are not substitutes for hand washing in all situations (see Box 10-3). Alcohol does not remove soil or dirt with organic material; however, it does produce antisepsis when the hands are visibly clean. Alcohol-based hand rubs remove microorganisms on the hands, including Gram-positive and Gram-negative bacteria, fungi, multidrug-resistant pathogens, and viruses. Because alcohol formulations have a brief rather than sustained antiseptic effect, however, nurses must reuse them over the course of a day.

Advantages of alcohol-based hand rubs over hand washing are that they (1) take less time considering drying does not require the use of paper towels; (2) are more accessible because they do not require sinks or water; (3) increase compliance because they are easier to perform; (4) provide convenience based on their location at the client's point of care; (5) provide the fastest and greatest reduction in microbial counts on the skin; (6) reduce costs by eliminating paper towels and waste management; and (7) are less irritating and drying than soap because they contain emollients. The Centers for Disease Control and Prevention (CDC) believes that with higher compliance, there is a greater potential for reducing the rate of health care–associated infections (see section "Standard Precautions and Infection Control Precautions", in Chapter 22).

Performing Surgical Hand Antisepsis

Surgical hand antisepsis, previously referred to as a surgical scrub, is a medically aseptic hand hygiene procedure that is performed before donning sterile gloves and garments when the nurse is actively involved in an operative or obstetric procedure. The purpose is to more extensively remove transient microorganisms from the nails, hands, and forearms. In fact, the cleanser should reduce microbial growth for increasingly longer periods when repeatedly performed. Table 10-3 lists several differences between surgical hand antisepsis and routine hand washing.

To maximally reduce the number of microorganisms, the fingernails must be short—no more than 1/4-in long, a length that does not extend beyond the tip of the fingers (CDC, 2022a). Artificial nails are prohibited. Nail polish is discouraged, especially if it is chipped, worn, or on for more than 4 days because it is conducive to harboring an increased number of microorganisms. All rings, watches, and jewelry are removed and safeguarded before surgical hand antisepsis (Skill 10-3).

Wearing Personal Protective Equipment

To reduce the transfer of microorganisms between themselves and clients, health care providers wear various garments including uniforms, scrub suits or gowns, masks, gloves, hair and shoe covers, and protective eyewear. They wear some of these items when caring for any client regardless of diagnosis or presumed infectious status (see Chapter 22).

Uniforms

Health care providers should wear their uniforms only while working with clients. Some nurses wear clean laboratory coats over their uniforms to reduce the spread of microorganisms onto or from the surface of clothing worn from home. When caring for clients, the nurse would wear a plastic apron or cover gown over the uniform if there is a potential for soiling it with blood or body fluids. When not wearing a cover, nurses take care to avoid touching the uniform with any soiled items such as bed linens. After work, they should change the uniform as soon as possible to avoid exposing their families and the public to the microorganisms present on work clothing.

Your 5 Moments
for Hand Hygiene

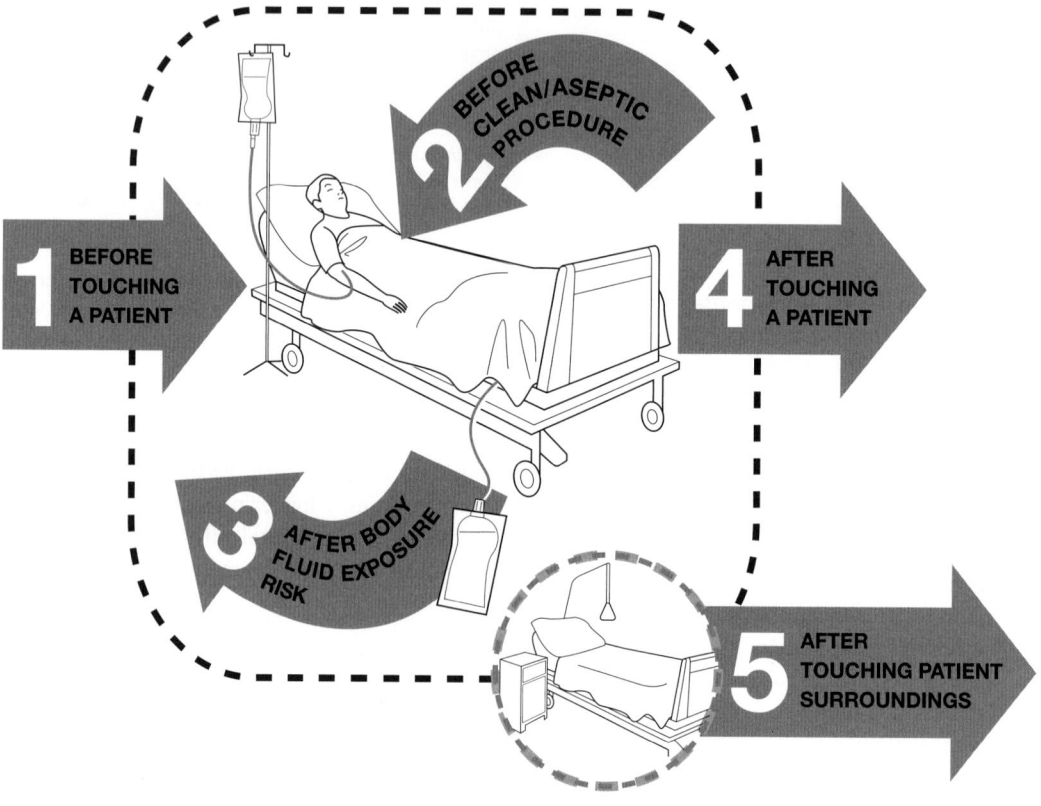

1	**BEFORE TOUCHING A PATIENT**	**WHEN?**	Clean your hands before touching a patient when approaching him/her.
		WHY?	To protect the patient against harmful germs carried on your hands.
2	**BEFORE CLEAN/ASEPTIC PROCEDURE**	**WHEN?**	Clean your hands immediately before performing a clean/aseptic procedure.
		WHY?	To protect the patient against harmful germs, including the patient's own, from entering his/her body.
3	**AFTER BODY FLUID EXPOSURE RISK**	**WHEN?**	Clean your hands immediately after an exposure risk to body fluids (and after glove removal).
		WHY?	To protect yourself and the health-care environment from harmful patient germs.
4	**AFTER TOUCHING A PATIENT**	**WHEN?**	Clean your hands after touching a patient and her/his immediate surroundings, when leaving the patient's side.
		WHY?	To protect yourself and the health-care environment from harmful patient germs.
5	**AFTER TOUCHING PATIENT SURROUNDINGS**	**WHEN?**	Clean your hands after touching any object or furniture in the patient's immediate surroundings, when leaving – even if the patient has not been touched.
		WHY?	To protect yourself and the health-care environment from harmful patient germs.

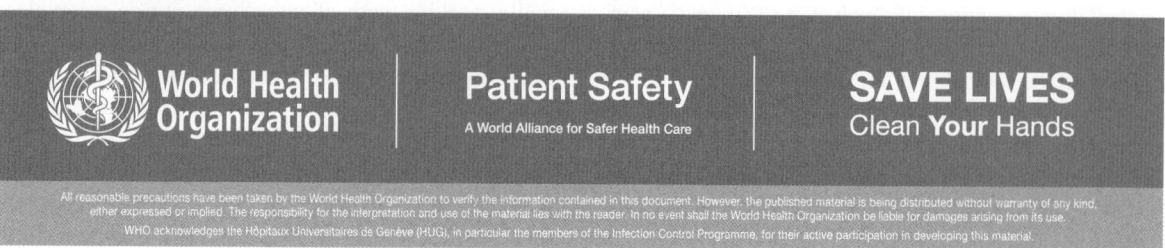

World Health Organization | **Patient Safety** A World Alliance for Safer Health Care | **SAVE LIVES** Clean **Your** Hands

FIGURE 10-3 *Your 5 Moments for Hand Hygiene*, a guide to improve the practice of hand hygiene. (World Health Organization. [2022]. *WHO guidelines on hand hygiene in healthcare.* Author.)

TABLE 10-3 Differences between Hand Washing and Surgical Hand Antisepsis

HAND WASHING	SURGICAL HAND ANTISEPSIS
Plain wedding band may be worn.	All hand jewelry, including watches, are removed.
Faucets with hand controls are used; elbow, knee, or foot controls are preferred.	Faucets are regulated with elbow, knee, or foot controls.
Liquid, bar, leaflet, or powdered soap or detergent is used.	Liquid antibacterial soap is used; devices such as sponges may be incorporated with antibacterial soap.
Washing lasts a minimum of 20 seconds.	Antisepsis lasts 2–6 minutes, depending on the antibacterial agent and time interval between subsequent repetitions.
Hands are held lower than the elbows during washing, rinsing, and drying.	Hands are held higher than the elbows during washing, rinsing, and drying.
Areas beneath fingernails are washed.	Areas beneath fingernails are cleaned with an orange stick or similar nail cleaner.
Friction is produced by rubbing the hands together.	Friction is produced by scrubbing with a brush or sponge.
Hands are dried with paper towels; the paper is used to turn off hand-regulated faucet controls.	Hands are dried with sterile towels.
Clean gloves are donned if the nurse has open skin or if there is a potential for contact with blood or body fluids.	Sterile gloves are donned immediately after the hands are dried.

Scrub Suits and Gowns

Scrub suits and gowns are hospital garments worn instead of a uniform. Their use is mandatory in some areas of a hospital, such as the nursery, the operating room, and the delivery room. These garments prevent health care providers from bringing microorganisms on their clothes into the working environment. Employees in other departments sometimes wear their own scrub suits or gowns because they are comfortable and practical. Providers who work in mandatory-wear areas put on scrub suits and gowns when they arrive for work. They wear cover gowns over the scrubs when taking breaks in other agency locations during their shift. Nurses discard mandatory-wear scrub suits and gowns in a laundry receptacle and change into street clothes before leaving the place of employment.

Masks

Masks are disposable, loose-fitting covers for the nose and mouth (Fig. 10-4). They help prevent droplet and airborne transmission of microorganisms by keeping splashes or sprays from reaching the wearer's nose and mouth. They are worn once and then discarded.

Respirators

To prevent the transmission of TB, the National Institute for Occupational Safety and Health (NIOSH, 2013) recommends the use of a disposable or replaceable particulate air filter respirator that fits snugly to the face. The minimum specification for a particulate air filter respirator is N95; N refers to "not resistant to oil" (i.e., it is effective at blocking particulate aerosols that are free of oil). An N95 air filter respirator (Fig. 10-5) can filter very small particles that may contain viruses with a minimum efficiency of 95%.

Particulate respirators are custom-sized and fitted for each health care provider to ensure that there is less than 10% leakage between the seal of the mask and the wearer's face. Once fitted, the health care provider can reuse their own N95 respirator as long as it remains intact and clean,

and the wearer does not grow facial hair, gain or lose 10 lb, or incur other facial changes that interfere with a tight facial seal (Nursing Guidelines 10-1).

In certain high-risk situations, such as when a bronchoscopy or autopsy is performed on a client with TB, a respirator that exceeds the minimum standard is used. In those cases, a nonpowered air-purifying respirator (APR) or powered air-purifying respirator (PAPR) is required (CDC, 2014). This type of respirator removes air contaminants by blowing them through a high-efficiency particulate air (HEPA) filter, thus providing purified air to enter a facepiece, hood, or helmet.

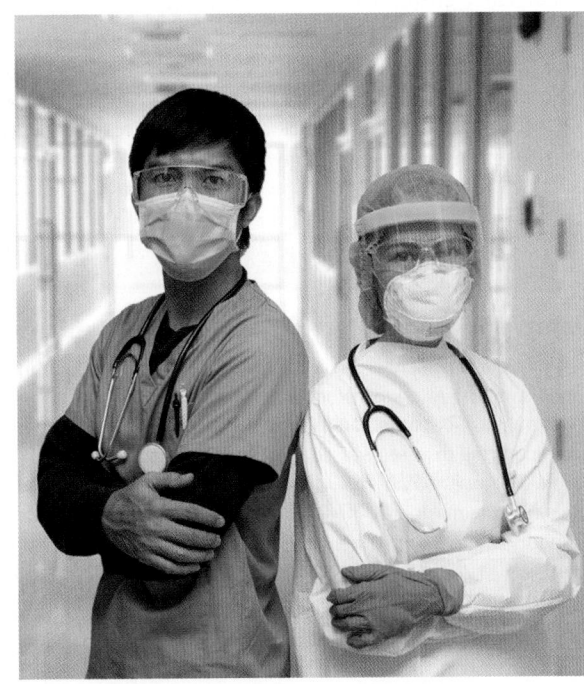

FIGURE 10-4 Various types of face masks. Earloop style and molded cup style.

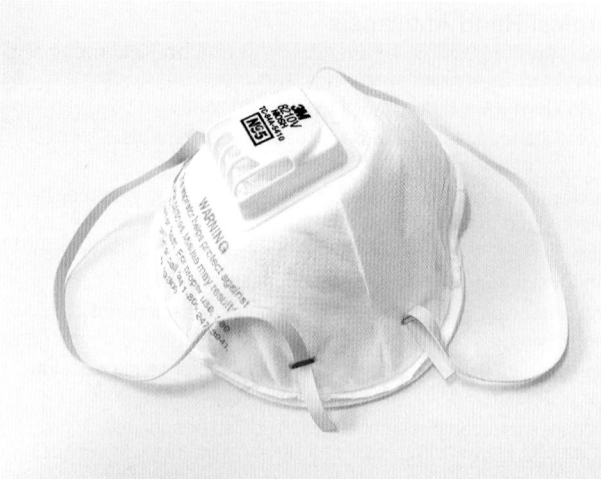

FIGURE 10-5 Example of an N95 respiratory face mask.

Gloves

Nurses wear clean gloves, sometimes called "examination gloves," in the following circumstances:

- As a barrier to prevent direct hand contact with blood, body fluids, secretions, excretions, mucous membranes, and nonintact skin
- As a barrier to protect clients from microorganisms transmitted from nursing personnel when performing procedures or care involving contact with the client's mucous membranes or nonintact skin
- When there is a potential transfer of microorganisms from one client or object to another during subsequent nursing care

Examination gloves are generally made of latex or vinyl, though other types are available (see Chapter 19). Latex and vinyl gloves are equally protective with nonvigorous use, but latex gloves have some advantages. They stretch and mold to fit the wearer almost like a second layer of skin, permitting greater flexibility with movement. Perhaps most importantly, they can reseal tiny punctures.

Unfortunately, some nurses and clients are allergic to latex. Reactions vary and range from annoying symptoms such as skin rash, flushing, itching and watery eyes, and nasal stuffiness to life-threatening swelling of the airway and low blood pressure. Nurses who are sensitive to latex can wear alternative types of gloves, or they can wear a double pair of vinyl gloves when the risk for contact with blood or body fluids is high. Gloves are changed if they become perforated, after a period of use, and between the care of clients. Hand hygiene is performed after removing gloves.

Hair and Shoe Covers

Hair and shoe covers reduce the transmission of pathogens present on the hair or shoes. Health care providers generally wear these garments during surgical or obstetric procedures. Shoe covers are fastened so that they cover the open ends of pant legs. Hair covers should envelop the entire head. Those with beards or long sideburns wear specially designed head covers that resemble a cloth or paper helmet. Even though hair covers are not required during general nursing care, health care providers should keep their hair short or contained with a clip, band, or some other means.

Protective Eyewear

Protective eyewear is essential when there is a possibility that body fluids will splash into the eyes. Goggles are worn along with a mask, or a multipurpose face shield is used (Fig. 10-6).

Confining Soiled Articles

Health care agencies use several medically aseptic practices to contain reservoirs of microorganisms, especially those on soiled equipment and supplies. They include using designated clean and dirty utility rooms and various waste receptacles.

Utility Rooms

Health care agencies have at least two utility rooms: one designated clean and the other considered dirty. Personnel must not place soiled articles in the clean utility room.

The dirty or soiled utility room contains covered waste receptacles, at least one large laundry hamper, and a flushable hopper. This room also houses equipment for testing stool

NURSING GUIDELINES 10-1

Using a Mask or Particulate Filter Respirator

- Wear a mask if there is a risk for coughing or sneezing within a radius of 3 ft. *The mask blocks the route of exit.*
- Wear a mask or particulate filter respirator if there is a potential for acquiring diseases caused by droplet or airborne transmission. *The mask blocks the port of entry.*
- Position the mask or respirator so that it covers the nose and mouth. *The mask provides a barrier to nasal and oral ports of entry.*
- Tie the upper strings of a mask snugly at the back of the head and the lower strings at the back of the neck. *Proper placement reduces the exit and entry routes for microorganisms.*
- Avoid touching the mask or respirator once it is in place. *Touching the mask transfers microorganisms to the hands.*
- Change the mask or respirator every 20 to 30 minutes or when it becomes damp; particulate filter respirators can be worn multiple times, but they must be rechecked for leakage and fit. *Changing the mask preserves its effectiveness.*
- Touch only the strings of the mask or the respirator strap during removal. *Touching the mask transfers microorganisms to the hands.*
- Discard used masks into a lined or waterproof waste container. *Proper disposal reduces the transmission of microorganisms to others.*
- Perform hand washing or hand antisepsis after removing a mask or respirator. *Hand washing and hand antisepsis remove microorganisms from the hands.*

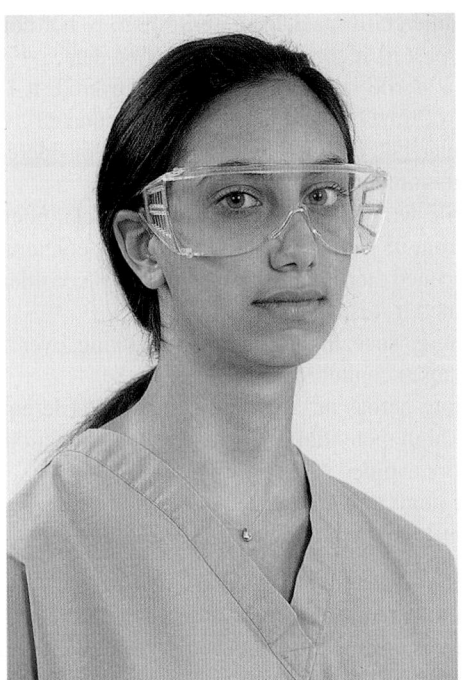

FIGURE 10-6 Protective goggles. (Photo by B. Proud.)

or urine. A sink is located in the soiled utility room for hand washing and for rinsing grossly contaminated equipment.

Waste Receptacles

Agencies rely on various methods to contain soiled articles until they can be discarded. Most clients have a paper bag at the bedside for tissues or other small, burnable items. Wastebaskets are generally lined with plastic. Suction and drainage containers are kept covered and emptied at least once during each shift. Most client rooms have a wall-mounted puncture-resistant container for needles or other sharp objects (Fig. 10-7).

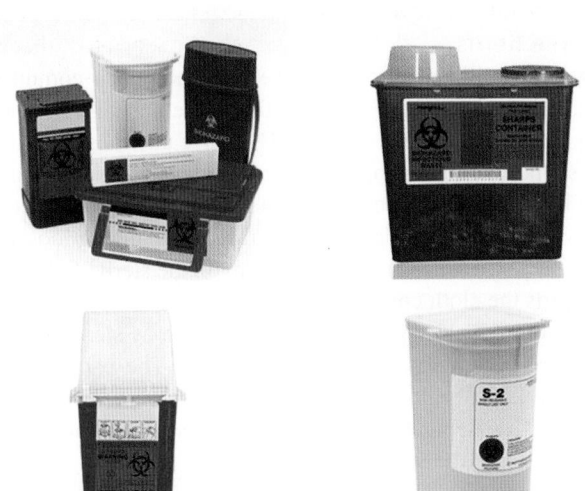

FIGURE 10-7 A sharps container. (U.S. Food and Drug Administration. [2021]. *Sharps disposal containers*. https://www.fda.gov/medical-devices/safely-using-sharps-needles-and-syringes-home-work-and-travel/sharps-disposal-containers)

Keeping the Environment Clean

Health agencies employ laundry staff and housekeeping personnel to assist with cleaning. In general, if soiled linen is bagged appropriately or handled with gloves, the detergents and heat from the water and the dryer are sufficient to rid linens of pathogenic organisms.

Housekeeping personnel are responsible for collecting and disposing of accumulated refuse and for performing concurrent and terminal disinfection. Housekeepers who follow the principles of medical asepsis carry out **concurrent disinfection** or measures that keep the client environment clean on a daily basis:

- They clean less soiled areas before grossly dirty ones.
- They wet-mop floors and damp-dust furniture to avoid dispersing microorganisms on dust particles and air currents.
- They frequently discard solutions used for mopping in a flushable hopper.
- They never place clean items on the floor.

Terminal disinfection is more thorough than concurrent disinfection and consists of measures used to clean a client's environment after discharge. It includes scrubbing the mattress surface and the insides of drawers and bedside stands.

Nurses who work in home health care can teach the client and the family simple aseptic practices for cleaning contaminated articles (Client and Family Teaching 10-1).

Client and Family Teaching 10-1
Cleaning Potentially Infectious Equipment

The nurse teaches the client and the family to:

- Wear waterproof gloves when handling heavily contaminated items or if there are open skin areas on the hands.
- Designate one container for the sole purpose of cleaning contaminated articles.
- Disassemble and rinse reusable equipment as soon as possible after use.
- Rinse grossly contaminated items first under cool, running water; hot water causes protein substances in body fluids to thicken or congeal.
- Soak reusable items in a solution of water and detergent or disinfectant if a thorough cleaning is not immediately possible.
- Use a sponge, scrub brush, or cloth to create friction and loosen dirt, body fluids, and microorganisms from the surface of contaminated articles.
- Force sudsy water through the hollow channels of items to remove debris.
- Rinse washed items well under running water.
- Drain rinsed equipment and air-dry.
- Wash hands for at least 20 seconds after cleaning equipment if the hands are visibly dirty, soiled with blood or other body fluids, or contaminated with proteinaceous material; substitute an alcohol-based hand rub in other circumstances.
- Store clean, dry items in a covered container or in a clean, folded towel.

Describe the methods of medical asepsis that are helpful in controlling the chain of infection of the common cold.

Surgical Asepsis

Surgical asepsis refers to those measures that render supplies and equipment totally free of microorganisms. **Sterile techniques** include practices that avoid contaminating microbe-free items. Both begin with the process of sterilization.

Sterilization

Sterilization consists of physical and chemical techniques that destroy all microorganisms, including spores. Sterilization of equipment is done within the health agency or by manufacturers of hospital supplies. Labels on commercially sterilized equipment identify a safe use date.

Physical Sterilization

Microorganisms and spores are destroyed physically through radiation or heat, boiling water, free-flowing steam, dry heat, and steam under pressure. Steam under pressure is the most dependable method for destroying all forms of organisms and spores. The *autoclave* is a type of pressure steam sterilizer that most health care agencies use. Pressure makes it possible to achieve much hotter temperatures (250° to 254°F) than the boiling point of water or free-flowing steam. Heat-sensitive tape that changes color or displays a pattern when exposed to high temperatures is used on sterilized packages as a visual indicator that the wrapped item is sterile.

Chemical Sterilization

Both gas and liquid chemicals are used to sterilize invasive equipment. Until chemicals were perfected as a sterilizing agent, sterilization using liquid chemicals was difficult and some questioned its reliability. Gas sterilization, using ethylene oxide gas, is a traditional method for destroying microorganisms if heat or moisture is likely to damage items or if no better method is available.

Principles of Surgical Asepsis

Surgical asepsis is based on the premise that once equipment and areas are free of microorganisms, they can remain in that state if contamination is prevented. Consequently, health care providers observe the following principles known as sterile technique:

- They preserve sterility by touching one sterile item with another that is sterile.
- Once a sterile item touches something that is not sterile, it is considered contaminated.
- Any partially unwrapped sterile package is considered contaminated.
- If there is a question about the sterility of an item, it is considered unsterile.
- The longer the time since sterilization, the more likely it is that the item is no longer sterile.

- A commercially packaged sterile item is not considered sterile past its recommended expiration date.
- Once a sterile item is opened or uncovered, it is only a matter of time before it becomes contaminated.
- The outer 1-in margin of a sterile area is considered a zone of contamination.
- A sterile wrapper, if it becomes wet, wicks microorganisms from its supporting surface, causing contamination.
- Any opened sterile item or sterile area is considered contaminated if it is left unattended.
- Coughing, sneezing, or excessive talking over a sterile field causes contamination.
- Reaching across an area that contains sterile equipment has a high potential for causing contamination and is therefore avoided.
- Sterile items that are located or lowered below waist level are considered contaminated because they are not within critical view.

Health care professionals observe the principles of surgical asepsis during surgery, when performing invasive procedures such as inserting urinary catheters, and when caring for open wounds. Practices that involve surgical asepsis include creating a sterile field, adding sterile items to the sterile field, and donning sterile gloves.

Creating a Sterile Field

A **sterile field** means a work area free of microorganisms. It is formed using the inner surface of a cloth or paper wrapper that holds sterile items, much like a table cloth. The field enlarges the area where sterile equipment or supplies are placed. When opening the sterile package, the nurse must be careful to keep the inside of the wrapper and its contents sterile. Refer to Skill 10-4.

Adding Items to a Sterile Field

Sometimes it is necessary to add sterile items or sterile solutions to the sterile field (see Skill 10-4).

Sterile Items

Agency-sterilized items or those that have been commercially prepared may be added to the sterile field. The former are generally wrapped in cloth. The nurse unwraps the cloth by supporting the wrapped item in one hand rather than placing it on a solid surface. The nurse holds each of the four corners to prevent the edges of the wrap from hanging loosely. The nurse places the unwrapped item on the sterile field and discards the cloth cover.

Commercially prepared supplies, such as sterile gauze squares, are enclosed in paper wrappers. The paper cover usually has two loose flaps that extend above the sealed edges. After separating the flaps, the nurse drops the sterile contents onto the sterile field.

Sterile Solutions

Sterile solutions, such as normal saline, come in various volumes. Some containers are sealed with a rubber cap or screw top. Either is replaced if the inside surface is contaminated.

To avoid contamination, the nurse places the cap upside down on a flat surface or holds it during pouring.

Before each use of a sterile solution, the nurse pours and discards a small amount from the mouth of the container to wash away airborne contaminants. This is called *lipping* the container. While pouring, the nurse holds the container in front of themselves. The nurse avoids touching any sterile areas within the field. They control the height of the container to avoid splashing the sterile field, causing a wet area of contamination. Agencies replace sterile solutions daily even if the entire volume is not used.

Putting on and Removing Sterile Gloves

When applied correctly, nurses can use sterile gloves to handle sterile equipment and supplies without contaminating them. Sterile gloves also provide a barrier against transmitting microbes to clients. Some packages of supplies include sterile gloves; they are also packaged separately in glove wrappers. Following principles of asepsis, nurses remove gloves without directly touching their more contaminated outer surface (Skill 10-5).

>>> **Stop, Think, and Respond 10-4**

What is the best action to take if, while donning sterile gloves, a nurse touches the thumb of an already gloved finger to their ungloved wrist?

Putting on a Sterile Gown

A sterile gown protects the client and the sterile equipment from microorganisms that collect on the surface of uniforms, scrub suits, or scrub gowns. Sterile gowns are required during surgery and childbirth. They are used during other sterile procedures as well.

Sterile gowns are usually made of cloth and are laundered and sterilized after each use. Before wrapping a gown for sterilization, it is folded so that the inside surface can be touched while putting it on. To avoid contamination, the nurse should follow the steps outlined in Nursing Guidelines 10-2.

NURSING IMPLICATIONS

Everyone is susceptible to infections, especially if sources of microorganisms among health care providers, clients, equipment, and the agency are not controlled. Nurses generally identify pertinent nursing diagnoses like those that follow when caring for particularly susceptible clients:

- Infection risk
- Surgical site infection risk
- Knowledge deficiency

Nursing Care Plan 10-1 illustrates how nurses incorporate guidelines for medical asepsis into a teaching plan for the nursing diagnosis of knowledge deficiency. Lippincott Advisor defines knowledge deficiency as insufficient cognitive information related to a specific topic.

 NURSING GUIDELINES 10-2

Donning a Sterile Gown

- Apply a mask and hair cover. *This sequence prevents contamination of the hands after they are washed.*
- Perform surgical hand antisepsis (see Skill 10-3). *This removes resident and transient microorganisms.*
- Pick up the sterile gown at the inner neckline. *This action preserves the sterility of the outer gown surface.*
- Hold the gown away from the body and other unsterile objects (Fig. A). *This prevents contamination.*

- Allow the gown to unfold while holding it high enough to avoid contact with the floor. *This prevents contamination.*
- Insert an arm within each sleeve without touching the outer surface of the gown. *This action maintains sterility.*
- Have an assistant pull at the inside of the gown to adjust the fit, expose the hands, and then tie it closed (Fig. B). *This action preserves the sterility of the front of the gown.*
- Don sterile gloves. *Wearing sterile gloves ensures the sterile condition of the hands and cuff of the gown.*

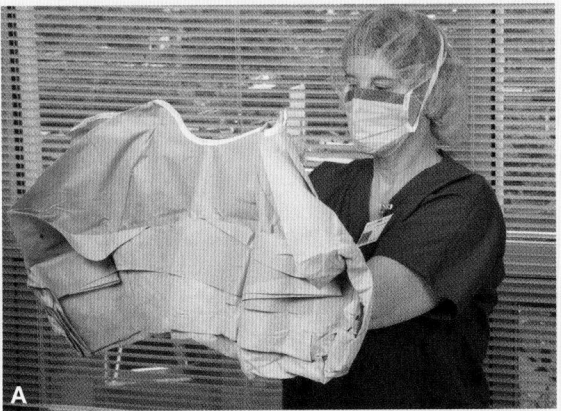

Unfolding a sterile gown.

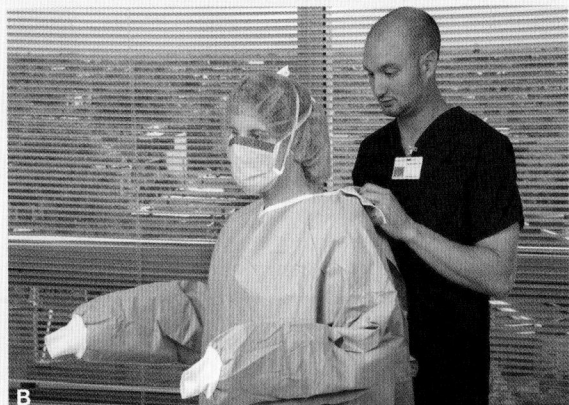

Assisting with putting on a sterile gown. (Photo by B. Proud.)

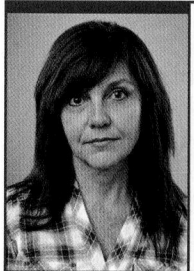

Clinical Scenario   A client is seeing the nurse who works in her primary care physician's office. The client is frantic after having received a notice from her daughter's school concerning a classmate who has been diagnosed with hepatitis A. This mother is seeking information about actions she should take with her daughter to prevent transmission of the disease.

■ What assessments are appropriate for the nurse to help identify a problem?

■ What nursing interventions would help the client with her issues?

See Nursing Care Plan 10-1 as a possible plan of care.

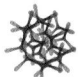

NURSING CARE PLAN 10-1   Deficient Knowledge

Assessment

- Explore the client's level of knowledge in a particular area of health care.
- Provide opportunities during which a client can request health-related information.

- Listen for statements that reflect inaccurate health information.
- Observe if a client performs health-related self-care incorrectly.
- Watch for signs of emotional distress that reflect inaccurate information.

Nursing Diagnosis. Deficient knowledge related to unfamiliarity with infectious disease (hepatitis A) transmission as evidenced by the statements, "The school nurse sent this note home saying there's been a case of hepatitis in my daughter's fifth grade class. Isn't that what people who use drugs get? Should I keep my daughter home from school? What will prevent her from catching it?"

Expected Outcome. The client will (1) state the difference in transmission of hepatitis A and hepatitis B, (2) list at least three signs and symptoms of hepatitis A, (3) verbalize how to avoid infection with hepatitis A, and (4) demonstrate how to wash hands appropriately after instruction.

Interventions	Rationales
Explain that hepatitis A is primarily transmitted from the stool of an infected person to the oral route of the susceptible person and that hepatitis B is spread by blood and body fluids.	This discussion provides accurate information concerning the mode of disease transmission.
Provide health-related information about hepatitis A, which includes: • The incubation period for hepatitis A is 25–30 days. • Signs and symptoms that may develop are low-grade fever, reduced activity, loss of appetite, nausea, abdominal pain, dark urine, light-colored stool, and yellowing of the skin and sclera of the eyes. • Hand washing is an excellent preventive measure especially when performed before eating and after using the toilet. • An injection of immune serum globulin is a method of providing temporary passive immunity when exposed to hepatitis A.	Specific information increases the client's knowledge, clarifies misinformation, and helps relieve anxiety.
Demonstrate hand washing and observe a return demonstration emphasizing the following: • Turn handles of the faucet on and let the water run. • Wet hands and lather with soap. • Rub lathered hands for at least 20 seconds. • Rinse, letting the water flow from wrists to fingers. • Dry hands with a paper towel. • Use the paper towel to turn the faucet off.	A demonstration provides health teaching by visual learning; returning a demonstration reinforces learning via a psychomotor activity.

Evaluation of Expected Outcomes

- The client identifies the mode of transmitting hepatitis A as the fecal/oral route.
- The client lists low fever, loss of appetite, and yellow sclera as indications of hepatitis A infection.
- The client states that frequent and thorough hand washing is a method for preventing the acquisition of hepatitis A.
- The client demonstrates appropriate hand washing and is prepared to teach her daughter the same skill.
- The client makes an appointment for her daughter to receive an injection of immune serum globulin.

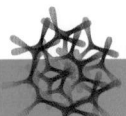

KEY POINTS

- Pathogens have a high potential for causing infectious diseases that can be transmitted to other people (e.g., measles, TB).
- Nonpathogens are pathogens that live on and in the body but do not cause disease (e.g., *Escherichia coli* that lives in the large intestine).
- Pathogens and nonpathogens include bacteria, viruses, fungi, rickettsiae, protozoans, mycoplasmas, helminths, and prions.
- Chain of infection: The sequence that enables the spread of disease-producing microorganisms that must be in place if pathogens are to be transmitted from one location or person to another:
  - An infectious agent
  - A reservoir for growth and reproduction
  - An exit route from the reservoir
  - A means of transmission
  - A portal of entry
  - A susceptible host

- Asepsis refers to those practices that decrease or eliminate infectious agents for transmission. It is the major method for preventing and controlling infection. Health care providers use medical and surgical asepsis to accomplish this goal.
  - Medical asepsis: Clean technique; those practices that confine or reduce the numbers of microorganisms (e.g., hygiene, using antimicrobial agents)
  - Surgical asepsis: Those measures that render supplies and equipment totally free of microorganisms; include practices that avoid contaminating microbe-free items (e.g., process of sterilization)
- Personal protective equipment: Various garments health care providers wear, including uniforms, scrub suits or gowns, masks, gloves, hair and shoe covers, and protective eyewear; some items are worn when caring for any client regardless of diagnosis or presumed infectious status.

CRITICAL THINKING EXERCISES

1. If the rate of infections increased on your nursing unit, what would you investigate to determine the contributing factors?
2. If the cause of health care–associated infections is related to inadequate hand washing among health care providers, what suggestions would you give for correcting the problem?
3. What methods could be used to evaluate if health care providers are performing hand hygiene appropriately?
4. What recommendations might you suggest to prevent transferring microorganisms from health care providers' homes to clients for whom they care?

NEXT-GENERATION NCLEX-STYLE REVIEW QUESTIONS

1. Before touching a client, what is the minimum amount of time the nurse should perform an alcohol-based hand rub?
   a. 5 seconds
   b. 10 seconds
   c. 15 seconds
   d. 20 seconds
   Test-Taking Strategy: Select the option that is similar to the time it takes to sing the song "Happy Birthday" twice.
2. A nurse needs to wear a mask while caring for a client. Which nursing actions are appropriate? Select all that apply.
   a. The mask is positioned to cover the nurse's nose and mouth.
   b. The nurse secures the ties at the back of the head and neck.
   c. The nurse adjusts the mask during the course of client care.

   d. The nurse avoids wearing the mask longer than 30 minutes.
   e. The nurse lowers the mask to the chest area during removal.
   f. The nurse discards the mask within a waterproof receptacle.
   Test-Taking Strategy: Consider if each option is true or false. Eliminate any false or incorrect options.
3. When caring for a client with an eye infection, what is the most important health teaching the nurse can provide to the client?
   a. Eat a well-balanced, nutritious diet.
   b. Wear sunglasses in bright light.
   c. Cease sharing towels and washcloths.
   d. Avoid products containing aspirin.
   Test-Taking Strategy: When some or all options seem appropriate, select one option that represents a priority. Consider an action that interrupts the chain of infection.
4. A nurse observes a newly employed nursing assistant perform hand washing. Which actions require more teaching? Select all that apply.
   a. The nursing assistant is wearing an engagement ring.
   b. The nursing assistant works a teaspoon of soap into a lather.
   c. The nursing assistant holds the hands downward during rinsing.
   d. The nursing assistant uses a paper towel to dry her hands.
   e. The nursing assistant turns the faucet off with her bare hands.
   f. The nursing assistant applies hand lotion to her dried hands.
   Test-Taking Strategy: Consider whether each option describes correct or incorrect actions when performing hand washing. In this question, select options that violate medically aseptic practices, in other words, the actions that are incorrect.

5. A nurse sets up a sterile field prior to changing a client's dressing. Which action is correct?

   a. The nurse first opens the sterile pack by unfolding the wrapper toward themselves.

   b. The nurse avoids adding supplies in the outer 1-in margin of the exposed field.

   c. The nurse sets a wrapped basin in the center of the sterile field.

   d. The nurse pours a sterile solution from 8 to 10 in above a sterile basin.

   Test-Taking Strategy: Eliminate options that have the potential for contamination.

NEXT-GENERATION NCLEX-STYLE CLINICAL SCENARIO QUESTIONS

Clinical Scenario:

A client is seeing the nurse who works in her primary care physician's office. The client is frantic after having received a notice from her daughter's school concerning a classmate who has been diagnosed with hepatitis A. This mother is seeking information about actions she should take with her daughter to prevent transmission of the disease.

1. Choose the most likely options for the information missing from the statements below by selecting from the list of options provided.

The mother is concerned about the hepatitis A diagnosis because it is a _____1_____. If her daughter is diagnosed with hepatitis A she will need to take _____2_____ precautions and her daughter would need _____3_____ medications.

OPTION 1	OPTION 2	OPTION 3
bacterial infection	airborne/respiratory	antifungal
fungal infection	body fluid	antibacterial
viral infection		antiviral

2. For each statement, use an "x" to indicate whether the intervention will be effective: help with expected outcomes, ineffective: did not help with the expected outcome, or unrelated: not related.

STATEMENT	EFFECTIVE	INEFFECTIVE	UNRELATED
A person who's infected with hepatitis A and uses needles can spread the virus by sharing them or not disposing of them safely.			
Wearing a facemask can help with avoiding transmission of hepatitis A.			
Hepatitis A can be transmitted by close personal contact with a person who is infected.			
Hepatitis A can be transmitted through food.			
A hepatitis A vaccine is available to help reduce hepatitis A virus.			

SKILL 10-1 Hand Washing

Suggested Action	Reason for Action
ASSESSMENT	
Review the medical record to determine whether it is appropriate to perform hand washing for longer than 20 seconds.	Demonstrates concern for immunosuppressed clients, newborns, or other susceptible hosts
Check that there are soap and paper towels near the sink and a waste receptacle nearby.	Promotes effective hand washing and disposal of paper towels; bar soap is supplied in small cakes, which are changed frequently and placed on a drainable holder to avoid colonization with microorganisms; liquid soap is stored in closed containers that are replaced, or cleaned, dried, and refilled on a regular schedule.
PLANNING	
Trim long fingernails so that they are less than 1/4 in long, a length at which the nails cannot be seen when the palms are held in front of the nose.	Reduces the reservoir where the majority of hand flora reside; prevents tearing gloves
Remove all jewelry; a plain, *smooth* wedding band can be worn; roll up long sleeves.	Facilitates removing transient and resident microorganisms; bacterial counts are higher when rings are worn during client care.
Explain the purpose for hand washing to the client.	Reinforces and demonstrates concern for client safety
IMPLEMENTATION	
Turn on the water using faucet handles; an automated faucet; or elbow, knee, or foot controls (Fig. A).	Serves as a wetting agent and facilitates lathering; using automated faucets, elbow, knee, or foot controls prevents recontamination of hands after they are washed

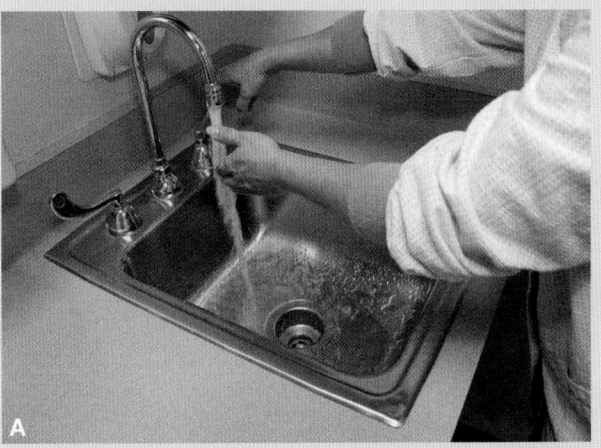

Turning on faucet.

If a lever-operated paper towel dispenser is available, activate it to dispense the paper towel.	Electronic sensors decrease hand contamination before and after hand washing, but they are not generally available in most health care agencies.
Wet your hands with comfortably warm water from the wrists toward the fingers (Fig. B).	Allows water to flow from the least contaminated area to the most contaminated area

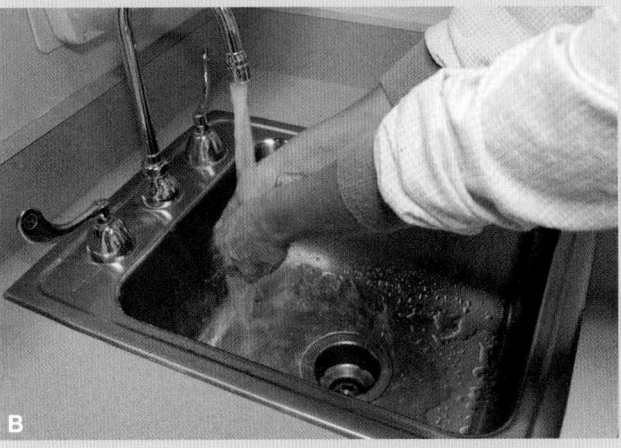

Wetting hands.

(continued)

SKILL 10-1 Hand Washing (*continued*)

Suggested Action	Reason for Action
Avoid splashing water from the sink onto your uniform.	Prevents transferring microorganisms to clothing via a wicking action
Dispense about 3–5 mL (1 tsp) of liquid soap into your hands.	Provides an agent for emulsifying body oils and releasing microorganisms
Work the soap into a lather and generate friction.	Expands the volume and distribution of the soap; begins to soften the keratin layer of the skin; loosens debris and directs soap into crevices of skin
Rub the lather vigorously over all surfaces of the hands including thumbs and backs of fingers and hands and under the fingernails for a minimum of 20 seconds—the time it takes to sing two rounds of the song "Happy Birthday" (Fig. C). 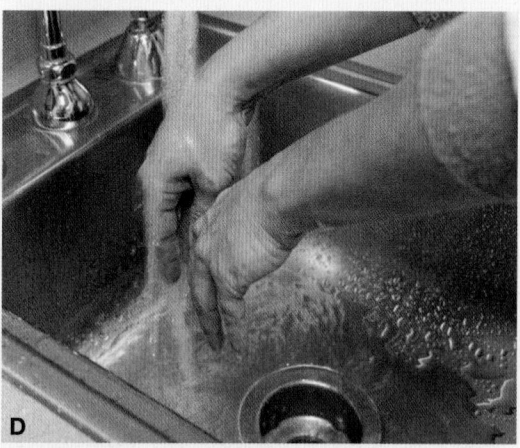 Cleaning backs of fingers.	Frees microorganisms that are lodged in skin creases and crevices
Rinse the soap from your hands by letting the water run from the wrists toward the fingers (Fig. D). D Rinsing hands.	Avoids transferring microorganisms to cleaner areas.
Stop the flow of water if it is controlled by an elbow or knee lever, or a foot pedal.	Terminates the flow of water without recontaminating the hands
Hold your draining hands lower than your wrists.	Promotes drainage by gravity flow toward the fingers
Dry your hands thoroughly with paper towels or similar items.	This prevents chapping. Cloth towels are the least desirable method of drying because they are prone to contamination. A warm air dryer (rarely available in client environments) is the best. Paper towels dispensed from a holder mounted high enough to avoid splash contamination are acceptable and effective.

SKILL 10-1 Hand Washing (*continued*)

Suggested Action	Reason for Action
Turn the hand controls of the faucet off using a paper towel (Fig. E).	Prevents recontamination of washed hands

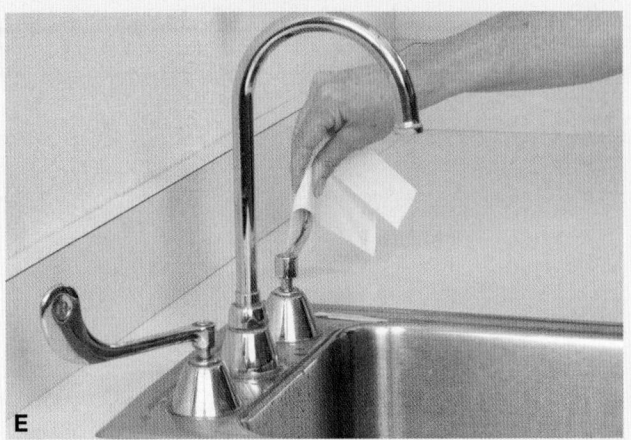

E

Turning off faucet.

Suggested Action	Reason for Action
Apply hand lotion from time to time.	Maintains the integrity of the skin because skin that becomes irritated and abraded from frequent hand washing increases the risk of acquiring pathogens by direct skin contact.

EVALUATION

- Hand washing has met time requirements.
- Hands are clean.
- Skin is intact.

DOCUMENT

Because hand washing is performed so frequently, it is not documented, but it is expected as a standard of care among all health care providers.

SKILL 10-2 Hand Antisepsis with an Alcohol-Based Rub

Suggested Action	Reason for Action
ASSESSMENT	
Determine that the hands are *not* visibly dirty or contaminated with proteinaceous material, blood, or other body fluids.	Hand washing is required when the hands are visibly soiled.
Identify the location of the alcohol-based dispenser.	Compliance increases when the dispenser is close to the point of client care such as at the entrance to the client's room or at the bedside.
PLANNING	
Prepare to perform routine hand antisepsis with at least a 60% alcohol-based product when the hands are not visibly soiled such as before and after touching a client, before and after performing a procedure, after touching a potential body fluid exposure, after touching items like side rails within the immediate vicinity of the client, and after removing gloves.	Hands acquire 100–1,000 colony-forming units, a measure of microbial load, during "clean activities." Products containing alcohol have better antimicrobial activity than soap (Boyce & Pittet, 2002).
IMPLEMENTATION	
Dispense approximately 3 mL of the alcohol-based product into a cupped palm (see figure).	Achieving effective antisepsis is related to a sufficient volume necessary to cover all hand and wrist surfaces.

(*continued*)

SKILL 10-2 Hand Antisepsis with an Alcohol-Based Rub (*continued*)

Suggested Action	Reason for Action
Accessing an alcohol-based product.	
Distribute and rub the alcohol-based product over all surfaces of the hands and fingers.	Effective antisepsis requires contact between the alcohol-based product and the skin surfaces where microorganisms reside.
Rub the back of each hand with the opposite palm.	Rubbing spreads the alcohol-based product over the dorsum of the hands and creates friction that loosens surface debris.
Spread the fingers and rub the webbed areas of exposed skin on each hand.	Microorganisms tend to collect and accumulate in the folds of skin.
Rub down the length of each thumb using a rotating motion.	A rotational movement ensures that the entire thumb is included.
Rub the tips of the fingers against the opposite palm on each hand in a circular fashion.	The areas that are cleaned less effectively during hand hygiene include the thumbs, fingertips, and webs between the fingers.
Rub the wrists of both hands in a rotating manner.	Cleaning the wrists is the final step in reducing surfaces in close proximity of clients.
Proceed with nursing activities after rubbing the hands until the hands are dry.	After sufficient rubbing and evaporation, bacterial counts on the hands are significantly reduced.

EVALUATION

Hand antisepsis is completed when the product containing alcohol has totally evaporated.

DOCUMENTATION

Hand hygiene is not documented, but it is expected to be performed conscientiously as a standard of care for all health care providers.

SKILL 10-3 Performing Surgical Hand Antisepsis

Suggested Action	Reason for Action
ASSESSMENT	
Locate the area designated for performing surgical hand antisepsis. Verify that the sink is deep and has a faucet with either a knee or a foot control. Ensure that there is a sufficient supply of liquid cleanser that can be dispensed with a foot pump; also check to see whether a hand sponge and nail cleaner are available.	This action reduces the potential for recontamination or repeating surgical hand antisepsis because of a lack of necessary supplies.
PLANNING	
Change from uniform or street clothes into a scrub gown or suit.	Changing attire decreases the number of microorganisms transferred from other areas of the health care agency.
Place uniform and valuables, which may include rings and a wristwatch, in a locker.	Storage ensures the safekeeping of items that contain abundant microorganisms.
Don a mask and hair and shoe covers.	These items prevent recontaminating the skin after the hands have been cleaned.
Verify that a sterile towel, gloves, and long-sleeved cover gown are in the operative or obstetric room adjacent to the cleansing area.	Checking ensures that clean hands can be dried and covered quickly to avoid transferring additional microbes to the cleansed areas.

SKILL 10-3 Performing Surgical Hand Antisepsis (*continued*)

Suggested Action	Reason for Action
IMPLEMENTATION	
Turn on the water to a comfortably warm temperature; wet the hands to the forearms and lather the liquid cleanser to all the wet areas, using friction for approximately 15 seconds.	This measure removes surface debris, oil, and some microorganisms before beginning surgical hand antisepsis.
Use a sponge or combination sponge–brush to scrub under the nails, around the cuticles, and in the creases in the palms.	A sponge may be used initially to remove superficial debris from the hands; there is no additional antimicrobial benefit in using a brush.
Clean beneath each fingernail with a nail file or orange stick (Fig. A); dispose of this item in a foot-operated waste container before rinsing.	This device removes deeper debris and microorganisms from beneath the nails.

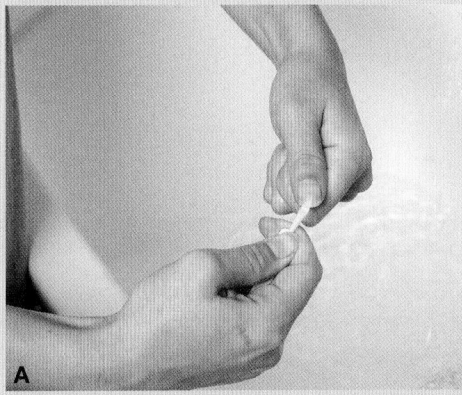

A

Cleaning the fingernails.

Rinse the lather while keeping the hands above the elbows.	Gravity prevents soiled lather from adhering to the hands.
Dispense the antimicrobial cleanser into the palm of a hand or use a wetted sponge that has been presaturated with the cleanser.	Doing so decreases microorganisms.
Using friction, wash the nails and all surfaces of each finger; proceed to the thumb, palm, and back of the hand (Fig. B).	These steps follow the principle of cleaning from most to least contaminated areas.

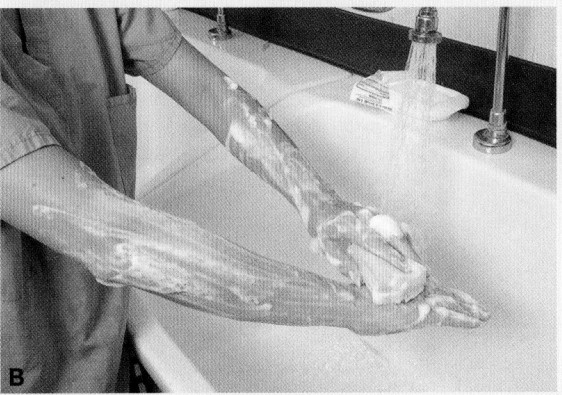

B

Washing all surfaces on the hands using friction.

Go over all areas with at least 10 strokes each; repeat on the other side.	This amount ensures adequate cleansing.
Avoid splashing water or lather onto the surface of the scrub gown or suit.	Wet areas wick microorganisms beneath the surface of the cover gown or suit to the surface.
Proceed to wash the forearms with circular strokes from lower to middle to upper areas.	Cleanse in the direction of cleaner areas of the body.
Ensure that washing continues for the time identified by the manufacturer of the cleansing agent, generally a total of 2–6 minutes.	Adequate time is necessary to reduce microorganisms. Current studies have shown that an alcohol-based hand rub for 3–5 minutes is as effective in killing bacteria as a scrub containing chlorhexidine soap.

(*continued*)

SKILL 10-3 Performing Surgical Hand Antisepsis (*continued*)

Suggested Action	Reason for Action
Drop the soapy sponge in the sink or discard it within a foot-operated waste container. Rinse lather by allowing the water to run from fingers to elbows (Fig. C).	These steps prevent touching unclean surfaces, as well as debris and loosened microorganisms from dripping over previously cleaned hands. Proceeding this way maintains cleanliness during relocation to the operating room or obstetric suite.

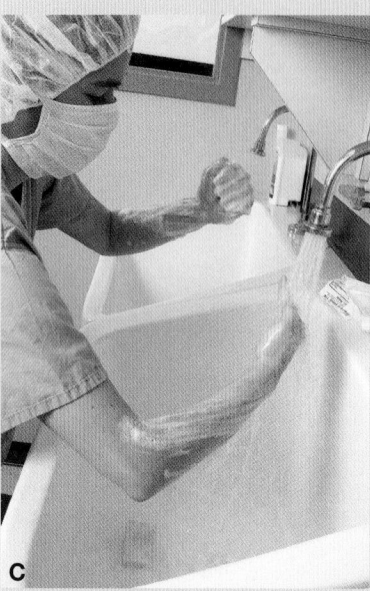

C
Rinse water flowing toward the elbows.

| Keep the hands elevated above the waist, well in front of the scrub gown or suit with the elbows flexed; enter the room where the sterile towel, gloves, and gown are located (Fig. D). | This step prevents transferring organisms from the scrub gown or suit to a sterile area. |

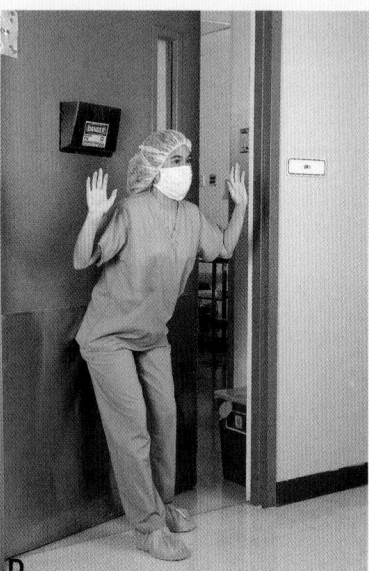

D
Holding the hands and arms upward and away from the body.

| Walk to the table containing an unwrapped sterile towel while keeping a slight distance from it. Pick up the sterile towel by its folded edge. After allowing it to unfold without touching anything, use one end to dry the hands and forearm in that order. Use the other end to dry the opposite hand and forearm (Fig. E). | This process avoids transferring organisms from an unclean to a clean area. |

SKILL 10-3 Performing Surgical Hand Antisepsis (*continued*)

Suggested Action	Reason for Action

Drying the hands with a sterile towel.

Suggested Action	Reason for Action
Discard the towel within a linen hamper.	Such disposal confines soiled items.
Pick up and don a sterile gown with assistance from another person (see Nursing Guidelines 10-2) and don sterile gloves.	This step keeps the front surface of the gown sterile and covers the clean hands.

EVALUATION

- Nails, hands, and forearms have been washed for the designated time.
- The sequence of cleansing supports principles of asepsis.
- The procedure and the use of equipment have followed principles to avoid recontamination.

DOCUMENT

Surgical hand antisepsis is not documented, but it is expected to be performed conscientiously following agency policies and procedures that are standards of care for all health care providers.

SKILL 10-4 Creating a Sterile Field and Adding Sterile Items

Suggested Action	Reason for Action
ASSESSMENT	
Inspect the work area to determine the cleanliness and orderliness of the surface on which you will work.	Working in a clean area is a principle of medical asepsis.
Obtain the prepared package that contains items needed for performing the clinical procedure.	Contents within a prepared package contain sterile items.
Check that the package is sealed and that its use date has not expired.	Items are not used if there is a question as to their sterility.
Determine whether additional sterile items are needed but not contained in the sterile package.	Gathering all necessary items facilitates organization and time management.
PLANNING	
Explain what is about to take place to the client.	Promotes understanding and cooperation
Plan to perform the procedure that requires a sterile field when the client is comfortable and there are no potential interruptions.	Once a sterile field is created, it has a potential for contamination when items are uncovered and the field is exposed for any length of time.
Remove objects from the area where the field will be created.	Removing unsterile items provides room for working and reduces the potential for accidental contamination.

(continued)

SKILL 10-4 Creating a Sterile Field and Adding Sterile Items (*continued*)

Suggested Action	Reason for Action
IMPLEMENTATION	
Perform hand washing or hand antisepsis with an alcohol-based rub.	Removes transient microorganisms and reduces the potential for transmitting infection
Place the wrapped package on a surface at or above waist level.	Placement above the waist keeps the sterile field and its contents within sight and reduces the potential for contamination.
Position the package so that the outermost triangular edge of the wrapper can be moved away from the front of the body (Fig. A).	This placement prevents reaching over the sterile area while the package is opened and reduces the potential for contamination.

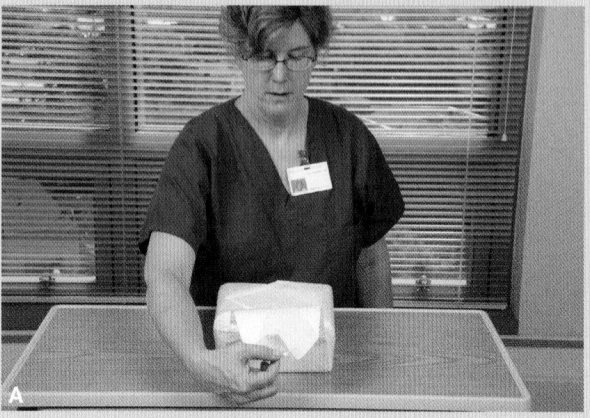

Unfolding away from the body.

Unfold each side of the wrapper by touching the area that will be in direct contact with the table or stand, or touch no more than the outer 1 in of the edge of the wrapper (Fig. B).	This action maintains a sterile area.

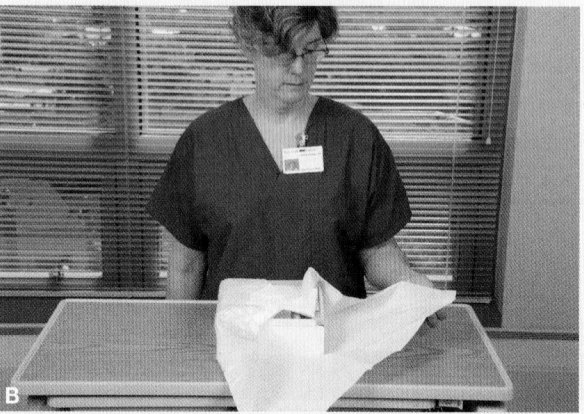

Unfolding the sides.

Unfold the final corner of the wrapper by pulling it toward the body (Fig. C).	This action avoids reaching over an uncovered sterile area, which has the potential for contaminating the sterile field and the items that rest upon it.

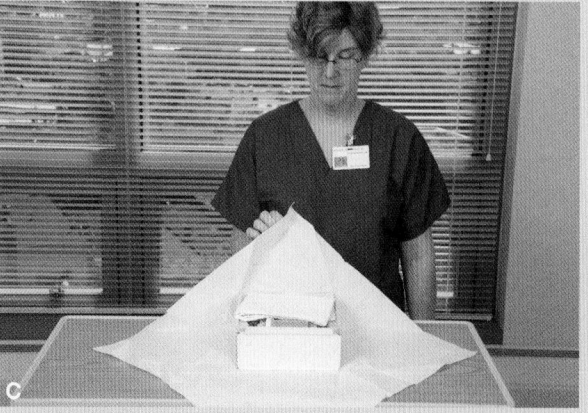

Unfolding toward the body.

SKILL 10-4 Creating a Sterile Field and Adding Sterile Items (*continued*)

Suggested Action	Reason for Action
Add additional wrapped sterile items by unwrapping them, securing the edges of the wrapper in one hand, and placing them on the sterile field (Fig. D).	Placing sterile items on a sterile field without touching anything that is unsterile preserves a sterile condition.

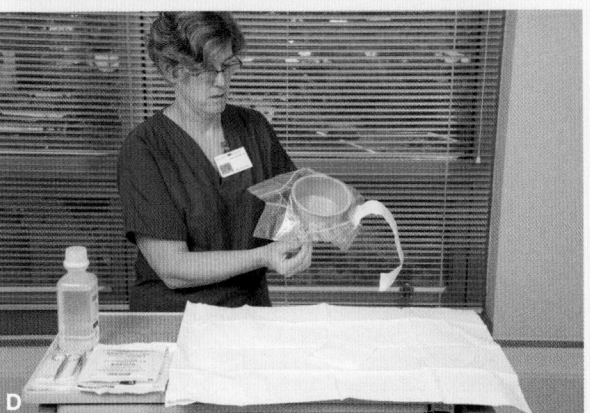

Adding an agency-sterilized item.

| Add additional paper-wrapped sterile items by separating the sealed flaps and dropping the contents onto the sterile field (Fig. E). | Placing sterile items on a sterile field without touching anything that is unsterile preserves a sterile condition. |

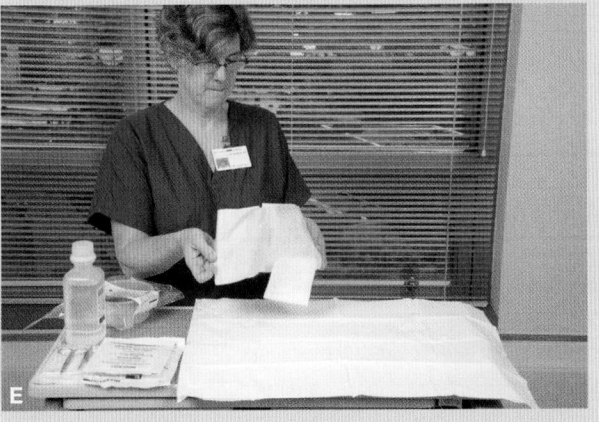

Adding sterile gauze.

Add a sterile solution to a sterile container, if it is needed, by:

- Opening the cap on the solution without touching the inner surface with anything that is unsterile
- Holding the labeled portion of the solution in the palm of the dominant hand
- Pouring and discarding a small amount into a waste container (Fig. F)

Placing sterile items on a sterile field without touching anything that is unsterile preserves a sterile condition.

This action keeps the label dry and prevents obliterating its contents.

Removes possible airborne contaminants from the rim of the container

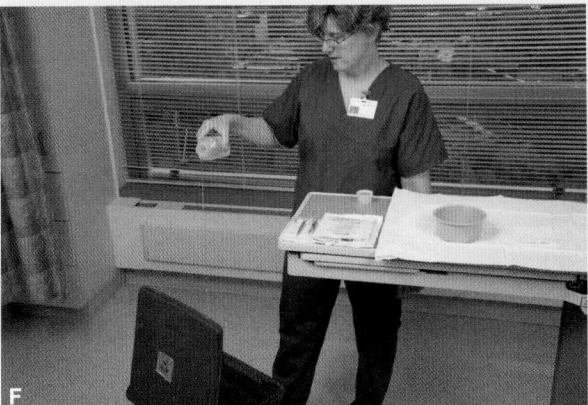

Lipping the container of solution.

(continued)

SKILL 10-4 Creating a Sterile Field and Adding Sterile Items (*continued*)

Suggested Action	Reason for Action
• Pouring the amount desired from a height of 4–6 in into the container on the sterile field without splashing the surface of the field (Fig. G)	Avoids splashing, thereby maintaining sterility of the work area

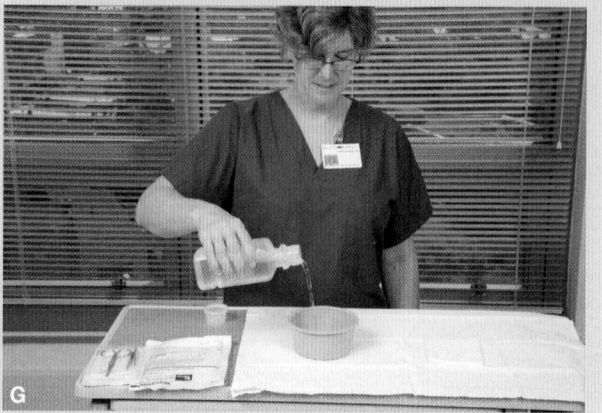

Adding sterile solution.

EVALUATION

• The exposed area of the field is sterile; nothing unsterile has touched the surface inside the 1-in outer margin.
• Additional items have been added to the sterile field in such a way as to preserve the sterility of the items and the surface of the sterile field.

DOCUMENT

Preparation of a sterile field and the addition of sterile items are not documented, but it is expected as a standard of care among all health professionals. The procedure that required the sterile field and the outcome of the procedure are documented (refer to the sample documentation that accompanies Skill 10-5).

SKILL 10-5 Putting on and Removing Sterile Gloves and Gowns

Suggested Action	Reason for Action
ASSESSMENT	
Determine whether the procedure requires surgical asepsis.	Complies with infection control measures
Read the contents of prepackaged sterile equipment to determine whether sterile gloves are enclosed.	Indicates whether extra supplies are needed
Discover how much the client understands about the subsequent procedure.	Provides a basis for teaching
PLANNING	
Explain what is about to take place to the client.	Promotes understanding and cooperation
Select a package of sterile gloves of the appropriate size.	Ensures ease when donning and using gloves
Remove unnecessary items from the overbed table or bedside stand.	Ensures an adequate, clean work space
IMPLEMENTATION	
Perform hand washing or hand antisepsis with alcohol-based rub.	Reduces the potential for transmitting microorganisms
Open the outer wrapper of the gloves (Fig. A).	Provides access to inner wrapper

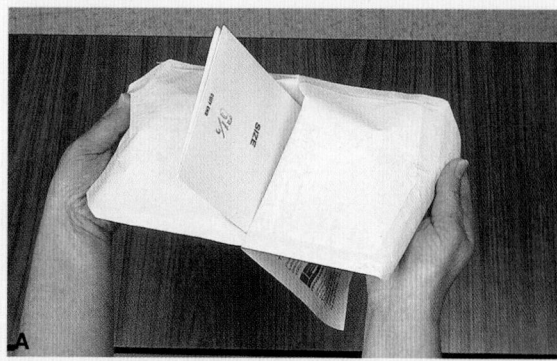

Opening the outer package.

SKILL 10-5 Putting on and Removing Sterile Gloves and Gowns (*continued*)

Suggested Action	Reason for Action
Carefully open the inner package and expose the sterile gloves with the cuff ends closest to you (Fig. B).	Facilitates donning gloves

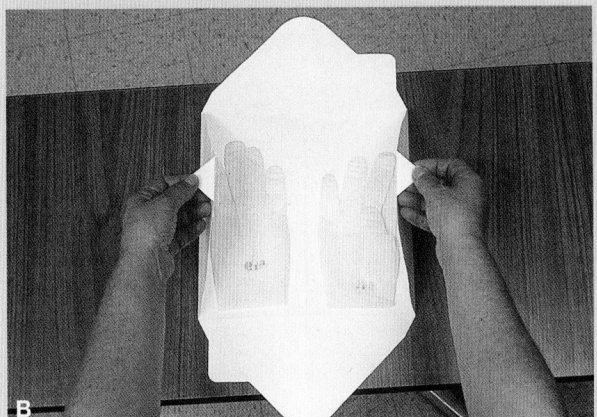
Positioning the inner wrapper.

Pick up one glove at the folded edge of the cuff using your thumb and fingers (Fig. C).	Avoids contaminating the outer surface of the glove

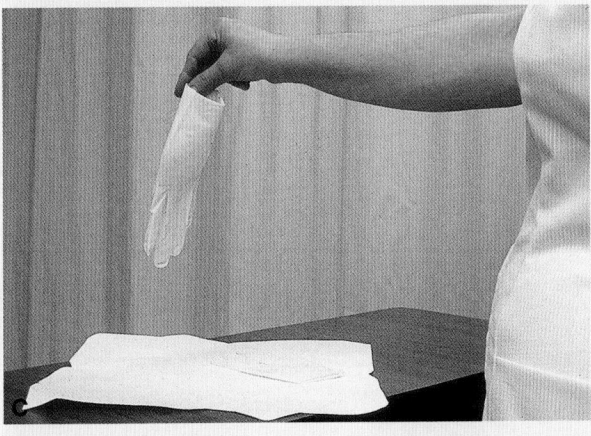
Picking up the first glove.

Insert your fingers while pulling and stretching the glove over your hand, taking care not to touch the outside of the glove to anything that is unsterile.	Avoids contaminating the outer surface of the glove
Unfold the cuff so that the glove extends above the wrist, but touch only the surface that will be in direct contact with the skin.	Extends the sterile area
Insert the gloved hand beneath the sterile folded edge of the remaining glove (Fig. D).	Maintains the sterility of each glove

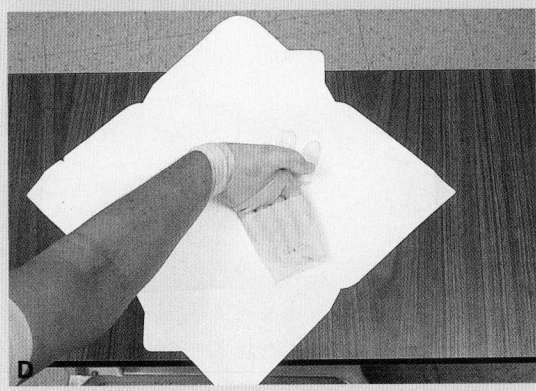
Picking up the second glove.

(continued)

SKILL 10-5 Putting on and Removing Sterile Gloves and Gowns (*continued*)

Suggested Action	Reason for Action
Insert the fingers within the second glove while pulling and stretching it over the hand (Fig. E).	Facilitates donning the glove

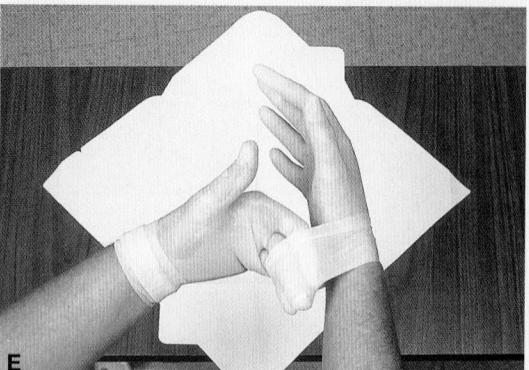

Pulling on the second glove.

Take care to avoid touching anything that is unsterile.	Maintains sterility
Maintain your gloved hands at or above waist level.	Prevents the potential for contamination
Repeat the procedure if contamination occurs.	Protects the client from acquiring an infection

REMOVING GLOVES ───────────────────────────────────

Grasp one of the gloves at the upper, outer edge at the wrist (Fig. F).	This position maintains a barrier between contaminated surfaces.

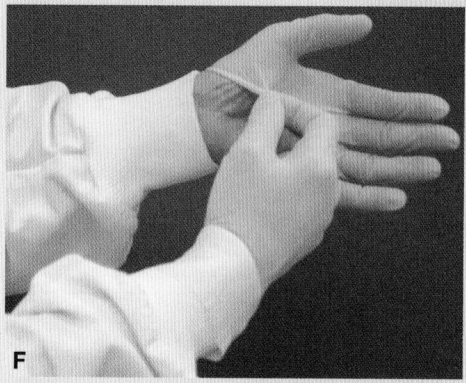

Pulling the cuff with the gloved hand.

Stretch and pull the upper edge of the glove downward while inverting the glove as it is removed (Fig. G).	This action encloses the soiled surface, blocking a potential exit route for microorganisms.

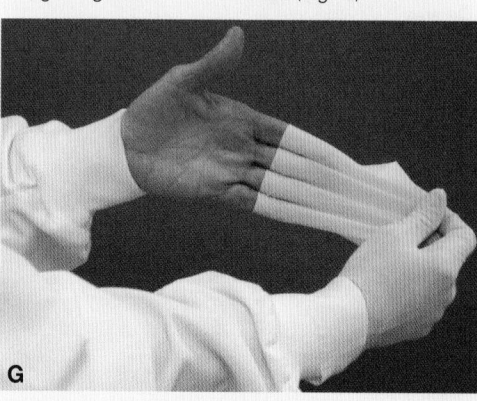

Pulling the glove off the hand inside out.

SKILL 10-5 Putting on and Removing Sterile Gloves and Gowns (*continued*)

Suggested Action	Reason for Action
Insert the fingers of the ungloved hand within the inside edge of the other glove (Fig. H). 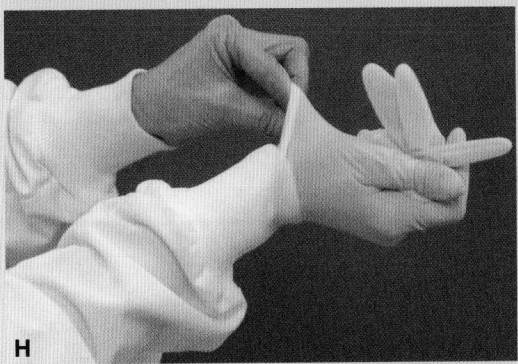 **H** Slipping the fingers of the ungloved hand under the wrist of the gloved hand.	The inside edge is the cleaner surface of the glove.
Pull the second glove inside out while enclosing the first glove within the palm (Fig. I). 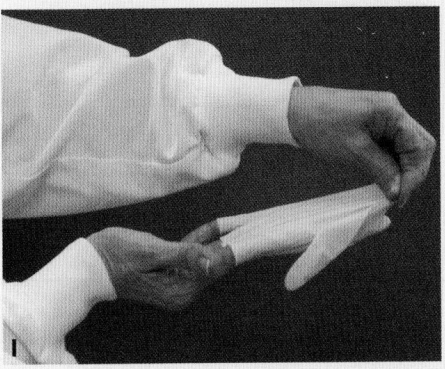 **I** Pulling the second glove inside out.	This action contains the reservoir of microorganisms.
Place the gloves within a lined waste container (Fig. J). 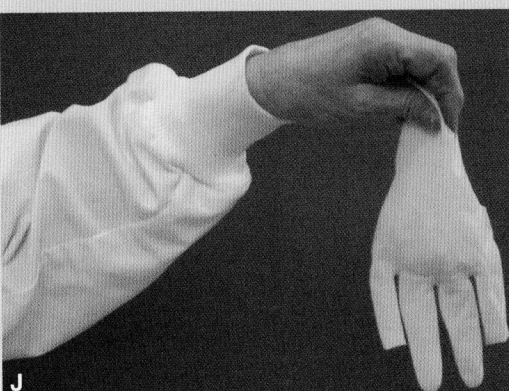 **J** Disposing of both gloves.	Proper disposal confines the reservoir of microorganisms.
Wash hands or perform hand antisepsis with an alcohol-based rub immediately after removing gloves.	Hand washing and hand antisepsis remove transient and resident microorganisms that have proliferated within the warm, dark, and moist environment inside the gloves.

(*continued*)

SKILL 10-5 Putting on and Removing Sterile Gloves and Gowns (*continued*)

Suggested Action	Reason for Action

EVALUATION

- Gloves are donned.
- Sterility is maintained.
- Gloves are removed keeping contaminated surfaces within the gloves.
- Glove removal is followed by hand hygiene.

DOCUMENT

- The procedure that was performed
- The outcome of the procedure

SAMPLE DOCUMENTATION

Date and Time Sterile dressing changed over abdominal incision. Wound edges are approximated, with no evidence of redness or drainage. _____ J. Doe, LPN

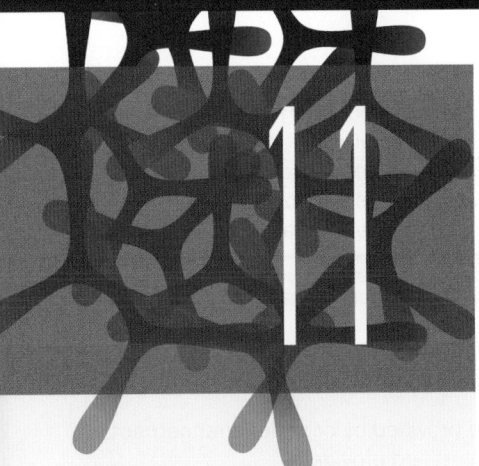

Admission, Discharge, Transfer, and Referrals

11

Words To Know

acute rehabilitation facility
admission
basic care facility
clinical résumé
continuity of care
discharge
discharge planning
extended care facility
home health care
intermediate care facility
long-term care facility
medication reconciliation
orientation
progressive care units
referral
skilled nursing facility
step-down units
transfer
transfer summary
transitional care units

Learning Objectives

On completion of this chapter, the reader should be able to:

1. List the major steps involved in the admission process.
2. Identify common psychosocial responses when clients are admitted to health agencies.
3. List the steps involved in the discharge process.
4. Give examples of the use of transfers in client care.
5. Describe the levels of care that nursing homes provide.
6. Discuss the purpose of a Minimum Data Set (MDS).
7. Explain the difference between transferring clients and referring clients.
8. Identify contributing factors to the increased demand for home health care.

INTRODUCTION

Everyone experiences health changes. Several levels of health care are available depending on the seriousness of the condition (see Chapter 4). Some people recover with self-treatment or by following health instructions from nurses or other health care team members.

This chapter describes skills used in caring for clients who become seriously ill, are injured, or have chronic health problems that require admission and temporary care in a facility, such as a hospital or extended care facility. This chapter also addresses nursing skills involved in the subsequent discharge, transfer, or referral of clients to community agencies that provide health care.

 Gerontologic Considerations

■ Many older adults fear that admission to a hospital or long-term care facility will eventually prevent their return to independent living. They may, therefore, minimize symptoms to protect their independent living status.

■ Aging directly correlates with increased incidence of acute disease and exacerbations of chronic conditions.

■ Pets are often an integral social support system and contribute to the general well-being of older adults. Those who live alone may be concerned about the welfare of pets. This should be considered during admission, with arrangements made for the care of the pet.

■ Detecting clues to elder abuse, neglect, or exploitation is an important nursing responsibility during the admission process for older adults. At least 10% of older adults are victims of elder abuse, which is most often perpetrated by trusted others (i.e., adult children, spouses, caregivers). Reports to Adult Protective Service organizations must be made when elder abuse is suspected, even if it is not confirmed.

■ Early discharge planning and the appropriate use of community resources may enable older adults to return to their own homes. Discharge planning for older adults should begin as soon as feasible and consider the needs of caregivers, which may include family, friends, or paid helpers. Delaying discharge planning or teaching until immediately before the discharge may not meet the educational needs of older clients and family members, which can result in readmissions.

■ Resources available to discharged older adults include senior centers, adult day care centers, faith-based organizations, churches, and care management services. In addition, support and education may come from advocacy groups, such as the Alzheimer's Association, Area Councils on Aging, Parkinson disease support groups, and the American Cancer Society.

■ Barriers to the use of community-based services by older adults include:

  ■ Lack of financial assets to pay for services

  ■ Reluctance to spend assets for services

  ■ Unwillingness to acknowledge or accept the need for services

  ■ Mistrust of service providers

  ■ Cultural differences

  ■ Lack of time, energy, or problem-solving ability to identify and select appropriate services

■ Nurses should allow additional time when admitting, discharging, or transferring older adults who have functional or cognitive impairments so they and their caregivers can process the information; nurses should allow additional time because of possible functional impairments.

■ Medicare requires that a client meet all the following five eligibility criteria for coverage of home care services:

  1. The services must be ordered by a primary care provider.

  2. The person must be homebound. Homebound status is met if leaving home requires a considerable and taxing effort, such as needing personal assistance or the help of a wheelchair or specialized van. Allowable activities include attendance at an adult day care center or religious service.

  3. The person needs skilled nursing care or rehabilitative services.

  4. The person requires intermittent, but not full-time, care.

  5. The care must be provided by or under arrangements with a Medicare-certified provider.

■ Some older adults have difficulty accepting help from others, or they may not recognize the need for it. It is important to identify methods to facilitate necessary changes and minimize any alterations when planning care for older adults.

■ Of the more than 55.8 million older adults in the United States (65 years or older), only 1.3 million live in nursing homes, representing 2.3% of the older adult population (Hallstrom, 2023). The range of housing options for older adults is increasing.

THE ADMISSION PROCESS

Admission means entering a health care agency for nursing care and medical or surgical treatment. It involves:

- Authorization from a physician that the person requires specialized care and treatment
- Collection of billing information by the admitting department of the health care agency
- Completion of the agency's admission database by nursing personnel
- Documentation of the client's medical history and findings from physical examination
- Development of an initial nursing care plan
- Initial medical orders for treatment

The various types of admissions are listed in Table 11-1.

TABLE 11-1 Types of Admissions

TYPE	EXPLANATION	EXAMPLE
Inpatient	Length of stay generally more than 24 hours	Acute pneumonia
Planned (nonurgent)	Scheduled in advance	Elective or required major surgery
Emergency admission	Unplanned; stabilized in emergency department and transferred to nursing care unit	Unrelieved chest pain, major trauma
Direct admission	Unplanned; emergency department bypassed	Acute condition such as prolonged vomiting or diarrhea
Outpatient	Length of stay <24 hours; possible return on a regular basis for continued care or treatment	Minor surgery, cancer therapy, physical therapy
Observational	Monitoring required; need for inpatient admission determined within 23 hours	Head injury, unstable vital signs, premature or early labor

Pharmacologic Considerations

Nonadherence to medication regimens accounts for more than 10% of older adult hospital admissions, nearly one fourth of nursing home admissions, and 20% of preventable adverse drug events among older persons in an ambulatory setting.

Medical Authorization

Before admission, a physician determines whether a client's condition requires special tests, technical care, or treatment. Some clients are scheduled for nonurgent care, such as some types of surgery, on a mutually agreeable date and time. Most clients, however, see a primary care or emergency department physician just before admission. The physician advises both the client and the nursing staff to proceed with the admission process.

The Admitting Department

In the admitting department of a hospital, clerical personnel begin to gather information from the prospective client or their family or caregiver (Fig. 11-1). They initiate the medical record with data obtained at this time. They prepare a form with the client's address, place of employment (if the client works), insurance carrier and policy numbers, Medicare information, and other personal data. The hospital's business office uses this information for record keeping and billing.

Clients who are extremely unstable or in severe discomfort may bypass the admitting department and go directly to the nursing unit. Personnel eventually will direct someone from the family to the admitting department on the client's behalf or go to the client's bedside to obtain the needed information.

Generally, the admissions clerk prepares an identification bracelet for the client, which contains the client's name, an identification number, and, in some cases, a barcode for computerized scanning purposes. Someone in the admitting department or the admitting nurse applies the bracelet

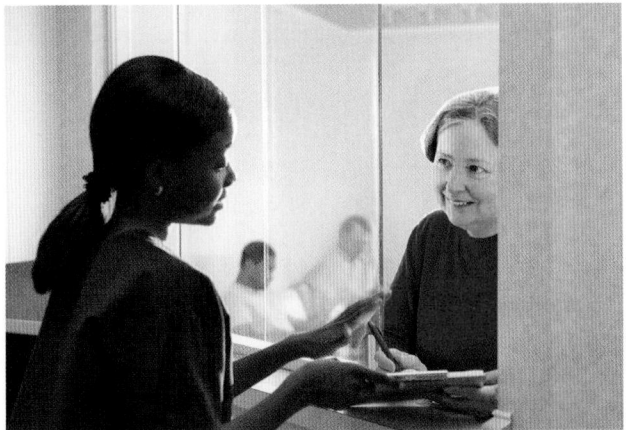

FIGURE 11-1 Obtaining information such as health insurance from a client prior to admission.

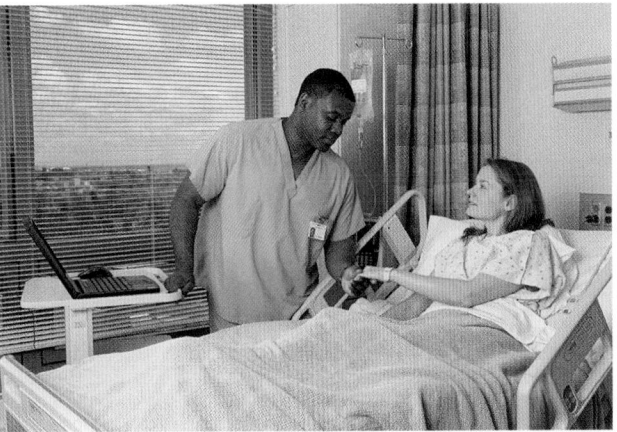

FIGURE 11-2 A nurse applies an identification bracelet to the client.

(Fig. 11-2). For the client's safety, the client must wear the bracelet throughout the stay. Along with asking a client's name and date of birth, the bracelet is the single most important method for identifying the client. If the identification bracelet is missing or has been removed, the nurse is responsible for replacing it as soon as possible.

Once personnel have collected preliminary data, they notify the nursing unit and escort the client to the site where they will receive care. They deliver the form initiated in the admitting department to the nursing unit. A computerized form with the client's information and physician orders accompanies the admission paperwork. Computer-generated labels will be printed and used for billing purposes, typically for specimens, medications, and special items such as dressing supplies used in the client's care.

Nursing Admission Activities
Preparing the Client's Room

When the admissions department informs the nursing unit that the client is about to arrive, nurses check the room to ensure it is clean and stocked with basic equipment for initial care (Box 11-1). They later provide personal care items such as soap, lotion, a toothbrush, toothpaste, razors, paper tissues, and denture containers for clients who need them. They also place oxygen administration equipment, a stand for supporting intravenous fluids, and anything else required at the time of initial treatment.

Welcoming the Client

One of the most important steps in admission is to make the client feel welcome. On arrival, the admitting nurse greets

BOX 11-1	Basic Room Supplies

Each bedside stand is generally stocked with:

- A wash basin
- A soap dish
- An emesis basin
- A water carafe
- A bedpan and a urinal

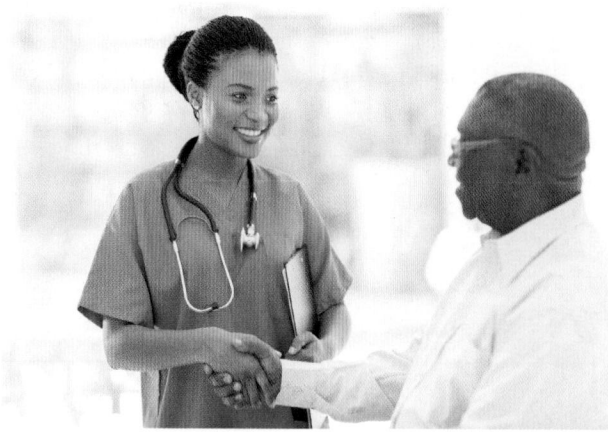

FIGURE 11-3 The nurse greets the client upon admission.

the client warmly with a smile and a handshake (Fig. 11-3). The nurse wears a nametag, introduces themself, and also introduces other personnel in the area. Being treated courteously helps the client relax. A client who feels unexpected or unwanted is likely to have a poor and lasting negative first impression of the unit.

Orienting the Client

Orientation (helping a person become familiar with a new environment) facilitates comfort and adaptation. When orienting a client, the nurse describes:

- The location of the nursing station, toilet, shower or bathing area, and lounge available to the client and visitors
- Where to store clothing and personal items
- How to call for nursing assistance from the bed and bathroom
- How to adjust the hospital bed
- How to regulate the room lights
- How to use the telephone and any policy about diverting incoming calls to the nursing station during the night
- How to operate the television
- The daily routine such as mealtimes or how to order food directly from the food service department
- When the doctor usually visits
- When surgery is scheduled
- When laboratory or diagnostic tests are performed

Some hospitals provide booklets with information about the agency, such as gift shop hours, newspaper deliveries, and the location of the chapel or name of the clergy. Such booklets, however, should never replace a nurse's individualized explanations.

Safeguarding Valuables and Clothing

Nurses give certain items, such as prescription and nonprescription medications, valuable jewelry, and large sums of money, to family members to take home. If this is not possible, *the nurse must carefully observe the agency's policies.* Some institutions provide clients who are not expected to stay longer than 24 hours with a locker to store personal effects. The nurse may be able to place the clients' valuables in the hospital's safe temporarily. The nurse notes in the medical record

the type of valuables and how they have been safeguarded. It is best to be as descriptive as possible. For example, rather than indicating that the nurse placed a ring in the safe, it is better to describe the type of metal and stones in the ring.

Losing a client's personal items can have serious legal implications for both the nurse and the health care agency. The client may sue, claiming the belongings were lost or stolen because of careless handling. Therefore, it is best to have a second nurse's, supervisor's, or security person's signature on the envelope containing the secured valuables.

One method for avoiding discrepancies between the items entrusted to the nurse and those eventually returned is to make an inventory (Fig. 11-4), which both the nurse and the client sign. The nurse gives one copy to the client and attaches another copy to the chart. When adding items or returning them to the client, the nurse revises the list and the client signs the new inventory. Problems with theft or loss may occur without subsequent documentation.

The nurse identifies client-owned equipment, such as a walker or wheelchair, with a large, easily read label. Labeling prevents confusing personal equipment with that belonging to the facility. Most agencies have places in the client's room for storing street clothing.

Because clients occasionally remove eyeglasses and dentures, such items may be lost or broken. Generally, the

CLOTHING LIST:
(Please check articles of clothing with client and describe.)

Dress	1 – Blue & white	Pants
Slip	1 – White (1/2 slip)	Shirt
Bra	1 – White	Undershirt
Panties	1 – White	Undershorts
Hose		Socks
Girdle		Tie
Slippers	1 – Pink	Shoes 1 – White
Nightgown	1 – Blue, 1 – Pink	Pajamas
Suit		Robe
Sweater		Coat
Slacks		Truss
Blouse		Back support
Shorts		Belt
Skirt		Hat

Other items not listed:

Check valuables below and describe if necessary:

Watch   Earrings

Medals   Rings – Type &   1 – Yellow, metal, plain
                                               Number   band
Other Jewelry

Dentures:	Yes ✔	No		Prosthesis:	Yes	No ✔
Contact Lenses:	Yes	No ✔		Glasses:	Yes ✔	No
Removed:	Yes	No		Hearing Aid:	Yes	No ✔

Wallet ✔	Color Red	With Pt. ✔	In Safe	To Family or Friend
Purse ✔	Color White	With Pt.	In Safe	To Family or Friend
Cash $25.00	With Pt.	In Safe ✔	To Family or Friend	
Checks/Check Book		With Pt.	In Safe	To Family or Friend

The above list is correct:
Client's Signature   Witness

Helen Jones   *Nancy Smith, L.P.N.*

Clothing taken home by

Relationship

Witness

Received by on Nursing Unit

FIGURE 11-4 An inventory of a client's personal belongings.

health care agency is responsible for replacing these items if the negligence of the staff causes accidental damage or loss.

Helping the Client Undress

To facilitate a physical examination, the client must undress. If the client cannot undress without the nurse's help, the nurse:

- Provides privacy
- Has the client sit on the edge of the bed, which has already been lowered
- Removes the client's shoes
- Gathers each stocking, sliding it down the leg and over the foot
- Helps the client lie down if weak or tired
- Releases fasteners such as zippers and buttons and removes the item of clothing in whatever way is most comfortable and least disturbing. For example, the nurse folds or gathers a garment and works it up and over the body. The nurse has the client lift the hips to slide clothes up or down.
- Lifts the client's head to guide garments over it
- Rolls the client from side to side to remove clothes that fasten up the front or back
- Covers the client with a bath blanket after removing the outer clothing, or puts a hospital gown on the client, explaining that hospital gowns fasten in the back

Compiling the Nursing Database

Upon admission, the nurse begins assessing the client and collecting information for the database (Fig. 11-5). Although the registered nurse (RN) is responsible for the admission assessment, the RN may delegate some aspects to the practical nurse, nursing student, or other ancillary staff. Physical assessment skills, which include taking vital signs, are discussed in more depth in Chapters 12 and 13.

Reconciling Medications

Medication reconciliation refers to obtaining and verifying the medications a client is currently taking. The name, dosage, frequency of administration, and route are necessary pieces of information to obtain. The information is collected on admission and readmission to a hospital, and before any transition in care such as to a long-term care facility, home

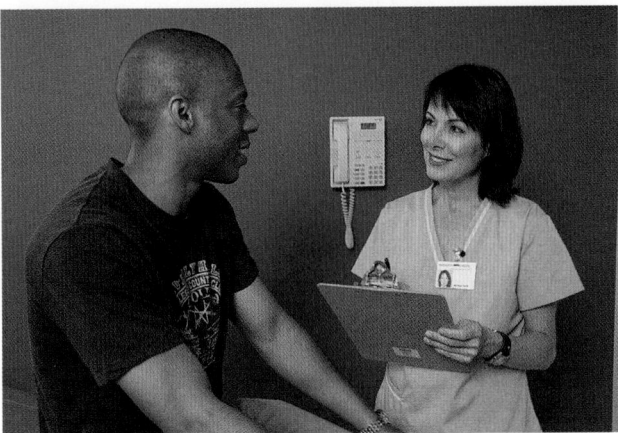

FIGURE 11-5 Beginning to compile the nursing database.

health services, or agency for rehabilitation. Any discrepancies are communicated to the client's physician.

Skill 11-1 describes the basic steps in admitting a client. Additions or modifications to the procedure depend largely on the client's condition and agency policies.

›› *Stop, Think, and Respond 11-1*

What aspects of admission could the registered nurse delegate to a practical nurse, a nursing student, or a nursing assistant? What are the responsibilities of the nurse who has delegated admission tasks?

 Pharmacologic Considerations

Medication reconciliation is one vitally important care process nurses use to help prevent medication errors. This involves reviewing patients' medication lists to make sure they are complete and accurate.

Initial Nursing Plan for Care

Once all admission data are collected, the nurse develops an initial plan for the client's care as soon as possible but no later than 24 hours following admission (see Chapter 2). The initial plan generally identifies priority problems and includes the client's projected needs for teaching and discharge planning. The nurse revises the care plan as more data accumulate or if the client's condition changes.

Medical Admission Responsibilities

The nurse notifies the physician once the admission procedure is completed. The physician provides medical orders for medications and other treatments, laboratory and diagnostic tests, activity, and diet. The physician also obtains a medical history and performs a physical examination within 24 hours of admission. The physician may delegate this task to another member of the medical team, such as a medical student, an intern, or a resident.

The medical history and physical examination generally include identifying data, reason for seeking care, history of present illness, personal history, past health history, family history, review of body systems, and conclusions (Box 11-2). If the physician is unsure of the actual medical diagnosis, they use the term *rule out* or the abbreviation *R/O* to indicate that the condition is suspected, but additional diagnostic data must be obtained before confirmation.

Common Responses to Admission

Nurses and physicians must remember that no matter how often they have admitted clients, it is a unique and possibly emotionally traumatic experience for each client. Leaving the security of the home and entering an unfamiliar environment compound the stress of physical illness and contribute to emotional and social distress.

Although specific responses to admission are unique, common reactions include anxiety, loneliness, decreased

| BOX 11-2 | Components of a Medical History and Physical Examination |

Identifying Data
- Age, gender, marital status
- General appearance
- Circumstances surrounding physician involvement
- Reliability of client as a historian
- Others providing information about the client's history

Chief Complaint
- Reason for seeking care (from client's perspective)

History of Present Illness
- Chronologic description of onset, frequency, and duration of current signs and symptoms
- Outcomes of earlier attempts at self-treatment and medical treatment

Medical History
- Childhood disease summary
- Physical injuries
- Major illnesses and surgeries
- Previous hospitalizations (medical or psychiatric)
- Drug history
- Alcohol and tobacco use
- Medical directives

Medications

Allergies

Personal History
- Occupation
- Primary language

Family History
- Health problems in immediate family members (living and deceased)
- Longevity and cause of death among deceased blood relatives (especially parents and grandparents)

Review of Body Systems

Results of Physical Examination

Assessment

Problem List and Recommendations
- Primary diagnosis (from chief complaint and physical examination)
- Secondary diagnoses reflecting stable or preexisting conditions, possibly affecting client's treatment

privacy, and loss of identity. In addition, the nurse may identify one or more of the following nursing diagnoses as a consequence of admission:

- Acute anxiety
- Fear
- Situational low self-esteem
- Altered health maintenance

Acute Anxiety

Acute anxiety is an uncomfortable feeling caused by insecurity. It can be defined as a vague, uneasy feeling of dread or discomfort that is accompanied by an autonomic response from the apprehension of perceived anticipation or danger.

Many adults do not manifest their anxiety in obvious ways. Observant nurses may note that adults appear sad or worried, are restless, have a reduced appetite, and have trouble sleeping (see Chapter 5). Because adults have a greater capacity to process information than children, it is helpful to acknowledge their uneasiness and to provide explanations and instructions before any new experience.

Nursing Care Plan 11-1 provides an example of how to use the nursing process when planning care for a client with anxiety.

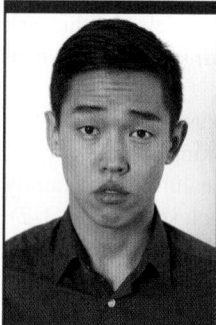

Clinical Scenario A 20-year-old client has a physician's appointment to discuss his inability to focus on his college courses. During the initial assessment, the nurse notes that the client is nervous. He asks the nurse to frequently repeat the assessment questions. He verbally rambles from topic to topic during the encounter. What further data may help the nurse identify the client's problem? What nursing suggestions could help the client at this time?

Refer to Nursing Care Plan 11-1.

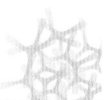

NURSING CARE PLAN 11-1 — Anxiety

Assessment
- Observe evidence of anxiety such as rapid heart rate, elevated blood pressure, sleep disturbance, restlessness, worry, irritability, facial tension, impaired attention, difficulty concentrating, talking excessively, crying, or being withdrawn.
- Encourage the client to validate observations by asking open-ended questions, such as "How are you feeling now?" If anxiety exists, ask the client to rate the level of anxiety, using a scale from 0 to 10 in which 0 represents no anxiety and 10 represents the most anxiety the client has ever experienced.
- Also ask the client to indicate the level at which they can tolerate or cope with anxiety.
- Inquire as to methods the client uses to control anxiety when it exists and the effectiveness of the identified methods.

Nursing Diagnosis. Acute anxiety related to the perception of danger as evidenced by a heart rate of 92 beats/min at rest, elevated blood pressure of 156/92, awareness of feelings of apprehension in the statement, "I feel like a rubber band that's stretched and ready to snap," and rating of 7 as the level of emotional discomfort.

Expected Outcome. The client's anxiety will be reduced to a self-rated level of tolerance of "5."

Interventions	Rationales
Encourage the client to use methods that have successfully relieved anxiety in the past.	Interventions that the client has relied upon and that have had beneficial outcomes can increase the potential for effectiveness in current and future episodes of anxiety.
Reduce external stimuli such as bright lights, noise, sudden movement, and unnecessary activity.	Numerous stimuli escalate anxiety because they interfere with attention and concentration. Dealing simultaneously with multiple stimuli can tax the client's energy and compromise the ability to cope.
Maintain a calm manner when interacting with the client.	People communicate anxiety to one another; an anxious nurse can increase anxiety in a client. Modeling a controlled state promotes a similar response in the client.
Take a position at least an arm's length away from the client.	Invading an anxious client's personal space may increase the client's discomfort.
Avoid touching the client without first asking permission.	An anxious client may misinterpret unexpected touching as threatening.
Establish trust by being available to the client and keeping promises.	Insecurity can be relieved if the client knows they can depend on assistance from the nurse.
Advise the client to seek out the nurse or another supportive person when feeling heightened anxiety.	The earlier the anxiety is deescalated, the sooner the client will experience relief of symptoms.
Stay with the client during periods of severe anxiety.	The nurse's presence can help the client stay in control or restore control to a more comfortable level.
Follow a consistent schedule for routine activities.	Unpredictability heightens anxiety; consistency helps a client manage time and cope with personal demands.
Encourage the client to identify what they perceive to be a threat to emotional equilibrium.	Processing situations verbally may give the client perspective on perceived threats so that they are more realistic and less exaggerated.
Use a soft voice, short sentences, and clear messages when exchanging information.	Anxious clients have a short attention span and reduced ability to concentrate; they may be unable to follow lengthy or complicated information.
Provide specific, succinct directions for tasks the client should complete or assist the client who becomes agitated.	Anxious clients have difficulty following instructions and performing tasks in correct sequence. Assistance relieves unnecessary distress.
Instruct and help the client with moderate or severe anxiety to perform one or more of the following until anxiety is within a tolerable level:	
• Count slowly backward from 100.	Distraction redirects the client's attention from distressing physiologic symptoms to a simple task.
• Breathe slowly and deeply in through the nose and out through the mouth.	Slowing respirations aborts hyperventilation and subsequent potential for fainting, peripheral tingling, and numbness from respiratory alkalosis.
• Offer a warm bath or backrub.	Sitting in warm running water promotes relaxation; massage relaxes tense muscles and possibly releases endorphins (natural chemicals that create a feeling of well-being).
• Help the client progressively relax groups of muscles from the toes to the head.	Consciously relaxing skeletal muscles relieves tension and fatigue.
• Suggest that the client repeat positive statements such as, "I am relaxed," "I am in control," and "I am safe."	Positive self-talk can be transformed into reality.
• Encourage the client to visualize a pleasant, relaxing place.	Imagery can transform a person's aroused state to one that is more relaxed.
• Have the client listen to a relaxation tape or soothing music.	Distraction helps refocus attention to less anxiety-provoking stimuli.
Advise the client to reduce dietary intake of substances that contain caffeine, such as colas and coffee.	Caffeine is a central nervous system stimulant that contributes to the symptoms the client experiences with anxiety.

Evaluation of Expected Outcomes

• The client deals with anxiety-provoking stimuli realistically and implements interventions that reduce anxiety.
• The client has extended periods during which their anxiety is at a tolerable level.
• The client has a reduced perception of being apprehensive.

Fear

The most common examples of situations in which the nurse may encounter patient fear are when treating a patient in the community, during diagnostic testing in an outpatient setting, or during hospitalization. The nurse's role is to identify when patients are experiencing fear and find ways to help them in a respectful way to face these feelings.

Situational Low Self-esteem

Self-esteem is defined as the way individuals think about themselves and how good they feel. Positive self-esteem develops when a person feels good and is capable of responding to challenges and stressors. Low self-esteem can reduce the quality of a person's life in many different ways, including negative feelings, fear, relationship problems, or low resilience. This change in self-esteem is a temporary phase in response to feeling helpless to control the current situation.

In a hospital setting, clients may feel a decrease in their self-esteem, related to their admission and their medical diagnosis. Nurses can help the client to understand their medical diagnosis and have them assist in the treatment associated with their hospitalization.

Altered Health Maintenance

Altered health maintenance is defined as an individualized plan of care, which is directed toward reducing risk factors and assisting the clients to achieve optimum levels of function and independence within the limits of defined health maintenance alterations. This nursing diagnosis is used when there is a change in the way a client is caring for themselves. Nurses can assist the clients in understanding ways to continue in their self-care and improving the way their health care is maintained.

>>> *Stop, Think, and Respond 11-2*

What actions are appropriate if a family member or significant other chooses to remain with the client after the client has been escorted to a room on the nursing unit at admission?

THE DISCHARGE PROCESS

Regardless of where or why clients are admitted, the goal is to keep the admission brief and to discharge clients to the home or to another health care facility of their choice as soon as possible. **Discharge** (the termination of care from a health care agency) generally consists of discharge planning, obtaining a written medical order, completing discharge instructions, notifying the business office, helping the client leave the agency, writing a summary of the client's condition at discharge, and requesting that the room be cleaned.

Discharge Planning

Discharge planning is a process that improves client outcomes by (1) predetermining the client's postdischarge needs in a timely manner and (2) coordinating the use of appropriate community resources to provide a continuum of care. If effective, discharge planning shortens the hospital stay, decreases the cost of in-hospital care, reduces the necessity for readmission, and eases the transition between the hospital and the next level of care.

Activities involved in discharge planning, which are incorporated within the plan of care, ideally begin at admission or shortly thereafter (Fig. 11-6). Although the discharge planner may be a nurse consultant or social worker, the planning often involves a multidisciplinary team of personnel from a skilled, intermediate, or basic care nursing facility, home health agency, and hospice provider; a physical, occupational, or speech therapist; a medical equipment supplier; and others. There are monetary penalties if clients with Medicare are readmitted to a hospital within 30 days of discharge.

Discharge planning is usually simple and routine. Clients with one or more of the following characteristics may have special considerations related to discharge planning:

- Age older than 75 years
- Multiple, chronic, or terminal health problems
- Cognitive impairment, motivational problems, or confusion
- Inability to perform self-care
- Impaired mobility
- Safety risks associated with independent living or that pose a burden to potential caregivers
- A treatment regimen involving multiple medications, dietary management, or complicated medical equipment
- History of multiple treatments in the emergency department

Obtaining Authorization for Medical Discharge

The physician determines when the client is well enough for discharge. Generally, the physician waits to write the medical order until after examining the client. Before leaving the nursing unit, the physician writes the discharge order, provides written prescriptions for the client, and indicates when and where a follow-up appointment should occur.

Leaving "against medical advice" (AMA) is a term that applies to situations when the client leaves before the physician authorizes the discharge. Many times, it happens because the client is unhappy with an aspect of care. In some cases, the nurse may negotiate a compromise or persuade the client to delay such action. In the meantime, the nurse informs the physician and nursing supervisor of the client's wish to leave.

If the client is determined to leave, the nurse asks them to sign a special form (see Chapter 3). This signed form may release the physician and agency from future responsibility for any complications, but it is not a guarantee. If the client refuses to sign, personnel still cannot prevent the client from leaving. They note in the client's medical record, however, that they presented the form and that the client subsequently refused it. It is a myth that the client's insurance provider will refuse to pay for the client's care following a discharge AMA.

Providing Discharge Instructions

When the nurse anticipates that a client will be discharged home, they establish the anticipated knowledge, skills, and community resources that the client will need to maintain a safe level of self-care. One discharge planning technique uses the acronym "METHOD" (Table 11-2). The nurse provides the teaching identified in the discharge plan periodically during the client's stay and documents it in the record (see Chapter 8).

Discharge Care Plan

Date & Sign.	**Plan and Outcome** *(check those that apply)*	Target Date:	**Nursing Interventions** *(check those that apply)*	Date Achieved:
	☐ The client/family's discharge planning will begin on day of admission including preparation for education and/or equipment.		☐ Assess needs of client/family beginning on the day of admission and continue assessment during hospitalization.	

	☐ On the day of discharge, the client/family will receive verbal and written instructions concerning:
	  - Medications
	  - Diet
	  - Activity
	  - Treatment
	  - Follow-up appointments
	  - Signs and symptoms to observe for (when to contact the doctor)
	  - Care of incisions, wounds, etc.
	
	☐ Other:
			☐ Anticipated needs/services:
			  - Respiratory equipment
			  - Hospital bed
			  - Wheelchair
			  - Walker
			  - Home health nurse
			  - Home PT/OT/ST
			
			☐ Involve client/family in the discharge process.
			
			☐ Discuss with physician the discharge plan and obtain orders if needed.
			
			☐ Contact appropriate personnel with orders.
			
			☐ Provide written and verbal instructions at the client/family's level of understanding.
			
			☐ Verbally explain instructions to client/family prior to discharge and provide client/family with a written copy.
			
			☐ Ascertain that client has follow-up care arranged at discharge.
			
			☐ Provide verbal and written information on what signs and symptoms to observe and when to contact the physician.
			
			☐ Assess if any community resources should be used (i.e., Home Health Nurse), and contact appropriate personnel.
			
			☐ Document all discharge teaching on Discharge Instruction Sheet and Nursing notes.
			
			☐ Other: _____	

Client/Significant other signature _____

RN signature _____

FIGURE 11-6 A sample discharge care plan. PT, physical therapist; OT, occupational therapist; RN, registered nurse; ST, speech therapist.

TABLE 11-2 The METHOD Discharge Planning Guide

TOPIC	NURSING ACTIVITY	EXAMPLE
M—Medications	Instruct the client about drugs that will be self-administered.	Insulin
E—Environment	Explore how the home environment can be modified to ensure the client's safety.	Remove scatter rugs
T—Treatments	Demonstrate how to perform skills involved in self-care and provide opportunities for returning the demonstration.	Dressing changes
H—Health teaching	Identify information that is necessary for maintaining or improving health.	Signs and symptoms of complications
O—Outpatient referral	Explain what community services are available that may ease the client's transition to independent living.	Physical therapy
D—Diet	Arrange for the dietitian to provide verbal and written instructions on modifying or restricting certain foods or suggestions for altering their methods of preparation.	Low-fat diet

Before the client leaves, the nurse reviews teaching that has been provided, gives the client prescriptions to have filled, and advises the client to make an office appointment for the date specified by the physician. The nurse provides a written summary of discharge instructions. The client signs and keeps the original; the nurse attaches a copy to the client's medical record.

Notifying the Business Office

Before the client leaves the agency, the nurse notifies the business office. At that time, clerical personnel verify that all insurance information is complete and that the client has signed a consent form authorizing the release of medical information to the insurance carrier. If records are incomplete or the client has no health insurance, the client may be asked to make arrangements for future financial payments before discharge.

Discharging a Client

When all the preliminary business is complete, the nurse helps the client gather their belongings, plan for transportation, and leave the agency.

Gathering Belongings

If necessary, the nurse helps the client repack personal items. The nurse uses the inventory of valuables to ensure that nothing has been lost or forgotten. Because most hospitals dispose of the plastic supplies (e.g., basin, bedpan, urinal), the nurse can offer them to the client; otherwise, the nurse discards them in the soiled utility room. A wheeled cart is helpful for transporting the client's belongings.

Arranging Transportation

The nurse informs clients about the agency's checkout time—the time before which they can avoid being charged for another full day. In most cases, the client contacts a family member or friend for assistance with transportation. If no transportation is available, the client may use public transportation, a taxi or ride service, or an ambulance to get home. Van transportation may be available for older adults through the local commission on aging, but 24-hour advance notification is usually required.

Escorting the Client

When the client is ready, the nurse takes them to the door in a wheelchair or allows the client to walk there, preferably with assistance. The client may choose to have discharge prescriptions filled at the hospital's pharmacy before leaving. Generally, the nurse remains with the client until they are safely inside a vehicle or waiting in the lobby for a ride. Skill 11-2 provides a step-by-step description of the discharge process.

Writing a Discharge Summary

After the client has left the health care agency, the nurse documents the discharge activities and client's condition (see Skill 11-2).

> **»» Stop, Think, and Respond 11-3**
> *What information is helpful to obtain to ensure a safe transition from a health agency to self-management before discharge?*

Terminal Cleaning

Except in unusual circumstances, housekeeping personnel prepare the client's room for the next admission. They strip the bed of its linens and clean it with disinfectant, and they restock the bedside cabinet with basic equipment. They then notify the admitting department that the unit is ready. These measures prevent assigning a client to a room that still requires cleaning.

THE TRANSFER PROCESS

A **transfer** (discharging a client from one unit or agency and admitting them to another without going home in the interim) may occur when a client's condition improves or worsens. Generally, a transfer has some advantage for the client. It may facilitate more specialized care in a life-threatening situation (Fig. 11-7), or it may reduce health care costs. Many hospitals are creating **step-down units, progressive care units,** or **transitional care units.** These units are for clients who were once in critical or unstable conditions but have recovered sufficiently to require less intensive nursing care.

Transfer Activities

Transferring a client to a different nursing unit is less complex than to another agency. In a transfer within the same agency, the nurse:

- Informs the client and family about the transfer
- Completes a **transfer summary** (a written review of the client's current status) briefly describing the client's current condition and reason for transfer (Fig. 11-8)
- Speaks with a nurse on the transfer unit to coordinate the transfer (the change of shift report in Chapter 9 can be used as a model)
- Transports the client and their belongings, medications, nursing supplies, and chart to the other unit

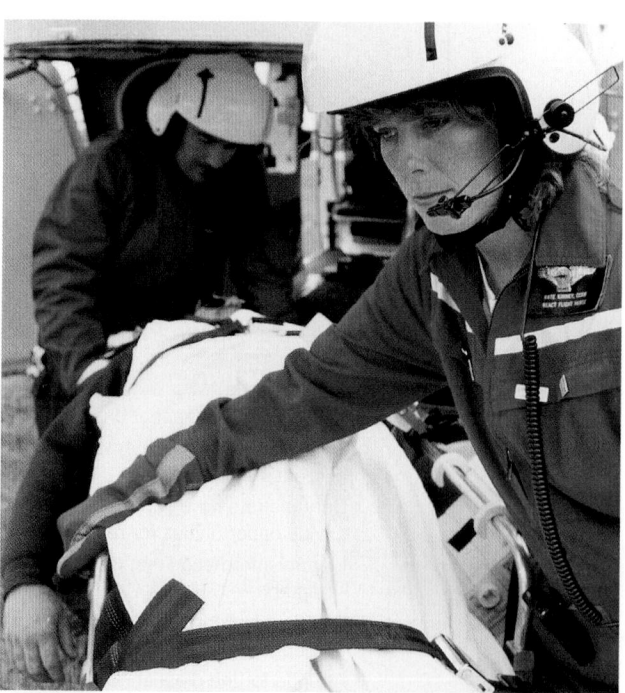

FIGURE 11-7 Transferring a client rapidly may be a life-saving measure.

PATIENT TRANSFER FORM
(INTER-AGENCY REFERRAL)

INSTRUCTIONS: The purpose of this form is to insure continuity of care in transfer from hospital to extended care facility or extended care facility to hospital. When writing, press firmly.

PATIENT'S LAST NAME | FIRST NAME | MI | DATE OF BIRTH

DECISION MAKER ❑ Self ❑ Durable POA (Health Care Proxy)
Name:_____
Relationship: _____

ADVANCE DIRECTIVES
Advance Directives: ❑ Yes, see attached ❑ No
DO NOT Resuscitate (DNR): ❑ Yes, see attached ❑ No

TRANSFERRING FACILITY
Facility Name: _____
Contact Name: _____
Contact Number: _____

REASON FOR TRANSFER (may include brief medical history)
_____
_____
_____
_____

DIAGNOSES (include mental health)
(a) Primary _____
_____

(b) Secondary _____
_____

SKIN CARE/ASSESSMENT
❑ No Wounds ❑ TAR attached ❑ See attached
Pressure Ulcer Risk Assessment:
Date of Assessment ____/____/____ Score ____ Scale (i.e., Braden)

VITALS AT TIME OF TRANSFER
Date Taken: _____/_____/_____ Time Taken: _____ ❑ AM ❑ PM
Ht._____ Wt._____ BP:_____ Temp.:_____
Pulse:_____ Resp.:_____ Pulse Ox:_____

ALLERGIES ❑ None known
Medication: ❑ Yes ❑ None known Food: ❑ Yes ❑ None known
Latex: ❑ Yes ❑ None known

AT RISK ALERTS ❑ None known
❑ Fall ❑ Harm to self ❑ Harm to others ❑ Seizure ❑ Elopement
❑ Aspiration ❑ Restraints ❑ Other _____

ISOLATION/PRECAUTION
❑ None ❑ Contact ❑ Droplet ❑ Airborne
❑ MRSA Date ___/___/___ Site:_____
❑ VRE Date ___/___/___ Site:_____
❑ ESBL Date ___/___/___ Site:_____
❑ Other Date ___/___/___ Site:_____
History of MDRO: ❑ No ❑ Yes Date ___/___/___
  MDRO type: _____
History of C-difficile? ❑ No ❑ Yes Date ___/___/___

IV ACCESS
❑ PICC: Size_____ Length_____ # of Lumens_____
❑ Heparin Lock ❑ Port-A-Catheter

Preventative Devises/Measures/Comments: _____
_____

Wound Site and Type	Stage/Size	Characteristics	Treatment Plan	Recent Status
Size:_____ ❑ Tear ❑ Trauma ❑ Surgical ❑ Vascular ❑ Diabetic ❑ Pressure related	1 2 3 4 US L W D	Odor: ❑ Yes ❑ No Drainage: ❑ Yes ❑ No Tunneling: ❑ Yes ❑ No Wound Color:_____		❑ Date of onset ___/___/___ ❑ Improving ❑ Unchanged ❑ Worsening
Size:_____ ❑ Tear ❑ Trauma ❑ Surgical ❑ Vascular ❑ Diabetic ❑ Pressure related	1 2 3 4 US L W D	Odor: ❑ Yes ❑ No Drainage: ❑ Yes ❑ No Tunneling: ❑ Yes ❑ No Wound Color:_____		❑ Date of onset ___/___/___ ❑ Improving ❑ Unchanged ❑ Worsening
Size:_____ ❑ Tear ❑ Trauma ❑ Surgical ❑ Vascular ❑ Diabetic ❑ Pressure related	1 2 3 4 US L W D	Odor: ❑ Yes ❑ No Drainage: ❑ Yes ❑ No Tunneling: ❑ Yes ❑ No Wound Color:_____		❑ Date of onset ___/___/___ ❑ Improving ❑ Unchanged ❑ Worsening
Size:_____ ❑ Tear ❑ Trauma ❑ Surgical ❑ Vascular ❑ Diabetic ❑ Pressure related	1 2 3 4 US L W D	Odor: ❑ Yes ❑ No Drainage: ❑ Yes ❑ No Tunneling: ❑ Yes ❑ No Wound Color:_____		❑ Date of onset ___/___/___ ❑ Improving ❑ Unchanged ❑ Worsening

FOLLOW-UP CARE/APPOINTMENT
_____
_____
_____
_____
_____
_____
_____
_____

DOCUMENTS ATTACHED
❑ Current Medication/Treatment Administration Record
❑ Current Medication Reconciliation Record ❑ Face Sheet
❑ Immunization Records ❑ Current Physician Orders, # of pages ____
❑ Other: _____

MEDICAL REPORTS, VALUES, PROCEDURES
(related to reasons for transfer)
Study Results (x-ray, ECG, CT, MRI, Scan, etc.): ❑ None
Lab Values: ❑ None ❑ See attached   ❑ See attached
Surgical Procedures: ❑ None ❑ See attached

Signature of Physician or Nurse:_____ Date: _____

39844 BRIGGS, Des Moines, IA 50306 (800) 247-2343 PRINTED IN U.S.A.   **PATIENT TRANSFER FORM**

Original: Keep with sending facility patient/resident records.   Copy: Send with patient/resident at time of transfer.

FIGURE 11-8 A transfer summary provides information that promotes continuity of care. BP, blood pressure; CT, computed tomography; ECG, electrocardiogram; ESBL, extended-spectrum beta-lactamases; IV, intravenous; MDRO, multidrug-resistant organism; MRI, magnetic resonance imaging; MRSA, methicillin-resistant *Staphylococcus aureus*; PICC, peripherally inserted central catheter; VRE, vancomycin-resistant enterococci.

NURSING GUIDELINES 11-1

Transferring a Client

- Be sure to inform the client and the family of the need for a transfer as early as possible. *Communication promotes cooperation.*
- If time permits and the client and family have some choice, encourage them to investigate various facilities and collaborate on the one they prefer. *The people most affected should make the decisions.*
- Communicate with the agency or unit where the client will be transferred. *Other personnel need time to prepare for the client's arrival.*
- Make a photocopy of the medical record. *A copy aids in continuity of care and avoids duplicating services.*
- Provide a written **clinical résumé**, which is a summary of previous care (see Fig. 11-8). It should include (1) the reason for the hospitalization, (2) significant findings, (3) the treatment rendered, (4) the current condition of the client, and (5) instructions, if any, to the client and family. Check that the client has been notified and given consent for the release of their personal health information. *To comply with privacy rules and data security standards set by the Health Insurance Portability and Accountability Act (HIPAA) in 1996 and further modified in 2001, 2002, and 2022 (see Chapter 9), the client must be informed and approve the release of health information among third parties for routine use in treatment.*

- Place the written information in a large manila envelope or send it via facsimile (fax) machine with a cover sheet. Call the transfer agency to let them how to momentarily expect the fax. *Under the revisions to the HIPAA privacy rules (2002), agencies must systematically protect the client's personal health information within and outside the institution.*
- Collect all the client's belongings. *Carelessness can lead to the loss of the client's clothing or valuables and can cause inconvenience in returning them.*
- Accompany emergency medical staff or paramedics to the client's room. *Seeing a familiar face may reduce the client's anxiety.*
- Help transfer the client onto the stretcher. *Assistance reduces the physical demands on the client.*
- Give the transfer personnel a copy of the medical record in a folder or envelope. *Enclosing the record protects confidentiality and prevents loss.*
- Complete the original medical record by adding a summary of the client's discharge. *Each medical record includes a discharge summary.*
- Send the completed chart within a file folder to the medical records department. *All charts are filed for future reference.*
- Notify the business office, admitting office, and housekeeping department of the client's transfer. *Each department has its own responsibilities when a client leaves.*

When transferring the client to a nursing home or other facility, the nurse conducts the process similarly to a discharge; the client is discharged from the hospital and admitted to the transfer facility. See Nursing Guidelines 11-1.

Extended Care Facilities

Older adults in particular may be transferred directly from an acute care hospital to a facility that provides extended care (Fig. 11-9). An **extended care facility** or long-term care facility (a health care agency that provides long-term care) is designed for people who do not meet the criteria for hospitalization. Although group homes for assisted living, acute rehabilitation units, adult day care centers, senior residential communities, home health care agencies, and hospice

organizations (see Chapter 38) all fit this description, extended care is generally associated with nursing homes.

Nursing homes are classified as skilled nursing facilities or those that provide intermediate or basic care (Table 11-3).

Skilled Nursing Facilities/Acute Rehabilitation Facilities

A nursing home licensed as a **skilled nursing facility**, or an **acute rehabilitation facility** provides 24-hour nursing care under the direction of an RN. The facility is reimbursed for the care of clients who require specific technical nursing skills, or intensive physical therapy treatment (Fig. 11-10). To qualify for skilled care, the client must be referred by a physician and must require daily skilled nursing care or

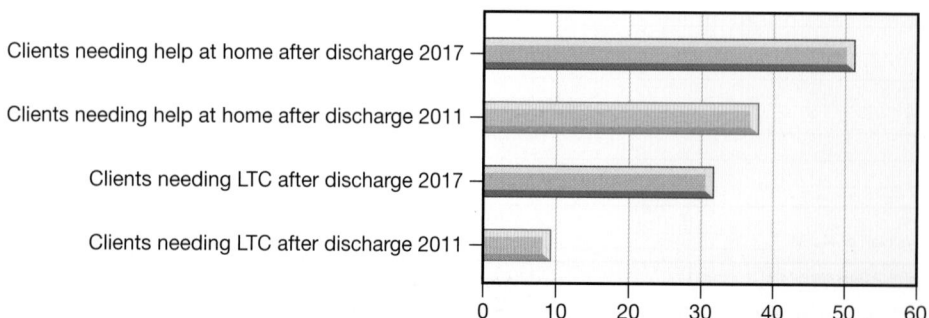

FIGURE 11-9 Seniors are getting discharged earlier from hospitals to recover at home. But is this best for all clients being discharged? LTC, long-term care. (MJH Life Sciences. [2021]. *Seniors are getting more help at home after hospitalization, but what are the costs?* https://www.chiefhealthcareexecutive.com/view/seniors-are-getting-more-help-at-home-after-hospitalization-but-what-are-the-costs-)

TABLE 11-3 10 Types of Senior Living Options 2022

INDEPENDENT LIVING OPTIONS		OPTIONS WITH ASSISTANCE	
Aging in place	A term used to describe when an older person keeps living in their current home instead of moving to a retirement facility	Nursing homes	Are senior living facilities that offer a high level of medical care. They have numerous amenities and help with basic activities, and they provide medication management and 24-hour supervision, leading to a more clinical environment.
55+ retirement communities	Age-restricted communities are housing options where residence is limited to people over a certain age.	Respite care	These are assisted living facilities or nursing homes that cater to individuals who need care for a short amount of time.
Continuing-care retirement communities (CCRCs)	Include several types of housing options for older people. CCRCs vary, but one might have senior apartments, assisted living facilities, and nursing homes all on the same property. Residents can move from one area to another as their needs change.	Assisted living	Are housing options that provide help with instrumental activities of daily living (IADLs), such as cooking and bathing, but not necessarily a lot of medical assistance. Residents usually have a private or semiprivate bedroom and bathroom, but they share all other areas.
Senior cohousing communities (SCCs)	Are one type of cohousing in which a group of seniors gets together to design and/or purchase a housing complex with private rooms or apartments and shared common areas	Memory care facilities	Are usually part of a nursing home or an assisted living community that is specifically for people with dementia. These facilities typically have a larger staff that offers more supervision.
Senior home sharing	There are different types of senior home-sharing: any arrangement where older adults share a living space. One type of arrangement involves an older adult renting out a room in a home or apartment they own to a college student or young single person to share housing costs and possibly receive help with tasks such as shopping, cooking, and housework in exchange for reduced rent. Another type of home sharing involves older adults pooling resources to rent or purchase a home where they can live together and support each other instead of moving into assisted living.	Hospice	Is a type of care for those with a terminal illness. People may receive *hospice care* in their home or in a nursing home. Hospice focuses on providing services like pain management to make the person's life as comfortable as possible.

Data from ConsumerAffairs. (n.d.). *10 types of senior living options.* https://www.consumeraffairs.com/health/senior-living-options.html

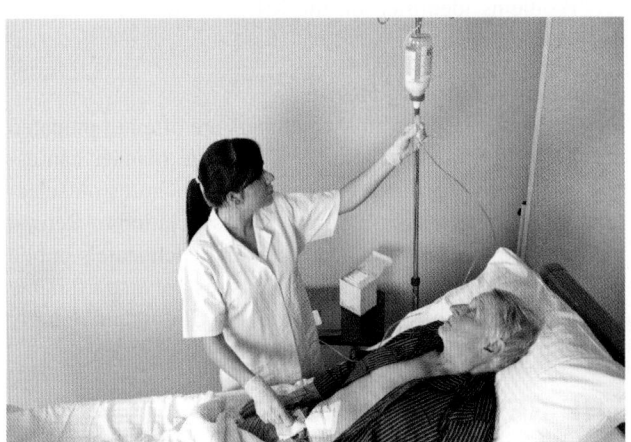

FIGURE 11-10 A client receives a gastric tube feeding in a skilled care facility.

physical therapy. The following are examples of common procedures that qualify:

- Care for a pressure ulcer
- Enteral feedings or intravenous fluids
- Bowel or bladder retraining
- Injectable medications
- Sterile dressing changes
- Tracheostomy care
- Stroke, surgery, accident, or significant illness recovery
- The client in need of physical or occupational therapy

Skilled care is provided from a multidisciplinary perspective. In addition to a 24-hour team of nurses, a skilled nursing facility must provide rehabilitation services, such as physical therapy and occupational therapy, pharmaceutical services, dietary services, diversional and therapeutic activities, and routine and emergency dental services. Many of the latter services are provided by qualified people on a contractual basis rather than through full-time employment.

To qualify for Medicare benefits in a nursing home, a person must have been hospitalized for 3 days or more within 30 days before needing skilled nursing care. Clients who meet the criteria are eligible for 60 days of assistance. On day 61, the client must pay co-insurance on days 61 to 90, until the end of the client's benefit. The client can receive up to 100 days of treatment before their Medicare Part A benefits are exhausted. Starting day 101, 100% of cost is the client's responsibility (Malzone, 2023). After clients have exhausted their own financial resources and those of a spouse, they may apply to the state for Medicaid or its equivalent.

Intermediate Care Facilities

A nursing home also may be licensed as an **intermediate care facility**. This type of agency provides health-related care and services to people who, because of their mental or physical condition, require institutional care, but not 24-hour nursing care. Clients who require intermediate care may need supervision because they tend to wander or are confused. They need assistance with oral medications, bathing, dressing, toileting, and mobility (Fig. 11-11).

Medicare does not provide reimbursement for intermediate care. Clients assume the costs. For low-income residents in some states, state programs such as Medicaid will pay. Some nursing homes do not accept Medicaid clients, however, because states fix the fees for reimbursement at much lower amounts than Medicare and private insurance provide.

Basic Care Facilities

A third type of nursing home is a **basic care facility** (an agency that provides extended custodial care). The emphasis is on providing shelter, food, and laundry services in a group setting. These clients assume much responsibility for their own activities of daily living, such as hygiene and dressing, preparing for sleep, and joining others for meals (Fig. 11-12). Intermediate and basic care may be provided at a skilled nursing facility but usually in separate wings.

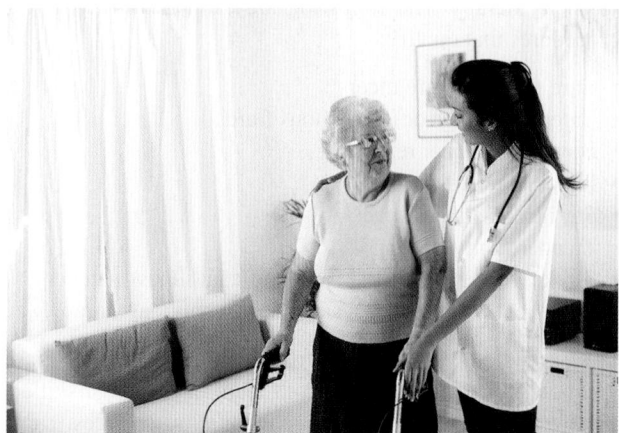

FIGURE 11-11 A nurse helps an older adult with mobility in an intermediate care facility.

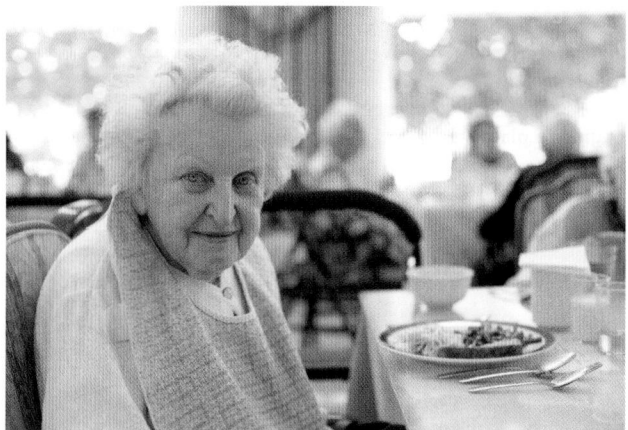

FIGURE 11-12 A client who resides in a basic care facility joins others for meals.

Determining the Level of Care

The level of care is determined at or prior to admission. Each client is assessed using a standard form developed by the Health Care Financing Association called a *Minimum Data Set (MDS) for Nursing Home Resident Assessment and Care Screening*. By federal law, the MDS is repeated every 3 months or whenever a client's condition changes. The MDS requires an assessment of:

- Cognitive patterns
- Communication and hearing patterns
- Vision patterns
- Physical functioning and structural problems
- Continence patterns in the last 14 days
- Psychosocial well-being
- Mood and behavior patterns
- Activity pursuit patterns
- Disease diagnoses
- Health conditions
- Oral and nutritional status
- Oral and dental status
- Skin condition
- Medication use
- Special treatments and procedures

Problems identified on the MDS are then reflected in the nursing care plan.

Selecting a Nursing Home

When the need arises, family members are often ill prepared for selecting a nursing home. A discharge planner can assist with arranging nursing home care. Brochures on selection are available from the American Association of Retired Persons, the Commission on Aging, and each state's public health and welfare departments. Websites are also available to provide valuable information. See Client and Family Teaching 11-1.

THE REFERRAL PROCESS

A **referral** is the process of sending someone to another person or agency for special services. Referrals generally

Client and Family Teaching 11-1
Selecting a Nursing Home

The nurse teaches the client or family to:

- Find out the levels of care (skilled, intermediate, or basic) that the nursing home is licensed to provide.
- Review inspection reports on each home. This information is available from the state's public health department on a fee-per-page basis.
- Ask others in the community, including the family physician, for recommendations.
- Visit nursing homes with and again without an appointment. Go at least once during a meal.
- Note the appearance of residents and how staff members respond to their needs.
- Observe the cleanliness of the surroundings and any unpleasant odors.
- Request brochures that identify medical care, nursing services, rehabilitation therapy, social services, activities programs, religious observances, and residents' rights and privileges.
- Clarify charges and billing procedures.
- Analyze the overall impression of the home to determine whether it is positive or negative.

TABLE 11-4 Common Community Services

ORGANIZATION	SERVICE
Commission on Aging	Assists older adults with transportation to medical appointments, outpatient therapy, and community meal sites
Hospice	Supports the family and clients with terminal illnesses who choose to stay at home
Visiting Nurses Association	Offers intermittent nursing care to homebound clients
Meals on Wheels	Provides one or two hot meals per day delivered either at home or at a community meal site
Homemaker services	Sends adults to the home to assist in shopping, meal preparation, and light housekeeping
Home health aides	Assist with bathing, hygiene, and medications
Adult protective services	Investigates and pursues accountability of individuals who are physically, socially, emotionally, or financially victimizing vulnerable adults
Respite care	Provides short-term, temporary relief to full-time caregivers of homebound clients
Older Americans' Ombudsman	Investigates and resolves complaints made by or on behalf of nursing home residents; at least one full-time ombudsman is mandated for each state.

are made to private practitioners or community agencies. Table 11-4 lists some common community services to which people with declining health, physical disabilities, or special needs are referred.

Considering Referrals

Considering referrals is part of good discharge planning. For example, a nurse, a case manager, or an agency discharge planner may help refer clients for home health care. Because planning, coordinating, and communicating take time, personnel initiate referrals as soon as possible once a need is identified. Early planning helps ensure **continuity of care** (uninterrupted client care despite a change in caregivers), thus avoiding any loss of progress that has been made.

Home Health Care

Home health care is health care provided in the home by an employee of a home health agency (Fig. 11-13). Public agencies (regional, state, or federal, such as the public health department) or private agencies may provide home health care.

The number of clients who receive home health care continues to rise, partly as an outcome of limitations imposed by Medicare and insurance companies on the number of hospital and nursing home days for which they reimburse care. Another factor is the growing number of chronically ill older adults in the population in need of assistance.

According to the National Center for Health Statistics, over 20% of the population over the age of 65 reported having one or more disabilities, such as hearing, vision, cognition, ambulation, self-care, or independent living (National

Center) (Fig. 11-14). Types of assistance older adults may need include basic activities of daily living (bathing, dressing, eating, and getting around the house), preparing meals, shopping, housework, managing money, using the phone, and taking medications.

Home care nursing services help shorten the time spent recovering in the hospital, prevent admissions to extended care facilities, and reduce readmissions to acute care facilities. Box 11-3 identifies the responsibilities assumed by home health nurses who provide community-based care.

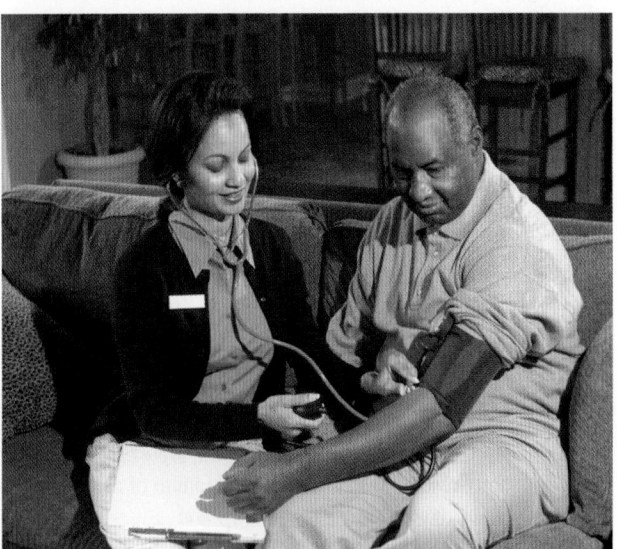
FIGURE 11-13 A home health care assessment.

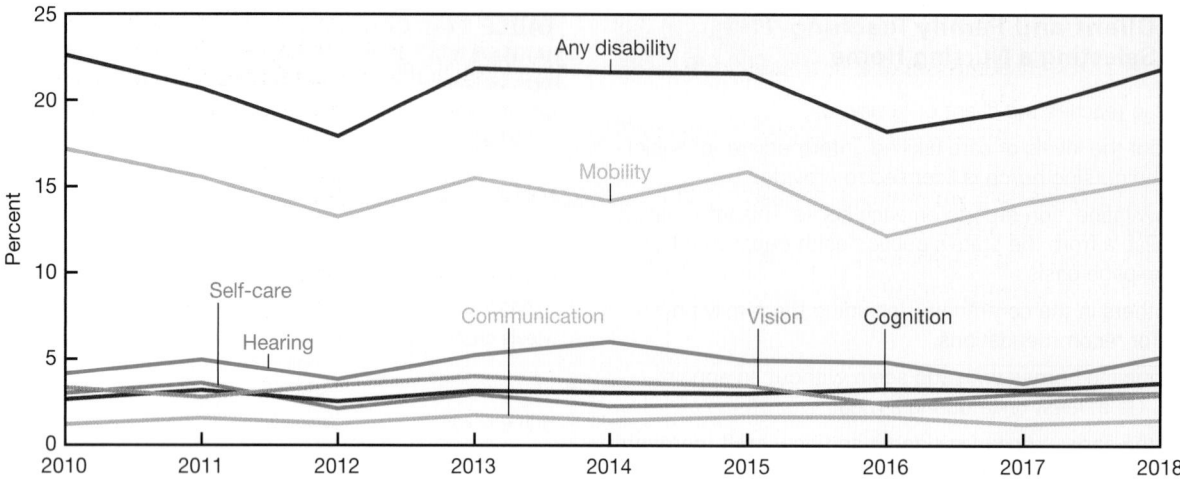

FIGURE 11-14 Percentage of people aged 65 years and over with a disability, by functional domain, 2010–2018. NOTE: *Disability* is defined as "a lot" or "cannot do/unable to do" when asked about difficulty with seeing, even if wearing glasses (vision); hearing, even if wearing hearing aids (hearing); walking or climbing steps (mobility); communicating, for example, understanding or being understood by others (communication); remembering or concentrating (cognition); and self-care, such as washing all over or dressing (self-care). Any disability is defined as having a lot of difficulty or being unable to do at least one of these activities. Reference population: These data refer to the civilian noninstitutionalized population. (National Center for Health Statistics, National Health Interview Survey.)

BOX 11-3 **Responsibilities of Home Health Nurses**

- Assess the readiness of the client and the home environment.
- Treat each client with respect, regardless of the person's standard of living.
- Identify health or social problems that require nursing, allied health, or supportive care services.
- Plan, coordinate, and monitor home care.
- Give skilled care to clients requiring part-time nursing services.
- Teach and supervise the client in self-care activities and family members who participate in the client's home care.

- Assess the safety of health practices that are being used.
- Observe, evaluate, and modify environmental and social factors that affect the client's progress.
- Evaluate the urgency and complexity of each client's changing health needs.
- Keep accurate written records and submit documentation to the agency for the purpose of reimbursement.
- Arrange for referrals to other health care agencies.
- Discharge clients who have reached a level of self-reliance.

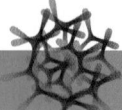

KEY POINTS

- Admission: Entering a health care agency for nursing care and medical or surgical treatment
  - Inpatient: Longer than 24 hours, planned (nonurgent), emergency admission, direct admission
  - Outpatient: Shorter than 24 hours, observational
- Nursing responsibilities for an admission
  - Setting up the room
  - Welcoming the client
  - Orienting the client
  - Safeguarding valuables and clothing
  - Helping the client undress
  - Compiling the nursing database
  - Reconciling medications
  - Initial nursing care plan
  - Medical admission responsibilities
- Discharge planning is a process that improves client outcomes by (1) predetermining clients' postdischarge needs in a timely manner and (2) coordinating the use of appropriate community resources to provide a continuum of care, and it is ideally begun during admission.
  - Obtaining authorization for medical discharge
  - Providing discharge instructions

- Notifying the business office
- Discharging a client
- Gathering belongings
- Arranging transportation
- Escorting the client
- Writing a discharge summary
- Determining the level of care for referral after discharge:
  - The level of care is determined at or prior to admission.
  - Each client is assessed using a standard form developed by the Health Care Financing Association called a *Minimum Data Set (MDS)* for Nursing Home Resident Assessment and Care Screening.
  - The MDS is repeated every 3 months or whenever a client's condition changes.
- Home health care: A wide range of health care services that can be provided in the home for an illness or injury; usually less expensive, more convenient, and just as effective as care in a hospital or skilled nursing facility

CRITICAL THINKING EXERCISES

1. Discuss how the admission of a child might differ from that of an adult.
2. Compare and contrast admission to a hospital and to a nursing home.
3. Describe the criteria you would use when selecting a nursing home for a relative.
4. If it becomes apparent that a relative cannot continue to live independently, what options would you pursue?

NEXT-GENERATION NCLEX-STYLE REVIEW QUESTIONS

1. Which nursing action is essential for complying with federal regulations that ensure the client's right to privacy?
   a. Addressing clients only by their first names
   b. Obtaining consent for releasing information
   c. Referring to the client as the person in Room 201
   d. Using a code number rather than a name in the medical record
   Test-Taking Strategy: Although all the options may protect the client's privacy, select the best option from among those provided.
2. Which information is essential for the nurse to obtain at the time of a client's admission to a health care agency?
   a. Social security number
   b. Medicare status
   c. Advance directive
   d. Health insurance policy
   Test-Taking Strategy: Eliminate options that identify information that is unnecessary or may be obtained by personnel in the business office. Select the option that correlates with information that is important to the nursing care of clients.
3. Which nursing observation is most suggestive that a newly admitted client is anxious?
   a. The client is unusually quiet and withdrawn.
   b. The client is restless and awakens frequently.
   c. The client eats little food at each meal.
   d. The client misses their spouse and children.
   Test-Taking Strategy: Select the option that is most representative of manifestations associated with stimulation of the sympathetic nervous system.
4. If the nurse suspects that an older adult in the community is the target of abuse, what agency would be appropriate to contact?
   a. Commission on Aging
   b. Visiting Nurse Association
   c. Older Americans' Ombudsman
   d. Adult Protective Services
   Test-Taking Strategy: Use the process of elimination to select the agency whose mandate is to ensure the safety of vulnerable adults.

5. Which type of extended care facility referral would be most appropriate for the nurse to recommend for an older adult who needs further rehabilitation for mobility at the time of discharge from an acute care facility?
   a. Skilled care facility
   b. Intermediate care facility
   c. Basic care facility
   d. Assisted living facility
   Test-Taking Strategy: Eliminate options that fail to correlate with the client's level of care.

NEXT-GENERATION NCLEX-STYLE CLINICAL SCENARIO QUESTIONS

Clinical Scenario:
A 20-year-old client has a physician's appointment to discuss his inability to focus on his college courses. During the initial assessment, the nurse notes that the client is nervous. He asks the nurse to frequently repeat the assessment questions. He verbally rambles from topic to topic during the encounter.

1. Choose the most likely options for the information missing from the statements below by selecting from the list of options provided.
   1. The client is maybe nervous due to his feelings of _____1_____. His _____2_____ may be the cause of his rambling answers.

OPTION 1	OPTION 2
self-assurance	anxiety
insecurity	resistance
safety	self-confidence

2. What nursing suggestions could help the client at this time?
   For each suggestion, use an "x" to indicate whether the interventions were effective (helped to meet the outcome), ineffective (did not help to meet the outcome), or unrelated (not related to the outcome).

SUGGESTION	EFFECTIVE	INEFFECTIVE	UNRELATED
Encourage relaxation techniques			
Educate the client on the importance of reducing outside stressors			
Tell the client that his sleep habits are unrelated to his anxiety			
Encourage the client to eat three meals a day			
Encourage the client to use coping strategies that have helped in the past			

SKILL 11-1 Admitting a Client

Suggested Action	Reason for Action
ASSESSMENT	
Obtain the name, admitting diagnosis, and condition of the client and the room to which they have been assigned.	Provides preliminary data from which to plan the activities that may be involved in admitting the client
Check the appearance of the room and the presence of basic supplies.	Demonstrates concern for cleanliness, order, and client convenience
PLANNING	
Assemble the needed equipment: admission assessment form, thermometer, blood pressure (BP) cuff (if not wall mounted), stethoscope, scale, and urine specimen container.	Enhances organization and efficient time management
Obtain special equipment, such as an intravenous pole or oxygen, that may be needed according to the client's needs.	Facilitates immediate care of the client without causing unnecessary delay or discomfort
Arrange the height of the bed to coordinate with the expected mode of arrival.	Reduces the physical effort in moving from a wheelchair or stretcher to the bed
Fold the top linen to the bottom of the bed if the client will be immediately confined to bed.	Reduces obstacles that may interfere with the client's comfort and ease of transfer
IMPLEMENTATION	
Greet the client by title and surname and demonstrate a friendly smile; extend a hand as a symbol of welcome.	Promotes feelings of friendliness and personal regard to help reduce initial anxiety
Introduce yourself to the client and those who have accompanied the client.	Establishes the nurse–client relationship on a personal basis
Observe the client for signs of acute distress.	Determines whether the admission process requires modification
Attend to urgent needs for comfort and breathing.	Demonstrates concern for the client's well-being
Introduce the client to others in the immediate environment.	Promotes a sense of familiarity to relieve social awkwardness; demonstrates concern for the client's emotional comfort
Offer the client a chair unless they require immediate bed rest.	Demonstrates concern for the client's physical comfort
Check the client's identification bracelet.	Enhances safety by accurately identifying the client
Orient the client to the physical environment of the room and the nursing unit.	Aids in adapting the client to unfamiliar surroundings
Demonstrate how to use the equipment in the room, such as the adjustments for the bed, how to signal for a nurse, and use of the telephone and television.	Promotes comfort and self-reliance; ensures safety
Explain the general routines and schedules that are followed for visiting hours, meals, and care.	Reduces uncertainty about when to expect activities
Explain the need to examine the client and ask personal health questions.	Prepares the client for what will follow next
Ask if the client would like family members to leave or remain.	Protects the client's right to privacy
Make provisions for privacy.	Demonstrates respect for the client's dignity
Request that the client undress and put on a hospital or examination gown; assist as necessary.	Facilitates physical assessment
Ask the client about the need to urinate at the present time, and obtain a urine specimen if ordered.	Shows concern for the client's immediate comfort; facilitates physical assessment of the abdomen
Weigh the client before helping them into bed.	Expedites the collection of a routine specimen for analysis; avoids disturbing the client once settled in bed
Assist the client to a comfortable position in bed.	Shows concern for the client's comfort; facilitates the examination
Take care of the client's clothing and valuables according to agency policy.	Provides safeguards for the client's possessions
Ask the client to identify allergies to food, drugs, or other substances and to describe the type of symptoms that accompany a typical allergic reaction.	Aids in preventing the potential for an allergic reaction during care; prepares staff for the manner in which the client reacts to the allergen

SKILL 11-1 Admitting a Client (*continued*)

Suggested Action	Reason for Action
Collect a list of medications the client currently takes and directions the client follows for administering them.	Ensures continuity of care in medication administration
Apply a second bracelet that is color coded to the client's arm that identifies the client's allergies.	Calls staff's attention to the fact that the client has allergies
Wash hands or perform hand antisepsis with an alcohol rub (see Chapter 10).	Reduces the direct transmission of microorganisms from the nurse's hands to the client
Obtain the client's temperature, pulse, respiratory rate, and BP.	Contributes to the initial database assessment
Place the signal cord where it can be conveniently reached.	Reduces the potential for accidents by ensuring that the client can make their needs known
Make sure the bed is in low position, and follow agency policy about raising the side rails on the bed.	Promotes safety; side rails are considered a form of physical restraint in a nursing home; their use may require written permission from the client
Remove the urine specimen if obtained at this time, attach a laboratory request form, and place it in the refrigerator or take it to the laboratory.	Ensures proper identification of the specimen, specifies the test to be performed, and prevents changes that may affect test results
Wash hands or perform hand antisepsis with an alcohol rub (see Chapter 10).	Removes microorganisms acquired from contact with the client or the urine specimen
Report the progress of the client's admission to the registered nurse, who may perform the nursing interview and physical assessment or delegate components at this time.	Complies with The Joint Commission standards; the entire admission assessment must be completed within 24 hours; parts of the assessment may be performed at periodic intervals until it is completed
Inform family or friends that they may resume visiting when the nursing activities are completed.	Facilitates the client's network of support

EVALUATION

- Client is comfortable and oriented to the room and to routines.
- Safety measures are implemented.
- Database assessments are initiated.
- Status and progress are communicated to nursing team.

DOCUMENT

- Date and time of admission
- Age and gender of client
- Overall appearance
- Mode of arrival to unit
- Room number
- Initial vital signs and weight
- List of allergies, if any; quote the client's description of a typical reaction or indicate if the client has no allergies by using the abbreviation "NKA" (no known allergies) or whatever abbreviation is acceptable.
- Disposition of urine specimen
- Present condition of client

SAMPLE DOCUMENTATION

Date and Time A 68-year-old female admitted to Room 258 by a wheelchair from admitting department with moderate dyspnea. O_2 running at 2 L per nasal cannula. Weighs 173 lb on bed scale wearing only a hospital gown. T 98.4°, P 92, R 32, BP 146/68 in R arm while sitting up. Cannot void at present. Allergic to penicillin, which causes "hives and difficulty breathing." Allergy bracelet applied. In high Fowler position at this time with a respiratory rate of 24 at rest. _____ J. Doe, LPN

SKILL 11-2 Discharging a Client

Suggested Action	Reason for Action
ASSESSMENT	
Determine that a medical order has been written.	Provides authorization for discharging the client
Check for written prescriptions and other medical discharge instructions.	Enables the client to continue self-care
Note if any new medical orders must be carried out before the client's discharge.	Ensures that the client will leave in the best possible condition
Review the nursing discharge plan.	Determines whether the client needs more health teaching or if instructions have been completed
PLANNING[a]	
Discuss the client's time frame for leaving the hospital.	Helps coordinate nursing activities within the client's schedule
Coordinate the discharge with the home health care agency, hospice organization, or company supplying oxygen or other medical equipment.	Facilitates continuity of care
Determine the client's mode of transportation.	Clarifies if the client needs the services of a cab company or other resource
[a]Notify the business office of the client's impending discharge.	Allows time for the clerical department to review the client's billing information and determine the necessity for further actions
[a]Inform the housekeeping department that the client will be leaving.	Alerts cleaning staff that the unit will need terminal cleaning
[a]Cancel any meals that the client will miss after discharge.	Avoids wasting food
[a]Notify the pharmacy of the approximate time of discharge.	Eliminates restocking drugs that will be unneeded
Plan to provide hygiene and medical treatments early.	Prevents delays in the client's departure
IMPLEMENTATION	
Wash hands or perform hand antisepsis with an alcohol rub (see Chapter 10).	Reduces transmission of microorganisms
Provide for hygiene but omit changing the bed linens.	Eliminates unnecessary work
Complete medical treatment and nursing interventions according to the plan for care.	Promotes continuation of nursing care
Help the client dress in street clothing or clothing appropriate for leaving the agency.	Demonstrates concern for the client's appearance and appropriateness for the weather
Review discharge instructions and complete health teaching.	Promotes safe self-care
Have the client sign the discharge instruction sheet, paraphrase the information it contains, and provide the client with the original form containing the discharge instructions and prescriptions that should be filled.	Validates that the client has understood instructions for maintaining health and can refer to the information at a future time
Assist the client with packing personal items; if appropriate, have the client sign the clothing inventory or valuables list.	Reduces claims that personal items were lost or stolen; signing a clothing inventory or valuables list is more likely to apply when a client is discharged from a nursing home or rehabilitation center
Obtain a cart for the client's belongings.	Eases the work of transporting multiple or heavy items
Assist the client in a wheelchair when transportation is available.	Reduces the potential for a fall if the client is weak or unsteady
Stop, if necessary, at the business office.	Complies with billing procedures
Escort the client to the waiting vehicle.	Promotes safety while still in the hospital
Return any forms from the business office.	Confirms that the client has left the hospital
Replace the wheelchair in its proper location on the nursing unit.	Makes equipment available for others to use
Wash hands or perform hand antisepsis with an alcohol rub (see Chapter 10).	Reduces the transmission of microorganisms
Complete a discharge summary in the medical record.	Closes the medical record for this admission

EVALUATION

- Health condition is stable (if being transferred in unstable condition, is accompanied by qualified personnel who have the knowledge and skills to intervene in emergencies).
- Client can paraphrase discharge instructions accurately.
- Business office indicates that billing records are in order.
- Client experiences no injuries during transport from room to vehicle.

SKILL 11-2 Discharging a Client (*continued*)

Suggested Action	Reason for Action

DOCUMENT

- Date and time of discharge
- Condition at the time of discharge
- Include a copy of discharge instructions.
- Mode of transportation
- Identity of person(s) who accompanied the client

SAMPLE DOCUMENTATION

Date and Time No fever or wound tenderness at this time. Sutures removed. Abdominal incision intact. No dressing applied. Given prescription for Keflex. Can repeat how many capsules to self-administer per dose, appropriate times for administration, and possible side effects. Repeated signs and symptoms of infection and the need to report them immediately. Instructed to shower as usual and temporarily avoid lifting objects over 10 lb. Informed to make follow-up appointment in 1 week with the physician as indicated on the discharge instruction sheet. Given a copy of written discharge instructions. Escorted to automobile in a wheelchair accompanied by spouse. Assisted into a private car without any unusual events. _____ J. Doe, LPN

^aActivities may be delegated to a clerk.

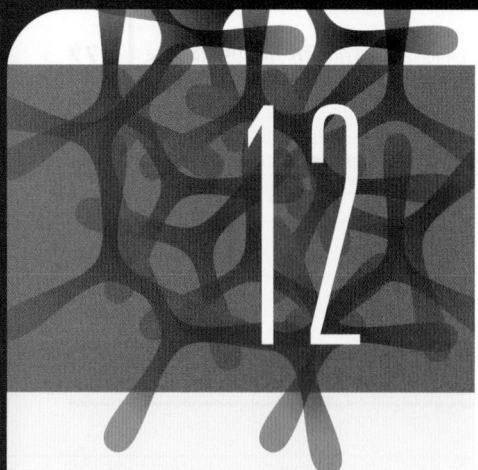

Vital Signs

Learning Objectives

On completion of this chapter, the reader should be able to:

1. List physiologic components measured during an assessment of vital signs.
2. Differentiate between shell and core body temperature.
3. Identify the scales used to measure temperature.
4. List temperature assessment sites and indicate the sites considered the closest to core temperature.
5. Name the types of clinical thermometers.
6. Discuss the difference between fever and hyperthermia.
7. Name the phases of a fever.
8. List signs or symptoms that accompany a fever.
9. Give reasons for using an infrared tympanic thermometer when body temperature is subnormal.
10. List signs and symptoms that accompany subnormal body temperature.
11. Identify characteristics noted when assessing a client's pulse.
12. Name the most commonly used site for pulse assessment and other assessment techniques that may be used.
13. Name and explain terms used to describe abnormal breathing characteristics.
14. Discuss the physiologic data that can be inferred from a blood pressure (BP) assessment.
15. Explain the difference between systolic and diastolic BP.
16. Name the pieces of equipment used to assess BP.
17. Describe the phases of Korotkoff sounds.
18. Identify alternative techniques for assessing BP.

INTRODUCTION

Vital signs (body temperature, pulse rate, respiratory rate, and blood pressure [BP]) are four objective assessment pieces of data that indicate how well or poorly the body is functioning. Pain is considered a fifth vital sign. A subjective pain assessment is performed at least daily and whenever vital signs are taken (see Chapter 20).

Vital signs are sensitive to alterations in physiology; therefore, nurses measure them at regular intervals (Box 12-1) or whenever they determine it is appropriate to assess a client's health status. This chapter describes how to obtain each component of the vital signs and explains what findings indicate based on established norms.

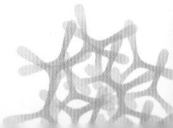

Words To Know (continued)

pulse rhythm
pulse volume
pyrexia
respiration
respiratory rate
set point
shell temperature
speculum
sphygmomanometer
stertorous breathing
stethoscope
stridor
systolic pressure
tachycardia
tachypnea
temperature translation
temporal artery thermometer
thermistor catheter
thermogenesis
training effect
ventilation
vital signs
white adipose tissue
white coat hypertension

BOX 12-1 **Recommendations for Measuring Vital Signs**

Vital signs are taken:
- On admission, when obtaining database assessments
- According to written medical orders
- Once per day when a client is stable
- At least every 4 hours when one or more vital signs are abnormal
- Every 5–15 minutes when a client is unstable or at risk for rapid physiologic changes such as after surgery
- Whenever a client's condition appears to have changed
- A second time, or more frequently, when there is a significant difference from the previous measurement
- When a client is feeling unusual
- Before, during, and after a blood transfusion
- Before administering medications that affect any of the vital signs and after to monitor the drug's effect

---

 Gerontologic Considerations

■ Older adults tend to have lower "normal" or baseline temperatures; therefore, a temperature in the normal range may actually be elevated for an older adult.

■ An older person's usual temperature should be assessed and documented to enable accurate comparison when assessing for elevations. Another age-related change that needs to be considered is that temperature elevations may not accompany infections.

■ Some older adults have a delayed and diminished febrile response to illnesses. A careful assessment is essential to identify temperature elevations or disease symptoms other than increased temperature. Often, a change in cognitive function, restlessness, or anxiety is the initial sign of infection.

■ Older adults are more susceptible to hypothermia and heat-related conditions. Environmental factors, such as extreme heat and cold conditions and inadequately heated or cooled living environments, pose additional risk factors for developing hypothermia and heat-related illnesses.

■ Some older adults have a wide pulse pressure because of a combination of elevated systolic pressure and normal diastolic pressure (the rising systolic pressure exceeds the rate of diastolic elevation). Such people have a higher incidence of hypertension.

■ Older adults can be taught to use home BP monitoring for initial and ongoing assessment, but the monitors should be validated for accuracy.

■ Current guidelines emphasize the importance of individualized medication management for older adults with hypertension to reach a goal of 130 to 139 mm Hg or lower systolic BP and 80 to 89 mm Hg or lower diastolic BP (American Heart Association [AHA], 2019).

■ Older adults may use self-monitoring devices or BP monitors in community settings, but these monitors should be validated for accuracy.

■ Older adults are more susceptible to postural and postprandial hypotension (a drop in BP of 20 mm Hg within 1 to 2 hours of eating a meal).

■ If hypotension is assessed in a client, plan for limited activities during the hour following eating or for frequent, smaller food consumption throughout the day.

■ Interventions for postural and postprandial hypotension include maintaining adequate fluid intake, eating smaller and more frequent meals, and avoiding sitting or standing still for prolonged periods, especially after meals.

BODY TEMPERATURE

Body temperature refers to the warmth of the human body. Body heat is produced primarily from exercise and metabolism of food. Heat is lost through the skin, the lungs, and the body's waste products through the processes of radiation, conduction, convection, and evaporation (Table 12-1).

The body's **shell temperature** (warmth at the skin surface) is usually lower than its **core temperature** (warmth in deeper sites within the body, such as the brain and heart). Core temperature is much more significant than shell temperature because there is a narrow range within which core temperature can fluctuate without resulting in negative outcomes.

Temperature Measurement

Physicists studying *thermokinetics*, or heat in motion, have developed various scales for measuring heat and cold. Some examples include Kelvin (K), Rankine (R), Fahrenheit (F), and centigrade (C) scales, all of which are based on increments at which water freezes and boils. The centigrade temperature scale is also known as *Celsius*. Health care providers commonly use the Fahrenheit and centigrade scales.

The **Fahrenheit scale** (a scale that uses 32°F as the temperature at which water freezes and 212°F as the point at which it boils) is generally used in the United States to measure and report body temperature. The **centigrade scale** (a scale that uses 0°C as the temperature at which water freezes and 100°C as the point at which it boils) is used more often in scientific research and in countries that use the metric system. Nurses are required to use both scales occasionally and to be able to convert between the two measurements (Box 12-2).

Normal Body Temperature

In healthy adults, shell temperature generally ranges from 96.6° to 99.3°F or 35.8° to 37.4°C; core body temperature ranges from 97.0° to 99.5°F or 36.0° to 37.5°C. If a client's temperature is above or below normal, the nurse records and

BOX 12-2	Temperature Conversion Formulas

To convert Fahrenheit to centigrade, use the formula:

$$°C = \frac{(°F - 32)}{1.8}$$

Example: Step 1: 98.6°F − 32 = 66.6
Step 2: 66.6 ÷ 1.8 = 37°C

To convert centigrade to Fahrenheit:

$$°F = (°C \times 1.8) + 32$$
Example: Step 1: 15°C × 1.8 = 27
Step 2: 27 + 32 = 59°F

reports the temperature, implements nursing and medical interventions for restoring a normal body temperature when appropriate, and reassesses the client frequently.

Temperature Regulation

The temperature of humans is considered *homeothermic*; that is, various structural and physiologic adaptations keep their body temperature within a narrow stable range regardless of the environmental temperature.

The **hypothalamus** (a structure within the brain that helps control various metabolic activities) acts as the center for temperature regulation. The anterior hypothalamus promotes heat loss through vasodilation and sweating. The posterior hypothalamus promotes two functions: *heat conservation* and *heat production*. It produces heat conservation by:

- Adjusting where blood circulates
- Causing **piloerection** (the contraction of arrector pili muscles in skin follicles), which stiffens body hairs and gives the appearance of what commonly is described as "goose flesh"
- Promoting a shivering response

TABLE 12-1 Mechanisms of Heat Transfer

	RADIATION	CONVECTION	EVAPORATION	CONDUCTION
Definition	The diffusion or dissemination of heat by electromagnetic waves	The dissemination of heat by motion between areas of unequal density	The conversion of a liquid to a vapor	The transfer of heat to another object during direct contact
Example	The body gives off waves of heat from uncovered surfaces.	An oscillating fan blows currents of cool air across the surface of a warm body.	Body fluid in the form of perspiration and insensible loss is vaporized from the skin.	The body transfers heat to an ice pack, causing the ice to melt.
Illustration				

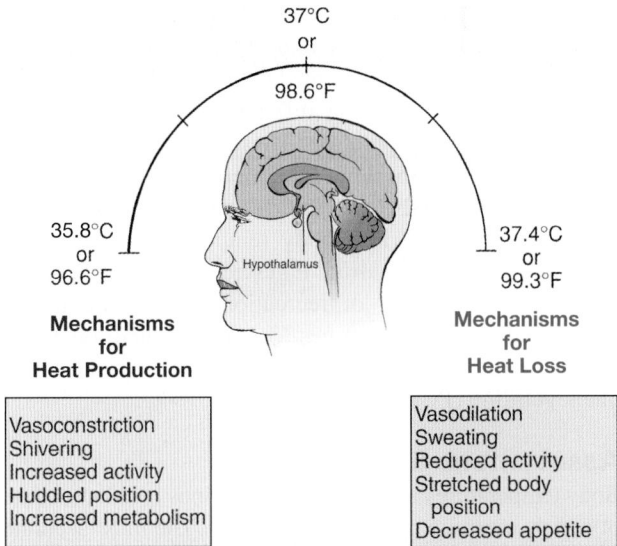

37°C
or
98.6°F

35.8°C
or
96.6°F

Hypothalamus

37.4°C
or
99.3°F

Mechanisms for Heat Production

Vasoconstriction
Shivering
Increased activity
Huddled position
Increased metabolism

Mechanisms for Heat Loss

Vasodilation
Sweating
Reduced activity
Stretched body position
Decreased appetite

FIGURE 12-1 The hypothalamus regulates body temperature.

The hypothalamus promotes heat production by increasing metabolism through secretion of thyroid hormone as well as epinephrine and norepinephrine from the adrenal medulla. When functioning appropriately, the hypothalamus maintains the core temperature **set point** (an optimal body temperature) within 1°C by responding to slight changes in the skin surface and blood temperatures. Other physiologic responses accompany the temperature-regulating mechanisms of the hypothalamus as shown in Figure 12-1.

Temperatures above 105.8°F (41°C) and below 93.2°F (34°C) indicate impairment of the hypothalamic regulatory center. According to Alexander (2022), the chance of survival is diminished when body temperatures exceed 109.4°F (43°C). Grimes (2022) reports, "When your core body temperature hits 91 degrees F (33 C), you might suffer amnesia. At 82 degrees F (28 C), you might lose consciousness. At 70 degrees F (21 C), you experience 'profound,' deadly hypothermia."

Factors Affecting Body Temperature

Various factors affect body temperature. Examples include food intake, age, climate, sex, exercise and activity, circadian rhythm, emotions, illness or injury, and medications.

Food Intake

Food intake, or lack of it, affects **thermogenesis** (heat production). When a person consumes food, the body requires energy to digest, absorb, transport, metabolize, and store nutrients. The process is sometimes described as the *specific dynamic action of food* or the *thermic effect of food* because it produces heat. Protein foods have the greatest thermic effect. Thus, both the amount and type of food eaten affect body temperature. Dietary restrictions can contribute to decreased body heat as a result of reduced processing of nutrients, which explains the low body temperature among those with anorexia nervosa, an eating disorder manifested by self-starvation.

Nutrition Notes

In a balanced diet consisting of a mix of carbohydrates, protein, and fat, specific dynamic action accounts for approximately 10% of the total calories expended daily. For example, approximately 200 calories are used to metabolize a balanced intake of 2,000 calories

Age

Infants and older adults have difficulty maintaining normal body temperature for several reasons. Both have limited subcutaneous **white adipose tissue (WAT)** that contains fat cells known as *adipocytes*. WAT provides heat insulation and cushioning of internal structures. The ability of both young and old people to shiver and perspire may also be inadequate, putting them at risk for abnormally low or high body temperatures. Another problem for both populations is an inability to independently forestall or reverse heat loss or gain without the assistance of a caregiver.

Newborns and young infants tend to experience temperature fluctuations because they have three times greater surface area from which heat is lost and a higher **metabolic rate** (use of calories for sustaining body functions) than adults. Older adults are compromised by progressively impaired circulation, which interferes with losing or retaining heat through the dilation or constriction of blood vessels near the skin. However, infants have the capacity to generate heat without shivering due to the presence of **brown adipose tissue (BAT)**. BAT contains brown adipocytes filled with mitochondria that raise body temperature by increasing metabolism (LogicalScience, 2022). BAT is usually located near the neck, the chest, and the upper back (Sisson, 2015). Although the amount of brown adipocytes decreases in adulthood, white adipocytes can be transformed into brown adipocytes by exposure to cold environmental temperatures (see section "Climate").

⟩⟩ *Stop, Think, and Respond 12-1*

Explain how infants and older adults are particularly vulnerable to alterations in temperature regulation.

Climate

Climate affects mechanisms for temperature regulation. Heat and cold produce neurosensory stimulation of thermal receptors in the skin, which transmit information through the autonomic nervous system to the hypothalamus. Cool environmental temperatures result in vasoconstriction of surface blood vessels with subsequent shunting of blood to vital organs. This physiologic phenomenon helps explain how brain cells are protected temporarily in cold water drownings.

People who live in predominately cold climates have more *brown adipocytes* uniquely adapted for nonshivering thermogenesis. Thermogenesis from brown fat occurs in the absence of shivering when norepinephrine triggers lipolysis (the breakdown of fat). Those who live in arctic regions are highly cold adaptive because they have increased brown adipocytes. They tend to have overall higher metabolic rates compared with those who live in geographic areas with less severe environmental temperatures. Conversely, those who live in the tropics have lower metabolic rates than those in milder climates.

Sex

Body temperature increases slightly in people of childbearing age during ovulation. This probably results from hormonal changes affecting metabolism or tissue injury and repair after the release of an ovum (egg). The change in body temperature is so slight that most people are unaware of it unless they are monitoring their temperature daily (to plan or avoid pregnancy).

Exercise and Activity

Both exercise and activity involve muscle contraction. As muscle groups and tendons repeatedly stretch and recoil, the friction produces body heat. Shivering is another example of contractile thermogenesis.

Muscles are also the largest mass of metabolically active tissue. This means that muscle activity generates additional heat from chemical reactions during the muscle cells' combustion of nutrients for cellular functions. To provide adequate calories that will give the energy necessary for muscle activity, the body adjusts its metabolic rate through endocrine hormones released from the pituitary, thyroid, and adrenal glands. In contrast, inactivity and reduced metabolism or nutrient intake may lead to lower body temperatures.

Circadian Rhythm

Circadian rhythms are physiologic changes, such as fluctuations in body temperature and other vital signs over 24-hour cycles. Body temperature fluctuates from 0.5° to 2.0°F (0.28° to 1.1°C) during a 24-hour period. It tends to be lowest from midnight to dawn and highest in the late afternoon to early evening. People who routinely work at night and sleep during the day have temperature fluctuations that cycle in reverse.

Emotions

Emotions affect metabolic rate by triggering hormonal changes through the sympathetic and parasympathetic pathways of the autonomic nervous system (see Chapter 5). People who tend to be consistently anxious and nervous are likely to have slightly increased body temperatures. Conversely, people who are apathetic or depressed are prone to have slightly lower body temperatures.

Illness or Injury

Diseases, disorders, or injuries that affect the function of the hypothalamus or mechanisms for heat production and loss alter body temperature, sometimes dramatically. Some examples include tissue injury, infections and inflammatory disorders, fluid loss, injury to the skin, impaired circulation, and head injury.

Medications

When a pyrogen (bacterium) is introduced, the body temperature is elevated. Drugs known as **antipyretics** (such as aspirin, acetaminophen, and ibuprofen) directly lower body temperature by acting on the hypothalamus. Yet, these drugs will not lower body temperature to subnormal levels. A number of medications will also impair thermoregulation or cause inflammation, which results in a raised body temperature. These drug classes include antibiotics, antiarrhythmics, antiepileptics, antihypertensives, antifungals, and interferons. Stimulants, such as ephedrine, may raise body temperature. Depending upon the amount of drug ingested, body temperature may rise when illicit or recreational drugs are taken. These include amphetamines, 3,4-methylenedioxymethamphetamine (MDMA or ecstasy), cocaine, marijuana, and phencyclidine (PCP).

Assessment Sites

Body temperature can be assessed at various locations, some of which are more practical than others. The most accurate locations for measuring core body temperature are the brain, heart, lower third of the esophagus, and the urinary bladder. Measuring the temperature in the brain is currently prohibitive because of a lack of technology. The temperature of blood circulating through the heart, esophagus, or bladder is measured using a **thermistor catheter** (heat-sensing device at the tip of an internally placed tube). The required skill for insertion and risks associated with the use of thermistor catheters, however, restricts their use to clients with highly acute illnesses.

The most practical and convenient temperature assessment sites are the tympanic membrane within the ear, skin over the temporal artery on the forehead to the lateral hairline and behind the ear, mouth, rectum, and axilla. These areas are anatomically close to superficial arteries containing warm blood, enclosed areas where heat loss is minimal, or both. Of the five sites, the ear and skin over the temporal artery are the peripheral sites that most closely reflect core body temperature.

Temperature measurements vary slightly depending on the assessment site (Table 12-2). To evaluate trends in body temperature, the nurse documents the assessment site as "O" for oral, "R" for rectal, "AX" for axillary, "T" for tympanic membrane, and "TA" for temporal artery. They take the temperature by the same route each time. Rectal and arterial temperatures are generally 1°F (0.5°C) higher than oral temperatures and 2°F (1°C) higher than axillary temperatures; axillary temperature is lower than any measured site. Report the temperature and site used.

TABLE 12-2 Equivalent Thermometer Measurements According to Site

ASSESSMENT SITE	FAHRENHEIT	CENTIGRADE
Oral	98.6°	37.0°
Rectal equivalent	99.5°	37.5°
Axillary equivalent	97.5°	36.4°
Tympanic membrane	99.5°	37.5°
Temporal artery	99.4°	37.4°

The Ear

Research indicates that the temperature near the tympanic membrane and the skin over the path of the temporal artery has the closest correlation to core temperature.

Tympanic Membrane Thermometry

The tympanic membrane is just 1.4 in (3.8 cm) from the hypothalamus; blood from the internal and external carotid arteries, the same vessels that supply the hypothalamus, also warms the tympanic membrane. For accuracy of temperatures obtained at this site, the thermometer must be inserted correctly (Fig. 12-2). Tympanic membrane temperatures are considered more reliable than those obtained at the oral and axillary sites. They also correlate closely with those taken at the rectal site. Because the tympanic membrane is fairly deep within the head, warm or cool air temperatures affect it less. Use of a tympanic membrane thermometer is not advised in children younger than 2 years of age because the diameter of the ear canal is smaller than the probe, resulting in an erroneously low reading.

Temporal Artery Thermometry

The superficial branch of the temporal artery, which receives blood from the aorta, lies less than 2 mm below the skin surface at the forehead. Because of this anatomic relationship, the temperature of blood flowing through the temporal artery is analogous to the temperature of blood within the heart, that is, core body temperature.

The **temporal artery thermometer** is the most noninvasive device when compared with others because it scans the artery at the skin surface, poses no risk for injury, and is suitable for nearly all ages. It is suitable for assessing the temperature of clients in whom oral temperatures are difficult to obtain, such as those having oral or facial trauma, oral surgery, or those who are uncooperative. Scanning from the forehead to the area behind the ear, described as the

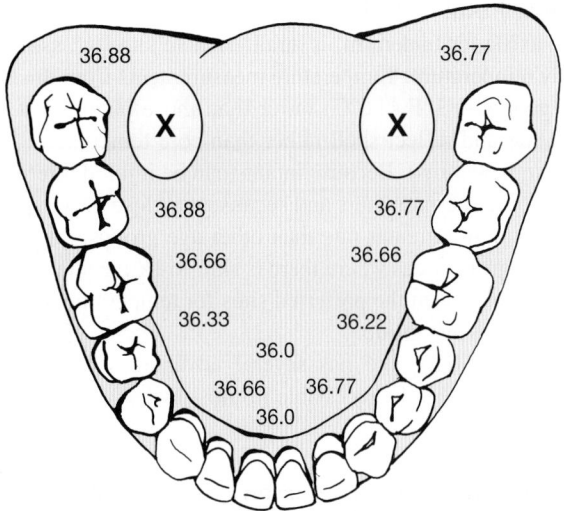

FIGURE 12-3 Temperature measurements vary with the placement of the oral thermometer. A thermometer placed at the rear sublingual pockets provides the most accurate measurement.

"perfume spot," facilitates an accurate reading, especially in clients who are diaphoretic. The skin over the forehead alone may be scanned in infants because vasodilation is more widespread in this age group.

Oral Site

The oral site, or mouth, is convenient. It generally measures temperatures 0.8° to 1.0°F (0.5° to 0.6°C) below the core temperature. The area under the tongue is in direct proximity to the sublingual artery. As long as the client keeps the mouth closed and breathes normally, the tissue remains at a fairly consistent temperature. Valid measurement also depends on accurate placement and maintenance of an oral thermometer in the rear sublingual pocket at the base of the tongue (Fig. 12-3). Poor placement or premature removal of the thermometer can result in inaccurate measurements, deviating by as much as 1.5°F (0.9°C) from the actual temperature.

The oral site is contraindicated for clients who are uncooperative, very young, unconscious, shivering, prone to seizures, or breathe through their mouths; those who have had oral surgery; and those who continue to talk during temperature assessment. To ensure accuracy, the nurse delays the oral temperature assessment for at least 30 minutes after the client has been chewing gum, smoking a cigarette, or eating hot or cold food or beverages.

Rectal Site

A rectal temperature differs only about 0.2°F (0.1°C) from the core temperature. It provides the best measurement for children less than 3 years of age, but care must be taken to avoid injuring a young child who is not cooperative. Rapid fluctuations in temperature may not be identified for as long as 1 hour, however, because this area retains heat longer than other sites. In addition, this site can be embarrassing and emotionally traumatic for alert clients. Furthermore, stool in the rectum, improper placement of the thermometer, and premature removal affect the accuracy of rectal temperature assessment.

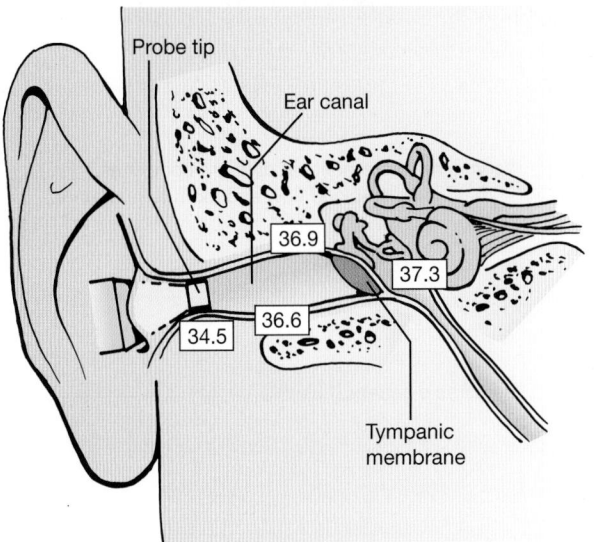

FIGURE 12-2 Obtain the most accurate tympanic temperature by aiming the probe toward the anterior inferior third of the ear canal.

Axillary Site

The axilla, or underarm, is an alternative site for assessing body temperature. Temperature measurements from this site are generally 1°F (0.6°C) lower than those obtained at the oral site and reflect shell rather than core temperature (except in newborns). Because infants can be injured internally with rectal thermometers and because they lose heat through their skin at a greater rate than other age groups, the axilla and the groin, areas where there is skin-to-skin contact, have traditionally been the preferred sites for temperature assessment in this age group.

The axillary site has several advantages for all age groups. It is readily accessible in most instances. It is safe. There is less potential for spreading microorganisms than with the oral and rectal sites, and it is less disturbing psychologically than the rectal site. This route, however, requires the longest assessment time of 5 minutes or longer depending on the electronic monitoring mode being used (discussed later). Poor circulation, recent bathing, or rubbing the axillary area dry with a towel also affects the accuracy of the axillary site.

Thermometers

There are several types of **clinical thermometers** (instruments used to measure body temperature): electronic, infrared, chemical, and digital (Table 12-3).

TABLE 12-3 Types of Clinical Thermometers

TYPE	ADVANTAGES	DISADVANTAGES
Electronic	Accurate No sterilization or disinfection needed Easy to use	Expensive Recharging is necessary. Probe needs to be held by the client or nurse. Interference with simultaneously taking the client's pulse while holding the probe with one hand and unit in the other
Infrared (tympanic)	Fast Convenient Close approximation of core temperature Less invasive Accuracy unaffected by eating, drinking, or breathing Sanitary	Expensive in comparison with others Battery recharging is necessary. Accuracy is affected by improper placement and probe size. Actual ear and core temperature ranges are slightly different from oral, rectal, and axillary sites. Tip requires cleaning with a paper tissue or alcohol swab. Extreme hot or cold environmental temperatures may affect electronics. No sterilization or disinfection is required.
Infrared (temporal artery)	Closest approximate of core temperature Most sanitary Most convenient for clients Records within 2 seconds Initial cost is similar to other types of electronic and tympanic membrane thermometers. Probe covers are not needed; decreases volume of disposal waste. Can be used over the femoral artery or lateral thoracic artery if the temporal artery is inaccessible due to bandaging or trauma	User error if the thermometer is moved too quickly across the skin Hair, clothing, or bandages between the probe and the skin can result in falsely high readings. Infrared probe requires cleaning between uses with an alcohol prep pad and dry swab.
Chemical	Inexpensive Safe; nonbreakable Sanitary Temperature registers in approximately 45 seconds to 3 minutes Resets in 30 seconds Cleans easily in hot soapy water Easily used by untrained people	Varying measurements at different body sites depending on blood flow and room temperature
Digital	Inexpensive Safe Memory displays last temperature. Fast; records in 1–3 minutes Audible signal during or after assessment Automatic shutoff to prolong battery Battery life of 200 hours Water resistant, which facilitates cleaning Large, lighted numerical display for ease of reading	Requires a battery (1.55 V)

Electronic Thermometers

An electronic thermometer (Fig. 12-4) uses a temperature-sensitive probe covered with a disposable sheath attached by a coiled wire to a display unit. Electronic thermometers are portable. They are recharged when not in use.

Electronic thermometers generally have two types of probes: one for oral or axillary use and the other for rectal use. Some models offer the option of providing the measurement in Fahrenheit or centigrade.

Electronic thermometers operate in either a *predictive mode* or a *monitor mode*. If used in the predictive mode, the thermometer takes multiple measurements that a computer chip processes in only a few seconds to determine what the temperature would be if the thermometer was left in place for several minutes. The monitor mode requires that the thermometer remain at the assessment site for a longer, more steady time to obtain the actual temperature. There is no significant difference in temperature measurements obtained by the predictive versus the monitor mode. The electronic unit senses when the temperature ceases to change and emits a beep. The audible signal alerts the nurse to remove the probe and read the displayed measurement.

Infrared (Tympanic) Thermometers

An infrared tympanic thermometer is a battery-operated device that contains an infrared sensor for detecting the warmth radiating from the tympanic membrane (eardrum) when a handheld covered probe is inserted into the ear canal (Fig. 12-5). When not in use, it rests in a base-charging unit referred to as its *cradle.*

A tympanic membrane thermometer converts the heat it detects into a temperature measurement in 2 to 5 seconds. The potential for transferring microorganisms from one client to another is reduced because the probe cover is changed after each use and because the ear does not contain mucous membranes or their accompanying secretions.

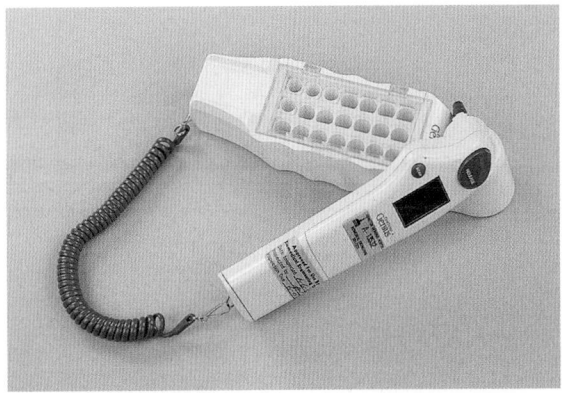

FIGURE 12-5 An infrared tympanic thermometer. (Photo by B. Proud.)

Despite the advantages of tympanic thermometers, infrared thermometers can produce inaccurate measurements in the following circumstances:

- The ear canal is not straightened appropriately.
- The probe, which measures 6 to 8 mm, is too large for the ear canal (a problem with infants and small children whose ear canals are 5 mm or smaller). The size difference alters the location where infrared light must be precisely directed. Consequently, use of a tympanic thermometer is contraindicated for children younger than 2 years.
- The sensor is directed at the ear canal rather than directly at the tympanic membrane.
- There is impacted **cerumen** (earwax), a common problem among older adults.
- There is fluid behind the tympanic membrane, a problem that occurs with middle ear infections.
- The **drawdown effect** (cooling of the ear when it comes in contact with the probe) occurs.

The first use of a tympanic thermometer after recharging is not always as accurate as a second reading. Another criticism of the tympanic temperature measurement is that currently, there is no standard for actual ear or core temperatures. At present, tympanic thermometers use internally calculated **offsets** (predictive mathematical conversions) for oral and rectal temperatures. These offsets vary among manufacturers.

Infrared Temporal Artery Thermometers

The temporal artery thermometer (Fig. 12-6) contains an infrared sensor that uses computerized algorithms to compute temperature measurements. It does so by calculating the difference between the heat radiating from the temporal artery at the center of the forehead and the heat loss at the skin. Because there may be evaporative cooling on the exposed skin on the forehead, *the thermometer is secondarily moved to scan the skin behind the ear lobe*, which tends to remain relatively dry (Nursing Guidelines 12-1). An assessment over the temporal artery in the forehead alone is sufficient for infants.

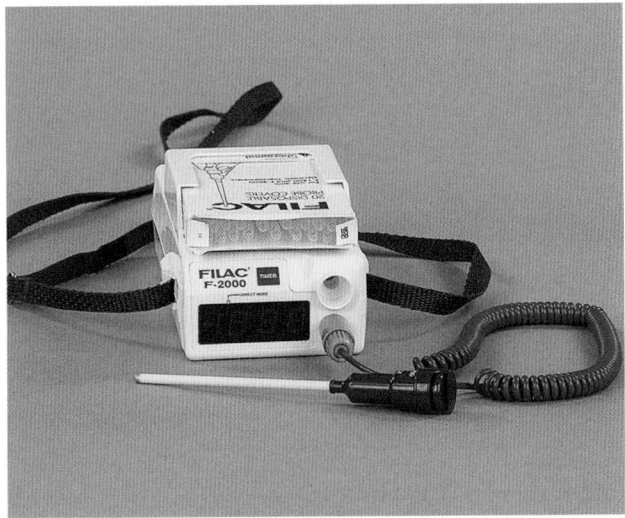

FIGURE 12-4 An electronic thermometer. (Photo by B. Proud.)

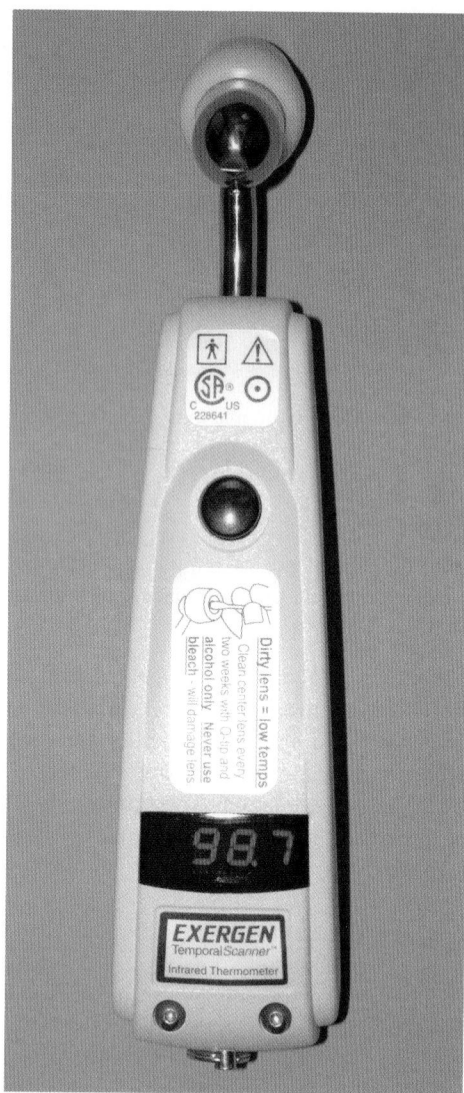

FIGURE 12-6 A temporal artery thermometer. (Photo by K. Timby.)

Chemical Thermometers
Various chemical thermometers are available. One example is a paper or plastic strip with chemically treated dots (Fig. 12-7). The oral temperature is determined by noting how many dots change color after the strip is held in the mouth. Chemical dot thermometers are discarded after one

use. They are used to assess the temperature of clients who require isolation precautions for infectious diseases. Their use eliminates the need to clean a multiuse electronic or infrared thermometer. Some physician's offices also use chemical dot thermometers because they are disposable.

A second type of chemical thermometer is made of heat-sensitive tape or patch applied to the abdomen or forehead (Fig. 12-8). The tape or patch changes color according to body temperature. Heat-sensitive tapes and patches can be reused several times before being thrown away.

Digital Thermometers
A plastic digital thermometer (Fig. 12-9) can be used at oral, axillary, and rectal sites. It has a sensing tip at the end of the stem, an on/off button, and a display area that lights up during use. The battery used to operate the thermometer requires occasional replacement.

Digital thermometers are designed for multiple uses; for this reason, they require cleaning after use. Digital thermometers are cleaned by wiping with isopropyl alcohol. Disposable plastic sheaths can be used to cover the probe with each use as an additional sanitary measure.

Automated Monitoring Devices
Some agencies use **automated monitoring devices** (equipment that allows for the simultaneous collection of multiple data). They may measure the temperature, BP, and pulse, as well as other information such as heart rhythm and pulse oximetry (Fig. 12-10). Some models can store and display the trends in vital signs. Their chief advantage is that they save time and money. Agencies favor the use of automated monitors for potentially unstable clients who require frequent assessments. To ensure reliable data, the accuracy of automated devices is compared with data measured with manual devices on a regular basis.

Continuous Monitoring Devices
Continuous temperature monitoring devices are used primarily in critical care areas. They measure body temperature using internal thermistor probes within the esophagus of anesthetized clients, inside the bladder, or attached to a pulmonary artery catheter. These measurements are generally required when caring for clients with extreme hypothermia or hyperthermia. Warming or cooling blankets are also

NURSING GUIDELINES 12-1

Using a Temporal Artery Thermometer
- Perform hand hygiene.
- Place the probe at the center of the forehead (Fig. A).
- Depress the sensing button on the thermometer throughout the procedure.
- Slide the thermometer laterally across the forehead to the hairline (Fig. B).
- Lift the probe while keeping the button depressed.
- Relocate the probe behind the ear.

- Slide the probe to the depression behind the ear lobe (Fig. C).
- Release the button.
- Read and record the displayed temperature.
- Wait 30 seconds if a sequential measurement is needed or use the opposite side.
- Clean the thermometer probe with an alcohol pad and a dry swab.
- Replace the 9 V alkaline battery when "BATT" display indicates the battery is low.

A

B

C

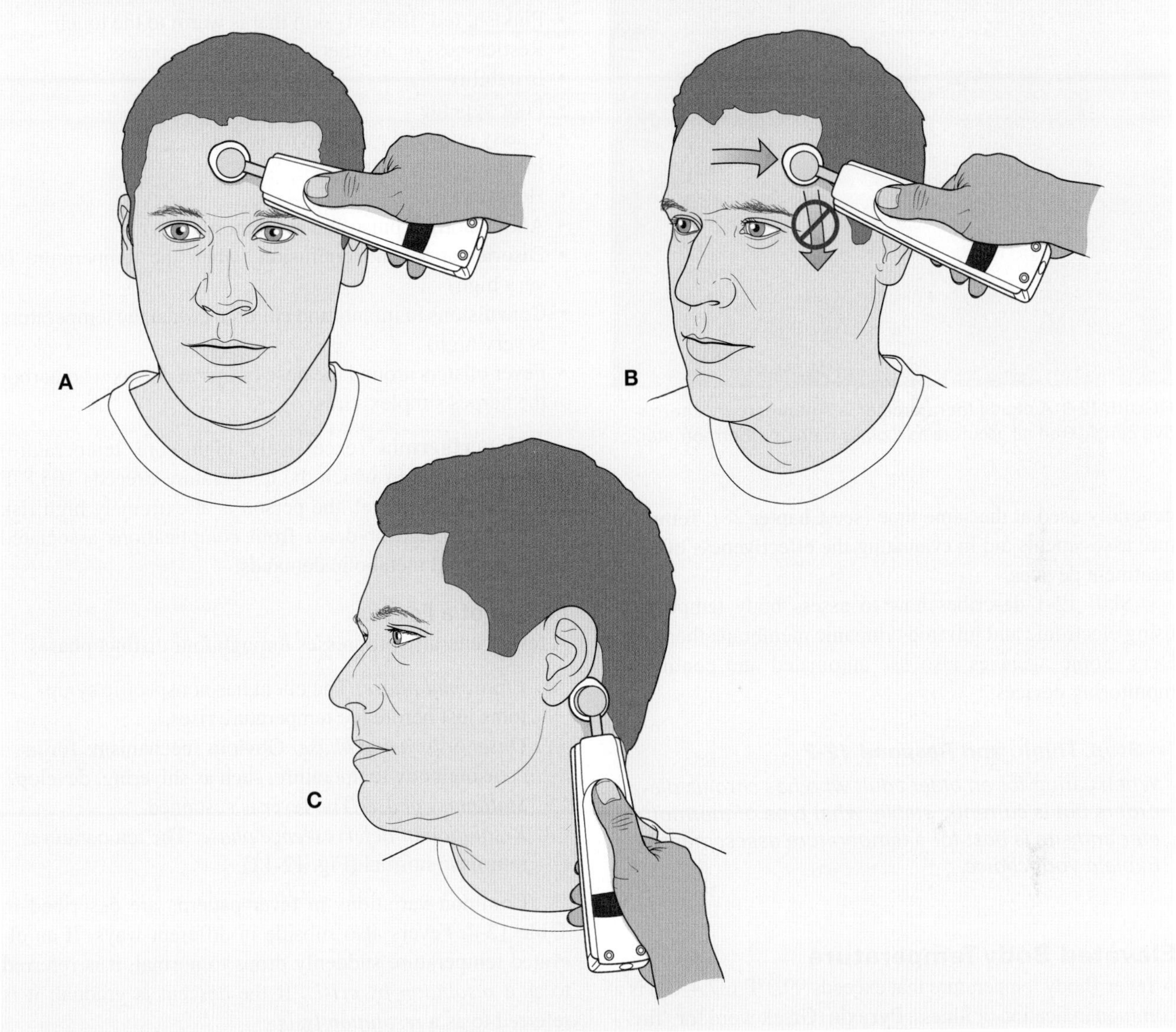

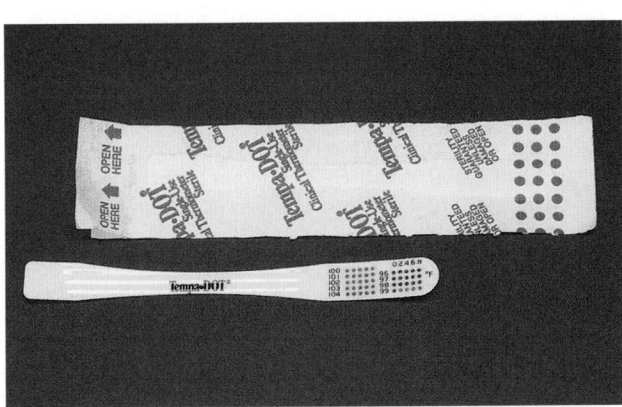

FIGURE 12-7 A chemical thermometer.

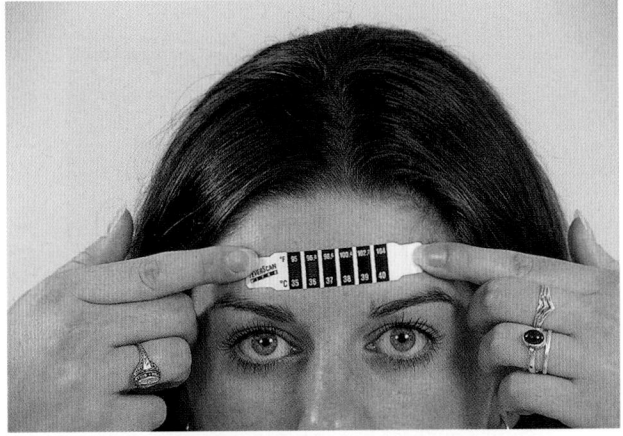

FIGURE 12-8 A disposable chemical thermometer with heat-sensitive liquid crystals. (Photo by B. Proud.)

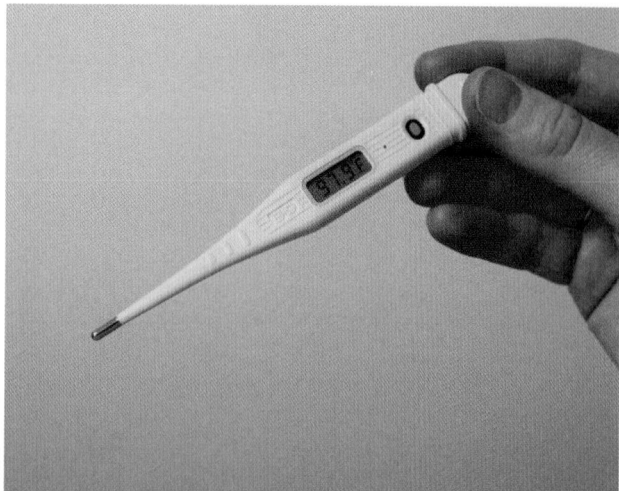

FIGURE 12-9 A digital thermometer is a nonmercury alternative considered as accurate as a glass mercury thermometer.

generally used at the same time (see Chapter 28). Temperature assessments aid in evaluating the effectiveness of these treatment devices.

Skill 12-1 describes how to assess body temperature using electronic and infrared tympanic membrane thermometers. Some agencies also use automated and continuous monitoring devices.

⟩⟩ *Stop, Think, and Respond 12-2*

When caring for an older adult who has chronic disorders but is currently stable, what type of thermometer and site is best for a temperature assessment? Explain your choice.

Elevated Body Temperature

A **fever** (body temperature that exceeds 99.3°F [37.4°C]) is a common indication of illness. **Pyrexia** (Greek word for "fire") is a term used to describe a warmer than normal set point. A person with a fever is said to be **febrile** (a condition in which the temperature is elevated) as opposed to **afebrile** (no fever).

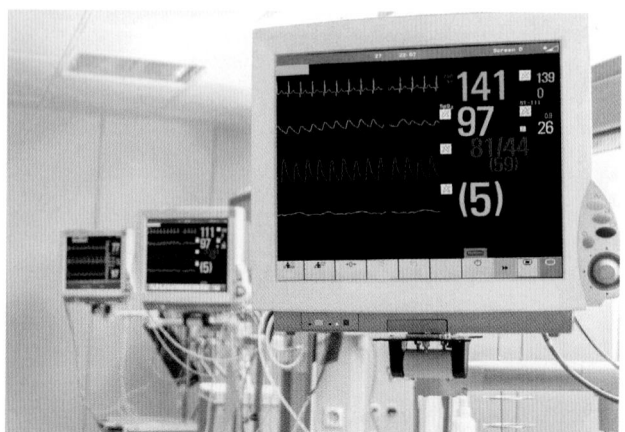

FIGURE 12-10 An automated monitoring device. (Beerkoff/Shutterstock)

The following are common signs and symptoms associated with fever:

- Pinkish, red (flushed) skin that is warm to the touch
- Restlessness or in others, excessive sleepiness
- Irritability
- Poor appetite
- Glassy eyes and a sensitivity to light
- Increased perspiration
- Headache
- Above-normal pulse and respiratory rates
- Disorientation and confusion (when the temperature is very high)
- Convulsions in infants and children (when the temperature is very high)
- Fever blisters around the nose or lips in clients who harbor the herpes simplex virus

Hyperthermia (excessively high core temperature) describes a state in which the temperature exceeds 105.8°F (40.6°C). At this level, the person is at extremely high risk for brain damage or death from complications associated with increased metabolic demands.

Phases of a Fever

A fever generally progresses through four distinct phases:

1. *Prodromal phase:* The client has nonspecific symptoms just before the temperature rises.
2. *Onset* or *invasion phase:* Obvious mechanisms for increasing body temperature, such as shivering, develop.
3. *Stationary phase:* The fever is sustained.
4. *Resolution* or *defervescence phase:* The temperature returns to normal (Fig. 12-11).

Common variations in fever patterns are described in Table 12-4. Fevers also subside in different ways. If an elevated temperature suddenly drops to normal, it is referred to as a *resolution by crisis.* If the descent is gradual, it is referred to as a *resolution lysis.*

Nursing Management

A fever is considered an important body defense for destroying infectious microorganisms. Therefore, as long as a fever remains below 102°F (38.9°C) and the person does not have a chronic medical condition, fluids or rest may be all that is necessary.

💊 Pharmacologic Considerations

Antipyretics (drugs that reduce fever), such as aspirin, acetaminophen, or ibuprofen, are helpful when a temperature is 102° to 104°F (38.9° to 40°C). To prevent liver damage, no more than 3,250 to 4,000 mg of acetaminophen should be taken per day.

Physical cooling measures are used for temperatures between 104° and 105.8°F (40° and 40.6°C). If the temperature is higher than 105.8°F (40.6°C) or if a high temperature is unchanged after a sufficient response time with conventional interventions, more aggressive treatment is warranted.

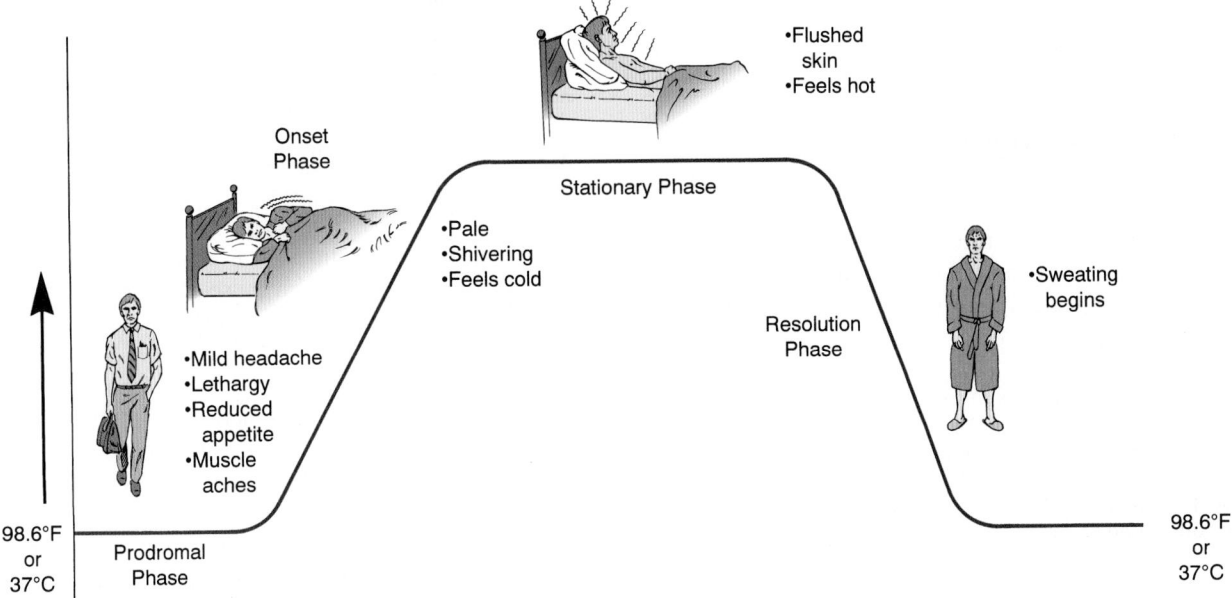

FIGURE 12-11 Phases of a fever and physiologic changes.

Subnormal Body Temperature

There are several ranges of **hypothermia** (a core body temperature less than 95°F [35°C]). A person is considered *mildly hypothermic* at temperatures of 95° to 93.2°F (35° to 34°C), *moderately hypothermic* at 93° to 86°F (33.8° to 30°C), and *severely hypothermic* below 86°F (30°C).

Cold body temperatures are best measured with a tympanic thermometer for two reasons. First, other clinical thermometers do not have the capacity to measure temperatures in hypothermic ranges. Second, the blood flow in the mouth, rectum, or axillae generally is so reduced that measurements taken from these sites are inaccurate.

The following are common signs and symptoms associated with hypothermia:

• Shivering until body temperature is extremely low
• Pale, cool, and puffy skin
• Impaired muscle coordination
• Listlessness
• Slow pulse and respiratory rates
• Irregular heart rhythm
• Decreased ability to think coherently and use good judgment
• Diminished ability to feel pain or other sensations

TABLE 12-4 Variations in Fever Patterns

TYPE OF FEVER	DESCRIPTION
Sustained fever	Remains elevated with little fluctuation
Remittent fever	Fluctuates several degrees but never reaches normal between fluctuations
Intermittent fever	Cycles frequently between periods of normal or subnormal temperatures and spikes of fever
Relapsing fever	Recurs after a brief but sustained period during which temperature has been normal

In some illnesses, such as hypothyroidism and starvation, the client typically has a subnormal temperature. Therefore, the nurse must assess clients just as closely when body temperature falls below normal ranges as when it is elevated.

Clients with severe hypothermia usually die. Nevertheless, clients have been known to live even with very low temperatures, as when nearly drowning in cold water and with exposure to extremely cold environments. Various supportive measures are implemented when clients have subnormal body temperatures (see Nursing Guidelines 12-2).

NURSING GUIDELINES 12-2

The Client with a Subnormal Temperature

• Raise the room temperature. *Doing so warms the body surface.*
• Remove wet clothing. *This measure reduces heat loss.*
• Apply layers of dry clothing and loosely woven blankets. *Layers trap body heat next to the skin.*
• Warm blankets and clothing in an oven or microwave if body temperature is quite low. *Heating raises the temperature of woven fabrics above ambient (room) temperature.*
• Position the client so that the arms are next to the chest and the legs are tucked toward the abdomen. *This position prevents heat loss.*
• Cover the head with a cap or towel. *Covering the head reduces heat loss.*
• Provide warm fluids. *Fluids conduct heat to internal organs.*
• Massage the skin unless it has been frostbitten. *Massage produces mechanical friction, which produces warmth.*
• Apply bags filled with warm water between areas of skin folds, or place an electronic warming pad beneath the back and hips (see Chapter 28) according to medical orders. *These measures transfer heat to the blood as it circulates through the skin.*

PULSE

A **pulse**, a wave-like sensation that can be palpated in a peripheral artery, is produced by the movement of blood during the heart's contraction. In most adults, the heart contracts 60 to 100 times per minute at rest.

Pulse Rate

The **pulse rate** (the number of peripheral pulsations palpated in 1 minute) is counted by compressing a superficial artery against an underlying bone with the tips of the fingers.

Rapid Pulse Rate

The pulse rate of adults is considered rapid if it exceeds 100 beats per minute (bpm) at rest. **Tachycardia** (100 to 150 bpm) is a fast heart rate, but heart and pulse rates can exceed 150 bpm. Rapid contraction, if sustained, tends to overwork the heart and may not oxygenate cells adequately because the heart has such little time between contractions to fill with blood.

The term **palpitation** (awareness of one's own heart contraction) can accompany tachycardia. Clients with rapid pulse rates are monitored closely, and the results are reported and recorded according to agency policy.

Slow Pulse Rate

The pulse rate of adults is considered slower than normal if it falls below 60 bpm. **Bradycardia** (less than 60 bpm) is less common than tachycardia; it merits prompt reporting and continued monitoring.

Factors Affecting Pulse and Heart Rates

Any factors that affect the rate of heart contraction also cause comparable effects on pulse rate. Because one depends on the other, the pulse rate can never be faster than the actual heart rate. Heart and pulse rates may vary depending on:

- *Age.* Some common rates are listed in Table 12-5.
- *Circadian rhythm.* Rates tend to be lower in the morning and increase later in the day.
- *Sex.* Male adults average approximately 60 to 65 bpm at rest; the average rate for female adults is about 7 or 8 bpm faster.
- *Body build.* Tall, slender people usually have slower heart and pulse rates than short, stout people.
- *Exercise and activity.* Rates increase with exercise and activity and decrease with rest. With regular aerobic

exercise, however, a **training effect** occurs in which the heart rate and consequently the pulse rate become consistently lower than average. This effect develops because the heart muscle becomes more efficient at supplying body cells with sufficient oxygenated blood with fewer beats. Those who are physically fit exhibit slower pulse rates, even during exercise.

- *Stress and emotions.* Stimulation of the sympathetic nervous system and emotions such as anger, fear, and excitement increase heart and pulse rates. Pain, which is stressful (especially when moderate to severe), can trigger faster rates.
- *Body temperature.* For every degree of Fahrenheit elevation, the heart and pulse rates increase by 10 bpm. With a fall in body temperature, the opposite effect occurs.
- *Blood volume.* Excessive blood loss causes the heart and pulse rates to increase. With decreased red blood cells or inadequate hemoglobin to distribute oxygen to cells, the heart rate accelerates in an effort to keep cells adequately supplied.
- *Drugs.* Certain drugs can slow or speed the rate of heart contraction. Digitalis preparations and sedatives typically slow the heart rate. Caffeine, nicotine, cocaine, thyroid replacement hormones, and epinephrine increase heart contractions and subsequently pulse rates.

 Pharmacologic Considerations

Older adults generally have more profound responses to cardiovascular medications than younger adults. Changes such as dizziness or fainting, diminished appetite, nausea, or visual changes may indicate the need for evaluation of cardiovascular medications.

Pulse Rhythm

The **pulse rhythm** (the pattern of the pulsations and the pauses between them) is normally regular. That is, the beats and the pauses occur similarly throughout the time the pulse is palpated.

An **arrhythmia** or **dysrhythmia** (an irregular pattern of heartbeats) with a consequently irregular pulse rhythm is reported promptly. Some types indicate potentially life-threatening cardiac dysfunctions that may warrant more sophisticated monitoring and treatment. Details about dysrhythmias and their causes can be found in textbooks that discuss cardiac disorders.

Pulse Volume

Pulse volume (the quality of palpated pulsations) is usually related to the amount of blood pumped with each heartbeat, or the force of the heart's contraction. When a pulse can be felt with mild pressure over the artery, it is described as being *strong*. A *feeble, weak,* or *thready pulse* refers to a pulse that is difficult to feel or, once felt, is obliterated easily with slight pressure. A rapid, thready pulse is usually a serious sign and should be reported promptly. A *bounding* or *full*

TABLE 12-5 Normal Pulse Rates per Minute at Various Ages

AGE	APPROXIMATE RANGE	APPROXIMATE AVERAGE
Newborn	120–160	140
1–12 months	80–140	120
1–2 years	80–130	110
3–6 years	75–120	100
7–12 years	75–110	95
Adolescence	60–100	80
Adulthood	60–100	80

TABLE 12-6 Identifying Pulse Volume

NUMBER	DEFINITION	DESCRIPTION
0	Absent pulse	No pulsation is felt despite extreme pressure.
1+	Thready pulse	Pulsation is not easily felt; slight pressure causes it to disappear.
2+	Weak pulse	Pulse is stronger than thready; light pressure causes it to disappear.
3+	Normal pulse	Pulsation is felt easily; moderate pressure causes it to disappear.
4+	Bounding pulse	Pulsation is strong and does not disappear with moderate pressure.

pulse produces a pronounced pulsation that does not easily disappear with pressure.

Another way to describe the volume or quality of the pulse is with corresponding numbers (Table 12-6). When documenting pulse volume, the nurse should follow the agency policy about using descriptive terms or a numbering system.

Assessment Sites

The arteries used for pulse assessment lie close to the skin. Most but not all are named for the bone over which they are located (Fig. 12-12). These pulse sites are collectively called "peripheral pulses" because they are distant from the heart. Of all the peripheral pulses, the radial artery, located on the inner (thumb) side of the wrist, is the site most often used for pulse assessment. Three alternative assessment techniques can be used instead of or in addition to the assessment of a peripheral pulse. These techniques include counting the apical heart rate, obtaining an apical–radial rate, and using a Doppler ultrasound device over a peripheral artery.

Apical Rate

The **apical heart rate** (the number of ventricular contractions per minute) is considered more accurate than the radial pulse for two reasons. First, the sound of each heartbeat is obvious and distinct. Second, sometimes, the heart contraction is not strong enough to be felt at a peripheral pulse site. Counting the apical rate, however, is less convenient than counting a radial pulse. An apical heart rate is generally assessed when the peripheral pulse is irregular or difficult to palpate because of a rapid rate or thready quality or when it is necessary to obtain an actual heart rate.

The apical heart rate is counted by listening at the chest with a stethoscope or by feeling the pulsations in the chest for 1 full minute at an area called the "point of maximum impulse." As the name suggests, the heartbeats are best heard or felt at the apex, or lower tip, of the heart. The apex in a healthy adult is slightly below the left nipple in line with the middle of the clavicle (Fig. 12-13).

When assessing the apical heart rate by listening to the chest—which is generally the more accurate technique—the nurse listens for the "lub-dub" sound. The lub sound is louder if the stethoscope has been correctly applied. These two sounds equal one pulsation at a peripheral pulse site. The rhythm is also evaluated.

Apical–Radial Rate

The **apical–radial rate** (the number of sounds heard at the heart's apex and the rate of the radial pulse during the same period) is counted by separate nurses at the same time using one watch or clock (Fig. 12-14). The apical and radial rates

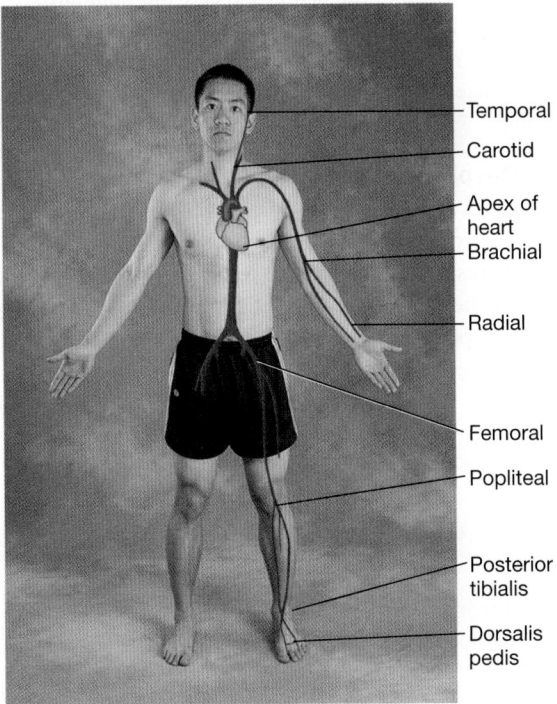

FIGURE 12-12 The peripheral pulse sites. (From LifeART © 2022, Lippincott Williams & Wilkins. All rights reserved.)

Temporal
Carotid
Apex of heart
Brachial
Radial
Femoral
Popliteal
Posterior tibialis
Dorsalis pedis

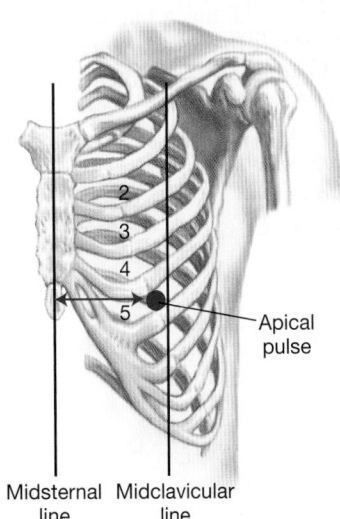

Midsternal line   Midclavicular line

FIGURE 12-13 Assess the apical heart rate to the left of the sternum at the interspace below the fifth rib in midline with the clavicle. (From Bickley, L. S., Szilagyi, P. G., Hoffman, R. M., & Soriano, R. P. [2020]. *Bates' guide to physical examination and history taking* [13th ed.]. Wolters Kluwer.)

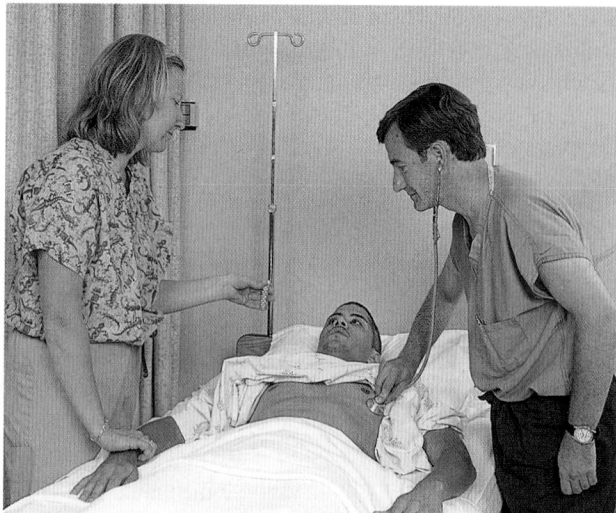

FIGURE 12-14 One nurse counts the radial pulse, while the other counts the apical rate. (Photo by B. Proud.)

should be the same, but in some clients, they are not. The **pulse deficit** (the difference between the apical and radial pulse rates) is noted. If a pulse deficit is significant—and the rates have been counted accurately—the nurse reports the findings promptly and documents them in the client's medical record.

Doppler Ultrasound Device

A Doppler ultrasound device is an electronic instrument that detects the movement of blood through peripheral blood vessels and converts the movement to a sound. This instrument is most helpful when slight pressure occludes pulsations or when arterial blood flow is severely compromised.

When the device is used, conductive gel is applied over the arterial site, and the probe is moved at an angle over the skin until a pulsating sound is heard (Fig. 12-15). The pulsating sounds are counted, much like the palpated pulsations. The nurse documents the assessment site and the rate, followed by the abbreviation D to indicate the use of a Doppler device.

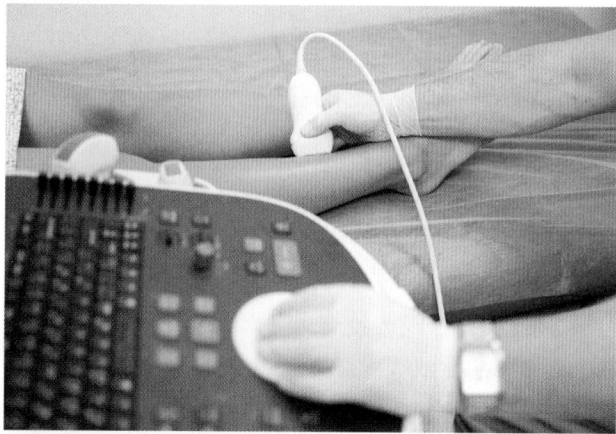

FIGURE 12-15 Using a Doppler ultrasound device. (YAKOBCHUK VIACHESLAV/Shutterstock)

Skill 12-2 describes how to assess the rate, rhythm, and volume of the pulse at the radial artery.

>>> *Stop, Think, and Respond 12-3*
If assessing the radial pulse is difficult or impossible, what alternative methods can be used?

RESPIRATION

Respiration is the exchange of oxygen and carbon dioxide. When it occurs between the alveolar and the capillary membranes, it is called *external* respiration. The exchange of oxygen and carbon dioxide between the blood and the body cells is called *internal or tissue* respiration.

Ventilation (the movement of air in and out of the chest) involves *inhalation* or *inspiration* (breathing in) and *exhalation* or *expiration* (breathing out). The medulla, which is the primary respiratory center in the brain, controls ventilation. The medulla is sensitive to the amount of carbon dioxide in the blood and adapts the rate of ventilations accordingly. Breathing can be voluntarily controlled to a certain extent.

Respiratory Rate

The **respiratory rate** (the number of ventilations per minute) varies considerably in healthy people, but normal ranges have been established (Table 12-7). Factors that influence pulse rate generally also affect respiratory rate. The faster the pulse rate, the faster the respiratory rate, and vice versa. The ratio of one respiration to approximately four or five heartbeats is fairly consistent in healthy adults.

Rapid Respiratory Rates

Resting respiratory rates that exceed the standards for a client's age are considered abnormal. **Tachypnea** (a rapid respiratory rate) often accompanies an elevated temperature or diseases that affect the cardiac and respiratory systems.

Slow Respiratory Rates

Bradypnea (a slower than normal respiratory rate at rest) can result from medications; for instance, morphine sulfate slows the respiratory rate. Slow respirations may also be observed in clients with neurologic disorders or who are experiencing hypothermia.

TABLE 12-7 Normal Respiratory Rates at Various Ages	
AGE	**AVERAGE RANGE**
Newborn	30–80
Early childhood	20–40
Late childhood	15–25
Adulthood	
Male	14–18
Female	16–20

Breathing Patterns and Abnormal Characteristics

Various breathing patterns and abnormal characteristics may be identified when assessing respiratory rates. *Cheyne–Stokes respiration* refers to a breathing pattern in which the depth of respirations gradually increases, followed by a gradual decrease, and then a period when breathing stops briefly before resuming the pattern again. Cheyne–Stokes respiration is a serious sign that may occur as death approaches.

Hyperventilation (rapid or deep breathing or both) and **hypoventilation** (diminished breathing) affect the volume of air entering and leaving the lungs. Changes in ventilation may occur in clients with airway obstruction or pulmonary or neuromuscular diseases.

Dyspnea (difficult or labored breathing) is almost always accompanied by a rapid respiratory rate as clients work to improve the efficiency of their breathing. Clients with dyspnea usually appear anxious and worried. The nostrils flare (widen) as the client fights to fill the lungs with air. They may use the abdominal and neck muscles to assist other muscles in breathing. When observing these clients, the nurse should note how much and what type of activity bring on dyspnea. For example, walking to the bathroom may bring on dyspnea associated with exertion, but sitting in a chair may not.

Orthopnea (breathing facilitated by sitting up or standing) occurs in clients with dyspnea who find it easier to breathe this way. The sitting or standing position causes organs in the abdominal cavity to fall away from the diaphragm with gravity. This gives more room for the lungs to expand within the chest cavity, allowing the person to take in more air with each breath.

Apnea (the absence of breathing) is life-threatening if it lasts more than 4 to 6 minutes. Prolonged apnea leads to brain damage or death. Brief periods of apnea lower oxygen levels in the blood and can trigger serious abnormal cardiac rhythms (see Chapter 21 for more on sleep apnea).

Terms such as **stertorous breathing** (noisy ventilation) and **stridor** (a harsh, high-pitched sound heard on inspiration when there is laryngeal obstruction) are used to describe sounds that accompany breathing. Infants and young children with croup often have stridor when breathing. The nurse uses a stethoscope to listen to the sounds of air moving through the chest. The assessment technique and the characteristics of lung sounds are described in Chapter 13.

Skill 12-3 lists techniques to use when counting the respiratory rate.

≫ Stop, Think, and Respond 12-4
What nursing actions are appropriate if a client has an abnormal respiratory rate?

BLOOD PRESSURE

Blood pressure is the force the blood exerts within the arteries. Several physiologic variables create BP:

- Circulating blood volume averages 4.5 to 5.5 L in female adults and 5.0 to 6.0 L in male adults. Lower than normal volumes decrease BP; excess volumes increase it.

- Contractility of the heart is influenced by the stretch of cardiac muscle fibers. Based on *Starling's law of the heart*, the force of heart contraction is related to **preload** (the volume of blood that fills the heart and stretches the heart muscle fibers during its resting phase). A common analogy is to compare the effect of preload and contractility with the snap of a rubber band stretched to various lengths—the longer the rubber band is stretched, the greater it snaps when released. Tissue damage that scars the heart, such as after a heart attack, impairs stretching and reduces contractility. Regular aerobic exercise increases the tone of the heart muscle, making it an efficient muscular pump.

- **Cardiac output** (the volume of blood ejected from the left ventricle per minute) is approximately 5 to 6 L (slightly more than a gallon) in adults at rest. It is estimated by multiplying the heart rate by the stroke volume (amount of blood that leaves the heart with each contraction). The average stroke volume in adults is 70 mL. With exercise, cardiac output can increase as much as five times the resting volume. Bradycardia can severely reduce cardiac output and thus BP.

- Blood viscosity (thickness) creates a resisting force when the heart contracts. The resistance compromises stroke volume and cardiac output. Blood thickens when there are more cells and proteins than water in plasma. Circulating viscous blood also causes cardiac fatigue and weakens the heart's ability to contract.

- Peripheral resistance, referred to as **afterload** (the force against which the heart pumps when ejecting blood), increases when the valves of the heart and arterioles (small subdivisions of arteries) are narrowed or calcified. Afterload is decreased when arteries dilate; constriction of arteries increases afterload.

In healthy people, the arterial walls are elastic and easily stretch and recoil to accommodate the changing volume of circulating blood. Measuring the BP helps assess the efficiency of the circulatory system. BP measurements reflect (1) the ability of the arteries to stretch, (2) the volume of circulating blood, and (3) the amount of resistance the heart must overcome when it pumps blood.

Factors Affecting Blood Pressure

Besides the physiologic variables that create BP, other factors that cause temporary or permanent alterations are as follows:

- *Age*: BP tends to become elevated with age as a result of arteriosclerosis, a process by which arteries lose their elasticity and become more rigid, and atherosclerosis, a process by which the arteries become narrowed with fat deposits. The rate of these conditions depends on heredity and lifestyle habits, such as diet and exercise.
- *Circadian rhythm*: BP tends to be lowest after midnight, begins rising at approximately 4 or 5 AM, and peaks during late morning or early afternoon.
- *Sex*: Female adults tend to have lower BP than male adults of the same age.
- *Exercise and activity*: BP rises during exercise and activity, when the heart pumps more blood. Regular exercise, however, helps maintain BP within normal levels.

• *Emotions and pain*: Strong emotional experiences and pain tend to increase BP from sympathetic nervous system stimulation.

• *Miscellaneous factors*: As a rule, a person has lower BP when lying down than when sitting or standing, though the difference in most people is insignificant. BP also seems to rise somewhat when the urinary bladder is full, when the legs are crossed, or when the person is cold. Drugs that stimulate the heart such as nicotine, caffeine, cocaine, and methamphetamine also tend to constrict the arteries and raise BP.

Pressure Measurements

When assessing BP, nurses obtain both systolic and diastolic measurements. **Systolic pressure** (pressure within the arterial system when the heart contracts) is higher than **diastolic pressure** (pressure within the arterial system when the heart relaxes and fills with blood). BP measurements are expressed as a fraction. The numerator is the systolic pressure, the pressure during systole, and the denominator is the diastolic pressure, the pressure during diastole (Fig. 12-16).

Currently, BP measurement is expressed in millimeters of mercury (mm Hg) because the mercury sphygmomanometer, an instrument for measuring BP using a graduated column of mercury, has been the standard for use. Thus, a recording of 118/78 means the systolic BP measured 118 mm Hg and the diastolic BP measured 78 mm Hg.

The **pulse pressure** (the difference between systolic and diastolic BP measurements) is computed by subtracting the smaller measurement from the larger. For example, when the BP is 126/88 mm Hg, the pulse pressure is 38. A pulse pressure between 30 and 50 is considered normal, with 40 being a healthy average.

Studies of healthy people show that BP can fluctuate within a wide range and still be normal. Because individual differences can be considerable, analyzing the usual ranges and patterns of BP measurements for each person is important. A rise or fall of 20 to 30 mm Hg in usual pressure is significant, even if it is well within the generally accepted range for normal.

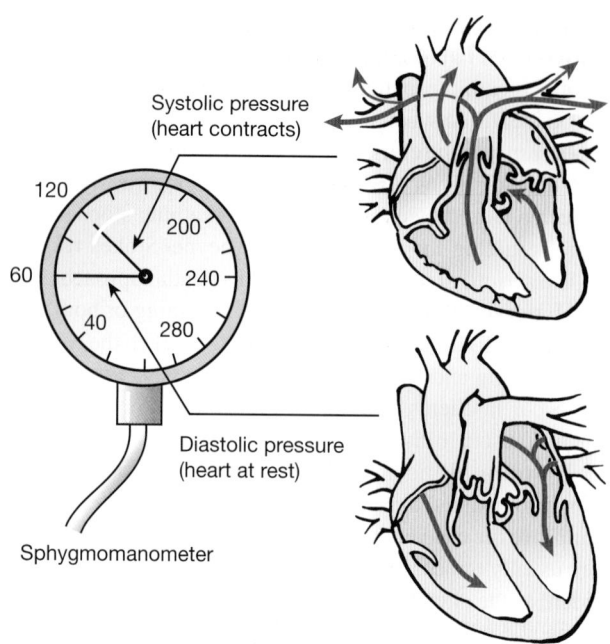

FIGURE 12-16 The pressure of blood in the arteries is higher during systole when the heart contracts and is lower during diastole when the heart muscle relaxes, hence the terms "systolic" and "diastolic" pressure, respectively.

Assessment Sites

BP is usually assessed over the brachial artery at the inner aspect of the elbow. It is also possible to use the lower arm and radial artery, the thigh and the popliteal artery, and the lower leg and the posterior tibial or dorsalis pedal artery (Fig. 12-17). There are situations in which the nurse must use an alternative to brachial or radial measurement, such as in the following circumstances:

• When the client's arms are missing
• When both of a client's breasts have been removed
• When a client has had vascular surgery (such as that which permits dialysis treatments for kidney failure)
• When plaster or fiberglass casts or dressings obscure the brachial and radial sites

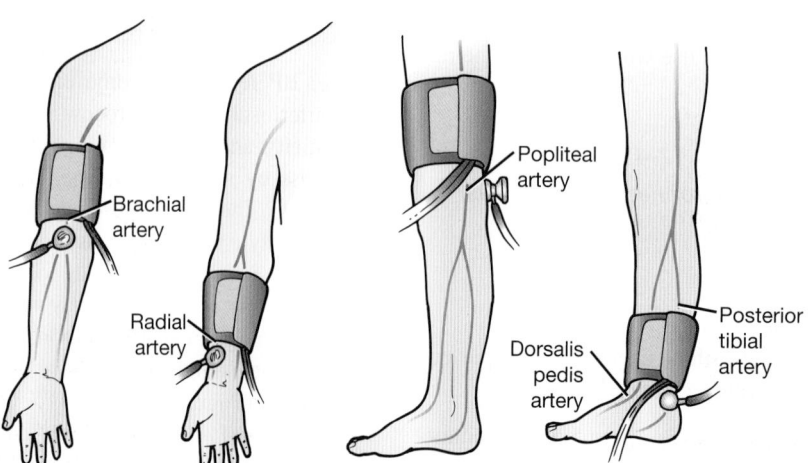

FIGURE 12-17 Arterial sites for measuring blood pressure.

In these and other unusual circumstances, BP can be measured over the popliteal artery behind the knee (see sections "Alternative Assessment Techniques" and "Measuring Thigh Blood Pressure"), the radial artery in the lower arm, or the posterior tibial or dorsalis pedis artery in the lower leg. Documentation of the site is essential because measurements vary depending on the site used.

Equipment for Measuring Blood Pressure

BP is most often measured with a **sphygmomanometer** (a device for measuring BP), an inflatable cuff, and a stethoscope.

Sphygmomanometer

A sphygmomanometer (shortened to *manometer*) is an instrument for measuring the pressure of a gas or liquid. It is attached to a cuff with an enclosed air bladder that is inflated manually with a pump or electronically (Fig. 12-18). Presently, two types of devices are available for measuring BP noninvasively: the aneroid and electronic oscillometric manometers.

Aneroid Manometer

An aneroid manometer (see Fig. 12-18), named from the French word *aneroide*, which means "no liquid," measures pressure using a spring mechanism. Its gauge features a needle that moves around a numbered dial. The numbers correspond to the measurements obtained with a mercury manometer. Before using an aneroid manometer, the needle on the gauge must be positioned at zero to ensure an accurate measurement.

Electronic Oscillometric Manometer

An electronic oscillometric manometer is battery operated or uses power from an electrical outlet (Fig. 12-19). Unlike an aneroid manometer, an electronic oscillometric manometer does not require a stethoscope for auscultating sounds that correspond to pressure measurements. It measures BP with a transducer within the cuff. The transducer is a device that receives sound waves, in this case, from the flow of blood within the artery. The device actually measures the mean arterial pressure and then electronically calculates the systolic and diastolic pressure using a preprogrammed formula.

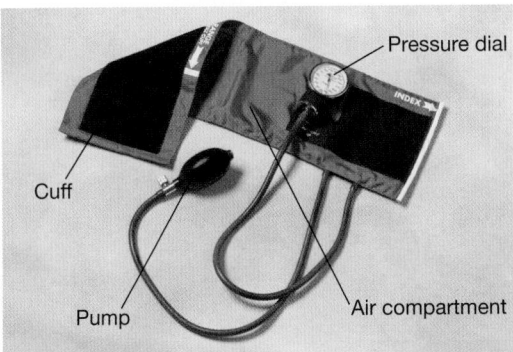

FIGURE 12-18 An aneroid manometer on a dial face is attached to a cuff with an enclosed air bladder that is inflated manually with a pump.

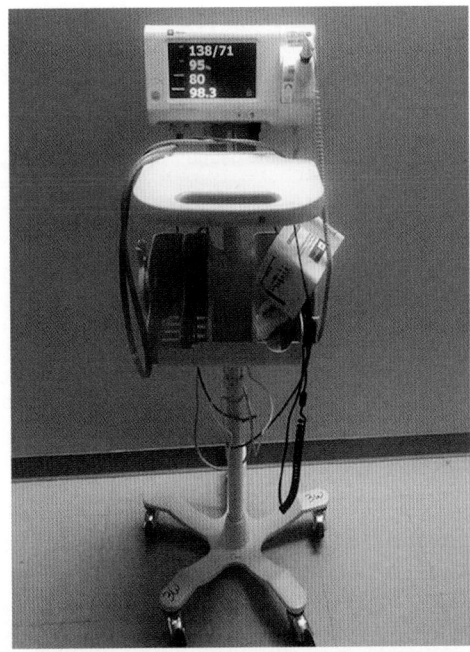

FIGURE 12-19 An oscillometric manometer inflates the air bladder electronically and displays pressure measurements digitally.

The calculated pressures are visually displayed. Models vary from those used in intensive care settings to others intended for home use.

Aneroid and electronic monitors have advantages and disadvantages (Table 12-8). Either can be used to assess BP, provided they are working properly and are used correctly.

Inflatable Cuff

The cuff contains an inflatable bladder to which two tubes are attached. One is connected to the manometer, which registers the pressure. The other is attached to a bulb that is used to inflate the bladder with air. A screw valve on the bulb allows the nurse to fill and empty the bladder. As the air escapes, the pressure is measured.

Cuffs come in various adult sizes, ranging from small adult arm, adult arm, large adult arm, and even adult thigh. A common guide is to use a cuff that has a bladder width of at least 40% and a length that is 80% to 100% of midlimb circumference (Fig. 12-20). *Note that it is not the width and length of the cuff itself, but rather the inflatable bladder that must be the correct size.*

If the cuff is too wide, the BP reading will be falsely low. If the cuff is too narrow, the BP reading will be falsely high. The most frequent error in measuring BP is using the wrong cuff size. The nurse must select a cuff with an appropriate bladder size for the body proportions of each client.

Stethoscope

A **stethoscope** (an instrument that carries sound to the ears) is composed of eartips, a brace and binaurals, and tubing leading to a chest piece that may be a bell, diaphragm, or both (Fig. 12-21). The eartips are generally rubber or plastic. When the stethoscope is used, the eartips are positioned downward and forward within the ears to produce the best

TABLE 12-8 Comparisons of Sphygmomanometer Equipment

TYPE	ADVANTAGES	DISADVANTAGES
Aneroid	Inexpensive Easy to carry and store Ability to read the gauge from any position	Delicate Periodic equipment checking against a second sphygmomanometer necessary for accuracy Gauge possibly clumsy to attach to cuff Stethoscope and accurate hearing necessary Calibration check and readjustment recommended yearly Manufacturer repair required
Electronic	Digital display of measurement No stethoscope required Accurate for people with hearing loss Facilitation of blood pressure measurement of newborns and infants in whom auscultation (listening with a stethoscope) is difficult	Expensive depending on quality Batteries necessary Body movements and improper cuff application can influence accuracy. Calibration check and readjustment recommended every 6 months Manufacturer repair needed

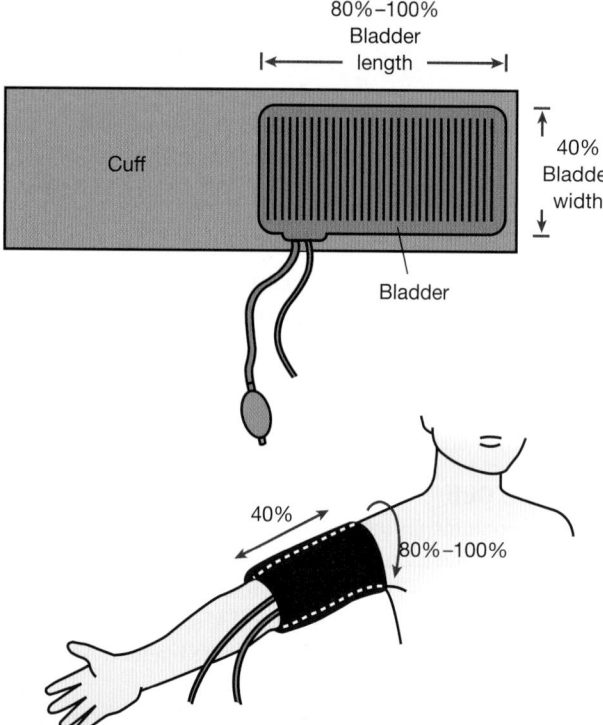

FIGURE 12-20 To determine the appropriate size of blood pressure cuff, the width of the bladder should be 40% of the midarm circumference and the length should be at least 80%.

sound perception. If various people are using stethoscopes in common, they must clean the eartips with alcohol pads between uses. Personal stethoscopes also need periodic cleaning to keep the eartips free of cerumen and dirt.

The brace and binaurals are generally made of metal. They connect the eartips to the tubing and chest piece. The brace prevents the tubing from kinking and distorting the sound. Stethoscope tubing is rubber or plastic. The best length for good sound conduction is about 20 in (50 cm).

The bell, or cup-shaped chest piece, is used to detect low-pitched sounds, such as those produced in blood vessels. The diaphragm, or disk-shaped chest piece, detects high-pitched sounds, such as those in the lungs, heart, or abdomen. A cracked diaphragm must be replaced. When the bell is used, care is taken to position it lightly over the anatomic area because pressure flattens the skin and creates the same effect as a diaphragm.

Measuring Blood Pressure

The first time BP is measured, it is assessed in each arm. The two BP measurements should not vary more than 5 to 10 mm Hg unless pathology (disease) is present. Some agency protocols specify that a BP assessment is taken with the client in lying, sitting, and standing positions for the initial database. Several variables can result in inaccurate BP measurements (Table 12-9).

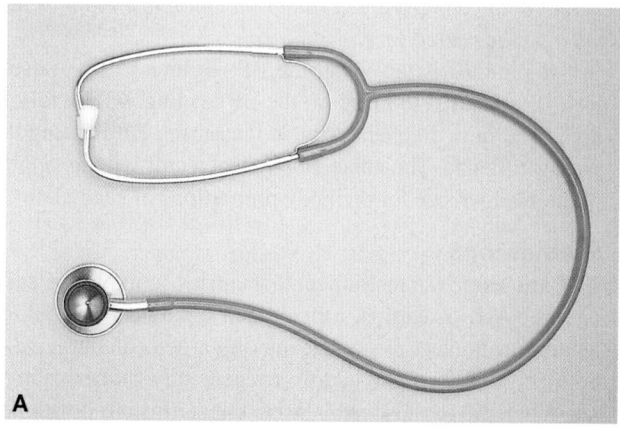

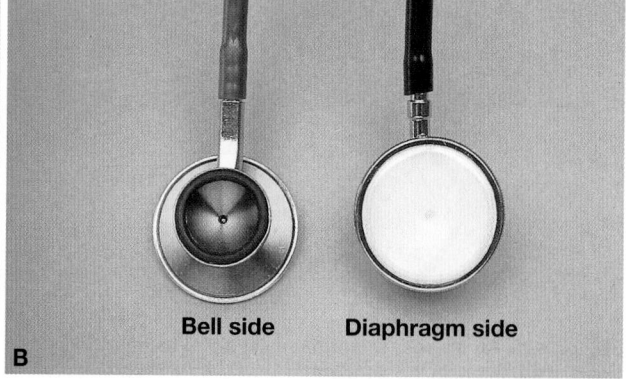

FIGURE 12-21 A stethoscope **(A)** and a chest piece **(B)**.

TABLE 12-9 Common Causes of Blood Pressure Assessment Errors

CAUSE	EFFECT	CORRECTION
Inaccurate manometer calibration	False high or low readings	Recalibrate, repair, or replace gauge.
Loosely applied cuff	High reading	Wrap snugly with equal pressure around extremity.
Cuff too small for extremity	High reading	Select appropriate size.
Cuff too large for extremity	Low reading	Select appropriate size.
Cuff applied over clothing	Creates noise or interferes with sound perception	Remove arm from sleeve or have client don a gown.
Tubing that leaks	Rapid loss of pressure	Replace or repair.
Improper positioning of eartips	Poor sound conduction	Reposition and retake blood pressure.
Impaired hearing	Altered sound perception	Use an alternative assessment technique or equipment.
Loud environmental noise	Interferes with sound perception	Reduce noise and reassess.
Impaired vision	Inaccurate observation of gauge	Correct vision; reposition gauge in adequate range.
Rapid cuff deflation	Inaccurate observation of gauge	Reassess and deflate at 2–3 mm Hg/sec.
Number bias	Falsely high or low measurements	Use an electronic sphygmomanometer.

Korotkoff Sounds

Most BP recordings are obtained indirectly. That is, they are determined by applying a BP cuff, briefly occluding arterial blood flow, and listening for **Korotkoff sounds** (sounds that result from the vibrations of blood within the arterial wall or changes in blood flow). BP measurements are determined by correlating the phases of Korotkoff sounds with the numbers on the sphygmomanometer. If Korotkoff sounds are difficult to hear, they can be intensified in one of two ways:

• Have the client elevate the arm before and during cuff inflation, then lower the arm after full inflation.
• Have the client open and close the fist after cuff inflation.

Korotkoff sounds have five unique phases (Fig. 12-22).

Phase I begins with the first faint but clear tapping sound that follows a period of silence as pressure is released from the cuff. When the first sound occurs, it corresponds to the peak pressure in the arterial system during heart contraction, or the systolic pressure measurement. It is recorded as the first number in the fraction.

The first sound, which is heard for at least two consecutive beats, may be missed if the cuff pressure is not initially pumped high enough. Palpating for the disappearance of a distal pulse when inflating the cuff helps ensure that the cuff pressure is above arterial pressure.

Phase I sounds may disappear briefly before they become reestablished, especially in older adults and in clients with high BP or peripheral arterial disease. An **auscultatory gap** (a period during which sound disappears) can range as much as 40 mm Hg. Failure to identify the first sound preceding an auscultatory gap results in an inaccurate BP assessment from undermeasurement of the systolic pressure.

 Concept Mastery Alert

Systolic Blood Pressure Sounds

Be careful not to confuse the first sound audible after the auscultatory gap as the systolic pressure. This sound constitutes the first diastolic sound and is typically not recorded when measuring an adult's BP. The systolic BP is the first faint but clear tapping sound that follows a period of silence as pressure is released from the cuff.

Consequently, hypertension may be unidentified and thus undiagnosed and untreated.

Phase II is characterized by a change from tapping sounds to swishing sounds. At this time, the diameter of the artery is widening, allowing more arterial blood flow.

Phase III is characterized by a change to loud and distinct sounds described as crisp knocking sounds. During this phase, blood flows relatively freely through the artery once more.

Phase IV sounds are muffled and have a blowing quality. The sound change results from a loss in the transmission of pressure from the deflating cuff to the artery. The point at which the sound becomes muffled is considered the first diastolic pressure measurement. It is generally preferred when documenting BP measurements in children.

Phase V is the point at which the last sound is heard, or the second diastolic pressure measurement. This is considered the best reflection of adult diastolic pressure because phase IV is often 7 to 10 mm Hg higher than direct diastolic pressure measurements. When recording adult BP measurements, the pressures at phases I and V are used.

Oscillometric devices have been proven that allow accurate BP measurement while reducing human errors associated with the auscultatory method. Fully automated oscillometric devices capable of taking continuous readings even without a viewer being present may provide a more accurate measurement of BP than auscultation. Directions for standard auscultatory BP measurements are given in Skill 12-4.

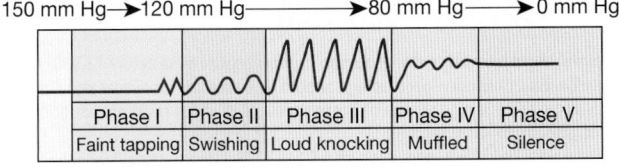

FIGURE 12-22 Characteristics of Korotkoff sounds.

Alternative Assessment Techniques

When Korotkoff sounds are difficult to hear in the usual manner no matter how conscientious the effort to augment them, nurses can assess BP using alternative methods. They can measure BP by palpation or by using a Doppler stethoscope. When BP requires frequent or prolonged assessment, an automated BP machine is necessary. When the brachial or radial artery is inaccessible in both arms or assessing BP at these sites is contraindicated, the thigh is an optional alternative.

Palpating the Blood Pressure

When palpating the BP, the nurse applies a BP cuff. Instead of using a stethoscope, however, the nurse positions the fingers over the artery while releasing the cuff pressure. The point at which the nurse feels the first pulsation corresponds to the systolic pressure. The diastolic pressure cannot be measured because there is no perceptible change in the quality of pulsations like there is in the sounds. When recording a BP taken this way, it is important to indicate that palpation was used.

Doppler Stethoscope

A **Doppler stethoscope** (Fig. 12-23) helps detect sounds created by the velocity of blood moving through a blood vessel. The sounds of moving blood cells are reflected toward the ultrasound receiver, producing a tone. The nurse notes the pressure at which the sound occurs. The onset of sound represents the peak pressure of arterial blood flow. A description of how Doppler is used was given earlier in this chapter. When documenting the pressure measurement, the nurse writes a "D" to indicate the use of Doppler.

Automatic Blood Pressure Monitoring

An automatic electronic BP monitoring device consists of a BP cuff attached to a microprocessing unit. Such devices diagnose unusual fluctuations in BP that single or sporadic monitoring cannot identify. When used, the device records the client's BP every 10 to 30 minutes or as needed over 24 hours. It stores the data in the microprocessor's memory. Measurements are printed or transferred by hand to a flow sheet for vital signs. Outpatients can wear a portable model

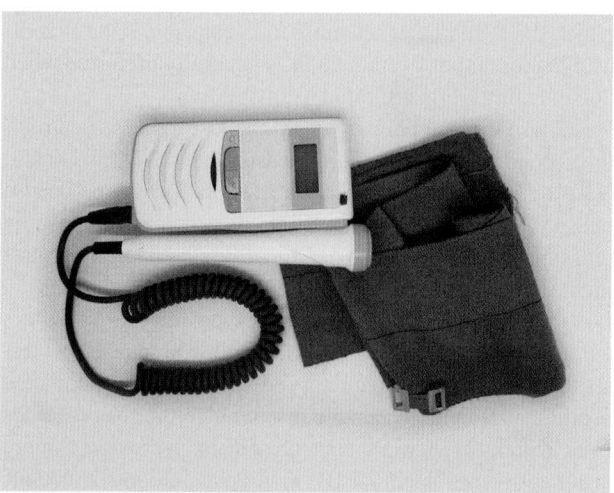

FIGURE 12-23 A Doppler stethoscope is used when Korotkoff sounds are difficult to hear. (Konokae/Shutterstock)

supported at either the shoulder or the waist to help diagnose conditions in which BP is altered.

Measuring Thigh Blood Pressure

The thigh is a structure that corresponds anatomically to the upper arm. Nurses use this site for BP assessment when they cannot obtain readings in either of the client's arms. Information varies regarding how thigh BPs compare with arm pressures. Readings tend to be 10% to 20% higher than readings taken in the arm. Skill 12-5 describes the technique for obtaining a thigh BP measurement.

>>> **Stop, Think, and Respond 12-5**
What suggestions would you offer to a nurse who has difficulty hearing Korotkoff sounds when assessing a client's blood pressure?

Abnormal Blood Pressure Measurements

BP above or below normal ranges may indicate significant health problems.

High Blood Pressure

Hypertension (high BP) exists when the systolic pressure, diastolic pressure, or both are sustained above normal levels for the person's age. For adults 18 years or older, a systolic pressure of less than 120 mm Hg and a diastolic pressure of less than 80 mm Hg are considered normal (AHA, 2024). Per the AHA, a systolic pressure of 120 to 129 130 mm Hg or higher and a diastolic pressure of less than 80 mm Hg are considered elevated BP (Table 12-10). An occasional elevation in BP does not necessarily mean a person has hypertension. It does mean that the BP should be monitored at various intervals depending on the significance of the measurements (Table 12-11). Monitoring is especially important to determine whether the elevated BP is sustained, changing, or the result of **white coat hypertension** (a condition in which the BP is elevated when taken by a health care provider but normal at other times).

TABLE 12-10 Classification of Adult Blood Pressure Measurements

CATEGORY	SYSTOLIC (mm Hg) (upper number)		DIASTOLIC (mm Hg) (lower number)
Normal[a]	<120	and	<80
Elevated[b]	120–129	and	<80
High blood pressure (hypertension) stage 1	130–139	or	80–89
High blood pressure (hypertension) stage 2	≥140	or	≥90
Hypertensive crisis (Consult your doctor immediately)	>180	and/or	>120

[a]Normal blood pressure with respect to cardiovascular risk is below 120/80 mm Hg. However, unusually low readings should be evaluated for clinical significance.
[b]Based on the average of two or more readings taken at each of two or more visits after an initial screening.
Healthy and unhealthy blood pressure ranges. (2024). From https://www.heart.org/en/health-topics/high-blood-pressure/understanding-blood-pressure-readings

TABLE 12-11 Recommendations for Follow-Up Based on Initial Set of Blood Pressure Measurements

INITIAL BLOOD PRESSURE (mm Hg)[a]		
SYSTOLIC	DIASTOLIC	RECOMMENDED FOLLOW-UP[b]
<120	<80	Promote healthy lifestyle[c] and recheck in 1 year
120–129	<80	Nonpharmacologic therapy and reassess in 3–6 months
130–139	80–89	Nonpharmacologic therapy and blood pressure lowering medication, reassess in 3–6 months
140–159 or greater	90–99 or greater	Nonpharmacologic therapy and blood pressure lowering medication, reassess 1 month

[a]If systolic and diastolic categories are different, follow recommendations for shorter follow-up (e.g., client with 160/86 mm Hg should be evaluated or referred to source of care within 1 month).
[b]Modify the scheduling of follow-up according to reliable information about past blood pressure measurements, other cardiovascular risk factors, or target organ disease.
[c]Provide advice about lifestyle modifications.
Data from American Heart Association. (2022). Hypertension guideline resources. https://www.heart.org/en/health-topics/high-blood-pressure/high-blood-pressure-toolkit-resources

Hypertensive BP measurements are often associated with:

- Anxiety
- Obesity
- Vascular diseases
- Stroke
- Heart failure
- Kidney diseases

 N u t r i t i o n   N o t e s

The Dietary Approaches to Stop Hypertension (DASH) diet is promoted by the National Heart, Lung, and Blood Institute (NHLBI) and the AHA as a healthy dietary pattern to prevent and treat hypertension. Eating a diet rich in fruit, vegetables, low-fat dairy products, and whole grains substantially lowers both systolic and diastolic BPs. The diet contains moderate amounts of poultry, fish, and nuts and is low in fat, red meat, and added sugar. Reducing sodium intake either alone or in combination with a DASH eating plan also lowers BP. In fact, this combination was found to lower systolic BP throughout multiple stages of hypertension, including in adults with the highest levels (150 mm Hg and above). Other nutrition interventions that effectively lower BP are to lose weight if overweight and limit alcohol intake to no more than two drinks a day for most men and no more than one drink a day for women and lighter weight men.

Low Blood Pressure

Hypotension (low BP) is when BP measurements are below the normal systolic values for the person's age. Having a consistently low pressure, 96/60 mm Hg, for example, seems to cause no harm. In fact, low BP is usually associated with efficient functioning of the heart and blood vessels. People with low BP, however, should continue to be monitored to evaluate its significance. Low BP measurements may indicate shock, hemorrhage, or side effects from drugs.

Postural Hypotension

Postural or **orthostatic hypotension** is a temporary drop in BP when rising from a reclining position after 3 to 5 minutes of rest. It is most common in those with circulatory problems—especially common in older adults, those who are dehydrated, and those who take diuretics or other drugs that lower BP.

A consequence of the decrease in BP is dizziness and fainting, putting those affected at a high risk for falls. Clients become symptomatic because approximately 500 to 1,000 mL of blood pools by gravity to the lower body when standing (Fig. 12-24). Under ordinary circumstances, a decrease in BP is accompanied by a response by **baroreceptors** sensory nerves in the walls of large arteries. A baroreceptor's function is to maintain arterial pressure. In clients who experience postural hypotension, there is a delay in the baroreceptor response, resulting in a brief inability to sufficiently raise the BP to restore adequate circulation to the brain.

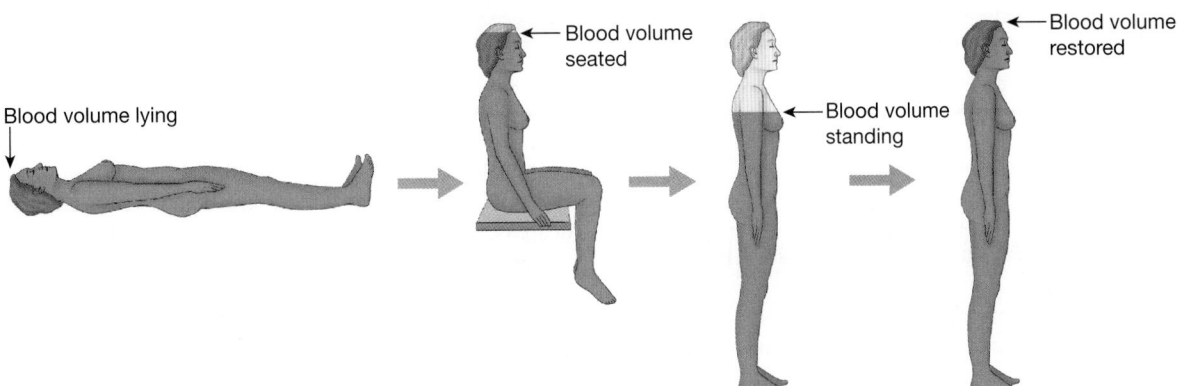

FIGURE 12-24 Influence of gravity on circulating blood volume.

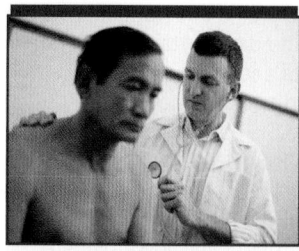

Clinical Scenario While assessing a client who has been admitted for dizziness, the nurse notes that when the client stood up, they almost fell. The client states that they have been very dizzy upon standing for the last few days. The nurse proceeds to assess the client's vital signs.

■ What additional data would contribute to identifying a nursing diagnosis?

■ What nursing measures are currently indicated?

See Nursing Care Plan 12-1.

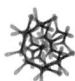 **NURSING CARE PLAN 12-1** | **Orthostatic Hypotension**

Assessment

Determine the following:

- Current vital signs including orthostatic vital signs
- Contributing factors such as dehydration, illness, history of cardio, neurological, or vascular disorders
- Current prescribed or over-the-counter (OTC) drugs that may have a cardiovascular effect
- Trend in blood pressure readings when sitting, standing, or lying down

Nursing Diagnosis. Orthostatic hypotension related taking prescribed cardiovascular medications and OTC medications for a cold

Expected Outcome. The client will not experience dizziness when going from a sitting position to a standing position within 24 hours of interventions.

Interventions	Rationales
Obtain and monitor the clients blood pressure: Sitting Standing Lying down	Have a baseline set of vital signs (blood pressure) including orthostatics. Have client purchase a home blood pressure machine in order to monitor blood pressure and vital signs at home. Observe the client's response to orthostatic blood pressure (vital signs).
Client has dizziness upon rising after 3–5 minutes of rest.	Advise client to hold on to something and rise slowly. Apply compression stockings to the lower extremities to reduce pooling of blood upon standing. Avoid sitting or standing for long periods of time, especially after meals. Limit alcohol intake.
Client is not drinking enough fluids and is dehydrated.	Restore adequate hydration by encouraging an increase in fluid intake (if not contraindicated). Increase consumption of foods containing sodium (if not contraindicated—e.g., hypertension). Limiting long baths or long walks in hot weather. Educate family regarding fluid intake.
Administer prescribed medications.	Medications that mimic aldosterone to help reduce the loss of sodium in the urine and to raise the blood volume, or a vasopressor, to constrict blood vessels causing an antihypotensive effect Review OTC medications for side effects that may cause dehydration and dizziness. Consult with provider regarding OTC medications for colds, etc.

Evaluation of Expected Outcome

The client did not experience any dizziness after following the use of the interventions.

 Pharmacologic Considerations

The first 3 weeks of antihypertensive drug therapy (especially diuretic use) is a critical time period for fall risk due to the side effects of lowering the BP. Clients over 60 years of age are at greatest risk.

Postural hypotension is validated by a fall in the standing systolic BP equal to or more than 20 mm Hg and or a decrease in diastolic BP equal to or more than 10 mm Hg within 2 minutes of standing when compared with the supine BP reading. An increase in the pulse rate of 15 to 30 bpm accompanying an upright position further supports the conclusion that the client experiences postural hypotension. Nursing Guidelines 12-3 describes how to assess clients for postural hypotension.

NURSING GUIDELINES 12-3

Assessing for Postural Hypotension

- Read the client's history for any reference to cardiac, vascular, or neurologic disorders.
- Review the list of prescribed drugs for any that may have cardiovascular effects.
- Gather equipment for assessing the client's blood pressure.
- Wait 30 minutes from the time the client has ingested caffeine, consumed a heavy meal, exercised vigorously, or taken a hot shower or bath.
- Explain to the client that the blood pressure and pulse will be taken after lying quietly for 3–5 minutes and again after standing for 1–3 minutes.
- Perform hand antisepsis.
- Apply the blood pressure cuff with the client in a supine position.
- Make sure that the client's legs are uncrossed so as not to affect the blood pressure.
- Support the cuffed arm maintaining the cuff at the level of the heart.
- Proceed to pump the air bladder 30 mm Hg above the measurement of where the pulse previously disappeared.

- Listen for Korotkoff sounds with the stethoscope as air is slowly released from the cuff.
- Note the systolic and diastolic measurements.
- Assess the client's pulse rate.
- Assist the client into a standing position.
- Steady the client should they become dizzy or faint.
- Repeat the blood pressure and pulse measurement within 3 minutes of standing.
- Subtract the standing systolic measurement from the supine measurement.
- Subtract the standing diastolic measurement from the supine measurement.
- Note the difference between the resting pulse rate and the standing pulse rate.
- Restore the client to a therapeutic position or one that provides comfort.
- Repeat hand antisepsis.
- Label and document the measurements in the client's medical record.
- Report the assessment findings verbally to the nurse in charge.

Once postural hypotension is confirmed, the nurse can reduce the client's risk for falling in the following ways: (1) ensure that the client remains seated after rising until dizziness passes, (2) restore adequate hydration if the client's fluid volume is low, (3) increase consumption of salty foods and those containing sodium providing the client is not hypertensive, (4) apply compression stockings to the lower extremities to reduce pooling of blood upon standing, and (5) administer prescribed medications such as a *synthetic mineralocorticoid* that mimics aldosterone, an adrenal hormone, to reduce the loss of sodium in urine thus raising blood volume, or a *sympathetic nervous system vasopressor*, a drug that constricts blood vessels, causing an antihypotensive effect.

 Pharmacologic Considerations

In extreme cases of symptomatic postural hypotension, administration of fludrocortisone (a synthetic mineralocorticoid) aids in sodium retention for better fluid balance and management of hypotensive episodes.

DOCUMENTING VITAL SIGNS

Once nurses have obtained vital sign measurements, they are documented in the medical record for analysis of patterns and trends (Fig. 12-25). They also may be entered as data, along with any other subjective or objective information elsewhere in the client's record, such as in the narrative nursing notes.

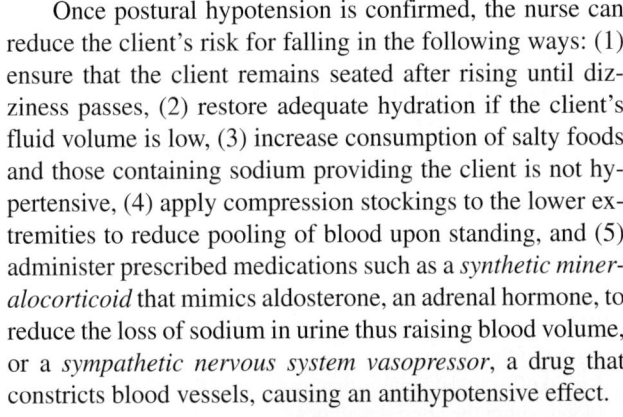
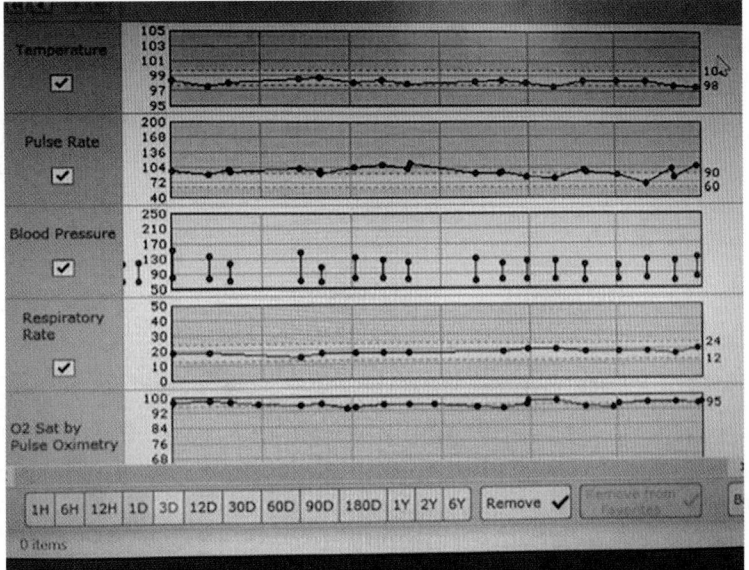

FIGURE 12-25 A graphic recording of vital signs.

NURSING IMPLICATIONS

Vital sign assessment is part of every client's care and forms the basis for identifying problems. Based on the analysis of assessment data, the nurse may identify one or more of the following nursing diagnoses:

- Altered breathing pattern
- Hypertension risk
- Hypotension risk
- Orthostatic hypotension
- Injury risk

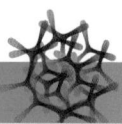

KEY POINTS

- Vital signs
  - Temperature: In healthy adults, temperature is 96.6° to 99.3°F.
    - Oral
    - Rectal equivalent
    - Axillary equivalent
    - Tympanic membrane
    - Temporal artery
  - Pulse: In most adults, the heart contracts 60 to 100 times per minute at rest. The pulse rate (the number of peripheral pulsations palpated in 1 minute) is counted by compressing a superficial artery against an underlying bone with the tips of the fingers.
  - Respirations: In most adults, the respiratory rate is 14 to 20 times per minute at rest.
  - BP: The force that the blood exerts within the arteries
- Factors affecting vital signs:
  - Age
  - Circadian rhythm
  - Sex
  - Exercise and activity
  - Emotions and pain
  - Climate
  - Illness or injury
  - Medications
  - Food intake
- Fever versus hyperthermia
  - Phases of a fever:
    - Prodromal phase: The client has nonspecific symptoms just before the temperature rises.
    - Onset or invasion phase: Obvious mechanisms for increasing body temperature, such as shivering, develop.
    - Stationary phase: The fever is sustained.
    - Resolution or defervescence phase: The temperature returns to normal.
  - Fever: A body temperature that exceeds 99.3°F (37.4°C); a common indication of illness; a person with a fever is said to be febrile.
  - Hyperthermia: A state in which the temperature exceeds 105.8°F (40.6°C); at this level, the person is at

extremely high risk for brain damage or death from complications associated with increased metabolic demands.
- When assessing a client's pulse, the nurse notes pulse rate, pulse rhythm, and pulse volume.
  - The most common site to take a pulse is the radial; located on the inner (thumb) side of the wrist.
  - The most accurate site is the apical pulse; best heard or felt at the apex, or lower tip, of the heart, the apex in a healthy adult is slightly below the left nipple in line with the middle of the clavicle.
- BP
  - The force that the blood exerts within the arteries. Several physiologic variables create BP:
    - Circulating blood volume
    - Contractility of the heart
    - Cardiac output
    - Blood viscosity (thickness)
    - Peripheral resistance
- Systolic pressure: Pressure within the arterial system when the heart contracts and is higher and diastolic BP; the numerator is the systolic pressure fraction.
- Diastolic pressure: Pressure within the arterial system when the heart relaxes and fills with blood; the denominator is the diastolic pressure fraction.
- BP is usually assessed over the brachial artery at the inner aspect of the elbow.
- Korotkoff sounds: Sounds that result from the vibrations of blood within the arterial wall or changes in blood flow that determines the BP
  - Phase I: First faint but clear tapping sound that follows a period of silence (systolic)
  - Phase II: Characterized by a change from tapping sounds to swishing sounds
  - Phase III: Characterized by a change to loud and distinct sounds described as crisp knocking sounds
  - Phase IV: Sounds are muffled and have a blowing quality (diastolic).
  - Phase V: The point at which the last sound is heard

CRITICAL THINKING EXERCISES

1. When visiting a friend with a fever, you see that the only thermometer available is made of glass and contains mercury. What suggestions for replacement would you offer when your friend feels better?

2. A neighbor with no medical experience asks how to tell if her 4-year-old child has a fever. What advice would you give?

3. An 80-year-old client explains that as an economy measure, she keeps her thermostat set at 65°F. What health information would be appropriate considering this woman's age?

4. While participating in a community health assessment, you discover a person with a blood pressure that measures 190/110 mm Hg. What actions are appropriate at this time?

NEXT-GENERATION NCLEX-STYLE REVIEW QUESTIONS

1. When assessing the temperature of a toddler who is 20 months old, which methods are appropriate? Select all that apply.
  a. Oral
  b. Rectal
  c. Tympanic
  d. Temporal
  e. Axillary
  Test-Taking Strategy: Use the process of elimination to select options that are considered accurate as well as anatomically and developmentally appropriate for a young pediatric client.

2. When delegating the task of taking an oral temperature on a client who has just finished eating breakfast, what instructions are best for the nurse to give the nursing assistant? Select all that apply.
  a. Assess the client's temperature at the rectal site.
  b. Postpone the assessment until before lunch.
  c. Take all of the vital signs, but omit the temperature.
  d. Assess the client's oral temperature in 30 minutes.
  e. Hold the thermometer in the client's mouth for 5 minutes.
  f. Inform the client when a temperature will be assessed.
  Test-Taking Strategy: Note the key word, "best." Analyze each option and select only those actions that support accuracy and conscientious care of the client.

3. What nursing action is best when a client with a temperature of 103.6°F is shivering?
  a. Offer the client a cup of hot soup.
  b. Cover the client with a light blanket.
  c. Direct a fan in the client's direction.
  d. Darken the room to provide rest.
  Test-Taking Strategy: Although some or all the options may have merit, based on the key term "best," select the option that represents a priority.

4. A nurse finds it difficult to palpate a radial pulse. Which other options are appropriate? Select all that apply.
  a. Assess the pulse rate at the ulnar artery.
  b. Use a Doppler stethoscope over a peripheral artery.
  c. Count the rate at the apex of the heart.
  d. Determine the apical–radial heart rate.
  e. Record the radial pulse as accurately as possible.

5. When assessing Korotkoff sounds, which of the below descriptions best describes the sound the nurse identifies as an adult's diastolic blood pressure measurement?
  a. A loud and distinct knocking sound is heard.
  b. A swishing sound occurs following tapping sounds.
  c. A muffled sound with a blowing quality is first detected.
  d. A faint but clear tapping sound is heard after a period of silence.
  Test-Taking Strategy: Use the process of elimination to select the option that is most appropriate when caring for the described client.

6. If the nurse detects that a client has symptoms associated with orthostatic hypotension, what is the best instruction the nurse can offer the client?
  a. Limit consumption of fluids during the day.
  b. Rise slowly from a lying or sitting position.
  c. Remain on bed rest throughout care in the health agency.
  d. Ambulate about the health agency at least four times a day.
  Test-Taking Strategy: Use the process of elimination to select the option that ensures the safety of the client without imposing unnecessary restrictions.

NEXT-GENERATION NCLEX-STYLE CLINICAL SCENARIO QUESTIONS

Clinical Scenario:
While assessing a client who has been admitted for dizziness, the nurse notes that when the client stood up, they almost fell. The client states that they have been very dizzy upon standing for the last few days. The nurse proceeds to assess the client's vital signs.

1. From the following list, select all of the answers that may play a factor in the client's situation.
  a. Medications
  b. Dehydration
  c. Hyperthermia
  d. Standing for long periods of time after a meal
  e. Eating a diet high in sodium

2. Choose the most likely options for the information missing from the statements below by selecting from the list of options provided.
  a. The client understands the need to _____1_____, and to increase ___2___ in their diet.

OPTION 1	OPTION 2
lay down	potassium
stand slowly	carbohydrates
walk	sodium

SKILL 12-1 Assessing Body Temperature

Suggested Action	Reason for Action
ASSESSMENT	
Determine when and how frequently to monitor the client's temperature (see Box 12-1) and the type of thermometer previously used.	Demonstrates accountability for making timely and appropriate assessments; ensures consistency in the technique for gathering data
Review previously recorded temperature measurements.	Aids in identifying trends and analyzing significant patterns
If using an oral electronic or digital thermometer:	
Observe the client's ability to support a thermometer within the mouth and breathe adequately through the nose with the mouth closed.	Shows consideration for accuracy because thermal energy is transferred from the oral cavity to the thermometer probe; escape of heat invalidates the measurement
Read the client's history for any reference to recent seizures or a seizure disorder.	Shows consideration for safety and identifies possible contraindication for oral site
Determine whether the client consumed any hot or cold substances or smoked a cigarette within the past 30 minutes.	Shows consideration for accuracy because the temperature in the oral cavity can be temporarily altered from substances recently placed within the mouth
PLANNING	
Arrange to take the client's temperature as near to the scheduled routine as possible.	Ensures consistency and accuracy
Gather supplies including a thermometer, watch, and probe cover or disposable sleeve if needed. Include lubricant, paper tissues, and gloves if using the rectal site or other route if there is a potential for contact with body secretions. (Use of gloves is determined on an individual basis. The virus that causes acquired immunodeficiency syndrome [AIDS] has not been shown to be transmitted through contact with oral secretions unless they contain blood; thorough hand hygiene or hand antisepsis is always appropriate before and after any client contact, and following the removal of gloves.)	Promotes efficiency, accuracy, and safety
IMPLEMENTATION	
Introduce yourself to the client if you have not done so during earlier contact.	Demonstrates responsibility and accountability
Explain the procedure to the client.	Reduces apprehension and promotes cooperation
Wash hands or perform hand antisepsis with an alcohol rub (see Chapter 10).	Reduces the spread of microorganisms
ELECTRONIC THERMOMETER	
Remove the electronic unit from the charging base.	Promotes portability
Select the oral or rectal probe depending on the intended site for assessment.	Ensures appropriate use
Insert the probe into a disposable cover until it locks into place (Fig. A).	Protects the probe from contamination with secretions containing microorganisms

Inserting the probe into a disposable cover. (Photo by Rick Brady.)

SKILL 12-1 Assessing Body Temperature (*continued*)

Suggested Action	Reason for Action
ORAL METHOD	
Place the covered probe beneath the tongue to the right or left of the frenulum (the structure that attaches the underneath surface of the tongue to the fleshy portion of the mouth) (Fig. B).	Locates the probe near the sublingual artery to ensure the correct location

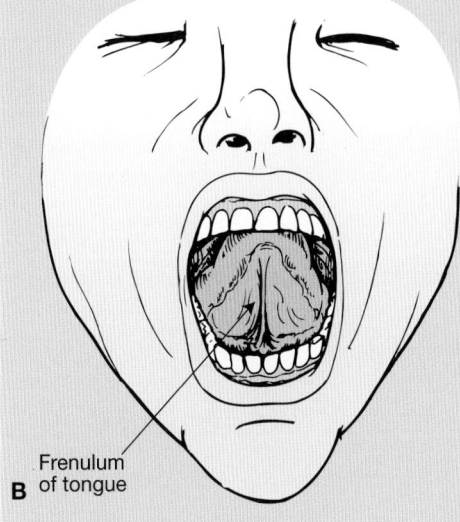

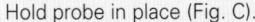
Frenulum of tongue
B

Location for oral temperature assessment.

| Hold probe in place (Fig. C). | Supports the probe so that it does not drift away from its intended location; ensures valid data collection |

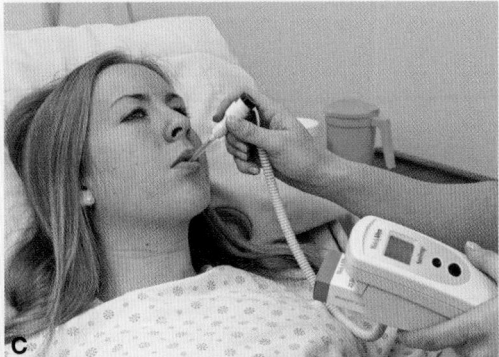
C

Maintaining the probe in position. (Photo by Rick Brady.)

Maintain the probe in position until an audible sound occurs.	Signals when the sensed temperature remains constant
Observe the numbers displayed on the electronic unit.	Indicates temperature measurement
Remove the probe and eject the probe cover into a lined receptacle (Fig. D).	Confines contaminated objects to an area for proper disposal without direct contact

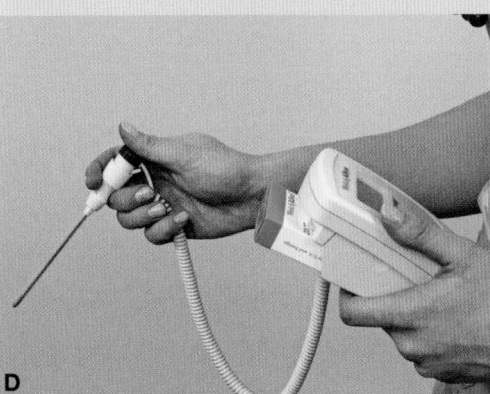
D

Releasing the probe cover. (Photo by Rick Brady.)

| Replace the probe in the storage holder within the electronic unit. | Prevents damage to the probe attachment |

(*continued*)

SKILL 12-1 Assessing Body Temperature (*continued*)

Suggested Action	Reason for Action
RECTAL METHOD	
Provide privacy.	Demonstrates respect for the client's dignity
Lubricate approximately 1 in (2.5 cm) of the rectal probe cover.	Promotes comfort and ease of insertion
Position the client on the side with the upper leg slightly flexed at the hip and knee (Sims position).	Helps to locate the anus and facilitate probe insertion
Instruct the client to breathe deeply.	Relaxes the rectal sphincter and reduces discomfort during insertion
Insert the thermometer approximately 1.5 in (3.8 cm) in an adult, 1 in (2.5 cm) in a child, and 0.5 in (1.25 cm) in an infant (Fig. E). **E**	Rectal thermometer insertion.
Maintain the probe in position until an audible sound occurs.	Signals when the sensed temperature remains constant
Observe the numbers displayed on the electronic unit.	Indicates temperature measurement
Remove the probe and eject the probe cover into a lined receptacle (see Fig. D).	Confines contaminated objects to an area for proper disposal without direct contact
Replace the probe in the storage holder within the electronic unit.	Prevents damage to the probe attachment
Wipe lubricant and any stool from around the client's rectum.	Demonstrates concern for the client's hygiene and comfort
Remove and discard gloves, if worn; wash hands or perform hand antisepsis with an alcohol rub (see Chapter 10).	Reduces the transmission of microorganisms
AXILLARY METHOD	
Insert the thermometer into the center of the axilla and lower the client's arm to enclose the thermometer between the two folds of skin (Fig. F). **F**	Confines the tip of the thermometer so that room air does not affect it
	Placement for an auxiliary temperature assessment.
Hold the probe in place.	Supports the probe so it does not drift away from its intended location; ensures valid data collection
Maintain the probe in position until an audible sound occurs.	Signals when the sensed temperature remains constant

SKILL 12-1 Assessing Body Temperature (*continued*)

Suggested Action	Reason for Action
Remove the probe and eject the probe cover into a lined receptacle (see Fig. D).	Confines contaminated objects to an area for proper disposal without direct contact
Replace the probe in the storage holder within the electronic unit.	Prevents damage to the probe attachment
Return the electronic unit to its charging base.	Facilitates reuse
Record the assessment measurement on the graphic sheet or flow sheet, or in the narrative nursing notes.	Provides documentation for future comparisons
Verbally report elevated or subnormal temperatures.	Alerts others to monitor the client closely and make changes in the care plan

INFRARED TYMPANIC THERMOMETER

Remove the thermometer component from its holding cradle (Fig. G).	Facilitates insertion of the tympanic **speculum** (funnel-shaped instrument used to widen and support an opening in the body)

A tympanic thermometer and cradle. (Photo by Rick Brady.)

Suggested Action	Reason for Action
Inspect the tip of the thermometer for damage and the lens for cleanliness.	Promotes safety and hygiene
Replace a cracked or broken tip; clean the lens with a dry wipe or lint-free swab moistened with a small amount of isopropyl alcohol, and then wipe to remove the alcohol film.	Ensures accurate data collection
Wait 30 minutes after cleaning with alcohol.	Allows the thermometer to readjust after the cooling effect created by alcohol evaporation
Cover the speculum with a disposable cover until it locks in place.	Maintains cleanliness of the tip
Press the mode button to select the choice of **temperature translation** (conversion of tympanic temperature into an oral, rectal, or core temperature).	Adjusts the tympanic measurement, norms for which have not been established, into more common frames of reference; the rectal equivalent is recommended for children younger than 3 years
Depress the mode button for several seconds to select either Fahrenheit or Centigrade.	Eliminates the need to calculate conversion measurements by hand
Hold the probe in your dominant hand.	Improves motor skill and coordination
Position the client with the head turned 90 degrees, exposing the ear with the hand holding the probe.	Promotes proper probe placement; if the right hand is holding the probe, the left ear is assessed
Wait for display of a "Ready" message.	Indicates offset has been programmed
Pull the external ear of adults up and back by grasping the external ear at its midpoint with your nondominant hand; for children aged 6 years and younger, pull the ear down and back.	Straightens the ear canal
Insert the probe into the ear, advancing it with a gentle back-and-forth motion until it seals the ear canal.	Seals the tip of the probe within the ear canal and confines the radiated heat within the area of the probe

(*continued*)

SKILL 12-1 Assessing Body Temperature (*continued*)

Suggested Action	Reason for Action
Point the tip of the probe in an imaginary line between the sideburn hair and the eyebrow on the opposite side of the face (Fig. H).	Positions the probe in direct alignment with the tympanic membrane; if pointed elsewhere, the infrared sensor detects the temperature of surrounding tissue rather than membrane temperature

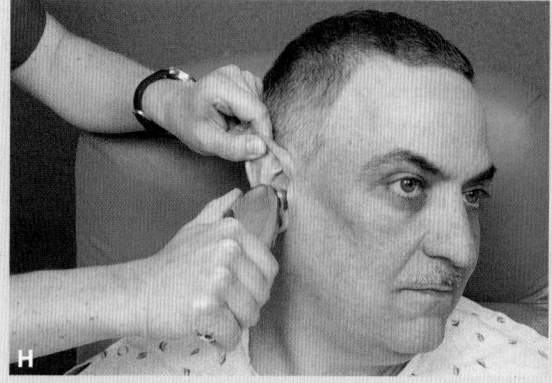

Placement of a probe for accurate tympanic assessment.

Suggested Action	Reason for Action
Press the button that activates the thermometer as soon as the probe is in position.	Initiates electronic sensing; for some models, this action must be done within 25 seconds of having removed the thermometer from its holding cradle
Keep the probe within the ear until the thermometer emits a sound or flashing light.	Indicates that the procedure is complete
Repeat the procedure after waiting 2 minutes if this is the first use of the tympanic thermometer since it was recharged.	Ensures accuracy with a second assessment
Read the temperature, remove the thermometer from the ear, and release the probe cover into a lined receptacle (Fig. I).	Controls the transmission of microorganisms

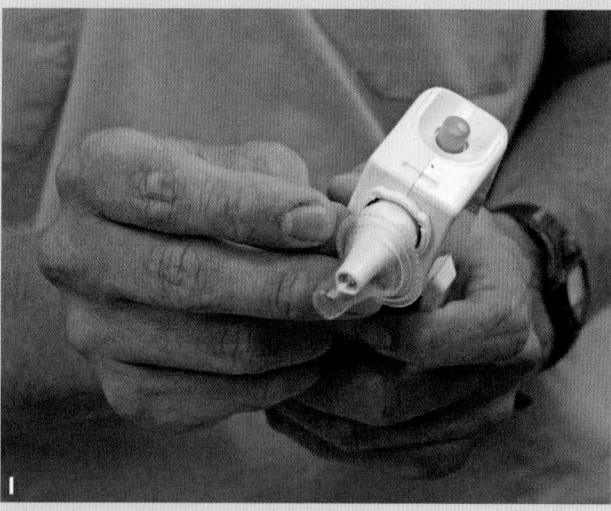

Disposing of the probe cover. (Photo by Rick Brady.)

Suggested Action	Reason for Action
Record the assessment measurement on the graphic sheet or flow sheet, or in the narrative nursing notes.	Provides documentation for future comparisons
Verbally report elevated or subnormal temperatures.	Alerts others to monitor the client closely and make changes in the plan for care

HOW TO TAKE A TEMPORAL TEMPERATURE

Suggested Action	Reason for Action
Remove the probe cover (some models have this) and place it on the device, if it requires one. Some devices do not have probe filters, but require a thorough cleaning after use.	Avoids cross-contamination
Turn on the thermometer.	Follow instructions for use.

SKILL 12-1 Assessing Body Temperature (*continued*)

Suggested Action	Reason for Action
Start on the center of the forehead, and sweep the thermometer across the forehead to the hairline (Fig. J).	Obtains most accurate results
J	Sweeping the thermometer across the forehead.
If the patient is sweaty, start on the center of the forehead and sweep the thermometer across the forehead to the hairline and then behind the base of the ear.	Keeps contact with the skin
Read temperature measurement.	Provides client data
Clean thermometer per facility's protocol.	Removes microbes, avoiding cross-contamination

EVALUATION

- Thermometer remained inserted the appropriate time.
- Level of temperature is consistent with accompanying signs and symptoms.
- Thermometer and surrounding tissue remain intact.

DOCUMENT

- Document
- Degree of heat to the nearest tenth
- Temperature scale
- Site of assessment
- Accompanying signs and symptoms
- To whom abnormal information was reported and the outcome of the interaction

SAMPLE DOCUMENTATION

Date and Time T 102.4°F (O). States, "I feel cold and my throat hurts." Pharynx looks beefy red. Reported to Dr. Washington. New orders for throat culture. _____ J. Doe, LPN

SKILL 12-2 Assessing the Radial Pulse

Suggested Action	Reason for Action
ASSESSMENT	
Determine when and how frequently to monitor the client's pulse (see Box 12-1).	Demonstrates accountability for making timely and appropriate assessments
Review data collected in previous assessments of the pulse or abnormalities in other vital signs.	Aids in identifying trends and analyzing significant patterns
Read the client's history for any reference to cardiac or vascular disorders.	Demonstrates an understanding of factors that may affect the pulse rate
Review the list of prescribed drugs for any that may have cardiac effects.	Helps in analyzing the results of assessment findings
PLANNING	
Arrange to take the client's pulse as near to the scheduled routine as possible.	Ensures consistency and accuracy
Make sure a watch or wall clock with a second hand is available.	Ensures accurate timing when counting pulsations

(*continued*)

SKILL 12-2 Assessing the Radial Pulse (*continued*)

Suggested Action	Reason for Action
Plan to assess the client's pulse after 5 minutes of inactivity.	Reflects the characteristics of the pulse at rest rather than data that may be influenced by activity
Plan to use the right or left radial pulse site unless it is inaccessible or difficult to palpate.	Provides consistency in evaluating data

IMPLEMENTATION ———————————————————————————————

Introduce yourself to the client if you have not done so earlier.	Demonstrates responsibility and accountability
Explain the procedure to the client.	Reduces apprehension and promotes cooperation
Raise the height of the bed.	Reduces musculoskeletal strain
Wash hands or perform hand antisepsis with an alcohol rub (see Chapter 10).	Reduces the spread of microorganisms
Help the client to a position of comfort	Avoids stress or pain from influencing the pulse rate
Rest or support the client's forearm with the wrist extended (Fig. A).	Provides access to the radial artery and relaxes the arm

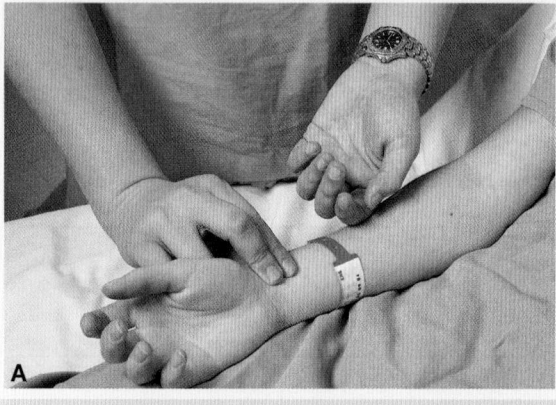

Locating the radial pulse.

Press the first and second fingertips toward the radius while feeling for a recurrent pulsation.	Ensures accuracy because the nurse may feel their own pulse if using the thumb; light palpation should not obliterate the pulse
Palpate the rhythm and volume of the pulse once it is located.	Provides comprehensive assessment data
Note the position of the second hand on the clock or watch.	Identifies the point at which the assessment begins
Count the number of pulsations for 15 or 30 seconds and multiply the number by 4 or 2, respectively. If the pulse is irregular, count for a full minute.	Provides pulse rate data; a regular pulse rate should not vary whether it is counted for a full minute or some portion thereof, while the rate of an irregular pulse may be significantly inaccurate if assessed for less than a full minute
Write down the pulse rate.	Ensures accurate documentation
Restore the client to a therapeutic position or one that provides comfort, and lower the bed.	Demonstrates responsibility for client care, safety, and comfort
Record the assessed measurement on the graphic sheet or the flow sheet, or in the narrative nursing notes.	Provides documentation for future comparisons
Verbally report rapid or slow pulse rates.	Alerts others to monitor the client closely and to make changes in the plan for care

EVALUATION ———————————————————————————————

- Pulse rate remained palpable throughout the assessment.
- Pulse rate is consistent with the client's condition.

DOCUMENT ———————————————————————————————

- Date and time
- Assessment site
- Rate of pulsations per minute, pulse volume, and rhythm
- Accompanying signs and symptoms, if appropriate
- To whom abnormal information was reported and the outcome of the interaction

SAMPLE DOCUMENTATION

Date and Time Radial pulse 88 bpm full and regular. _____ J. Doe, LPN

SKILL 12-3 Assessing the Respiratory Rate

Suggested Action	Reason for Action
ASSESSMENT	
Determine when and how frequently to monitor the client's respiratory rate (see Box 12-1).	Demonstrates accountability for making timely and appropriate assessments
Review data collected in previous assessments of the respiratory rate and other vital signs.	Aids in identifying trends and analyzing significant patterns
Read the client's history for any reference to respiratory, cardiac, or neurologic disorders.	Demonstrates an understanding of factors that may affect the respiratory rate
Review the list of prescribed drugs for any that may have respiratory or neurologic effects.	Helps in analyzing the results of assessment findings
PLANNING	
Arrange to count the client's respiratory rate as close to the scheduled routine as possible.	Ensures consistency and accuracy
Make sure a watch or wall clock with a second hand is available.	Ensures accurate timing
Plan to assess the client's respiratory rate after a 5-minute period of inactivity.	Reflects the characteristics of respirations at rest rather than under the influence of activity
IMPLEMENTATION	
Introduce yourself to the client if you have not done so previously.	Demonstrates responsibility and accountability
Explain the procedure to the client.	Reduces apprehension and promotes cooperation
Raise the height of the bed.	Reduces musculoskeletal strain
Wash hands or perform hand antisepsis with an alcohol rub (see Chapter 10).	Reduces the spread of microorganisms
Help the client to a sitting or lying position.	Facilitates the ability to observe breathing
Note the position of the second hand on the clock or watch.	Identifies the point at which assessment begins
Choose a time when the client is unaware of being watched; it may help to count the respiratory rate while appearing to count the pulse or while the client holds a thermometer in the mouth.	Discourages conscious control of breathing or talking during the assessment of the rate of breathing
Observe the rise and fall of the client's chest for a full minute if breathing is unusual. If breathing appears noiseless and effortless, count ventilations for a fractional portion of 1 minute and then multiply to calculate the rate.	Determines the respiratory rate per minute
Write down the respiratory rate.	Ensures accurate documentation
Restore the client to a therapeutic position or one that provides comfort, and lower the bed.	Demonstrates responsibility for client care, safety, and comfort
Record the assessed measurement on the graphic sheet or flow sheet, or in the narrative nursing notes.	Provides documentation for future comparisons
Verbally report rapid or slow respiratory rates or any other unusual characteristics.	Alerts others to monitor the client closely and make changes in the plan for care

EVALUATION

- Respiratory rate is counted for an appropriate time.
- Respiratory rate is consistent with the client's condition.

DOCUMENT

- Date and time
- Rate per minute
- Accompanying signs and symptoms, if appropriate
- To whom abnormal information was reported and the outcome of the interaction

SAMPLE DOCUMENTATION

Date and Time Respiratory rate of 20/minute at rest. Breathing is noiseless and effortless. _____ J. Doe, LPN

SKILL 12-4 Assessing Blood Pressure

Suggested Action	Reason for Action
ASSESSMENT	
Determine when and how frequently to monitor the client's blood pressure (see Box 12-1).	Demonstrates accountability for making timely and appropriate assessments
Review the data collected in previous assessments.	Aids in identifying trends and analyzing significant patterns
Determine in which arm and in what position previous assessments were made.	Ensures consistency when evaluating data
Read the client's history for any reference to cardiac or vascular disorders.	Demonstrates an understanding of factors that may affect the blood pressure
Review the list of prescribed drugs for any that may have cardiovascular effects.	Helps in analyzing the results of assessment findings
PLANNING	
Gather the necessary supplies: blood pressure cuff, sphygmomanometer, and stethoscope.	Promotes efficient time management; a recently calibrated aneroid or a validated electronic device can be used
Select an appropriately sized cuff for the client.	Ensures valid assessment findings
Arrange to take the client's blood pressure as near to the scheduled routine as possible.	Ensures consistency
Plan to assess the blood pressure after at least 5 minutes of inactivity unless it is an emergency.	Reflects the blood pressure under resting conditions
Wait 30 minutes after the client has ingested caffeine or used tobacco.	Avoids obtaining a higher than usual measurement from arterial constriction
Plan to use the right or left arm unless inaccessible.	Provides consistency in evaluating data
IMPLEMENTATION	
Introduce yourself to the client if you have not done so earlier.	Demonstrates responsibility and accountability
Explain the procedure to the client.	Reduces apprehension and promotes cooperation
Raise the height of the bed.	Reduces musculoskeletal strain
Wash hands or perform hand antisepsis with an alcohol rub (see Chapter 10).	Reduces the spread of microorganisms
Help the client to a sitting position or one of comfort.	Relaxes the client and reduces elevations caused by stress or discomfort
Support the client's forearm at the level of the heart with the palm of the hand upward.	Ensures collecting accurate data and facilitates locating the brachial artery
Expose the inner aspect of the elbow by removing clothing or loosely rolling up a sleeve.	Facilitates application of the blood pressure cuff and optimum sound perception
Center the cuff bladder so that the lower edge is about 1–2 in (2.5–5 cm) above the inner aspect of the elbow (Fig. A).	Places the cuff in the best position for occluding the blood flow through the brachial artery

Applying the pressure cuff. (Photo by B. Proud.)

Wrap the cuff snugly and uniformly about the circumference of the arm.	Ensures the application of even pressure during inflation

SKILL 12-4 Assessing Blood Pressure (*continued*)

Suggested Action	Reason for Action
Make sure the aneroid gauge can be clearly seen.	Prevents errors when observing the gauge
Palpate the brachial pulse (Fig. B).	Determines the most accurate location for assessing and hearing Korotkoff sounds

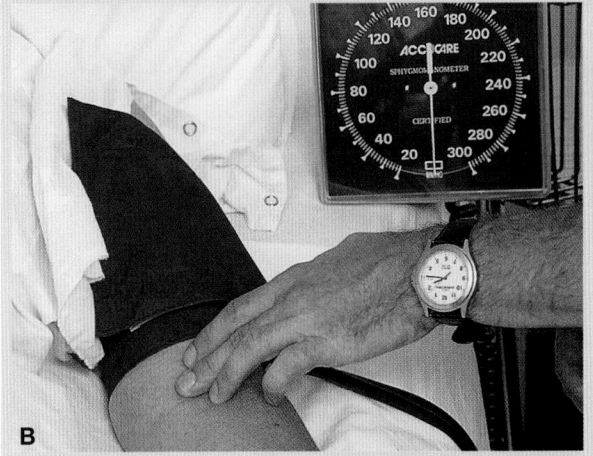

Palpating the brachial artery. (Photo by B. Proud.)

B

Suggested Action	Reason for Action
Tighten the screw valve on the bulb (Fig. C).	Prevents loss of pumped air

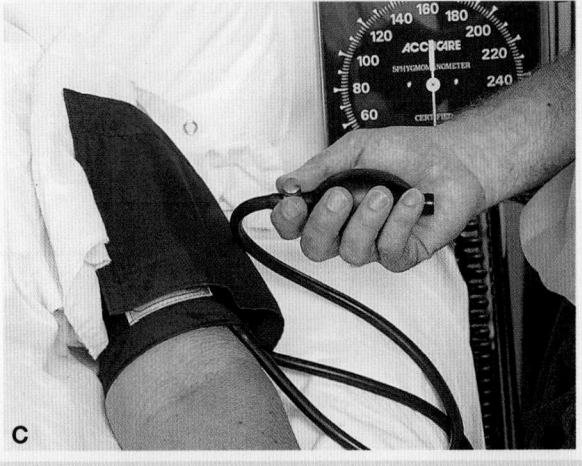

Tightening the screw valve. (Photo by B. Proud.)

C

Suggested Action	Reason for Action
Compress the bulb until the pulsation within the artery stops and note the measurement at that point.	Provides an estimation of systolic pressure
Deflate the cuff and wait 15–30 seconds.	Allows the return of normal blood flow
Place the eartips of the stethoscope within the ears and position the bell of the stethoscope lightly over the location of the brachial artery (Fig. D). The diaphragm may be used, but it is not preferred.	Ensures accurate assessment

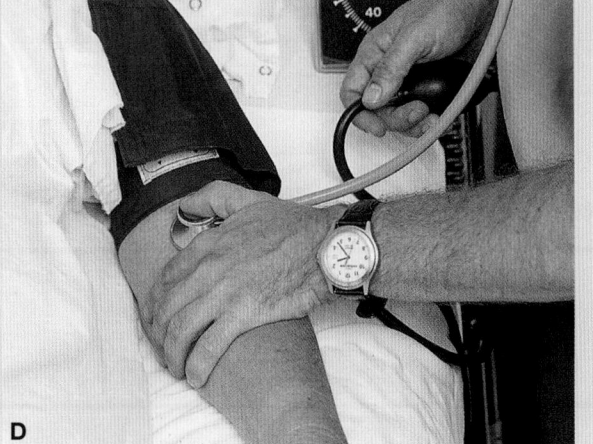

Placing the stethoscope. (Photo by B. Proud.)

D

(*continued*)

SKILL 12-4 Assessing Blood Pressure (*continued*)

Suggested Action	Reason for Action
Keep the tubing free from contact with clothing.	Reduces sound distortion
Pump the cuff bladder to a pressure that is 30 mm Hg above the point where the pulse previously disappeared (Fig. E).	Facilitates identifying phase I of Korotkoff sounds
E	Pumping the bulb. (Photo by B. Proud.)
Loosen the screw on the valve.	Releases air from the cuff bladder
Control the release of air at a rate of approximately 2–3 mm Hg/sec.	Ensures an accurate assessment between the perception of a sound and noting the numbers on the gauge
Listen for the onset and changes in Korotkoff sounds.	Aids in determining the systolic and diastolic pressures
Read the manometer gauge to the closest even number when phase I, IV, or V is noted.	Follows recommended standards for children or adults
Release the air quickly when there has been silence for at least 10 mm Hg.	Indicates phase V is complete
Write down the blood pressure measurements.	Ensures accurate documentation
Repeat the assessment after waiting at least 1 minute if unsure of the pressure measurements.	Allows time for the arterial pressure to return to baseline before another assessment
Restore the client to a therapeutic position or one that provides comfort, and lower the bed.	Demonstrates responsibility for client care, safety, and comfort
Wash hands or perform hand antisepsis with an alcohol rub (see Chapter 10).	Reduces the spread of microorganisms
Record the assessed measurement on the graphic sheet or flow sheet, or in the narrative nursing notes.	Provides documentation for future comparisons
Verbally report elevated or low blood pressure measurements.	Alerts others to monitor the client closely and make changes in the plan for care

EVALUATION

• Korotkoff sounds are heard clearly.
• Blood pressure is consistent with the client's condition.

DOCUMENT

• Date and time
• Systolic and diastolic pressure measurements
• Assessment site
• Position of the client
• Accompanying signs and symptoms, if appropriate
• To whom abnormal information was reported and the outcome of the interaction

SAMPLE DOCUMENTATION

Date and Time BP 136/72 in R arm while in sitting position. _____ J. Doe, LPN

SKILL 12-5 Obtaining a Thigh Blood Pressure

Suggested Action	Reason for Action
ASSESSMENT	
Determine when and how frequently to monitor the client's blood pressure (see Box 12-1).	Demonstrates accountability for making timely and appropriate assessments
Review the data collected in previous assessments.	Aids in identifying trends and analyzing significant patterns
Determine on which thigh previous assessments were made.	Ensures consistency when evaluating data
Read the client's history for any reference to cardiac or vascular disorders.	Demonstrates an understanding of factors that may affect blood pressure
Review the list of prescribed drugs for any that may have cardiovascular effects.	Helps in analyzing the results of assessment findings
PLANNING	
Gather the necessary supplies: thigh blood pressure cuff, sphygmomanometer, and stethoscope.	Promotes efficient time management and ensures an accurate measurement when a wider and longer blood pressure cuff is used
Plan to assess blood pressure after the client has been reclining for at least 10 minutes.	Promotes conditions for obtaining accurate measurements
Wait 30 minutes from the time the client has ingested caffeine, used tobacco, consumed a heavy meal, exercised vigorously, or taken a hot shower or bath.	Eliminates factors that contribute to the constriction or dilation of blood vessels
IMPLEMENTATION	
Introduce yourself to the client if you have not done so earlier.	Demonstrates responsibility and accountability
Explain the procedure to the client.	Reduces apprehension and promotes cooperation
Provide privacy.	Demonstrates respect for the client's dignity
Raise the height of the bed.	Reduces musculoskeletal strain
Wash hands or perform hand antisepsis with an alcohol rub (see Chapter 10).	Reduces the spread of microorganisms
Place the client in either the supine or the prone position, with the knee slightly flexed and the hip abducted (Fig. A).	Facilitates application of the blood pressure cuff

Application of blood pressure cuff to the thigh.

Suggested Action	Reason for Action
Make sure the manometer can be seen clearly.	Prevents observational errors
Palpate the popliteal pulse.	Determines the most accurate location for hearing Korotkoff sounds
Warn the client that they may experience discomfort when the cuff is inflated but that remaining still will facilitate accuracy.	Prepares the client for sensation and provides an explanation for its necessity
Tighten the screw valve on the bulb.	Prevents the loss of air from the cuff bladder
Compress the bulb until the pulsation within the artery stops and note the pressure measurement.	Provides an estimation of systolic pressure
Deflate the cuff and wait 15–30 seconds.	Allows the return of normal blood flow
Place the eartips of the stethoscope within the ears, and position the bell of the stethoscope lightly over the location of the popliteal artery. (Note: The diaphragm of the stethoscope may be used, but it is not preferred.)	Ensures an accurate assessment

(continued)

SKILL 12-5 Obtaining a Thigh Blood Pressure (*continued*)

Suggested Action	Reason for Action
Keep the tubing free from contact with clothing and bed linens.	Reduces sound distortion
Pump the cuff bladder to a pressure that is 30 mm Hg above the point where the pulse previously disappeared.	Facilitates identifying phase I of Korotkoff sounds
Loosen the screw on the valve.	Releases air from the cuff bladder
Control the release of air at a rate of approximately 2–3 mm Hg/sec.	Ensures accurate assessment between perception of the sound and noting the numbers on the gauge
Listen for the onset and changes in Korotkoff sounds.	Aids in determining systolic and diastolic pressure
Read the manometer when phases I, IV, and V are noted.	Follows recommended standards for adults or children
Release the air quickly when there has been silence for at least 10 mm Hg.	Indicates that phase V is complete
Write down the blood pressure measurements.	Ensures accurate documentation
Restore the client to a therapeutic position or one that provides comfort.	Demonstrates responsibility for client care, safety, and comfort
Wash hands or perform hand antisepsis with an alcohol rub (see Chapter 10).	Reduces the spread of microorganisms
Record assessed measurements on the graphic sheet or the flow sheet, or in the narrative nursing notes.	Provides documentation for future comparisons
Verbally report blood pressure measurements to the nurse in charge.	Alerts others to monitor the client closely or to modify the client's plan of care

EVALUATION

- Korotkoff sounds are heard clearly.
- Blood pressure is consistent with the client's condition.

DOCUMENT

- Date and time
- Systolic and diastolic pressure measurements
- Assessment site
- Accompanying signs and symptoms, if appropriate
- To whom abnormal information was reported, and the outcome of the interaction

SAMPLE DOCUMENTATION

Date and Time BP 176/88 at popliteal artery of left thigh. States, "It hurts when the blood pressure cuff gets tight."
_____ J. Doe, LPN

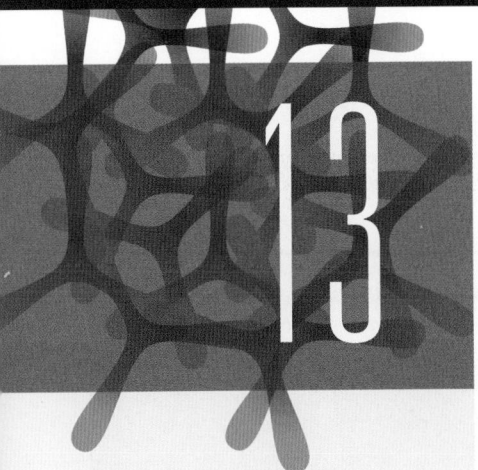

Physical Assessment

13

Learning Objectives

On completion of this chapter, the reader should be able to:

1. List the purposes of a physical assessment.
2. Name assessment techniques.
3. List items needed when performing a basic physical assessment.
4. Describe criteria for an appropriate assessment environment.
5. Identify assessments that can be obtained during the initial survey of clients.
6. State reasons for draping clients.
7. Differentiate a head-to-toe and a body systems approach to physical assessment.
8. List ways in which the body may be divided for organizing data collection.
9. Identify self-examinations nurses should teach their adult clients.

INTRODUCTION

The first step in the nursing process is assessment, or gathering of information. The **physical assessment** (a systematic examination of body structures) is one method for gathering health data. This chapter describes how to perform a physical assessment from a generalist's or beginning nurse's point of view and identifies common assessment findings. Students can learn advanced physical assessment skills through additional education and experience or by consulting specialty texts.

 Gerontologic Considerations

■ The nurse shows consideration for alterations in hearing, vision, or mobility before starting the examination. Before the physical assessment, the nurse may ask, "Is there anything you want me to know before we begin?" or "How can I make you as comfortable as possible during this examination?"

■ For example, if the person is hearing impaired, the limitations are identified, the nurse makes appropriate adjustments to the examination, such as speaking into the ear with the best hearing, reducing background noise as much as possible, and making sure the person can see the nurse's face.

■ Physical limitations from chronic diseases (e.g., difficulty breathing, limited movement, weakness) may require modifying assessment techniques during the examination.

OVERVIEW OF THE PHYSICAL ASSESSMENT

Health care providers use various techniques and equipment to perform a physical assessment. Although the settings for a physical assessment vary, each environment must facilitate accurate data collection and be conducive to the client's privacy and comfort.

Purposes

The overall goal of a physical assessment is to gather objective data about a client. To achieve this goal, nurses thoroughly examine clients on admission, briefly at the start of each shift, and any time a client's condition changes. The purposes of assessment are:

- To evaluate the client's current physical condition
- To detect early signs of developing health problems
- To establish a baseline for future comparisons
- To evaluate the client's responses to medical and nursing interventions

Cultural Competence

Cultural competence (see Chapter 6) is essential when performing physical assessments. "Cultural competence in healthcare refers to the ability of practitioners in the system to address the health issues of people from diverse backgrounds effectively by applying knowledge, empathy, and insight into the views on health that those backgrounds present" (Study.com, 2022). Consequently, educators and students in the health care field must use proper assessment tools in order to provide culturally competent care and better outcomes to diverse populations. Cultural competence assessment tools include understanding biases in health care and the need for medical information as well as instructions in a variety of languages.

Techniques

The four basic physical assessment techniques are inspection, percussion, palpation, and auscultation.

Inspection

Inspection (purposeful observation) is the most frequently used assessment technique. It involves examining particular body parts and looking for specific normal and abnormal characteristics (Fig. 13-1A). With advanced instruction, some nurses learn to use special instruments to inspect parts of the body, such as the interior of the eyes, that are potentially inaccessible to ordinary vision and inspection techniques.

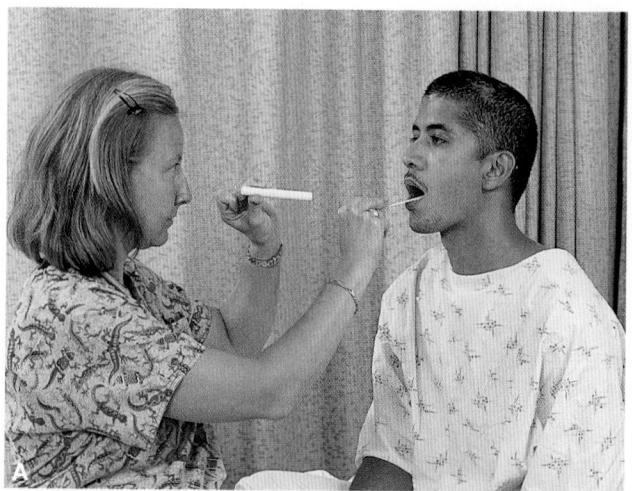
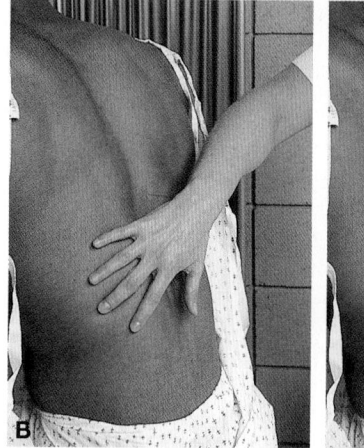
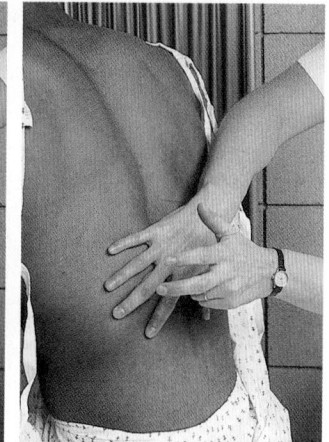

FIGURE 13-1 A. Inspection. (Photo by B. Proud.) **B.** Percussion. (Copyright Ken Kasper.)

Percussion

Percussion, the least used assessment technique by nurses, is striking or tapping a part of the client's body with the fingertips to produce vibratory sounds (see Fig. 13-1B, Table 13-1). The quality of the sounds aids in determining the location, size, and density of underlying structures. A sound different from that expected suggests a pathologic change in the area being examined. If percussion is performed correctly, the client experiences no discomfort. Pain could indicate a disease process or tissue injury.

Palpation

Palpation involves lightly touching or applying pressure to the body. *Light palpation* involves using the

TABLE 13-1 Percussion Sounds

SOUND	INTENSITY	DESCRIPTIVE TERM	COMMON LOCATIONS
Muted	Soft	Flat	Muscle, bone
Thud	Soft to moderate	Dull	Liver, full bladder, and tumorous mass
Empty	Moderate to loud	Resonant	Normal lung
Cavernous	Loud	Tympanic	Intestine filled with air
Booming	Very loud	Hyperresonant	Barrel-shaped chest overinflated with trapped air as a result of chronic lung disease

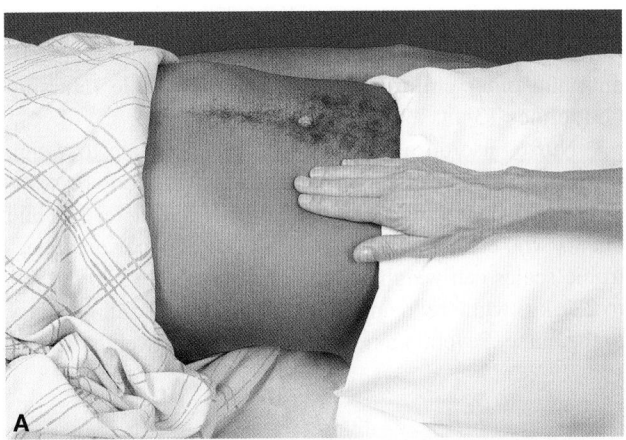

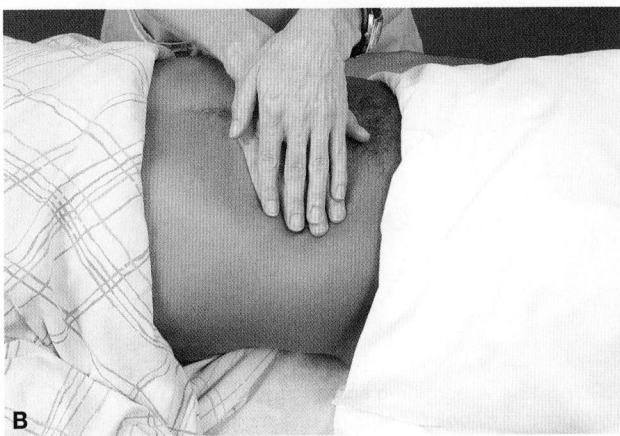

FIGURE 13-2 Palpation techniques. **A.** Light palpation. **B.** Deep palpation. (From Craven, R. F., Henshaw, C. M., & Hirnle, C. J. [2020]. *Fundamentals of nursing* [9th ed.]. Lippincott Williams & Wilkins.)

fingertips, the back of the hand, or the palm of the hand (Fig. 13-2A). It is best used when feeling the surface of the skin, structures that lie just beneath the skin, pulsations from peripheral arteries, and vibrations in the chest. *Deep palpation* is performed by depressing tissue approximately 1 in (2.5 cm) with the forefingers of one or both hands (Fig. 13-2B).

Palpation provides information about:

- The size, shape, consistency, and mobility of normal tissue and unusual masses
- The symmetry or asymmetry of bilateral (both sides of the body) structures, such as the lobes of the thyroid gland
- Skin temperature and moisture
- Any tenderness
- Unusual vibrations

Auscultation

Auscultation (listening to body sounds) is used frequently, most often to assess the heart, lungs, and abdomen. A stethoscope is required to hear most internal sounds (Fig. 13-3), but, in some cases, loud sounds, such as those associated with intestinal hyperactivity, are audible with gross hearing (i.e., listening without any instrumentation).

Nurses must practice auscultation repeatedly on various healthy and ill people to gain proficiency with the equipment

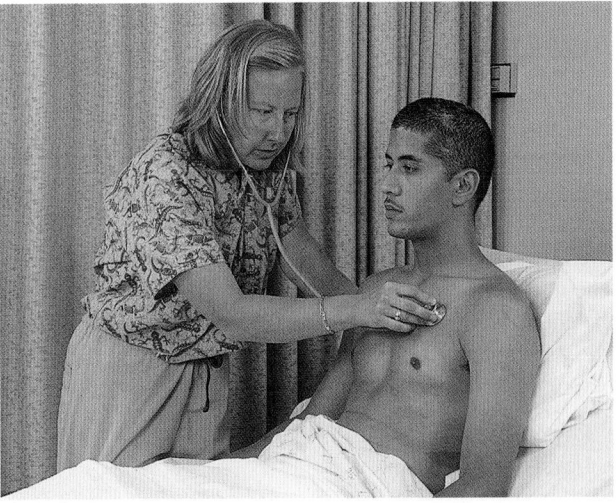

FIGURE 13-3 Auscultation. (Photo by B. Proud.)

and experience in interpreting data. To ensure the accuracy of findings, it is best to eliminate or reduce environmental noise as much as possible.

Equipment

The items generally needed for a basic physical assessment are listed in Box 13-1. More advanced practitioners may use additional examination equipment.

Environment

Nurses assess clients in a special examination room or at the bedside. Regardless of the assessment location, the area should have easy access to a restroom; a door or curtain that ensures privacy; adequate warmth for client comfort; a padded, adjustable table or bed; sufficient room for moving to either side of the client; adequate lighting; facilities for hand hygiene; a clean counter or surface for placing examination equipment; and a lined receptacle for soiled articles.

 Concept Mastery Alert

Client Comfort
Client comfort is essential when performing an assessment, especially when the assessment involves touching the client. To promote maximum client comfort, be sure your hands and any equipment are warmed prior to touching the client.

BOX 13-1	Physical Assessment Equipment

For a basic physical assessment, the nurse needs the following:
- Gloves
- Examination gown
- Cloth or paper drapes
- Scale
- Stethoscope
- Sphygmomanometer
- Thermometer
- Penlight or flashlight
- Tongue blade
- Assessment form and pen

PERFORMING A PHYSICAL ASSESSMENT

Basic activities involved in a physical assessment include gathering general data, draping and positioning the client, selecting a systematic approach for collecting data, and examining the client.

Gathering General Data

The nurse obtains general data during the first contact with the client. At this time, the nurse appraises the client's overall condition. By observing and interacting with the client before the actual physical examination, the nurse notes:

- Physical appearance with regard to clothing and hygiene
- Level of consciousness
- Body size
- Posture
- Gait and coordinated movement (or lack of it)
- Use of ambulatory aids
- Mood and emotional tone

The nurse also gathers some preliminary data, such as vital signs (see Chapter 12), weight, and height, at this time.

The nurse documents the client's weight and height because they provide more reliable data than a subjective assessment of body size or asking the client to provide the information. The recorded measurements are extremely important in assessing trends in future weight loss or gain. For hospitalized clients, health care providers also use weight and height to calculate the dosages of some drugs. In most cases, nurses weigh and measure adult clients and older children using a standing scale (Nursing Guidelines 13-1).

Nurses use an electronic bed or chair scale to weigh medically unstable clients, clients who have a body mass index (BMI) greater than 40 (see Fig. 15-6 in Chapter 15), and clients who cannot stand (Fig. 13-4). Battery-powered electronic scales can weigh people who are 400 to 500 lb (181 to 227 kg) while reducing the risk of a client's fall or injury to the nurse. Several models store the client's weight in their

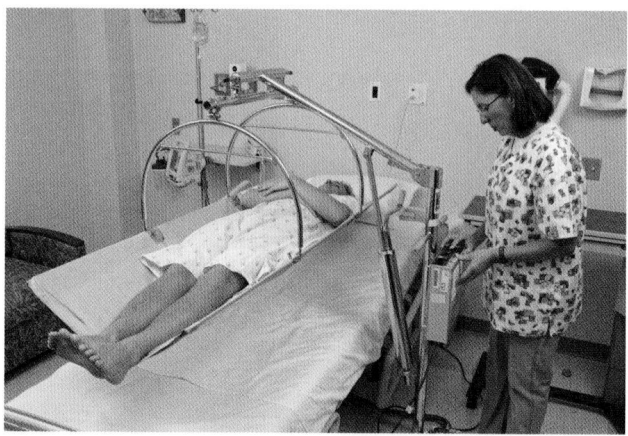

FIGURE 13-4 A bed-sling scale. (From Carter, P. [2019]. *Lippincott textbook for nursing assistants* [5th ed.]. Lippincott Williams & Wilkins.)

 NURSING GUIDELINES 13-1

Obtaining Weight and Height

- Check to see that the scale is calibrated at zero. *Doing so ensures accuracy.*
- Ask or assist the client in removing shoes and all but a minimum of clothing. *Doing so facilitates measuring body weight.*
- Place a paper towel on the scale before the client stands on it with bare feet. *This helps reduce contact with microorganisms on equipment that other people use.*
- Assist the client onto the scale. *Doing so helps prevent injury should the client become dizzy or unstable.*
- Position the heavier weight in a calibrated groove of the scale arm. *Doing so provides a rough approximation of the gross body weight.*
- Move the lighter weight across the calibrations for individual pounds and ounces until the bar balances in the center of the scale. *This positioning correlates with the actual weight.*
- Read the weight and write it down. *Doing so ensures accurate documentation.*
- Raise the measuring bar well above the client's head. *This provides room for positioning the client without injury* (see figure).
- Ask the client to stand straight and look forward. *Doing so facilitates measuring height.*
- Lower the measuring bar until it lightly touches the top of the client's head. *This positioning correlates with actual height.*
- Note the height and write it down. *This ensures accurate documentation.*

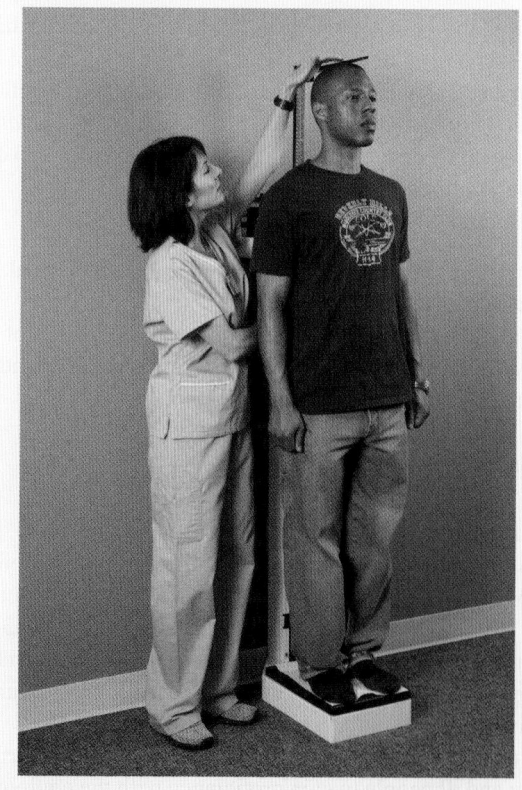

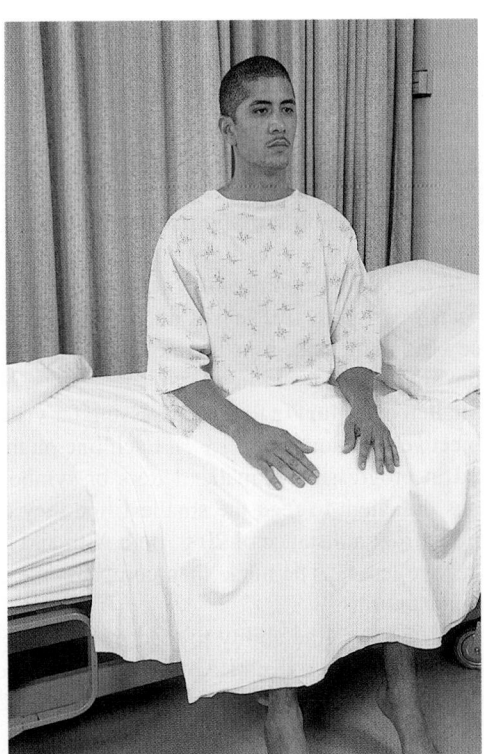

FIGURE 13-5 A client is prepared for examination. (Photo by B. Proud.)

memory, allowing it to be automatically recalled until another client is weighed. Electronic scales can be transported from storage to a client's room when needed.

Draping and Positioning

Because assessment takes place while clients are naked (or wearing only a loose examination gown), they generally appreciate being covered with a **drape** (a sheet of soft cloth or paper). A drape provides more modesty than warmth.

The examination usually begins with the client standing or sitting (Fig. 13-5). Some components of the physical assessment require the client to recline and turn from side to side. Specific positions for special examinations are described and illustrated in Chapters 14 and 23.

Selecting an Approach for Data Collection

Once the client is draped and positioned, selection of a systematic, organized pattern facilitates further data collection. Two common approaches are the head-to-toe approach and the body systems approach. The objective of both methods is to obtain the same basic data. Consequently, each nurse develops their own order and sequence for examining clients or uses an assessment form as a guide. Nurses should conduct the assessment consistently each time to avoid omitting essential information.

Head-to-Toe Approach

A **head-to-toe approach** means assessing the client from the top of the head down to the feet. This has three advantages:

1. It prevents overlooking some aspects of data collection.
2. It reduces the number of position changes required of the client.

3. It generally takes less time because the nurse is not constantly moving around the client in what may appear to be a haphazard manner.

Body Systems Approach

A **body systems approach** means assessing the client according to the functional systems of the body. It involves examining the structures in each system separately. For example, the nurse assesses the skin, mucous membranes, nails, and hair because they are all parts of the integumentary system. When assessing the cardiovascular system, the nurse palpates peripheral pulses, listens to heart sounds, and so on. One advantage of this method is that findings tend to be clustered, making problems more easily identifiable. Disadvantages are that the nurse examines the same areas of the body several times before completing the assessment; also, frequent position changes during the examination may tire the client.

Examining the Client

The procedure for performing a physical assessment is described in Skill 13-1. Specific assessment techniques, their purposes, and the data they provide are described later in the chapter.

 Nutrition Notes

■ Dietitians use data obtained through the nurse's physical examination to help diagnose malnutrition.

■ Physiologic changes can adversely affect the nutritional status of adults, such as sensory functions including taste, smell, and vision as well as diminishing muscle mass and strength decline, along with the immune system gradually deteriorating (Norman, K., Haß, U., & Pirlich M., 2021).

>>> *Stop, Think, and Respond 13-1*

You have been asked to assess two new clients. One arrived by wheelchair and has been walking around the nursing unit. The other was transported by ambulance, has intravenous fluid infusing, and is receiving oxygen. Which client would you assess first? Why? What differences might you use in the physical assessment of each client?

DATA COLLECTION

When collecting data, the nurse may divide the body into six general areas: the head and neck, the chest, the extremities, the abdomen, the genitalia, and the anus and rectum. The following discussion identifies structures commonly assessed, specific techniques used, and common findings.

Head and Neck

Head

The nurse begins at the client's head by assessing their mental status and the symmetry and function of craniofacial structures (eyes, ears, nose, and mouth). The nurse also assesses the client's skin, oral and nasal mucous membranes, hair, and scalp.

Mental Status Assessment

A **mental status assessment** (a technique for determining the level of a client's cognitive functioning) provides information about a client's attention, concentration, memory, and ability to think abstractly. For most clients, documenting that they are alert and oriented to person, place, time, and circumstances is all that is necessary. More objective assessment data are important, however, when caring for the following clients:

• Clients who were previously unconscious
• Clients who were recently resuscitated
• Clients with periods of confusion
• Clients with head injuries
• Clients who overdosed on drugs
• Clients with histories of chronic alcohol use disorder
• Clients with psychiatric diagnoses

Eyes

When examining the head, one of the most obvious assessments is the appearance of the eyes, which are generally of similar size and distance from the center of the face. Each iris is the same color. The sclerae (plural of sclera) appear white, or in clients with dark skin, the sclerae may normally appear yellow as a result of the presence of melanin, a brown pigment, or carotene, a yellow-orange pigment deposited in subconjunctival fat. The corneas are clear, and eyelashes are present along the margins of each eye. More advanced practitioners use an instrument called an **ophthalmoscope** (Fig. 13-6) to examine structures within the eye. After gross inspection, the nurse assesses functions such as visual acuity, pupil size and response, and ocular movements.

Visual acuity (the ability to see both far and near) is not assessed in every client. It is always appropriate, however, to ask if a client wears glasses or contact lenses, has a prosthetic eye, or considers themself blind.

To assess far vision grossly, the nurse asks the client to cover one eye at a time and, from a distance of approximately 20 ft, count the number of fingers the nurse raises. Clients can wear corrective lenses during this assessment. For close vision, the nurse asks literate clients to read newsprint from approximately 14 in away.

A **Snellen eye chart** (a tool for assessing far vision) is a more objective technique (Fig. 13-7). Each line on the chart is printed in progressively smaller letters or symbols. The nurse asks the client to read the smallest line they can see comfortably from a distance of 20 ft, both with and without any corrective lenses. The nurse then compares the client's vision against norms.

Normal vision is the ability to read printed letters that most people can see at a distance of 20 ft without prescription lenses. This number is written as a fraction (e.g., 20/20). If, at 20 ft from the chart, a person sees only the first line—one that people with normal vision can see from 200 ft away—the client's visual acuity is recorded as 20/200. The nurse tests near vision using a **Jaeger chart**, a visual assessment tool with small print or newsprint with varying sizes of letters (Fig. 13-8).

The size of each pupil is estimated in millimeters under normal light conditions (Fig. 13-9). Normal pupils are round and equal in size. There is also a **consensual response** (a brisk, equal, and simultaneous constriction of both pupils when one eye and then the other is stimulated with light). In addition, the nurse assesses the pupils for **accommodation** (the ability to constrict when looking at a near object and dilate when looking at an object in the distance). The nurse documents normal findings using the abbreviation **PERRLA**: *p*upils *e*qually *r*ound and *r*eactive to *l*ight and *a*ccommodation (Nursing Guidelines 13-2).

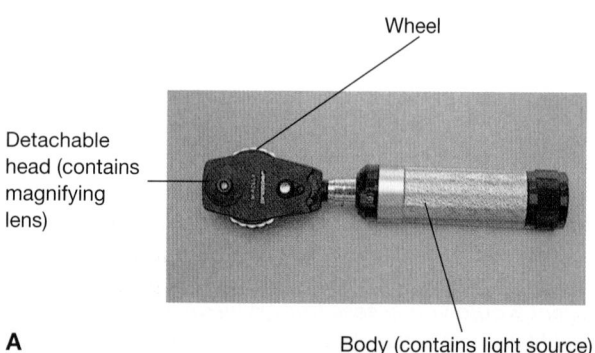

Wheel

Detachable head (contains magnifying lens)

Body (contains light source)

A

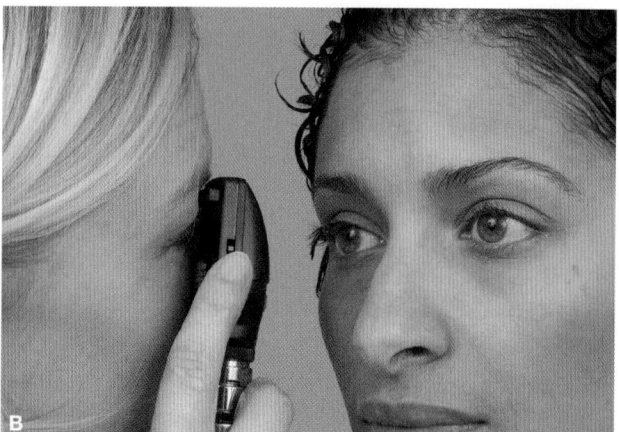

FIGURE 13-6 **A.** Components of an ophthalmoscope. **B.** Performing an ophthalmoscopic examination. (From Craven, R. F., Henshaw, C. M., & Hirnle, C. J. [2020]. *Fundamentals of nursing* [9th ed.]. Lippincott Williams & Wilkins.)

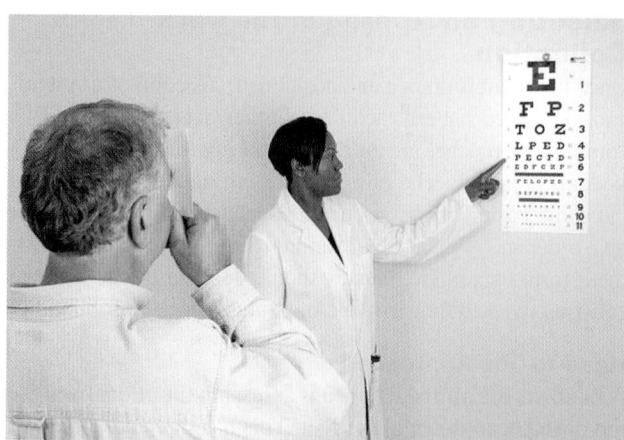

FIGURE 13-7 Distant visual acuity is tested with a Snellen chart. (From Weber, J. R., & Kelley, J. H. [2022]. *Health assessment in nursing* [7th ed.]. Lippincott Williams & Wilkins.)

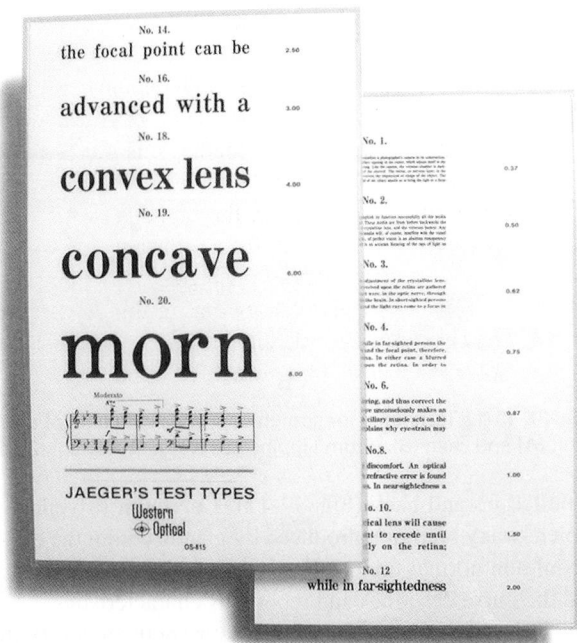

FIGURE 13-8 A Jaeger reading test card used for assessing near visual acuity. (Western Ophthalmics, Lynnwood, WA. http://www.west-op.com)

The nurse observes **extraocular movements**, which are eye movements controlled by several pairs of eye muscles. To do this, the nurse asks the client to focus on and track the nurse's finger or some other object as it moves in each of six positions (Fig. 13-10). During the assessment, both eyes should move in a coordinated manner. No movement in one eye may indicate cranial nerve damage; irregular or uncoordinated movement may suggest other neurologic pathology.

A **visual field examination** is the assessment of peripheral vision and continuity in the visual field. The nurse may perform a gross assessment (Fig. 13-11) or test using more sophisticated ophthalmic equipment. For gross assessment, the nurse stands directly in front of the client, and each person covers their eye. The nurse instructs the client to look straight ahead and indicate when they sees a light or the nurse's finger as the nurse brings it from several sectors of the periphery toward the center. If the client's and the nurse's visual fields are normal, they see the object at the same time. Certain eye and neurologic disorders are associated with changes in the visual field.

Ears

The nurse inspects and palpates the external ears. More advanced practitioners use an **otoscope**, an instrument used to examine the tympanic membrane, or eardrum.

Grading pupil size

 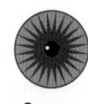 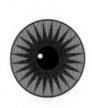 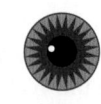 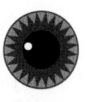 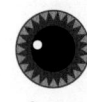 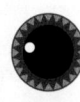 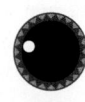 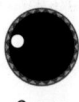

| 1 mm | 2 mm | 3 mm | 4 mm | 5 mm | 6 mm | 7 mm | 8 mm | 9 mm |

FIGURE 13-9 Pupil size assessment guide. (From *Lippincott's nursing procedures and skills* [9th ed.]. [2022]. Lippincott Williams & Wilkins.)

NURSING GUIDELINES 13-2

Assessing Pupillary Response

• Dim the lights in the examination area and instruct the client to stare straight ahead. *Doing so facilitates pupil dilation* (Fig. A).

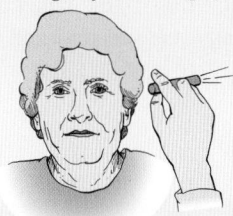

A

• Bring a narrow beam of light, like that from a penlight or small flashlight, from the temple toward the eye. *This step provides a direct stimulus for pupil constriction* (Fig. B).

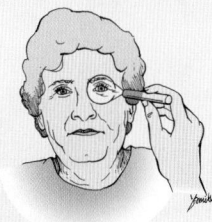

B

• Observe the pupil of the stimulated eye as well as the unstimulated pupil. The response should be the same. *This assessment indicates the status of brain function.*

• Repeat the assessment by directly stimulating the opposite eye. *Doing so provides comparative data.*

• Ask the client to look at a finger or object approximately 4 in (10 cm) from their face. *This measure produces a situation in which the pupils should get smaller* (Fig. C).

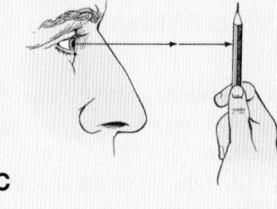

C

• Tell the client to look from the near object to another that is more distant. *This measure produces a situation in which the pupils should get larger* (Fig. D).

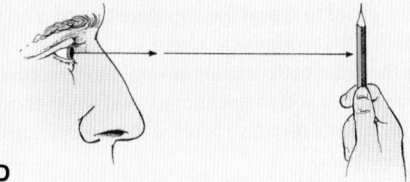

D

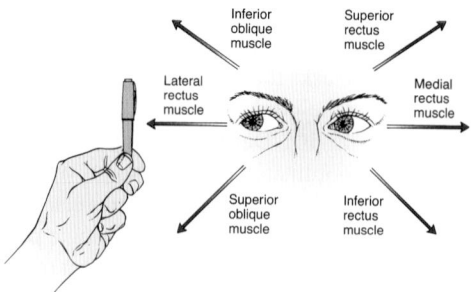

FIGURE 13-10 Assessing extraocular movements.

The nurse performs a gross examination of the ear by observing the appearance of the ears. Both should be similar in size, shape, and location. The nurse moves the skin behind and in front of the ears as well as the underlying cartilage to determine whether there is any tenderness. The nurse shines a penlight or other light source within each ear to illuminate the ear canal. For optimal visualization, the nurse straightens the curved ear canal as much as possible. For children, this is done by pulling the ear down and back; for an adult, the ear

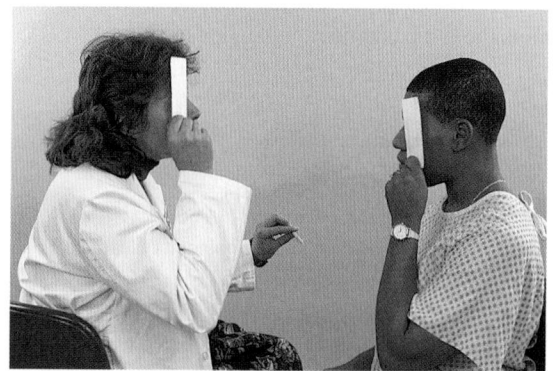

FIGURE 13-11 A gross examination of the visual field. (From Weber, J. R., & Kelley, J. H. [2022]. *Health assessment in nursing* [7th ed.]. Lippincott Williams & Wilkins.)

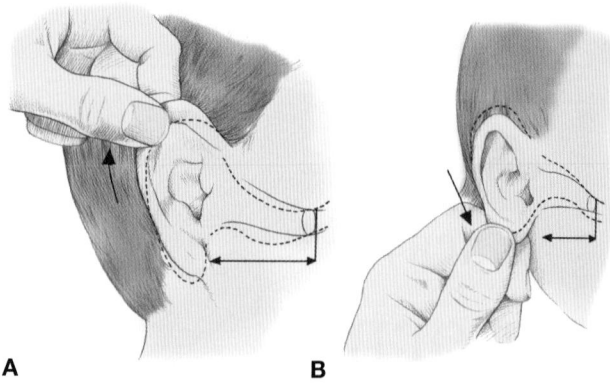

A　　　　　　　　　　**B**

FIGURE 13-12 Technique for straightening the ear canal of an adult **(A)** and child **(B)**. (From Lippincott's Nursing Advisor, 2022.)

is pulled up and back (Fig. 13-12). **Cerumen** (a yellowish brown, waxy secretion produced by glands within the ear) is a common normal finding. Any other drainage is abnormal, and the nurse describes and reports its characteristics.

The nurse may discover changes in **hearing acuity** (the ability to hear and discriminate sound) by performing a voice/whisper test or the Weber or Rinne test (Nursing Guidelines 13-3). If the client relies on a hearing aid to amplify sound, the nurse notes that information on the assessment form.

The Weber and Rinne tests help determine hearing impairment resulting from sensory nerve damage or disorders that interfere with sound conduction through the ear. To perform the **Weber test** (an assessment technique for determining equality or disparity of bone-conducted sound), the nurse strikes a tuning fork on their palm and places the vibrating stem in the center of the client's head (Fig. 13-13). The nurse then asks the client if the sound is audible equally in both ears. A positive response indicates either a normal finding or that hearing in both ears is equally diminished. Hearing the sound louder in one ear is a sign of unequal bone-conducted hearing (hearing loss greater in one ear).

 NURSING GUIDELINES 13-3

Performing a Voice/Whisper Test for Hearing Acuity

- Stand approximately 2 ft behind and to the side of the client. *This placement simulates the distance between most people during social interaction and prevents the client from observing visual cues.*
- Instruct the client to cover the ear on the opposite side (see figure). *This step facilitates sound conduction to the tested ear only.*
- Whisper a color, number, or name toward the uncovered ear. *Doing so delivers a high-pitched sound, the most common type of hearing loss, toward the tested ear.*
- Instruct the client to repeat the whispered word. *This reveals the client's ability to discriminate sound.*
- Continue the same pattern using several more words; increase the volume from a soft to medium to loud whisper or spoken voice if the client's response is inaccurate. *Variations provide more reliable data.*
- Repeat the test on the opposite ear. *Doing so provides separate assessment findings for each ear.*

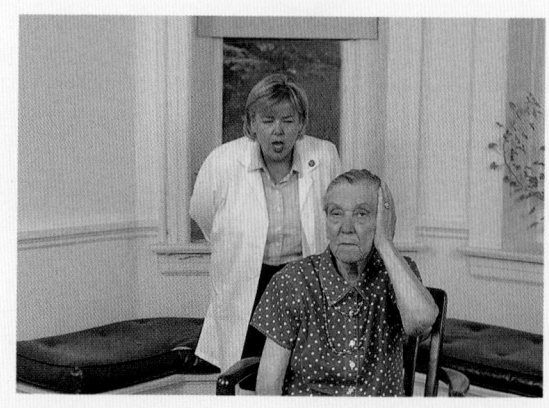

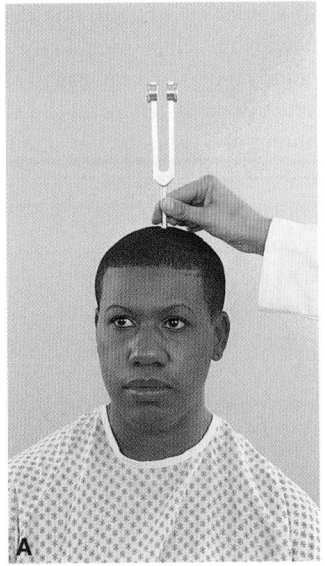

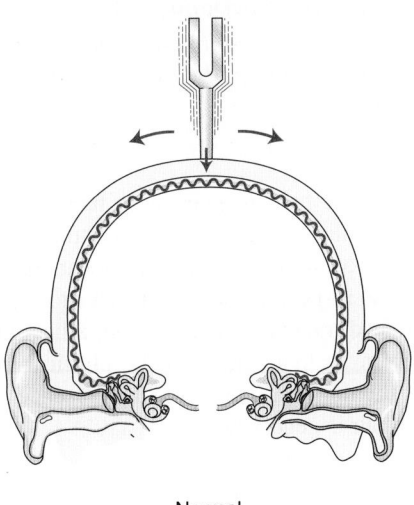

Normal

B

FIGURE 13-13 For the Weber test, place the tuning fork centered on the client's head **(A)**. The sound should be equally audible in both ears **(B)**. (From Jones, R. [2015]. *Patient assessment in pharmacy practice* [3rd ed.]. Lippincott Williams & Wilkins.)

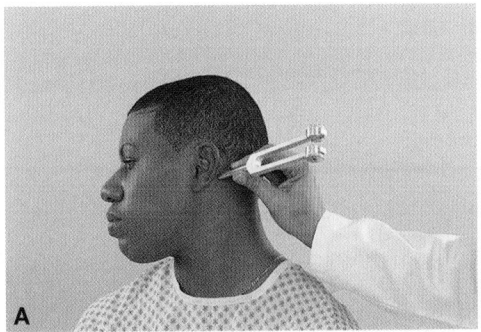

A

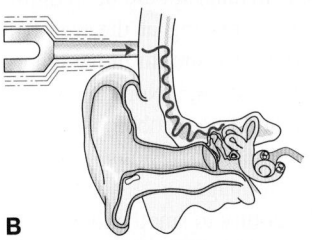

B

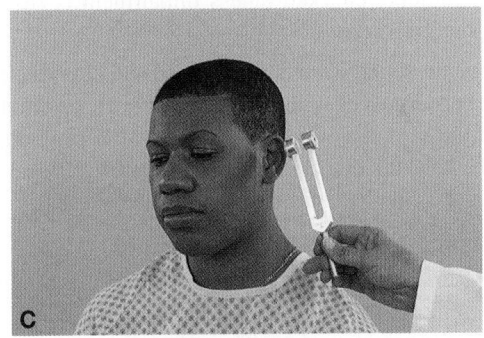

C

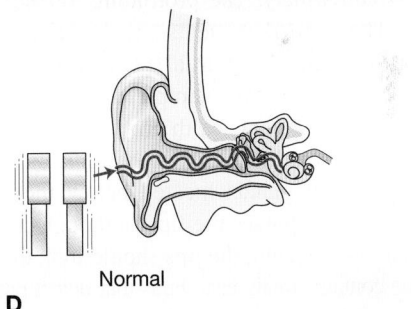

Normal

D

FIGURE 13-14 For the Rinne test, the tuning fork base is placed first on the mastoid process **(A, B)** to test bone conduction of sound after which the prongs are moved to the front of the external auditory canal **(C, D)** to test air conduction of sound. **(A** and **C**, Photos by B. Proud; **B** and **D**, From Jones, R. [2015]. *Patient assessment in pharmacy practice* [3rd ed.]. Lippincott Williams & Wilkins.)

A tuning fork is also necessary in the **Rinne test** (an assessment technique for comparing air vs. bone conduction of sound). First, the nurse strikes the tuning fork and then places the stem on the client's mastoid area behind the ear (Fig. 13-14) to assess bone conduction of sound waves in the tested ear. The client reports when the sound stops. Next, the nurse moves the tines of the still-vibrating tuning fork near the ear canal and asks the client if they perceive sound. This assesses air conduction of sound through the ear canal to the middle and inner ear. Both ears are assessed separately. Normally, sound is heard longer by air conduction. If the client does not continue to hear sound when the tuning fork is beside the ear, it indicates a problem with the ear structures that collect air and transmit sound to the auditory nerve in the inner ear.

Audiometry measures hearing acuity at various sound frequencies. An *audiologist* is a professional trained to test hearing with standardized instruments. Audiometric hearing tests measure exact pitch and volume deficits. They measure hearing in decibels (intensity of sound); the greater the intensity required for the client to perceive the sound, the more impaired the hearing (Table 13-2).

Nose

The nurse inspects the nose and nasal passages by having the client assume a "sniffing" position. The septum (the

TABLE 13-2 Hearing Acuity Levels

HEARING LEVEL	DECIBEL RANGE (DB)
Normal	0–25
Mildly impaired	26–30
Moderately impaired	31–55
Moderately to severely impaired	56–70
Severely impaired	71–90
Profoundly impaired	≥91

tissue that divides the nose in half) should be in midline with equal-sized nasal passages. Pressing at the tip of the nose facilitates deeper inspection. Air should move fairly quietly through the nose during breathing. Normal nasal mucous membrane is pink, moist, and free of obvious drainage. The nurse documents a deviated septum, lesions, growths, flaring of the nostrils, or unusual drainage.

Smelling acuity (the ability to smell and identify odors) is not commonly checked unless impairment is suspected. To test smelling acuity:

1. Have the client occlude one nostril and close their eyes.
2. Place substances with strong odors, such as lemon, vanilla extract, coffee, peppermint, or alcohol, one at a time beneath the patient's (open) nostril.
3. Ask the client to sniff and identify the substance.

Mouth and Oral Mucous Membranes

The lips surround the mouth, which contains the tongue and teeth. The nurse inspects these structures by having the client open the mouth widely. The protruding tongue is normally midline. The nurse documents any dentures, missing or malpositioned teeth, or a partial plate. Some unusual breath odors are diagnostic. For example, the odor of alcohol or acetone suggests additional health problems.

Normal oral mucous membranes are pink, intact, and kept moist by salivary glands located below the tongue. When the client smiles, purses the lips as though preparing to whistle, or shows the teeth, the lips should look the same.

The tongue contains many taste buds that detect particular taste characteristics. Although assessing taste is rarely done, it is facilitated by placing substances on the tongue and asking the client to identify them with the eyes closed. To ensure valid results, the nurse instructs the client to sip water between assessments.

Facial Skin

The nurse notes characteristics of the facial skin while assessing the head. Although skin assessment begins here, it continues as the nurse examines other body areas. Regardless

of location, skin should be smooth, unbroken, of uniform color consistent with the client's ethnicity or race, warm, and elastic. It should not be wet or unusually dry. Diagnostic variations in skin color are listed in Table 13-3.

While examining the skin, the nurse may detect one or more alterations in its integrity:

- A *wound* is a break in the skin.
- An *ulcer* is an open, crater-like area.
- An *abrasion* is an area that has been rubbed away by friction.
- A *laceration* is a torn, jagged wound.
- A *fissure* is a crack in the skin, especially in or near mucous membranes.
- A *scar* is a mark left by the healing of a wound or lesion.

Other common skin lesions and their characteristics are described in Table 13-4. Additional skin assessments are described later as related to other body areas.

››› Stop, Think, and Respond 13-2

A nurse has documented that a client has maculopapular skin lesions over their body. Describe how these would appear.

Hair

Assessment of the hair includes scalp hair, eyebrows, and eyelashes. The nurse notes the color, texture, and distribution (presence or absence in unusual locations for sex or age). They also inspect the hair for debris such as blood in a client with head trauma, nits (eggs from a lice infestation), or scales from scalp lesions. As the physical assessment progresses, the nurse also observes the presence or absence where body hair is generally located.

Scalp

The nurse assesses the scalp by randomly separating the hair and inspecting the skin surface. They look for signs that the scalp is smooth, intact, and free of lesions. The nurse also palpates the skull for any unusual contour.

Neck

The neck supports the head midline. The client should be able to bend the head forward, backward, and to either side, as well as to rotate it 180 degrees. The trachea (windpipe) should be in the center of the neck. Pulsations in the carotid arteries (see Chapter 12) are visible and easy to palpate. There should be no unusual bulges or fullness in the neck. Some nurses lightly palpate the lymph nodes in the neck area or assess anteriorly for an enlarged thyroid gland.

TABLE 13-3 Common Skin Color Variations

COLOR	TERM	POSSIBLE CAUSES
Pale, regardless of race	Pallor	Anemia, blood loss
Red	Erythema	Superficial burns, local inflammation, carbon monoxide poisoning
Pink	Flushed	Fever, hypertension
Purple	Ecchymosis	Trauma to soft tissue
Blue	Cyanosis	Low tissue oxygenation
Yellow	Jaundice	Liver or kidney disease, destruction of red blood cells
Brown	Tan	Ethnic variation, sun exposure, pregnancy, Addison disease

TABLE 13-4 Common Skin Lesions

TYPE OF LESION	DESCRIPTION	EXAMPLE	ILLUSTRATION
Macule	Flat, round, colored, nonpalpable area	Freckles	
Papule	Elevated, palpable, solid	Wart	
Vesicle	Elevated, round, filled with serum	Blister	
Wheal	Elevated, irregular border, no free fluid	Hives	
Pustule	Elevated, raised border, filled with pus	Boil	
Nodule	Elevated, solid mass, deeper and firmer than papule	Enlarged lymph node	
Cyst	Encapsulated, round, fluid-filled or solid mass beneath the skin	Tissue growth	

Chest and Spine

The chest is a cavity surrounded by the ribs and vertebrae and houses the heart and lungs. The nurse observes the chest's shape and movement with breathing, notes the curved appearance of the spine, and assesses skin turgor, breasts, heart sounds, and lung sounds.

Turgor (the resiliency of the skin; fullness or lack thereof) is a combination of the elastic quality of the skin and the pressure exerted on it by the fluid within it. To assess skin turgor, the nurse gently pinches the client's skin over the sternum or below the clavicle (Fig. 13-15) in an attempt to lift it from the underlying tissue. The area over the chest is a good assessment location because the skin in other areas tends to loosen with age. When the nurse releases the tissue, it should return quickly to its original position. Prolonged

"tenting" indicates dehydration. When documenting skin turgor, it could be described as elastic if it resumes its previous position when the fold of skin is released or nonelastic if the fold of skin remains longer than 3 seconds.

Chest Shape and Movement

In healthy adults, the lateral dimension of the chest is approximately twice the anterior–posterior dimension. Various musculoskeletal abnormalities, cardiac or respiratory diseases, or trauma can cause changes in shape (Fig. 13-16). With normal breathing, the chest expands equally on both sides. To assess chest expansion, the nurse places their thumbs side by side over the client's posterior vertebrae at about the level of the 10th rib (Fig. 13-17). As the client inhales, the nurse notes how far the thumbs separate; normally the distance is 1 to 2 in (3 to 5 cm).

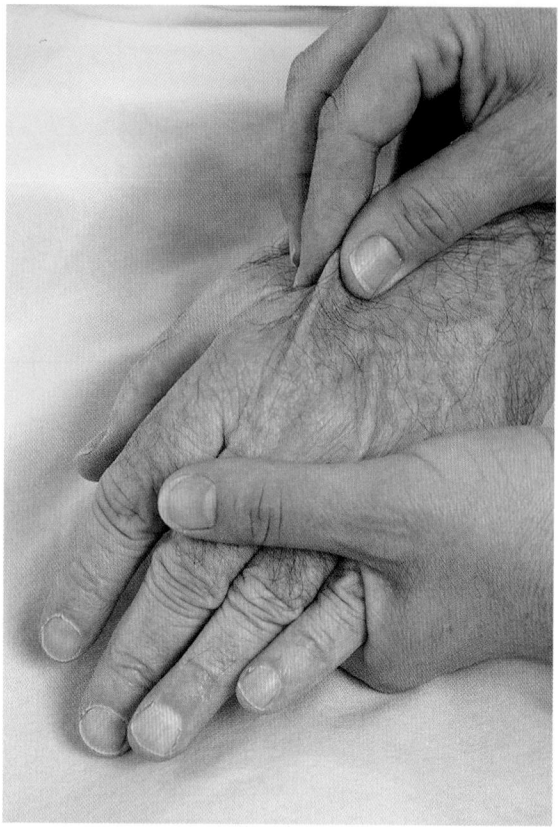

FIGURE 13-15 Assessing skin turgor. (Jensen, S. [2022]. *Nursing health assessment.* Wolters Kluwer Health and Pharma.)

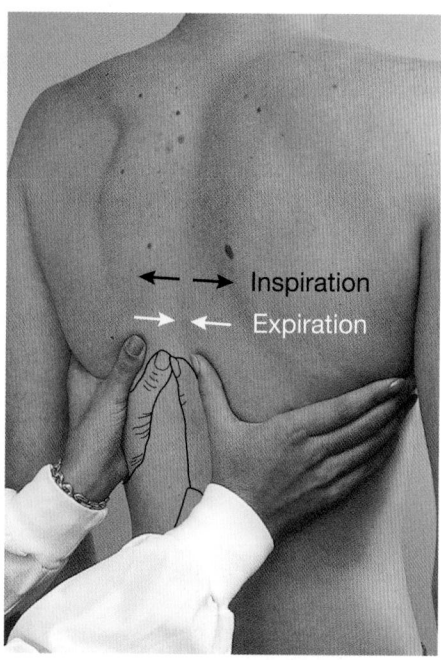

FIGURE 13-17 Palpation of thoracic excursion. In the posterior approach, the nurse places the hands at the level of the 10th rib and observes for equal movement as the client inhales.

Spine

The spine, or vertebral column, appears midline with gentle concave and convex curves when viewed from the side. The shoulders are at equal height. Some common deviations may be noted (Fig. 13-18). *Lordosis* is an exaggerated natural lumbar curve of the spine. *Kyphosis* is an increased thoracic curve. *Scoliosis* is a pronounced lateral curvature of the spine.

Breasts

Although breast abnormalities such as tumors can occur in men, they are more common in women. Usually, more advanced practitioners examine the breasts manually. In January 2016, the U.S. Preventive Services Task Force recommended biennial screening mammography for women aged 50 to 74 years. The recommendation for women aged 40 to 49 years is based on average risk and family history of breast cancer. However, the Society of Breast Imaging, the American College of Radiology, and the American Cancer Society (2019) continue to advocate that mammography screening should begin at age 40 and continue yearly as long as women do not have chronic health problems. Furthermore, the American

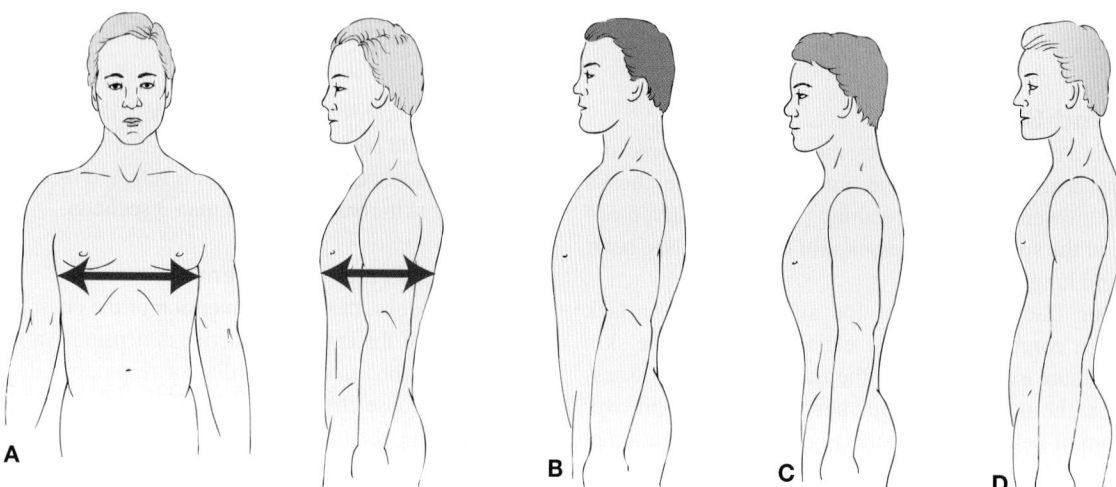

FIGURE 13-16 **A.** Normal chest size and shape; anterolateral dimension is twice the anteroposterior dimension. **B.** Barrel chest. **C.** Pigeon chest. **D.** Funnel chest.

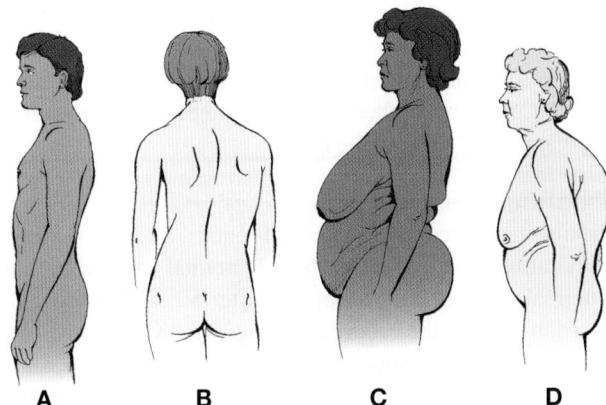

FIGURE 13-18 Variations in spinal curves: normal (**A**), scoliosis (**B**), lordosis (**C**), and kyphosis (**D**).

Cancer Society recommends that although breast self-examination plays a small role in finding breast cancer, its benefit beginning at age 20 lies in helping women assess the look and feel of their breasts to detect changes. For those women who wish to perform breast self-examination, nurses are the ideal health provider to teach this self-assessment technique (Client and Family Teaching 13-1, Table 13-5).

Client and Family Teaching 13-1
Breast Self-Examination

The nurse teaches the client as follows:

- Examine the breasts monthly about 1 week after the menstrual period or on a specific date postmenopause.
- Begin the examination in the shower.

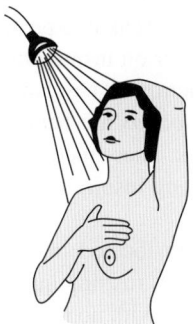

- Next, stand in front of a mirror.

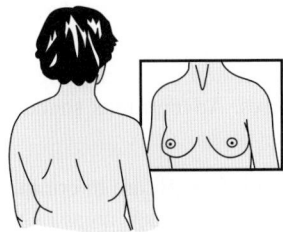

- Look at both breasts with the arms relaxed at the side, with the hands pressing on the hips, and with the hands elevated above the head.

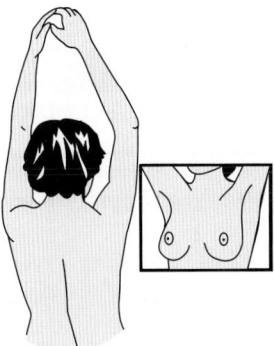

- Look for dimpling in the skin or retraction of either nipple.
- Lie down for the remainder of the examination.
- Put a pillow or folded towel under the shoulder on the side where the first breast will be examined; reverse the pillow before examining the second breast.

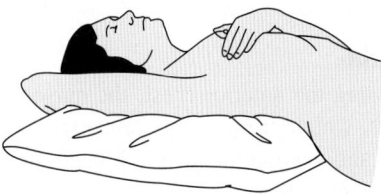

- Use the right hand to examine the left breast and the left hand to examine the right breast.
- Use the flat surface of the fingers in an up-and-down pattern from the underarm and across the breast from the clavicle to the base of the ribs to feel for changes in any area of the breast.

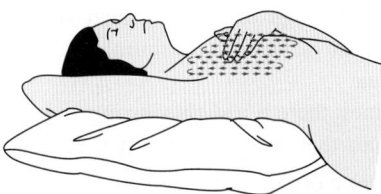

- Feel upward toward the axilla of each arm.
- Determine whether there are any lumps or hard or thickened areas. Squeeze the nipple gently between the thumb and the index finger to determine whether there is any clear or bloody discharge.

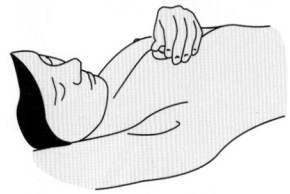

- Repeat the examination on the opposite breast and axilla.
- Report any unusual findings or changes to a physician.
- Breast self-examination may be combined with a clinical examination and mammography to ensure early diagnosis and treatment of cancerous tumors (see Table 13-5).

Casanova, R., Goepfert, A., Hueppchen, N.A., Weiss, P.M., Connolly, A.M., (2023). Beckmann and Ling's Obstetrics and Gynecology (9th ed.). Lippincott Williams & Wilkins.

TABLE 13-5 Breast Examination Guidelines

TECHNIQUE	AGE	FREQUENCY
Self-examination (optional)	≥20 years	Once per month
Clinical examination by a nurse or physician	20–39 years	Every 3 years
	≥40 years	Every year
Mammography	40 years	First examination and yearly thereafter
	>50 years	Optional every other year (2017)
Clinical examination, mammography, magnetic resonance imaging (MRI)	Any age, high risk	Yearly

Data from American Cancer Society. (2022). *American Cancer Society screenings recommendations for women at average breast cancer risk.* https://www.cancer.org/cancer/breast-cancer/screening-tests-and-early-detection/american-cancer-society-recommendations-for-the-early-detection-of-breast-cancer.html

Heart Sounds

When assessing the anterior chest, the nurse listens to the heart sounds, which presumably are caused by the closing of the atrial and ventricular valves. A beginning nurse may limit assessment to the apical area (see Chapter 12). Experienced nurses expand their skills to auscultate at the aortic, pulmonic, tricuspid, and mitral areas (Fig. 13-19).

Normal Heart Sounds

The two normal heart sounds are S1 and S2. The first heart sound, S1, correlates with the "lub" sound and is louder at the apex or mitral area when using the diaphragm of a stethoscope. Although the second heart sound, S2, or the "dub" sound, can be heard in the mitral area, it is louder over the aortic area.

Sometimes, there is a slight slurring, or splitting, of one or both sounds that lasts just a fraction of a second longer.

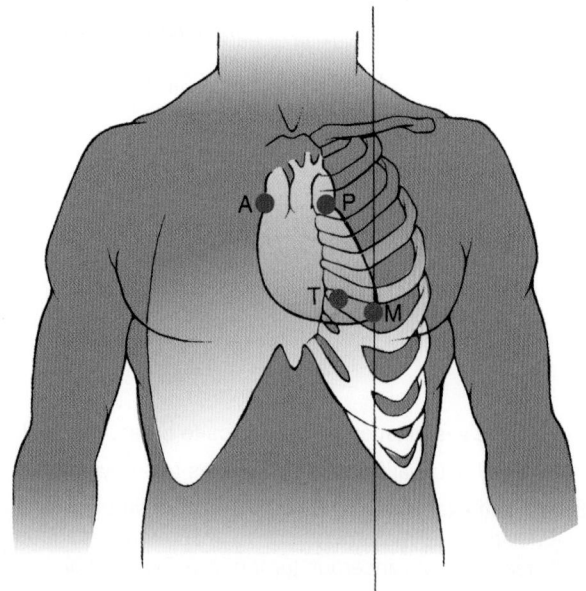

FIGURE 13-19 Locations for assessing heart sounds: A, aortic area; M, mitral area; P, pulmonic area; T, tricuspid area.

It may sound like "lubba-dub" or "lub-dubba." Split sounds are generally attributed to the fact that the valves between the atria (or ventricles) do not always close in exact unison. Splitting, if heard at all, is generally noted with the stethoscope at point P or T on the chest.

Abnormal Heart Sounds

The nurse may hear two additional sounds, S3 and S4, when auscultating the chest. S3, which is normal in children but abnormal in most adults, appears after S2. S3 sounds like "lub-dub-dub" or the cadence of sounds in "Ken-tuck-y." An S3 is much more pronounced than a split second sound. S4 is heard just before S1. It may sound like "lub-lub-dub" or the syllables in "Ten-nes-see."

Identifying abnormal heart sounds—S3, S4, heart murmurs, clicks, and rubs—is a skill that nurses master after they become proficient at distinguishing S1 from S2. A beginning nurse should consult with an experienced nurse or physician if there are any unusual characteristics in a client's S1 and S2 heart sounds.

Lung Sounds

Listening to the lungs is another skill that requires frequent and repeated practice because some sounds are normal and others are abnormal (Nursing Guidelines 13-4).

Normal Lung Sounds

Normal lung sounds occur when air moves in and out of passageways. The sounds vary in pitch and duration in relation to the size and location of the air passages (Fig. 13-20). There are four normal lung sounds:

- *Tracheal sounds* are loud and coarse. They are equal in length during inspiration and expiration and are separated by a brief pause.
- *Bronchial sounds*, heard over the upper sternum anteriorly and between the scapulae posteriorly, are harsh and loud. They are shorter on inspiration than expiration with a pause between them.
- *Bronchovesicular sounds* are heard on either side of the central chest or back. These medium-range sounds that are equal in length during inspiration and expiration have no noticeable pause.
- *Vesicular sounds* are located in the periphery of all the lung fields. Their soft, rustling quality is longer on inspiration than expiration with no pause between.

Abnormal Lung Sounds

Abnormal lung sounds, known as *adventitious sounds*, are those heard in addition to normal lung sounds. Most adventitious sounds are created by air moving through secretions or narrowed airways. Adventitious sounds are divided into four categories:

- *Crackles*, also called *rales*, are intermittent, high pitched, popping, and heard in distant areas of the lungs, primarily during inspiration. They resemble the sound of crisped rice cereal when milk is added. They are attributed to the opening of partially collapsed alveoli (terminal air sacs) or

NURSING GUIDELINES 13-4

Assessing Lung Sounds

- Wash hands or perform hand antisepsis with an alcohol rub (see Chapter 10). *These measures reduce the spread of infection.*
- Provide privacy. *Doing so demonstrates concern for client modesty.*
- Raise the bed to a comfortable position for you. *Doing so reduces strain on the musculoskeletal system.*
- Assist the client into a sitting position if possible. *This position facilitates auscultating the anterior, posterior, and lateral aspects of the chest with minimal client exertion.*
- Remove or loosen the client's upper clothing. *Doing so aids in identifying anatomic landmarks.*
- Reduce or eliminate environmental noise such as suction motors and oxygen equipment. *Quiet conditions promote the accurate identification of lung sounds.*
- Ask the client to refrain from talking. *Talking interferes with concentration and distorts lung sounds.*
- Warm the diaphragm of the stethoscope in the palm of your hand. *Warmth reduces discomfort when the diaphragm is applied to the chest.*
- Instruct the client to breathe in and out through an open mouth deeply but slowly. *This type of breathing reduces noise from air turbulence and prevents hyperventilation.*
- Apply the chest piece to the upper back, but avoid placement over the scapulae or ribs. *This method facilitates hearing sounds in the upper and lower lobes and reduces competing sounds from the heart.*
- Listen for one complete ventilation (inspiration and expiration) at each area auscultated. *This method ensures hearing characteristics during each phase of ventilation.*
- If body hair causes noise, wet it or press harder with the chest piece. *This technique reduces sound distortion.*
- Move the diaphragm from side to side from the apices (top) to the bases (bottom) of the lungs. *This sequence facilitates comparison of sounds (Fig. A).*

- Auscultate the lateral and anterior chest in a similar manner. *Doing so ensures a comprehensive assessment (Figs. B and C).*

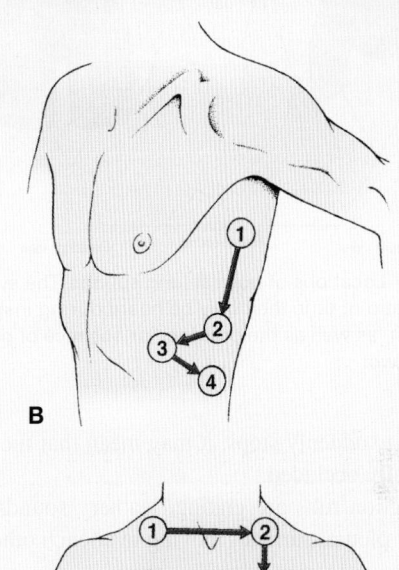
B

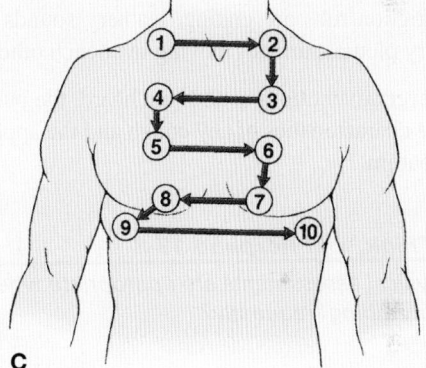
C

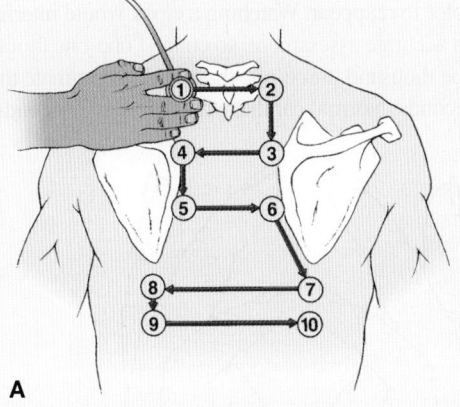
A

- Ask the client to cough or breathe deeply if crackles or gurgles are audible. *This method helps clear the air passages and open the alveoli.*
- Reapply clothing and lower the bed. *Doing so restores comfort and safety.*
- Wash hands or perform hand antisepsis with an alcohol rub (see Chapter 10). *Doing so reduces the spread of microorganisms.*
- Record assessment findings. *Documented data can be used for future comparisons.*
- Repeat lung sound assessments according to agency policy or the client's condition. *Doing so demonstrates responsibility, accountability, and good clinical judgment.*

the movement of air over minute amounts of fluid in the periphery of the lungs during deep inspiration. Crackles may be described as fine if they are soft and brief or coarse if they are louder and last longer.

- *Gurgles*, also called *rhonchi*, are low pitched, continuous, bubbling, and heard in larger airways. They are more prominent during expiration. Some describe gurgles as

sounding like wet snoring. Gurgles may clear with deep breathing or coughing.

- *Wheezes* are whistling or squeaking sounds caused by air moving through a narrowed passage. They can be heard anywhere in the chest during inspiration or expiration. Wheezes may be audible without a stethoscope. Coughing and deep breathing do not usually alter a wheeze; in fact,

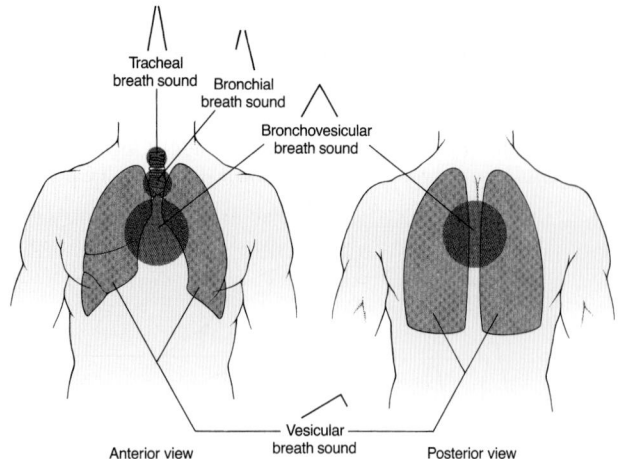

FIGURE 13-20 Locations of normal lung sounds. The symbols indicate the ratio of time they may be heard during inspiration and expiration, as well as the presence or absence of pauses between the two.

if wheezing suddenly stops, it may mean that the air passage is totally occluded.

• Pleural friction rubs are grating, leathery sounds caused by two dry pleural surfaces moving over each other.

Whenever adventitious sounds are heard, the nurse also assesses the characteristics of any cough and the appearance of raised sputum.

>>> ***Stop, Think, and Respond 13-3***
What physical assessments are appropriate when a client is coughing frequently?

Extremities

The nurse notes the alignment, mobility, and strength of the extremities and compares their sizes. They feel the skin temperature, note the characteristics of the nails, time the capillary refill, palpate local peripheral pulses (see Chapter 12), check for edema, and may test the perception of skin sensations. Advanced practitioners assess deep tendon reflexes with a reflex hammer.

Muscle Strength

The nurse assesses all four extremities separately to determine muscle strength. They ask the client to grasp, squeeze, and release the nurse's fingers. As the nurse pulls and pushes on the forearm and upper arm, they instruct the client to resist. To test strength in the lower extremities, the nurse has the client push and pull against resistance (Fig. 13-21).

Fingernails and Toenails

Changes in the shape and thickness of the fingernails and toenails are often signs of chronic cardiopulmonary disease (Fig. 13-22) or fungal infections. The nurse documents any unusual characteristics of the nails or surrounding tissues.

Capillary refill time (the time it takes blood to resume flowing in the base of the nail beds) is normally less than 3 seconds after compression and release of the nail bed. To assess capillary refill time:

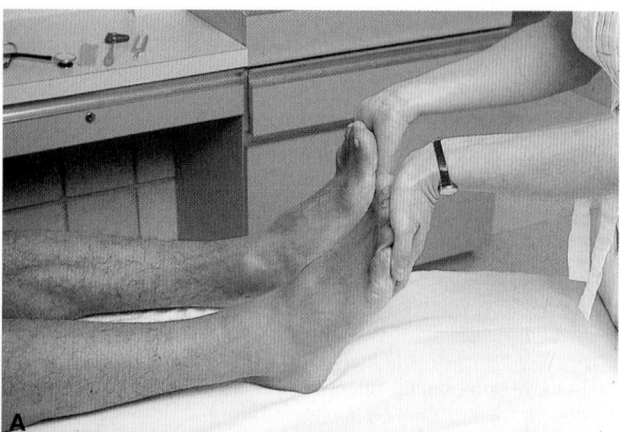
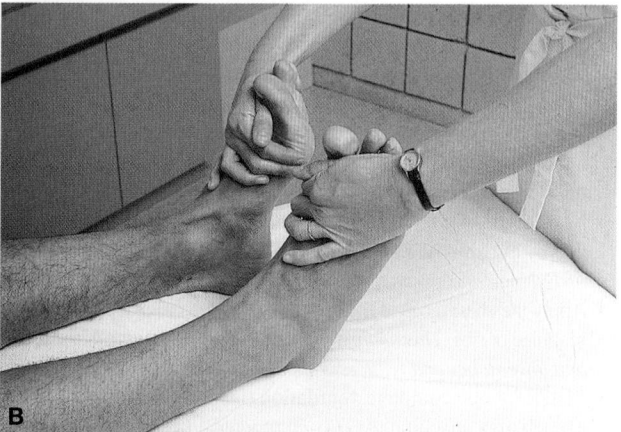

FIGURE 13-21 Assessing muscle strength of lower extremities. **A.** Resisting the push of a nurse. **B.** Resisting the pull by a nurse.

1. Observe the color in the nail bed.
2. Depress the nail bed, displacing capillary blood.
3. Release the pressure.
4. Note how many seconds it takes for the preassessment color to reappear. Watching a clock would interfere with an accurate assessment, so count, "one-one thousand, two-one thousand, three-one thousand" to estimate the time in seconds. Normal capillary refill time is 2 seconds or less.

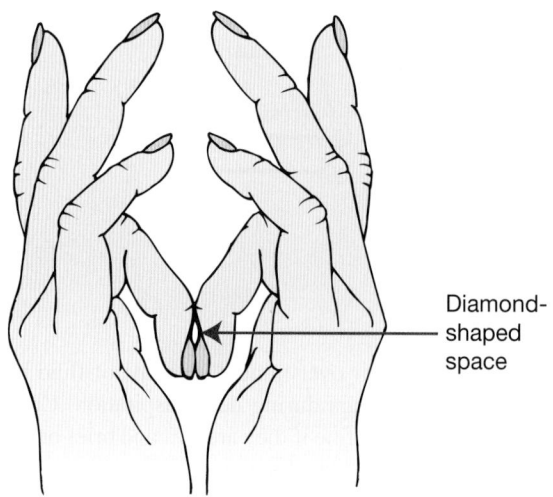

Diamond-shaped space

FIGURE 13-22 A technique for assessing clubbed fingernails. A diamond-shaped space between the nails of the ring fingers is normal.

Edema

Edema is excessive fluid within tissue and signifies abnormal fluid distribution. Clients with cardiovascular, liver, and kidney dysfunction are prone to edema. Subtle signs of edema include weight gain, tight rings, and patterns in the skin after removing socks or shoes. To determine the extent of any edema, the nurse presses a thumb or finger into the tissue over a bone. If an indentation remains (*pitting edema*), the nurse attempts to quantify its severity (Box 13-2).

Skin Sensation

During a comprehensive rather than a basic assessment, the nurse tests the client's ability to differentiate between light touch, warmth, cold, sharp, dull, and vibration (Nursing Guidelines 13-5).

Abdomen

Most gastrointestinal and accessory digestive organs lie within the abdomen. The bladder, if distended, may rise into the abdomen.

For assessment purposes, the abdomen is divided into four quadrants (Fig. 13-23). *The abdomen is always inspected and then auscultated in that sequence before using palpation or percussion techniques.* Touching or manipulating the abdomen can alter bowel sounds, thus producing invalid findings.

Bowel Sounds

Wave-like muscular contractions of the large and small intestines that move fluid and intestinal contents toward the rectum produce bowel sounds. The nurse routinely assesses a client's bowel sounds on admission and once per shift.

BOX 13-2	Criteria for Estimating Pitting Edema

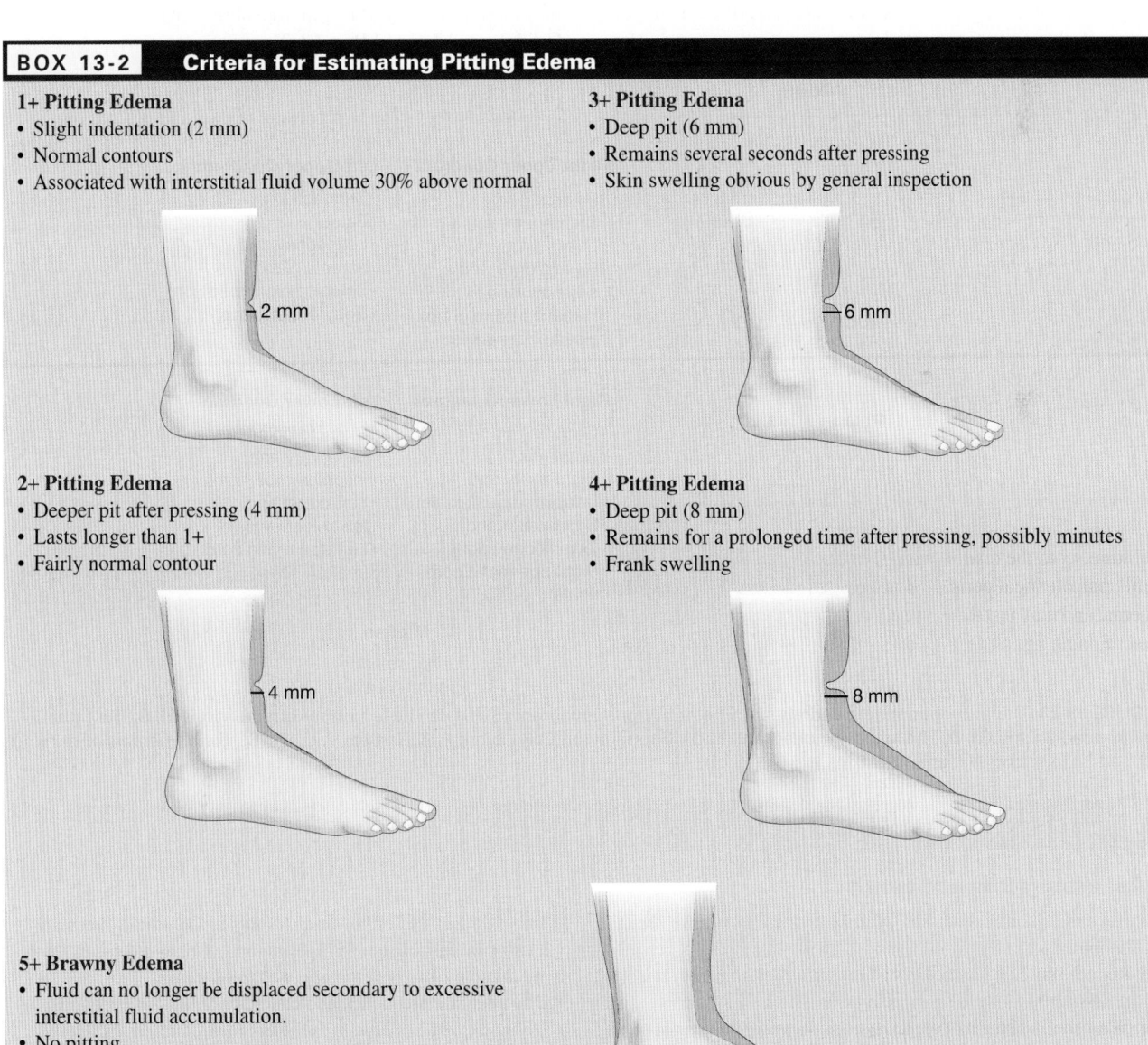

1+ Pitting Edema
- Slight indentation (2 mm)
- Normal contours
- Associated with interstitial fluid volume 30% above normal

2 mm

2+ Pitting Edema
- Deeper pit after pressing (4 mm)
- Lasts longer than 1+
- Fairly normal contour

4 mm

3+ Pitting Edema
- Deep pit (6 mm)
- Remains several seconds after pressing
- Skin swelling obvious by general inspection

6 mm

4+ Pitting Edema
- Deep pit (8 mm)
- Remains for a prolonged time after pressing, possibly minutes
- Frank swelling

8 mm

5+ Brawny Edema
- Fluid can no longer be displaced secondary to excessive interstitial fluid accumulation.
- No pitting
- Tissue palpates as firm or hard.
- Skin surface shiny, warm, moist

NURSING GUIDELINES 13-5

Assessing Sensory Skin Perception

- Gather a cotton ball, a safety pin, or other pointed object; a small container of warm water and one of ice water; and a tuning fork. *These materials provide for a variety of test resources.*
- Instruct the client to shut both eyes. *Doing so reduces the potential for gathering invalid data.*
- Explain that you will touch the skin with test objects at various places and on both sides of the body and that you will ask the client to identify the location and characteristics of the sensation. *This information identifies the test method and how the client is expected to respond.*

- Touch the client with the test objects in a random pattern. *A random pattern prevents the potential for correct guessing.*
- Use both the pointed and curved ends of the safety pin to determine whether the client can discriminate between sharp and dull. Take care not to puncture the skin. *Doing so prevents injury.*
- Stroke the skin with the cotton ball; touch areas with the warm and cold containers. *These tests assess the client's ability to identify fine touch and differences in temperature.*
- Strike a tuning fork and place the stem against bony areas, such as the wrists and along the length of the shins. *This tests the client's ability to sense vibration.*

Normal bowel sounds resemble clicks or gurgles and occur 5 to 34 times a minute (Bickley, 2012). They are more frequent after eating. Bowel sounds are described as *hyperactive* if they are frequent, *hypoactive* if they occur after long intervals of silence, and *absent* if no sound is heard for 2 to 5 minutes. Occasionally, the nurse also detects the sound of blood pulsating through the abdominal aorta (Nursing Guidelines 13-6 and Box 13-3).

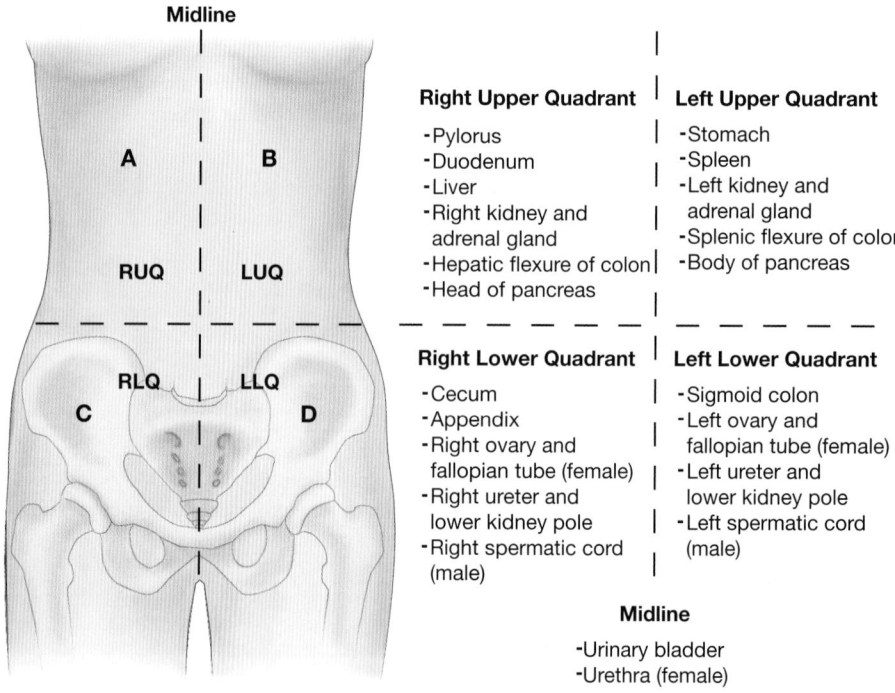

Midline

Right Upper Quadrant
- Pylorus
- Duodenum
- Liver
- Right kidney and adrenal gland
- Hepatic flexure of colon
- Head of pancreas

Left Upper Quadrant
- Stomach
- Spleen
- Left kidney and adrenal gland
- Splenic flexure of colon
- Body of pancreas

Right Lower Quadrant
- Cecum
- Appendix
- Right ovary and fallopian tube (female)
- Right ureter and lower kidney pole
- Right spermatic cord (male)

Left Lower Quadrant
- Sigmoid colon
- Left ovary and fallopian tube (female)
- Left ureter and lower kidney pole
- Left spermatic cord (male)

Midline
- Urinary bladder
- Urethra (female)

FIGURE 13-23 The four abdominal quadrants. **A.** The right upper quadrant (RUQ). **B.** The left upper quadrant (LUQ). **C.** The right lower quadrant (RLQ). **D.** The left lower quadrant (LLQ). (From Taylor, C. R., Lynn, P., & Bartlett, J. L. [2018]. *Fundamentals of nursing* [9th ed.]. Lippincott Williams & Wilkins.)

NURSING GUIDELINES 13-6

Assessing Bowel Sounds

- Have the client recline. *This position provides access to the abdomen.*
- Reduce noise. *A quiet environment facilitates an accurate assessment.*
- Warm the diaphragm of the stethoscope. *Warmth promotes comfort.*
- Place the diaphragm lightly in the right lower quadrant (RLQ) and listen for clicks or gurgles. Move the chest piece over all four quadrants in a clockwise pattern from the RLQ to the right upper quadrant (RUQ) to the left upper quadrant (LUQ),

and ending at the left lower quadrant (LLQ). If no sounds are audible initially, listen for 2–5 minutes. *This sequence follows the anatomic areas of the upper to lower bowel.*
- Document the frequency and character of the bowel sounds. *Doing so provides data for problem identification and future comparisons.*
- Once you have finished the auscultation, note the softness or firmness of the abdomen and feel for palpable masses (see Box 13-3).

BOX 13-3	Characteristics of Palpated Masses
Characteristic	**Description**
Mobility	Fixed—does not move
	Mobile—can be moved with palpation
Shape	Round—resembles a ball
	Tubular—is elongated
	Ovoid—resembles an egg
	Irregular—has no definite shape
Consistency	Edematous—leaves indentation when palpated
	Nodular—feels bumpy to touch
	Granular—feels gritty to touch
	Spongy—feels soft to touch
	Hard—feels firm to touch
Size	Measured in centimeters (1 cm = approximately 0.4 in)
Tenderness	Amount of discomfort when palpated—none, slight, moderate, or severe

Abdominal Girth

If the abdomen appears unusually large, the nurse checks its girth (circumference) daily by using a tape measure around the largest diameter. To ensure that they always measure from the same location, the nurse makes guide marks on the skin with an indelible pen (Fig. 13-24).

Genitalia

In most cases, the nurse only inspects the genitalia. If contact with genital structures or secretions is required, the nurse puts on gloves. To eliminate the possibility of being falsely accused of sexual impropriety, it is a good practice to ask someone of the client's sex to be present when the nurse touches the genitalia.

During inspection, the nurse notes the condition of the skin and the distribution and characteristics of pubic hair (lice may infest pubic hair), as well as the presence of lesions. A physician or nurse with advanced skills examines females internally with an instrument called a *speculum* (see Chapter 14); in males, the prostate gland is palpated during a digital rectal examination.

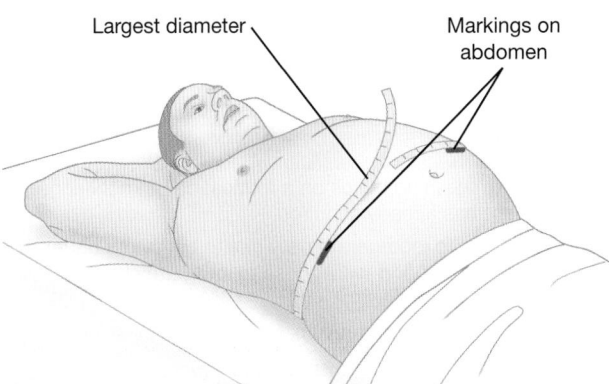

FIGURE 13-24 Measuring abdominal girth.

The nurse observes if the male is circumcised and if the scrotum appears to be of normal size. Whenever possible, they instruct male clients how to examine their testicles (Client and Family Teaching 13-2).

Client and Family Teaching 13-2
Testicular Self-Examination

The nurse teaches the client as follows:

- Examine the testes monthly at a time when the testicles are warm and positioned loosely within the scrotum (e.g., during bathing or showering).
- Elevate the penis with one hand.
- Gently roll each testicle within the scrotum between the thumb and the index finger.
- Feel each testicle horizontally (Fig. A).
- Feel each testicle vertically (Fig. B).
- Check for any unusual lumps; cancerous lumps are located most often on the upper and outer sides of the testes.
- Continue palpation following the spermatic cord from the testicle to where it ascends into the abdomen (Fig. C).
- Report any unusual findings to a physician as soon as possible; an early diagnosis carries a better prognosis.

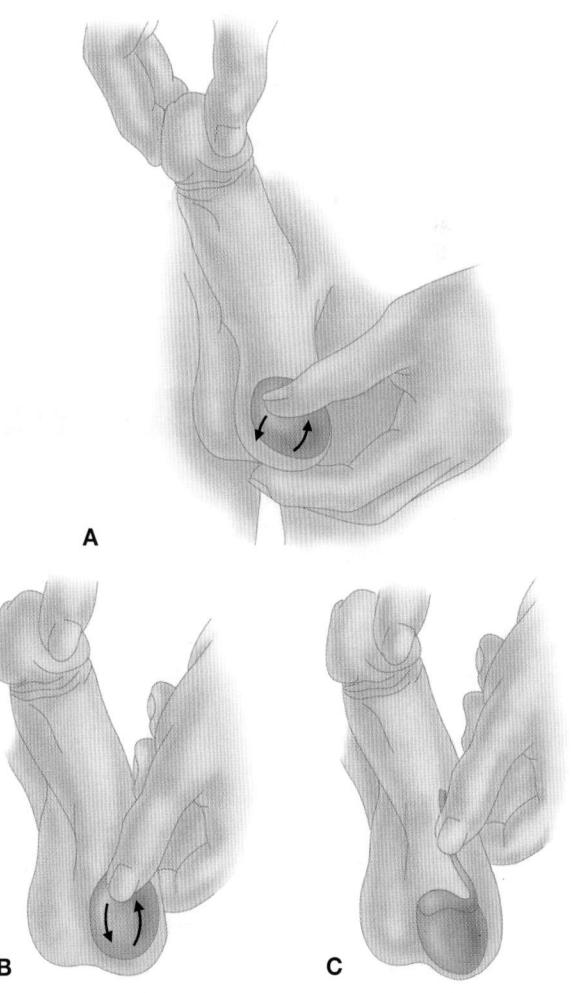

Adapted from Testicular Cancer Society. (2023). *Testicular self-exam.* https://testicularcancersociety.org/pages/self-exam-how-to

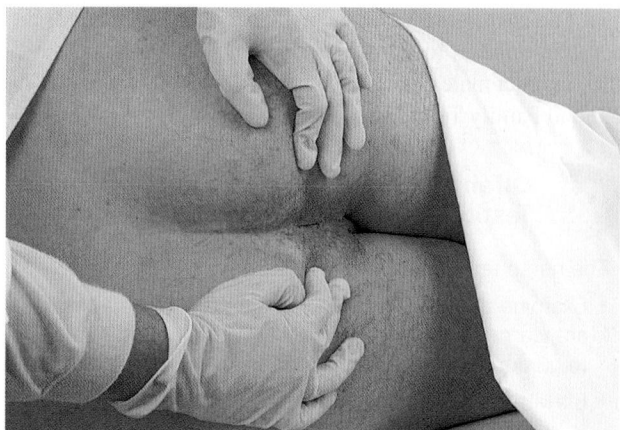

FIGURE 13-25 An inspection of the anus.

Anus and Rectum

Unless a client has specific symptoms, the nurse only inspects the anus. If touching is required, gloves are necessary. To examine the anus, the nurse positions the client on the side with the knees bent. The nurse separates the client's buttocks and inspects the external orifice (Fig. 13-25). The area should appear intact but more pigmented than adjacent skin; it should be moist and hairless. External hemorrhoids

(saccular protrusions filled with blood) may extend beyond the external sphincter muscle. There may be rectal fissures (cracks) if the client has a history of chronic constipation. Trauma may also be present if the client has anal intercourse.

NURSING IMPLICATIONS

Assessment findings form the basis for identifying health problems. Often during a physical assessment, clients reveal situations that caused their health to fail, or they indicate a desire for more health information. The following are some nursing diagnoses that may apply:

- Risky health behavior
- Knowledge deficiency
- Nonadherence
- Altered health maintenance
- Altered health seeking behavior

Nursing Care Plan 13-1 is an example of how the nursing process is used when a client has the nursing diagnosis of risky health behavior. Assisting the patient in identifying poor health behaviors and their consequences is "a pattern of regulating and integrating into daily living a therapeutic regimen for the treatment or illness and its sequelae, which can be strengthened"(Lippincott Advisor, 2022).

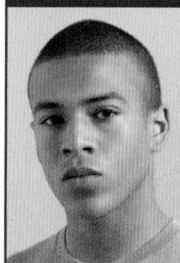

Clinical Scenario Prior to being discharged from the hospital, a 20-year-old client reveals that he has been having unprotected sex with multiple female partners. He is concerned about the risk for acquiring sexually transmitted infections (STIs) or becoming involved in an unplanned pregnancy.

See Nursing Care Plan 13-1.

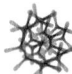

NURSING CARE PLAN 13-1 — Risky Health Behavior

Assessment
- Interact with the client to determine whether they express a desire to seek a higher level of wellness or manifest a lack of knowledge about health promotional activities.
- Other evidence that validates the nursing diagnosis of readiness for enhanced health management is that the client voices an interest in making choices in daily living that are appropriate for meeting goals that reduce health risk factors and prevent illness.

Nursing Diagnosis. Risky health behavior related to prevention of sexually transmitted infections (STIs) and pregnancy as evidenced by the following statements: "I've been having sex with many women. None of them has gotten pregnant, and I haven't caught any diseases as far as I know. But I don't want to take chances anymore."

Expected Outcome. The client will describe safer sexual practices within 24 hours (time of anticipated discharge) following a surgical repair of an inguinal hernia.

Interventions	Rationales
Determine the client's knowledge regarding various common STIs and how they are transmitted.	Effective health teaching builds on a foundation of knowledge that the client has already acquired.
Explore the client's views concerning nonpermanent measures that men can implement to reduce the potential for pregnancy.	The client's ability to incorporate new health behaviors depends on an acceptance of and willingness to integrate changes.
Provide pamphlets and written materials that describe birth control measures and illustrate the technique for applying a condom to prevent STIs.	Information from an authoritative resource provides scientifically based information.

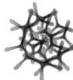

NURSING CARE PLAN 13-1   Risky Health Behavior (*continued*)

Interventions	Rationales
Give the client a supply of free condoms.	An initial supply of condoms facilitates implementation of new health behaviors until the client acquires a personal supply.
Reduce sexual partners to one noninfected, monogamous person.	Sex with a monogamous, disease-free partner reduces the potential for acquiring an STI.
Use a latex condom and apply nonoxynol-9 either over the tip of the condom or as a vaginal application.	A condom provides a barrier for sperm and microorganisms. Nonoxynol-9 is a chemical spermicide.
Roll the condom completely over the erect penis while pinching a space at the condom tip (Fig. A).	Leaving a space provides an area where semen can collect without breaking the condom.

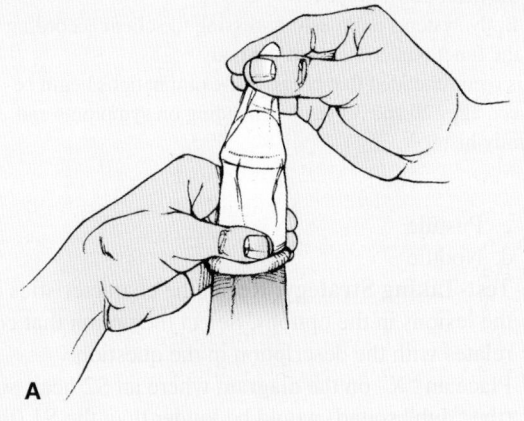

(A) To apply, roll the condom completely over the erect penis while pinching the space at the condom tip.

A

Hold the condom at the base of the penis and promptly remove the condom-covered penis from the vagina before the penis becomes limp (Fig. B).	Prompt removal of a condom reduces the potential for leaking sperm within the vagina, which can lead to pregnancy.

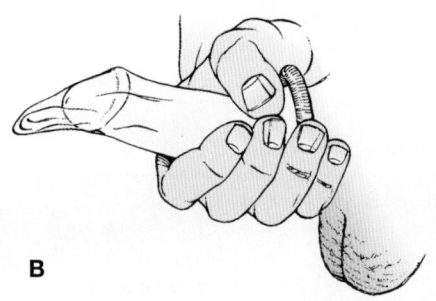

(B) Hold the condom at the base of the penis during its removal from the vagina.

B

Do not have sexual contact again unless another condom is applied.	For maximum effectiveness, condoms are recommended for single use.
If a condom breaks or leaks, urinate immediately and wash the penis with soap and water.	Urination helps eliminate microorganisms that cause STIs through the male urethra. Washing with soap and water removes microorganisms from the surface of the penis.

Evaluation of Expected Outcomes

- The client reads the written materials provided.
- The client states, "Condoms are inconvenient, but they're better than getting a disease. They're also cheaper than babies. I plan to use them from now on until I find the right life partner."

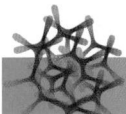

KEY POINTS

- Purpose of the physical assessment: Overall goal is to gather objective data about a client
  - To evaluate the client's current physical condition
  - To detect early signs of developing health problems
  - To establish a baseline for future comparisons
- Four assessment techniques, performed in this order:
  - Inspect
  - Percuss
  - Palpate
  - Auscultate
- Equipment needed for an assessment:
  - Gloves
  - Scale
  - Stethoscope
- Sphygmomanometer
- Thermometer
- Penlight or flashlight
- Tongue blade
- Collecting physical assessment data:
  - Observe and interact with the client.
  - Provide privacy.
  - Head-to-toe approach: Assessing the client from the top of the head down to the feet
  - Body systems approach: Assessing the client according to the functional systems of the body
- It is recommended that breast self-examinations begin between ages 20 and 30 years depending on symptoms and family history.

CRITICAL THINKING EXERCISES

1. A client reports he has not had a bowel movement for 3 days, which is unusual for him. Discuss the physical assessments important to perform at this time.
2. Describe the characteristics of lung sounds normally heard at the midchest area below the nipple line.
3. What action is appropriate if an older adult becomes fatigued during a physical assessment?
4. What information could the nurse provide to a female client who is confused about changes in the breast examination guidelines?

NEXT-GENERATION NCLEX-STYLE REVIEW QUESTIONS

1. Place the following assessment techniques in the sequence that should be used when assessing a client's abdomen.
   a. Auscultation
   b. Percussion
   c. Inspection
   d. Palpation
   Test-Taking Strategy: Read the list of options and place them in the order they are performed from the first to last.
2. When assessing a client with a cough, besides documenting the characteristics of the cough, what other assessment information is essential?
   a. The client's family history of respiratory disease
   b. A current assessment of the client's heart rate
   c. The appearance of respiratory secretions
   d. Any self-treatment the client is using
   Test-Taking Strategy: Note the key word, "essential," indicating one answer is better than any other. Select the option that is most important to assess.
3. Which term is most accurate when documenting the appearance of a skin lesion that is elevated, round, and filled with serum?
   a. Papule
   b. Vesicle

c. Pustule
d. Nodule
Test-Taking Strategy: Recall the characteristics of the lesions in the options. Select the option that correlates with the description in the question.

4. Place an "X" on the diagram where an S2 heart sound (the "dub" sound) would be louder than the S1 (the "lub" sound) when auscultating heart sounds.

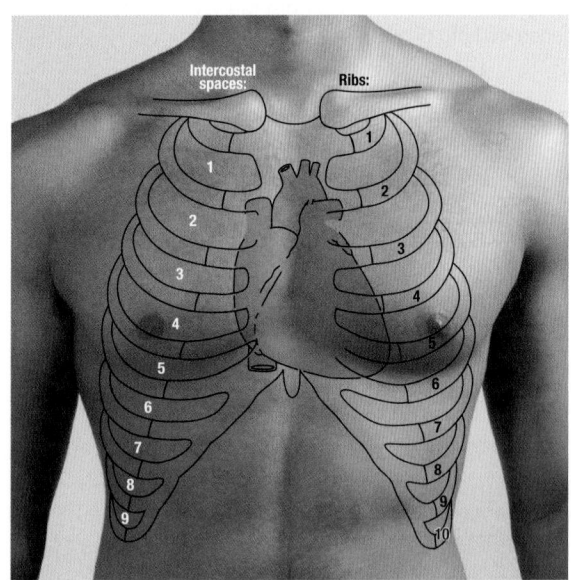

5. When the nurse assesses a client's distant visual acuity, which are required? Select all that apply.
   a. Penlight
   b. Snellen chart
   c. Newsprint
   d. Ophthalmoscope
   e. Mark at 20 ft
   f. Jaeger chart
   Test-Taking Strategy: Note the key words, "distant visual acuity." Read the choices carefully. Select options that correlate with assessing the ability to see distant objects clearly.

NEXT-GENERATION NCLEX-STYLE CLINICAL SCENARIO QUESTIONS

Clinical Scenario:

Prior to being discharged from the hospital, a 20-year-old client reveals that he has been having unprotected sex with multiple female partners. He is concerned about the risk for acquiring sexually transmitted infections (STIs) or becoming involved in an unplanned pregnancy. Client states "I've been having sex with many women. None of them has gotten pregnant, and I haven't caught any diseases as far as I know. But I don't want to take chances anymore."

1. Place an "x" under effective to identify methods that will help the client with understanding the risks of STIs and preventing the client from getting an STI. Place an "x" under ineffective ways that would hinder understanding and prevention of STIs.

METHODS	EFFECTIVE	INEFFECTIVE
Provide pamphlets and material regarding STIs		
Preaching abstinence		
Give the client a supply of free condoms		
Show the client pictures of STI infections		
Tell the client to follow up with the local health clinic		

SKILL 13-1 Performing a Physical Assessment

Suggested Action	Reason for Action
ASSESSMENT	
Identify the client.	Ensures that the assessment is being performed on the correct person
Determine the client's age, gender, and race.	Forms the basis for planning techniques for physical assessment
Observe the client's state of alertness and ability to move.	Aids in determining the best location for the assessment and if the nurse, client, or both will require assistance
Ask the client's opinion about their health status and any current or recent signs and symptoms.	Helps to focus attention during the assessment on particular structures and their functions
PLANNING	
Give the client a specimen container, if a urine sample is needed.	Takes advantage of an opportunity when the client's bladder contains urine
Have the client empty their bladder before undressing.	Facilitates the examination and reduces discomfort
Pull the curtain or close the door and give the client a drape or examination gown to put on after undressing.	Prepares the client for an accurate assessment and ensures privacy
Gather assessment equipment and supplies (see Box 13-1 for basic necessities).	Promotes organization and efficient time management
Decide to examine the client using either a head-to-toe or a body systems approach.	Establishes the plan for assessment and ensures that comprehensive data will be gathered
IMPLEMENTATION	
Explain how the assessment will be conducted.	Reduces anxiety
Explain that all information will be kept confidential among those involved in the client's care.	Encourages the client to be honest and open in identifying health problems
Wash hands or perform hand antisepsis with an alcohol rub (see Chapter 10), preferably in the client's presence.	Provides reassurance that the nurse is clean and conscientious about controlling the spread of microorganisms
Warm your hands before touching the client.	Demonstrates concern for the client's comfort
Obtain the client's height, weight, and vital signs.	Contributes to the general survey of the client
Assist the client to sit at the bottom of the examination table.	Facilitates examination of the upper body without requiring the client to change positions
Modify the client's position if the examination is being conducted in locations other than an examination room.	Demonstrates adaptability
Explain each assessment technique before performing it.	Reduces anxiety
Try to avoid tiring the client and apologize if the client experiences discomfort.	Demonstrates concern for the client's comfort
Help the client resume sitting after the examination.	Places the client in the best position for communicating
Wash hands or perform hand antisepsis with an alcohol rub (see Chapter 10) once again.	Shows responsibility for controlling the spread of microorganisms
Review pertinent findings, both normal and abnormal, without making medical interpretations.	Demonstrates compliance with the client's right to information
Offer the client an opportunity to ask questions.	Encourages active participation in learning and decision-making
Begin organizing assessment findings outside the examination room while the client dresses or dons a bathrobe.	Ensures privacy
Help the client leave the examination room.	Demonstrates courtesy and concern for the client's safety
Dispose of soiled equipment, restore cleanliness and order to the examination room, and restock used supplies.	Shows consideration for the next person who uses the examination room

SKILL 13-1 Performing a Physical Assessment (*continued*)

EVALUATION

• All aspects of the assessment have been carried out, and comprehensive data have been collected.
• The client remained safe, warm, and comfortable.
• The client's questions or concerns have been addressed.

DOCUMENT

• Date and time
• Normal and abnormal findings
• Any unexpected outcomes during the procedure and the nursing actions taken
• To whom abnormal findings were verbally reported and the outcome of the interaction

SAMPLE DOCUMENTATION

Date and Time A 67-year-old man transported from bed to examination room by wheelchair for physical assessment. Can cooperate without distress. Refer to assessment form for examination findings. _____ J. Doe, LPN

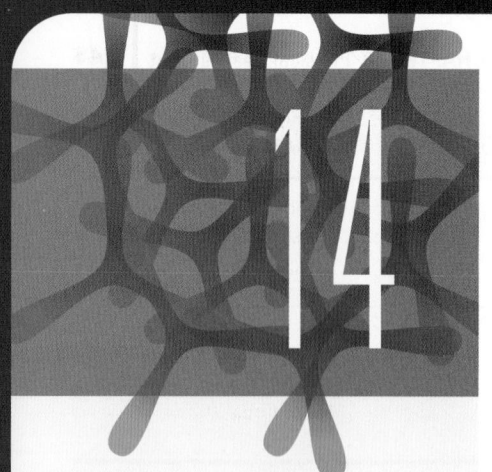

14

Special Examinations and Tests

Words To Know

cold spot
computed tomography
contrast medium
culture
diagnostic examination
dorsal recumbent position
echography
electrocardiography
electroencephalography
electromyography
endoscopy
fluoroscopy
glucometer
Gram staining
hot spot
insulin pumps
knee–chest position
laboratory test
lithotomy position
lumbar puncture
magnetic resonance imaging
modified standing position
nuclear medicine department
Papanicolaou (Pap) test
paracentesis
pelvic examination
positron emission tomography
prone position
radiography
radionuclides
roentgenography
Sims position
specimens
speculum
spinal tap
supine position
transducer
ultrasonography

Learning Objectives

On completion of this chapter, the reader should be able to:

1. Differentiate between an examination and a test.
2. Identify word endings and their meanings that provide clues as to how tests and examinations are performed.
3. Discuss factors to consider when performing examinations and tests on older adults.
4. List general nursing responsibilities related to assisting with special examinations and tests.
5. Name positions commonly used during tests and examinations.
6. List commonly performed categories of tests and examinations.
7. Explain what is involved in a pelvic examination and a Papanicolaou (Pap) test.
8. Describe the following diagnostic tests: paracentesis, lumbar puncture, throat culture, and measurement of capillary blood glucose.

INTRODUCTION

In addition to obtaining a health history and performing a physical assessment, the nurse gains assessment data by evaluating the results of special examinations and tests. This chapter gives an overview of some common diagnostic examinations and tests and related nursing responsibilities. Tests involving the collection of urine and stool specimens are discussed in Chapters 30 and 31, respectively.

 Gerontologic Considerations

■ Some laboratory values change minimally or not at all with age. Parameters are often determined by using averaged statistics. Failure to consider age-related differences in laboratory values can lead to inaccurate and inappropriate treatment.

■ Because many prescription and over-the-counter medications, as well as vitamins, minerals, and herbal products, can affect laboratory values, it is important to review all medications and other bioactive substances when considering laboratory procedures.

■ Knowing the usual range of laboratory results for older adults who have chronic conditions is important. Test results that are outside the normal range may be normal or acceptable for people with chronic conditions. It is also important to compare the client's previous results for the diagnostic test with current findings.

■ When working with an older adult who is cognitively compromised (e.g., dementia), consider including the person who has a medical durable power of attorney. Include the caregiver or family member in the procedure as much as possible and with the client's permission.

■ Older adults, especially those who are medically frail, may have difficulty tolerating the withholding of food or fluids for long periods before tests or examinations. Assessment of urinary output, blood pressure, and mental status provides data on how well an older adult is tolerating a fasting state.

■ When older adults must abstain from food or fluid before a test or examination, administration of their prescribed medications with a small amount of water may be allowed based on consultation with the physician.

■ Frail older adults fatigue easily; therefore, coordinate tests and examinations with diagnostic personnel to eliminate long periods of fasting or waiting in uncomfortable environments.

■ Older adults may need additional clothing, slippers, and extra covers to keep them warm in waiting rooms and examination areas.

■ After a diagnostic examination, offer older adults food and fluid and a period of rest. Encourage fluids because older adults may have a diminished thirst sensation and may not realize the need for fluid replacement.

■ Some older adults become exhausted by preparations for gastrointestinal examinations that require the use of laxatives and enemas. Harsh laxatives or multiple enemas may also deplete electrolyte balance, leading to weakness or dizziness.

■ Providing a bedside commode and hands-on assistance is helpful for older adults, especially those with impaired mobility, when they are undergoing preparation for gastrointestinal examinations.

■ Dehydration is common in older adults and can cause false elevations of laboratory tests, such as hematocrit, blood urea nitrogen (BUN), and urine osmolality.

EXAMINATIONS AND TESTS

A **diagnostic examination** is a procedure that involves the physical inspection of body structures and evidence of their functions. It is facilitated through the use of technical equipment and techniques, such as:

- Radiography (X-rays)
- Endoscopy (optical scopes)

BOX 14-1	**General Nursing Responsibilities for Examinations and Tests**

- Determine the client's understanding of the procedure.
- Witness the client's signature on a consent form.
- Teach or follow test preparation requirements.
- Obtain equipment and supplies.
- Arrange the examination area.
- Position and drape the client.
- Assist the examiner.
- Provide the client with physical and emotional support.
- Care for specimens.
- Record and report appropriate information.

- Radionuclide imaging (radioactive chemicals)
- Ultrasonography (high-frequency sound waves)
- Electrical graphic recordings

By learning root words and suffixes (word endings), which are primarily of Latin and Greek origin, it is possible to decipher many unfamiliar names of diagnostic examinations and tests (Table 14-1).

A **laboratory test** is a procedure that involves the examination of body fluids or specimens. It involves comparing the components of a collected specimen with normal findings. A diagnostic examination may or may not include the collection of specimens.

General Nursing Responsibilities

When clients undergo diagnostic examinations and laboratory tests, nurses have specific responsibilities before, during, and after the procedures (Box 14-1).

Preprocedural Care

Before a client agrees to a procedure, the nurse determines whether the client understands its purpose and the activities involved. Once the client's consent for a diagnostic test is obtained, the nurse prepares the client, obtains the equipment and supplies, and prepares the examination area.

Clarifying Explanations

In some cases, a signed consent form is required before performing examinations or tests. Legally, consent must contain three elements: *capacity*, *comprehension*, and *voluntariness* (Box 14-2).

TABLE 14-1 Deciphering Diagnostic Terms

SUFFIX	MEANING	EXAMPLES	DESCRIPTION
-graphy	To record	Angiography	Test that records an image of blood vessels
-gram	An image	Angiogram	The actual image recorded during angiography
-scopy	To see	Sigmoidoscopy	Test in which the lower intestine is inspected
-scope	Examination instrument	Sigmoidoscope	A tube with a light and lens for looking within the lower intestine
-centesis	To puncture	Thoracentesis	Procedure in which a needle is used to puncture the thorax and withdraw fluid
-metry	To measure	Pelvimetry	Procedure in which the pelvis is measured
-meter	Instrument for obtaining measurements	Glucometer	Instrument for measuring glucose

BOX 14-2	Elements of Informed Consent
Capacity	Indicates that the client has the ability to make a rational decision; if not, a spouse, parent, or legal guardian must do so.
Comprehension	Indicates that the client understands the physician's explanation of the risks, benefits, and alternatives that are available[a]
Voluntariness	Indicates that the client is acting of their own free will without coercion or the threat of intimidation

[a]Sedative drugs or the effects of anesthesia may temporarily affect capacity and comprehension.

Concept Mastery Alert

Informed Consent

Although nurses are often involved in repeating, simplifying, clarifying, or expanding explanations to promote informed consent, *ultimately*, it is the responsibility of the physician to provide the information for informed consent.

Although physicians are responsible for giving clients sufficient information to obtain informed consent, not all clients fully understand the information. Some are too anxious to process details, others feel too insecure to ask questions, and still others express additional concerns after the physician has left. Often, the nurse must repeat, simplify, clarify, or expand the original explanation.

There are no exact rules for clarifying explanations. In general, it is best to find out how much of the physician's explanation the client understands and use the client's questions as a guide for providing further information. Nurses should follow the suggestions for teaching and providing emotional support given in Chapter 8.

Preparing Clients

Some examinations and tests require special preparation of the client, such as withholding food and fluids or modifying the diet.

Because test preparation requirements vary among health care agencies, the nurse refers to written protocols in the agency's manual rather than relying on memory. Once they understand the specific requirements for a test, the nurse provides directions to the client, nursing staff, and other hospital departments, such as the dietary department involved in the test. Everyone involved must cooperate to ensure test accuracy. The nurse reports any incorrect test preparations promptly because the procedure may need to be canceled and rescheduled. Because many tests and examinations are done on an outpatient basis, the nurse must understand the client's responsibilities and instruct them accordingly (Client and Family Teaching 14-1).

Regardless of the type of examination or test, the nurse helps the client change into an examination gown, ensures there is an identification bracelet, takes vital signs, and suggests that the client empty their bladder (unless a full bladder

Client and Family Teaching 14-1
Preparation for Special Examinations or Tests

The nurse teaches the client who is not hospitalized to:

- Call (specify the number) if test preparation instructions are not clearly understood or cannot be followed.
- Refrain from eating or drinking anything for at least 8 hours before a test or examination that requires a fasting state.
- Follow all dietary specifications for eating or omitting certain foods exactly as directed.
- Check with the physician about taking or readjusting the time schedule for taking prescribed medications on the day of the test or examination.
- Bathe or shower as usual on the day of the test or examination.
- Dress casually and in layers so that items of clothing can be removed or added to maintain comfort in the test environment.
- Ask a friend or family member to provide transportation to and from the site if there is a potential for drowsiness, lingering pain, or weakness after the procedure.
- Arrive at least 30 minutes before the test is scheduled.
- Identify oneself at the information or appointment desk upon arrival.
- Bring information to verify insurance or Medicare coverage.

is required for the test). The nurse continues to monitor the condition of waiting clients who can experience adverse effects from fatigue, delayed food consumption, or medical symptoms.

Obtaining Equipment and Supplies

If an examination or test is performed at the bedside or in an examination room on the nursing unit, the nurse obtains equipment and supplies ahead of time. Nurses are relieved of this responsibility if the examination or test is carried out in other locations or when a special technician performs the procedure.

Some items that nurses may need are in packaged kits (such as a lumbar puncture kit) kept in a clean utility room (Fig. 14-1) or may be obtained from a central supply department (also called "materials management" in some health care agencies). If using a packaged kit, the nurse checks the list of contents to determine what, if any, additional items are needed. Clean gloves, goggles, masks, and gowns are required to prevent direct contact with blood or body secretions (see section "Standard Precautions" in Chapter 22).

Arranging the Examination Area

If the procedure is performed at the bedside, the nurse removes unnecessary articles from the area and provides privacy. Many nursing units contain an examination room that is clean, well lit, and stocked with frequently used equipment and supplies. The nurse covers the examination table

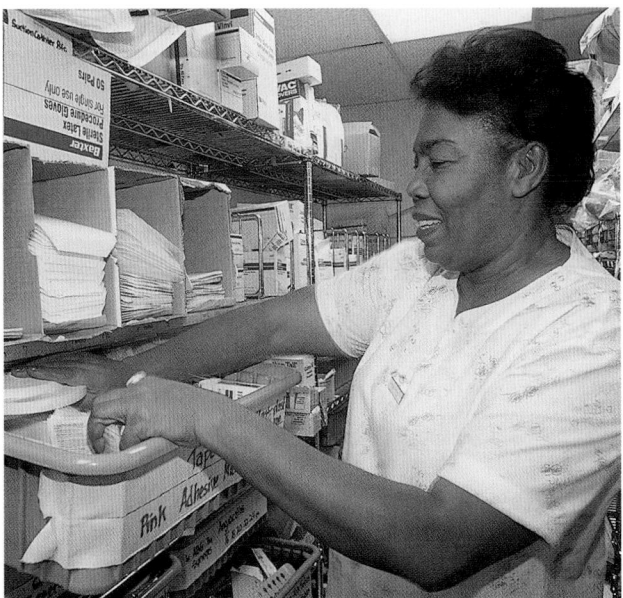

FIGURE 14-1 Obtaining equipment from the supply room. (Photo by Sharon Guynup.)

with a sheet or paper dispensed from a roll. A lined receptacle is nearby for the disposal of soiled items.

The nurse arranges equipment and supplies for easy access by the examiner (Fig. 14-2). Sterile items remain wrapped or covered until just before their use. Before the examiner arrives, nurses check instruments that require electric power, batteries, or lights so that they can replace nonfunctioning equipment.

Procedural Responsibilities

During the examination or test, the nurse positions and drapes the client, provides the examiner with technical assistance, and supports the client physically and emotionally.

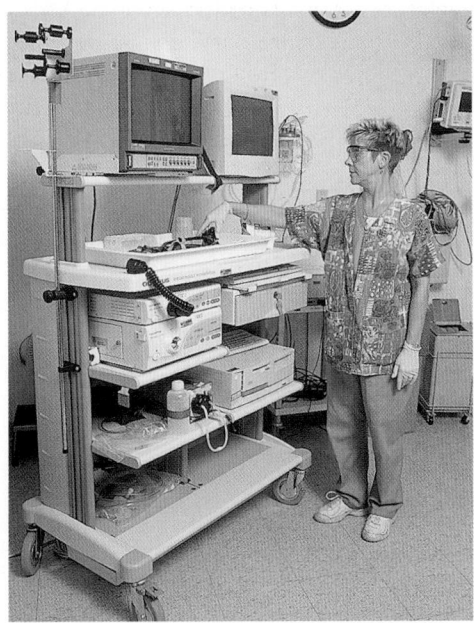

FIGURE 14-2 The nurse arranges supplies and equipment in an endoscopic examination room. (Photo by B. Proud.)

Positioning and Draping

Seven positions are commonly used depending on the type of examination, the condition of the client, and the preference of the examiner. They include the supine position, prone position, dorsal recumbent position, Sims or left lateral position, lithotomy position, knee–chest or genupectoral position, and modified standing position (Table 14-2).

The **supine position** is one in which the client is lying flat with the face up. The arms and legs are extended. The client may wear a paper or cloth examination gown and be further covered with a drape. The surface of the table is covered with paper for hygiene purposes.

The **prone position** is opposite of the supine position. The client lies on their abdomen with the head turned to one side. The arms may be above the head or at the sides of the body. A drape covers the body.

The **dorsal recumbent position** is a reclining position with the knees bent, hips rotated outward, and feet flat. It is commonly used for various examinations. The nurse uses a bath blanket to drape the client and places examination paper or a disposable pad under the client's buttocks to absorb drainage.

The **lithotomy position** is a reclining position with the feet in metal supports called *stirrups*. It is used to facilitate gynecologic (female reproductive), urologic, and, sometimes, rectal examinations. The nurse uses a drape to cover the client's exposed perineum and legs.

In the **Sims position**, the client lies on the left side with the chest leaning forward, the right knee bent toward the head, the right arm forward, and the left arm extended behind the body. Indications are similar to those for the lithotomy position. It is an alternative gynecologic or urologic position when a client cannot abduct the hips (move the legs outward from midline) because of restricted joint movement, such as that caused by arthritis. This position also provides access to the anus and rectum when the client requires rectal administration of medication or the instillation of an enema solution.

In the **knee–chest position**, also called a "genupectoral position," the client rests on the knees and chest. The client turns the head, which is supported on a small pillow, to one side. The nurse places a pillow under the client's chest for added comfort. The arms are above the head or bent at the elbows so that they rest alongside the client's head. The nurse places a drape to cover the client's back, buttocks, and thighs. This position is difficult for most clients—especially older adults—to assume for any length of time. Therefore, the nurse waits to place the client in this position until just before the examination. Some examination tables have movable sections that facilitate maintaining this position without much client effort.

In the **modified standing position**, the client stands with the upper half of the body leaning forward. It is used primarily for examining the prostate gland. For comfort and safety, the draped client stands in front of the examination table and leans forward from the waist.

Assisting the Examiner

The nurse must be familiar with the examination equipment and the order of its use. They place instruments and equipment on the side of the examiner's dominant hand, if possible.

TABLE 14-2 Indications for Common Examination Positions

POSITION	USES
Supine position (Fig. A) 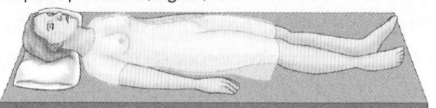	Examinations of the head, neck, chest, abdomen, and extremities
Prone position (Fig. B) 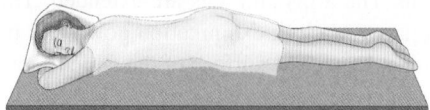	Examinations of the posterior head, back, buttocks, and extremities
Dorsal recumbent position (Fig. C) 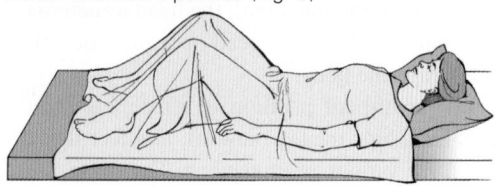	• External genitalia inspection • Vaginal examination • Rectal examination • Urinary catheter insertion
Lithotomy position (Fig. D) 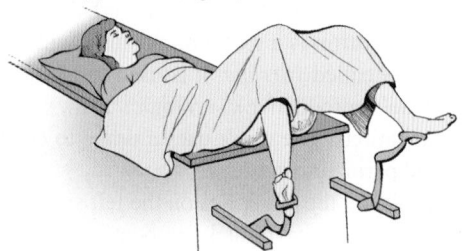	• Internal pelvic examination (female) • Obstetric delivery • Cystoscopic (bladder) examination • Rectal examination
Sims position (Fig. E) 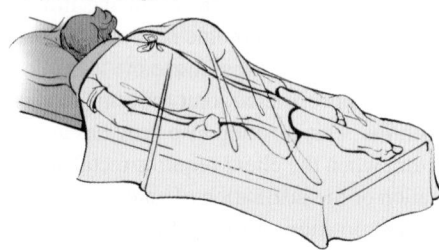	• Rectal examination • Vaginal examination • Rectal temperature assessment • Suppository insertion • Enema administration
Knee–chest position (Fig. F) 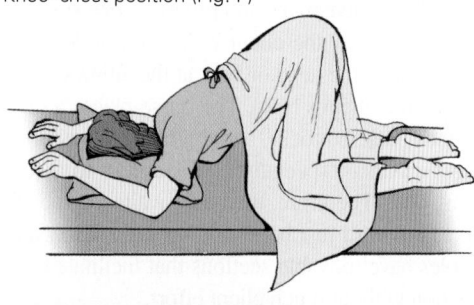	• Rectal and lower intestinal examinations • Prostate gland examination
Modified standing position (Fig. G) 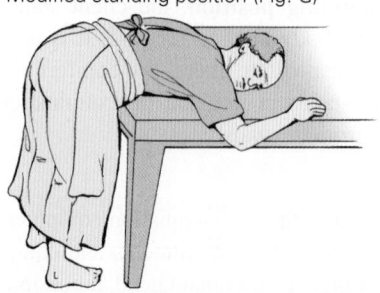	Prostate gland examination

If not, the nurse anticipates what will be needed during the procedure and hands the examiner one item at a time.

If the skin and underlying tissue require local anesthesia, the nurse holds a container of the medication as the physician withdraws some of its contents. The nurse always carefully checks the drug name and concentration on the label. A second method for ensuring the use of the correct drug is to hold the container so that the examiner can read the label.

If the nurse is responsible for performing the test or examination, they cannot leave the client to obtain equipment and supplies. If they need assistance or additional equipment, the nurse summons help with a wearable wireless call system, telephone, or call light in the examination room.

Providing Physical and Emotional Support

Throughout any examination or test, the nurse continuously observes the client's physical and emotional reactions and responds accordingly. For example, comfort measures are in order if the client is cold or in pain. Holding the client's hand and offering words of encouragement help the client to endure temporary discomfort. The nurse communicates assessments of the client to the examiner, who may choose to shorten or modify the examination in some manner.

Postprocedural Care

After the completion of an examination and/or test, the nurse attends to the client's comfort and safety, cares for specimens, and records and reports pertinent data.

Attending to the Client

First, the nurse helps the client into a position of comfort. They recheck vital signs to verify that the client's condition is stable. The nurse cleans any substances from the client that caused soiling. They offer hospitalized clients a clean gown or direct outpatients to dress in their own clothing. When it is safe to do so, the nurse escorts clients to their rooms or to the discharge area and provides instructions for follow-up care.

Caring for Specimens

Sometimes, **specimens** (samples of tissue or body fluids) are collected during an examination or test. To ensure their accurate analysis, the nurse does the following:

- Collects the specimen in an appropriate container
- Labels the specimen container with the correct information
- Attaches the proper laboratory request form
- Ensures that the specimen does not decompose before it can be examined
- Delivers the specimen to the laboratory as soon as possible

Box 14-3 lists factors that often interfere with accurate examinations or that invalidate test results.

Recording and Reporting Data

The nurse must document certain information whenever a client undergoes a special examination or test. General information includes:

- Date and time
- Pertinent preexamination assessments and preparations

BOX 14-3	Common Factors That Invalidate Examination or Test Results

- Incorrect diet preparation
- Failure to remain fasting
- Insufficient bowel cleansing
- Drug interactions
- Inadequate specimen volume
- Failure to deliver specimen in a timely manner
- Incorrect or missing test requisition

- Type of test or examination
- Who performed the test or examination
- Where the test or examination was performed
- Response of client during the examination and afterward
- Type of specimen obtained, if any
- Appearance, size, or volume of specimen
- Where the specimen was transported

In addition to the documented account of the examination, the nurse reports significant information to other nursing team members. This may include that the examination has been completed, the client's reactions during and immediately after the procedure, and any delayed reactions. When the nursing team stays aware of current events and changes in the client's condition, they can revise and keep the plan of care current.

Common Diagnostic Examinations

Many types of diagnostic examinations are performed commonly to assess and evaluate clients. Some of the most common are discussed in this section. Additional information can be found in laboratory and test manuals and courses in which specific diseases are studied; beginning nurses also gain experience with these examinations in the clinical setting.

Pelvic Examination

A **pelvic examination** is the physical inspection of the vagina and the cervix with palpation of the uterus and the ovaries. A physician, a physician's assistant, or a nurse practitioner usually performs a pelvic examination. They often collect a specimen of cervical secretions for a **Papanicolaou (Pap) test**. This test, also called a *Pap smear*, screens for abnormal cervical cells, the status of reproductive hormone activity, and normal or infectious microorganisms within the vagina or uterus (Table 14-3).

When a pelvic examination is being used to screen for cervical cancer, the American Cancer Society and the American College of Obstetricians and Gynecologists (ACOG) recommend the revised guidelines (2022) in Box 14-4 for cancer screening.

Related Nursing Responsibilities

Skill 14-1 identifies the nursing responsibilities involved in assisting with a pelvic examination and collecting cervical secretions for a Pap test.

TABLE 14-3 Pap and HPV Test Results

HPV test results

Negative HPV test result: High-risk HPV was not found. You should have the next test in 5 years. You may need to come back sooner if you had abnormal results in the past.

Positive HPV test result: High-risk HPV was found. Your health care provider will recommend follow-up steps you need to take, based on your specific test result.

Pap test results

Normal Pap test results: No abnormal cervical cells were found. A normal test result may also be called a **negative** test result or negative for intraepithelial lesion (area of abnormal growth) or malignancy.

Unsatisfactory Pap test results: The lab sample may not have had enough cells, or the cells may have been clumped together or hidden by blood or mucus. Your health care provider will ask you to come in for another Pap test in 2–4 months.

Abnormal Pap test results: An abnormal test result may also be called a *positive* test result. Some of the cells of the cervix look different from the normal cells. An abnormal test result does not mean you have cancer. Your health care provider will recommend monitoring, more testing, or treatment.

HPV, human papillomavirus.
HPV and Pap Test Results: Next Steps after an Abnormal Cervical Cancer Screening Test. (2022). https://www.cancer.gov/types/cervical/screening/abnormal-hpv-pap-test-results

Radiography

Radiography, or **roentgenography** (a general term for procedures that use roentgen rays, or X-rays), produces images of body structures. The actual film image is technically called a "roentgenogram" but is commonly known as an *X-ray.* Roentgen rays produce electromagnetic energy that

BOX 14-4	Cervical Cancer Screening Guidelines
<21	No screening
21–29	Pap every 3 years or human papillomavirus (HPV) 25–29//Pap are preferred.
30–65	Choose one of the three options: Pap and HPV every 5 years Pap every 3 years HPV every 5 years
>65	No screening, if no history of cervical changes, and either three negative Pap tests in a row or two negative co-tests (Pap and HPV) in a row for 10 years

American College of Obstetricians and Gynecologists. (2022). *Cervical cancer screening.* https://www.acog.org/womens-health/infographics/cervical-cancer-screening

passes through body structures, leaving an image of dense tissue on special film. Table 14-4 lists common radiographic examinations and indications for their use.

X-rays cannot be seen or felt, but cells absorb the energy. Repeated exposure to X-rays, even at small doses, or a single exposure to a high dose causes cell damage that can lead to cancerous cell changes. Consequently, practitioners tend to be cautious about the number of X-ray studies that they request. X-rays are avoided during pregnancy if at all possible because a developing fetus is at greater risk for cellular damage from X-rays. **Magnetic resonance imaging** (MRI) is a technique for producing an image by using atoms subjected to a strong electromagnetic field. This diagnostic alternative does not involve exposure to the type of radiation produced with roentgenography (Fig. 14-3).

TABLE 14-4 Common Radiographic Examinations

EXAMINATION	EXPLANATION AND INDICATIONS OF EXAM
Computed tomography (CT), also known as a computed axial tomography (CAT) scan, including CT angiography	Combines a series of X-ray images taken from different angles around your body and uses computer processing to create cross-sectional images (slices) of the bones, blood vessels and soft tissues inside your body
Fluoroscopy, including upper GI, lower GI and barium enema	Aids in diagnosis of ulcers, GI tumors, narrowing of the esophagus, and helps in diagnosis of polyps or tumors of the bowel, intestinal obstruction, and structural changes within the intestine
Magnetic resonance imaging (MRI) and **magnetic resonance angiography** (MRA)	An MRI creates detailed images of organs and tissues. An MRA focuses more on the blood vessels than the tissue surrounding it.
Mammography	An X-ray imaging to detect for the presence of tumor or lump in breast
Nuclear medicine, which includes tests such as a **bone scan, thyroid scan, and thallium cardiac stress test**	A nuclear medicine scan uses small amounts of radiation to create pictures of tissues, bones, and organs inside the body. The radioactive material collects in certain areas of your body, and special cameras find the radiation.
X-rays, which includes chest x-ray	Detects pneumonia, broken ribs, lung tumors, enlarged heart, and fractures
Positron emission tomography, also called PET imaging, PET scan	An imaging test that checks your body for diseases by using radiotracers to assess organ and tissue functions
Ultrasound	Ultrasound, also called *sonography,* is an imaging method that uses sound waves to produce images of structures within your body.

GI, gastrointestinal.
MedlinePlus. (2021). Imaging and radiology. https://medlineplus.gov/ency/article/007451.htm#:~:text=The%20most%20common%20types%20of%20diagnostic%20radiology%20exams,Plain%20x-rays%2C%20which%20includes%20chest%20x-ray%20More%20items; Mayo Clinic. (2022). *CT scan.* https://www.mayoclinic.org/tests-procedures/ct-scan/about/pac-20393675; Sawyers, T. (2022). *MRI vs MRA.* https://www.healthline.com/health/mri-vs-mra; Frysh, P. (2022). *Nuclear medicine scan.* https://www.webmd.com/cancer/nuclear-medicine-scan; Mayo Clinic. (2022). Ultrasound. https://www.mayoclinic.org/tests-procedures/ultrasound/about/pac-20395177

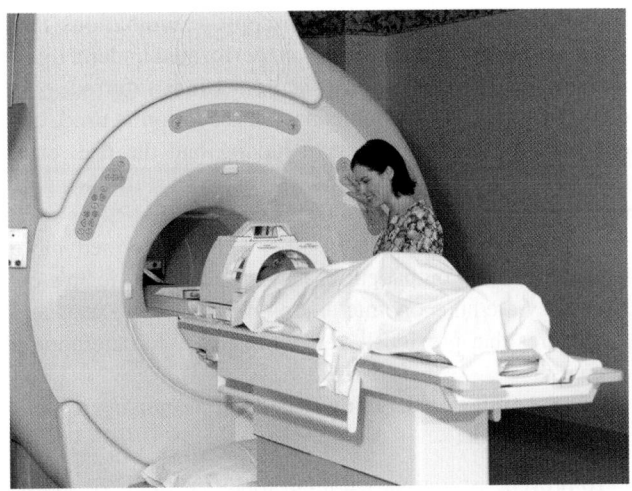

FIGURE 14-3 Magnetic resonance imaging.

Some hospitals offer MRIs that are open or partially open as opposed to completely enclosing the client within a tube. Claustrophobic and anxious clients prefer the open system, which is also ideal for pediatric clients and clients weighing more than 500 lb. Some metal devices that are within the body prohibit performing an MRI; metal objects on a client's person must be removed before an MRI (Box 14-5). MRIs can now be done on clients with metal joint implants, but it requires the radiologist to use an adjustment called *metal artifact reduction sequence* (MARS) to avoid radiographic distortion of the image.

Contrast Medium

A **contrast medium** is a substance, such as barium sulfate or iodine, that adds density to a body organ or cavity. It makes hollow body areas appear more distinct when imaged on X-ray film. Some people are sensitive to substances used in contrast media and have an immediate allergic reaction to them.

Contrast media are administered orally or rectally or injected intravenously. **Fluoroscopy** is a form of radiography that displays an image in real time. It is used to observe the movement of contrast media—for example, as it is being swallowed, instilled, or injected. **Computed tomography** (CT) scanning is a form of roentgenography that shows planes of tissue. This and other types of X-ray examinations use contrast media. The CT contrast medium makes it possible to identify differences in tissue density when obtaining X-ray images from various angles and levels in the body (Fig. 14-4).

Related Nursing Responsibilities

For the client undergoing a radiographic examination, nursing responsibilities include:

- Assess vital signs before the examination to provide a baseline and to help detect changes in the client's condition during or after the procedure.
- Remove any metal items such as a religious medal or clothing that contains metal such as the hooks and eyes on a bra. Metal produces a dense image that may be confused with a tissue abnormality.
- Request a lead apron or collar to shield a fetus or vulnerable body parts during X-rays.
- If the radiographic study involves administration of a contrast medium, ask the client about allergies, especially to seafood or iodine, or previous adverse reactions such as a vasovagal response (reflex that occurs when circulating blood is diverted to the legs rather than the head, resulting in dizziness and fainting) during a diagnostic examination. A reaction can range from mild nausea and vomiting to shock and death.

BOX 14-5	Metal Devices That Prohibit a Magnetic Resonance Imaging
Within the Body	**On the Body (Must Be Removed)**
Metallic spinal rod	Purse, wallet, money clip, credit cards, cards with magnetic strips
Plates, pins, screws, or metal mesh used to repair a bone or joint	Electronic devices such as beepers, cell phones, smartphones, and tablets
Joint replacement or prosthesis	External hearing aids
Metallic jewelry including those used for body piercing or body modification	Metallic jewelry and watches
Some tattoos or tattooed eyeliner (these alter MRI, and there is a chance of skin irritation or swelling; black and blue pigments are the most troublesome)	Pens, paper clips, keys, coins
Makeup (such as eye shadow and eyeliner), nail polish, or other cosmetic that contains metal	Hair barrettes, hairpins, hair clips, and some hair ointments
Dental fillings or braces (while usually unaffected by the magnetic field, these may distort images of the facial area or brain; the same is true for orthodontic braces and retainers)	Shoes, belt buckles, safety pins
	Any article of clothing that has metallic fibers or threads, metal-based antibacterial compounds, metallic zippers, buttons, snaps, hooks, or underwire

RadiologyInfo.org. (2024). *MRI safety*. https://www.radiologyinfo.org/en/info/safety-mr#:~:text=Objects%20that%20may%20interfere%20with%20 image%20quality%20if,blue%20pigments%20are%20the%20most%20troublesome%29%20More%20items

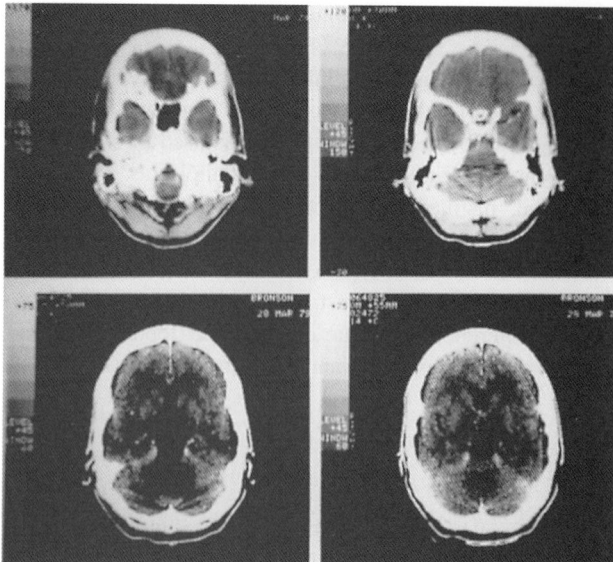

FIGURE 14-4 Cross sections of a cranial computed tomography scan. (Photo by K. Timby.)

- Know the location of emergency equipment and drugs in case there is an unexpected allergic reaction to the contrast medium.
- To avoid interference with subsequent visual imaging, schedule procedures requiring iodine before those that use barium.
- To promote urinary excretion, encourage the client to drink a large amount of fluid after an examination involving iodine to promote its excretion.
- Check on bowel elimination and stool characteristics for at least 2 days after the administration of an oral barium contrast medium. Barium retention can lead to constipation and bowel obstruction. Report an absence of bowel elimination beyond 2 days. The administration of a prescribed laxative is often necessary.

Endoscopic Examinations

Endoscopy (a visual examination of internal structures) is performed using optical scopes. Endoscopes have lighted mirror–lens systems attached to a tube and are quite flexible so that they can be advanced through curved structures.

Endoscopic examinations are named primarily for the structure being examined (Box 14-6). In addition to allowing the examiner to inspect the appearance of a structure, endoscopes also have attachments that permit various forms of treatment or the collection of specimens

---

BOX 14-6   **Examples of Endoscopic Examinations**

- *Bronchoscopy*—inspection of the bronchi
- *Gastroscopy*—inspection of the stomach
- *Colonoscopy*—inspection of the colon
- *Esophagogastroduodenoscopy*—inspection of the esophagus, stomach, and duodenum
- *Laparoscopy*—inspection of the abdominal cavity
- *Cystoscopy*—inspection of the urinary bladder

---

for microscopic analysis. Endoscopic examinations that produce discomfort or anxiety are performed under a light, short-acting form of anesthesia, sometimes referred to as *conscious sedation*. When conscious sedation is used, clients may have no memory of having had the test, even though they communicate and interact with staff during its performance.

Endoscopic examinations are being performed more frequently on an outpatient basis and in the physician's office. They are an economic alternative to invasive tests and procedures that previously required surgery to determine a diagnosis.

For the client undergoing an endoscopy, nursing responsibilities include:

- To prevent aspiration, withhold food and fluids or advise the client to do so for at least 6 hours before any procedure in which an endoscope is inserted into the upper airway or upper gastrointestinal tract.
- If conscious sedation is used, monitor the client's vital signs, breathing, oxygen saturation (using pulse oximetry; see Chapter 21), and cardiac rhythm. Have oxygen and resuscitation equipment readily available.
- If topical anesthesia is used to facilitate the passage of an endoscope into the airway or upper gastrointestinal tract, withhold food or fluids for at least 2 hours after the procedure and until swallow, cough, and gag reflexes return.
- Relieve the client's sore throat with ice chips, fluids, or gargles when it is safe to do so.
- Confirm that a bowel preparation using laxatives and enemas has been completed before endoscopic procedures of the lower intestine.
- Report difficulty in arousing a client or any sharp pain, fever, unusual bleeding, nausea, vomiting, or difficulty with urination after any endoscopic examination.

>>> **Stop, Think, and Respond 14-1**
Explain why it is important for clients to have a sigmoidoscopy.

Skill 14-2 describes the nurse's role when assisting with a sigmoidoscopy.

Radionuclide Imaging

Radionuclides are elements that have molecular structures that are altered to produce radiation. They are identified by a superscript number followed by a chemical symbol, such as ^{131}I (radioactive iodine) and ^{99}Tc (radioactive technetium). When radionuclides are instilled in the body, usually by the intravenous route, particular tissues or organs absorb them. A scanning device that detects radiation creates an image of the size, shape, and concentration of the organ containing the radionuclide. The terms **hot spot** (area where the radionuclide is intensely concentrated) and **cold spot** (area with little if any radionuclide concentration) refer to the amount of radiation that the tissue absorbs. **Positron emission tomography** (PET) combines the technology of radionuclide scanning with the layered analysis of tomography.

Radionuclide imaging offers two advantages over standard radiography; it visualizes areas within organs and tissues that are not possible with standard X-rays, and it involves less exposure to radiation than with roentgenography. Tests using radionuclides, however, are contraindicated for clients who are pregnant or breastfeeding; the energy released is harmful to the rapidly growing cells of an infant or fetus.

For the client undergoing radionuclide imaging, nursing responsibilities include:

- Inquire about a client's menstrual and obstetric history. Notify the **nuclear medicine department** (the unit responsible for radionuclide imaging) if the client is pregnant, could possibly be pregnant, or is breastfeeding.
- Ask about the allergy history because iodine is commonly used in radionuclide examinations.
- Assist the client with a gown, robe, and slippers. Make sure that the client has no internal metal devices or external metal objects because these interfere with diagnostic findings.
- Obtain an accurate weight because the dose of radionuclide is calculated according to weight.
- Inform the client that they will be radioactive for a brief period (usually less than 24 hours) but that body fluids, such as urine, stool, and emesis, can be safely flushed away.
- Instruct premenopausal clients to abstain from intercourse or use an effective contraceptive method for the short period during which radiation continues to be present.

Ultrasonography

Ultrasonography (a soft tissue examination that uses sound waves in ranges beyond human hearing) is also known as **echography**. During ultrasonography, which is similar to the echolocation used by bats, dolphins, and sonar devices on submarines, a handheld probe called a **transducer** projects sound through the body's surface. The sound waves cause vibrations within body tissues, producing images as the waves are reflected back toward the machine. The reflected sound waves are converted into a visual image called an *ultrasonogram*, *sonogram*, or *echogram*, which can be viewed in real time on a monitor and recorded for future analysis. Doppler ultrasound, discussed in Chapter 12, is a variation of this type of technology.

Ultrasound examinations are used to visualize breast, abdominal, and pelvic organs; male reproductive organs; structures in the head and neck; the heart and valves; and structures within the eyes. Air-filled structures such as the lungs or the intestines and extremely dense tissue such as bones do not image well. This type of examination is used in obstetrics to determine the fetal size, more than one fetus, and the location of the placenta. The outline of fetal anatomy during pregnancy is sometimes visible on ultrasound, allowing the client to find out the sex of the fetus prior to birth. Because ultrasound examinations do not involve radiation or contrast media, they are extremely safe diagnostic tools.

For the client undergoing ultrasonography, nursing responsibilities include:

- Schedule abdominal and pelvic ultrasonography before any examinations that use barium for the best visualization.

- Instruct clients undergoing an abdominal ultrasonography to drink five to six full glasses of fluid approximately 1 to 2 hours before the test. To ensure a full bladder, urination should be avoided until after the test is completed.
- Explain that acoustic gel, which may feel cold, is applied over the area where the transducer is placed.

Electrical Graphic Recordings

Machines can record electrical impulses from structures such as the heart, brain, and skeletal muscles. These tests are identified by the prefix "electro-" as in **electrocardiography** (ECG or EKG, an examination of the electrical activity in the heart); **electroencephalography** (EEG, an examination of the energy emitted by the brain); and **electromyography** (EMG, an examination of the energy produced by stimulated muscles).

To detect electrical activity, wires called *electrodes* are attached to the skin (or muscle in the case of an EMG). They transmit electrical activity to a machine that converts it into a series of waveforms (Fig. 14-5). Except for an awareness of the electrodes, the client undergoing an ECG or EEG usually does not experience any other sensations. Occasionally, there is slight discomfort during an EMG.

For the client undergoing an ECG, nursing responsibilities include:

- Clean the skin and clip hair in the area where the electrode tabs will be placed to ensure adherence and to reduce discomfort on removal.
- Attach the adhesive electrode tabs to the skin where the electrode wires will be fastened.
- Avoid attaching the adhesive tabs over bones, scars, or breast tissue.

For the client undergoing an EEG, nursing responsibilities include:

- Instruct the client to shampoo the hair the evening before the procedure to facilitate firm attachment of the electrodes. They should shampoo the hair after the test to remove adhesive from the scalp.
- Withhold coffee, tea, and cola beverages for 8 hours before the procedure. Consult with the physician about withholding scheduled medications, especially those that affect neurologic activity.

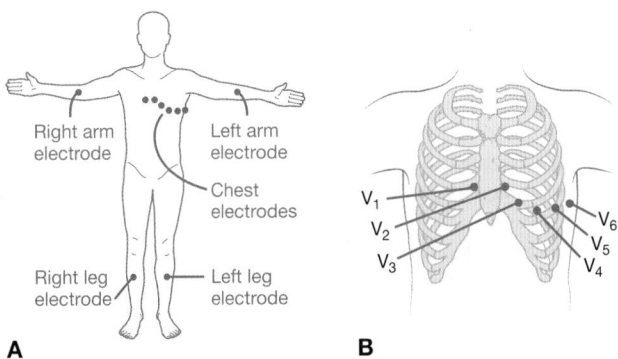

A   **B**

FIGURE 14-5 Placement of electrocardiogram electrodes. **A.** Standard positions. **B.** Close-up view of chest electrode placement, at the standard positions.

- If a sleep-deprived EEG is scheduled, instruct the client that they must stay awake after midnight before the examination.

  For the client undergoing an EMG, nursing responsibilities include:

- Tell the client they will be instructed to contract and relax certain muscles during the examination.
- Explain that electrical current is applied to muscles during an EMG but that the sensation is not usually painful. Also, a muscle electrode is inserted with a small-gauge needle in 10 or more locations, but the experience is painless unless it touches a terminal nerve in the area.

Diagnostic Laboratory Tests

Nurses, laboratory personnel, and physicians collect specimens such as blood, urine, stool, sputum, intestinal secretions, spinal fluid, and drainage from wounds or infected tissue. They repeat tests on collected specimens at intervals to monitor the progress of clients. Students can refer to laboratory manuals to learn the purpose of specific tests and the associated nursing responsibilities.

Several examples of specimen collection are discussed in future chapters where they are more pertinent. Nursing responsibilities for assisting with a paracentesis and a lumbar puncture, collecting a specimen for a throat culture, and measuring capillary blood glucose are followed.

Assisting with a Paracentesis

A **paracentesis** is a procedure for withdrawing fluid from the abdominal cavity. A physician always performs it with the assistance of a nurse. A paracentesis is done most commonly to relieve abdominal pressure and to improve breathing, which generally becomes labored when fluid crowds the lungs. Sometimes, paracentesis removes 1 L (approximately 1 qt) or more of fluid. The physician may send a specimen of the fluid to the laboratory for microscopic examination (Nursing Guidelines 14-1).

 NURSING GUIDELINES 14-1

Assisting with a Paracentesis

- Explain the procedure or clarify the physician's explanation to the client. *Explanations prepare the client for an unfamiliar experience or promote a clearer understanding.*
- Ensure that the client has signed the consent form if needed. *A consent form provides legal protection.*
- Measure and record the client's weight, blood pressure, and respiratory rate; measure abdominal girth at its widest point with a tape measure. *These data serve as a basis for postprocedural comparisons.*
- Obtain a prepackaged paracentesis kit along with a vial of local anesthetic. *Gathering supplies promotes efficient time management.*
- Make sure that extra gloves, a gown, a mask, and goggles are available. *These items protect against contact with microorganisms, such as human immunodeficiency virus (HIV), that may be in the blood or other body fluids.*
- Encourage the client to empty the bladder just before the procedure. *An empty bladder prevents accidental puncture of the bladder.*
- Place the client in a sitting position. *This position pools abdominal fluid in the lower areas of the abdomen and displaces the intestines posteriorly.*
- Hold the container of local anesthetic so the physician can withdraw a sufficient amount. *Doing so prevents contaminating the physician's sterile gloves.*
- Offer the client support as an area of the abdomen is anesthetized, then pierced with an instrument called a *trocar*, and a hollow sheath called a *cannula* is inserted (see figure). *Empathetic concern helps to relieve anxiety.*
- Reassess the client periodically after the cannula insertion; expect that blood pressure and respiratory rate may decrease. *Assessment indicates the client's response.*
- Place a Band-Aid or small dressing over the puncture site after withdrawal of the cannula. *The dressing acts as a barrier to microorganisms and absorbs drainage.*
- Assist the client into a position of comfort. *Doing so demonstrates concern for the client's welfare.*

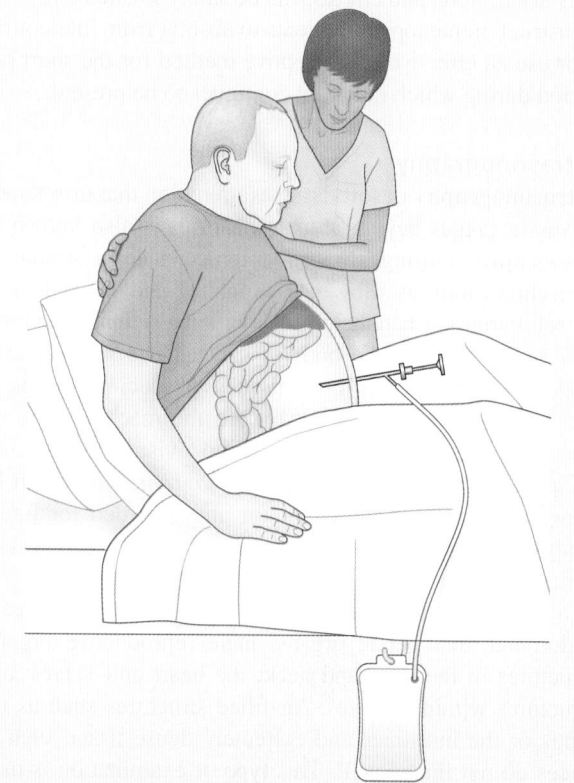

The nurse offers support during an abdominal paracentesis.

- Measure the volume of fluid withdrawn. *This measurement contributes to an accurate assessment of fluid volume.*
- Label the specimen, if ordered, and send it to the laboratory with the appropriate requisition form. *Doing so facilitates an appropriate analysis.*
- Document pertinent information such as the appearance and volume of the fluid, client assessments, and disposition of the specimen. *Such documentation adds essential data to the client's medical record.*

Assisting with a Lumbar Puncture

The physician requires nursing assistance when performing a **lumbar puncture or spinal tap**. This procedure involves inserting a needle between lumbar vertebrae in the spinal canal but below the spinal cord itself. The physician advances the tip of the needle until it is beneath the middle layer of the membrane surrounding the spinal cord. They measure the spinal fluid pressure and then withdraw a small amount of fluid.

This test is performed for various reasons. It is used to diagnose conditions that raise the pressure within the brain, such as brain or spinal cord tumors, or infections such as meningitis. Spinal fluid also is withdrawn before instilling a contrast medium for X-rays of the spinal column. Finally, the treatment of some conditions requires the instillation of drugs directly into the spinal fluid after withdrawing a similar amount (Nursing Guidelines 14-2).

Collecting a Specimen for a Throat Culture

A **culture** (an incubation of microorganisms) is performed by collecting body fluid or substances suspected of containing infectious microorganisms, growing the living microorganisms in a nutritive substance, and examining their characteristics with a microscope. Cultures are performed

NURSING GUIDELINES 14-2

Assisting with a Lumbar Puncture

- Explain the procedure or clarify the physician's explanation to the client. *Explanations prepare the client for an unfamiliar experience or promote a clearer understanding.*
- Ensure the client has signed the consent form if needed. *A consent form provides legal protection.*
- Perform a basic neurologic examination including the client's pupil size and response and muscle strength and sensation in all four extremities. *This information provides a baseline for future comparisons.*
- Encourage the client to empty the bladder. *An empty bladder promotes comfort during the procedure.*
- Administer a sedative drug if ordered. *Sedatives reduce anxiety.*
- Obtain a prepackaged lumbar puncture kit along with a vial of local anesthetic. *Gathering supplies promotes efficient time management.*
- Make sure that extra gloves, a gown, a mask, and goggles are available. *These items offer protection from contact with microorganisms, such as human immunodeficiency virus (HIV), that may be present in the blood or other body fluids.*
- Place the client on their side with the knees and neck acutely flexed (see figure) or in a sitting position, bent from the hips. *These positions separate the bony vertebrae.*
- Instruct the client that once the needle is inserted, they must avoid movement. *This prevents injury.*

- Hold the container of local anesthetic so the physician can withdraw a sufficient amount. *Doing so prevents contaminating the physician's sterile gloves.*
- Stabilize the client's position at the neck and knees. *This reinforces the need to remain motionless.*
- Support the client emotionally as the needle is inserted and the skin is injected with local anesthesia. *Empathetic concern helps relieve anxiety.*
- Tell the client that it is not unusual to feel pressure or a shooting pain down the leg. *This information prepares the client for expected sensations.*
- Perform a *Queckenstedt test*, if asked, by compressing each jugular vein separately for approximately 10 seconds while pressure is being measured. *A Queckenstedt test helps demonstrate if there is an obstruction in the circulation of spinal fluid. If so, the pressure remains unchanged, rises slightly, or takes longer than 20 seconds to return to baseline.*
- Observe that the physician fills three separate numbered containers with 5 to 10 mL in their appropriate sequence if laboratory analysis is desired. *In this way, if blood is present but in the least amount in the third container, its source is most likely trauma from the procedure rather than central nervous system pathology.*
- Place a Band-Aid or small dressing over the puncture site after the needle has been withdrawn. *The dressing acts as a barrier to microorganisms and absorbs drainage.*
- Position the client flat on the back or abdomen; instruct the client to remain flat and roll from side to side for the next several hours. *These measures reduce the potential for severe headache.*
- Reassess the client's neurologic status. Check the puncture site for bleeding or clear drainage. *Comparative data help the nurse evaluate changes in the client's condition.*
- Offer oral fluids frequently. *They restore the volume of spinal fluid.*
- Label the specimens, if ordered, and send them to the laboratory with the appropriate requisition form. *Doing so facilitates an appropriate analysis.*
- Document pertinent information such as the appearance of the fluid, client assessments, and disposition of the specimen. *Doing so adds essential data to the client's medical record.*

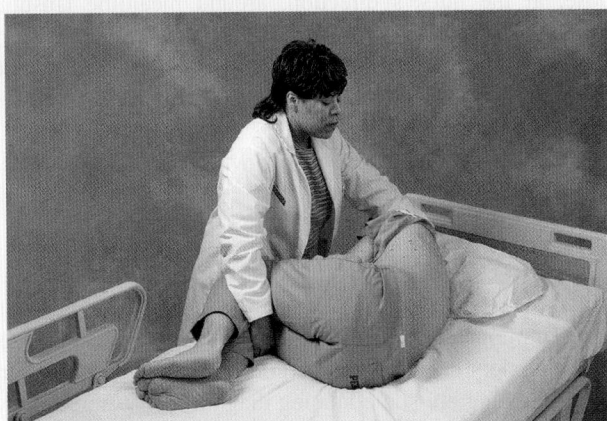

Positioning for lumbar puncture. (Photo by B. Proud.)

commonly on urine, blood, stool, wound drainage, and throat secretions.

To identify and treat the cause of a throat infection (commonly streptococcal bacteria), the nurse obtains a specimen from the throat. An abbreviated test that takes approximately 10 minutes is performed on throat specimens in many doctors' offices and student health clinics. A rapid preliminary diagnosis is made so that appropriate treatment can be initiated immediately. If the quick test is not clearly negative and symptoms strongly suggest a streptococcal infection, a follow-up specimen is obtained and sent to the laboratory for culturing. Conclusive results of a bacterial culture generally require 24 to 72 hours for sufficient microbial growth to take place.

Once bacteria grow within the nutritive medium, they are identified microscopically by their shape and by the color they acquire when stained with special dyes. **Gram staining** (a process of adding a dye to a microscopic specimen) is named after the Danish physician who developed the technique. The Gram stain helps determine whether bacteria are Gram positive or Gram negative. *Gram-positive bacteria* appear violet after staining. Those that repel the violet dye but appear red, the color of a counterstain, are called *Gram-negative bacteria* (Fischbach, Fischbach & Stout, 2021). *Streptococci* are round, grow in chains, and are Gram-positive bacteria.

When there is evidence of microbial growth and the infectious microorganism is identified, the most appropriate treatment can be provided. A throat culture is performed most often on young children who are susceptible to complications from upper respiratory infections and infection of the tonsils. Adults who tend to harbor infectious microorganisms in the pharynx, however, are also tested. A culture may be repeated after a course of treatment to determine its effectiveness (Nursing Guidelines 14-3).

Measuring Capillary Blood Glucose

Glucose is the type of sugar in blood that results from eating carbohydrates. A certain amount is always present to supply cells with a source of instant energy. The American Diabetes Association (2023) recommends that the amount of blood glucose before meals should range between 80 and 130 mg/dL (milligrams per deciliter) and less than 180 mg/dL within 1 to 2 hours after the beginning of a meal when using a blood sample drawn from a finger. The body produces the hormones glucagon and insulin, which regulate glucose metabolism and maintain normal blood glucose levels.

People with diabetes have an impaired ability to produce or utilize insulin and have difficulty regulating blood glucose levels. They control their disease with diet, exercise, and, in some cases, medications. People with diabetes may experience low or high blood glucose levels, both of which can have life-threatening consequences. Therefore,

many clients with diabetes measure their own capillary blood glucose levels rather than having venous blood drawn for laboratory analysis.

A **glucometer** is an instrument that measures the amount of glucose in capillary blood. It operates by assessing the amount of light reflected through a chemical test strip (Fig. 14-6). Based on the amount of measured glucose in the blood, clients with diabetes adjust their intake of food or medication.

Because diabetes is so common, nurses frequently are called on to teach people who have been recently diagnosed how to test their own blood glucose levels. Nurses measure blood glucose levels for clients with diabetes who are hospitalized or being cared for in long-term care facilities. There are several important points to remember about measuring blood glucose:

1. Several types of glucometers are available. The user must follow the manufacturer's instructions for accurate use.
2. The blood glucose level is usually measured about 30 minutes before eating and before bedtime to determine what are likely to be the lowest levels of glucose. This allows time for the client to increase or decrease food consumption or, if insulin dependent, to administer additional prescribed insulin (see Chapter 34), referred to as *coverage*.
3. Measuring blood glucose involves a risk for contact with blood. Because blood may contain infectious viruses, nurses *always* wear gloves when performing this test.

Because piercing the skin to obtain a sample of blood is uncomfortable, some people with diabetes avoid testing their blood glucose levels as often as they should. The **insulin pump** is a solution to decrease the need for continuous piercing of the skin (Fig. 14-7). Insulin pumps measure sugar levels in the body and send data to the pump. The insulin pump then delivers insulin to the body through a thin, flexible tube called an *infusion set* as needed. The devices can deliver insulin in two ways: in a steady measured and continuous dose (the "basal" insulin), or as a surge ("bolus") dose, at the nurse's direction, around mealtime (Insulin Pumps, 2022).

Some devices can be paired with a smartphone app. The client is able to view blood sugar levels, and insulin doses without removing the device.

Skill 14-3 presents the steps involved in using a lancet and LifeScan glucometer.

NURSING IMPLICATIONS

Most clients who undergo special examinations and tests have emotional needs from the stress of a potential diagnosis or the anxiety created by undergoing something unfamiliar. The following are some nursing diagnoses that nurses may

NURSING GUIDELINES 14-3

Collecting a Specimen for a Throat Culture

- Check with the physician about proceeding with the throat culture if the client is taking antibiotics. *Antibiotics affect test results.*
- Delay collecting a specimen if the client has recently used an antiseptic gargle. *Such gargles affect the test's diagnostic value.*
- Explain the purpose of and technique for obtaining the culture. *Explanations help reduce anxiety and promote cooperation.*
- Collect supplies: sterile culture swab, glass slide, tongue blade, gloves, mask if the client is coughing, paper tissues, and an emesis basin if the client gags. *Doing so facilitates organization and efficient time management.*
- Have the client sit where light is optimal. *Light enhances inspection of the throat anatomy.*
- Put on gloves and a mask if necessary. *Their use reduces the potential for transferring microorganisms.*
- Loosen the cap on the tube in which the swab is located. *Doing so facilitates hand dexterity.*
- Tell the client to open the mouth wide, stick out the tongue, and tilt the head back. *This position promotes access to the back of the throat.*
- Depress the middle of the tongue with a tongue blade in your nondominant hand (Fig. A). *Doing so opens the pathway for the swab.*
- Rub and twist the tip of the swab around the tonsil areas and the back of the throat without touching the lips, teeth, or tongue. *Doing so transfers microorganisms from the inflamed tissue to the swab* (Fig. B).

- Be prepared for the client's gagging. *Stroking the back of the throat stimulates the gag reflex.*
- Remove the swab and discard the tongue blade in a lined receptacle. *This measure controls the spread of microorganisms.*
- Spread the secretions on the swab across the glass slide. *Doing so prepares a specimen for quick staining and microscopic examination.*
- Replace the swab securely within the tube, taking care not to touch the outside of the container. *This method avoids collecting unrelated microorganisms and provides containment for the collected specimen.*
- Crush the packet in the bottom of the tube. *Crushing releases nourishing fluid to promote bacterial growth.*
- Remove gloves, discard them in a lined receptacle, and wash your hands or perform hand antisepsis with an alcohol rub (see Chapter 10). *These steps reduce the transmission of microorganisms.*
- Label the culture tube with the client's name, the date and time, and the source of the specimen. *These steps provide laboratory personnel with essential information.*
- Attend to the staining and examination of the prepared glass slide if appropriate. *Doing so provides tentative identification of streptococcal bacteria.*
- Deliver the sealed culture tube to the laboratory or refrigerate it if there will be a delay of longer than 1 hour. *These steps ensure that the microorganisms will grow when transferred to other culture media.*

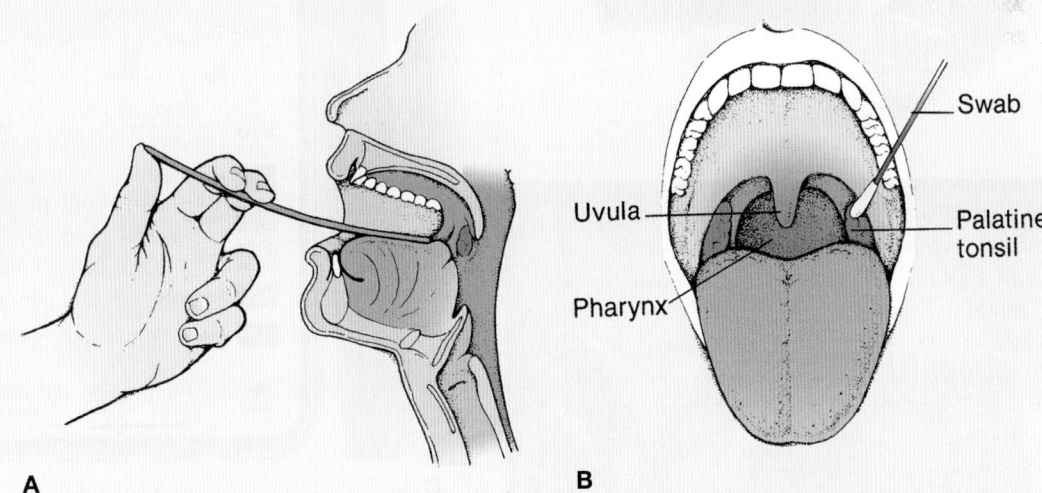

A   **B**

A throat culture. **A.** Depressing the tongue. **B.** Obtaining a specimen.

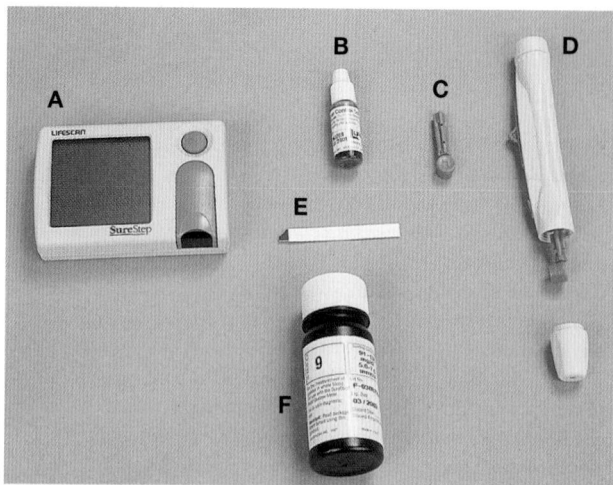

FIGURE 14-6 Equipment used to perform capillary blood glucose testing: a glucometer **(A)**, control solution **(B)**, a lancet **(C)**, a lancet holder **(D)**, a test strip **(E)**, and a container of test strips **(F)**. (Photo by B. Proud.)

identify during preprocedural and postprocedural stages of examinations and tests:

- Acute anxiety
- Fear
- Altered health maintenance
- Knowledge deficiency

Discuss the nursing management for a client facing this life-altering situation. See Nursing Care Plan 14-1.

Nursing Care Plan 14-1 illustrates the nursing process as it relates to the nursing diagnosis of Acute anxiety, defined by the American Psychiatric Association (APA) as persistent worry, uncertainty about the course of action to be taken when choice among competing actions involves risk, loss, or challenge to values and beliefs.

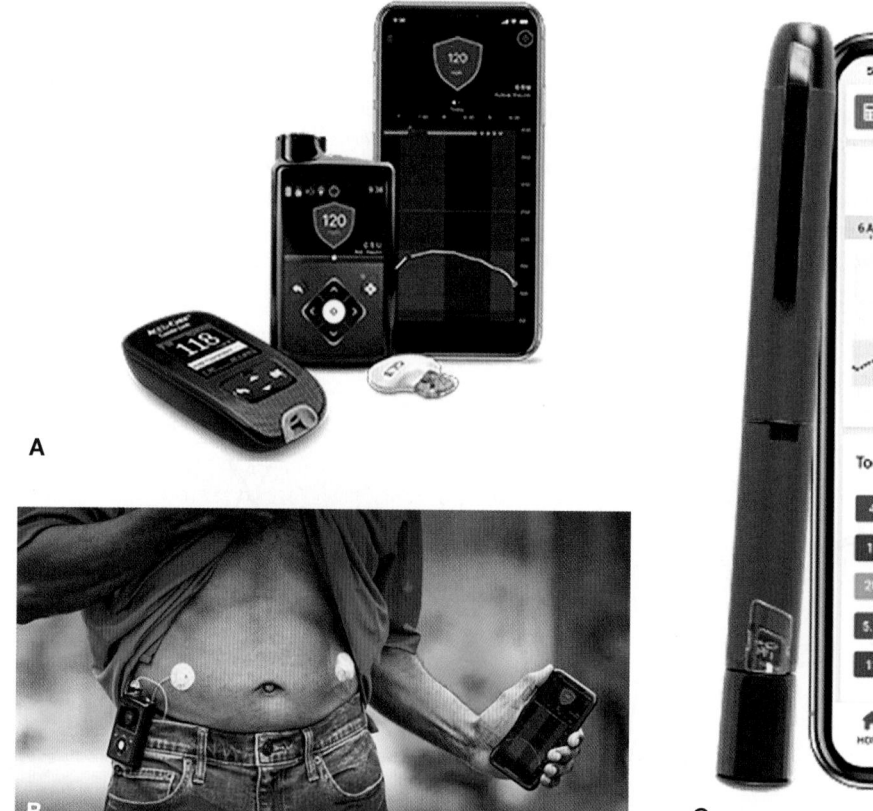

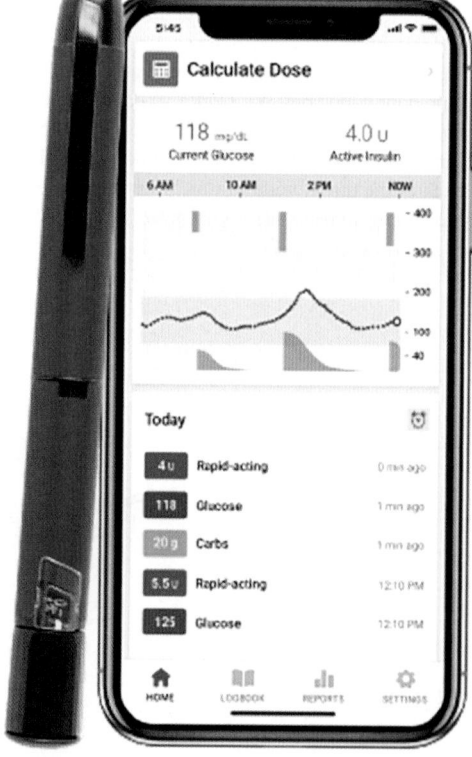

FIGURE 14-7 Insulin pump. **A.** Equipment used for an insulin pump. **B.** Example of the placement of the insulin pump on the body. **C.** Smartphone app. (A & C Insulin pump therapy. [2022]. *Medtronic 770G system.* https://www.medtronicdiabetes.com/treatments/insulin-pump-therapy. B. Taylor's Clinical Nursing Skills [2022].)

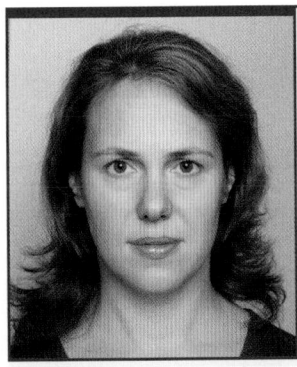

Clinical Scenario A healthy 32-year-old female is in her 16th week of an unplanned pregnancy. A previous ultrasound indicated that the fetus might have a possible chromosomal defect. The client is scheduled for an amniocentesis, a procedure in which a sample of amniotic fluid is obtained from the pregnant uterus, in this case, to diagnose genetic defects. The client's parents live in another state and are not supportive of this pregnancy. The father of the fetus has severed his relationship with the client. Caring for an infant with a disability would result in the client either having to change her employment or become dependent on government assistance. Depending on the results of the amniocentesis, the client must decide whether to carry the fetus to term or undergo an elective abortion before 20 weeks of gestation.

See Nursing Care Plan 14-1.

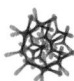

NURSING CARE PLAN 14-1   Acute Anxiety

Assessment
Determine the following:
- Signs of distress, such as restlessness, tachycardia, increased muscle tension, and rapid respirations
- Values and beliefs about terminating a pregnancy

- Remarks indicating uncertainty about subsequent choices pending the outcome of the amniocentesis
- Feelings of anguish or ambivalence regarding the decision to either carry the fetus to term or abort it

Nursing Diagnosis. Acute anxiety related to birthing options as evidenced by tearfulness, sleep disturbance, heart rate of 90–100 bpm at rest, request for visitation from a clergyperson, reading their Bible, and statement, "I don't feel I can make a decision about this."

Expected Outcome. The client will make an informed choice about the outcome of the current pregnancy within 1 week when the results of the amniocentesis are known.

Interventions	Rationales
Acknowledge the client's distress.	Empathy demonstrates awareness of the client's emotional state.
Convey an accepting nonjudgmental attitude.	An unbiased approach enhances the open expression of feelings.
Offer referrals to pro-choice and right-to-life groups and organizations that provide information about the disorder that may affect the client's child.	Consulting others helps clarify issues and decreases feelings of helplessness.
Encourage the client to discuss concerns with other significant people.	Sharing concerns with others helps the client perceive conflicts more realistically and facilitates implementation of a subsequent plan.
Suggest that the client compose a written list of the advantages and disadvantages to possible choices before the return appointment.	Identifying the pros and cons of alternatives is the first step in formulating a decision.
Give verbal recognition for efforts made to reach a solution.	Acknowledgment improves the client's ability to cope with the burden of a difficult decision.
Support the client's decision even if it would not be your personal choice.	Clients have the right to autonomy and self-determination.

Evaluation of Expected Outcome

Client makes a decision with the support of significant others to continue pregnancy carrying a fetus that will have cystic fibrosis.

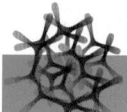

KEY POINTS

- Diagnostic examination: A procedure that involves the physical inspection of body structures and evidence of their functions
- Laboratory test: A procedure that involves the examination of body fluids or specimens
- Nurses have general responsibilities related to examinations and testing according to each facility's protocol. These may include:
  - Teaching clients
  - Assisting clients
  - Assisting physicians
- Procedures require differing positions for the clients. Be sure to explain them and know the specific positions related to the procedure.
- Nurse responsibilities for specimens collected during an examination:
  - Collects the specimen in an appropriate container

- Labels the specimen container with the correct information
- Attaches the proper laboratory request form
- Ensures that the specimen does not decompose before it can be examined
- Delivers the specimen to the laboratory as soon as possible
- Nurses must consider the implications of examinations and tests when caring for the gerontologic population:
  - Consider the mentation of the client and if they need help understanding the procedures.
  - The client may need extra blankets or clothing due to cold waiting rooms or examination areas.
  - Examination preparation may leave the client weak and dizzy.
  - After examinations or testing, encourage fluids because diminished thirst sensation can put the client at risk for dehydration.

CRITICAL THINKING EXERCISES

1. Discuss how the procedure for a sigmoidoscopy or another test or examination may differ if performed on an outpatient basis rather than in a hospital.
2. How might diminished mentation (the capacity to understand), reduced strength and stamina, and pain affect the performance of a diagnostic examination or test?
3. How might a pelvic examination be different if the person being examined is a survivor of rape?
4. How can a nurse respond to a client who is uncertain about having a lumbar puncture because of a fear of paralysis from trauma to the spinal cord?

NEXT-GENERATION NCLEX-STYLE REVIEW QUESTIONS

1. Following the nurse's preparation of a client who is scheduled for a sigmoidoscopy, which of the following indicates that a client needs more teaching?
   a. The client says an anesthetic will be given before the examination.
   b. The client says a light meal is allowed the evening before the examination.
   c. The client says a flexible scope will be inserted into the rectum.
   d. The client says prescribed medications may be taken in the morning.
   Test-Taking Strategy: Analyze the information the question asks. In this question, select the client's statement that is incorrect.

2. Which nursing action is essential before performing a chest roentgenogram?
   a. Make sure that the client does not eat food.
   b. Remove the client's metal necklace.
   c. Have the client swallow contrast dye.
   d. Administer a dose of pain medication.
   Test-Taking Strategy: Use the key word "essential" to identify an option that represents a priority.

3. Which nursing instruction is most appropriate if a specimen for a Pap test will be obtained at the time of a pelvic examination?
   a. Do not douche for several days before your appointment.
   b. Stop using any and all forms of contraception temporarily.
   c. Drink at least 1 qt of liquid 1 hour before your appointment.
   d. Take a mild laxative the night before your scheduled appointment.
   Test-Taking Strategy: Use the key word and modifier "most appropriate" to select the one option that is better than any of the others.

4. Which nursing actions are correct when measuring a client's capillary blood glucose? Select all that apply.
   a. Plan to perform the test 1 hour before a meal.
   b. Check that the test strip code matches the one programmed in the glucometer.
   c. Have the client wash their hands with soap and water before the test.
   d. Pierce the central pad of the thumb or fingers with the lancet.
   e. Cover the test spot on the test strip completely with a drop of blood.
   Test-Taking Strategy: Analyze the options and select those that are accurate.

5. When assisting with a pelvic examination during which a Pap smear will be obtained, place the steps the nurse should follow in the order in which they are performed.
   a. Hand the examiner a brush applicator.
   b. Deposit the applicator in a chemical fixative solution.
   c. Place the client in a lithotomy position.
   d. Lubricate the examiner's gloved fingers.
   e. Provide the examiner with a vaginal speculum.
   Test-Taking Strategy: Arrange the nursing actions in the sequence the nurse would follow when assisting with a pelvic examination and collection of cervical and endocervical cells.

NEXT-GENERATION NCLEX-STYLE CLINICAL SCENARIO QUESTIONS

Clinical Scenario:

A healthy 32-year-old female is in her 16th week of an unplanned pregnancy. A previous ultrasound indicated that the fetus might have a possible chromosomal defect. The client is scheduled for an amniocentesis, a procedure in which a sample of amniotic fluid is obtained from the pregnant uterus, in this case, to diagnose genetic defects. The client's parents live in another state and are not supportive of this pregnancy. The father of the fetus has severed his relationship with the client. Caring for an infant with a disability would result in the client either having to change her employment or become dependent on government assistance. Depending on the results of the amniocentesis, the client must decide whether to carry the fetus to term or undergo an elective abortion before 20 weeks of gestation.

1. Place an "x" under "effective" to identify methods that will show support for the client's decisions. Place an "x" under "ineffective" to identify unsupportive behavior.

METHODS	EFFECTIVE	INEFFECTIVE
Convey a judgmental attitude.		
Encourage the client to discuss concerns with significant others.		
Give verbal recognition for making decisions.		
Relate pros and cons of possible choices.		
Give the client pamphlets with information and send them home.		

SKILL 14-1 Assisting with a Pelvic Examination

Suggested Action	Reason For Action
ASSESSMENT	
Determine the identity of the client on whom the examination will be performed.	Prevents errors
Determine whether a Pap test is needed.	Indicates the need for additional equipment and supplies
Find out whether the client has had a pelvic examination before.	Provides a basis for teaching
Ask whether the client is currently menstruating or has had intercourse within the last 48 hours.	Blood, semen, and lubricant are three substances that obscure and distort cells, making it difficult to determine whether they are atypical and interfering with the microscopic examination of collected specimens. The examiner may wish to delay obtaining a specimen.
Inquire whether the client has douched or used vaginal hygiene products in the last 24 hours.	Suggests a need to reschedule the Pap test because an adequate sample of cells and secretions may not be available
Ask the client's age, date of the last menstrual period, number of pregnancies and live births, and description of symptoms such as bleeding or drainage, itching, or pain.	Provides data to determine the possibility of pregnancy, to compare cellular specimens with hormonal activity, and to provide clues as to possible pathology and the need for additional tests
Determine whether and what type of birth control the client is using if is the client is premenopausal. For oral contraceptives, identify the name of the drug and the dosage.	Correlates the influence of prescribed hormones on cellular specimens
Ask menopausal patients whether they are taking hormone replacement, and the brand name and dosage.	Correlates the influence of prescribed hormones on cellular specimens
Observe for impaired strength or joint limitation.	Suggests the need to modify the examination position
PLANNING	
Explain the procedure and give the client an opportunity to ask questions.	Tends to reduce anxiety
Provide an examination gown and direct the client to empty the bladder.	Facilitates palpation of the uterus and ovaries
Place a **speculum** (a metal or a disposable plastic instrument for widening the vagina), gloves, examination light, lubricant, and the following materials for the Pap smear: long soft applicators and spatula and at least three glass slides, a chemical fixative, and a container for holding the slides on the counter or on a tray in the examination room (Fig. A). (The liquid-based cytology [ThinPrep Pap Test], an alternative technique of specimen preservation approved by the U.S. Food and Drug Administration, eliminates using slides; instead, it involves rinsing the collection tool within a liquid transport medium.)	Promotes efficient time management; metal specula (plural of speculum) are reused after sterilization; select an appropriate size according to the individual client. Use of a liquid medium for transporting specimens eliminates debris that adheres to slides and increases the accuracy of a diagnostic assessment of cells.

A

Equipment used for a pelvic examination

Mark one slide with an E for endocervical, another with a C for cervical, and the last with a V for vaginal.	Identifies the location from which the specimens are taken; *endocervical* means inside the cervix; the cervix is the lower portion of the uterus, or womb.
Arrange for a female nurse to be with the client during the examination, especially if the examiner is male.	Reduces the potential for claims of sexual impropriety

SKILL 14-1 Assisting with a Pelvic Examination (*continued*)

Suggested Action	Reason For Action
Plan to assist with the collection of the vaginal and cervical secretions for the Pap test before the examiner proceeds to palpate the internal organs.	Prevents lubricant used during palpation from interfering with a microscopic examination of the specimens

IMPLEMENTATION

Suggested Action	Reason For Action
Place the client's legs in stirrups to facilitate a lithotomy position (Fig. B); use an alternative position, such as Sims or dorsal recumbent, if the client is disabled.	Provides access to the vagina

Lithotomy position

Suggested Action	Reason For Action
Cover the client with a cotton or paper drape.	Maintains modesty and privacy
Introduce the examiner to the client if the two are strangers.	Tends to reduce anxiety
Fold back the drape just before the examination begins.	Exposes the genitalia while minimizing client exposure
Direct the examination light from behind the examiner's shoulder toward the vaginal opening.	Illuminates the area, facilitating inspection
Wet the speculum with warm water; if a Pap smear will not be obtained, apply water-soluble lubricant to the speculum blades.	Eases and provides comfort during insertion
Prepare the client to expect the momentary insertion of the speculum. Explain that the client will hear a loud click as it locks in place.	Tends to reduce anxiety and aids in relaxation
Hand the examiner a soft-tipped applicator, spatula, and brush applicator in that order (Fig. C).	Facilitates collection of secretions for the Pap smear

Insertion of speculum and spatula. (From Mayo Clinic. [2023]. *Pap smear*. https://www.mayoclinic.org/tests-procedures/pap-smear/about/pac-20394841. Used with permission of Mayo Foundation for Medical Education and Research, all rights reserved.)

Suggested Action	Reason For Action
Position the lined receptacle so the examiner can dispose of the collection device and the speculum after use.	Controls the spread of microorganisms
If using the liquid-based cytology technique, immerse the sampling device in the container of solution, cap it, and discard the tool	Disperses the cells and breaks up blood, mucus, and nondiagnostic debris

(*continued*)

SKILL 14-1 Assisting with a Pelvic Examination (*continued*)

Suggested Action	Reason For Action
Lubricate the gloved fingers of the examiner's dominant hand and prepare the client for an internal vaginal (and, in some cases, rectal) examination.	Reduces friction; keeps the client informed of the progress of the examination
Put on gloves and clean the skin of lubricant when the examination is completed; then remove the gloves.	Prevents the transmission of microorganisms; promotes comfort and hygiene
Wash hands or perform hand antisepsis with an alcohol rub (see Chapter 10).	Reduces microorganisms on the hands
Lower both feet simultaneously from the stirrups and assist the client to sit up.	Reduces strain on abdominal and back muscles
Assist the client from the room after client has dressed.	Maintains client safety

EVALUATION

- Client demonstrated understanding of the purpose for the examination.
- Client assumed and was maintained in a satisfactory position for examination.
- Client privacy, comfort, and safety were maintained.
- Specimens were collected, identified, and preserved.

DOCUMENT

- Date and time
- Pertinent preassessment data, if any
- Type of examination, including any specimens collected
- Examiner and/or location
- Condition of the client after the examination
- Disposition of specimens

SAMPLE DOCUMENTATION

Date and Time Taken to examination room by wheelchair for pelvic examination by Dr. Wood. Able to assume lithotomy position without difficulty. Smears of endocervical, cervical, and vaginal specimens obtained and sent to lab. Returned to room by wheelchair and assisted into bed. _____ J. Doe, LPN

SKILL 14-2 Assisting with a Sigmoidoscopy

Suggested Action	Reason for Action
ASSESSMENT	
Identify the client on whom the examination will be performed.	Prevents errors
Check for a signed consent form.	Provides legal protection
Ask the client to describe the procedure.	Indicates the accuracy of the client's understanding and provides an opportunity to clarify the explanation
Inquire about the client's current symptoms and family history of significant diseases.	Provides information about the purpose for performing the procedure and an opportunity for reinforcing the need for future regular sigmoidoscopic examinations
Ask for a description of the client's dietary and fluid intake and bowel cleansing protocol and results.	Indicates whether the client complied with proper preparation for the procedure
Assess the client's vital signs and obtain other physical assessments according to agency policy, such as weight or bowel sounds.	Provides a baseline for future comparisons
Ask for an allergy history and a list of medications being taken.	Influences drugs that may be prescribed and alerts staff to other medical problems
PLANNING	
Direct the client to undress, put on an examination gown, and use the restroom.	Facilitates the examination and gives the client an opportunity to empty the bowel and bladder again

SKILL 14-2 Assisting with a Sigmoidoscopy (*continued*)

Suggested Action	Reason for Action
Prepare for the examination by placing a sigmoidoscope (Fig. A), gloves, gown, mask, goggles, lubricant, suction machine, and containers for biopsied tissue in the examination room.	Promotes efficient time management

A

Flexible sigmoidoscope

Suggested Action	Reason for Action
Check that the light at the end of the sigmoidoscope and the suction equipment are operational.	Avoids delay, inconvenience, and discomfort once the examination is in progress

IMPLEMENTATION

Suggested Action	Reason for Action
Help the client assume a Sims position if a flexible sigmoidoscope will be used, or a knee–chest position if a rigid sigmoidoscope, which is less common, is used.	Facilitates passage of the scope; an endoscopic table may be used in lieu of a self-maintained knee–chest position.
Cover the client with a cotton or paper drape.	Maintains modesty and privacy
Introduce the examiner to the client if the two are strangers.	Tends to reduce anxiety
Lubricate the examiner's gloved fingers.	Reduces discomfort when the fingers are used to dilate the anal and rectal sphincters
Prepare the client for the introduction of the examiner's fingers followed by the insertion of the sigmoidoscope (Fig. B).	Tends to reduce anxiety by keeping the client informed of each step and the progress being made

B

The sigmoidoscope is advanced to the proximal sigmoid colon. (Designua/Shutterstock.)

Suggested Action	Reason for Action
Acknowledge any discomfort that the client may be experiencing; explain that it should be short-lived.	Indicates that the nurse empathizes with the client's distress
Inform the client if and before suction is used, air is introduced, or a sample of tissue is obtained.	Prepares the client for unexpected sensations or temporary increases in discomfort
Open the specimen container, cover the specimen with preservative, and recap the container.	Prevents the loss and decomposition of the specimen
Inform the client when the scope will be withdrawn.	Keeps the client informed of progress
Put on gloves and clean the skin of lubricant and stool after the examination is completed; remove the gloves.	Prevents the transmission of microorganisms; promotes comfort and hygiene

(*continued*)

SKILL 14-2 Assisting with a Sigmoidoscopy (*continued*)

Suggested Action	Reason for Action
Wash hands or perform hand antisepsis with an alcohol rub (see Chapter 10).	Reduces microorganisms
Assist the client from the room to an area where their clothing is located or provide a clean gown.	Maintains client safety and dignity
Explain that there may be slight abdominal discomfort until the instilled air has been expelled and that the client may observe some rectal bleeding if a biopsy was taken.	Provides anticipatory health teaching
Stress that if severe pain occurs or bleeding is excessive, the client should notify the physician.	Identifies significant data to report
Advise that the client may consume food and fluids as desired.	Clarifies dietary guidelines
Clean the sigmoidoscope and any other soiled equipment according to agency and infection control guidelines.	Prevents the transmission of microorganisms
Restore order and cleanliness to the examination room; restock supplies.	Prepares the room for future use
Complete the laboratory requisition form, label the specimen, and ensure that the specimen is transported to the laboratory for analysis.	Facilitates microscopic examination

EVALUATION

- Client demonstrated understanding of the purpose for the examination.
- Appropriate dietary and bowel preparations were carried out.
- Client assumed required position.
- Comfort and safety were maintained.
- Postprocedural instructions were given.
- Specimen was preserved, identified, and delivered appropriately.

DOCUMENT

- Date and time
- Pertinent preassessment data, if any
- Type of examination and specimen collected, if any
- Examiner and/or location
- Condition of the client after the examination
- Instructions provided
- Disposition of specimens

SAMPLE DOCUMENTATION

Date and Time   Arrived ambulatory for routine sigmoidoscopic examination. No current symptoms, no known allergies. Takes atenolol for hypertension. Last dose was @0700. BP 142/90 in the right arm while sitting. T—98.2°; P—90; R—22. Bowel sounds active in all four quadrants. Has eaten lightly this morning and self-administered two enemas last night with good results and one this morning with very little stool expelled. Placed in Sims position for examination. Biopsy omitted. Instructed to resume eating and taking fluid as desired. Explained that gas pains are possible and that walking about will help, but to notify Dr. Ross if the discomfort is prolonged or severe. Discharged ambulatory accompanied by wife. _____ J. Doe, LPN

SKILL 14-3 Using a Glucometer

Suggested Action	Reason for Action
ASSESSMENT	
Determine that a test using one or more control solutions has been performed on the glucometer since midnight in a health agency. Identify the client on whom the examination will be performed.	Determines that the glucometer is functioning accurately; complies with an agency's policies for quality assurance and prevents errors
Find out whether the client has ever had a blood glucose level measured with a glucometer or whether the client has any questions.	Provides a basis for teaching
Review previous blood glucose level and trends that may be obvious.	Helps evaluate the reliability of the assessed measurement when it is obtained

SKILL 14-3 Using a Glucometer (*continued*)

Suggested Action	Reason for Action
Check to see whether insulin coverage has been ordered if glucose levels are higher than normal.	Aids in quickly reducing high blood glucose levels
Check the date on the container of test strips; discard if the date has expired.	Determines whether test strips are still appropriate for use
Discard unused test strips stored in a vial 4 months after they are opened.	Ensures accuracy
Observe the code number on the container of test strips; compare it with the code number programmed into the glucometer (Figs. A and B).	Code numbers range from 1 to 16; if the numbers do not match, the meter number is changed.
	Comparing the code number on a test strip bottle to the glucometer code number. (Photo by B. Proud.)
	Finger inspection
Inspect the client's fingers and thumb for a nontraumatized area (Fig. B); some meters can use blood from the forearm, thigh, or fleshy part of the hand (Diabetes.org., 2024).	Avoids secondary trauma

PLANNING

Test the machine's calibration with a control strip or solution supplied by the manufacturer if it has not been done since midnight.	Verifies the machine's accuracy
Arrange care so that the test is performed approximately 30 minutes before a meal and at bedtime.	Ensures consistency in obtaining data and facilitates the detection of trends
Collect the necessary equipment and supplies: a glucometer, lancets, test strips, and gloves.	Promotes efficient time management

(*continued*)

SKILL 14-3 Using a Glucometer (*continued*)

Suggested Action	Reason for Action
IMPLEMENTATION	
Ask the client to wash their hands with soap and warm water and towel dry.	Reduces microorganisms on the skin; warmth dilates the capillaries and increases blood flow; swabbing with alcohol is not necessary and can alter the results if not totally evaporated.
Turn on the machine; observe the last blood glucose reading, current test strip code, and the message "Insert strip."	Prepares the machine for testing the blood sample; the machine retains the last glucose measurement in its memory.
Put on clean gloves after washing your hands or performing hand antisepsis with an alcohol rub (see Chapter 10).	Provides a barrier against contact with blood
Select a nontraumatized side of a client's finger or thumb; avoid the central pads (Fig. C).	Avoids puncturing an area with sensitive nerve endings

Appropriate puncture sites

C

Apply the lancet firmly to the side of the finger and press the release button (Fig. D).	Opens a path for blood

The lancet is pressed into the test site.

D

Hold the finger or thumb so that a large hanging drop of blood forms (Fig. E).	Uses gravity to aid in collecting blood

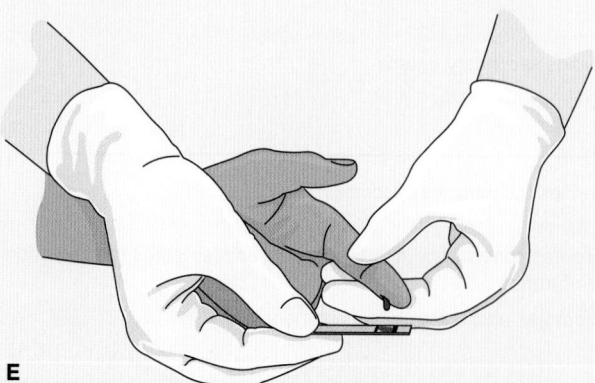

Obtaining a hanging drop of blood. (From LifeART image © [2015] Lippincott Williams & Wilkins.)

E

SKILL 14-3 Using a Glucometer (*continued*)

Suggested Action	Reason for Action
Touch the hanging drop of blood to the test spot on the strip, making sure that the spot is completely covered and stays wet during the test (Fig. F).	Saturates the test spot to ensure accurate test results
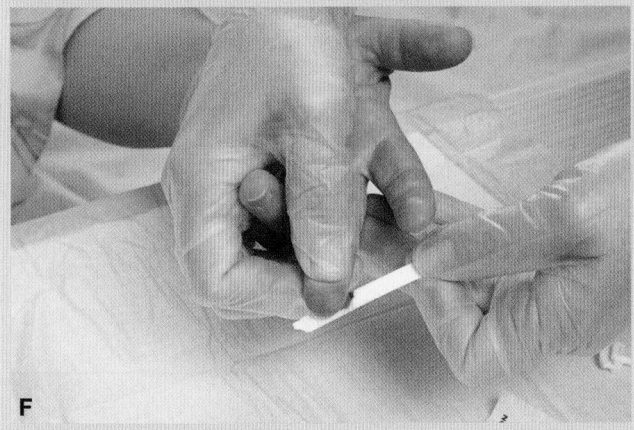 F	A drop of blood is applied to the test strip.
Insert the test strip into the glucometer (Fig. G).	Allows glucometer to gather data
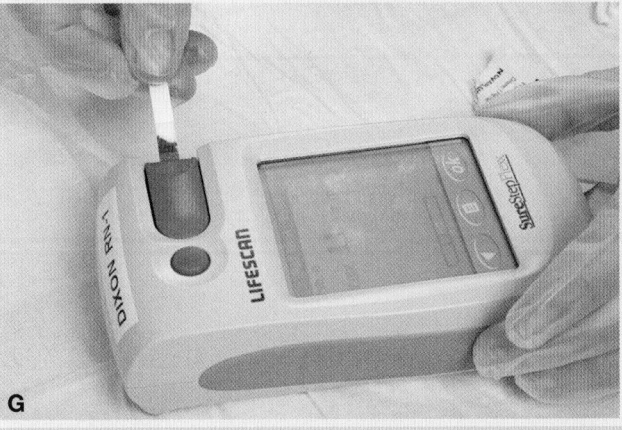 G	The test strip is inserted into the glucometer.
Listen for the meter to beep followed by a series of beeps 45 seconds later.	Activates the timing mechanism
Read the display on the meter after the series of beeps.	Identifies the client's blood glucose level
Turn the machine off.	Extends the life of the battery
Offer the client a Band-Aid, paper tissue, or gauze square (Fig. H).	Absorbs blood and controls bleeding
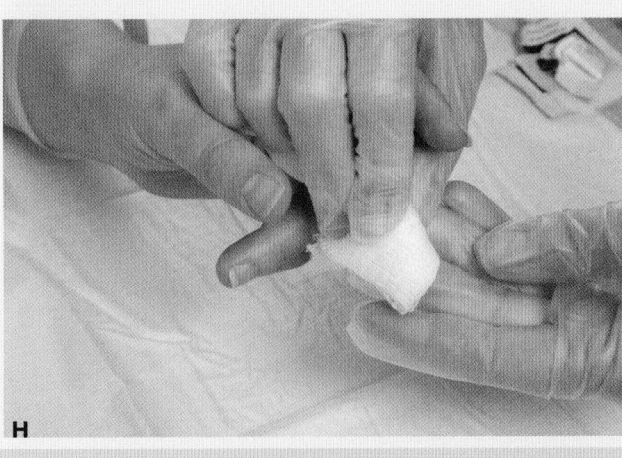 H	Controlling the bleeding
Place the test strip and lancet into a puncture-resistant container.	Prevents the potential for a needlestick injury and transmission of blood-borne infectious microorganisms

(*continued*)

SKILL 14-3 Using a Glucometer (*continued*)

Suggested Action	Reason for Action
Clean the opening of the test strip holder with a cotton swab or damp cloth to remove dirt, blood, or lint at least once a week.	Keeps the equipment free of debris that can impair light detection
Remove gloves and immediately wash your hands or perform hand antisepsis with an alcohol rub (see Chapter 10).	Reduces microorganisms
Remove equipment from the bedside if it does not belong to the client.	Facilitates the use of equipment that may be needed for other clients
Store the test strips in a cool dry place at 37–85°F (1.7–30°C).	Prevents decomposition from heat and humidity
Record the glucose measurement in the client's diabetic record.	Documents essential data
Report the blood glucose level to the nurse in charge.	Communicates information for making treatment decisions

EVALUATION

- Client demonstrates understanding of the purpose for the examination.
- Adequate blood is obtained.
- Results are consistent with the client's present condition, previous trends, and concurrent treatment.
- Additional treatment is provided depending on glucose measurement.

DOCUMENT

- Date and time
- Pertinent preassessment data, if any
- Results obtained when using the glucometer; in most agencies, the test data are recorded on a diabetic flow sheet rather than charted in narrative nursing notes.
- Treatment provided based on abnormal test results

SAMPLE DOCUMENTATION

Date and Time   Blood glucose level 210 mg/dL per glucometer. 5 units of Humulin R insulin given subcutaneously as coverage.
_____ J. Doe, LPN

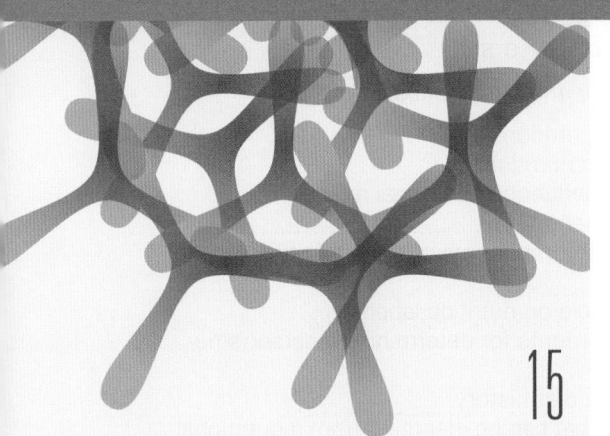

UNIT 5

Assisting with Basic Needs

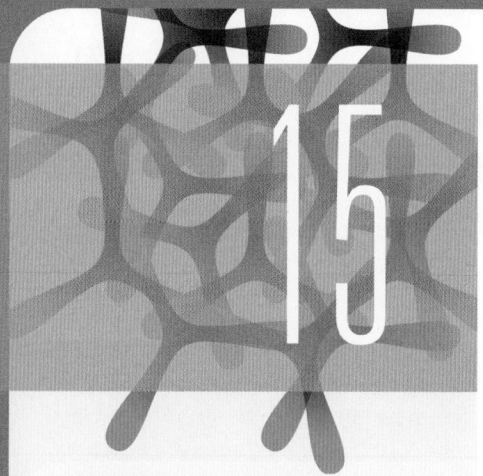

Nutrition

Learning Objectives

On completion of this chapter, the reader should be able to:

1. Define nutrition and malnutrition.
2. List components of basic nutrition.
3. Identify five factors that influence nutritional needs.
4. Explain protein complementation.
5. Discuss the purpose and components of the MyPlate food guidelines.
6. Describe the facts available on nutrition labels.
7. Identify objective assessments for determining a person's nutritional status.
8. Discuss the purpose of a diet history.
9. List common problems that can be identified from a nutritional assessment.
10. Plan nursing interventions for resolving problems caused or affected by nutrition.
11. Describe common hospital diets and their characteristics.
12. Discuss nursing responsibilities for meeting clients' nutritional needs.
13. Identify facts a nurse must know about a client's diet.
14. Describe and demonstrate techniques for feeding clients.
15. Explain how to meet the nutritional needs of clients with dysphagia, visual impairment, and dementia.
16. Discuss unique aspects of nutrition that apply to older adults.

INTRODUCTION

In general, healthy people are becoming increasingly selective about the quantity and quality of their daily food intake. However, in a country of affluence, Americans are both undernourished and overweight. According to Mechanick et al. (2020), one fifth of the adult population, an estimated 47 million people, in the United States either has cardiometabolic disease or is at high risk for cardiometabolic syndrome. **Cardiometabolic syndrome**, also known as *metabolic syndrome*, *syndrome X*, *insulin resistance syndrome*, and *other diagnostic terms*, is a cluster of modifiable risk factors that can potentially lead to cardiovascular diseases and type 2 diabetes mellitus if uncontrolled. The syndrome includes combinations of obesity (particularly abdominal fat), hypertension, elevated blood glucose (insulin resistance), abnormal blood fat levels, smoking, and inflammatory markers.

This chapter includes information about normal nutrition for promoting health. It also provides suggestions that nurses may offer clients about what and how much to eat, the dangers of food fads and unsafe dieting, and techniques for managing the care of clients whose ability to eat, digest, absorb, or eliminate food is impaired.

Gerontologic Considerations

■ Because older adults need fewer calories, it is important to teach them and their caregivers about the consumption of nutrient-dense foods such as meat, fruits, vegetables, soy-based proteins, dairy products, and whole-grain foods.

■ Older adults often consume diets high in carbohydrates. Reasons include changes in taste, changes in the ability to prepare or obtain foods, limited accessibility, or financial limitations related to increased cost of health care and other expenses on a fixed income.

■ Some older adults have difficulty obtaining and preparing nutritious meals because of socioeconomic barriers, such as low income and an inability to get to the grocery store.

■ Additional considerations include appropriate food storage (e.g., outdated food, proper storage temperature) and access to cupboards due to physical limitations.

■ Because age-related changes occur gradually, it is important to evaluate an older adult's nutritional status at least annually and more frequently if indicated by weight gain or loss of 10% within 6 months or 5% within 1 month.

■ Medical conditions, adverse medication effects, functional impairments, and psychosocial conditions (e.g., dementia, depression, social isolation) commonly affect the nutritional status of older adults.

■ Oral and dental problems, such as missing teeth and poorly fitting dentures, are common in older adults and can interfere with adequate nutrition. Encourage older adults to get dental care every 6 months and to practice good dental hygiene daily.

■ Psychosocial impairments such as dementia or depression interfere with food preparation, consumption, and enjoyment. An important initial sign of these changes may be weight loss.

■ Homebound older adults may benefit from home-delivered meals. The nutrition of older adults who are isolated, depressed, or cognitively impaired may improve with participation in a group meal program. Home-delivered meals and group meal programs are widely available and are funded through the Older Americans Act. The National Eldercare Locator can provide information.

■ Refer low-income older adults to their local Council on Aging for assistance in accessing federally funded programs.

■ Diminished senses of smell and taste, which may occur with normal aging, can interfere with appetite and intake.

■ A variety of nutritional supplements are available for increasing an older client's intake of calories and nutrients. Protein-based liquid supplements will not provide the needed fiber and should not be relied on as the main source of protein.

■ Encourage older adults to participate in appropriate physical activity as an intervention for improving appetite and overall health.

■ Older adults who have functional limitations may benefit from adaptive utensils for eating and food preparation.

■ Dysphagia among older adults often results from neurologic conditions (e.g., stroke, dementia), esophageal disorders, or increased abdominal pressure. Referrals for swallowing evaluations can provide helpful information about techniques to improve the person's ability to eat and drink safely.

■ Dry mouth (xerostomia) is common in older adults and is often caused by medications or the effects of disease. It interferes with chewing, swallowing, and enjoying meals. Encourage people with dry mouth to drink adequate noncaffeinated and nonalcoholic beverages or to chew sugarless gum to promote salivation.

■ Oral infections, poorly fitting dentures, or vitamin deficiencies can cause a painful or burning tongue, ulcers on the gums, or other difficulties that interfere with eating.

Nutrition Notes

Dark chocolate is a rich source of antioxidants and minerals, and it generally contains less sugar than milk chocolate. Research suggests that dark chocolate may help lower the risk of heart disease, reduce inflammation and insulin resistance, increase the diversity of the gut microbiome, and improve brain function. People interested in adding dark chocolate to their diet should keep in mind that it is high in fat and calories, so moderation is key. The research also suggests that eating 85% dark chocolate may have a positive correlation with mood (Medical News Today, 2022).

OVERVIEW OF NUTRITION

Eating is a basic need. It is the chief mechanism by which nutrients are obtained. An optimal nutritional status provides (1) sufficient energy for daily activities, (2) maintenance and replacement of body cells and tissues, and (3) restoration of health following illness or injury. Because the type and amount of nutrients consumed affect health, it is important to understand basic **nutrition,** or the process by which the body uses food. Chronic, inadequate nutrition leads to **malnutrition** (a condition resulting from a lack of proper nutrients in the diet). Evidence of malnutrition is common among people living in low-income, resource-limited countries; however, it also occurs among people living in countries known for their prosperity, like the United States. Examples of those in the United States at risk for an inadequate nutritional intake include:

• Older adults who are socially isolated or living on fixed incomes
• People experiencing homelessness
• Children with low socioeconomic status
• Pregnant teenagers
• People with substance use problems, such as alcohol use disorder
• Clients with eating disorders, such as anorexia nervosa and bulimia nervosa

Human Nutritional Needs

Increasing data support the connections between nutritional status and health and well-being. Consequently, an emphasis on improving nutrition to prevent and treat disease is also growing. All humans have basic nutritional needs. Through scientific study, researchers have determined standards for the recommended daily amounts of:

- Calories that provide the body with energy
- Proteins, carbohydrates, and fats that supply calories and are substances needed for the growth and repair of body structures
- Vitamins and minerals that do not supply calories but are essential for regulating and maintaining the physiologic processes necessary for health
- Water, which is also necessary for life (discussed in Chapter 16)
- Although standards have been established for the types and amounts of dietary components necessary to sustain health, individual nutritional needs are influenced by and may require adjustment according to:
  - Age
  - Weight and height
  - Growth periods
  - Activity
  - Health status

Calories

Food is the source of energy for humans. Some nutrients produce more energy than others. By using a calorimeter, a device for measuring heat, the nutrients in food are burned in a laboratory and then analyzed to quantify their energy value.

The energy, or heat equivalent, of food is measured in calories. A **calorie** (cal), the amount of heat that raises the temperature of 1 g of water by 1°C, is one way to express the energy value of food. Sometimes, the energy equivalent of food is expressed in **kilocalories** (kcal) (1,000 cal, or the amount of heat that raises the temperature of 1 kg of water by 1°C).

When proteins, carbohydrates, and fats are metabolized, they produce energy. Proteins yield 4 kcal/g, carbohydrates yield 4 kcal/g, and fats yield 9 kcal/g. Alcohol yields 7 kcal/g but is not considered an essential nutrient.

The number of calories a person needs depends on age, body size, physical condition, and physical activity. The U.S. Department of Health and Human Services (2019) recommends requirements of 1,600 to 2,400 cal/day for adult women and 2,000 to 3,000 cal/day for adult men; the lower end of the range is for sedentary individuals, whereas the higher end is for active individuals. Unless the caloric intake includes an appropriate mix of proteins, carbohydrates, and fats, the person may be marginally nourished or malnourished. In other words, consuming 2,400 calories of chocolate, exclusive of any other food, is not adequate to sustain a healthy state. Fortunately, most foods contain a variety of nutrients, vitamins, and minerals.

Proteins

Protein, a component of every living cell, is a nutrient composed of *amino acids*, which are chemical compounds composed of nitrogen, carbon, hydrogen, and oxygen. Amino acids are responsible for building and repairing cells. Twenty-two amino acids have been identified so far. Of these, nine are referred to as **essential amino acids**, which are protein components that must be obtained from food because the body cannot synthesize them. **Nonessential amino acids** are protein components manufactured within the body; however, this term is misleading. "Nonessential" refers to the fact that these amino acids are not dependent on dietary intake, not that they are unnecessary for health.

The body uses proteins primarily to build, maintain, and repair tissue. The body spares protein from being used for energy as long as calories are available from carbohydrates and fats.

Dietary proteins are obtained from animal and plant food sources, which include milk, meat, fish, poultry, eggs, soy, legumes (peas, beans, and peanuts), nuts, and components of grains. Generally, animal sources provide **complete proteins** (proteins that contain adequate amounts and proportions of all the essential amino acids); plant sources contain **incomplete proteins** (proteins that contain insufficient quantities of one or more essential amino acids). **Protein complementation** (combining plant sources of protein so that amino acids that are missing in one are compensated by those contained in another) helps a person to acquire all essential amino acids from nonanimal sources than plant sources alone would provide (Fig. 15-1). Protein complementation is discussed later in relation to vegetarian diets.

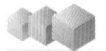 **Concept Mastery Alert**

Incomplete Proteins

Proteins derived from plant sources, such as peanut butter, are considered incomplete proteins. To ensure that the client consumes the required essential amino acids, it is important for the client to combine an incomplete protein with a complementary protein. For example, combining peanut butter with milk, an animal protein that is considered a complementary protein, would achieve this goal.

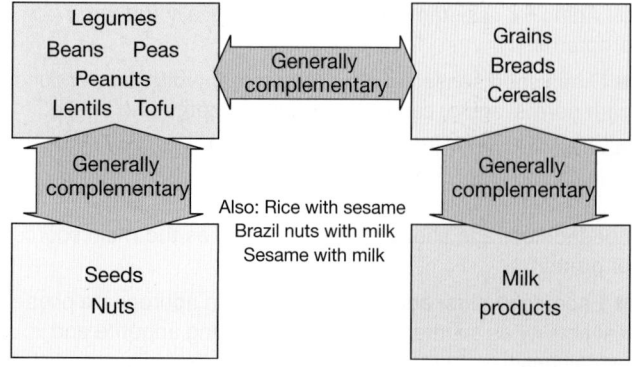

FIGURE 15-1 A complementary protein guide for meatless meals.

Carbohydrates

Carbohydrates are nutrients that contain molecules of carbon, hydrogen, and oxygen and are generally found in plant food sources. They are classified according to the number of sugar (saccharide) units they contain. Carbohydrates are subdivided into *monosaccharides*, *disaccharides*, and *polysaccharides* (starches).

Carbohydrates, the chief component of most diets, are the body's primary source for quick energy. In addition to providing calories, carbohydrates may contain fiber (complex polysaccharides that humans are unable to digest). **Cellulose** is a type of fiber in the stems, skins, and leaves of fruits and vegetables, which forms intestinal bulk to promote bowel elimination. Other types of fiber help lower serum cholesterol levels and delay the rise in serum glucose after eating.

Sources of carbohydrates include cereals and grains such as rice, wheat and wheat germ, oats, barley, corn, and corn meal; fruits and vegetables; and sweeteners. Milk is the only significant animal source of carbohydrates. Box 15-1 lists terms on food labels that identify ingredients that are essentially sugar. Foods containing added sugar as a major ingredient tend to supply calories but few, if any, other nutrients.

Fats

Fats, nutrients that contain molecules composed of glycerol and fatty acids called *glycerides*, are part of a family of compounds known collectively as *lipids*. Depending on the number of fatty acids that make up a fat molecule, fats are referred to as *monoglycerides*, *diglycerides*, or *triglycerides*.

Fats are a concentrated energy source, supplying more than twice the calories per gram than either proteins or carbohydrates. Although fats are high in calories, they should not be eliminated from the diet. Fats provide energy and are necessary for many chemical reactions in the body. They are also necessary for the absorption of some vitamins. Fats also add flavor to food, and because they leave the stomach slowly, they promote a feeling of having satisfied appetite and hunger. Food sources that contain fat include meat, fish, and poultry; butter, margarine, and vegetable oils; egg yolks;

BOX 15-1 — Label Ingredients That Represent Sugar

- Sucrose (table sugar)
- Fructose
- Glucose (dextrose)
- Brown sugar
- Corn sweetener
- Corn syrup
- High-fructose corn syrup
- Fruit juice concentrate
- Honey
- Invert sugar
- Lactose
- Maltose
- Brown rice syrup
- Caramel
- Carob syrup
- Dehydrated cane juice
- Xylose
- Sorghum/sorghum syrup
- Treacle
- Palm sugar
- Malt
- syrup
- Raw sugar
- Molasses

---

whole milk and cheese; peanut butter; salad dressings; avocados; chocolate; nuts; and most desserts.

Role of Cholesterol

Cholesterol is transported through the blood in molecules of **lipoproteins** (a combination of fats and proteins). Lipoproteins vary in their proportions of protein to cholesterol. The more protein a molecule contains, the higher is its density. High-density lipoprotein (HDL) is referred to as "good cholesterol" because the cholesterol is delivered to the liver for removal. Low-density lipoprotein (LDL) is called "bad cholesterol" because the cholesterol is deposited within the walls of arteries, which can eventually result in cardiovascular disease.

Types of Fats

All fats in food are a mixture of saturated and unsaturated fats. **Saturated fats** are lipids that contain as much hydrogen as their molecular structure can hold and are generally solid. Saturated fats are the predominant type of fat in red meats, full-fat dairy products, and palm and coconut oils. Cholesterol is only present in foods of animal origin, but the body also synthesizes cholesterol. **Unsaturated fats** are missing some hydrogen. They are a healthier form of fats and are liquid at room temperature or congeal slightly when refrigerated. Unsaturated fats are the predominant type of fat in fish, poultry, nuts, and most plant oils, such as corn, safflower, olive, peanut, and soybean. **Trans fats**, also known as partially hydrogenated oils (PHOs), are unsaturated fats that have been *hydrogenated*, a process in which hydrogen is added to the fat. Hydrogenation changes the unsaturated fat to a more saturated form that remains solid at room temperature. An example includes the hydrogenation of vegetable oil to create margarine or shortening. Hydrogenation reduces the rate at which a fat becomes rancid, thus increasing the shelf life of food items that contain it (e.g., cake mixes). The U.S. Food and Drug Administration has determined that PHOs are no longer recognized as safe in any human food. Food supplies and products cannot have added PHOs and had to be in compliance with this regulation by January 1, 2020 (U.S. Food and Drug Administration, 2022).

Health Risks Related to Fat and Cholesterol

Generally, Americans consume more fats than people do in most other countries. The relationship between fat consumption and obesity to disorders such as cardiometabolic syndrome, heart disease, hypertension, diabetes, and some cancers is well documented. Although the creation of trans fats has improved the marketing of convenience foods, health-concerned agencies like the American Heart Association (AHA) indicate that consumption of trans fats increases the risk for coronary heart disease. Health care providers use cholesterol, lipoprotein, and triglyceride levels to assess clients' risks for cardiac and vascular diseases (Table 15-1). Cardiac risk can also be estimated by dividing the total serum cholesterol level, which should be less than 200 mg/dL, by the HDL level. A result greater than 5 suggests that a client has a potential for coronary artery disease.

TABLE 15-1 Cardiac Risk Associated with Blood Fat Levels

	TOTAL CHOLESTEROL	HDL CHOLESTEROL	LDL CHOLESTEROL	TRIGLYCERIDES
Good	<200 (but the lower the better)	Ideal is ≥60; ≥40 for men and ≥50 for women is acceptable.	<100; <70 if coronary artery disease is present	<149; ideal is <100.
Borderline	200–239	NA	130–159	150–199
High	≥240	≥60	≥160; 190 is considered very high.	≥200; 500 is considered very high.
Low	NA	<40 for men and <50 for women	NA	NA

HDL, high-density lipoprotein; LDL, low-density lipoprotein.
MedlinePlus. (2020). *Cholesterol levels: What you need to know.* National Library of Medicine. https://medlineplus.gov/cholesterollevelswhatyouneedtoknow.html

Pharmacologic Considerations

Many medications, such as hydroxymethylglutaryl-coenzyme A (HMG-CoA) reductase inhibitors (statins), fibrates, and bile acid sequestrants, are available for reducing cholesterol and triglyceride levels. Liver function and blood glucose levels for people for whom statins are prescribed must be assessed periodically. Some experience muscle pain when taking statins, resulting in discontinuing the medication.

Nutrition Notes

■ Omega-3 fatty acid (fish oil), a natural substance, may be used by some to prevent or manage dyslipidemia. Omega-3 fatty acid (fish oil) is believed to lower triglycerides and very low-density lipoprotein (VLDL) levels.

■ Dietary sources that can provide omega-3 fatty acids include fish such as salmon, halibut, sardines; olive oil; flaxseed; walnuts; and beans such as soybeans, navy beans, and kidney beans.

⟫⟫ Stop, Think, and Respond 15-1

Which client has the lowest cardiac risk factor?

- *Client A: Total cholesterol level is 224 mg/dL; high-density lipoprotein (HDL) level is 38 mg/dL.*
- *Client B: Total cholesterol level is 198 mg/dL; HDL level is 35 mg/dL.*
- *Client C: Total cholesterol level is 210 mg/dL; HDL level is 55 mg/dL.*

Minerals

Minerals (noncaloric substances in food that are essential to all cells) help regulate many of the body's chemical processes, such as blood clotting and the conduction of nerve impulses. Table 15-2 lists some of the body's major and trace minerals, their chief functions, and common dietary sources.

As a national policy, specified amounts of certain minerals and vitamins are added to some processed foods. For example, enriched flour and bread contain iron, thiamine, riboflavin, and niacin to replace what is lost when the grain

TABLE 15-2 Common Dietary Minerals

MINERAL	CHIEF FUNCTIONS	COMMON DIETARY SOURCES
Sodium	Maintenance of water and electrolyte balance Neuromuscular activity Enzyme reactions	Table salt Processed meat
Potassium	Maintenance of electrolyte balance Neuromuscular activity Enzyme reactions	Bananas Oranges Potatoes
Chloride	Maintenance of fluid and electrolyte balance	Table salt Processed meat
Calcium	Formation of teeth and bones Neuromuscular activity Blood coagulation Cell wall permeability	Milk Milk products
Phosphorus	Buffering action Formation of bones and teeth	Eggs Meat Milk
Iodine	Regulation of body metabolism Promotion of normal growth	Seafood Iodized salt
Iron	Component of hemoglobin Assistance in cellular oxidation	Liver, clams, and oysters Egg yolks, soybeans, and tofu Red meat Swiss chard, spinach
Magnesium	Neuromuscular activity Activation of enzymes Formation of teeth and bones	Whole grains Milk Meat
Zinc	Constituent of enzymes and insulin	Seafood Liver

is ground into flour. Fortified foods have nutrients added that either were not naturally present in the food or were present in insignificant amounts.

Vitamins

Vitamins are chemical substances necessary in minute amounts for normal growth, the maintenance of health, and the functioning of the body (Table 15-3). They were originally named with letters; numbers were subsequently added to some letters as more vitamins were identified. Chemical names are now replacing the letter–number system of identification.

Water-soluble vitamins (B complex and C) are eliminated with body fluids and so require daily replacement. **Fat-soluble vitamins** (A, D, E, and K) are stored in the body as reserves for future needs.

TABLE 15-3 Vitamins

VITAMIN	CHIEF FUNCTIONS	COMMON DIETARY SOURCES
A (retinol) Not destroyed by ordinary cooking temperatures	Growth of body cells Promotion of vision, healthy hair and skin, and integrity of epithelial membranes Prevention of xerophthalmia, a condition characterized by chronic conjunctivitis	Animal fats Butter, cheese, and cream Egg yolks Whole milk Fish liver oil and liver Dark green, leafy vegetables Deep orange fruits and vegetables
B_1 (thiamine) Not readily destroyed by ordinary cooking temperatures	Carbohydrate metabolism Functioning of the nervous system Normal digestion Prevention of beriberi, a condition caused by neuritis	Fish Pork Lean meat and poultry Glandular organs Milk Whole, fortified, and enriched breads, cereals, and grains Peas, beans, and peanuts
B_2 (riboflavin) Not destroyed by heat, except in the presence of alkali	Formation of certain enzymes Normal growth Light adaptation in the eyes	Eggs Green, leafy vegetables Lean meat Milk Whole grains Dried yeast
B_3 (niacin)	Carbohydrate, fat, and protein metabolism Enzyme component Prevention of appetite loss Prevention of pellagra, a condition characterized by cutaneous, gastrointestinal, neurologic, and mental symptoms	Lean meat and liver Fish Peas and beans Whole-grain cereals Peanuts Yeast Eggs Liver
B_6 (pyridoxine) Destroyed by heat, sunlight, and air	Healthy gums and teeth Red blood cell formation Carbohydrate, fat, and protein metabolism	Whole-grain cereals and wheat germ Vegetables Yeast Meat Bananas Blackstrap molasses
B_9 (folic acid)	Protein metabolism Red blood cell formation Normal intestinal tract functioning	Green, leafy vegetables Glandular organs Yeast
B_{12} (cyanocobalamin)	Protein metabolism Red blood cell formation Healthy nervous system tissues Prevention of pernicious anemia, a condition characterized by decreased red blood cells	Liver and kidney Dairy products Lean meat Milk Salt water fish and oysters
C (ascorbic acid) Readily destroyed by cooking temperatures	Healthy bones, teeth, and gums Formation of blood vessels and capillary walls Proper tissue and bone healing Facilitation of iron and folic acid absorption Prevention of scurvy, a condition characterized by bleeding and abnormal bone and teeth formation	Citrus fruits and juices Tomatoes Berries Cabbage Green vegetables Potatoes

(continued)

TABLE 15-3 Vitamins (*continued*)

VITAMIN	CHIEF FUNCTIONS	COMMON DIETARY SOURCES
D (calciferol) Relatively stable with refrigeration	Absorption of calcium and phosphorus Prevention of rickets, a condition characterized by weak bones	Milk Egg yolks Butter Liver Oysters Formed in the skin by exposure to sunlight
E (α-tocopherol) Heat stable in the absence of oxygen	Protection of essential fatty acids Important for normal reproduction in experimental animals (i.e., rats)	Wheat germ oil Margarine Brown rice
Pantothenic acid	Metabolism	Liver Egg yolks Milk
H (biotin) Heat sensitive	Enzyme activity Metabolism of carbohydrates, fats, and proteins	Egg yolks Green vegetables Milk Liver and kidney Yeast
K (menadione)	Production of prothrombin	Liver Eggs Green, leafy vegetables Synthesized in the gastrointestinal tract by bacteria

With the exception of vitamin D, vitamin K (menadione), and biotin, the body does not manufacture vitamins. People can easily meet their vitamin requirements, however, by eating a variety of foods. Cooking, processing, and lack of refrigeration can deplete the content of some vitamins in food. Some commercially packaged foods such as margarine, milk, and flour have been vitamin enriched or fortified to promote health.

Generally, vitamin and mineral supplements are not necessary if a person eats a well-balanced diet. Consuming **megadoses** (amounts exceeding those considered adequate for health) of vitamins and minerals can be dangerous. Some athletes and people with terminal diseases choose to follow unconventional diets and take large doses of nutritional supplements. Athletes are motivated by a desire to alter their muscle mass, strength, and endurance; people with terminal diseases seek attempts for cure. Although various deficiency diseases develop from inadequate nutrition, no conclusive evidence at this time supports consuming excessive nutrients, vitamins, or minerals as a safe substitute for healthy eating or as a singular established treatment for disease.

Nutritional Strategies

Healthy People 2030, a national effort to improve the health of Americans, provides recommendations to enhance nutrition and weight status (Box 15-2). Other nutritional strategies include using the U.S. Department of Agriculture's MyPlate, referring to the nutrition labels on processed and packaged foods, and understanding standard definitions for the terms used on food labels.

Healthier Food Access

Healthy People 2030 aims to have an increased number of healthy food outlets, such as farmers' markets and healthier foods on display by food retailers. With the increase in healthier foods, another objective is to promote availability and accessibility for people to use food as an incentive program for a healthier diet, including whole grains and fruits and vegetables.

Availability of Recreational Facilities

Where we live affects our health in multiple ways. Poor health measures are focused in neighborhoods that are most disadvantaged by society's social, economic, and housing inequities, which lead to higher incidence of chronic disease.

Studies show that people who live close to recreational areas experience better mental health and that frequency of exercise by adults and children and having fresh produce available is associated with healthier lifestyles (Healthy People 2030, 2020).

BOX 15-2   Overarching Goals for *Healthy People 2030*

- Attain healthy, thriving lives and well-being, free of preventable disease, disability, injury, and premature death.
- Eliminate health disparities, achieve health equity, and attain health literacy to improve the health and well-being of all.
- Create social, physical, and economic environments that promote attaining full potential for health and well-being for all.
- Promote healthy development, healthy behaviors, and well-being across all life stages.
- Engage leadership, key constituents, and the public across multiple sectors to take action and design policies that improve the health and well-being of all.

HealthyPeople.gov. (2020). *Healthy people 2030 framework*. Retrieved February 18, 2020, from https://www.healthypeople.gov/2020/About-Healthy-People/Development-Healthy-People-2030/Framework

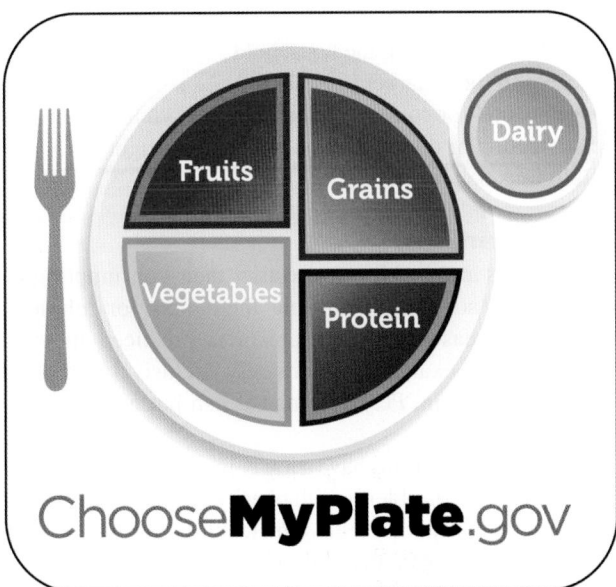

FIGURE 15-2 MyPlate is color coded to show the five groups of foods that should be consumed each day in the following proportions: 30% grains, of which half are preferably whole grains; 30% vegetables; 20% fruits; 20% protein; accompanied by low-fat/nonfat milk or other reduced fat dairy products. (USDA, ChooseMyPlate.gov.)

Nutrition Facts

Serving Size 1/2 cup (114 g)
Servings Per Container 4

Amount Per Serving	
Calories 90	Calories from Fat 30

	% Daily Value*
Total Fat 3 g	5
Saturated Fat 0 g	0
Trans Fat 1 g	
Cholesterol 0 mg	0
Sodium 300 mg	13
Total Carbohydrate 13 g	4
Dietary Fiber 3 g	12
Sugars 3 g	
Protein 3 g	

Vitamin A	80%	Vitamin C	60%
Calcium	4%	Iron	4%

* Percent Daily Values are based on a 2,000 cal diet. Your daily values may be higher or lower depending on your caloric needs:

		Calories	2,000	2,500
Total Fat	Less than		65 g	80 g
Sat Fat	Less than		20 g	25 g
Cholesterol	Less than		300 mg	300 mg
Sodium	Less than		2,400 mg	2,400 mg
Total Carbohydrate			300 g	375 g
Fiber			25 g	30 g

Calories per gram:
Fat 9 • Carbohydrate 4 • Protein 4

FIGURE 15-3 A sample label with nutritional information. (From Taylor, C. R., Lynn, P. B., & Bartlett, J. L. [2018]. *Fundamentals of nursing: The art and science of nursing care* [9th ed.]. Lippincott Williams & Wilkins.)

MyPlate

MyPlate, introduced in 2011 by the U.S. Department of Agriculture, replaces the previously used Food Pyramid and MyPyramid. MyPlate is an improved simplified tool for promoting a healthful daily intake of food (Fig. 15-2). Its advantage is that the recommended percentages of consumed food from among five food group categories promote healthy nutrition. Nutritionists also advocate reducing salt consumption and substituting water for sugary beverages. Following MyPlate guidelines promotes the achievement of the dietary recommendations set by the U.S. Department of Health and Human Services and the U.S. Department of Agriculture's Dietary Guidelines for Americans.

Children, adolescents, pregnant people, and those who are breastfeeding require more servings per day of certain food groups, particularly the dairy group. Recommendations for specific populations can be accessed at the website for the Department of Health and Human Resources: Dietary Guidelines for Americans.

⟫ Stop, Think, and Respond 15-2

Using MyPlate, what percentage of whole grains should an adult consume each day?

Nutritional Labeling

Nutritional information has appeared on food labels since 1974. Today, all packages of fresh meat and poultry must provide printed disease prevention guidelines. There have also been major changes in the way nutritional information is provided on approximately 90% of processed and packaged food labels (Fig. 15-3). The labels identify the amounts of each nutrient per serving, identified in household measurements. To interpret the information accurately, however, consumers must become familiar with a variety of terms, such as daily value (DV). DVs are calculated in percentages based on standards set for total fat, saturated fat, cholesterol, sodium, carbohydrate, and fiber in a 2,000-cal diet. The standards are as follows:

- Total fat: less than 65 g
- Saturated fat: less than 20 g
- Cholesterol: less than 300 mg
- Sodium: less than 2,400 mg
- Total carbohydrate: 300 g
- Dietary fiber: 25 g

People consuming diets of more or less than 2,000 cal must adjust the percentage of DVs. The required calculation may be difficult for the average consumer. An expanded table showing the DV equivalents for both a 2,000- and 2,500-cal diet appears on some, but not all, food labels. Because the requirements for vitamins and minerals do not depend on calories, those amounts are uniform to all consumers.

Additional regulations affect food labels. For example, the federal Nutrition Labeling and Education Act requires companies to comply with standard definitions if they use health-related claims such as "low-fat" on their labels (Box 15-3).

> **BOX 15-3** **Regulations for Labeling Terms**
>
> Based on figures per serving:
> - Calorie free: <5 cal
> - Low calorie: ≤40 cal
> - Reduced calorie: at least 25% fewer calories than the standard product
> - Light or "lite:" one-third fewer calories or 50% less fat than the regular product
> - Fat free: <0.5 g fat; example: skim milk
> - Low fat: ≤3 g fat; example: 1% milk
> - Reduced fat: at least 25% less fat than the regular product; example: 2% milk
> - Cholesterol free: <2 mg cholesterol and ≤2 g saturated fat
> - Low cholesterol: ≤20 mg cholesterol and ≤2 g saturated fat
> - Sugar free: <0.5 g sugar
> - Reduced sugar: <25%
> - Sodium free: <5 mg
> - Low sodium: <140 mg
> - Reduced sodium: <25%
> - Imitation: new food that resembles a traditional food and contains less protein or less of any essential vitamin or mineral than the traditional food (e.g., imitation cheese)

U. S. Food and Drug Administration. (2013). *Guidance for industry: food labeling guide.* https://www.fda.gov/regulatory-information/search-fda-guidance-documents/guidance-industry-food-labeling-guide

NUTRITIONAL PATTERNS AND PRACTICE

Influences on Eating Habits

Most people learn their eating habits early in life. Cultural (Fig. 15-4), economic, emotional, and social variables influence the kinds of food a person consumes and their eating habits. Some influential factors include:

- Food preferences acquired during childhood
- Established patterns for meals
- Attitudes about nutrition
- Knowledge of nutrition
- Income level

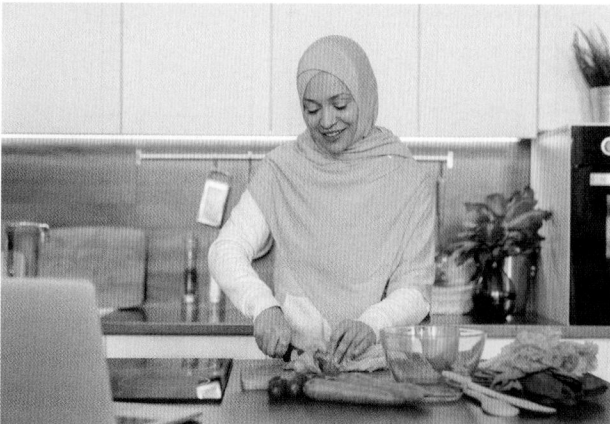

FIGURE 15-4 Cultural influences affect eating habits. (Inside Creative House/Shutterstock.)

- Time available for food preparation
- Number of people in the household
- Access to food markets
- Use of food for comfort, celebration, or symbolic reward
- Satisfaction or dissatisfaction with body weight
- Religious beliefs

Vegetarianism

Vegetarians are people who restrict their consumption of animal food sources, modifying their diets for religious or personal reasons. Vegetarianism is practiced in various forms. For example, **vegans** rely exclusively on plant sources for protein. Pescatarians eat fish but no other animal meat.

Overall, vegetarians have a lower incidence of colorectal cancer and fewer problems with obesity and diseases associated with a high-fat diet (Harvard Health Publishing, 2015). Nevertheless, a vegan diet, unless skillfully planned, can be inadequate in protein, calcium, vitamins B_{12} and D, iron, zinc, and omega-3 fatty acids. Thus, it is helpful to teach vegans about protein complementation if they are unfamiliar with the practice. Protein complementation involves eating a variety of incomplete plant proteins over the course of the day to provide adequate amounts and proportions of all the essential amino acids present in animal protein sources (see Fig. 15-1 and Client and Family Teaching 15-1 for more information).

**Client and Family Teaching 15-1
Vegetarian Diets**

The nurse teaches the vegetarian client and their family as follows:

- Plan menus 1 day or week at a time.
- Eat a wide variety of foods.
- Eat a variety of different plant proteins every day.
- Include fortified ready-to-eat cereals, soy foods, dried fruit, molasses, and dried peas for iron.
- Enhance absorption of iron by including a good source of vitamin C (e.g., orange juice) with each meal.
- Use fortified ready-to-eat cereals and fortified soy milk to obtain vitamin B_{12}, vitamin D, and zinc.
- Choose calcium-fortified orange juice; fortified soy yogurt, milk, and tofu; and bok choy, broccoli, collards, kale, okra, and turnip greens for calcium.
- Select plant sources of omega-3 fatty acids, such as canola oil, ground flaxseed, walnuts, and soybeans.
- Breast-feed infants if possible.
- Consider taking cod liver oil as a source of vitamin D.
- Purchase meat analogs, products with the taste and appearance of meat, poultry, or fish that are made from textured vegetable protein. Such analogs are available in health food and grocery stores.
- Contact a Seventh Day Adventist church, whose members practice vegetarianism, for information on sources for meatless products and food preparation classes.

NUTRITIONAL STATUS ASSESSMENT

Because eating is a basic need, nurses must identify any current or potential client problems associated with nutrition. They obtain subjective information by asking clients focused questions on a diet history. Nurses gather objective data using physical assessment techniques.

 Pharmacologic Considerations

Interaction of certain foods can make medications less effective. Be alert for reports of antibiotics, antidepressants, and antihypertensives that can interact with select foods.

Subjective Data

A **diet history** is an assessment technique for obtaining facts about a client's eating habits and factors that affect nutrition. The findings add to the database of nutritional information. Common components in a diet history include:

- The level of appetite
- Unintentional weight loss or gain of 10% in the past 6 months
- The number of meals the client eats per day
- Foods (in approximate household measurements) that the client has eaten in the previous 24 hours
- Time when the client generally eats meals
- Frequency with which the client eats meals alone
- Food likes, dislikes, allergies, intolerances, and cultural beliefs about food
- The amount of alcohol the client consumes daily or weekly
- Vitamin or mineral supplements the client takes routinely
- Any problems with eating, digestion, or elimination
- Special diets that have been medically prescribed or self-imposed
- The use of over-the-counter (OTC) drugs, such as antacids or laxatives
- Food supplements or restrictions and the reasons for them
- The desire to improve nutritional intake or to gain or lose weight

Objective Data

The body is composed of water, fat, bone, and muscle. The nurse uses physical assessments and laboratory data, anthropometric data, and a person's body measurements to help determine a client's nutritional status.

Anthropometric Data

Anthropometric data are measurements pertaining to body size and composition. The nurse obtains them by measuring height and weight, calculating body mass index (BMI), and measuring midarm circumference, triceps skinfold thickness, and **abdominal circumference** waist-to-hip ratio. Eating disorder clinics and fitness centers use more sophisticated tests such as bioelectrical impedance analysis (Fig. 15-5) that calculate lean body mass, body fat, and total body water based on changes in conduction of an applied electrical current.

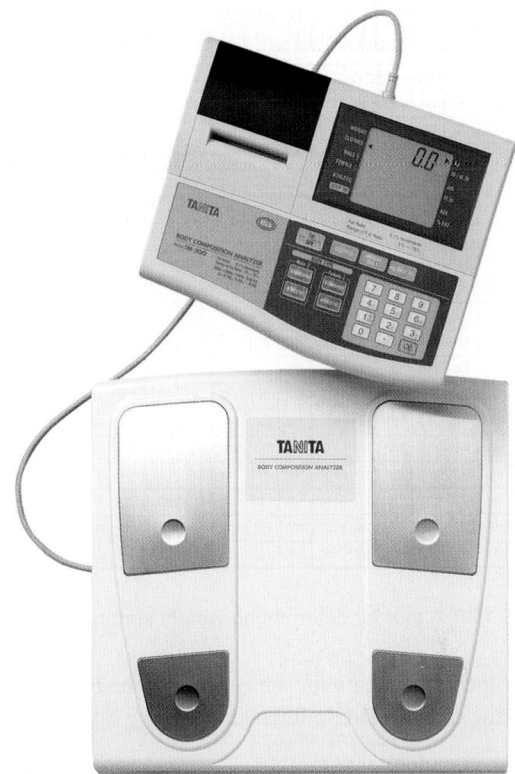

FIGURE 15-5 A bioelectric analyzer resembles a bathroom scale. When standing on the device, electrodes in the footplates send electrical impulses through the body that result in a calculation of body weight and body fat content in less than a minute.

Obtaining the client's height and weight generally provides sufficient anthropometric data unless a severe nutritional problem is suspected or long-term therapy is anticipated. An actual weight, rather than the client's estimate, is essential. The nurse uses a standing, chair, or bed scale depending on the client's condition. They record the date and time, the type of scale, and the clothing the client wears. It is important to duplicate all these factors when taking subsequent weights for comparison. The nurse measures the client's height without shoes. A gross assessment tool using weight and height is shown in Figure 15-6.

⟩⟩ Stop, Think, and Respond 15-3

Using the graph in Figure 15-6 and the formula in Box 15-4, what is your analysis of a person who is 5 ft 7 in and weighs 185 lb?

Body mass index (BMI) provides numeric data to compare a person's size in relation to established norms for the adult population. It is calculated using height and weight (Box 15-4).

Midarm circumference helps determine skeletal muscle mass. This technique, combined with other body measurements, helps assess a client's nutritional status. The measurement is based on the assumption that muscle is

Height (in)	Normal						Overweight					Obese										Extreme Obesity														
BMI	19	20	21	22	23	24	25	26	27	28	29	30	31	32	33	34	35	36	37	38	39	40	41	42	43	44	45	46	47	48	49	50	51	52	53	54
58	91	96	100	105	110	115	119	124	129	134	138	143	148	153	158	162	167	172	177	181	186	191	196	201	205	210	215	220	224	229	234	239	244	248	253	258
59	94	99	104	109	114	119	124	128	133	138	143	148	153	158	163	168	173	178	183	188	193	198	203	208	212	217	222	227	232	237	242	247	252	257	262	267
60	97	102	107	112	118	123	128	133	138	143	148	153	158	163	168	174	179	184	189	194	199	204	209	215	220	225	230	235	240	245	250	255	261	266	271	276
61	100	106	111	116	122	127	132	137	143	148	153	158	164	169	174	180	185	190	195	201	206	211	217	222	227	232	238	243	248	254	259	264	269	275	280	285
62	104	109	115	120	126	131	136	142	147	153	158	164	169	175	180	186	191	196	202	207	213	218	224	229	235	240	246	251	256	262	267	273	278	284	289	295
63	107	113	118	124	130	135	141	146	152	158	163	169	175	180	186	191	197	203	208	214	220	225	231	237	242	248	254	259	265	270	278	282	287	293	299	304
64	110	116	122	128	134	140	145	151	157	163	169	174	180	186	192	197	204	209	215	221	227	232	238	244	250	256	262	267	273	279	285	291	296	302	308	314
65	114	120	126	132	138	144	150	156	162	168	174	180	186	192	198	204	210	216	222	228	234	240	246	252	258	264	270	276	282	288	294	300	306	312	318	324
66	118	124	130	136	142	148	155	161	167	173	179	186	192	198	204	210	216	223	229	235	241	247	253	260	266	272	278	284	291	297	303	309	315	322	328	334
67	121	127	134	140	146	153	159	166	172	178	185	191	198	204	211	217	223	230	236	242	249	255	261	268	274	280	287	293	299	306	312	319	325	331	338	344
68	125	131	138	144	151	158	164	171	177	184	190	197	203	210	216	223	230	236	243	249	256	262	269	276	282	289	295	302	308	315	322	328	335	341	348	354
69	128	135	142	149	155	162	169	176	182	189	196	203	209	216	223	230	236	243	250	257	263	270	277	284	291	297	304	311	318	324	331	338	345	351	358	365
70	132	139	146	153	160	167	174	181	188	195	202	209	216	222	229	236	243	250	257	264	271	278	285	292	299	306	313	320	327	334	341	348	355	362	369	376
71	136	143	150	157	165	172	179	186	193	200	208	215	222	229	236	243	250	257	265	272	279	286	293	301	308	315	322	329	338	343	351	358	365	372	379	386
72	140	147	154	162	169	177	184	191	199	206	213	221	228	235	242	250	258	265	272	279	287	294	302	309	316	324	331	338	346	353	361	368	375	383	390	397
73	144	151	159	166	174	182	189	197	204	212	219	227	235	242	250	257	265	272	280	288	295	302	310	318	325	333	340	348	355	363	371	378	386	393	401	408
74	148	155	163	171	179	186	194	202	210	218	225	233	241	249	256	264	272	280	287	295	303	311	319	326	334	342	350	358	365	373	381	389	396	404	412	420
75	152	160	168	176	184	192	200	208	216	224	232	240	248	256	264	272	279	287	295	303	311	319	327	335	343	351	359	367	375	383	391	399	407	415	423	431
76	156	164	172	180	189	197	205	213	221	230	238	246	254	263	271	279	287	295	304	312	320	328	336	344	353	361	369	377	385	394	402	410	418	426	435	443

Body weight (lb)

FIGURE 15-6 A tool for determining weight status. (https://www.nhlbi.nih.gov/health/educational/lose_wt/BMI/bmi_tbl.pdf)

usually located in anatomic areas, such as the biceps. When measuring midarm circumference:

- Use the nondominant arm.
- Find the midpoint of the upper arm between the shoulder and the elbow.
- Mark the midarm location.
- Position the arm loosely at the client's side.
- Encircle the arm with a tape measure at the marked position.
- Record the circumference in centimeters.

Triceps skinfold measurement adds additional data for estimating the amount of subcutaneous fat deposits (Fig. 15-7). The skinfold thickness measurement relates to total body fat. To measure triceps skinfold thickness:

- Use the same arm as for the midarm circumference measurement.

- Grasp and pull the skin separate from the muscle at the previously marked location.
- Place the calipers around the skinfold.
- Record the measurement in millimeters.

To calculate how much of the midarm circumference is the actual muscle (midarm muscle circumference), multiply the triceps skinfold measurement by 0.314. To interpret the significance of the midarm circumference measurement and triceps skinfold thickness, the nurse compares measurements with averages provided in standardized charts (Table 15-4). Skinfold thickness norms do not exist for adults older than 75 years.

BOX 15-4 Body Mass Index Calculation and Interpretation

Calculation
1. Divide pounds (lb) by 2.2 = kilograms (kg).
2. Divide height in inches (in) by 39.4 = meters (m).
3. Square the answer in step 2 by multiplying the number times itself.
4. Divide weight in kg by m².

INTERPRETATION	BMI
Underweight	<18.5
Normal	18.5–24.9
Overweight	25.0–29.9
Obesity Class 1	30.0–34.9
Obesity Class 2	35.0–39.9
Obesity Class 3	≥40

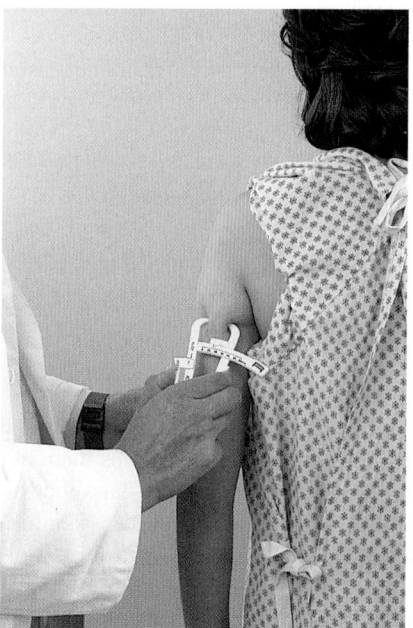

FIGURE 15-7 Measuring triceps skinfold thickness with calipers. (Photo by B. Proud.)

TABLE 15-4 Anthropometric Measurements for Adults

MEASUREMENT	SEX	NORMAL RANGE[a]
Triceps skinfold	Male	12.5–7.3 mm
	Female	16.5–9.9 mm
Waist-to-hip ratio	Male	0.90–0.95
	Female	0.80–0.86
Waist circumference	Male	<31.5 in (<80 cm)
	Female	<27.5 in (<70 cm)

[a]Anthropomorphic measurements for adults.
Adapted from American Council on Exercise. (2021). *Anthropometric measurements: When to use this assessment.* https://www.acefitness.org/fitness-certifications/ace-answers/exam-preparation-blog/3815/anthropometric-measurements-when-to-use-this-assessment/

Waist-to-hip ratio looks at health risks based on where a person carries their weight. When a person carries excess fat around the midsection (sometimes called having an "android" or "apple-shaped" body), it is called *abdominal obesity*. This fat is called "visceral fat"; it surrounds the liver and other organs found in the abdominal area. Visceral fat causes inflammation in the body sent by hormones and fatty acids and also causes an increase in cholesterol, blood pressure, and blood glucose. Carrying the fat in the hips, buttocks, and thighs (sometimes called having a "gynoid" or "pear-shaped" body) is different from the visceral fat and is called *subcutaneous fat*. It is the fat found just under the skin. Having some subcutaneous fat is healthy; it protects the muscles and bones and helps to control body temperature (Cleveland Clinic, 2024). This is the fat that is measured by skinfold calipers. Healthwise, it is much better to carry some weight as subcutaneous fat in the hips and thighs than as visceral fat in the belly (Table 15-4).

Accumulation of centrally located adipose tissue indicates a predisposition for diabetes and cardiovascular disease. To facilitate accuracy, the client should be (1) wearing underwear or light clothing to avoid including bulky fabric in the measurement and (2) standing upright with the legs spread 10 to 12 in apart. The tape measure should be placed around the client at the iliac crest of the pelvis without compressing the soft tissue and read to the nearest quarter inch (Fig. 15-8). Increases or decreases in abdominal measurements correlate with changes in risk factors for diabetes and cardiovascular disease. Health risks increase for males whose abdominal circumference measures more than 40 in and for females whose abdominal circumference is greater than 35 in (Mayo Clinic, 2022).

Physical Assessment

In addition to anthropometric data, the nurse assesses:

- General appearance
- Integrity of the mouth
- Condition of the teeth
- Ability to chew and swallow
- Gag reflex
- Characteristics of skin and hair
- Joint flexibility
- Hand strength
- Attention and concentration

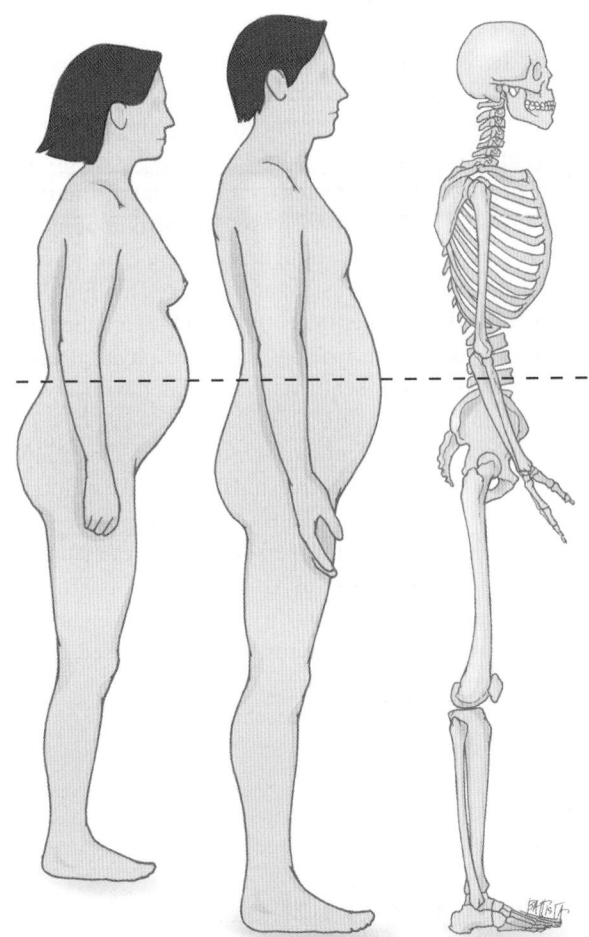

FIGURE 15-8 The location for measuring abdominal circumference in adults. (From Taylor, C. R., Lynn, P. B., & Bartlett, J. L. [2018]. *Fundamentals of nursing: The art and science of nursing care* [9th ed.]. Lippincott Williams & Wilkins.)

Laboratory Data

Laboratory tests used in nutritional assessment include hemoglobin and hematocrit; glucose; serum albumin and transferrin levels that indicate protein status; and cholesterol, triglyceride, and lipoprotein levels that may reflect a need to adjust the amount of fat the client eats.

MANAGEMENT OF PROBLEMS INTERFERING WITH NUTRITION

Based on the assessment data, the nurse may identify one or more of the following nursing diagnoses:

- Malnutrition risk
- Feeding activities of daily living (ADL) deficit
- Aspiration risk

If a nutritional problem is beyond the scope of independent nursing practice, the nurse consults with the physician. If the problem can be resolved through independent nursing measures, the nurse may proceed by collaborating with the dietitian, selecting the appropriate nursing interventions, and continuing to monitor the client to evaluate the effectiveness of the nursing care plan.

Obesity

Obesity is a condition in which a person's BMI equals or exceeds 30 or the triceps skinfold measurement exceeds 15 mm. Obesity indicates the need for healthy weight reduction measures. Research indicates that excess abdominal fat is a great health risk factor (National Heart, Lung, and Blood Institute, 2024). An increased proportion of abdominal fat is associated with a higher incidence of heart and vascular disease, hypertension, and diabetes mellitus. People with a BMI of greater than 40 (Box 15-4) are medically evaluated to determine whether there are physical etiologies for the disorder or health risks associated with a weight loss program.

To lose 1 lb, the client must reduce their caloric intake by 3,500 cal/week. Thus, decreasing one's intake of food by 500 cal/day will produce a 1-lb weight loss per week. By omitting 1,000 cal/day, the person will lose 2 lb/week. Generally, a sustained loss of 1 to 2 lb/week is a healthy goal. The nurse advises clients trying to lose weight about healthy eating and the hazards of unsupervised weight loss techniques, such as fasting, fad diets, or diet drugs (Fig. 15-9; Client and Family Teaching 15-2).

Pharmacologic Considerations

■ Rapid weight gain can occur when atypical antipsychotic medications are taken. Weight gain also occurs among those who are prescribed insulin to manage diabetes mellitus.

■ A number of drugs now on the market inhibit the enzyme lipase to promote weight loss. Lipase inhibition reduces absorption of dietary fat and fat-soluble vitamins. Consequently, vitamin supplementation with fat-soluble vitamins is necessary. These drugs should only be used when the patient's BMI is above 30.

■ Weight loss medications are also known to result in drug–drug interactions when taken with antihypertensive medications, some types of antidepressants, as well as cough, cold, and allergy medications containing pseudoephedrine.

Emaciation

Progressive or prolonged weight loss resulting in a BMI less than 16 can have serious consequences. **Emaciation** (excessive leanness) and **cachexia** (general wasting away

United States Department of Agriculture

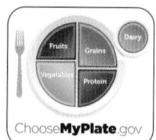
MyPlate Daily Checklist
Find your Healthy Eating Style

Everything you eat and drink matters. Find your healthy eating style that reflects your preferences, culture, traditions, and budget—and maintain it for a lifetime! The right mix can help you be healthier now and into the future. The key is choosing a variety of foods and beverages from each food group—*and making sure that each choice is limited in saturated fat, sodium, and added sugars.* Start with small changes—**"MyWins"**—to make healthier choices you can enjoy.

Food Group Amounts for 2,000 Calories a Day

 Fruits	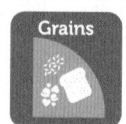 Vegetables	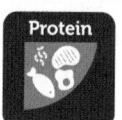 Grains	Protein	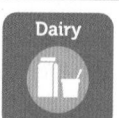 Dairy
2 cups	**2 1/2 cups**	**6 ounces**	**5 1/2 ounces**	**3 cups**
Focus on whole fruits	Vary your veggies	Make half your grains whole grains	Vary your protein routine	Move to low-fat or fat-free milk or yogurt
Focus on whole fruits that are fresh, frozen, canned, or dried.	Choose a variety of colorful fresh, frozen, and canned vegetables—make sure to include dark green, red, and orange choices.	Find whole-grain foods by reading the Nutrition Facts label and ingredients list.	Mix up your protein foods to include seafood, beans and peas, unsalted nuts and seeds, soy products, eggs, and lean meats and poultry.	Choose fat-free milk, yogurt, and soy beverages (soy milk) to cut back on your saturated fat.

 **Limit**

Drink and eat less sodium, saturated fat, and added sugars. Limit:
• Sodium to **2,300 milligrams** a day.
• Saturated fat to **22 grams** a day.
• Added sugars to **50 grams** a day.

Be active your way: Children 6 to 17 years old should move **60 minutes** every day. Adults should be physically active at least **2 1/2 hours** per week.
Use SuperTracker to create a personal plan based on your age, sex, height, weight, and physical activity level.

SuperTracker.usda.gov

FIGURE 15-9 MyPlate's 2,000-cal daily food plan.

Client and Family Teaching 15-2
Promoting Weight Loss

The nurse teaches the client who needs to lose weight and their family as follows:

- When using MyPlate, follow the food plan for the appropriate calorie allowance based on the individual's sex, age, and activity level (Fig. 15-9).
- Count portions from each group based on MyPlate serving sizes:
  - Grains—one slice of bread, 1 cup of ready-to-eat cereal, or a 1/2 c of cooked pasta, rice, or cooked cereal is a 1 oz equivalent
  - Vegetables—2 c of raw leafy vegetables, 1 c of other raw or cooked vegetables, or 1 c of vegetable juice counts as 1 c
  - Fruits—1 c of fruit or 100% fruit juice or 1/2 c dried fruit counts as 1 c
  - Milk—1 c of milk or yogurt, 1.5 oz of natural cheese, or 2 oz of processed cheese counts as 1 c
  - Meat and beans—1 oz of lean meat, poultry, or fish, 1/4 c of cooked dry beans, one egg, 1 tbsp of peanut butter, or 1/2 oz of nuts or seeds equals 1 oz of meat
- Use fats, oils, and sugar sparingly.
- Eliminate junk food (contributes calories but not much nutrition) and alcoholic beverages.
- Eat small but more frequent meals rather than three large meals per day. Any nutrients not used from large meals are stored as fat.
- Sit at the table to eat. Do not read or do other tasks while eating; distraction often fools the brain into thinking that food has not been consumed.
- Increase fiber in the diet from fresh fruits, vegetables, and whole grains. Fiber is not digested and may provide a full feeling without a large number of calories.
- Participate in some regular, active form of exercise. Exercise raises the **metabolic rate** (the speed at which the body uses calories) while suppressing appetite. Information on activity and exercise is located in Chapter 23.

of body tissue) are consistent with severe malnourishment. States of severe malnourishment require collaboration with a physician, who will prescribe measures to ensure the client's nutrition using gastric or enteral tube feedings or parenteral nutrition if oral intake is inadequate (see Chapter 29).

Independent nursing interventions, including client teaching, are appropriate for people who are approximately 10% below their ideal body weight. To gain 1 lb, a person must consume 3,500 cal more than their metabolic needs per week. This is best done gradually (Client and Family Teaching 15-3).

Client and Family Teaching 15-3
Promoting Weight Gain

The nurse teaches the client who needs to gain weight and their family as follows:

- Eat a variety of foods from MyPlate, but increase the number of servings or serving sizes.
- Eat small amounts frequently.
- Eat with others.
- Snack on high-calorie but nutritious foods, such as hard cheese, milkshakes, and nuts.
- Disguise extra calories by fortifying foods with powdered milk, gravies, or sauces.
- Garnish food with cubed or grated cheese, diced meat, nuts, or raisins.
- Rest after eating.

Pharmacologic Considerations

■ The drug megestrol, a synthetic female hormone belonging to the progesterone group, can be used to stimulate appetite for the purpose of promoting weight gain. Its prescription is generally reserved for clients who are emaciated due to a serious illness like cancer or acquired immunodeficiency syndrome (AIDS).

■ Medical marijuana (cannabis), which contains tetrahydrocannabinol (THC), may also be used to increase appetite in states where it is legally available from regulated dispensaries.

Anorexia

Anorexia (a loss of appetite) is associated with multiple factors: illness, altered taste and smell, oral problems, and tension and depression. Simple anorexia is generally a short-lived symptom that requires no medical or nursing intervention. Anorexia nervosa, a psychobiologic disorder, is associated with a 20% to 25% loss in previously stable body weight. No matter what the etiology, the nurse never ignores that a client is not eating. If food is uneaten, the nurse assesses the client for physiologic, emotional, cultural, or social etiologies that may be the contributing factors (Nursing Guidelines 15-1).

⟩⟩ Stop, Think, and Respond 15-4
How can the nurse make food and its presentation visually attractive to entice a client to eat?

Nausea

Nausea usually precedes vomiting and is produced when gastrointestinal sensations, sensory data, and drug effects

NURSING GUIDELINES 15-1

Overcoming Simple Anorexia

- Cater to the client's food preferences. *The client will more likely consume food they select.*
- Serve nutrient-dense foods (foods loaded with calories). *They may compensate for a low intake of food.*
- Offer small servings of food frequently. *Eating small amounts frequently may result in a cumulative intake within acceptable nutritional levels.*
- Ensure that the client is rested before meals. *A lack of energy may overpower the desire to eat.*
- Provide an opportunity for oral hygiene before meals. *Mouth care stimulates salivation and potentiates the pleasure from eating.*
- Help the client into a sitting position. *Seeing food stimulates the appetite center; sitting also promotes access to the food.*
- Arrange for the client to eat with others. *Because eating is a social activity, the client may eat more when with a group.*
- Serve food attractively. *A visual presentation of food stimulates appetite.*
- Suggest adding spices and herbs to foods. *Intensifying flavors and aromas may stimulate a desire to eat; however, it may have the opposite effect as well. When experimenting, add new seasonings to small amounts of food.*
- Serve foods at their appropriate temperature. *The client may eat more food if hot foods are hot and cold foods are cold.*
- Serve cool, bland foods to clients with a mouth irritation. *Hot or spicy foods intensify the irritation of oral structures.*

stimulate a portion of the medulla that contains the vomiting center. Nausea may be associated with feeling faint or weak. Often, dizziness, perspiration, skin pallor, a rapid pulse rate, and headache are present. The nurse consults the physician when the measures presented in Nursing Guidelines 15-2 are unsuccessful for overcoming nausea. Prescribed medications may be necessary.

Once nausea is relieved, assisting the client in resuming fluid intake and nourishment becomes a priority. The nurse

NURSING GUIDELINES 15-2

Relieving Nausea

- Check to see if something as simple as an annoying odor or sight is contributing to nausea. *Offensive sensory data can stimulate the vomiting center in the brain.*
- Assist the client with taking deep breaths. *Distraction can overcome nausea by directing conscious attention away from the unpleasant sensation.*
- Limit the client's abrupt movements and activities. *Movement may shift gastrointestinal structures and their contents, intensifying stimulation of the vomiting center.*
- Limit the client's intake of food and fluid temporarily until nausea subsides. *Distention of the stomach is a common trigger of the vomiting center.*
- Avoid making negative comments about food. *Verbal comments create visual images that may cause psychogenic stimulation of the vomiting center.*

starts this process gradually, offering sips of clear fluids first. If the client tolerates fluids, the nurse adds soft, bland foods in small amounts.

Vomiting

Vomiting (a loss of stomach contents through the mouth) commonly accompanies nausea. **Emesis** or **vomitus** (the substance that is vomited) is readily visible. **Retching** (the act of vomiting without producing vomitus) may occur if the stomach is empty. **Regurgitation** (bringing stomach contents to the throat and mouth without the effort of vomiting) occurs commonly among infants after eating. **Projectile vomiting** (vomiting that occurs with great force) is associated with certain disease conditions, such as increased pressure in the brain or gastrointestinal bleeding. Nausea may be present, but it often is not (Nursing Guidelines 15-3).

The nurse describes the emesis in the client's medical record. If possible, the nurse measures the amount of emesis and records the volume. Documentation includes the amount, color, appearance, and any unusual odor such as the odor of fecal material or alcohol. If the characteristics of the emesis are unusual, the nurse saves a specimen for the physician to examine. If there are any doubts about whether to discard or save the emesis, it is best to check with a more experienced nurse. The nurse always consults the physician when vomiting is prolonged. It may be necessary to administer prescribed medications for relief.

Stomach Gas

Gas in the stomach is primarily a result of swallowing air. It becomes a problem only when it accumulates. **Eructation** (belching) is a discharge of gas from the stomach through the mouth. **Flatus** is gas formed in the intestine and released from the rectum when eructation does not occur. Nursing guidelines for relieving intestinal gas are discussed in Chapter 31 (see Nursing Guidelines 15-4).

Pharmacologic Considerations

■ Nausea, stomach gas, and heartburn are frequently self-treated with OTC medications, such as Beano, which contains an enzyme that breaks down vegetables containing polysaccharides (starches), or products containing simethicone, such as Gas-X, Mylicon, and Mylanta Gas. Instruct the client to contact the physician if the condition persists or does not respond to self-treatment.

■ Prescription drugs are available to manage nausea and vomiting for a variety of conditions accompanied by vomiting such as emesis due to cancer chemotherapy.

Nutrition Notes

Avoiding gas-forming foods in the diet such as beans, onions, cucumbers, cabbage and similar cruciferous vegetables such as broccoli, and carbonated beverages can reduce gastrointestinal gas, eructation, and flatus.

NURSING GUIDELINES 15-3

Managing the Care of a Vomiting Client

- Temporarily limit the client's food intake. *Adding contents to an already upset stomach may prolong episodes of vomiting.*
- Lean the client's head forward over a container or the toilet. *Tilting the chin toward the chest reduces the possibility that vomitus will enter the lungs.*
- Adjust light, sound, ventilation, and temperature to a comfortable level. *Minimizing sensory stimulation may reduce the urge to vomit.*
- Apply a cool washcloth to the client's forehead or back of the neck. *Increased perspiration and a clammy feeling to the skin may accompany vomiting.*
- Help the client rinse the mouth, offer mouthwash, or provide mouth care as soon as possible after vomiting. *Gastric acid is harmful to tooth enamel. Emesis usually produces an unpleasant aftertaste.*

- Turn a vomiting client who is unconscious or weak onto the abdomen or side. *Gravity helps emesis drain from the mouth rather than remain in the throat, where the client could aspirate it into the lungs.*
- Use a suction machine to clear vomitus from the mouth and throat of a weak or unconscious client. *Suctioning pulls fluid from the oral cavity and airway, thus preventing choking and aspiration* (see Chapter 36).
- Provide firm support with the hands or a pillow to the abdominal incision if the client has had abdominal surgery. An abdominal binder may also help support the incision (see Chapter 28). *Strong muscle contractions may pull on stitches and increase pain and discomfort.*
- Remove the container of emesis from the bedside as soon as possible. Provide ventilation to remove any lingering odors. *The appearance and odor of vomitus may stimulate more vomiting.*

MANAGEMENT OF CLIENT NUTRITION

Common Hospital Diets

Common hospital diets include:

- Regular or general: allows unrestricted food selections
- Light or convalescent: differs from regular diet in preparation; typically omits fried, fatty, gas-forming, and raw foods and rich pastries
- Soft: contains foods soft in texture; is usually low in residue and readily digestible; contains few or no spices or condiments; provides fewer fruits, vegetables, or meats than a light diet
- Mechanical soft: resembles a light diet but is used for clients with chewing difficulties; provides cooked fruits and vegetables and ground meats

- Full liquid: contains fruit and vegetable juices, creamed or blended soups, milk, ice cream, yogurt without bits of fruit, pudding, milkshakes, gelatin, junket, custards, and cooked cereals
- Clear liquid: consists of items that may be colored, but are generally transparent and do not contain any pulp or bits of food; examples include water, broth, fruit juices, flavored gelatin, popsicles, clear soft drinks, tea, and coffee
- Special therapeutic: consists of foods prepared to meet special needs, such as low in sodium, fat, calories, or fiber

Most health care agencies have a dietitian who plans the meals and a centralized food service that prepares clients' meals. Nurses are generally responsible for ordering and canceling diets for clients, serving and collecting meal trays, helping clients eat, and recording the percentage of food that

NURSING GUIDELINES 15-4

Preventing and Relieving Stomach Gas

- Suggest that the client chew food with the mouth closed. *Laughing and talking while eating increase the amount of swallowed air.*
- Advise against using a straw. *Each swallow of liquid also contains the air in the straw.*
- Advise against chewing gum and smoking cigarettes. *Chewing gum increases salivation and results in swallowing both secretions and air. The client actually may swallow a portion of inhaled cigarette smoke.*
- Limit or restrict foods that contain large volumes of air such as soufflés, yeast breads, and carbonated beverages. *Swallowing air trapped within food and drinking beverages that contain dissolved gas distend the stomach.*

- Recommend that when under stress, the client avoid eating. *Emotions delay stomach emptying, which prevents the movement of gas to the intestine.*
- Propose walking if uncomfortable. *Activity helps gas to rise to its highest point in the stomach, making belching easier.*
- Consult with the physician about the use of medications that relieve gas accumulation. Instruct clients who purchase over-the-counter (OTC) drugs to follow label directions for their use. *Simethicone is an ingredient in several nonprescription antacids. Drugs containing simethicone facilitate the elimination of gas by reducing the surface tension of gas bubbles trapped in the gastrointestinal tract.*

clients eat. Nurses must know the type of diet prescribed for each client, the purpose for the diet, and its characteristics. They take care to ensure that clients receive the correct diet and that restricted foods are withheld.

Meal Trays

Meals are usually served at the bedside, but some health care institutions have dining rooms or cafeterias for ambulatory clients. Some hospitals allow clients to call the dietary department and place their orders from a printed menu. Clients in nursing homes generally eat together in small groups unless they physically cannot. Nurses and dietary personnel work together to ensure that clients receive food at mealtimes and that trays are collected afterward. The nursing responsibilities for serving and removing trays are identified in Skill 15-1.

Feeding Assistance

Some clients need help with eating (Fig. 15-10). Skill 15-2 provides suggested actions for feeding clients who can bite, sip, chew, and swallow but cannot cut food or use utensils for eating. Suggestions for helping clients with **dysphagia** (difficulty swallowing), for helping clients who are blind or have both eyes patched, and for promoting self-feeding in those with dementia (impairment of intellectual functioning) follow.

Feeding the Client with Dysphagia

Nurses use the following techniques when caring for clients who have difficulty chewing and swallowing food:

- Always have equipment for oral and pharyngeal suctioning at the bedside (see Chapter 36).
- Remain with the client throughout eating when there is a potential for aspiration.
- If the client has a tracheostomy tube or endotracheal tube, make sure the cuff is inflated (see Chapter 36).
- Place the client in a sitting position.
- Ensure that the client is rested and that you have their attention.
- Give short, simple instructions to prompt the client to eat and swallow.
- Limit distracting stimuli; turn off the television and reduce or eliminate activities taking place in the area.
- Request a full liquid or mechanically soft diet for the client who has missing teeth or has recently had oral surgery.
- Provide small frequent meals if efforts to eat and swallow tire the client.
- Modify eating or feeding equipment to facilitate the client's safety and independence.

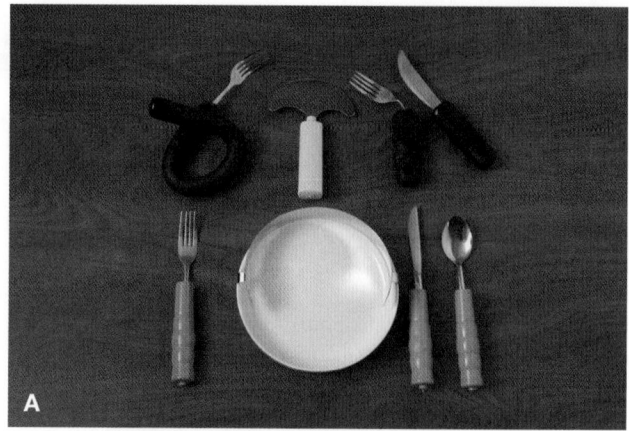

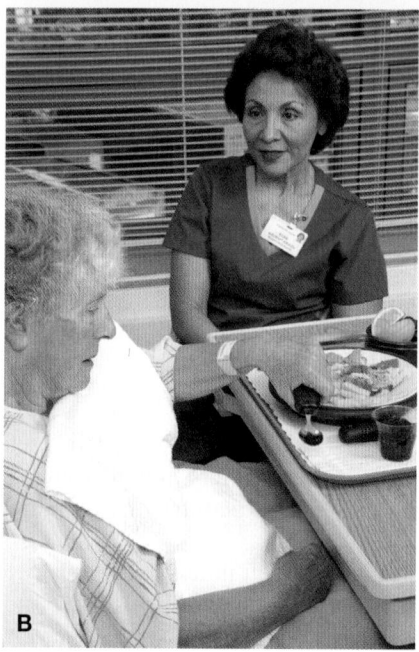

FIGURE 15-10 A. Assistive feeding devices make it easy for patients to grasp and get food on utensils. **B.** Assistive feeding devices may be required for patients who are weak, fatigued, or paralyzed or have neuromuscular impairment (From Hinkle, J. L., Cheever, K. H., & Overbaugh, K. [2021]. *Brunner & Suddarth's textbook of medical-surgical nursing* [15th ed.]. Lippincott Williams & Wilkins.)

- Determine that the client has swallowed one portion of food before offering another.
- Encourage repeated swallowing attempts if there is wet, gurgly vocalization, a sign that food is in the esophagus and not in the stomach.

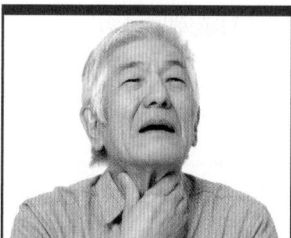

Clinical Scenario An 82-year-old client who has had a stroke tells the nurse that he has difficulty swallowing. He explains that he has choked on food and liquids in the past. Refer to Nursing Care Plan 15-1 for an example of how the nurse can manage the care of a client with impaired swallowing. *Aspiration risk* is defined as abnormal functioning of the swallowing mechanism associated with deficits in oral, pharyngeal, or esophageal structure or function.

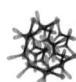
NURSING CARE PLAN 15-1 | Aspiration Risk

Assessment

- Note if there is coughing, choking, or drooling from the mouth when the client swallows saliva, liquids, or food.
- Look for asymmetry of the mouth.
- Ask the client to extend the tongue; observe if it deviates from a midline position.
- Determine whether the oral mucous membranes are moist or dry.
- Check for the gag reflex by stimulating the posterior oral pharynx with a cotton-tipped swab.

- Inspect the mouth and buccal cavities for retained food, the condition of the teeth, and evidence of tissue irritation, swelling, or injury.
- Observe the client's ability to understand and follow verbal instructions.
- Review the results of a fluoroscopic swallowing study as ordered by the physician.

Nursing Diagnosis. Aspiration risk related to left hemiparesis secondary to cerebrovascular accident (stroke) as manifested by incomplete swallowing of food, occasional coughing while eating, and the statement, "I'm losing weight. I've almost given up trying to eat. I get more on me than in me since my stroke."

Expected Outcome. The client will swallow more effectively as evidenced by an empty mouth after each mastication and attempt at swallowing.

Interventions	Rationales
Maintain a suction machine, a suction catheter, and an oxygen mask at the bedside.	Equipment for suctioning the airway and improving oxygenation may be necessary if the airway becomes obstructed.
Place the client in a sitting position.	An upright position uses gravity to move food from the pharynx to the esophagus and stomach.
Provide oral hygiene before each meal.	Oral hygiene moistens the mouth, making it easier to swallow a bolus of food.
Request that the dietary department initially avoid dry foods such as crackers and sticky foods such as bananas.	Dry and sticky foods are more difficult for a client to masticate and swallow.
Request semisolid foods with some texture such as oatmeal, poached eggs, and mashed potatoes.	Semisolids are easier to swallow than liquids and watery pureed food.
Add a commercial thickener such as Thick-It or SimplyThick to oral liquids, or thicken liquids with powdered mashed potatoes or baby rice cereal.	Thickeners create a consistency that the tongue can manipulate more easily against the pharynx.
Help the client load a spoon or fork with 1/4 tsp to 1/2 tsp of food.	Smaller amounts of food are more easily swallowed; the amount of food increases as the client demonstrates effective swallowing.
Place the food on the nonparalyzed (right) side of the mouth.	Chewing and swallowing require neuromuscular function.
Encourage the client to chew food thoroughly.	Chewing compresses food and mixes it with saliva to facilitate swallowing.
Instruct the client to lower the chin to the chest and swallow repeatedly without breathing in between.	A chin-to-chest position closes the pathway to the trachea and reduces the potential for aspiration. Repeated swallowing uses muscular contraction to move the food bolus into the esophagus.
Have the client raise the chin after swallowing efforts, clear the throat, and resume breathing.	Raising the chin, clearing the throat, and breathing improve ventilation.
Inspect the client's mouth after each swallowing attempt; encourage the client to do so as well by looking in the mouth with a handheld mirror.	Inspection helps identify retained food.
Have the client use the tongue or finger to sweep retained food from the cheek and repeat the swallowing technique; if the client is unsuccessful, apply finger pressure on the outside of the client's cheek.	Mechanical movement relocates the food to an area of the mouth where it can be manipulated and swallowed.
Keep the client in a sitting or semi-sitting position for at least a half hour.	The potential for aspiration is reduced once food leaves the stomach.

Evaluation of Expected Outcomes

The client demonstrates techniques for clearing the mouth of food.
The client consumes sufficient calories to maintain weight.
The client swallows food completely.

Feeding the Visually Impaired Client

When caring for clients who are temporarily or permanently sightless:

- Place a thick towel across the client's chest and over the lap.
- If the client can eat independently, consider using dishes with rims or bowls to prevent spilling.
- Arrange as much as possible to have finger foods (foods that may be eaten with the hands) prepared for the client.
- Describe the food and indicate its location on the tray.
- Guide the client's hand to reinforce the location of food and utensils.
- Prepare the food by opening cartons, cutting bite-size pieces, adding salt and pepper, buttering bread, and pouring coffee.
- Use the analogy of a clock when describing where the client may find food on the plate. For example, "The potatoes are at 3 o'clock."
- If the client needs to be fed, tell them what kind of food you are offering with each mouthful.
- Devise a system by which the client can indicate when they are ready for more food or drink, such as asking or raising a finger.
- Do not rush the client; eating should be done at a leisurely pace.

Assisting the Client with Dementia

Dementia refers to the deterioration of previous intellectual capacity. It is a common problem among those with neurologic conditions, such as Alzheimer disease. These clients often can retain their ability to carry out ADLs, such as self-feeding, by maintaining attention and concentration and repeating actions. Therefore, the following are useful nursing actions:

- Have the same staff person help the client, if possible, to develop a rapport with the client and promote continuity of care.
- Be consistent with the time and place for eating.
- Reduce or eliminate environmental distractions to promote concentration on the task at hand.
- Place the food tray close to the client, not the staff person, to communicate visually and spatially that the client is to eat the food.
- Remove wrappers, containers, and food covers to reduce confusion.
- Pour milk from the carton into a glass so that it is easily recognizable.
- Encourage the client's participation by offering finger foods and utensils to stimulate awareness and memory.
- Ensure that the client can see at least one other person who is also eating. This serves as a model for the desired behavior.
- Guide the hand with food to the client's mouth.
- Reinforce a desired response by praising, touching, and smiling at the client.
- Remain with the client. Do not begin feeding, leave, and then return, because this interrupts the client's attention and concentration.

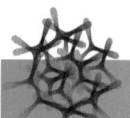

KEY POINTS

- Nutrition: The process by which the body uses food
- Malnutrition: A condition resulting from a lack of proper nutrients in the diet
- Components of basic nutrition
  - Calories: Provide the body with energy
  - Proteins: A component of every living cell; a nutrient composed of *amino acids*, which are chemical compounds composed of nitrogen, carbon, hydrogen, and oxygen that are responsible for building and repairing cells
  - Carbohydrates: The body's primary source for quick energy; contain fiber
  - Fats: A concentrated energy source, supplying more than twice the calories per gram than either proteins or carbohydrates; high in calories but should not be eliminated from the diet
  - Minerals: Noncaloric substances in food that are essential to all cells; help regulate many of the body's chemical processes, such as blood clotting and the conduction of nerve impulses
  - Vitamins: Chemical substances necessary in minute amounts for normal growth, the maintenance of health, and the functioning of the minerals
  - Water: Also necessary for life

- Five factors that influence nutritional needs
  - Age
  - Weight and height
  - Growth periods
  - Activity
  - Health status
- Healthy cholesterol values
  - Total cholesterol: less than 200 mg/dL
  - LDL: less than 100 mg/dL
  - HDL: 60 mg/dL or more
  - Triglyceride: less than 150 mg/dL
- Recommended DVs available on nutrition labels
  - Total fat: less than 65 g
  - Saturated fat: less than 20 g
  - Cholesterol: less than 300 mg
  - Sodium: less than 2,400 mg
  - Total carbohydrate: 300 g
  - Dietary fiber: 25 g
- Subjective assessments for determining a person's nutritional status include a diet history
- Objective assessments for determining a person's nutritional status
  - Anthropometric data
    - BMI
    - Midarm circumference

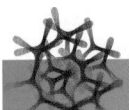

KEY POINTS

- Triceps skinfold measurement
- Abdominal circumference
- Physical assessment
- Laboratory data
- Emaciation: Excessive leanness caused by progressive or prolonged weight loss resulting in a BMI less than 16; can have serious consequences
- Cachexia: General wasting away of body tissue; consistent with severe malnourishment
- Anorexia: A loss of appetite associated with multiple factors that may include illness, altered taste and smell, oral problems, and tension and depression

- Management of client nutrition
  - Common hospital diets
    - Regular
    - Light
    - Soft
    - Mechanical soft
    - Full liquid
    - Clear liquid
    - Special therapeutic
- Feeding assistance is sometimes required for clients with dysphagia, visual impairment, and dementia.

CRITICAL THINKING EXERCISES

1. Describe appropriate nursing actions if a client eats none or only some food served.
2. A client tells the nurse that she eats the following every day: cereal, milk, and banana for breakfast; a sandwich made with processed meat, mayonnaise, and a soft drink for lunch; a candy bar in the late afternoon; and meat, potatoes, a vegetable, and a glass of milk for dinner. In the late evening, she snacks on potato chips. What recommendations should the nurse make to improve this client's nutrition?
3. When a client reports experiencing nausea for the past few weeks, what questions would be appropriate for the nurse to ask to determine possible causes?
4. After calculating that a client's BMI is 32 and measured abdominal circumference is 42 in, what information is appropriate for the nurse to provide?

NEXT-GENERATION NCLEX-STYLE REVIEW QUESTIONS

1. When caring for a client whose oral mucous membranes are irritated and sore, which item is best for the nurse to withhold from the dietary tray?
   a. Tomato soup
   b. Lime gelatin
   c. Canned peaches
   d. Rice pudding
   Test-Taking Strategy: Note the key word, "best." Review the options and select the food item that would create the most discomfort.
2. A nurse notes that a client coughs and chokes while eating. What initial nursing recommendation is best?
   a. Have the dietary department send baby foods from now on.
   b. Tell the client to chew their food thoroughly.

   c. Advise the client to drink more liquids between bites of food.
   d. Withhold milk and other dairy products in the future.
   Test-Taking Strategy: Note the key words, "best" and "initial." Select the option that should be implemented first before any other measures.
3. Which piece of information is the best evidence that a client with anorexia as a result of cancer is responding to the nutritional regimen developed by the nurse and dietitian?
   a. The client remains alert.
   b. The client gains weight.
   c. The client feels hungry.
   d. The client is pain free.
   Test-Taking Strategy: Note the key word and modifier, "best evidence." Select the option that demonstrates the result of improved nutrition better than any other options.
4. When a client on a clear liquid diet asks for some nourishment, which items are appropriate for the nurse to provide? Select all that apply.
   a. Skim milk
   b. Vanilla pudding
   c. Chicken broth
   d. Lime gelatin
   e. Apple juice
   f. Egg custard
   Test-Taking Strategy: Recall and select items on a clear liquid diet that are transparent.
5. When a nurse reviews lipid laboratory test results with a client, which value is the nurse correct in identifying as falling within a desirable range?
   a. Total cholesterol: 175 mg/dL
   b. HDL: 55 mg/dL
   c. LDL: 135 mg/dL
   d. Triglyceride: 210 mg/dL
   Test-Taking Strategy: Recall normal ranges of common laboratory values and apply them to the options.

NEXT-GENERATION NCLEX-STYLE CLINICAL SCENARIO QUESTIONS

An 82-year-old client who has had a stroke tells the nurse that he has difficulty swallowing. He explains that he has choked on food and liquids in the past. Aspiration risk is defined as abnormal functioning of the swallowing mechanism associated with deficits in oral, pharyngeal, or esophageal structure or function.

1. Place an "x" under "effective" to identify methods to decrease the client's risk for aspiration. Place an "x" under "ineffective" that may increase the client's risk of aspiration.

METHODS	EFFECTIVE	INEFFECTIVE
Have client sit up in bed when eating.		
Give sedative medications prior to meals.		
Provide thin liquids to the client.		
Provide a rest period prior to the meal.		

SKILL 15-1 Serving and Removing Meal Trays

Suggested Action	Reason for Action
ASSESSMENT	
Check on the usual time for meals.	Facilitates planning nursing care
Determine which clients are undergoing tests or must have food withheld for some other reason.	Ensures that eating does not affect therapeutic outcomes
Note the type of diet currently prescribed for each client.	Follows the client's therapeutic management plan
Review the health record for information concerning clients' food allergies or food intolerances.	Reduces the potential for adverse reactions
PLANNING	
Prepare clients so that they are ready to eat at the designated time.	Ensures food is served at its appropriate temperature
Meet clients' needs for comfort, hygiene, and elimination before the meal arrives.	Promotes appetite and eating
Help clients to a sitting position (Fig. A).	Assists ambulatory clients to a comfortable position
	Raise the head of the bed to reduce the risk of aspiration and choking.
IMPLEMENTATION	
Wash hands or perform hand antisepsis with an alcohol rub (see Chapter 10) before serving trays.	Prevents the transmission of microorganisms
Provide supplies for the client to perform hand hygiene (Fig. B).	Prevents the transmission of microorganisms
	Facilitate the client's hand hygiene before a meal.

(continued)

SKILL 15-1 Serving and Removing Meal Trays (*continued*)

Suggested Action	Reason for Action
Protect the client's hospital gown with a napkin or towel (Fig. C).	Maintains cleanliness
 C	Protect garments and bed linen from spills.
Deliver trays, one by one, as soon as possible.	Facilitates the enjoyment of eating through prompt delivery of food at its intended temperature
Compare the name on the tray with the name on the client's identification bracelet, or ask the client to identify themself by name.	Avoids dietary errors
Place the tray in such a way that the client can see it.	Provides ease of access to food
Uncover the food and check its appearance.	Ensures that the tray is complete, orderly, and tidy
Assist the client, if necessary, in opening cartons and prepare food (Fig. D).	Demonstrates consideration and facilitates independence
 D	Prepare the client's food for ease of consumption.
Replace food that is objectionable or request special additional items from the dietary department.	Demonstrates respect for unique needs
Before leaving the room, check whether the client has any further requests, such as an adjustment of pillows or donning eyeglasses.	Reduces inconveniences during mealtime
Make sure the signal cord is handy in case a need arises later.	Provides a means for summoning assistance
Check the client's progress from time to time.	Indicates a willingness to provide assistance
Remove the food tray after the client has finished eating.	Restores order and cleanliness to the environment
Record the amount of fluid consumed from the dietary tray on the bedside flow sheet if the client's fluid intake is being monitored.	Ensures accurate fluid assessment
Note the percentage of food that the client has eaten.[a]	Ensures documentation of dietary intake according to The Joint Commission standards rather than the use of vague terms, such as "good," "fair," and "poor"
Assist the client in brushing and flossing the teeth, if desired.	Removes food residue that may support microbial growth
Place the client in a position of comfort.	Demonstrates care and concern

SKILL 15-1 Serving and Removing Meal Trays (*continued*)

Suggested Action	Reason for Action

EVALUATION
- Client states that hunger is satisfied.
- Most food is consumed.

DOCUMENT

Type of diet and percentage of food consumed

SAMPLE DOCUMENTATION[a]

Date and Time Ate 100% of mechanical soft diet with need for assistance. _____ J. Doe, LPN

[a]Many agencies mandate that nurses should record the percentage of consumed food on a flow sheet or checklist. Nurses record other pertinent data within the medical record.

SKILL 15-2 Feeding a Client

Suggested Action	Reason for Action
ASSESSMENT	
Compare the dietary information in the medical record.	Ensures accuracy in therapeutic management
Verify that food or fluids are not being temporarily withheld.	Prevents delaying or having to cancel diagnostic tests
Determine whether the client's fluid intake is being measured.	Ensures the accurate documentation of data
Assess the client to determine what or how much assistance is necessary.	Aids in identifying specific problems and selecting nursing interventions
Review the medical record to see how well and how much the client has eaten during previous meals; note weight trends.	Helps establish realistic goals and to evaluate progress
Review the characteristics of the diet order.	Helps determine whether the correct food is being served
Analyze the purpose for the prescribed diet.	Assists in evaluating therapeutic responses
Assess the client's needs for elimination or relief from pain, nausea, and fatigue.	Identifies unmet physiologic needs
Check the medication record for drugs that must be administered before or with meals.	Facilitates optimal drug absorption and reduces drug side effects
PLANNING	
Set realistic goals for how much food the client will eat and how much the client will participate with self-feeding.	Establishes criteria for evaluating client responses
Select appropriate nursing measures to promote client comfort, such as administering an analgesic.	Helps resolve problems that, if ignored, may interfere with eating
Complete priority responsibilities for assigned clients.	Allows a period of uninterrupted feeding
Provide oral hygiene and hand washing before serving the tray.	Controls the transmission of microorganisms; promotes appetite and aesthetics
Prepare medications that must be given before or with meals, or delegate that responsibility.	Coordinates drug and nutritional therapy
Clear clutter and soiled articles from the eating area.	Promotes orderliness and a sanitary environment
IMPLEMENTATION	
Wash hands or perform hand antisepsis with an alcohol rub (see Chapter 10) before preparing food.	Prevents the transmission of microorganisms
Obtain or clean special utensils or containers that have been adapted for use by a client with a physical disability, for example, a fork to which a handgrip has been attached.	Promotes independence and self-reliance

(continued)

SKILL 15-2 Feeding a Client (*continued*)

Suggested Action	Reason for Action
Raise the head of the bed to a sitting position, or assist the client into a chair (see figure).	Promotes safety by facilitating swallowing

Feeding a client

Suggested Action	Reason for Action
Check that you serve the correct diet and tray to the correct client.	Indicates responsibility and accountability for therapeutic management
Cover the client's upper chest and lap with a napkin or towel.	Protects clothes and bed linens
Sit beside or across from client.	Promotes socialization and communication
Uncover the food, open cartons, and season food.	Increases gastric secretions and motility
Encourage the client to assist to the limit of their abilities.	Maintains or supports independence and self-care
Avoid rushing.	Communicates a relaxed atmosphere while eating
Collaborate with the client on which foods they desire before loading a fork or spoon.	Accommodates individual preferences
Provide manageable amounts of food with each bite.	Prevents choking or airway obstruction
For a client with a stroke, direct the food toward the nonparalyzed side of the mouth.	Places food in an area where there is feeling and muscle control for chewing and swallowing
Give the client time to chew thoroughly and swallow.	Chewing aids digestion by grinding the food and mixing it with saliva and enzymes.
Let the client indicate when they are ready for more food or a sip of beverage.	Promotes an independent locus of control
Talk with the client about pleasant subjects.	Combines eating with socialization
Record fluid intake if the client's intake is being measured.	Documents essential assessment data
Remove the tray and make the client comfortable. It is best for clients to remain sitting or semi-sitting for at least 30 minute after eating unless there is a medical reason to do otherwise.	A sitting position prevents the reflux of stomach contents into the esophagus and reduces the potential for aspiration.
Offer the client an opportunity for oral hygiene.	Removes sugar and starches that support microbial growth and tooth decay
Estimate the amount of food that the client has eaten.	Provides data for determining current and future nutritional needs

EVALUATION

- Client eats approximately 75% of meal.
- Client maintains body weight.
- Client participates at maximum capacity.

DOCUMENT

- Type of diet
- Percentage of food consumed
- Tolerance of food
- Client's ability to participate
- Problems encountered with chewing or swallowing
- Approaches taken to resolve problems

SAMPLE DOCUMENTATION

Date and Time Stated "I'm full" after consuming 75% of full liquid diet. Unable to hold spoon or glass but could direct straw into mouth. _____ J. Doe, LPN

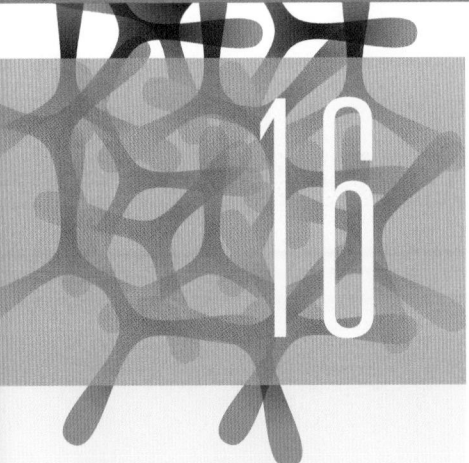

16

Fluid and Chemical Balance

Learning Objectives

On completion of this chapter, the reader should be able to:

1. Name the components of body fluid.
2. List physiologic transport mechanisms for distributing fluid and its constituents.
3. Name assessments that provide data about a client's fluid status.
4. Explain the purpose for assessing intake and output and circumstances when it is warranted.
5. Describe methods for maintaining or restoring fluid volume.
6. Describe methods for reducing fluid volume.
7. List reasons for administering intravenous (IV) fluids.
8. Differentiate between crystalloid and colloid solutions, and give examples of each.
9. Explain the terms "isotonic," "hypotonic," and "hypertonic" when used in reference to IV solutions.
10. List factors that affect the choice of tubing used to administer IV solutions.
11. Name techniques for infusing IV solutions.
12. Discuss criteria for selecting a vein when administering IV fluid.
13. List complications associated with IV fluid administration.
14. Discuss purposes for inserting an intermittent venous access device.
15. Name the types of transfusion reactions.
16. Explain the concept of parenteral nutrition.
17. Identify differences between administering blood and crystalloid solutions.

INTRODUCTION

Body fluid is a mixture of water, chemicals called electrolytes and nonelectrolytes, and blood cells. Water, the vehicle for transporting the chemicals, is the essence of life. Because water is not stored in any great reserve, daily replacement is the key to maintaining survival. This chapter discusses the mechanisms for maintaining fluid balance and restoring fluid volume and the components in body fluid.

Words To Know (*continued*)
pulmonary embolus
third spacing
thrombus formation
total parenteral nutrition
venipuncture
volumetric controller

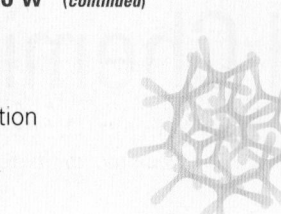

 Gerontologic Considerations

■ Mobility limitations, cognitive impairments, and difficulty performing activities of daily living (ADLs) can lead to fluid and electrolyte deficits in older adults.

■ Dehydration in older adults may be a consequence or indicator of abuse or neglect.

■ Older adults may need to be encouraged to drink fluids, even at times when they do not feel thirsty, because age-related changes may diminish the sensation of thirst.

■ Rather than asking older adults if they would like a drink, it is important to identify their preferences and offer small amounts of their preferred liquids at frequent intervals. This intervention will assist in keeping oral mucosa moist and providing hydration needs.

■ To maintain adequate consumption of nutrients, it is best to offer fluids to older adults at times other than meals. Distending the stomach with liquids creates a sensation of satiety (fullness) and reduces the consumption of food.

■ When older adults must fast before certain procedures, emphasize the need to increase oral fluid intake in the hours before beginning fluid restrictions to prevent dehydration.

■ Encourage older adults to drink noncaffeinated beverages because of the diuretic effect of caffeine or to replace the volume of caffeinated beverages by consuming the same volume of noncaffeinated fluids per day.

■ Because skin elasticity diminishes with aging, skin turgor is best assessed over the sternum. In addition to decreased skin turgor, indicators of dehydration in older adults include mental status changes; increases in pulse and respiratory rates; a decrease in blood pressure; dark, concentrated urine with a high specific gravity; dry mucous membranes; warm skin; furrowed tongue; low urine output; hardened stools; and elevated hematocrit, hemoglobin, serum sodium, and blood urea nitrogen.

■ Older adults may restrict their fluid intake under the mistaken notion that this will reduce urinary incontinence. This practice can contribute to the problem by increasing bladder irritability and increases the risks for urinary tract infection, postural hypotension, falls, and injuries. An assessment of fluid and electrolyte imbalances is important for any older adult who has a change in mental status.

■ It may be possible and advantageous to avoid using a tourniquet when accessing a vein that is visually prominent on an older adult. Use of a tourniquet may result in bursting the vein, sometimes referred to as "blowing the vein," when it is punctured with a needle.

■ Nurses need to closely monitor the response of older adults to intravenous (IV) infusions because they may have difficulty tolerating volumes that are safe for younger adults.

BODY FLUID

Water
Depending on age and sex, the human body comprises approximately 45% to 75% of water. Body water is normally supplied and replenished from three sources: drinking liquids, consuming food, and metabolizing nutrients. Once the water is absorbed, it is distributed among various locations, called *compartments*, within the body.

Fluid Compartments
Body fluid is located in two general compartments. **Intracellular fluid** (ICF; fluid inside the cells) represents the greatest proportion of water in the body. The remaining body fluid is **extracellular fluid** (ECF; fluid outside the cells). ECF is further subdivided into **interstitial fluid** (fluid in the tissue space between and around cells) and **intravascular fluid** (the watery plasma, or serum, portion of blood) (Fig. 16-1). The percentage of water in these compartments varies according to age and sex (Table 16-1).

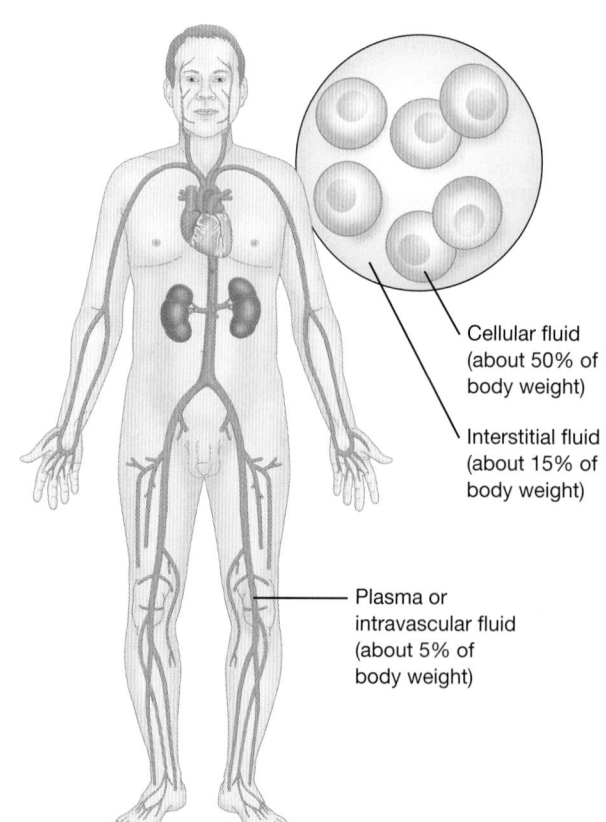

Cellular fluid (about 50% of body weight)

Interstitial fluid (about 15% of body weight)

Plasma or intravascular fluid (about 5% of body weight)

FIGURE 16-1 The average distribution of body fluid.

TABLE 16-1 Percentages of Body Fluid According to Age and Sex

FLUID COMPARTMENT	INFANTS (%)	ADULT MALES (%)	ADULT FEMALES (%)	OLDER ADULTS (%)
Intravascular	4	4	5	5
Interstitial	25	11	10	15
Intracellular	48	45	35	25
Total	77	60	50	45

Electrolytes

Electrolytes are chemical compounds, such as sodium and chloride, that possess an electrical charge when dissolved, absorbed, and distributed in body fluid. They are essential for maintaining cellular, tissue, and organ functions. For example, electrolytes affect fluid balance and complex chemical activities, such as muscle contraction and the formation of enzymes, acids, and bases (see discussion of minerals in Chapter 15).

Electrolytes are obtained from dietary sources of food and beverages but may be provided through pharmaceutical supplements for clients who are not eating or cannot do so. Electrolytes are decreased, for example, through malnutrition or an altered state of health such as vomiting and diarrhea, severe burns, disorders such as renal disease, and even medications like diuretics.

Collectively, electrolytes are called **ions** (substances that carry either a positive or a negative electrical charge). **Cations** (electrolytes with a positive charge) and **anions** (electrolytes with a negative charge) are present in equal amounts overall, but their distribution varies in each body fluid compartment (Table 16-2). For example, more potassium ions are present inside the cells than outside them.

Electrolytes are measured in the serum of blood specimens, and the amount is reported in milliequivalents (mEq). When one or more cations or anions become excessive or deficient, an electrolyte imbalance occurs. Significant imbalances can lead to dangerous physiologic problems. In many situations, electrolyte imbalances accompany changes in fluid volumes.

Nonelectrolytes are chemical compounds that remain bound together when dissolved in a solution and do not possess an electrical charge. The chemical end products of carbohydrates, proteins, and fat metabolism—namely, glucose, amino acids, and fatty acids—provide a continuous supply of nonelectrolytes.

In the absence of metabolic disease, a stable amount of nonelectrolytes circulates in body fluid as long as a person consumes adequate nutrients. Deficiency states occur when body fluid is lost or when the ability to eat is compromised.

Blood

On average, blood consists of 3 L of plasma, or fluid, and 2 L of blood cells for an average total circulating volume of 5 L. Blood cells include erythrocytes, or red blood cells; leukocytes, or white blood cells; and platelets, also known as *thrombocytes*. For every 500 red blood cells, there are approximately 30 platelets and one white blood cell (Fischbach et al., 2021).

Any disorder that alters the volume of body fluid, whether it is fluid retention or loss, also affects the plasma volume of blood. Examples include chronic bleeding or hemorrhage, infection, chemicals or conditions that destroy the blood cells once they have been produced, and disorders that affect the bone marrow's production of blood cells. Deficits in either fluid or cell volume are treated by administering fluid, whole blood or packed red blood cells, or individual blood components.

Fluid and Electrolyte Distribution Mechanisms

Although fluid compartments are identified separately, water and the substances dissolved therein continuously circulate throughout all areas of the body. Physiologic transport mechanisms such as osmosis, filtration, passive diffusion, facilitated diffusion, and active transport govern the movement and relocation of water and substances within body fluid (Fig. 16-2).

Osmosis

Osmosis helps regulate the distribution of water by controlling the movement of fluid from one location to another. Under the influence of osmosis, water moves through a semipermeable membrane like those surrounding body cells, capillary walls, and body organs and cavities, from an area where the fluid is more dilute to another area where the fluid is more concentrated (see Fig. 16-2A). Once the fluid is of equal concentration on both sides of the membrane, the transfer of fluid between compartments does not change appreciably, except volume for volume.

TABLE 16-2 Major Serum Electrolytes

ELECTROLYTE	CHEMICAL SYMBOL	CATION/ANION	NORMAL SERUM LEVEL (mEq/L)	PREDOMINANT COMPARTMENT
Sodium	Na	Cation	135–148	ECF
Potassium	K	Cation	3.5–5.0	ICF
Chloride	Cl	Anion	90–110	ECF
Phosphate	PO_4	Anion	1.7–2.6	ICF
Calcium	Ca	Cation	4.5–5.5	ICF
Magnesium	Mg	Cation	1.3–2.1	ICF
Bicarbonate	HCO_3	Anion	22–26	ICF

ECF, extracellular fluid; ICF, intracellular fluid.

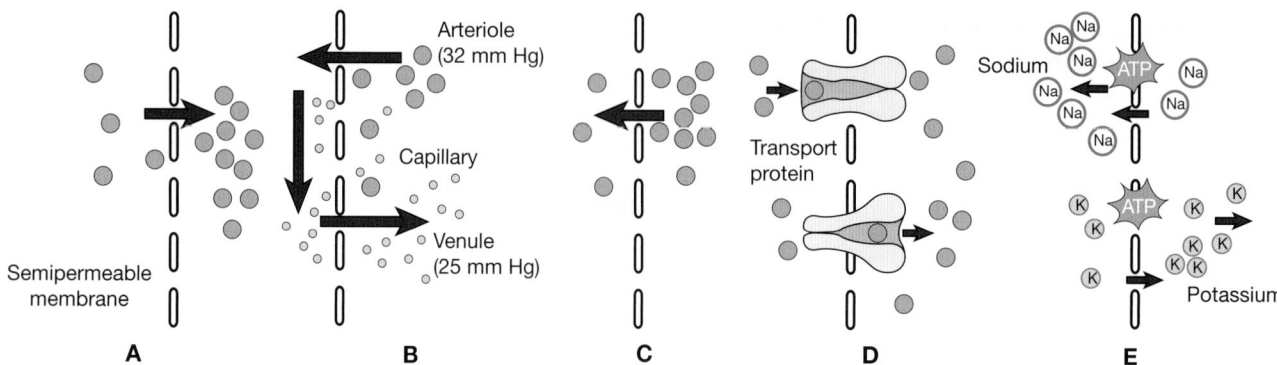

FIGURE 16-2 A. Osmosis. **B.** Filtration. **C.** Passive diffusion. **D.** Facilitated diffusion. **E.** Active transport. ATP, adenosine triphosphate.

The presence and quantity of colloids on either side of the semipermeable membrane influence osmosis. **Colloids** are undissolved protein substances such as albumin and blood cells within body fluids that do not readily pass through membranes. Their very presence produces **colloidal osmotic pressure** (the force for attracting water) that influences fluid volume in any given fluid location.

Filtration

Filtration, another mechanism that influences fluid distribution, regulates the movement of water and substances from a compartment where the pressure is higher to one where the pressure is lower. The force of filtration is referred to as **hydrostatic pressure** (the pressure exerted against a membrane). For example, because of contraction of the left ventricle, the fluid pressure is higher at the arterial end of a capillary than at the venous end. Consequently, fluid and dissolved substances are forced into the interstitial compartment at the capillary's arterial end. Water is then reabsorbed from the interstitial fluid in comparable amounts at the venous end of the capillary because of colloidal osmotic pressure (see Fig. 16-2B). Filtration also governs how the kidney excretes fluid and wastes and then selectively reabsorbs water and substances that need to be conserved.

Passive Diffusion

Passive diffusion is the physiologic process by which dissolved substances, such as electrolytes and gases, move from an area of higher concentration to an area of lower concentration through a semipermeable membrane (see Fig. 16-2C). It occurs without any expenditure of energy—hence the modifier *passive*. Passive diffusion facilitates **electrochemical neutrality** (an identical balance of cations with anions) in any given fluid compartment. Like osmosis, passive diffusion remains fairly static once equilibrium is achieved.

Facilitated Diffusion

Facilitated diffusion is the process by which certain dissolved substances require the assistance of a carrier molecule to pass from one side of a cellular membrane to the other (see Fig. 16-2D). Facilitated diffusion distributes substances from an area of higher concentration to one that is lower. Glucose is an example of a substance that requires facilitated diffusion because once in the bloodstream, glucose

cannot permeate cell walls. Glucose is made available to cells in combination with insulin and glucose transport (GLUT) proteins located within cellular membranes. Without insulin, GLUT is very low; in the presence of insulin, GLUT is rapidly stimulated. The GLUT proteins (a) bind with glucose in plasma on the outside of the cell membrane, then (b) the GTUTs face the inner area of the cell and (c) the glucose moves into the cell (Moosmosis, 2020).

Active Transport

Active transport, a process of chemical distribution that requires an energy source, involves a substance called *adenosine triphosphate* (ATP) (see Fig. 16-2E). ATP provides energy to drive the dissolved chemicals against the concentration gradient. In other words, it allows chemical distribution from an area of low concentration to one that is higher—the opposite of passive diffusion.

An example of active transport is the *sodium–potassium pump system* on cellular membranes, which regulates the movement of potassium from lower concentrations in the ECF into cells where it is more highly concentrated. It also moves sodium, which has a lower concentration within the cells, to ECF where it is more abundant.

Fluid Regulation

In healthy adults, fluid intake generally averages approximately 2,500 mL/day, but it can range from 1,800 to 3,000 mL/day with a similar volume of fluid loss (Table 16-3). Normal mechanisms for fluid loss are urination, bowel elimination, perspiration, and breathing. Losses from the skin in areas other than where sweat glands are located and from the vapor in exhaled air are referred to as *insensible losses* because for practical purposes, they are unnoticeable and unmeasurable.

Under normal conditions, several mechanisms maintain a match between fluid intake and output (I&O). For example, as body fluid becomes concentrated, the brain triggers the sensation of thirst, which then stimulates the person to drink. As fluid volume expands, the kidneys excrete a proportionate volume of water to maintain or restore proper balance. There are circumstances, however, in which oral intake or fluid losses are altered. Therefore, nurses assess clients for signs of fluid deficit or excess, particularly in those prone to fluid imbalances (Box 16-1).

TABLE 16-3 Daily Fluid Intake and Losses

SOURCES OF FLUID		MECHANISMS OF FLUID LOSS	
Oral liquids	1,200–1,500 mL/day	Urine	1,200–1,700 mL/day
Food	700–1,000 mL/day	Feces	100–250 mL/day
Metabolism	200–400 mL/day	Perspiration	100–150 mL/day
		Insensible losses	
		Skin	350–400 mL/day
		Lungs	350–400 mL/day
Total	2,100–2,900 mL/day	**Total**	2,100–2,900 mL/day
Average intake	2,500 mL/day	**Average loss**	2,500 mL/day

FLUID VOLUME ASSESSMENT

Nurses assess fluid status using a combination of a physical assessment (Table 16-4) and a measurement of I&O volumes.

Intake and output (I&O) is one tool to assess fluid status by keeping a record of a client's fluid intake and fluid loss over a 24-hour period. Agencies often specify the types of clients that are placed automatically on I&O; generally, they include:

- Clients who have undergone surgery until they are eating, drinking, and voiding in sufficient quantities
- Clients receiving IV fluids
- Clients receiving tube feedings
- Clients with some type of wound drainage or suction equipment
- Clients with urinary catheters until it can be determined that output is adequate or they are voiding well after removal of the catheter
- Clients undergoing diuretic drug therapy

In addition, many agencies allow nurses to independently order an I&O assessment for clients who have or are at risk for a fluid imbalance problem. The nurse discontinues the nursing order when the assessment is no longer indicated but consults with the physician if it has been medically ordered. Each agency has a specific I&O form kept at the bedside so that nurses can conveniently record the type of fluid and amounts that are consumed and lost throughout the day (Fig. 16-3). The nurse subtotals the amounts at the end of each shift or more frequently in critical care areas. They document the grand total in a designated area in the medical record, for example, on the graphics sheet with other vital sign information.

Fluid Intake

Fluid intake is the sum of all fluid volume that a client consumes or is instilled into the client's body, including:

- All the liquids a client drinks
- The liquid equivalent of melted ice chips, which is half of the frozen volume

BOX 16-1 **Conditions That Predispose Clients to Fluid Imbalances**

Fluid Deficit
- Starvation
- Impaired swallowing
- Vomiting
- Gastric suction
- Diarrhea
- Laxative misuse
- Potent diuretics
- Hemorrhage
- Major burns
- Draining wounds
- Fever and sweating
- Exercise and sweating
- Environmental heat and humidity

Fluid Excess
- Kidney failure
- Heart failure
- Rapid administration of intravenous fluid or blood
- Administration of albumin
- Corticosteroid drug therapy
- Excessive intake of sodium
- Pregnancy
- Premenstrual fluid retention

TABLE 16-4 Signs of Fluid Imbalance

ASSESSMENT	FLUID DEFICIT	FLUID EXCESS
Weight	Weight loss ≥2 lb/24 hours	Weight gain ≥2 lb/24 hours
Blood pressure	Low	High
Temperature	Elevated	Normal
Pulse	Rapid, weak, thready	Full, bounding
Respirations	Rapid, shallow	Moist, labored
Urine	Scant, dark yellow	Light yellow
Stool	Dry, small volume	Bulky
Skin	Warm, flushed, dry	Cool, pale, moist
	Poor skin turgor	Pitting edema
Mucous membranes	Dry, sticky	Moist
Eyes	Sunken	Swollen
Lungs	Clear	Crackles, gurgles
Breathing	Effortless	Dyspnea, orthopnea
Energy	Weak	Fatigues easily
Jugular neck veins	Flat	Distended
Cognition	Reduced	Reduced
Consciousness	Sleepy	Anxious

- Foods that are liquid by the time they are swallowed, such as gelatin, ice cream, and thin-cooked cereal
- Fluid infusions, such as IV solutions
- Fluid instillations, such as those administered through feeding tubes or tube irrigations

Fluid volumes are recorded in milliliters (mL). The approximate equivalent for 1 oz is 30 mL, a teaspoon is 5 mL, and a tablespoon is 15 mL. Packaged beverage containers such as milk cartons usually indicate the specific fluid volume on the label. Hospitals and nursing homes

INTAKE AND OUTPUT RECORD

DATE _____   NAME _____

Equivalents:
1 oz = 30 cc
Juice cup, serving of jello, ice cream, sherbet = 4 oz = 120 cc
Soup = 6 oz = 180 cc
Milk carton, coffee mug, plastic cold cup = 8 oz = 240 cc
Styrofoam cups 6 oz = 180 cc; 7 oz = 210 cc
Soft drinks: 12 oz can = 360 cc; 10 oz bottle = 300 cc; 16 oz bottle = 480 cc

Record for Intake:
Water, milk, Ensure, soup, coffee, tea, Kool-Aid, soft drinks, fruit juices, ice cream, sherbet, gelatin, and IV fluids

Record for Output:
Urine, vomitus, excessive perspiration, blood, and wound drainage, liquid stools
For urine output, record time voided or time found wet for incontinent persons.

TIME (11-7)	INTAKE AMOUNT IN CCs	TYPE OF INTAKE	TIME	* OUTPUT AMOUNT IN CCs	TYPE OF OUTPUT
TOTAL					
TIME (7-3)					
TOTAL					
TIME (3-11)					
TOTAL					
24 HR TOTAL					

* **Record amount of urine/void only if ordered by M.D.**
If person does not urinate/void for 8 hours, call your nurse or supervisor.

Outreach Services of Indiana   OR-FN-HS-NU-36(11-9-09)

*If Client does not void for 12 hours, call your Nurse.   4/07

FIGURE 16-3 Intake and output volumes are recorded throughout a 24-hour period and subtotaled at the end of each 8-hour shift.

BOX 16-2	Volume Equivalents for Common Containers
Container	**Volume (mL)**
Teaspoon	5
Tablespoon	15
Juice glass	120
Drinking glass	240
Coffee cup	210
Milk carton	240
Water pitcher	900
Paper cup	180
Soup bowl	200
Cereal bowl	120
Ice cream cup	120
Gelatin dish	90

commonly identify the volume equivalents contained in the cups, glasses, and bowls used to serve food and beverages from the dietary department (Box 16-2). If an equivalency chart is not available, the nurse uses a calibrated container (Fig. 16-4) to measure specific amounts; estimated volumes are considered inaccurate.

》》 *Stop, Think, and Respond 16-1*

Use Box 16-2 to calculate the volume of fluid intake for the following: a glass of orange juice, a half-pint carton of milk, a bowl of tomato soup, a dish of lime gelatin, a cup of coffee, and a 100-mL infusion of intravenous antibiotic solution.

Fluid Output

Fluid output is the sum of liquid eliminated from the body, including:

- Urine
- Emesis (vomitus)

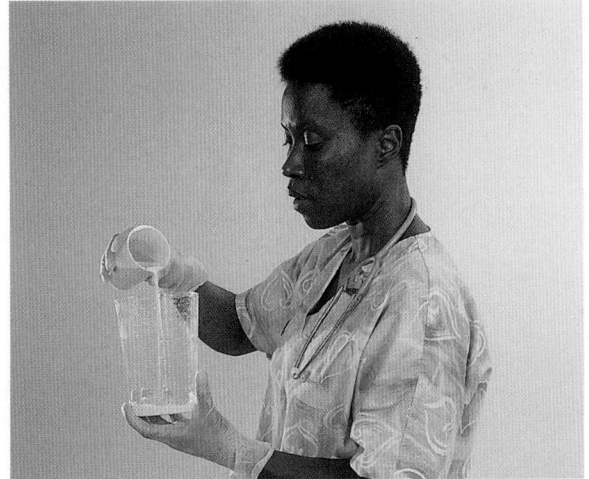

FIGURE 16-4 Calibrated containers used to measure liquid volumes. (Photo by B. Proud.)

 ### Client and Family Teaching 16-1
Recording Intake and Output

The nurse teaches the client or family as follows:

- Write down the amount or notify the nurse whenever oral fluid is consumed.
- Use a common household measurement, such as one glass or cup, to describe the volume consumed, or refer to an equivalency chart.
- Do not let a staff person remove a dietary tray until the fluid amounts have been recorded.
- Do not empty a urinal or urinate directly into the toilet bowl.
- Make sure that a measuring device is in the toilet bowl if the bathroom is used for voiding (see figure).

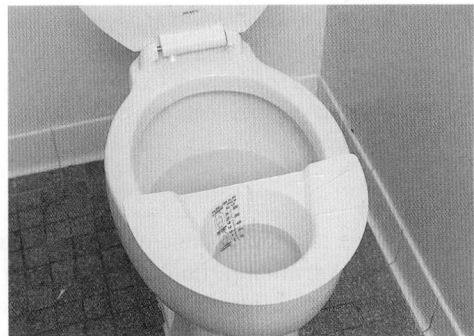

- If a urinal needs to be emptied, call the nurse or empty its contents into a calibrated container.
- Use a container such as a bedpan or bedside commode if diarrhea occurs. Notify the nurse to measure the contents before it is emptied.
- If vomiting occurs, use an emesis basin rather than the toilet.

- Blood loss
- Diarrhea
- Wound or tube drainage
- Aspirated irrigations

In cases in which an accurate assessment is critical to a client's treatment, the nurse weighs wet linens, pads, diapers, or dressings and subtracts the weight of a similar dry item. An estimate of fluid loss is based on the equivalent: 1 lb (0.47 kg) = 1 pint (475 mL).

Client cooperation is needed for accurate I&O records. Therefore, the nurse informs clients whose I&O volumes are being recorded about the purpose and goals for fluid replacement or restrictions and the ways they can assist in the procedure (Client and Family Teaching 16-1). Suggested actions for maintaining an I&O record are provided in Skill 16-1.

COMMON FLUID IMBALANCES

Fluid imbalance is a general term describing any of several conditions in which the water content of the body is not in the proper volume or location within the body. It can be life-threatening. Common fluid imbalances include hypovolemia, hypervolemia, and third spacing.

NURSING GUIDELINES 16-1

Increasing Oral Intake

- Explain to the client the reasons for increasing consumption of oral fluids. *Knowledge facilitates client cooperation.*
- Compile a list of the client's preferences for beverages. *Involving the client facilitates individualized collaboration with the dietary department.*
- Obtain a variety of beverages on the client's list. *Catering to client preferences promotes compliance.*
- Develop a schedule for providing small portions of the total fluid volume over a 24-hour period. *Scheduling ensures that the final goal is reached by meeting short-term goals.*
- Plan to provide the bulk of the projected fluid intake at times when the client is awake. *Providing a higher proportion of fluid during waking hours avoids disturbing sleep.*
- Offer verbal recognition and frequent feedback, or design a method for demonstrating the client's progress, such as a bar

graph or pie chart. *Positive reinforcement encourages adherence and maintains goal-directed efforts.*
- Keep fluids handy at the bedside and place them in containers the client can handle. *Availability and convenience promote compliance.*
- Vary the types of fluid, serving glass, or container frequently. *Variety reduces boredom and maintains interest in working toward the goal.*
- Serve fluids in small containers and in small amounts. *Small portions avoid overwhelming the client.*
- Ensure that fluids are at an appropriate temperature. *Palatability promotes pleasure and enjoyment.*
- Include gelatin, popsicles, ice cream, and sherbet as alternatives to liquid beverages if allowed. *Varying the liquid's consistency and techniques for consumption offers an alternative to items that are sipped from a glass.*

Hypovolemia

Hypovolemia refers to a low volume of ECF. If untreated, it may result in **dehydration** (a fluid deficit in both extracellular and intracellular compartments). Mild dehydration is present when there is a 3% to 5% loss of body weight; moderate dehydration is associated with a 6% to 10% loss of body weight; and severe dehydration, a life-threatening emergency, occurs with a loss of more than 9% to 15% of body weight. In addition to weight loss, dehydration is evidenced by decreased skin turgor.

Causes of fluid volume deficits include:

- Inadequate fluid intake
- Fluid loss in excess of fluid intake
- Translocation of large volumes of intravascular fluid to the interstitial compartment or to areas with only potential spaces, such as the peritoneal cavity, pericardium, and pleural space

Fluid balance is restored by treating the cause of hypovolemia, increasing oral intake, administering IV fluid replacements, controlling fluid losses, or a combination of these measures (Nursing Guidelines 16-1).

Pharmacologic Considerations

An increased risk of hypovolemia can result with medication use. For example, diuretic medications used to treat cardiovascular and kidney disorders are prescribed to remove excess water and may result in fluid and potassium depletion. Overuse of laxatives and enemas can cause fluid and electrolyte depletion.

Hypervolemia

Hypervolemia means a higher than normal volume of water in the intravascular fluid compartment and is another example of a fluid imbalance. **Edema** develops when excess fluid is distributed to the interstitial space (Fig. 16-5). When fluid

accumulates in dependent areas of the body (those influenced by gravity), the tissue pits (forms indentations) when compressed (see Chapter 13). Edema does not usually occur unless there is a 3 L excess in body fluid. Hypervolemia can lead to **circulatory overload** (severely compromised heart function) if it remains unresolved.

Control of edema is an important nursing priority. Fluid balance is restored by:

- Treating the disorder contributing to the increased fluid volume
- Restricting or limiting oral fluids
- Reducing salt consumption (Box 16-3)
- Discontinuing IV fluid infusions or reducing the infusing volume
- Administering drugs that promote urine elimination
- Using a combination of these interventions

See Nursing Guidelines 16-2.

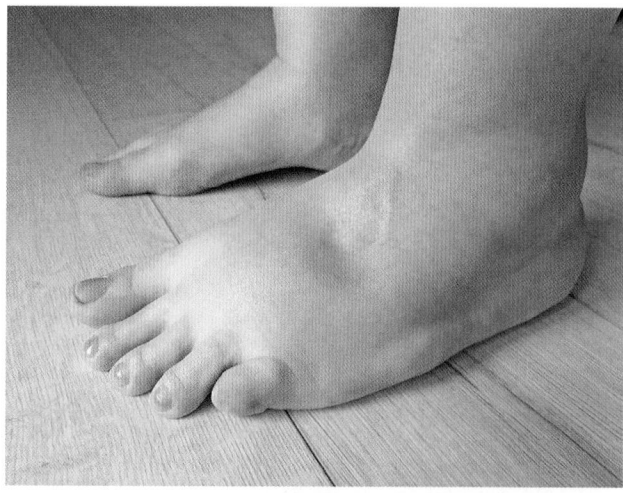

FIGURE 16-5 An example pitting edema, caused by fluid retention. (PJs Panda/Shutterstock.)

BOX 16-3	**Foods High in Sodium**

- Processed meats such as frankfurters and cold cuts
- Smoked fish
- Frozen egg substitutes
- Peanut butter
- Dairy products, especially hard cheeses like American, cheddar
- Powdered cocoa or hot chocolate mixes
- Canned vegetables, especially sauerkraut
- Pickles
- Tomato and tomato-vegetable juice
- Canned soup and bouillon
- Boxed casserole mixes
- Baking mixes
- Salted snack foods
- Seasonings such as ketchup, gravy mixes, soy sauce, monosodium glutamate, pickle relish, and tartar sauce

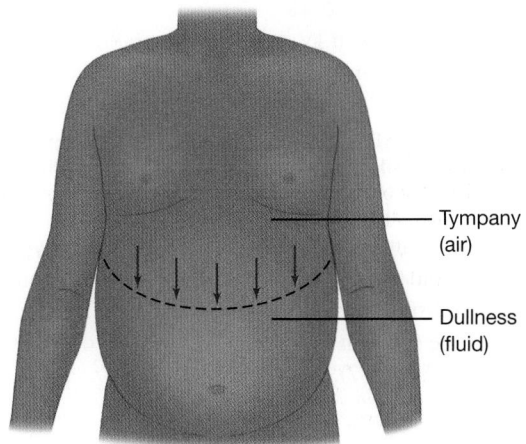

FIGURE 16-6 Fluid accumulation within the peritoneal cavity. Dullness on percussion indicates fluid, whereas tympany indicates air.

Third Spacing

Third spacing is the movement of intravascular fluid to nonvascular fluid compartments, where it becomes trapped and useless. It is generally manifested by tissue swelling or fluid that accumulates in a body cavity, such as the peritoneum (Fig. 16-6). Third spacing is associated commonly with disorders in which albumin, a plasma protein, levels are low because albumin facilitates colloidal osmotic pressure, retaining fluid within the vascular system. Causes of **hypoalbuminemia** (a deficit of albumin in the blood) include liver disease, chronic kidney disease, and disorders in which capillary and cellular permeability are altered, such as burns and severe allergic reactions.

Depletion of fluid in the intravascular space may lead to hypotension and shock; thus, fluid therapy becomes critical. The priority is to restore the circulatory volume by providing IV fluids, sometimes in large volumes at rapid rates. Blood transfusions or the administration of albumin by IV infusion is also used to restore colloidal osmotic pressure to pull the trapped fluid back into the intravascular space. When this occurs, clients who were previously hypovolemic can suddenly become hypervolemic. The nurse closely monitors clients who receive albumin replacement for signs of circulatory overload.

INTRAVENOUS FLUID ADMINISTRATION

Policies and practices vary concerning how much responsibility practical/vocational nurses assume with IV fluid therapy. The discussion that follows is provided to meet the needs of those nurses who have been trained and have demonstrated competencies for administering IV fluids.

Intravenous fluids are solutions infused into a client's vein to:

- Maintain or restore fluid balance when oral replacement is inadequate or impossible
- Maintain or replace electrolytes
- Administer water-soluble vitamins
- Provide a source of calories
- Administer drugs (see Chapter 35)
- Replace blood and blood products

 NURSING GUIDELINES 16-2

Restricting Oral Fluids

- Explain the purpose for the restrictions. *Knowledge facilitates client cooperation.*
- Identify the total amount of fluid the client may consume using measurements with which the client is familiar. *An explanation helps the client understand the extent of the restrictions.*
- Work out a plan for distributing the permitted volume over a 24-hour period with the client. *Including the client in planning promotes cooperation.*
- Ration the fluid so that the client can consume beverages between meals as well as at mealtimes. *Distributing opportunities to drink fluid helps minimize thirst.*
- Avoid sweet drinks and foods that are dry or salty. *This reduces thirst and the desire for fluid.*

- Serve liquids at their proper temperature. *This demonstrates concern for the client's pleasure and enjoyment.*
- Offer ice chips as an occasional substitute for liquids. *Ice chips appear to contain more liquid than they actually do, and holding them within the mouth prolongs the time over which the fluid is consumed.*
- Provide water or other fluid in a plastic squeeze bottle or spray atomizer. *These devices provide only a small volume of fluid.*
- Help the client with frequent oral hygiene. *Oral hygiene relieves thirst, moistens oral mucous membranes, and prevents drying and chapping of lips.*
- Allow the client to rinse their mouth with water but not swallow it. *Rinsing reduces thirst and keeps the mouth moist.*

Types of Solutions

There are two types of IV solutions: crystalloid and colloid. **Crystalloid solutions** are made of water and other uniformly dissolved crystals, such as salt and sugar. **Colloid solutions** are made of water and molecules of suspended substances, such as blood cells and blood products (such as albumin).

Crystalloid Solutions

Crystalloid solutions are classified as isotonic, hypotonic, and hypertonic (Table 16-5), depending on the concentration of dissolved substances in relation to plasma. The concentration of the solution influences the osmotic distribution of body fluid (Fig. 16-7).

Isotonic Solutions

An **isotonic solution** contains the same concentration of dissolved substances normally found in plasma. Isotonic solutions are generally administered to maintain fluid balance in clients who may not be able to eat or drink for a short period. Because of its equal concentration, an isotonic solution does not cause any appreciable redistribution of body fluid.

>>> **Stop, Think, and Respond 16-2**

Identify the net effect when the following intravenous solutions are infused: 0.45% NaCl, Ringer's solution, and 50% glucose.

Hypotonic Solutions

A **hypotonic solution** contains fewer dissolved substances than normally found in plasma. It is administered to clients

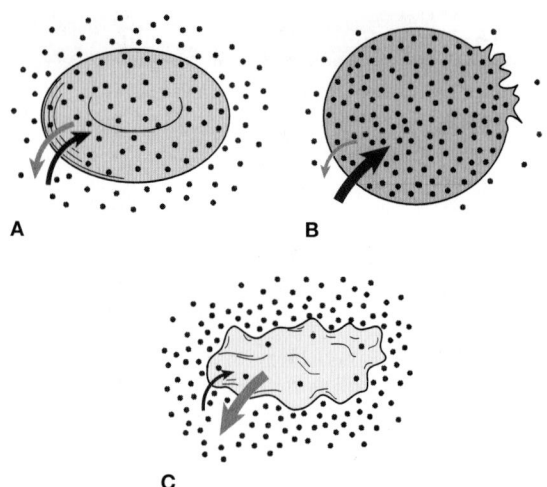

FIGURE 16-7 A. Isotonic solutions. **B.** Hypotonic solutions. **C.** Hypertonic solutions.

with fluid losses in excess of fluid intake, such as those who have diarrhea or vomiting. Because hypotonic solutions are dilute, the water in the solution passes through the semipermeable membrane of blood cells, causing them to swell. This temporarily increases blood pressure as it expands the circulating volume. The water also passes through capillary walls and becomes distributed within other body cells and the interstitial spaces. Hypotonic solutions, therefore, are an effective way to rehydrate clients experiencing fluid deficits.

TABLE 16-5 Types of Crystalloid Intravenous Solutions

SOLUTION	COMPONENTS	SPECIAL COMMENTS
Isotonic Solutions		
0.9% saline, also called normal saline	0.9 g of NaCl/100 mL of water	Amounts of sodium and chloride are physiologically equal to those found in plasma.
5% dextrose and water, also called D_5W	5 g of dextrose (glucose/sugar)/100 mL of water	Isotonic when infused but the glucose metabolizes quickly, leaving a solution of dilute water.
Ringer's solution or lactated Ringer's	Water and a mixture of sodium, chloride, calcium, potassium, bicarbonate, and, in some cases, lactate	Electrolyte replacement in amounts similar to those found in plasma; when present, lactate helps maintain acid–base balance.
Hypotonic Solutions		
0.45% NaCl, also called half-strength saline	0.45 g of NaCl/100 mL of water	Smaller ratio of sodium and chloride than found in plasma, causing it to be less concentrated in comparison
0.33% NaCl	0.33 g of NaCl/100 mL of water	Smaller ratio of sodium and chloride than found in plasma, used to allow kidneys to retain the needed amounts of water
5% dextrose in 0.45% saline	5 g of dextrose and 0.45 NaCl/100 mL of water	A quick source of energy from sugar, leaving a hypotonic salt solution
Hypertonic Solutions		
10% dextrose in water, also called $D_{10}W$	10 g of dextrose/100 mL of water	Twice the concentration of glucose as in plasma
3% saline	3 g of NaCl/100 mL of water	Dehydration of cells and tissues from the high concentration of salt in the plasma
20% dextrose in water	20 g of dextrose/100 mL water	Rapid increase in the concentration of sugar in the blood, causing a fluid shift to the intravascular compartment

Hypertonic Solutions

A **hypertonic solution** is more concentrated than body fluid and draws cellular and interstitial water into the intravascular compartment. This causes cells and tissue spaces to shrink. Hypertonic solutions are used infrequently, except in extreme cases when it is necessary to reduce cerebral edema or to expand the circulatory volume rapidly.

Colloid Solutions

Colloid solutions are used to replace circulating blood volume because the suspended molecules pull fluid from other compartments. Examples are blood, blood products such as albumin, and solutions known as *plasma expanders*.

Blood

Whole blood and packed cells are probably the most common colloid solutions. One unit of whole blood contains approximately 475 mL of blood cells and plasma plus 60 to 70 mL of preservative and anticoagulant (Hinkle & Cheever, 2021). Packed cells have most of the plasma removed and are preferred for clients who need cellular replacement but do not need or may be harmed by the administration of additional fluid.

Most blood given to clients comes from public donors. In some cases, for example, when a person anticipates the potential need for blood in the near future or when procedures are used to reclaim blood from wound drainage, the client's own blood may be reinfused (see Chapter 27).

Blood Products

Several blood products are available for clients who need specific substances but do not need all the fluid or cellular components in whole blood (Table 16-6).

Blood Substitutes

Blood substitutes are fluids that, when transfused, carry and distribute oxygen to cells, tissues, and organs. Many practitioners feel blood substitutes should be more accurately called **oxygen therapeutics** because they do not replace all the functions of human blood.

Finding a safe blood substitute could have many advantages: (1) it would benefit those with medical conditions that require long-term blood transfusions; (2) it could be used as donor organ preservatives; (3) it would be an acceptable alternative for people, such as Jehovah's Witnesses, who object to receiving blood transfusions based on their religious beliefs; (4) the risks for blood-borne diseases, such as hepatitis and acquired immune deficiency syndrome (AIDS), and transfusion reactions from transfused human blood could be eliminated; (5) there would be a greater potential for saving the lives of military casualties in locations lacking resources; and (6) it could be used in disasters and major trauma cases while awaiting transfusable human blood.

Currently, oxygen therapeutics fall into two categories: *perfluorocarbons* (PFCs) and *hemoglobin-based oxygen carriers* (HBOCs). PFCs are solutions containing fluorine and carbon, the liquid PFC could be a perfect breathing medium, due to its highly efficient capability of dissolving oxygen, but can also act as an antiinflammatory for human tissue (Kakaei et al., 2023). HBOCs are derived from three sources: (1) hemoglobin harvested from outdated human blood or (2) bovine (cattle) blood and (3) cultured from bacteria in which the gene for human hemoglobin is inserted (recombinant technology), much like human insulin is produced.

Because PFCs have a smaller molecular size than red blood cells, it is possible that they could deliver oxygen-carrying molecules to blood vessels that have been narrowed as a result of blood clots, thus relieving impaired circulation after a stroke or heart attack. That same property could be used to treat clients during a sickle cell crisis; their pain could be relieved by oxygenating tissues in which sickled red blood cells have obstructed blood flow. In addition, PFCs could prolong the preservation of organs for transplantation and could improve the oxygenation of cancer cells, making them more vulnerable to standard treatments.

According to Cardinale et al. (2017), "[HBOCs] have the potential to increase blood oxygen content in patients with life-threatening anemia in whom red blood cell transfusion is not an option." There are ongoing clinical trials to identify the potential use of HBOCs.

Plasma Expanders

Various nonblood solutions are used to pull fluid into the vascular space. Two examples are dextran 40 (Rheomacrodex) and hetastarch (Hespan). These two substances are polysaccharides—large, insoluble complex carbohydrate molecules. When mixed with water, they form colloidal solutions. Because the suspended particles cannot move through semipermeable membranes when given IV, they

TABLE 16-6 Types of Blood Products

BLOOD PRODUCT	DESCRIPTION	PURPOSE FOR ADMINISTRATION
Platelets	Disk-shaped cellular fragments that promote coagulation of blood	Restores or improves the ability to control bleeding
Granulocytes	Types of white blood cells	Improves the ability to overcome infection
Plasma	Serum minus blood cells	Replaces clotting factors or increases intravascular fluid volume by increasing colloidal osmotic pressure
Albumin	Plasma protein	Pulls third-spaced fluid by increasing colloidal osmotic pressure
Cryoprecipitate	Mixture of clotting factors	Treats blood clotting disorders, such as hemophilia

attract water from other fluid compartments. The desired outcome is to increase the blood volume and raise the blood pressure. Consequently, plasma expanders are used as economic and virus-free substitutes for blood and blood products when treating hypovolemic shock.

Preparation for Administration

Regardless of the prescribed solution, the nurse prepares the solution for administration, performs a venipuncture, regulates the rate of administration, monitors the infusion, and discontinues the administration when fluid balance is restored.

Solution Selection

IV solutions are commonly stored in plastic bags containing 1,000, 500, 250, 100, and 50 mL of solution. A few solutions are stocked in glass containers. The physician specifies the type of solution, additional additives, and the volume (in mL) and duration of the infusion. To reduce the potential for infection, IV solutions are replaced every 24 hours even if the total volume has not been completely instilled.

Before preparing the solution, the nurse inspects the container and determines that:

• The solution is the one prescribed by the physician.
• The solution is clear and transparent.
• The expiration date has not elapsed.
• No leaks are apparent.
• A separate label is attached, identifying the type and amount of other drugs added to the commercial solution.

Tubing Selection

All IV tubing consists of a spike for accessing the solution, a drip chamber for holding a small amount of fluid, a length of plastic tubing with one or more ports for adding IV medications (see Chapter 35), and a roller or slide clamp to regulate the rate of infusion (Fig. 16-8). The nurse then selects from several options:

• Primary (long) or secondary (short) tubing
• Vented or unvented tubing
• Microdrip (small drops) or macrodrip (large drops) chamber

• Unfiltered or filtered tubing
• Needle or needleless access ports

Primary versus Secondary Tubing

Primary tubing is approximately 110 in (2.8 m), and secondary tubing is 37 in (94 cm) long. These measurements vary among manufacturers. Primary tubing is used when the tubing must span the distance from a solution that hangs several feet above the infusion site. Secondary tubing, which is shorter, is used to administer smaller volumes of solution into a port within the primary tubing.

Vented versus Unvented Tubing

Vented tubing draws air into the container, while unvented tubing does not (Fig. 16-9). The choice depends on the type of container in which the solution is packaged. Vented tubing is necessary for administering solutions packaged in rigid glass containers; if unvented tubing is inserted into a glass bottle, the solution will not leave the container. Plastic bags of IV solutions do not need vented tubing because the container collapses as the fluid infuses.

Drop Size

Drop size refers to the size of the opening through which the fluid is delivered into the tubing. The nurse determines whether it is more appropriate to use macrodrip tubing, which produces large drops, or microdrip tubing, which produces very small drops. When a solution infuses at a fast rate, such as 125 mL/hour, it is generally easier to count fewer, larger drops than many smaller ones. When the solution must infuse precisely or at a slow rate, smaller drops are preferred.

Microdrip tubing, regardless of the manufacturer, delivers a standard volume of 60 drops/mL. Macrodrip tubing manufacturers, however, have not been consistent in designing the size of the opening. Therefore, the nurse must read the package label to determine the **drop factor** (number of drops/mL). Some common drop factors are 10, 15, and 20 drops/mL. The drop factor is important in calculating the infusion rate when it is instilled by gravity (e.g., without an electronic infuser) and is discussed later in this chapter.

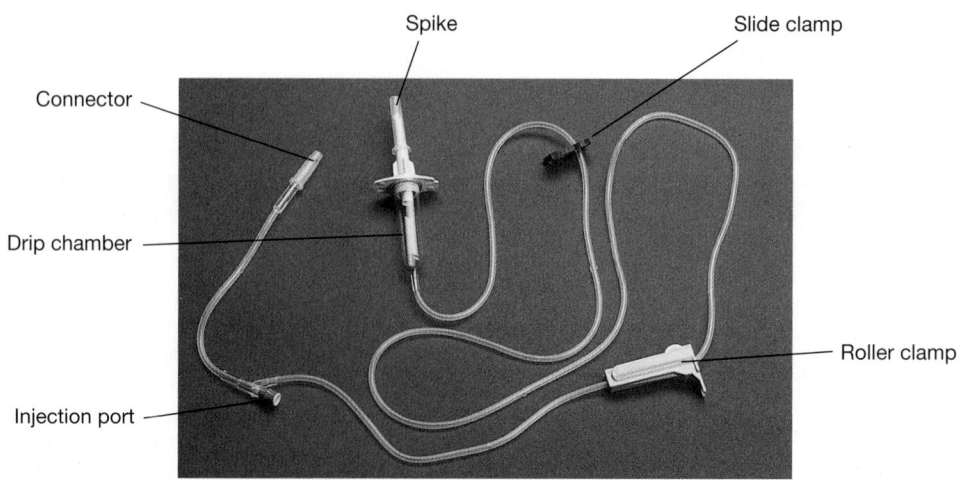

FIGURE 16-8 Basic intravenous tubing. (Nisitmicrostock/Shutterstock.)

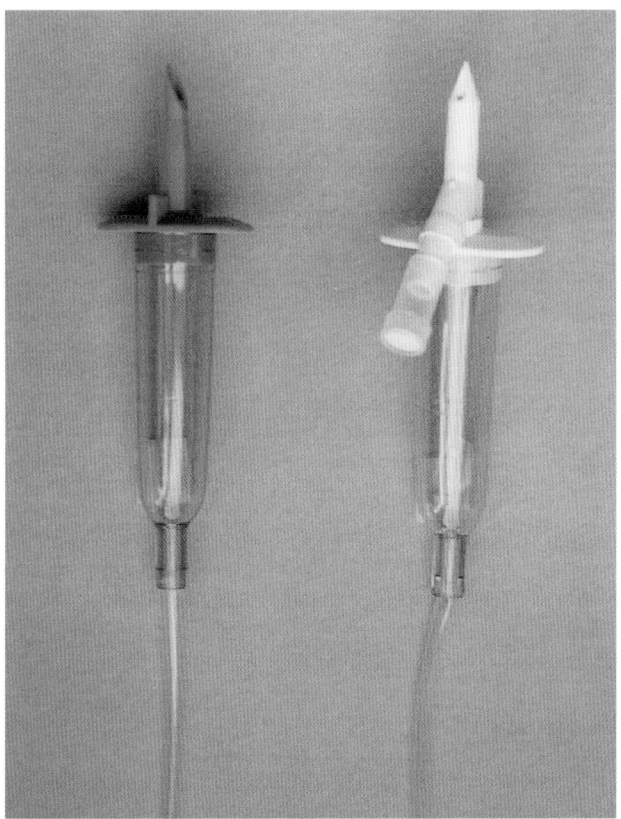

FIGURE 16-9 Unvented (left) and vented (right) tubing. (Photo by K. Timby.)

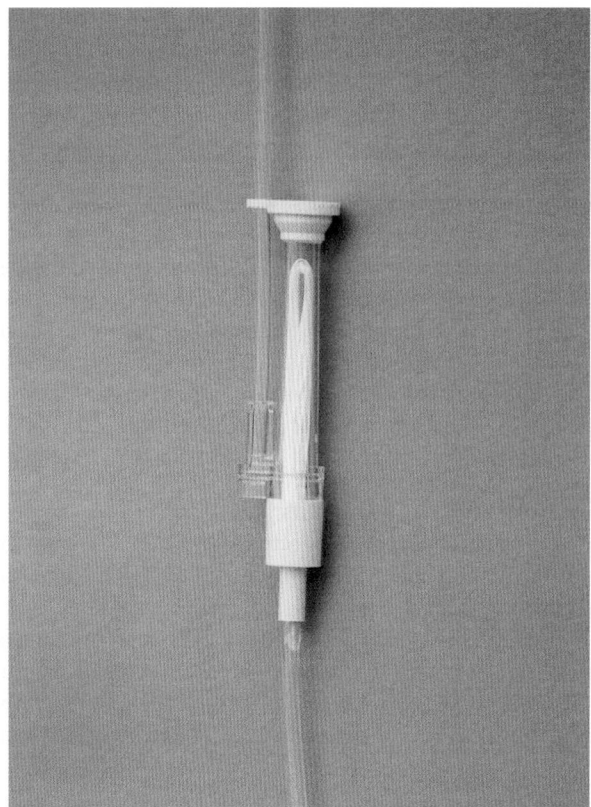

FIGURE 16-10 An in-line filter. (Photo by K. Timby.)

Filters

An in-line filter (Fig. 16-10) removes air bubbles as well as undissolved drugs, bacteria, and large substances. Filtered tubing generally is used when:

- Administering parenteral nutrition
- The client is at high risk for infection
- Infusing IV solutions to pediatric clients
- Administering blood and packed cells

Needle or Needleless Access Ports

Traditionally, the **ports** (sealed openings) in an IV tubing were designed for access with a needle. This method, however, contributes to the many needlestick injuries in the United States each year, with nurses accounting for a large percentage of those injuries under a variety of circumstances (Box 16-4). Prevention of needlestick injuries is an area of competency established by the Quality and Safety Education for Nurses (QSEN), an initiative developed by leaders from schools of nursing to minimize the risk of harm to clients and health care providers.

To reduce the incidence of work-related injuries and the potential for infection with blood-borne pathogens, **needleless systems** (IV tubing that eliminates the need for access needles) are preferred. Other recommended equipment includes safe needle devices used for administering injections (see Chapter 34), IV insertion equipment, and equipment used for blood specimen collection. With a needleless system, the nurse uses a blunt cannula to pierce the resealable port each time it is necessary to enter the tubing (Fig. 16-11; see Chapter 35).

BOX 16-4 **Conditions That Contribute to Needlestick Injuries**

- Reduced staff
- Difficult client care situations
- Reduced environmental light
- New staff or students
- Improperly disposed needles
- Emptying sharps disposal containers

SlideShare. (2014). *Needle-stick injuries among health care workers.* Retrieved July 2015, from http://www.slideshare.net/cetdmgh/14-needlestick-injuries-among-health-care-workers

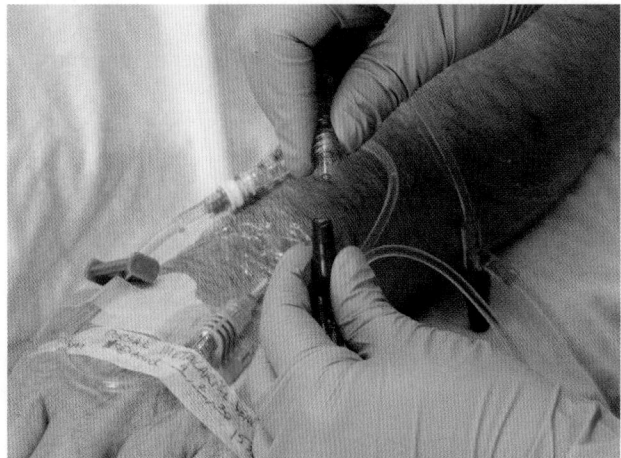

FIGURE 16-11 Needleless systems allow resealable ports to be penetrated with a needleless syringe or a secondary intravenous tubing connection.

Infusion Techniques

IV infusions are administered either by gravity alone or with an **infusion device**—an electric or battery-operated machine that regulates and monitors the administration of IV solutions. The use of an infusion device may affect the type of tubing used.

Gravity Infusion

Generally, most basic types of tubing can be used for infusing a solution by gravity. The height of the IV solution rather than the tubing is the most important factor affecting gravity infusions.

To overcome the pressure within the client's vein, which is higher than atmospheric pressure, the solution is elevated at least 18 to 24 in (45 to 60 cm) above the site of the infusion. The height of the solution affects the rate of flow; the higher the solution, the faster the solution infuses, and vice versa.

Electronic Infusion Devices

The two general types of electronic infusion devices are infusion pumps and volumetric controllers. Both are programmed to deliver a preset volume per hour. They trigger audible and visual alarms if the infusion is not progressing at the rate intended. They also sound an alarm when the infusion container is nearly empty, air is detected within the tubing, or obstruction or resistance occurs in delivering the fluid.

Infusion Pumps

An **infusion pump** (an electronic infusion device that uses pressure to infuse solutions) requires special tubing that contains a device such as a cassette to create sufficient pressure to push fluid into the vein (Fig. 16-12). The machine adjusts the pressure according to the resistance it meets. This can be a disadvantage because if the catheter or needle within the vein becomes displaced, the pump continues to infuse fluid into the tissue until the machine's maximum preset pressure limit is reached.

Volumetric Controllers

A **volumetric controller** (an electronic infusion device that instills IV solutions by gravity) mechanically compresses the tubing at a certain frequency to infuse the solution at a precise, preset rate. Volumetric controllers may or may not require special tubing. Some models allow the nurse to program the infusion of more than one simultaneous infusion of solutions. In some cases, when one container of fluid finishes

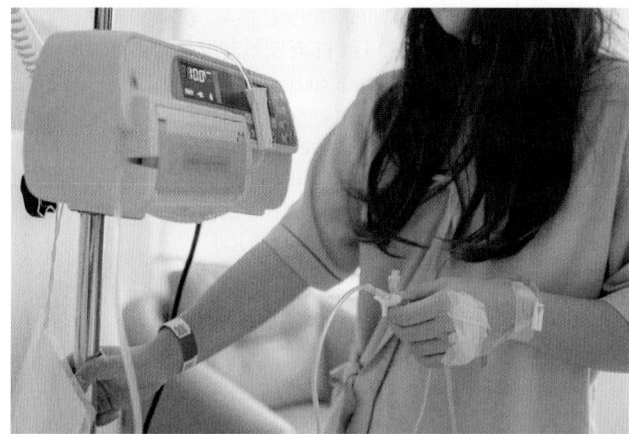

FIGURE 16-12 Electronic infusion device. (Winnievinzence/Shutterstock.)

infusing, the controller automatically resumes infusing another solution. The solution and tubing are prepared before accessing the vein with a needle or catheter. Skill 16-2 describes how to prepare IV solution for administration.

Venipuncture

Venipuncture (accessing the venous system by piercing a vein with a needle) is a nursing responsibility when a peripheral vein (one distant from the heart) is used. When performing a venipuncture, the nurse assembles the needed equipment, inspects and selects an appropriate vein, and inserts the venipuncture device.

Venipuncture Devices

Devices used to access a vein include a butterfly needle, an over-the-needle catheter (most common), or a through-the-needle catheter (Fig. 16-13).

Venipuncture devices are available in various diameters or gauges; the larger the gauge number, the smaller the diameter. The diameter of the venipuncture device should always be smaller than the vein into which it is inserted to reduce the potential for occluding blood flow. An 18-, 20-, or 22-gauge is the size most often used for adults.

In addition to a device for puncturing the vein, the following items are needed: clean gloves, a tourniquet, antiseptic swabs to cleanse the skin, a transparent dressing to cover

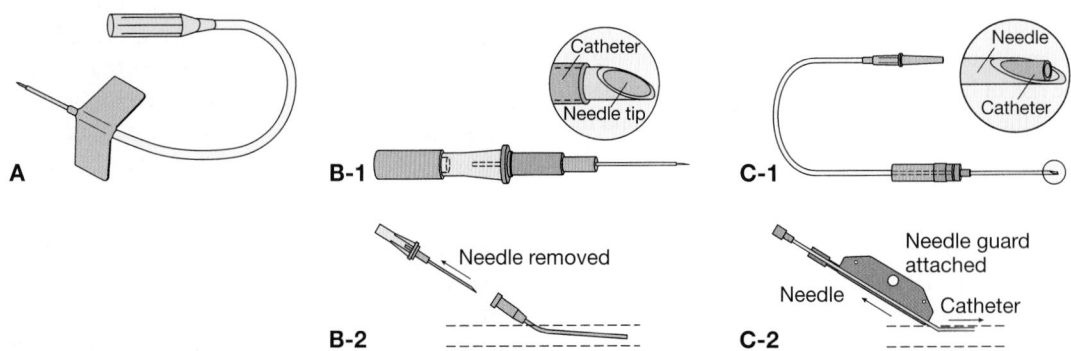

FIGURE 16-13 Venipuncture devices. **A.** A butterfly needle. **B-1.** An over-the-needle catheter. **B-2.** The needle removed. **C-1.** A through-the-needle catheter. **C-2.** A needle guard covers the tip of the needle, which remains outside the skin.

the puncture site, and adhesive tape to secure the venipuncture device and tubing. Do not use antibiotic or antimicrobial ointment at the site because it may promote fungal infections or antibiotic resistance (Centers for Disease Control and Prevention, 2017). An arm board may be needed to prevent the client from dislodging the venipuncture device.

Vein Selection
The veins in the hand and forearm are most commonly used for inserting a venipuncture device (Fig. 16-14); scalp veins are used for infants and small children (Nursing Guidelines 16-3).

Once the general site is selected, the nurse applies a tourniquet to select a specific vein. Box 16-5 identifies several techniques for promoting vein distention. A blood pressure cuff can be substituted for a rubber tourniquet. Whichever technique is used, the radial pulse should be palpable to indicate that arterial blood flow is being maintained.

Venipuncture Device Insertion
Skill 16-3 describes the technique for inserting an over-the-needle catheter within a vein.

Infusion Monitoring and Maintenance
Once the venipuncture is performed and the solution is infusing, the nurse regulates the rate of infusion, assesses for complications, cares for the venipuncture site, and replaces equipment as needed.

Regulating the Infusion Rate
The nurse is responsible for calculating, regulating, and maintaining the rate of infusion according to the physician's order. If an infusion device is used, the electronic equipment is programmed in milliliters per hour. If the solution is infused without an electronic infusion device (i.e., by gravity), the rate is calculated in drops (gtt) per minute. Formulas for calculating infusion rates are provided in Box 16-6.

For gravity infusions, the nurse counts the number of drops falling into the drip chamber per minute. By adjusting the roller clamp, the number of drops is increased or decreased until the infusion rate matches the calculated rate.

>>> ***Stop, Think, and Respond 16-3***
Calculate the rate of infusion for the following two medical orders:

1. *Infuse 1,000 mL of 0.9% NaCl over 12 hours using an electronic infusion device.*
2. *Infuse 500 mL of 5% dextrose and 0.45% NaCl in 8 hours by gravity infusion; your tubing delivers 15 gtt/mL.*

Assessing for Complications
Complications associated with the infusion of IV solutions (Table 16-7) are circulatory overload (an intravascular volume that becomes excessive), **infiltration** (the escape of IV fluid into the tissue), **phlebitis** (inflammation of a vein), **thrombus formation** (a stationary blood clot), **pulmonary embolus** (a blood clot that travels to the lung), infection (growth of microorganisms at the site or within the bloodstream), and **air embolism** (a bubble of air traveling within the vascular system).

 Pharmacologic Considerations

Some medications (such as diazepam, phenytoin, dopamine, and selected chemotherapy agents) can injure soft tissue if the IV solution leaks from the vein. Supplies and protocols for treatment should be readily available when these IV drugs are used.

The minimum quantity of air that may be fatal to humans is not known. Animal research indicates that fatal volumes of air are much larger than the quantity present in the entire length of infusion tubing. The average infusion tubing holds about 5 mL of air, an amount not ordinarily considered dangerous. Clients, however, are often frightened when they see air in the tubing, and nurses must make every effort to remove air bubbles (Nursing Guidelines 16-4).

Caring for the Site
Because venipuncture is a type of wound, it is important to inspect the site routinely. The nurse documents its appearance in the client's record. A common practice is to change the dressing over the venipuncture site every 24 to 72 hours according to the agency's infection control policy (see Chapter 28).

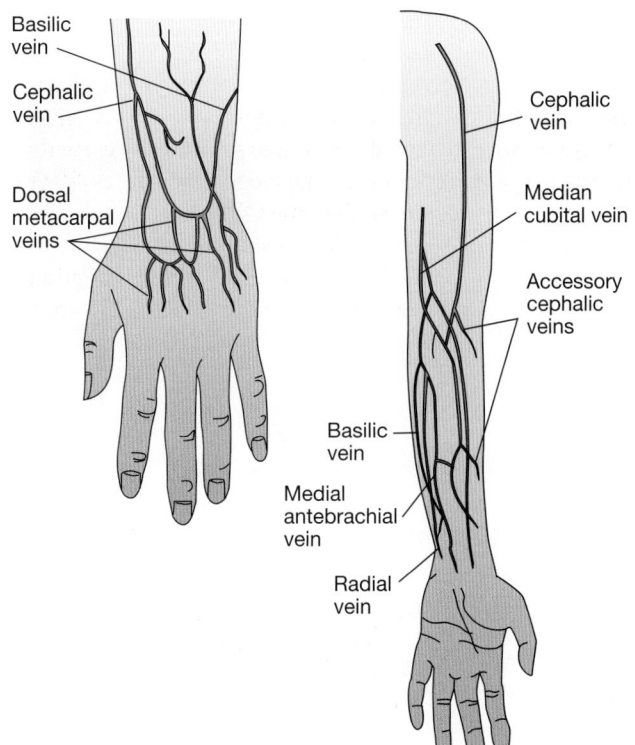

FIGURE 16-14 Potential venipuncture sites.

NURSING GUIDELINES 16-3

Selecting a Venipuncture Site

- Collect a latex tourniquet and other items needed for performing a venipuncture (see Skill 16-3). *A tourniquet is necessary to help distend veins.*
- Ask the client to identify their name and birthdate. *Obtaining two forms of identification prevents performing a procedure on the wrong client.*
- Perform hand hygiene. *Hand hygiene reduces the potential for transmitting infectious microorganisms.*
- Check if the client has any scars, lesions, inflammation, edema, or hematomas (blood that has seeped within tissue) in either arm, has had a previous mastectomy, or has a fistula for kidney dialysis. *Puncturing a vein with an injury or a vascular purpose creates a potential for infection, further compromises circulation, and has the potential for poor healing.*
- Eliminate veins in the foot or leg. *Using foot and leg veins restricts mobility and increases the potential for blood clots.*
- Inquire as to whether the client is right- or left-handed. *Initially, the nondominant upper extremity is preferred to facilitate activities.*
- Extend the arm on the nondominant side and place it in a dependent position. *Lowering the arm promotes the gravitational filling of blood within veins.*
- Place the tourniquet under the nondominant arm approximately 2 to 4 in above the elbow, and pull the ends of the tourniquet in opposite directions (Fig. A). *This location helps assess veins in the antecubital fossa (elbow location) and veins in the distal arm and hand.*
- Pull one end of the tourniquet tightly while stabilizing the opposite end and tuck the stretched end of the tourniquet beneath the other so both ends of the tourniquet point upward (Fig. B). *This gradually traps blood within the veins and facilitates the loosening or removal of the tourniquet.*
- Ensure that an arterial pulse is still palpable. *Circulation of oxygen-carrying arterial blood should not be obstructed.*
- Ask the client to pump their fist several times. *Contraction of skeletal muscles helps distend veins with blood.*
- Palpate the veins on the nondominant side for their characteristic spongy elastic feeling. Exclude any blood vessels in which a pulsation can be felt. *This action helps to differentiate veins from arteries.*
- Choose a vein in a location unaffected by joint movement. *A venipuncture device in such a location could become displaced more easily.*
- Look for a large vein if a large-gauge needle or catheter is necessary. *Matching the needle and vein size prevents compromising circulation.*
- Avoid using veins on the inner surface of the wrist. *This area is likely to cause pain and discomfort.*
- Look for a vein proximal to a running intravenous (IV) if a current site must be changed or in the opposite hand or arm. *This promotes healing and decreases the risk of fluid leaking from the vein into the tissue.*
- Feel and look for a fairly straight vein. *It is easier to thread the venipuncture device into a straight vein.*
- Do not keep the tourniquet applied for longer than 1 minute. *Stasis of blood has the potential for clot formation and*

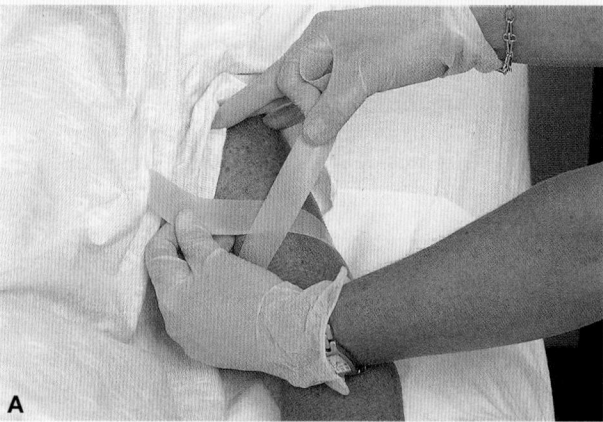

A

To apply a tourniquet, the ends are pulled tightly in opposite directions. (Photo by B. Proud.)

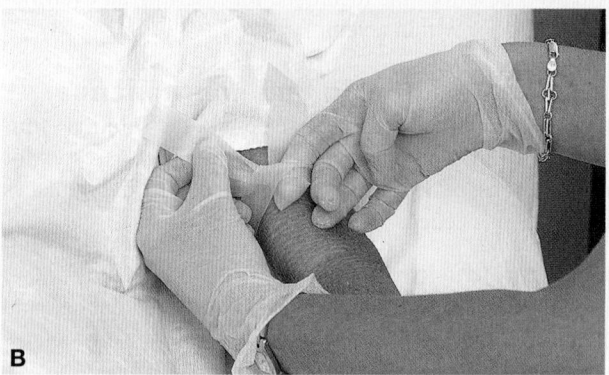

B

One end of the tourniquet is tucked beneath the other. (Photo by B. Proud.)

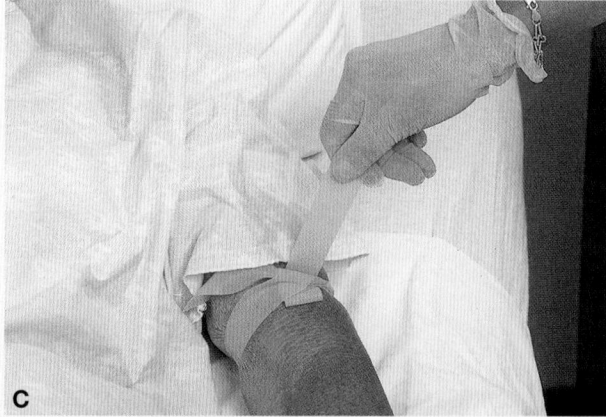

C

The tourniquet can be released easily by pulling one of the free ends. (Photo by B. Proud.)

the tightness of the tourniquet contributes to the client's discomfort.
- Release the tourniquet by pulling one of its free ends (Fig. C). *Releasing the tourniquet restores the circulation of venous blood.*

<table>
<tr><td>**BOX 16-5**</td><td>**Techniques for Promoting Vein Distention**</td></tr>
</table>

- Apply a tourniquet or blood pressure cuff tightly around the arm.
- Have the client make a fist and pump the fist intermittently.
- Tap the skin over the vein several times.
- Lower the client's arm to promote distal pooling of blood.
- Stroke the skin in the direction of the fingers.
- Apply warm compresses for 10 minutes to dilate veins and then reapply the tourniquet.

<table>
<tr><td>**BOX 16-6**</td><td>**Formulas for Calculating Infusion Rates**</td></tr>
</table>

When using an infusion device:

$$\frac{Total\ volume\ in\ mL}{Total\ hours} = mL/hour$$

When infusing by gravity:

$$\frac{Total\ volume\ in\ mL}{Total\ time\ in\ minutes} \times drop\ factor^a = gtt/minute$$

Example:

$$\frac{1,000\ mL}{8\ hours} = 125\ mL/hour$$

$$\frac{1,000\ mL}{480\ minutes} \times 20 = 42\ gtt/min$$

^{a}Drop factor is associated with the tubing set.

Replacing Equipment

Solutions are replaced when they finish infusing or every 24 hours, whichever occurs first (Skill 16-4). IV tubing is changed every 72 hours, depending on agency policy, with some exceptions. Tubing used to instill parenteral nutrition is replaced daily. Tubing used to administer whole blood can be reused for a second unit if one unit is administered immediately after the other. Whenever tubing is changed, it is more convenient to replace both the solution and the tubing at the same time. Skill 16-5 describes how to replace just the tubing, which is generally more difficult.

Discontinuation of an Intravenous Infusion

IV infusions are discontinued when the solution has infused and no more is scheduled to follow. Skill 16-6 is a procedure for removing a venipuncture device when IV infusions are no longer needed. When the client needs occasional infusions of solutions or the administration of IV medications, the venipuncture is temporarily capped but kept patent with the use of an intermittent venous access device also known as a *medication lock*.

Insertion of an Intermittent Venous Access Device

An **intermittent venous access device** (a sealed chamber that provides a means for administering IV medications or solutions periodically; Fig. 16-15) is inserted into a venipuncture device. An intermittent peripheral venous access

TABLE 16-7 Complications of Intravenous Therapy

COMPLICATION	SIGNS AND SYMPTOMS	CAUSE(S)	ACTION
Infection	Swelling Discomfort	Growth of microorganisms	Change site. Apply antiseptic and dressing to the previous site.
		Redness at site	
	Drainage from site		Report findings.
Circulatory overload	Elevated blood pressure Shortness of breath Bounding pulse Anxiety	Rapid infusion Reduced kidney function Impaired heart contraction	Slow the IV rate. Contact the physician. Elevate the client's head. Give oxygen.
Infiltration	Swelling at the site Discomfort	Displacement of the venipuncture device	Restart the IV. Elevate the arm. Decrease in infusion rate Cool skin temperature at the site
Phlebitis	Redness, warmth, and discomfort along the vein	Administration of irritating fluid Prolonged use of the same vein	Restart the IV. Report findings.
			Apply warm compresses.
Thrombus formation	Swelling Discomfort Slowed infusion	Stasis of blood at the catheter, needle tip, or vein	Restart the IV. Report findings. Apply warm compresses.
Pulmonary embolus	Sudden chest pain Shortness of breath Anxiety	Movement of a previously stationary blood clot to the lungs	Stay with the client. Call for help. Administer oxygen. Rapid heart rate Drop in blood pressure
Air embolism	Same as a pulmonary embolus	Failure to purge air from the tubing	Same as for a pulmonary embolus, but also place the client's head lower than the feet. Position the client on their left side.

IV, intravenous.

NURSING GUIDELINES 16-4

Removing Air Bubbles from Intravenous Tubing

- Flush the line with IV solution before inserting the adaptor into the venipuncture device. *This action purges air from the tubing.*
- Tighten the roller clamp if small bubbles are observed. *This action prevents continued forward movement of the air.*
- Tap the tubing below the air bubbles (Fig. A). *Doing so promotes upward movement of the air above the fluid in the drip chamber.*
- Milk the air in the direction of the drip chamber or filter if one is incorporated within the tubing. *Doing so pushes the air physically to an area where it can be trapped or released.*
- Wrap the tubing around a circular object, like a pencil, starting below the trapped air (Fig. B). *This moves the air toward the drip chamber where it can escape from the liquid into the empty air space.*

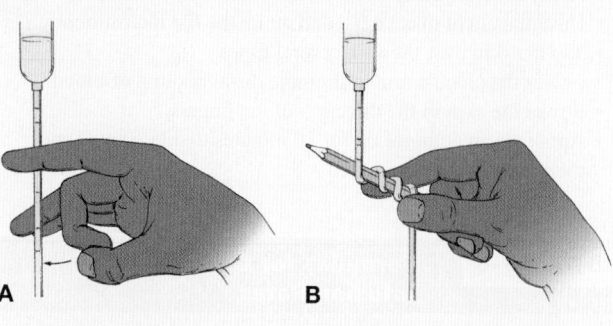

A   B

- Insert the barrel of a syringe within a port below the air and open the roller clamp. *This siphons fluid and air from the tubing as it passes by the bevel of the needle.*

device is also called a "saline lock" because the chamber is filled and periodically flushed with sterile normal saline to prevent blood from clotting at the tip of the catheter or needle. Central venous catheters are usually kept patent by flushing the device with heparinized saline. Intermittent venous access devices are used when the client:

- No longer needs continuous infusions of fluid
- Needs intermittent administrations of IV medication
- May need emergency IV fluid or medications if their condition deteriorates

These devices are replaced when the venipuncture site is changed. Skill 16-7 describes how to insert an intermittent venous access device and ensure its patency. The use of a medication lock when administering IV drugs is discussed in Chapter 35.

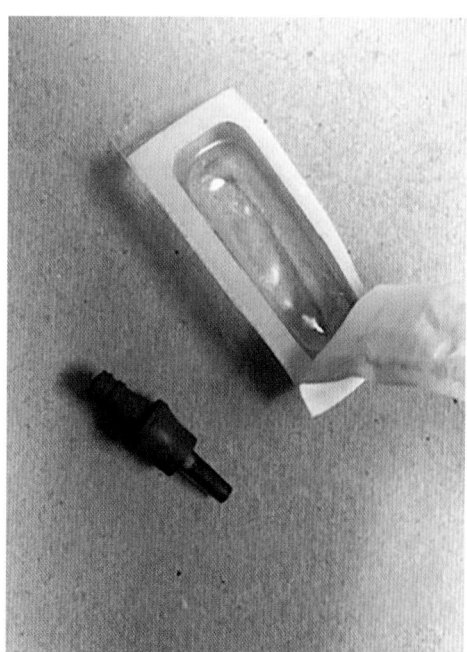

FIGURE 16-15 Venous access device. (Picture by L. Moreno.)

BLOOD ADMINISTRATION

Blood is collected, stored, and checked for safety and compatibility before it is administered as a transfusion.

Blood Collection and Storage

Blood donors are screened to ensure that they are healthy and will not be endangered by the temporary loss in blood volume. Refrigerated blood can be stored for 21 to 35 days, after which it is discarded.

Blood Safety

Once collected, the donated blood is tested for syphilis, hepatitis, and human immunodeficiency virus (HIV) antibodies to exclude administering blood that may transmit these blood-borne diseases. Blood that tests positive is discarded. Unfortunately, disease-carrying viruses may remain undetected if the antibodies have not reached a level high enough to be measured.

The U.S. Blood Safety Council, a division of the Department of Health and Human Services, has policies regarding potential hepatitis C infection by blood transfusions. All blood collection agencies must notify people who received blood before 1987 if the donation came from a donor who has tested positive for hepatitis C since 1990. This policy is being implemented to promote early diagnosis and treatment of infected but asymptomatic transfusion recipients.

The American Red Cross has a policy concerning blood donations to eliminate the potential transmission of neurologic infectious microorganisms known as *prions*. Prions cause various brain disorders, one of which is bovine spongiform encephalopathy ("mad cow disease") detected in people who live in the United Kingdom. Because blood is one possible mode of transmitting prions from animals to humans and humans to humans, the collection of blood is banned from anyone who has lived in the United Kingdom for a total of 3 months or longer since 1980, lived anywhere in Europe for a total of 6 months since 1980, or received a blood transfusion in the United Kingdom.

America's Blood Centers and the American Red Cross ask prospective blood donors who may have been exposed to someone with Ebola to refrain from donating blood for 21 days following their last contact with the infected person. It is recommended that a person who recently or currently has the Ebola virus would be indefinitely deferred as a blood donor (Food and Drug Administration, 2017). If diagnosed with the Zika virus, the wait time to donate blood is 120 days after symptoms resolve (American Red Cross, 2020).

Blood Compatibility

There are several hundred differences among the proteins in the blood of a donor and a recipient. They can cause minor or major transfusion reactions. One of the most dangerous differences involves the antigens, or protein structures, on membranes of red blood cells. Antigens determine the characteristic blood group—A, B, AB, and O—and Rh factor. Rh positive means the protein is present; Rh negative means the protein is absent.

Before donated blood is administered, the blood of the potential recipient is typed and mixed, or crossmatched, with a sample of the stored blood to determine whether the two are compatible (Fig. 16-16). To avoid an incompatibility reaction, it is best to administer the same blood group and Rh factor. Exceptions are listed in Table 16-8.

Type O blood is considered the universal donor because it lacks both A and B blood group markers on its cell membrane. Therefore, type O blood can be given to anyone because it will not trigger an incompatibility reaction when given to recipients with other blood types. Individuals with type AB blood are referred to as *universal recipients* because their red blood cells have proteins compatible with types A, B, and O. Rh-positive individuals may receive Rh-positive or Rh-negative blood because the latter does not contain the sensitizing protein. Rh-negative individuals, however, should never receive Rh-positive blood.

››› *Stop, Think, and Respond 16-4*
Which blood type or types are compatible for clients who are blood types B Rh positive and O Rh negative?

Blood Transfusion

Before administering blood, the nurse obtains and documents the client's vital signs to provide a baseline for comparison should the client have a transfusion reaction. Each client who receives blood has a color-coded bracelet with identifying numbers that must correlate with those on the unit of blood. IV medications are never infused through tubing being used to administer blood.

Blood Transfusion Equipment

There are certain standards for the gauge of the catheter or needle and the type of tubing used to transfuse blood.

Catheter or Needle Gauge

Because blood contains cells in addition to water, it is generally infused through a 16- to 20-gauge—preferably an 18-gauge—catheter or needle. Using a smaller gauge increases the potential for prolonging the infusion beyond 4 hours, and 4 hours is the maximum safe period for administering one unit of blood.

Blood Transfusion Tubing

Blood is administered through tubing referred to as a *Y-set* (Fig. 16-17). Two branches are at the top of the tubing; one is used to administer normal saline solution, and the other is used to administer blood. Normal saline (0.9% NaCl) is the only solution used when administering blood because other solutions destroy red blood cells. The two branches of the Y-set join above a filter that removes clotted blood and dead cell debris. The normal saline is always administered before the blood is hung and follows after the blood has been infused. It is also used during the infusion if the client has a transfusion reaction (Skill 16-8).

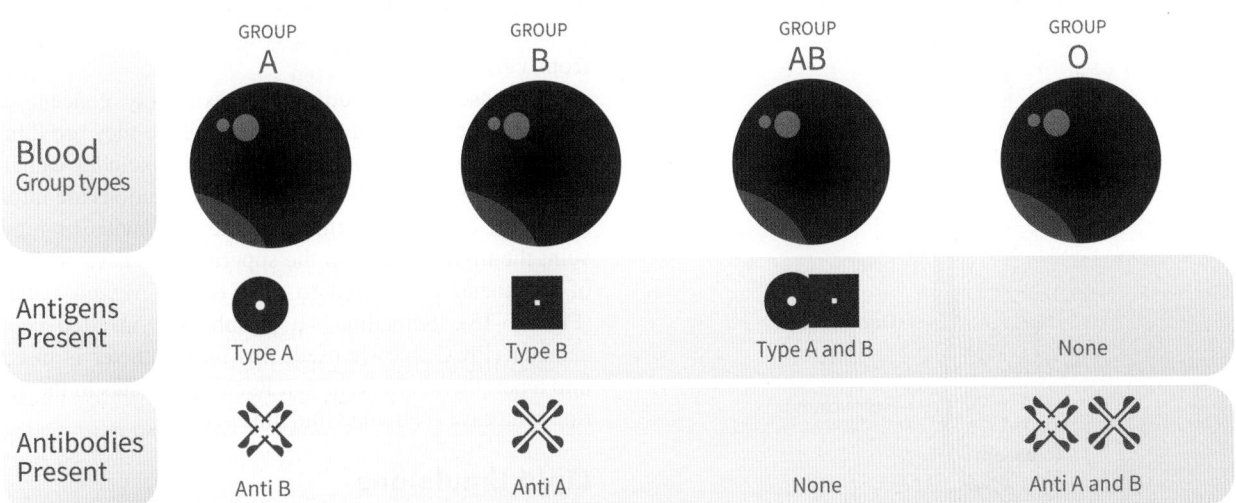

FIGURE 16-16 Blood type donor and recipient compatibility. (Anshuman Rath/Shutterstock.)

TABLE 16-8 Most Common Blood Type by Ethnicity

In the United States, 38% of the population has O-positive blood, making it the most common blood type. According to the American Red Cross, the following statistics show the most common blood types in the United States based on the donor population:

RACE	O POSITIVE (%)	A POSITIVE (%)	B POSITIVE (%)	AB NEGATIVE (%)	B NEGATIVE (%)	A NEGATIVE (%)
African American	47	24	18	0.3	1	25
Latin American	53	29	9	0.2	1	2 AB positive
Asian	39	27	25	0.1	0.4	0.5
White	37	33	9	1	2	3 AB positive only

Data from Dresden, D. (2024). What are the rarest and most common blood types? *Medical News Today.* https://www.medicalnewstoday.com/articles/most-common-blood-type-by-race

Transfusion Reactions

Life-threatening transfusion reactions generally occur within the first 5 to 15 minutes of the infusion, so the nurse or someone designated by the nurse usually remains with the client during this critical time. Because a transfusion reaction can occur at any time, however, nurses monitor clients frequently during a transfusion and instruct them to call for assistance if they feel any unusual sensations (Table 16-9).

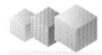 Concept Mastery Alert

Transfusion Reactions

Whenever a transfusion reaction is suspected or identified, the nurse's first step is to stop the transfusion, thereby limiting the amount of blood to which the client is exposed.

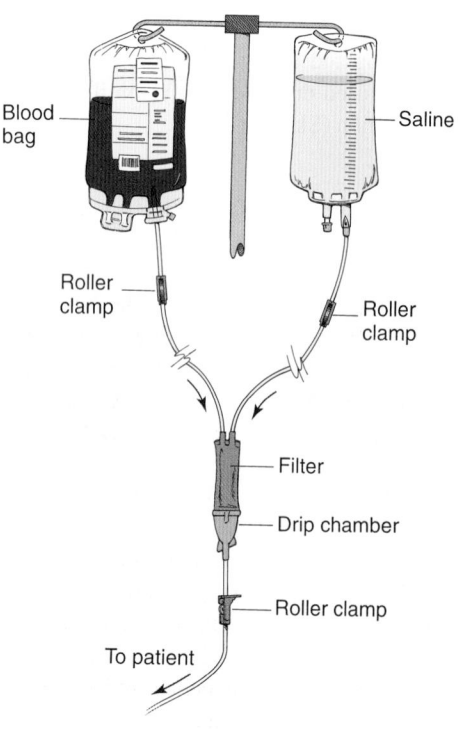

FIGURE 16-17 Blood transfusion tubing.

PARENTERAL NUTRITION

The term *parenteral* means "a route other than enteral or intestinal." Therefore, **parenteral nutrition** (nutrients such as protein, carbohydrate, fat, vitamins, minerals, and trace elements administered IV) is provided by routes other than the oral route. Depending on the concentration of these substances, parenteral nutrition is administered through an IV catheter that terminates in a central vein near the heart.

Peripheral Parenteral Nutrition

Peripheral parenteral nutrition (an isotonic or hypotonic IV nutrient solution instilled in a vein distant from the heart) is not extremely concentrated and consequently can be infused through peripheral veins. It provides temporary nutritional support of approximately 2,000 to 2,500 calories daily. It can meet a person's metabolic needs when oral intake is interrupted for 7 to 10 days, or it can be used as a supplement during a transitional period as the client begins to resume eating.

Total Parenteral Nutrition

Total parenteral nutrition (TPN; a hypertonic solution of nutrients designed to meet almost all caloric and nutritional needs) is preferred for clients who are severely malnourished or may not be able to consume food or liquids for a long period. Box 16-7 lists clients who may benefit from TPN.

Because TPN solutions are extremely concentrated, they must be delivered into an area where they are diluted in a fairly large volume of blood. This excludes catheters that terminate in peripheral veins. TPN solutions are infused through a catheter inserted into the subclavian or jugular vein; the tip terminates in the superior vena cava. This type of a catheter is referred to as a *central venous catheter* (Fig. 16-18). Sometimes, a peripherally inserted central catheter (PICC line) is used; this long catheter is inserted into a peripheral arm vein, but its tip terminates in the superior vena cava (Nursing Guidelines 16-5).

Lipid Emulsions

An **emulsion** (a mixture of two liquids, one of which is insoluble in the other) can be administered parenterally.

TABLE 16-9 Transfusion Reactions

TYPE OF REACTION	SIGNS AND SYMPTOMS	CAUSE(S)	ACTION
Incompatibility	Hypotension, rapid pulse rate, difficulty breathing, back pain, flushing	Mismatch between donor and recipient blood groups	Stop the infusion of blood. Infuse saline at a rapid rate. Call for assistance. Administer oxygen. Raise the feet higher than the head. Be prepared to administer emergency drugs. Send first urine specimen to laboratory. Save the blood and tubing.
Febrile	Fever, shaking chills, headache, rapid pulse, muscle aches	Allergy to foreign proteins in the donated blood	Stop the blood infusion. Start the saline. Check vital signs. Report findings.
Septic	Fever, chills, hypotension	Infusion of blood that contains microorganisms	Stop the infusion of blood. Start the saline. Report findings. Save the blood and tubing.
Allergic	Rash, itching, flushing, stable vital signs	Minor sensitivity to substances in the donor blood	Slow the rate of infusion. Assess the client. Report findings. Be prepared to administer an antihistamine.
Moderate chilling	No fever or other symptoms	Infusion of cold blood	Continue the infusion. Cover and make the client comfortable.
Overload	Hypertension, difficulty breathing, moist breath sounds, bounding pulse	Large volume or rapid rate of infusion; inadequate cardiac or kidney function	Reduce the rate. Elevate the head. Give oxygen. Report findings. Be prepared to give a diuretic.
Hypocalcemia (low calcium)	Tingling of fingers, hypotension, muscle cramps, convulsions	Multiple blood transfusions containing anticalcium agents	Stop the blood infusion. Start saline. Report findings. Be prepared to give antidote (calcium chloride).

The combination allows a vehicle for administering lipids, or fat, which is often missing from parenteral nutritional solutions. A parenteral lipid emulsion is a mixture of water and fats in the form of soybean or safflower oil, egg yolk phospholipids, and glycerin.

BOX 16-7 Candidates for Total Parenteral Nutrition

- Clients who have not eaten for 5 days and are not likely to eat during the next week
- Clients who have had a 10% or more loss of body weight
- Clients exhibiting self-imposed starvation (anorexia nervosa)
- Clients with cancer of the esophagus or stomach
- Clients with postoperative gastrointestinal complications
- Clients with inflammatory bowel disease in an acute stage
- Clients with major trauma or burns
- Clients with liver and renal failure

Lipid solutions, which look milky white, are given intermittently with TPN solutions. They provide additional calories and promote adequate blood levels of fatty acids. Lipid solutions are administered peripherally or in a port in the central catheter below the filter and close to the vein. If the lipid solution is squeezed or mixed with TPN solutions in larger volumes than those moving through the catheter, the lipid molecules tend to "break" and separate in the solution.

The client receiving an administration of lipids may have an adverse reaction within 2 to 5 hours of the infusion (Dudek, 2021). Common manifestations include fever, flushing, sweating, dizziness, nausea, vomiting, headache, chest and back pain, dyspnea, and cyanosis. Delayed reactions (up to 10 days later) are characterized by enlargement of the liver and spleen accompanied by jaundice, reduced white blood cell and platelet counts, elevated blood lipid levels, seizures, and shock.

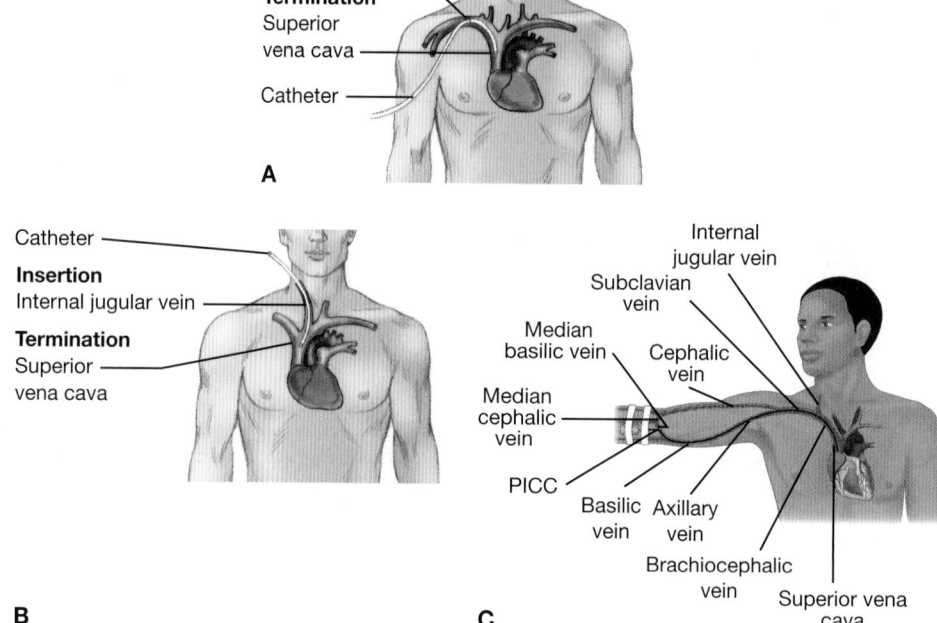

FIGURE 16-18 A central venous catheter inserted into the subclavian **(A)** threaded into the superior vena cava **(B)**, jugular **(C)**, and basilic vein. PICC, peripherally inserted central catheter.

NURSING IMPLICATIONS

Clients who have fluid, electrolyte, blood, and nutritional imbalances are likely to have one or more of the following nursing diagnoses:

- ADL deficit
- Fluid overload
- Risk for fluid overload
- Hypovolemia
- Risk for altered skin integrity
- Deficient knowledge

Nursing Care Plan 16-1 illustrates the nursing process as applied to a client with hypovolemia, defined as decreased intravascular fluid, interstitial fluid, and/or ICF.

NURSING GUIDELINES 16-5

Administering Total Parenteral Nutrition

- Weigh the client daily. *A record of the client's weight assists with monitoring their response to treatment.*
- Use tubing that contains a filter. *Filters absorb air and bacteria, two potential complications associated with the use of central venous catheters.*
- Change TPN tubing daily. *Doing so reduces the potential for infection.*
- Tape all connections in the tubing and central catheter. *Taping prevents accidental separation and reduces the potential for an air embolism.*
- Clamp the central catheter and have the client bear down whenever separating the tubing from its catheter connection. *This action prevents an air embolism.*
- Use an infusion device to administer TPN solution. *An infusion device monitors and regulates precise fluid volumes.*
- Infuse initial TPN solutions gradually (25–50 mL/hour). *Gradual administration allows time for physiologic adaptation.*
- Never increase the rate of infusion to make up for an uninfused volume unless the physician has been consulted. *Speeding up the infusion tends to increase blood glucose levels.*
- Monitor intake and especially urine output. *High blood glucose levels can trigger diuresis (increased urine excretion), resulting in output greater than intake.*
- Monitor capillary blood glucose levels (see Chapter 14). *Blood glucose may not be adequately metabolized without the additional administration of insulin.*
- Wean the client from TPN gradually. *Weaning prevents a sudden drop in blood glucose levels.*

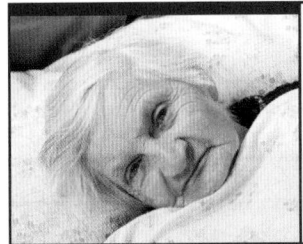

Clinical Scenario A home health nurse has been called by the family to assess their 85-year-old grandmother who has been experiencing nausea, vomiting, and diarrhea for several days. They explain that as a consequence, she has not been consuming food and fluids. She has become quite weak and remained in bed, except to use the toilet. After assessing the older woman, the visiting nurse recommends that the client be evaluated in the emergency department of the hospital. She is subsequently admitted as an inpatient. The admitting nurse develops the following nursing care plan.

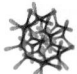

NURSING CARE PLAN 16-1   Hypovolemia

Assessment

- Monitor intake and output (I&O) each shift, and total the sum every 24 hours.
- Assess for unusual loss of fluid via emesis, diarrhea, wound drainage, intestinal suction, blood loss, etc.
- Weigh the client consistently on the same scale, at the same time, and in similar clothing and compare the findings.
- Note the color and odor of urine.
- Check vital signs every 4 hours while the client is awake.

- Assess skin turgor over the sternum each shift.
- Note the color and warmth of the skin and the degree of moisture in the mucous membranes each shift.
- Ask the client to identify any thirst, weakness, or fatigue.
- Determine the client's level of consciousness and evidence of confusion or disorientation.
- Review laboratory data such as specific gravity of urine, hematocrit, and electrolyte concentration.

Nursing Diagnosis. Hypovolemia related to inadequate oral fluid intake and increased fluid loss as manifested by intake of 1,000 mL in previous 24 hours, urine output of 750 mL in previous 24 hours, dry oral mucous membranes, dark yellow urine with strong odor, oral temperature of 100°F, weak pulse rate of 100 beats/minute (bpm), respiratory rate of 28 breaths/minute, blood pressure (BP) of 118/68 mm Hg, and dry skin that tents for more than 3 seconds

Expected Outcome. The client's fluid volume will be adequate as evidenced by an oral intake of 1,500 to 3,000 mL in the next 24 hours (8/15) with a urine output nearly the same volume as oral intake.

Interventions	Rationales
Administer the prescribed antiemetic and antidiarrheal medication as ordered.	Medications help control vomiting and diarrhea.
Explain the need to increase oral fluid intake to the client and the process of recording the volume of fluid I&O.	Teaching helps facilitate the client's cooperation in reaching the goal.
Place an I&O record form at the client's bedside.	Having a form for recording I&O promotes an accurate assessment.
Put a device for collecting urine inside the bowl of the toilet; explain its purpose to the client.	Placing a device for collecting voided urine helps prevent accidental flushing of urine that needs to be measured.
Instruct the client to record fluids and amounts consumed and to remind nursing personnel to do likewise.	Periodic recording facilitates accuracy.
Inform the client to use the signal light when there is a need to use the toilet.	The client is at risk for a fall and potential injury.
Ask the client to turn on the signal light after using the toilet or bedpan.	Measuring urine output after each voiding or stool and recording the amount ensure accuracy.
Compile a list of fluid likes and dislikes.	Catering to the client's personal preferences facilitates increasing oral fluid intake.
Provide a minimum of 100 to 200 mL of preferred oral fluid every hour over the next 16 hours (day and evening shifts).	An oral fluid intake of 100 mL/hour for 16 hours will meet the minimum target of 1,500 mL.
Offer oral fluid if the client awakens during the night, but avoid disturbing the client if asleep and if the oral intake from the previous shifts is adequate.	Ensuring sleep is a priority as long as the goals for fluid intake are met.
Request that the dietary department include foods that are good sources of sodium, such as milk, cheese, bouillon, and ham.	Sodium attracts water.

Evaluation of Expected Outcomes

- Total oral intake for 24 hours is 2,250 mL.
- Total urine output for 24 hours is 1,975 mL.
- Oral temperature is 98.2°F, pulse is 88 bpm and strong, respirations are 18 breaths/minute at rest, and BP is 128/84 mm Hg in right arm while lying down.
- Weight remains at admission weight of 118 lb.
- Urine is light yellow and free of strong odor.
- Oral mucous membranes are pink and moist.
- Skin is warm and elastic.
- The client is alert and oriented.
- The client is not thirsty, weak, or unusually fatigued.

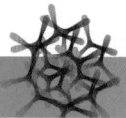

- Four components of body fluid
  - Water
  - Electrolytes
  - Nonelectrolytes
  - Blood cells
- Fluid compartments
  - Intracellular: Fluid inside the cells
  - Extracellular: Fluid outside the cells
  - Interstitial: Fluid in the tissue space between and around cells
  - Intravascular: The watery plasma, or serum, portion of blood
- Fluid volume assessment
  - Intake
  - Output
- Fluid imbalances
  - *Hypovolemia* refers to a low volume of ECF. If untreated, it may result in dehydration.
  - *Hypervolemia* means a higher than normal volume of water in the intravascular fluid compartment and is another example of a fluid imbalance. Edema develops when excess fluid is distributed to the interstitial space.
  - Third spacing is the movement of intravascular fluid to nonvascular fluid compartments, where it becomes trapped and useless. It is generally manifested by tissue swelling or fluid that accumulates in a body cavity, such as the peritoneum.
- IV fluid administration
  - Maintain or replace electrolytes.
  - Administer water-soluble vitamins.
  - Provide a source of calories.
  - Administer drugs.
  - Replace blood and blood products.
- Types of IV solutions
  - Crystalloids: Made of water and other uniformly dissolved crystals, such as salt and sugar
    - Isotonic: Sodium and chloride equal to those found in plasma
    - Hypotonic: Sodium and chloride less than found in plasma, less concentrated
    - Hypertonic: Twice the concentration of glucose than found in plasma
- Colloids: Made of water and molecules of suspended substances, such as blood cells and blood products
  - Whole blood
  - Packed cells
  - Blood substitutes
- Solution selection: Before preparing the solution, the nurse inspects the container and determines that:
  - The solution is the one prescribed by the physician.
  - The solution is clear and transparent.
  - The expiration date has not elapsed.
  - No leaks are apparent.
  - A separate label is attached, identifying the type and amount of other drugs added to the commercial solution.
- Tubing selection
  - Primary (long) or secondary (short) tubing
  - Vented or unvented tubing
  - Microdrip (small drops) or macrodrip (large drops) chamber
  - Unfiltered or filtered tubing
  - Needleless access ports
- Venipuncture
  - Venipuncture device
  - Vein selection
- Infusion rate regulation: The nurse is responsible for calculating, regulating, and maintaining the rate of infusion according to the physician's order.
- Assessing for venipuncture complications
  - Infection
  - Circulatory overload
  - Infiltration
  - Phlebitis
- Blood administration
  - Blood collection and storage
  - Blood safety
  - Blood compatibility: O, A, B, AB, and the Rh factor
  - Blood transfusion
  - Blood transfusion equipment
  - Blood transfusion reactions: Incompatibility, allergic, febrile, chilling, septic, fluid overload
- Parenteral nutrition: Means "a route other than enteral or intestinal"; nutrients such as protein, carbohydrate, fat, vitamins, minerals, and trace elements, administered IV, provided other than by the oral route

CRITICAL THINKING EXERCISES

1. When calculating a client's I&O, you find she has had a total 24-hour intake of 1,000 mL and output of 750 mL. What other assessment findings are you likely to observe?

2. A client whose oral intake is being limited to 1,000 mL/24 hours is experiencing thirst and asks for assistance in relieving his discomfort. What nursing actions could be taken?

3. While assessing a client's IV infusion that is instilling by gravity, you note that it is infusing at a significantly slower rate than when it was originally regulated. What actions are appropriate to take?

4. A client will be receiving a blood transfusion. The registered nurse who hangs the unit of blood and initiates the administration of the blood asks you to assess the client during its infusion. What assessments are appropriate to monitor?

NEXT-GENERATION NCLEX-STYLE REVIEW QUESTIONS

1. When the nursing care plan indicates that a client is to be weighed regularly, what is most important to consider?
   a. When the client was weighed before
   b. When the client last took a drink of fluid

c. How much the client has eaten so far today

d. Whether the client feels like being weighed

Test-Taking Strategy: Note the key term and modifier, "most important." Use the process of elimination to determine which option is better than any of the others.

2. A nurse is most accurate in identifying which items that a client on a low-sodium diet should avoid? Select all that apply.

a. Soy sauce

b. Lemon juice

c. Cheddar cheese

d. Maple syrup

e. Onion powder

f. Smoked salmon

Test-Taking Strategy: Use the process of elimination to select items that are high in sodium that would be restricted on a low-sodium diet.

3. When a client asks how a transfusion of packed red blood cells differs from the usual whole blood transfusion, which nursing explanation is most correct?

a. A unit of packed red blood cells has the same number of red blood cells in less fluid volume.

b. A unit of packed red blood cells contains more red blood cells in the same amount of fluid volume.

c. A unit of packed red blood cells is less likely to cause an allergic transfusion reaction.

d. A unit of packed red blood cells will stimulate the bone marrow to make more red blood cells.

Test-Taking Strategy: Note the key word and modifier, "most correct." Analyze the options to determine which answer is accurate among others that contain incorrect information.

4. When sent to the blood bank to obtain a unit of blood for a client with type A, Rh-positive blood, if all the following units of blood are available, which is the nurse correct to refuse?

a. Type A, Rh negative

b. Type O, Rh positive

c. Type O, Rh negative

d. Type AB, Rh positive

Test-Taking Strategy: Note that the question asks for the unit of blood that would be hazardous or fatal if administered to this client. Eliminate the units of blood that would be safe to administer.

5. When the nurse monitors a client receiving a blood transfusion, which is most indicative that the client is experiencing a transfusion reaction during the first 15 minutes of the infusion?

a. The client feels an urgent need to urinate.

b. The client's blood pressure becomes low.

c. Localized swelling develops at the infusion site.

d. The skin is pale at the site of the infusing blood.

Test-Taking Strategy: Note the key word and modifier, "most indicative." Use the process of elimination to select the manifestation that correlates with a transfusion reaction better than any other answer.

NEXT-GENERATION NCLEX-STYLE CLINICAL SCENARIO QUESTIONS

Clinical Scenario:

A home health nurse has been called by the family to assess their 85-year-old grandmother who has been experiencing nausea, vomiting, and diarrhea for several days. They explain that as a consequence, she has not been consuming food and fluids. She has become quite weak and remained in bed except to use the toilet. After assessing the older woman, the visiting nurse recommends that the client be evaluated in the emergency department of the hospital. She is subsequently admitted as an inpatient.

1. From the following list, select some of the factors that may be contributing to the hypovolemia.

a. Nausea

b. Pitting edema

c. Diarrhea

d. Decrease intake of fluid

e. Age

f. Decrease food intake

g. Bed rest

2. Choose the most likely options for the missing information from the following statement by selecting from the list of options provided.

Hypovolemia is due to a decrease in fluid intake. ___1___ may also be depleted with fluids, causing hypovolemia, which could lead to___2___.

OPTION 1	OPTION 2
White blood cells	insulin shock
Sodium	increased urination
Bile	confusion

SKILL 16-1 Recording Intake and Output

Suggested Action	Reason for Action
ASSESSMENT	
Check the medical record or listen in report to determine whether an assigned client is on I&O.	Ensures adherence to the plan for care
Verify during the report how much intravenous (IV) fluid has been accounted for from any currently infusing solution.	Indicates the credited volume for calculating fluid intake at the end of the shift
Review the nursing care plan for any previously identified fluid problem and nursing orders for specific interventions.	Promotes continuity of care
Review the client's medical record and analyze trends in I&O, vital sign measurements, laboratory findings, and weight records.	Aids in analyzing trends in fluid status
Perform a physical assessment to obtain data that reflect the client's fluid status (see Table 16-4).	Provides current data
Inspect all tubings and drains to ensure they are patent (open).	Ensures that methods for instilling or removing fluids are functional
Notice whether all suction containers or drainage containers were emptied at the end of the previous shift.	Ensures accurate recordkeeping
Determine how much the client understands about I&O measurements, fluid intake goals, or fluid restrictions.	Verifies whether additional teaching is needed
Look for a calibrated container and bedside I&O record.	Facilitates keeping accurate data
Obtain a collection device inside the toilet (see Client and Family Teaching 16-1) if the client has none and uses the toilet for urinary elimination.	Facilitates measuring voided urine
Measure the amount of water in the client's bedside carafe at the beginning of the shift.	Provides a baseline for measuring fluid consumed in addition to that served at regular mealtimes
PLANNING	
Place the client on I&O or plan to measure I&O if the client is at high risk for fluid imbalance or the assessment data suggest a problem.	Demonstrates safe and appropriate nursing care
Identify the goal for fluid intake or restriction. A minimum of 1,000 mL in 8 hours is not unrealistic for a client in fluid deficit. An amount prescribed by the physician or an intake equal to the client's previous hourly output may be used as a guideline for fluid restrictions.	Provides a target for client care
IMPLEMENTATION	
Explain or reinforce the purpose and procedures that will be followed for measuring I&O.	Facilitates client cooperation
Record the volume for all fluids consumed from the dietary tray and other sources of oral liquids.	Contributes to accurate assessment records
Make sure that all IV fluids or tube feedings are being administered at the prescribed rate.	Ensures adherence to medical therapy
Ensure that the nurse who adds additional IV fluid containers also records the volume when the infusion is complete or replaced.	Ensures accurate recordkeeping
Keep track of the fluid volumes used to irrigate drainage tubes or flush feeding tubes.	Ensures accurate recordkeeping
Measure and record the volume of voided urine. Although urine is not considered a vehicle for the transmission of blood-borne microorganisms, gloves are worn as standard precautions.	Ensures accurate recordkeeping and reduces the transmission of microorganisms

SKILL 16-1 Recording Intake and Output (*continued*)

Suggested Action	Reason for Action
Measure and record the volume of urine collected in a catheter drainage bag near the end of the shift (see figure).	Ensures accurate recordkeeping

Urine drainage bag (Photo by B. Proud.)

Suggested Action	Reason for Action
Wear gloves to measure liquid stool or other body fluids and record their measured amounts.	Prevents the transmission of microorganisms and provides assessment data
Wash hands or perform hand antisepsis with an alcohol rub (see Chapter 10) after removing and disposing of the gloves.	Reduces the presence and potential transmission of microorganisms
Check the volume remaining in currently infusing IV fluids; subtract the remaining volume from the credit provided at the beginning of the shift.	Ensures accurate assessment data
Total all fluid intake volumes and all fluid output volumes for the current 8-hour shift; record the amounts.	Ensures accurate recordkeeping
Compare the data to determine whether the I&O is approximately the same and if the goals for fluid intake or restrictions have been met.	Demonstrates concern for safe and appropriate care
Report major differences in I&O to the nurse in charge or the client's physician.	Demonstrates concern for safe and appropriate care
Review the plan of care and make revisions if the goals have not been met or if additional nursing interventions seem appropriate.	Demonstrates responsibility and accountability
Report the I&O volumes, IV fluid credit amount, and any other pertinent data to the nurse who will be assuming responsibility for the client's care.	Demonstrates responsibility and accountability

EVALUATION

- Intake approximates output.
- Goals for fluid intake or restriction have been met.
- Significant data have been reported.
- The client's fluid status justifies continuing the care as planned, or the care plan has been revised.

DOCUMENT

- Date and time
- I&O volumes for the previous 8 hours

SAMPLE DOCUMENTATION

Date and Time Fluid intake for the previous 8 hours is 1,200 mL and output is 1,000 mL. _____ J. Doe, LPN

SKILL 16-2 Preparing Intravenous Solutions

Suggested Action	Reason for Action
ASSESSMENT	
Check the medical order for the type, volume, and projected length of fluid therapy.	Ensures accuracy and guides the selection of equipment
Determine whether the solution is in a bag or bottle and if the infusion will be administered by gravity or infusion device.	Affects the selection of tubing
Review the client's medical record for information on the risk for infection.	Determines the need for filtered tubing
Read the label on the solution at least three times.	Helps prevent errors
IMPLEMENTATION	
Wash hands or perform hand antisepsis with an alcohol rub (see Chapter 10).	Reduces the transmission of microorganisms
Select the appropriate tubing and stretch it once it has been removed from the package.	Straightens the tubing by removing bends and kinks
Tighten the roller clamp (Fig. A).	Aids in filling the drip chamber

Tightening the roller clamp. (Photo by B. Proud.)

Suggested Action	Reason for Action
Remove the cover from the access port.	Provides access for inserting the spike
Insert the spike by puncturing the seal on the container (Fig. B).	Provides an exit route for fluid

Inserting the spike. (Photo by B. Proud.)

Suggested Action	Reason for Action
Hang the solution container from an IV pole or suspended hook.	Inverts the container
Squeeze the drip chamber, filling it no more than half full.	Leaves space to count the drops when regulating the rate of infusion
Release the roller clamp.	Flushes air from the tubing
Invert ports within the tubing as the solution approaches.	Displaces air that may be trapped in the junction
Tighten the roller clamp when all the air has been removed.	Prevents a loss of fluid

SKILL 16-2 Preparing Intravenous Solutions (*continued*)

Suggested Action	Reason for Action
Attach a piece of tape or a label on the tubing giving the date, time, and your initials.	Provides a quick reference for determining when the tubing needs to be changed
Take the solution and tubing to the client's room.	Facilitates administration

EVALUATION
- Solution and tubing are properly labeled.
- Tubing has been purged of air.

DOCUMENT
- Date and time
- Type and volume of solution
- Rate of infusion once venipuncture has been performed
- Location of venipuncture site

SAMPLE DOCUMENTATION

Date and Time 1,000 mL of 5% D/W infusing at 125 mL/hour through IV in L. forearm. _____ J. Doe, LPN

SKILL 16-3 Starting an Intravenous Infusion

Suggested Action	Reason for Action
ASSESSMENT	
Check the identity of the client.	Prevents errors
Review the client's medical record to determine whether there are any allergies to iodine or tape.	Influences supplies that will be used and modifications in the procedure
Inspect and palpate several potential venipuncture sites (Fig. A).	Provides an alternative if the first attempt is unsuccessful

A

Palpating veins. (Photo by B. Proud.)

PLANNING	
Bring all the necessary equipment to the bedside.	Promotes organization and efficient time management
Position the client on their back or in a sitting position.	Promotes comfort and facilitates inspection of the arm
Place an absorbent pad beneath the hand or arm.	Prevents having to change the bed linen if the site bleeds
Select a site most likely to facilitate the purpose for the infusion and comply with the criteria for vein selection.	Facilitates continuous fluid administration and minimizes potential complications
Clip body hair at the site if it is excessive.	Facilitates visualization and reduces discomfort when adhesive tape is removed
Apply topical anesthetic.	Provides local anesthesia to the insertion site to minimize pain associated with a needlestick

(*continued*)

SKILL 16-3 Starting an Intravenous Infusion (*continued*)

Suggested Action	Reason for Action
Tear strips of tape, and open the package with the venipuncture device and transparent dressing.	Saves time and ensures that the venipuncture device is not displaced once inserted. Transparent dressings facilitate site assessment.

IMPLEMENTATION —————————————————————————————————————

Suggested Action	Reason for Action
Wash hands or perform hand antisepsis with an alcohol rub (see Chapter 10).	Reduces the number of microorganisms
Apply a tourniquet or a blood pressure cuff 2–4 in (5–10 cm) above the vein that will be used.	Distends the vein
Use an antimicrobial solution and/or alcohol to cleanse the skin, starting at the center of the site outward 2–4 in (Fig. B).	Reduces the potential for infection

B

Swabbing the site. (Photo by B. Proud.)

Suggested Action	Reason for Action
Allow the antiseptic to dry.	Potentiates the effectiveness of antiseptic and prevents burning when the needle is inserted
Put on clean gloves.	Provides a barrier for blood-borne viruses
Use the thumb to stretch and stabilize the vein and soft tissues about 2 in (5 cm) below the intended site of entry (Fig. C).	Helps straighten the vein and prevents it from moving around underneath the skin

C

Stabilizing the vein. (Photo by B. Proud.)

Suggested Action	Reason for Action
Position the venipuncture device with the bevel up and at approximately a 45-degree angle above or to the side of the vein (Fig. D).	Facilitates piercing the vein

Bevel

Lumen

D

Placing the bevel up.

SKILL 16-3 Starting an Intravenous Infusion (*continued*)

Suggested Action	Reason for Action
Warn the client just before inserting the needle.	Prepares the client for discomfort
Feel for a change in resistance and look for blood to appear behind the needle.	Indicates the vein has been pierced
Once blood is observed, advance the needle about 1/8 to 1/4 of an inch (Fig. E).	Positions the catheter tip within the inner wall of the vein

Advancing the needle tip. (Photo by B. Proud.)

E

Withdraw the needle slightly so that the tip is within the catheter.	Prevents puncturing the outside of the vein wall
Slide the catheter into the vein until only the end of the infusion device can be seen.	Ensures full insertion of the catheter
Release the tourniquet.	Reduces venous pressure and restores circulation
Apply pressure over the internal tip of the catheter.	Limits blood loss
Remove the protective cap covering the end of the IV tubing and insert it into the end of the venipuncture device.	Facilitates infusing the solution
Release the roller clamp and begin infusing the solution slowly.	Clears blood from the venipuncture device before it can clot
Cover the site with a transparent dressing according to agency policy (Fig. F).	Reduces the potential for infection

Applying a transparent dressing. (From Nettina, S. M. [2013]. *Lippincott manual of nursing practice* [10th ed.]. Lippincott Williams & Wilkins.)

F

SKILL 16-3 Starting an Intravenous Infusion (*continued*)

Suggested Action	Reason for Action
Apply tape, taking care to loop and secure the tubing (Fig. G).	Prevents tension on the tubing that may cause displacement

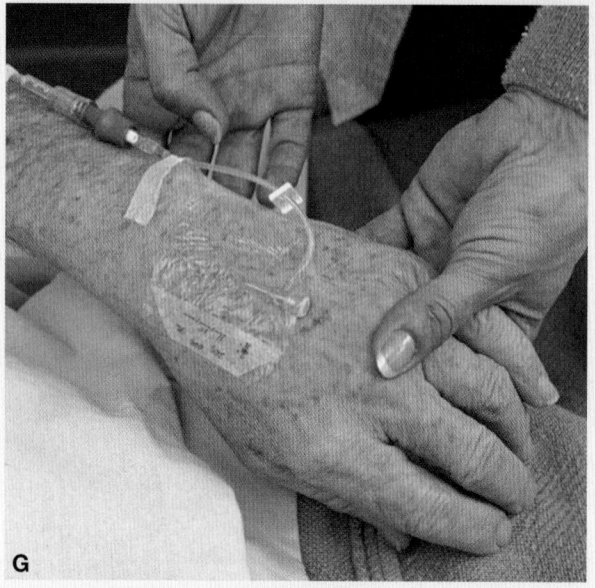

G

	Prevents catheter displacement.
Write the date, time, gauge of the catheter, and your initials on the site dressing or the outer piece of tape.	Provides a quick reference for determining when the site must be changed
Tighten or release the roller clamp to regulate the rate of fluid infusion.	Facilitates compliance with the medical order

EVALUATION

- A flashback of blood was observed before advancing the catheter.
- Minimal discomfort and blood loss occurred.
- Fluid is infusing at the prescribed rate.

DOCUMENT

- Date and time
- Gauge and type of venipuncture device
- Site of venipuncture
- Type and volume of solution
- Rate of infusion

SAMPLE DOCUMENTATION

Date and Time No. 20 gauge over-the-needle catheter inserted into vein in L. forearm. 1,000 mL 0.9% saline infusing at 42 gtt/minute. _____ J. Doe, LPN

SKILL 16-4 Changing Intravenous Solution Containers

Suggested Action	Reason for Action
ASSESSMENT	
Assess the volume that remains in the infusing container and the rate at which it is infusing.	Helps establish when the solution will need to be replaced
Check the medication record or physician's orders to determine what solution is to follow the current infusion.	Ensures adherence to the medical order
PLANNING	
Obtain the replacement solution well in advance of needing it.	Ensures that the infusion will be uninterrupted
Organize client care to change the container when the current infusion becomes low.	Demonstrates efficient time management

SKILL 16-4 Changing Intravenous Solution Containers (*continued*)

Suggested Action	Reason for Action
IMPLEMENTATION	
Check the identity of the client by asking the client's name and birthdate.	Prevents errors
Wash hands or perform hand antisepsis with an alcohol rub (see Chapter 10).	Reduces the transmission of microorganisms
Tighten the roller clamp slightly or slow the rate of infusion on an infusion device.	Slows the rate of infusion so that the drip chamber remains filled with solution
Remove the almost empty solution container from the suspension hook with the tubing still attached.	Facilitates separating the tubing from the container
Invert the empty solution container and pull the spike free.	Prevents minor loss of remaining solution
Deposit the empty bag in a lined waste receptacle.	Keeps the environment clean and orderly
Remove the seal from the replacement solution container.	Provides access to the port
Insert the spike into the port of the new container.	Provides a route for infusing fluid
Hang the new container from the suspension hook on the IV standard or infusion device.	Restores height to overcome venous pressure
Inspect for the presence of air within the tubing; remove it if air is present.	Reduces the potential for air embolism or an alarm from an infusion device detecting air
Readjust the roller clamp or reprogram the infusion device to restore the prescribed rate of infusion.	Demonstrates compliance with the medical order

EVALUATION

- Solution container is replaced.
- Infusion continues.

DOCUMENT

- Volume infused from the previous container on intake and output (I&O) record
- Time, volume, type of solution, and signature on the medication record or wherever the agency specifies documenting the administration of IV solutions
- Condition of the client

SAMPLE DOCUMENTATION

Date and Time   1,000 mL lactated Ringer's instilling at 42 gtt/minute. Dressing over venipuncture is dry and intact. No swelling or discomfort in the area of the infusing fluid. _____ J. Doe, LPN

SKILL 16-5 Changing Intravenous Tubing

Suggested Action	Reason for Action
ASSESSMENT	
Determine the agency's policy for changing IV tubing.	Demonstrates responsibility for complying with infection control policies
Check the date and time on the label attached to the tubing.	Determines the approximate time when the tubing must be changed
Determine whether the solution container will need to be replaced before the time expires on the tubing.	Facilitates changing both the container and the tubing at the same time
PLANNING	
Obtain appropriate replacement tubing and supplies for changing the dressing.	Ensures that equipment will be available and ready when needed
Attach a new label to the tubing indicating the date and time the tubing is changed and your initials.	Provides a quick reference for determining when the tubing must be changed again
IMPLEMENTATION	
Wash hands or perform hand antisepsis with an alcohol rub (see Chapter 10).	Reduces the transmission of microorganisms

(continued)

SKILL 16-5 Changing Intravenous Tubing (*continued*)

Suggested Action	Reason for Action
Prepare dressing materials and strips of tape, and place them in a convenient location.	Facilitates dexterity later in the procedure
Open the new package containing the tubing, stretch the tubing, and tighten the roller clamp.	Prepares the tubing for insertion into the solution container
Remove the solution container from the suspension hook with the tubing still attached.	Facilitates separating the tubing from the container
Invert the solution container and pull the spike free.	Prevents the minor loss of remaining solution
Secure the spike to the IV pole with a strip of previously torn tape, avoiding any contamination.	Facilitates continued infusion
Insert the spike from the new tubing into the container of solution.	Provides a route for the fluid
Squeeze the drip chamber to fill it half full, open the roller clamp, and purge the air from the tubing.	Prepares the tubing for use
Remove the dressing from the venipuncture site and any tape securing the expired tubing to the arm.	Provides access to the venipuncture device and frees the expired tubing
Put on gloves.	Provides a barrier from contact with blood
Tighten the roller clamp on the expired tubing.	Temporarily interrupts the infusion
Stabilize the hub of the venipuncture device and separate the tubing from it.	Prevents accidental removal of the catheter or needle from the vein
Remove the cap from the end of the new tubing and attach it to the end of the venipuncture device.	Connects the venipuncture device to the tubing without contaminating the tip of the tubing
Continue to hold the venipuncture device with one hand while releasing the roller clamp on the new tubing.	Reestablishes the infusion
Replace the dressing on the venipuncture site and secure the tubing.	Covers the site and keeps the tubing and venipuncture device from being pulled out
Readjust the rate of infusion.	Adheres to the medical order
Write the date, time, and your initials on the new dressing, and include the gauge of the venipuncture device and the original date of insertion.	Provides a quick reference for determining future nursing responsibilities for infection control
Dispose of the expired tubing in a lined receptacle.	Maintains a clean and orderly environment

EVALUATION

- Tubing is replaced.
- Solution continues to infuse at the prescribed rate.

DOCUMENT

- Date and time
- Assessment findings of venipuncture site
- Dressing change

SAMPLE DOCUMENTATION

Date and Time   No redness, swelling, or tenderness at venipuncture site in L. forearm. Dressing changed following replacement of IV tubing. _____ J. Doe, LPN

SKILL 16-6 Discontinuing an Intravenous Infusion

Suggested Action	Reason for Action
ASSESSMENT	
Confirm that the physician has written an order to discontinue the infusion of IV fluid.	Demonstrates responsibility and accountability for carrying out medical orders
Check the client's identity by obtaining the client's name and birthdate.	Prevents errors
PLANNING	
Assemble necessary equipment, which includes clean gloves, sterile gauze, and tape.	Promotes organization and efficient time management

SKILL 16-6 Discontinuing an Intravenous Infusion (*continued*)

Suggested Action	Reason for Action
IMPLEMENTATION	
Wash hands or perform hand antisepsis with an alcohol rub (see Chapter 10).	Reduces the spread of microorganisms
Clamp the tubing and remove any tape and dressing over the venipuncture.	Facilitates removal without leaking fluid
Put on gloves.	Prevents contact with blood
Press a gauze square gently over the site where the venipuncture device enters the skin.	Helps absorb blood
Remove the catheter or needle by pulling it out without hesitation following the course of the vein.	Prevents discomfort and injury to the vein
Apply pressure to the site of the venipuncture for 30–45 seconds while elevating the forearm.	Pressure and elevation control bleeding.
Secure the gauze with tape.	Acts as a dressing to reduce the potential for infection
Dispose of the venipuncture device in a sharp container if it is a needle.	Prevents accidental needlestick injuries and the transmission of blood-borne infectious microorganisms
Enclose a catheter used for venipuncture within a glove as they are removed and discarded within a lined waste container.	Facilitates disposal and prevents contact with blood
Wash hands or perform hand antisepsis with an alcohol rub (see Chapter 10) after glove disposal.	Removes transient microorganisms
Encourage the client to flex and extend the arm or hand several times.	Helps the client to regain sensation and mobility
Record the amount of IV fluid the client received before discontinuing the infusion on the intake and output (I&O) sheet.	Contributes to an accurate record of fluid intake
Document the time the infusion was discontinued and the condition of the venipuncture site.	Demonstrates responsibility and accountability for the client's care

EVALUATION

- Site appears free of inflammation.
- Bleeding is controlled.
- Discomfort is minimized or absent.
- Equipment is disposed in a manner to prevent injury and transmission of infection.

DOCUMENT

- Date and time
- Condition of venipuncture site
- Volume of infused solution

SAMPLE DOCUMENTATION

Date and Time Infusion of Ringer's lactate discontinued per physician's order following administration of 1,000 mL. No. 22 gauge angiocatheter removed from L. forearm. No redness, swelling, or drainage evident at site of venipuncture. Venipuncture site covered with a dry sterile dressing. _____ J. Doe, LPN

SKILL 16-7 Inserting a Medication Lock

Suggested Action	Reason for Action
ASSESSMENT	
Confirm that the physician has written an order to discontinue the continuous infusion of intravenous (IV) fluid and insert a medication lock.	Demonstrates responsibility and accountability for carrying out medical orders
Check the client's identity by asking the client's name and birthdate.	Prevents errors
Inspect the site for signs of redness, swelling, or drainage.	Provides data indicating whether the site can be maintained or a new venipuncture should be performed
Observe whether the infusion is instilling at the predetermined rate.	Indicates whether the vein and catheter are patent (open)
Determine whether the client understands the purpose and technique for inserting a medication lock.	Indicates the need for client teaching

(continued)

SKILL 16-7 Inserting a Medication Lock (*continued*)

Suggested Action	Reason for Action
PLANNING	
Assemble necessary equipment, which includes the medication lock, syringe containing 2 mL of sterile normal saline (0.9% NaCl, depending on the agency's policy), alcohol swabs, gloves, and supplies for changing or reinforcing the dressing over the site.	Promotes organization and efficient time management
IMPLEMENTATION	
Wash hands or perform hand antisepsis with an alcohol rub (see Chapter 10).	Reduces the spread of microorganisms
Fill the chamber of the medication lock with saline solution.	Displaces air from the empty chamber
Loosen the dressing to expose the connection between the hub of the catheter or needle and the tubing adapter; also remove the tape that is stabilizing the tubing to the client's arm.	Facilitates removing the tubing from the client
Loosen the protective cap from the end of the medication lock.	Maintains sterility while preparing for the insertion of the lock
Put on clean gloves.	Provides a barrier from contact with blood
Tighten the roller clamp on the tubing and stop the infusion pump or controller if one is being used.	Prevents leakage of fluid when the tubing is removed
Apply pressure over the tip of the catheter or needle (Fig. A).	Controls or prevents blood loss
A	Applying pressure over the catheter tip. (Photo by B. Proud.)
Remove the tip of the tubing from the venipuncture device and insert the medication lock (Fig. B).	Seals the opening in the catheter or needle
B	Inserting the device. (Photo by B. Proud.)
Screw the lock onto the end of the catheter or needle.	Stabilizes the connection
Swab the rubber port on the medication lock with alcohol.	Cleanses the port
Pierce the port with the blunt needleless adapter and gradually instill 2 mL of saline until the syringe is almost empty (Fig. C).	Clears blood from the venipuncture device and lock before it can clot

SKILL 16-7 Inserting a Medication Lock (*continued*)

Suggested Action	Reason for Action
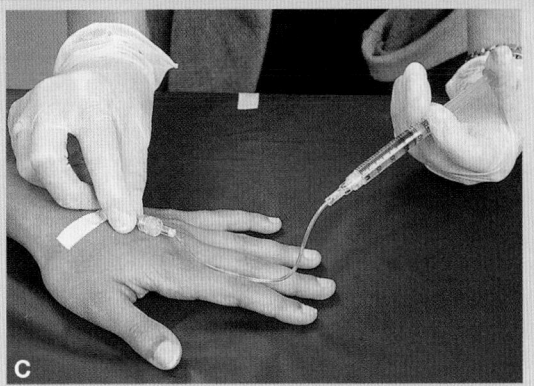	Instilling saline solution. (Photo by B. Proud.)
Begin to remove the syringe from the port as the last volume of solution is instilled; clamp or pinch the tubing, or press over the venipuncture device before removing a needleless adapter.	Continues the application of positive pressure (pushing effect) rather than negative pressure (pulling effect) during the time the syringe is removed; negative pressure pulls blood into the catheter or needle tip, which may cause an obstruction
Reapply a dressing.	Reduces the possibility that the lock and catheter may be accidentally dislodged
Plan to flush the lock after each use or at least every 8 hours with 1 or 2 mL of flush solution depending on agency policy.	Ensures continued patency

EVALUATION

- Site appears free of inflammation.
- Patency is maintained.
- Flush solution instills easily.
- Device is stabilized.

DOCUMENT

- Date and time
- Discontinuation of infusing solution
- Volume of infused IV solution
- Insertion of medication lock
- Volume and type of flush solution
- Assessment findings

SAMPLE DOCUMENTATION

Date and Time Infusion of 5% D/W discontinued. 700 mL of IV solution infused. Medication lock inserted into IV catheter in R. hand and flushed with 2 mL of normal saline. No redness, swelling, or discomfort at site. _____ J. Doe, LPN

SKILL 16-8 Administering a Blood Transfusion

Suggested Action	Reason for Action
ASSESSMENT	
Check the client's identity using two forms of identification, such as asking the client's name and birthdate.	Prevents errors
Determine whether a special signed consent is required.	Complies with legal responsibilities
Check the gauge of the current venipuncture device if an intravenous (IV) is infusing.	Indicates whether another venipuncture must be performed
Review the medical record for results of type and cross-match.	Indicates whether blood is available in the blood bank
Take temperature (T), pulse (P), respirations (R), and blood pressure (BP) within 30 minutes of obtaining blood.	Provides a baseline for comparison during the transfusion

(*continued*)

SKILL 16-8 Administering a Blood Transfusion (*continued*)

Suggested Action	Reason for Action
PLANNING	
Complete major nursing activities before starting the infusion of saline unless the blood must be given immediately.	Avoids disturbing the client once the blood is administered
Plan to perform a venipuncture or start the infusion of saline just before obtaining the unit of blood from the blood bank.	Prevents administering fluid unnecessarily
Obtain necessary equipment including a 250-mL container of normal saline (0.9% NaCl) and a Y-set.	Adheres to the standards of care for administering blood
Tighten the roller clamp on one branch of the Y-tubing and the roller clamp below the filter (see Fig. 16-17).	Prepares the tubing for purging with saline
Insert the unclamped branch of the Y-set into the container of saline.	Moistens the filter and fills the upper portion of the tubing with saline
Squeeze the drip chamber until it and the filter are half full. Release the lower clamp and flush air from the remaining section of tubing.	Reduces the potential for infusing a bolus of air
IMPLEMENTATION	
Perform the venipuncture or connect the Y-set to the present venipuncture device if it is a 16–20 gauge.	Provides access to the venous circulation and ensures that blood will move freely through the catheter or needle
Begin the infusion of saline.	Ensures that the site is patent and that there will be no delay once the unit of blood is obtained
Go to the blood bank to pick up the unit of blood, making sure to take a form identifying the client.	Prevents mistaken identity when releasing the matched blood
Double-check the information on the blood bag with the cross-matched information on the lab slip with the blood bank personnel.	Prevents releasing the wrong unit of blood or blood that is not a compatible blood group and Rh factor
Check that the blood has not passed the expiration date.	Ensures maximum benefit from the transfusion
Inspect the container of blood and reject the blood if it appears dark black or has obvious gas bubbles inside.	Indicates deteriorated or tainted blood
Plan to give the blood as soon as it is brought to the unit.	Demonstrates an understanding that blood must be totally infused within 4 hours after being released from the blood bank
Rotate the blood, but do not shake or squeeze the container if the serum has separated from the cells.	Avoids damaging intact cells
At the bedside, check the label on the blood bag with the numbers on the client's wristband with a second nurse; sign in the designated areas on the transfusion record.	Reduces the potential for administering incompatible blood
Spike the container of blood.	Provides a route for administering the blood
Tighten the roller clamp on the saline branch of the tubing and release the roller clamp on the blood branch.	Fills the tubing and filter with blood
Regulate the rate of infusion at no more than 50 mL/hour for the first 15 minutes (check the drop factor to determine the rate in gtt/minute).	Establishes a slow rate of infusion so that the nurse can monitor for and respond to signs of a transfusion reaction
Increase the rate after the first 15 minutes to complete the infusion in 2–4 hours if a second assessment of vital signs is basically unchanged and no signs of a reaction have occurred.	Increases the rate of administration to infuse the unit within a safe period
Assess the client at 15- to 30-minute intervals during the transfusion.	Ensures client safety
Clamp the tubing from the blood and release the clamp on the saline when the blood has infused.	Flushes blood cells from the tubing
Take vital signs one more time.	Documents the condition of the client at the completion of the blood administration
Tighten the roller clamp below the filter when the tubing looks reasonably clear of blood.	Prevents leaking when the IV is discontinued
Put on gloves.	Provides a barrier from contact with blood

SKILL 16-8 Administering a Blood Transfusion (*continued*)

Suggested Action	Reason for Action
Loosen the dressing covering the venipuncture site and remove the catheter, or remove the blood tubing and reconnect the previously infusing solution.	Discontinues the infusion or restores previous fluid therapy
Apply a dressing over the venipuncture site if the IV is discontinued.	Prevents infection
Dispose of the blood container and tubing according to agency policy.	Blood is a biohazard and requires special bagging to ensure that others will not accidentally come in direct contact with the blood.

EVALUATION

- Entire unit of blood is administered within 4 hours.
- Client demonstrates no evidence of transfusion reaction.
- Reactions have been minimized by appropriate interventions.
- Infusion is discontinued or previous orders are resumed.

DOCUMENT

- Venipuncture procedure, if initiated for the administration of blood
- Preinfusion vital signs
- Names of nurses who checked the armband and blood bag container
- Time blood administration began
- Rate of infusion during the first 15 minutes and remaining period of time
- Signs of reaction, if any, and nursing actions
- Periodic vital sign assessments
- Time blood infusion completed
- Volume of blood and saline infused
- Vital signs after transfusion is completed

SAMPLE DOCUMENTATION

Date and Time No. 18 gauge over-the-needle catheter inserted into L. forearm and connected to 250 mL of 0.9% saline infusing at 21 mL/hour. T—98°F (tympanic), P—90, R—22, BP 116/64 in R. arm while lying flat. One unit of type O+ whole blood No. 684381 obtained from the blood bank and checked by E. Rogers, RN, and D. Baker, RN. Blood bag and wristband information found to be compatible. Blood infusing at 50 mL/hour for 15 minutes. Rate increased to 125 mL/hour during remainder of infusion. Blood transfusion completed at 1,600. No evidence of transfusion reaction. T—98°F (tympanic), P—86, R—20, BP 122/70 in R. arm at end of transfusion. Total of 100 mL of saline and 475 mL of blood infused before IV discontinued. _____ J. Doe, LPN

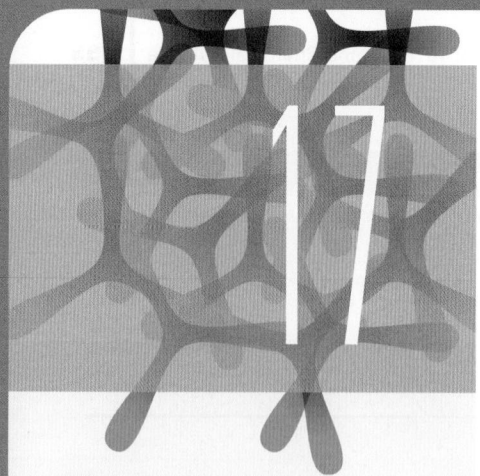

17

Hygiene

Learning Objectives

On completion of this chapter, the reader should be able to:

1. Define hygiene.
2. Name hygiene practices that most people perform regularly.
3. Provide reasons why a partial bath is more appropriate than a daily bath for older adults.
4. List the advantages of towel or bag baths.
5. Name the situations in which shaving with a safety razor is contraindicated.
6. List items recommended for oral hygiene.
7. Identify methods to prevent the chief hazard when providing oral hygiene to an unconscious client.
8. Describe techniques for preventing damage to dentures during cleaning.
9. Describe methods for removing hair tangles.
10. Name types of clients for whom nail care is provided with extreme caution.
11. Identify visual and hearing devices.
12. List alternatives for clients who cannot insert or care for their own contact lenses.
13. Discuss reasons for sound disturbances experienced by people who wear hearing aids.
14. Describe an infrared listening device (IRLD).

INTRODUCTION

Hygiene includes practices that promote health through personal cleanliness. People foster hygiene through activities such as bathing, performing oral care, cleaning and maintaining fingernails and toenails, and shampooing and grooming hair. Hygiene also includes care and maintenance of devices such as eyeglasses and hearing aids to ensure continued and proper function. Hygiene practices and needs differ according to age, inherited characteristics of the skin and hair, cultural values, and state of health.

This chapter provides suggestions for carrying out hygiene practices when providing client care. Principles that refer to the client's environment, such as bed-making skills, are discussed in Chapter 18.

 Gerontologic Considerations

■ Benign skin lesions such as seborrheic keratoses (tan to black raised areas) and senile lentigines (brown, flat patches on the face, hands, and forearms) are common in older adults (Fig. 17-1).

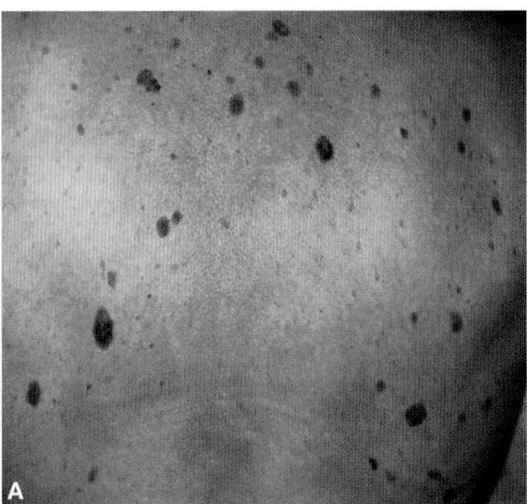 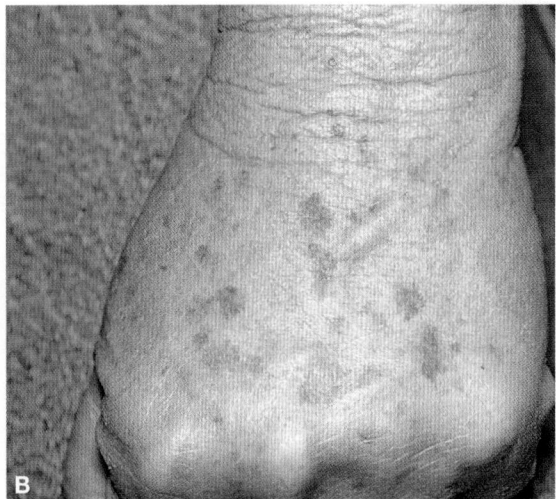

FIGURE 17-1 **A.** An example of keratoses on the back of an older man. **B.** An example of lentigines, colloquially known as *liver spots*.

■ The skin and integument are also affected by multiple disorders among older adults as well as those in other age groups (Table 17-1).

■ Tooth loss is common in older adults as a result of conditions such as periodontal disease, poor dental care, and chronic illnesses.

■ Poor hygiene and grooming in older adults can be indicators of conditions such as visual impairment, functional limitations, dementia, depression, abuse, or neglect.

■ To reduce the risk of falls in older adults when bathing, there are a variety of safety measures that can be provided such as the following:

■ Nonskid strips on the floor of tubs and showers are helpful.

■ Grab bars should be placed at arm level and within reach of the dominant hand.

■ A tub or shower seat is an important safety measure for adults who have mobility limitations or difficulty maintaining balance.

■ Diminished ability to sense temperature changes may occur with aging. The temperature of bath water should be checked with the wrist before immersing older adults.

■ Long-handled bath sponges or handheld shower attachments help older adults with limited range of motion to maintain independence.

■ Older adults should use soap sparingly because it is extremely drying to the skin. A mild, superfatted, nonperfumed soap may be preferable.

■ Because older adults have thin skin, decreased skin elasticity, and increased fragility of blood vessels in the dermis, gentle patting motions rather than harsh rubbing motions should be used when drying the skin.

■ One should thoroughly inspect the feet of older adults for ulcerations or other lesions of which they are unaware.

■ Bath oils can be added to a water basin when administering a bed bath to an older adult. Oils are not used in showers or bathtubs, however, because they increase the risk of falls.

■ Avoid the use of skin care products containing alcohol or perfumes when caring for older adults because these products tend to aggravate dry skin conditions and cause allergic reactions.

■ Increasing oral fluid intake or adding humidity to the air reduces the discomfort of dry skin experienced by older adults.

■ Encourage older adults to purchase sturdy shoes and to replace or repair them as they become worn to prevent skin and nail impairment in the lower extremities.

■ Older adults are more susceptible to impacted cerumen (ear wax)—a common cause of hearing loss. Over-the-counter eardrops can be used to prevent and treat this condition. Irrigation of the ear with body temperature tap water followed by instillation of a drying agent such as 70% alcohol may remove impacted cerumen.

THE INTEGUMENTARY SYSTEM

The word **integument** (covering) refers to the collective structures that cover the surface of the body and its openings. Most hygiene practices are based on maintaining or restoring a healthy **integumentary system**, which includes the skin, mucous membranes, hair, and nails. Because the mouth, or oral cavity (which is lined with mucous membrane), contains teeth, this chapter also discusses these accessory structures.

Skin

The skin consists of the epidermis, dermis, and subcutaneous layer (Fig. 17-2). The *epidermis*, or outermost layer, contains dead skin cells that form a tough protein called *keratin*. Keratin protects the layers and structures within the lower portions of the skin. The cells in the epidermis are shed continuously and replaced by the *dermis*, or true skin, which contains most of the secretory glands (Table 17-2). The *subcutaneous layer* separates the skin from skeletal muscles.

TABLE 17-1 Examples of Integumentary Disorders

CONDITION	DESCRIPTION	CLIENT TEACHING
Acne	Inflammation of sebaceous glands and hair follicles on the face, upper chest, and back	Keep the face clean. Refrain from touching or squeezing lesions. Avoid the use of oily cosmetics.
Contact dermatitis	Allergic sensitivity evidenced by red skin rash and itching	Avoid scratching or wearing clothing made of irritating fibers, such as wool. Use tepid water and hypoallergenic or glycerin soap when bathing. Pat the skin dry; do not rub.
Furuncle (boil)	Raised pustule, usually in the neck, axillary, or groin area that feels hard and painful	Keep hands away from the infected lesion. Use separate face cloth and towels from the rest of the family; launder personal bath items in hot water and bleach. Wash hands thoroughly before and after applying medication to the skin.
Psoriasis	Noninfectious chronic skin disorder that appears as elevated silvery scales that shed over elbows, knees, trunk, and scalp; acute episodes occur between periods of relief.	Follow a medical regimen, which may be lifelong. Be wary of advertised remedies that promise a cure or quick relief, because they rarely do.
Pediculosis (lice infestation)	Brown crawling insects that move over the scalp and skin and deposit yellowish white eggs on hair shafts, including pubic area; skin bite causes itching.	Inspect the skin carefully as adult lice move quickly from light. Look for eggs (nits) on hairs 1/4 to 1/2 in from the scalp or skin surface. Do not share clothing, combs, and brushes; lice are spread by direct contact. Use a pediculicide (chemical that kills lice) in addition to a lice comb and manual removal. Do not use hair conditioner; it coats the hair and protects the nits.
Scabies	Infestation with an itch mite that burrows within the webs and sides of fingers, around arms, axilla, waist, breast, lower buttocks, and genitalia	Bathe thoroughly in the morning and at night. Apply prescribed medication after bathing. Don clean clothes after bathing. Avoid skin-to-skin contact with uninfected people.
Tinea capitis, pedis, corporis, and cruris	Fungal infection in the scalp, feet, body, or groin that appears as a ring or cluster of papules or vesicles that cause itching and become scaly, cracked, and sore	Use separate bathing and grooming articles. Keep body areas dry, especially in the folds of the skin. Wear clothing that promotes evaporation of perspiration.
Skin cancer	Newly pigmented growth or change in the existing skin lesion, especially where the skin is chronically exposed to sun	See a physician for examination and possible biopsy. Avoid direct sun exposure between 10 AM and 4 PM. Recommend using a sunscreen with an SPF of ≥15. Wear a wide-brimmed hat on sunny days. Do not use artificial tanning facilities.
Fungal nail infection	Thick, yellowed, rough-appearing toenails or fingernails that can spread from one nail to others	Consult a physician about prescription drugs, which are approximately 50% effective. Wear leather shoes, and alternate pairs to reduce damp shoe conditions. Be aware that unsanitary utensils used in the application of artificial fingernails can spread the fungus. Seek professional nail care from a podiatrist.
Candidiasis	Yeast infection of the mouth or vagina; oral candidiasis appears as white patches or red spots on the tongue, gums, or throat; vaginal candidiasis appears as a thick, cottage cheese–like discharge that causes itching and burning.	Follow directions for oral or topical antifungal medications. Swish antifungal mouth rinses, retain the solution in the mouth as long as possible, and then swallow the rinse. Avoid simple sugars and alcohol because they promote the growth of yeast. Eat yogurt that contains live *Lactobacillus acidophilus* to restore a balance of helpful to harmful microbes.

SPF, sun protection factor.

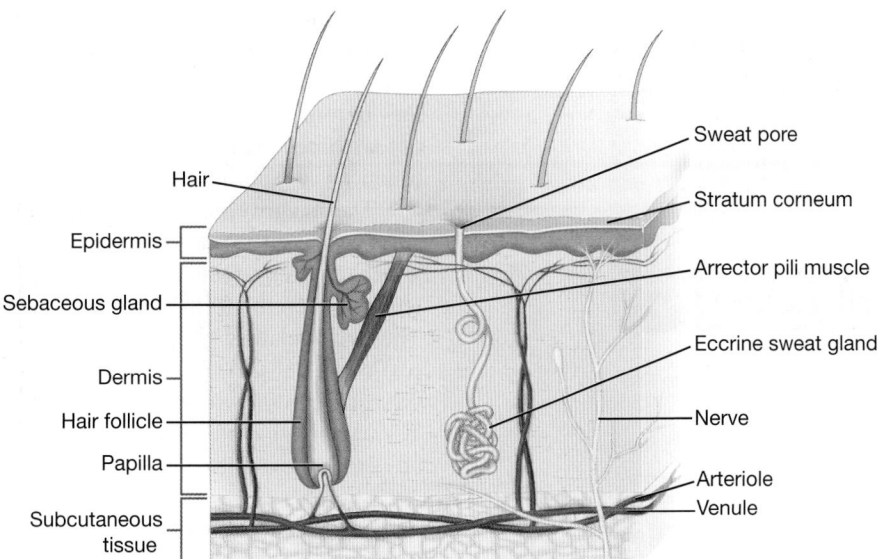

FIGURE 17-2 A cross section of the skin.

It contains fat cells, blood vessels, nerves, and the roots of hair follicles and glands.

Skin structures:

1. Protect inner body structures from injury and infection.
2. Regulate body temperature.
3. Maintain fluid and chemical balance.
4. Provide sensory information such as pain, temperature, touch, and pressure.
5. Assist in converting precursors to vitamin D when exposed to sunlight.

Mucous Membranes

The mucous membranes are continuous with the skin. They line body passages, such as the digestive, respiratory, urinary, and reproductive systems. Mucous membranes also line the conjunctiva of the eye. Goblet cells in the mucous membranes secrete *mucus,* a slimy substance that keeps the membranes soft and moist.

Hair

Each hair is a thread of *keratin,* a protein substance. Hair is formed from the cells at the base of a single follicle. Although hair covers the entire body, its amount, distribution, color, and texture vary considerably according to location and among males and females, infants and adults, and ethnic groups.

In addition to contributing to a person's unique appearance, hair helps prevent heat loss. As heat escapes from the skin, it gets trapped in the air between the hairs. The contraction of small arrector pili muscles around hair follicles, commonly described as goosebumps, further generates body heat.

Sebaceous glands in the hair follicles release sebum, an oily secretion that adds weight to the shafts of hair, causing them to flatten against the skull. Oily hair further attracts dust and debris.

The texture, elasticity, and porosity of hair are inherited characteristics influenced by the amount of keratin and sebum produced. To alter the basic genetically inherited structure, some people use chemicals to style their hair.

Nails

Fingernails (Fig. 17-3) and toenails are also made of keratin, which is in concentrated amounts, giving them their tough texture. Fingernails and toenails provide some protection to the digits. Healthy nails are thin, pink, and smooth. The free margin ordinarily extends from the end of each finger or toe, and the skin around the nails is intact. Changes in the shape, color, texture, thickness, and integrity of the nails provide evidence of local injury or infection and even systemic diseases (see Chapter 13).

Teeth

Teeth, the enamel of which is a keratin structure, are present beneath the gums at birth. The exposed portion of each tooth is referred to as the *crown*; the portion within the gum is the root (Fig. 17-4).

TABLE 17-2 Types of Skin Glands

GLAND	LOCATION	SECRETION	PURPOSE
Sudoriferous	Throughout the dermis and subcutaneous layers, especially in the axilla and groin	Sweat	Regulate body temperature. Excrete body waste.
Ceruminous	Ear canals	Cerumen	Perform protective functions; cerumen has antimicrobial properties.
Sebaceous	Throughout the dermis	Sebum	Lubricate skin and hair.
Ciliary	Eyelids	Sweat and sebum	Protect lid margin and lubricate eyelash follicles.

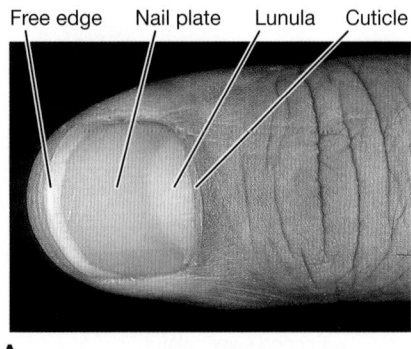

A

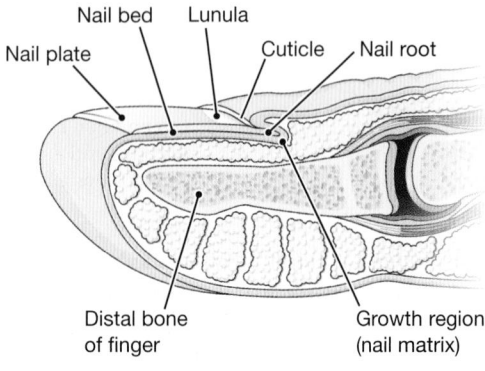

B

FIGURE 17-3 The external and cross-sectional views of a nail. **A.** External nail structures. **B.** Internal and external nail structures.

The teeth begin to erupt at about 6 months of age and continue to do so for 2 to 2.5 more years. As the jaw grows, the *deciduous teeth* (baby teeth) are replaced by *permanent teeth*. Adults have 28 to 32 permanent teeth, depending on whether the third molars (wisdom teeth) are present.

Healthy teeth are firmly fixed within the gums. Their alignment, which is related to jaw structure, is generally a result of heredity. Although the teeth are originally white, they become discolored from chronic consumption of coffee or tea, tobacco use, or certain drugs such as tetracycline antibiotics taken during childhood.

The integrity of the teeth largely depends on the person's oral hygiene practices, diet, and general health. Saliva, which moistens food and begins the digestive processes, tends to keep the teeth clean and inhibits bacterial growth. The accumulation of food debris, especially sugar, and **plaque** (a substance composed of mucin and other gritty substances in saliva) supports the growth of mouth bacteria. The combination of sugar, plaque, and bacteria may eventually erode the tooth enamel, causing **caries** (cavities).

Nutrition Notes

Although sugars are widely known to contribute to dental caries, starches are also to blame. Mouth bacteria ferment both of these types of carbohydrates to an acid that erodes teeth enamel. Therefore, although whole grain crackers are more nutritious than soft drinks, their potential damage to teeth is the same. How often carbohydrates are consumed, what they are eaten with, and how long after eating brushing occurs may be more important than whether they are sweet or sticky.

Tartar (hardened plaque) is more difficult to remove and may lead to **gingivitis** (inflammation of the gums). Pockets of gum inflammation promote **periodontal disease**, a condition that results in the destruction of the tooth-supporting structures and bones that make up the jaw.

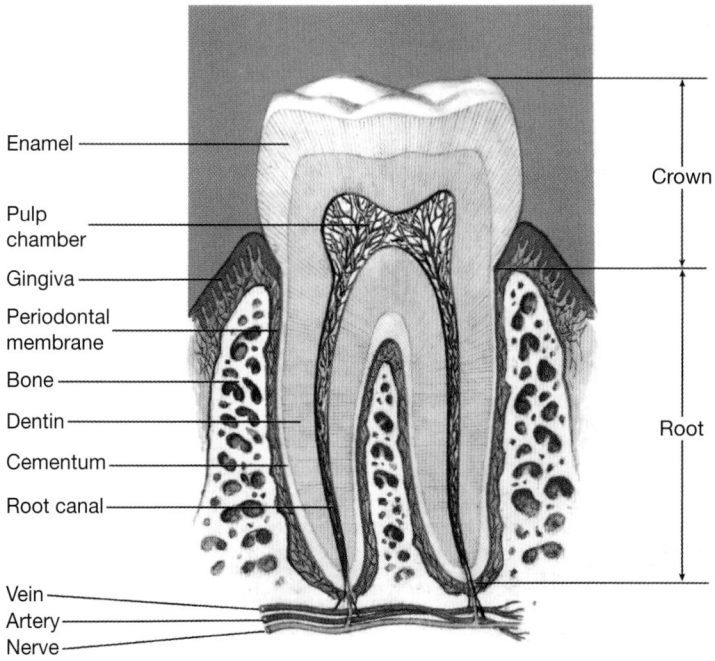

FIGURE 17-4 A cross section of a tooth. (From Cohen, B., & Jones, S. [2020]. *Medical terminology: An illustrated guide* [9th ed.]. Jones and Bartlett Learning.)

HYGIENE PRACTICES

The integument contains many secretory glands that produce odors and attract debris, and the teeth are prone to decay without proper care. Therefore, hygiene measures are beneficial for maintaining personal cleanliness and healthy integumentary structures. Although hygiene practices vary widely, most Americans routinely perform bathing, shaving, brushing teeth, shampooing, and caring for their nails.

Bathing

Bathing is a hygiene practice in which a person uses a cleansing agent such as soap and water to remove sweat, oil, dirt, and microorganisms from the skin. Although restoring cleanliness is the primary objective, bathing has several other benefits:

• Eliminating body odor
• Reducing the potential for infection
• Stimulating circulation
• Providing a refreshed and relaxed feeling
• Improving self-image

In addition to bathing for hygiene purposes, other types of bathing serve different functions (Table 17-3). In general, however, most bathing is done in a tub or shower, at a sink, or at the bedside.

>> *Stop, Think, and Respond 17-1*

How might a nurse respond to a client who believes daily bathing is unnecessary or even unhealthy?

Tub Bath or Shower

If the safety risks are negligible and there are no contraindications, the nurse encourages clients to bathe independently in a tub or shower (Skill 17-1). Most hospitals and nursing homes equip bathing facilities with various rails and handles to promote client safety (Fig. 17-5).

Partial Bath

A daily bath or shower is not always necessary—in fact, for older adults, who perspire less than younger adults and are prone to dry skin, frequent washing with soap further depletes oil from the skin. Therefore, partial or less frequent

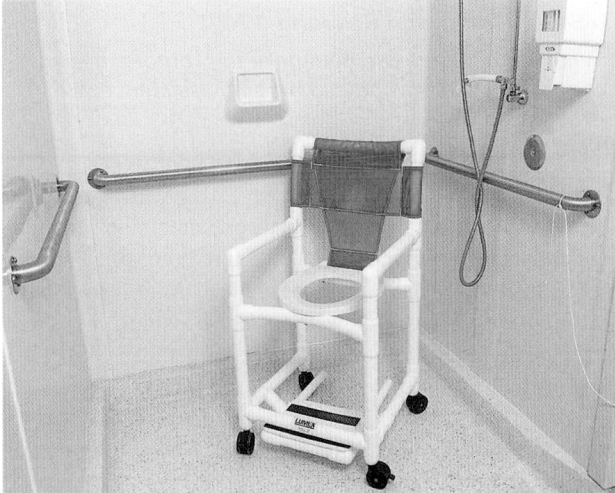

FIGURE 17-5 Simple adaptations such as an open shower, shower chair, grab bars to help a client stand, and a handheld shower spray promote safety while bathing older adults and those with disabilities.

bathing is sometimes appropriate. A **partial bath** means washing only those body areas that are subject to the greatest soiling or that are the sources of body odor—generally, the face, hands, axillae, and perineal area. Partial bathing is done at a sink or with a basin at the bedside.

Sometimes, the *perineum*, the area around the genitals and rectum, requires special or frequent cleansing in addition to bathing. **Perineal care** (also called *pericare*, techniques used to cleanse the perineum) is especially important after a vaginal delivery or gynecologic or rectal surgery so that the impaired skin remains as clean as possible. It is also appropriate whenever male or female clients have bloody drainage, urine, or stool collected in this area.

When providing perineal care, nurses must:

• Prevent direct contact between themselves and any secretions or excretions; this is generally accomplished by wearing clean gloves (see "Standard Precautions" in Chapter 22).
• Cleanse so that secretions and excretions are removed from less soiled to more soiled areas.

These principles help prevent the transfer of infectious microorganisms to the nurse and to uncontaminated areas on or within the client (Skill 17-2).

TABLE 17-3 Therapeutic Baths

TYPE	DESCRIPTION	PURPOSE
Sitz bath	Immersion of the buttocks and perineum in a small basin of continuously circulating water	Removes blood, serum, stool, or urine Reduces local swelling Relieves discomfort
Sponge bath	Applications of tepid water to the skin	Reduces a fever
Medicated bath	Soaking or immersing in a mixture of water and another substance, such as baking soda (sodium bicarbonate), oatmeal, or cornstarch	Relieves itching or a rash
Whirlpool bath	Warm water that is continuously agitated within a tub or tank	Improves circulation Increases joint mobility Relieves discomfort Removes dead tissue

>>> *Stop, Think, and Respond 17-2*

What suggestions can you make to promote the dignity of clients who need nursing assistance with perineal care?

Bed Bath

Clients who cannot take a tub bath or cannot shower independently may be given any one of three types of baths: a bed bath, a towel bath, or a bag bath. During a **bed bath** (washing with a basin of water at the bedside), the client may actively assist with some aspects of bathing. Skill 17-3 explains how to give a bed bath.

Some agencies use two variations of the traditional bed bath—the towel bath and the bag bath—because they save time and expense.

Towel Bath

With a **towel bath**, the nurse uses a single large towel to cover and wash a client. It requires a towel or bath sheet measuring 3 × 7.5 ft, but no basin or soap. The nurse prefolds and moistens the towel or bath sheet with approximately 1/2 gal (2 L) of water heated to 105° to 110°F (40° to 43°C) and 1 oz (30 mL) of no-rinse liquid cleanser. They unfold the towel so that it covers the client and use a separate section to wipe each part of the body, beginning at the feet and moving upward. The nurse folds the soiled areas of the towel to the inside as they bathe each area and allow the skin to air-dry for 2 to 3 seconds. After washing the front side of the body, the nurse positions the client on the side and repeats the procedure. They unfold the towel so that the clean surface covers the client. The nurse bathes the client's back and buttocks. When the towel bath is complete, the nurse changes the bed linens.

Bag Bath

A **bag bath** involves the use of a commercially packaged kit with 8 to 10 premoistened, disposable cloths in a plastic bag or container (Fig. 17-6). The cloths contain a no-rinse *surfactant* (a substance that reduces the surface tension between the skin and the surface contaminants) and an *emollient/humectant* (a substance that attracts and traps moisture in the skin),

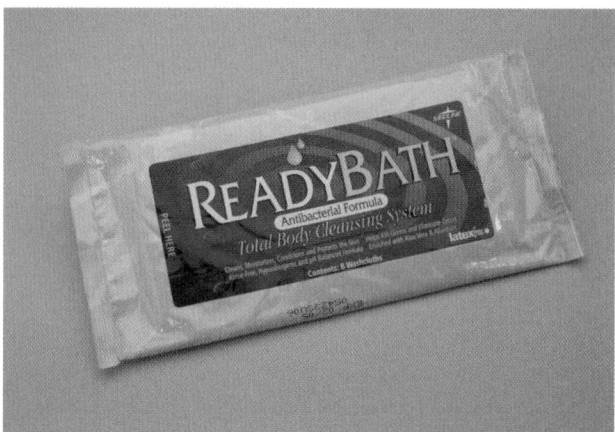

FIGURE 17-6 A commercially prepared bag bath kit contains supplies for an alternative to a traditional bath. The package is warmed prior to use.

| BOX 17-1 | Advantages of Commercial Bag Baths |

- Reduce the potential for skin impairment because the non-rinsable cleanser lubricates rather than dries the skin.
- Prevent the transmission of microorganisms that may be growing in wash basins.
- Reduce the spread of microorganisms from one part of the body to another because separate cloths or regions of the towel are used.
- Preserve the integrity of the skin because friction is not used while drying the skin.
- Promote self-care among clients who may lack the strength or dexterity to wet, wring, and lather a washcloth.
- Save time compared to conventional bathing.
- Promote comfort because the moist towel or cloths are used so quickly, and they are warmer when applied.

but no soap. The nurse warms the container and its contents in a microwave or warming unit or sets them in a container of warm water before use. At the bedside, the nurse uses separate cloths to wash each part of the client's body. Rinsing is not required. Air-drying circumvents the need for a towel. The advantages of bag baths are outlined in Box 17-1.

>>> *Stop, Think, and Respond 17-3*

Which method of bathing (shower, tub bath, bed/towel/bag bath) is appropriate for (1) a 75-year-old woman with arthritis of the hips, (2) a 60-year-old man with frequent seizures, (3) a 65-year-old man who becomes short of breath with exertion, and (4) a 72-year-old woman recovering from pneumonia? Explain the reasons for your answers.

Shaving

Shaving removes unwanted body hair. The nurse respects personal or cultural differences and asks each client about their preferences before assuming otherwise.

Shaving is accomplished with an electric or a safety razor. In some circumstances, the use of a safety razor is contraindicated (Box 17-2) and an electric or battery-operated razor is used instead. When the client cannot shave, the nurse assumes responsibility for this hygiene practice (Nursing Guidelines 17-1).

| BOX 17-2 | Contraindications to Using a Safety Razor |

Use of a safety razor is contraindicated for clients:
- Receiving anticoagulants (drugs that interfere with clotting)
- Receiving thrombolytic agents (drugs that dissolve blood clots)
- Taking high doses of aspirin
- With blood disorders such as hemophilia
- With liver disease who have impaired clotting
- With rashes or elevated or inflamed skin lesions on or near the face
- Who are suicidal

NURSING GUIDELINES 17-1

Shaving Clients

- Prepare a basin of warm water, soap, a face cloth, and a towel. *These supplies are necessary for wetting, rinsing, and lathering the face (or other area that requires shaving).*
- Wash the skin with warm, soapy water. *Washing removes oil, which helps raise hair shafts.*
- Lather the skin with soap or shaving cream (Fig. A). *The use of soap or shaving cream reduces surface tension as the razor is pulled across the skin.*

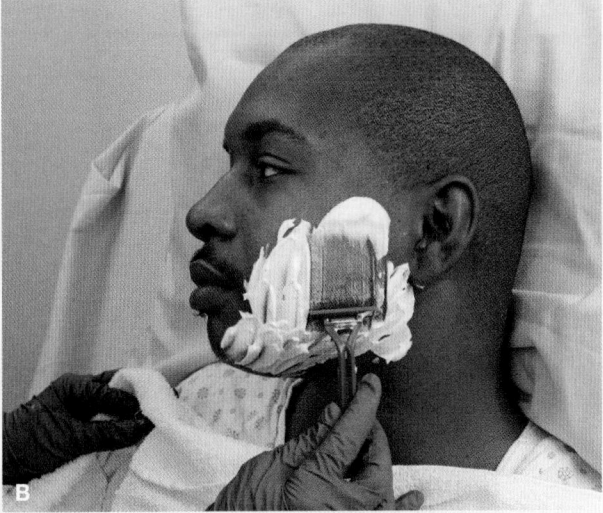

Begin shaving the upper areas of facial growth.

- Apply aftershave lotion, cologne, or cream to the shaved area if the client desires it. *The alcohol in lotion and cologne reduces and retards microbial growth in the tiny abrasions caused by the razor; cream restores oil to the skin.*

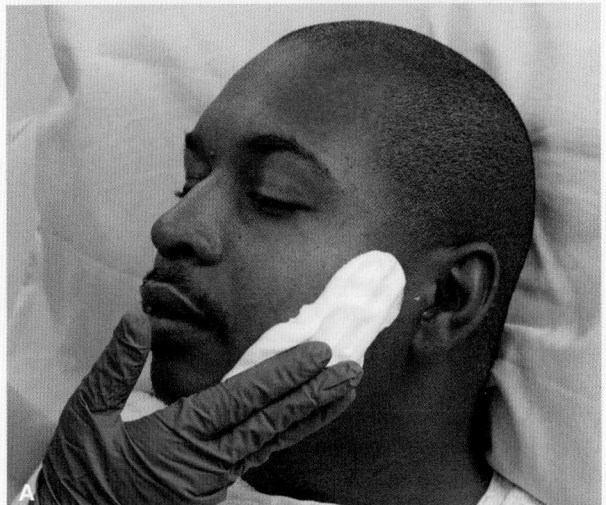

Lathering the face.

- Start at the upper areas of the face (or other area that requires shaving) and work down (Fig. B). *This progression provides more control of the razor.*
- Pull the skin taut below the area to be shaved. *This evens the level of the skin.*
- Pull the razor in the direction of hair growth. *Shaving with the hair reduces the potential for irritation.*
- Use short strokes. *They provide more control of the razor.*
- Rinse the razor after each stroke or as hair accumulates. *Rinsing keeps the cutting edge of the razor clean.*
- Rinse the remaining soap or shaving cream from the skin (Fig. C). *Rinsing reduces the potential for drying the skin.*
- Apply direct pressure to areas that bleed or apply alum sulfate (styptic pencil) at the site of bleeding. *Pressure or alum helps to promote clotting.*

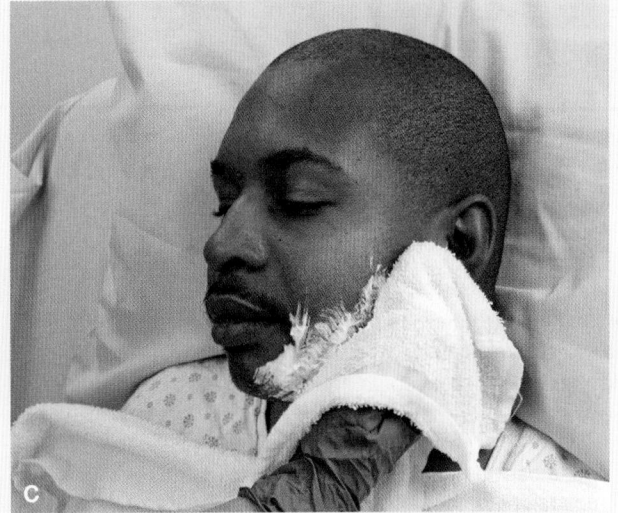

Removing residue.

Oral Hygiene

Oral hygiene consists of those practices used to clean the mouth, especially brushing and flossing the teeth. Dentures and bridges also require special cleaning and care.

Toothbrushing and Flossing

Clients who are alert and physically capable generally attend to their own oral hygiene. For clients confined to a bed, the nurse assembles the necessary items—a toothbrush, toothpaste, a glass of water, an emesis basin, and floss.

Most dentists recommend using a soft-bristled or electric toothbrush and toothpaste twice a day. For the advantages

of electric toothbrushes, see Box 17-3. Flossing removes plaque and food debris from the surfaces of teeth that a manual or electric toothbrush may miss. The choice of unwaxed or waxed floss is personal. Waxed floss is thicker and more difficult to insert between teeth; unwaxed floss frays more easily.

Although conscientious oral hygiene does not prevent dental problems completely, it reduces the incidence of tooth and gum disease. Therefore, clients need to learn how to maintain the structure and integrity of their natural teeth (Client and Family Teaching 17-1).

| BOX 17-3 | Advantages of Electric Toothbrushes |

- Last longer than manual toothbrushes.
- Promote a full 2 minutes or longer of toothbrushing.
- Can reach all corners and angles of the mouth.
- Remove 30% more plaque than manual toothbrushing.
- Have a higher reduction of gingivitis compared with manual toothbrushing.
- Decrease gingival trauma and gum recession because of less force used in brushing.
- Facilitate self-care among clients with disabilities or reduced manual dexterity.

 Client and Family Teaching 17-1
Reducing Dental Disease and Injuries

The nurse teaches the client or family to brush and floss the teeth as soon as possible after each meal, using the following techniques:

- Moisten the toothbrush and apply toothpaste.
- Hold a manual toothbrush at a 45-degree angle to the teeth (Fig. A).

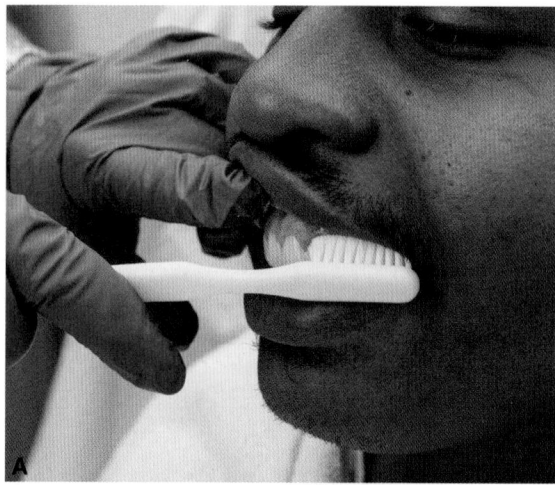

Start at the gums and then go down to the teeth.

- Brush the front and back of all teeth from the gum line toward the crown (Fig. B) using circular motions.
- Brush back and forth over the chewing surfaces of the molars.
- Brush the tongue (Fig. C) gently.
- Rinse the mouth (Fig. D) periodically to flush loosened debris.
- Have the client deposit the rinse solution within an emesis basin.
- Wrap an 18-in length of floss around the middle fingers of each hand.
- Slide the floss between two teeth until it is next to the gum.
- Move the floss (Fig. E) back and forth.
- Repeat flossing with new sections of the floss until all the teeth have been flossed including the outer surface of the last molar.
- Use a tartar-control toothpaste or a rinse containing fluoride.

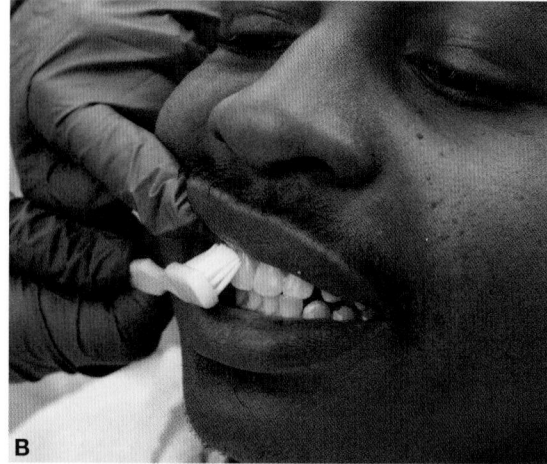

Brushing from gum to crown of each tooth.

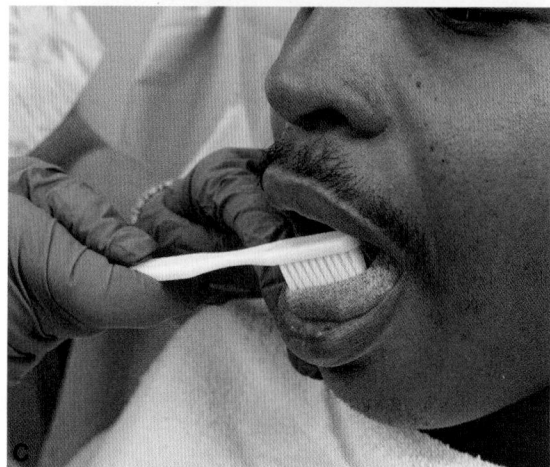

Brushing the tongue.

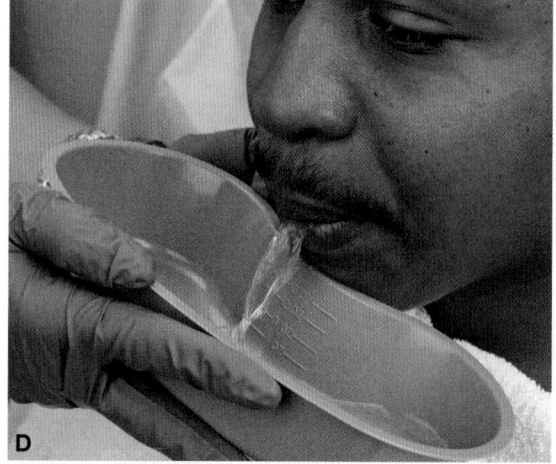

Rinsing the mouth.

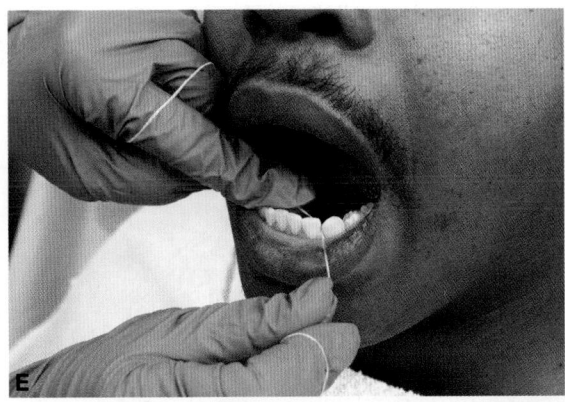

Inserting floss between the teeth.

- If brushing is impossible, rinse the mouth with water after eating.
- Use a battery-operated oral irrigating device, which uses pulsating jets of water to flush debris from teeth, bridges, or braces.

- Eat fewer sweets such as soft drinks containing sugar, candy, gum that contains fructose or another form of sugar, pastries, and sweet desserts.
- Eat more raw fruits and vegetables that naturally remove plaque and other food as they are chewed.
- Eat two or three servings of dairy products per day to provide calcium.
- If antacids are used, select ones with calcium.
- Use frozen orange juice concentrate fortified with calcium.
- Do not use the teeth to open packages or containers.
- Use scissors rather than the teeth to cut thread.
- Do not chew ice cubes or crushed ice.
- Avoid chewing unpopped or partially popped kernels of popcorn.
- Have dental checkups at least every 6 months.

Oral Care for Unconscious Clients

Oral hygiene cannot be neglected because the client is unconscious. In fact, because unconscious clients are not salivating in response to seeing, smelling, and eating food, they need oral care even more frequently than conscious clients. **Sordes** (dried crusts containing mucus, microorganisms, and epithelial cells shed from the mucous membrane) are common on the lips and teeth of unconscious clients.

Toothbrushing is the preferred technique for providing oral hygiene to unconscious clients (Skill 17-4). Clients who are not alert, however, are at risk for aspirating (inhaling) saliva and liquid oral hygiene products into their lungs. Aspirated liquids predispose clients to pneumonia. Therefore, the nurse uses special precautions to avoid getting fluid in the client's airway.

In addition to toothbrushing, the nurse moistens and refreshes the client's mouth with oral swabs. They use various substances for oral hygiene depending on the circumstances and assessment findings for each client (Table 17-4).

 Pharmacologic Considerations

Anticoagulant therapy—even daily low-dose aspirin—increases the risk of bleeding. Using an electric shaver, in place of a safety razor, and a soft bristle toothbrush will reduce bleeding during care of skin and gums.

Denture Care

Dentures (artificial teeth) substitute for a person's lower or upper set of teeth, or both. A **bridge**—a dental appliance that replaces one or several teeth—is fixed permanently to other natural teeth so that it cannot be removed, or it is fastened with a clasp that allows it to be detached from the mouth.

For clients who cannot remove their own dentures, the nurse puts on gloves and uses a dry gauze square or clean face cloth to grasp and free the denture from the mouth (Fig. 17-7). They clean dentures and removable bridges with a toothbrush, denture cleanser or toothpaste, and cold or tepid water. The nurse takes care to hold dentures over a plastic basin or towel so that they will not break if dropped.

Dentists recommend that dentures and bridges remain in place, except during cleaning. Keeping dentures and bridges out for long periods permits the gum lines to change, affecting the fit. If a nurse removes a client's bridge or dentures during the night, they store them in a covered cup. Plain water is used most often to cover dentures when they are not in the mouth, but some add mouthwash or denture cleanser to the water.

TABLE 17-4 Optional Substances for Oral Care

SUBSTANCE	USE
Antiseptic mouthwash diluted with water	Reduces bacterial growth in the mouth and freshens breath
Equal parts of baking soda and table salt in warm water, or baking soda mixed with normal saline	Removes accumulated secretions
One part hydrogen peroxide to 10 parts water	Releases oxygen and loosens dry, sticky particles; prolonged use may damage tooth enamel.
Milk of magnesia	Reduces oral acidity; dissolves plaque, increases flow of saliva, and soothes oral lesions
Lemon and glycerin swabs	Increases salivation and refreshes the mouth; glycerin may absorb water from the lips and cause them to become dry and cracked if used for more than several days.
Petroleum jelly	Lubricates lips

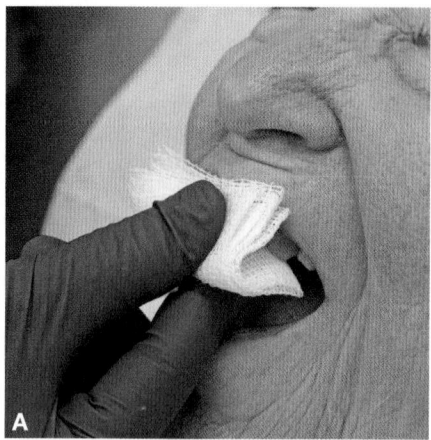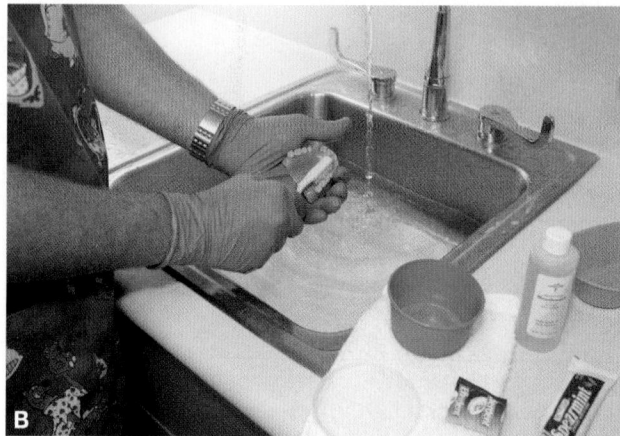

FIGURE 17-7 **A.** Removing an upper denture. **B.** Cleaning dentures.

>>> *Stop, Think, and Respond 17-4*
Compare independent oral hygiene performed by a client and that administered by a nurse. How are they similar, and how are they different?

Hair Care

Sometimes, clients need assistance with grooming or shampooing their hair.

Hair Grooming

The following are recommendations for grooming a client's hair:

- Try to use a hairstyle the client prefers.
- Brush the hair slowly and carefully to avoid damaging the hair.
- Brush the hair to increase circulation and distribution of sebum.
- Use a wide-toothed comb, starting at the ends of the hair rather than from the crown downward if the hair is matted or tangled.
- Apply a conditioner or alcohol to loosen tangles.
- Use oil on the hair if it is dry. Many preparations are available, but pure castor oil, olive oil, and mineral oil are satisfactory.
- Braid the hair to help prevent tangles.
- If hair loss occurs from cancer therapy or some other disease or medical treatment, provide the client with a turban or hat.
- Avoid using hairpins or clips that may injure the scalp.
- Obtain the client's or family's permission before cutting the hair if it is hopelessly tangled and cutting seems to be the only solution to provide adequate grooming.

Shampooing

Hair should be washed as often as necessary to keep it clean. A weekly shampoo is sufficient for most people, but shampooing more or less will not damage the hair. Long-term health care facilities often employ beauticians and barbers, but if professional services are unavailable, the nurse or delegated nursing staff member shampoos the client's hair (Skill 17-5). Dry shampoos, which are applied to the hair as a powder, aerosol spray, or foam, are available for occasional use. The nurse applies the cleaning agent to the hair, massages it thoroughly to distribute, and brushes or towels it from the hair afterward.

Nail Care

Nail care involves keeping the fingernails and toenails clean and trimmed. Clients who have diabetes, impaired circulation, or thick nails are at risk for vascular complications secondary to trauma. The services of a **podiatrist** (a person with special training in caring for feet) are often indicated. It is best to check with the client's physician before cutting fingernails or toenails.

If there are no contraindications, the nurse cares for the client's nails as follows:

- Soak the hands or feet in warm water to soften the keratin and loosen trapped debris (Fig. 17-8).
- Clean under the nails with a wooden orange stick or other sturdy but blunt instruments (Fig. 17-9).
- Push **cuticles** (thin edge of skin at the base of the nail) downward with a soft towel or cuticle pusher stick (Fig. 17-10).

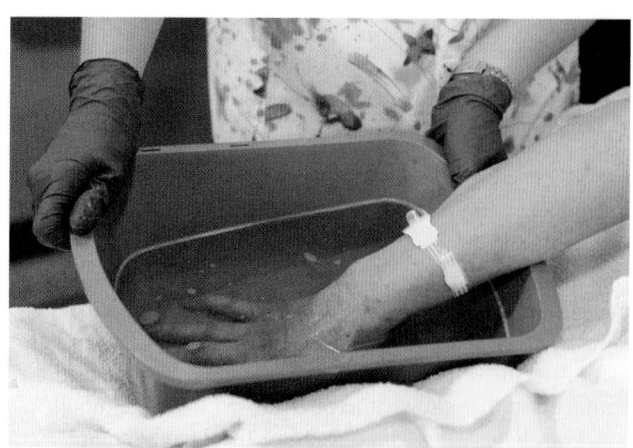

FIGURE 17-8 Soaking a hand before proceeding with nail care.

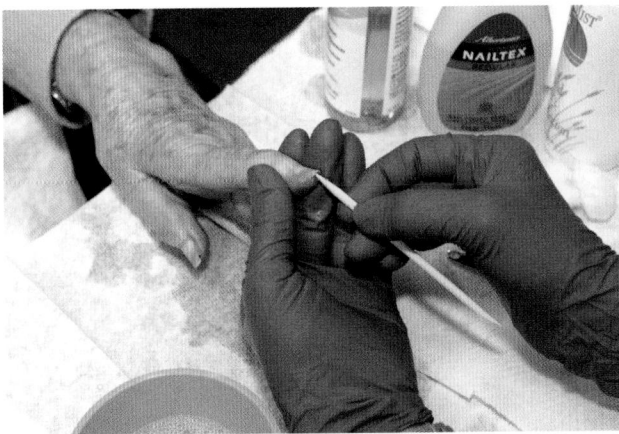

FIGURE 17-9 Cleaning beneath the nail edge with an orange stick.

- Use a handheld electric rotary file or an emery board to reduce the length of long fingernails or toenails.
- Avoid sharp or jagged points that may injure the adjacent skin.

To keep the skin and nails soft and supple, the nurse applies lotion or an emollient cream after bathing and nail care. If foot perspiration is a problem, they use a prescribed antifungal, deodorant powder. Because impaired skin, especially on the feet, is often slow to heal and is susceptible to infection, the nurse immediately reports any abnormal assessment findings. To avoid injuring the feet, clients should wear sturdy slippers or clean socks with nonskid soles and supportive shoes.

VISUAL AND HEARING DEVICES

Eyeglasses and hearing aids improve communication and socialization. Both represent a considerable financial investment. If they become damaged or broken, the temporary loss deprives clients of full sensory perception. Therefore, they should be well maintained and safely stored when not in use.

Although eyeglasses and hearing aids are not body structures, they are worn in close contact with the body for long periods. Consequently, they tend to collect secretions, dirt, and debris that may interfere with their function and

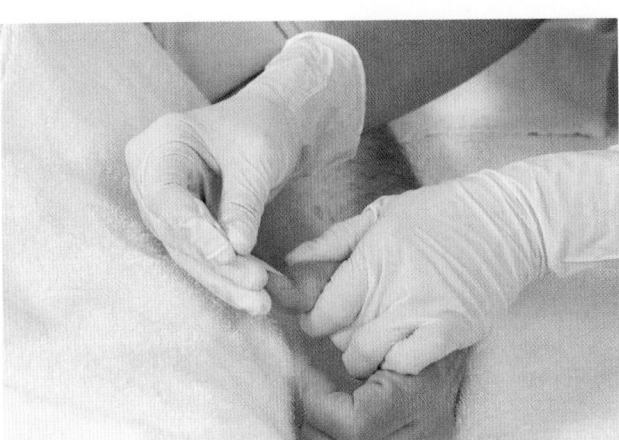

FIGURE 17-10 Pushing the cuticles from the base of the nail.

use. Therefore, the nurse cares for these devices when providing other hygiene measures.

Eyeglasses

Prescription lenses are made of glass or plastic. Plastic lenses weigh much less but are more easily scratched. Glass lenses are more likely to break if dropped. When not in use, eyeglasses are stored in a soft case or rested on the frame.

The nurse cleans glass and plastic lenses as follows:

- Hold the eyeglasses by the nose or ear braces.
- Run tepid water over both sides of the lenses (hot water can damage plastic lenses).
- Wash the lenses with soap or detergent.
- Rinse with running tap water.
- Dry with a clean, soft cloth, such as a handkerchief. Do not use paper tissues because some contain wood fibers, and pulp can scratch the lenses.

Some prefer to use a commercial glass cleaner, but this is not necessary.

Contact Lenses

A contact lens is a small plastic disc placed directly on the cornea. Clients usually wear contact lenses in both eyes, but some clients who have had cataract surgery on one eye wear a single contact lens or a single contact lens and eyeglasses. The nurse should not assume that someone who wears eyeglasses does not use contact lenses, and vice versa.

Several types of contact lenses are available: hard, soft, and gas permeable (Fig. 17-11). All contact lenses, even the disposable types, need removal for cleaning, eye rest, and disinfection. People who are not conscientious about following a routine for contact lens care risk infection, eye abrasion, and permanent damage to the cornea.

When caring for a client who wears contact lenses, the nurse asks the client to remove and insert the lenses and to care for them according to the client's established routine. For clients who cannot do so, the nurse may assist with the removal of the lenses or should consult the client's **ophthalmologist** (a medical doctor who treats eye disorders) or **optometrist** (a person who prescribes corrective lenses) about alternatives to promote adequate vision and safety. Some people, when ill, resume wearing eyeglasses temporarily, use a magnifying glass, or do without any visual aid.

 Concept Mastery Alert

Contact Lens Care

Regardless of the type of contact lenses worn, proper care and cleaning are critical to preventing eye infections and trauma.

Contact Lens Removal

Before removing contact lenses, the nurse obtains an appropriate storage container. Commercial containers are available. Because the lens prescriptions may differ for each eye, the nurse labels the container "left" and "right." The nurse

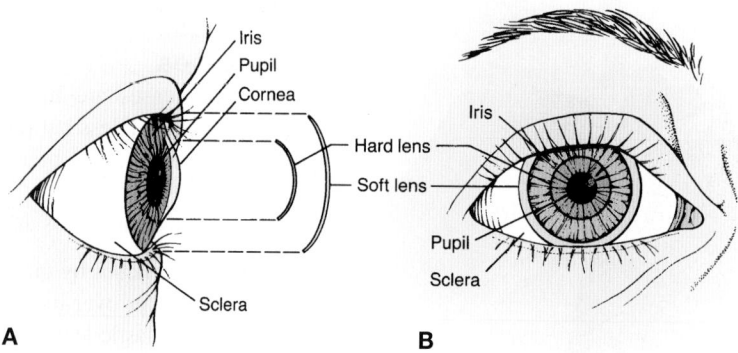

FIGURE 17-11 The location and size of hard and soft contact lenses. **A.** Side view. **B.** Front view.

elevates the client's head and places a towel over the chest to prevent loss or damage to the contact lenses. The technique for removing soft contact lenses is different than for hard contact lenses.

Soft Lenses

To remove a soft contact lens, the nurse moves the lens from the cornea to the sclera by sliding it into position with a clean, gloved finger as the client looks upward (Fig. 17-12). The nurse then gently grasps the repositioned loosened lens between the thumb and the forefinger for removal (Fig. 17-13). Soft lenses dry and crystallize if exposed to air, so the nurse immediately places them in a soaking solution in the storage container (Fig. 17-14).

Hard Lenses

To remove a hard contact lens, the blink method is the most common technique. The nurse positions and prepares the client similarly as for removing soft contact lenses, leaving the lens in place on the cornea. They place the thumb and a finger on the center of the upper and lower lids (Fig. 17-15). The nurse applies slight opposing pressure to the lids while instructing the client to blink, which separates the hard lens from the cornea. If the blink method is unsuccessful, the nurse places an ophthalmic suction cup on the lens and, with

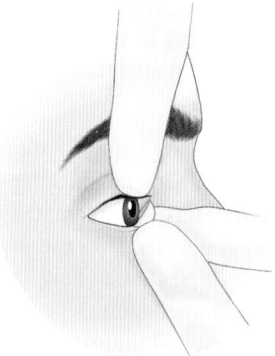

FIGURE 17-13 A soft lens is pinched between the forefinger and the thumb to free it from the sclera. (From Lynn, P. [2022]. *Taylor's clinical nursing skills* [6th ed.]. Lippincott Williams & Wilkins.)

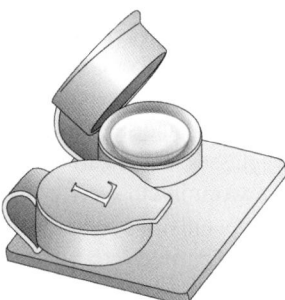

FIGURE 17-14 Contact lenses are stored in a solution-filled container labeled "R" and "L" for the right and left lens, respectively.

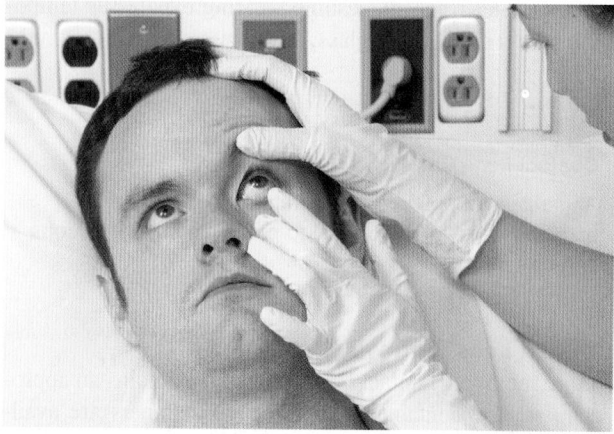

FIGURE 17-12 The nurse removes a soft contact lens from the client's eye.

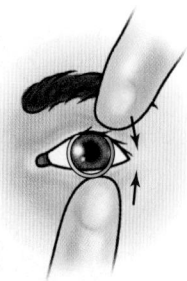

FIGURE 17-15 Moving the eyelids toward one another loosens the hard contact lens from the cornea surface when the client blinks.

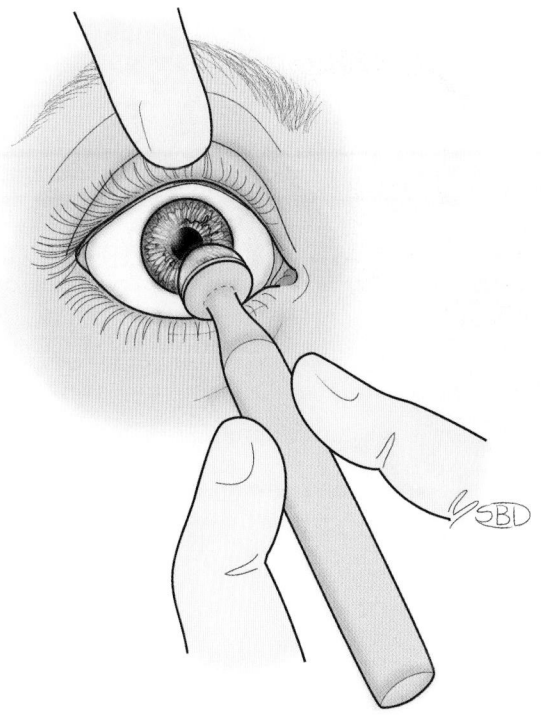

FIGURE 17-16 A suction device is used to remove a hard contact lens.

gentle suction, lifts the lens from the eye (Fig. 17-16). After removal, the nurse soaks the lenses in the storage container.

Prosthetic Eyes

A prosthetic eye is a plastic shell that acts as a cosmetic replacement for the natural eye (Fig. 17-17). There is no way to restore vision once the natural eye is removed. The prosthetic eye and the socket into which it is placed need occasional cleaning. If the client cannot care for the prosthetic eye, the nurse removes it by depressing the lower eyelid until the lid margin is wide enough to allow the prosthetic shell to slide free. The nurse irrigates the eye socket with water or saline before reinserting the prosthetic eye.

Hearing Aids

There are four types of hearing aids:

- In-the-ear devices are small, self-contained aids that fit in the outer ear.
- Canal aids fit deep within the ear canal and are largely concealed. Because of their small size, they may be difficult to remove and adjust.

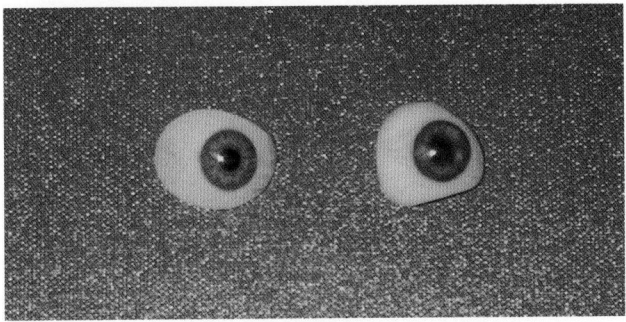

FIGURE 17-17 Examples of scleral shell eye prostheses.

- Behind-the-ear devices consist of a microphone and an amplifier worn behind the ear that delivers sound to an internal receiver.
- Body-aid devices use electrical components enclosed in a case carried somewhere on the body to deliver sound through a wire connected to an ear mold receiver (Fig. 17-18).

In-the-ear and behind-the-ear models are most common. Hearing aids for the right ear will be marked with an R or will have a red dot; hearing aids for the left ear will be marked with an L or will have a blue dot.

Behind-the-ear models can be attached to an eyeglass frame. The use of body aids is most common for those with severe hearing loss or those who cannot care for a small device. Hearing aids are powered by small mercury or zinc batteries that need to be replaced after 100 to 200 hours of use.

Most clients insert and remove their own hearing aids, but the nurse may need to assess and troubleshoot problems that develop (Table 17-5). Clients and their families need to know how to maintain the hearing aid (Client and Family Teaching 17-2).

Assistive Listening Systems

Assistive listening systems are various types of devices that increase the volume of sound to a level that is comparable to that of people with normal hearing. They amplify sounds, reduce the effect of distance between persons with hearing loss and the sound source, minimize background noise, and compensate for poor acoustics. Assistive listening systems are useful for persons who have mild hearing loss as well as those who use hearing aids or have cochlear implants.

There are three types of assistive listening devices (ALDs): frequency modulated (FM), infrared, and induction loop. *FM devices* use radio waves to transmit sound from a building's antenna to a receiver wearing earphones. It is a feature that may be used in churches, museums, theaters,

---

Client and Family Teaching 17-2
Maintaining a Hearing Aid

The nurse teaches the client and family as follows:

- Keep a supply of extra batteries on hand.
- Avoid exposing the electrical components to extreme heat, water, cleaning chemicals, or hair spray.
- Wipe the outer surface of a body aid or behind-the-ear case occasionally.
- Clean cerumen that has become embedded in the earpiece with a special instrument that comes with the hearing aid. If this is not available, use a thin needle as a substitute.
- Turn the hearing aid off when not in use to prolong the life of the battery.
- Check the battery before inserting a hearing aid by slowly turning the volume to high, placing a hand over the hearing aid, and listening for feedback.
- Store the hearing aid in a safe place where it will not fall or get lost.

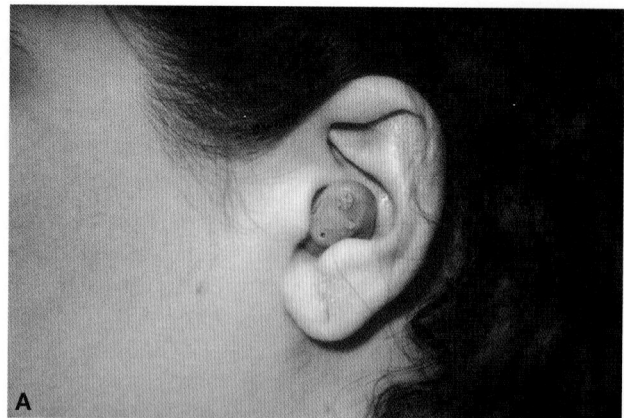

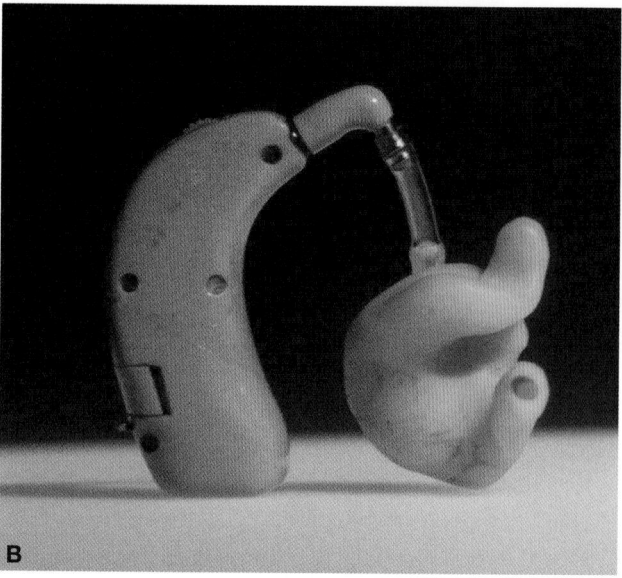

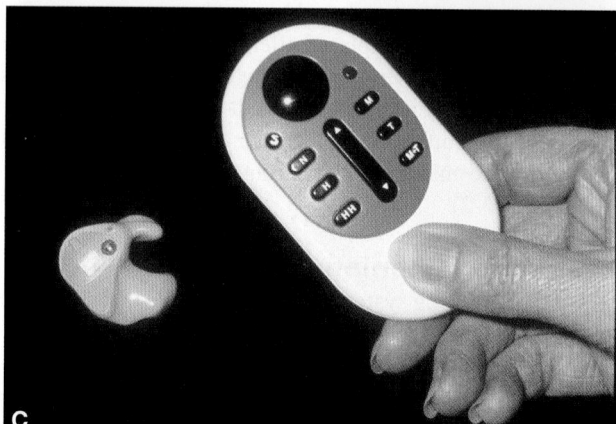

FIGURE 17-18 Examples of assistive hearing devices: in-the-ear **(A)**, behind-the-ear **(B)**, and one whose volume, pitch, and noise reduction can be controlled by a handheld remote control **(C)**.

TABLE 17-5 Troubleshooting Hearing Aid Problems

PROBLEM	POSSIBLE CAUSES	ACTION
Reduced or absent sound	Weak or dead battery	Test and replace battery.
	Incorrect battery position	Match the positive pole of the battery to the positive symbol in the case.
	Cracked tubing leading to the receiver	Repair tubing.
	Broken wire between body aid and receiver	Repair wire.
	Accumulation of cerumen in the ear	Clean the ear.
	Cerumen plugging the receiver	Remove cerumen with an instrument called a *wax loop*, or by using the tip of a pin, or the needle on a syringe.
	Ear congestion from an upper respiratory infection	Consult the physician about administering a decongestant.
	Damaged electrical components	Have the device inspected by a person who services hearing aids.
Shrill noise, called *feedback*, caused by conditions that return sound to the microphone	Malposition or failure to insert the receiver fully in the ear	Remove and reinsert.
	Kinked receiver tubing	Remove and untwist.
	Excessive volume	Reduce volume control.
	Hearing aid left on while being removed from the ear	Turn hearing aid off or replace it in the ear.
Garbled sound	Poor battery contact	Check battery for correct size; make sure the battery compartment is closed; clean metal contact points with an emery board.
	Dirty components	Clean with a soft cloth.
	Debris in the on/off switch	Move the switch back and forth several times.
	Corroded battery	Remove and replace.
	Cracked case	Repair or replace.

and so on. *IRLDs* convert sound into infrared light and send it through a wall- or ceiling-mounted receiver to the person wearing the listening device. The light is converted back into an auditory stimulus. People who need help hearing lectures, television, or live performances may use IRLDs. Some geriatric centers are installing IRLDs in rooms used for social and recreational activities. An *induction loop device* uses a magnetic field of copper loops installed within the floor of a building. Sound travels from a speaker's microphone through the loop to a person wearing a hearing aid equipped with a telecoil that picks up the sound from the speaker.

NURSING IMPLICATIONS

Clients who require assistance with personal hygiene may have a variety of nursing diagnoses:

- ADL deficit
- Altered skin integrity risk
- Bathing/hygiene ADL deficit
- Corneal injury risk
- Dressing ADL deficit
- Activity intolerance

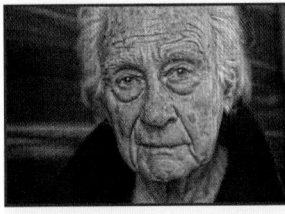

Clinical Scenario After visiting his father who has been a widower for several years, it has become apparent to the son that his father is no longer attending to his physical needs, such as bathing regularly, shaving, laundering, preparing meals, and maintaining the household. Arrangements are made to admit him to a basic care nursing home. The nurse assigned to the client upon admission has developed an initial plan for his nursing care. See Nursing Care Plan 17-1 for a client with a nursing diagnosis of bathing/hygiene ADL deficit, defined as impaired ability to accomplish or complete bathing activities for self.

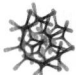

NURSING CARE PLAN 17-1 — Bathing/Hygiene ADL Deficit

Assessment
- Observe client's motor skills, strength, and coordination to determine the extent to which they can perform hygiene skills.
- Determine whether the client's mental status is sufficient to follow directions, complete tasks required for hygiene, and ensure safety.
- Assess client's level of endurance to accomplish hygiene activities such as changes in respiratory and heart rate, increased blood pressure, pain, or fatigue when performing self-care.

Nursing Diagnosis. Bathing/hygiene activities of daily living (ADL) deficit related to impaired ability to wash body secondary to progressive total body weakness as evidenced by failure to regularly bathe and perform hygiene practices and wearing clothing that is soiled and smells of body odor

Expected Outcomes. The client will receive assistance with bathing biweekly and oral hygiene on a daily and p.r.n. (as needed) basis.

Interventions	Rationales
Assist with a shower twice a week at a convenient time for the client.	Scheduling hygiene according to the client's preferences and avoiding conflicts with other components of care and treatment meets the client's individualized needs and avoids unnecessary interruptions
Use castile soap that the client prefers.	Demonstrates organization and respect for the client's personal choices
Let the client assist with bathing to whatever level is possible; areas that the client cannot wash must be completed by nursing staff.	Facilitates participation in care and maintains self-esteem
Apply the client's deodorant and body lotion located in the bedside cabinet after bathing is completed.	Demonstrates respect for the client's choices in hygiene products; ensures a feeling of well-being and confidence in social interactions
Assist the client with putting on personal clothing.	Promotes cleanliness and personal identity
Help the client shave following bathing or during bathing if desired.	Improves self-image
Provide supplies for oral hygiene.	Promotes self-care
Arrange for a haircut every 3 weeks.	Raises self-esteem and self-identity
Deposit soiled clothing in agency laundry.	Promotes cleanliness and reduces the potential for detectable body odor

Evaluation of Expected Outcome

- The client's hygiene needs for bathing and oral care are completed.
- The client assists with hygiene needs to the extent possible.
- The client states, "I feel so much better after I've gotten cleaned up."

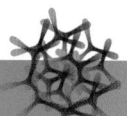

- Hygiene: Practices that promote health through personal cleanliness; includes care and maintenance of devices such as eyeglasses and hearing aids to ensure continued and proper function; practices and needs differ according to age, inherited characteristics of the skin and hair, cultural values, and state of health
- Hygiene practices:
  - Bathing
  - Tub bath or shower
  - Partial bath
  - Bed bath
    - Towel bath
    - Bag bath
  - Shaving
  - Oral hygiene

- Toothbrushing
- Flossing
- Dentures
- Hair care
  - Hair grooming
  - Shampooing
- Nail care
- Visual and hearing devices: Because eyeglasses and hearing aids are worn in close contact with the body for long periods, they tend to collect secretions, dirt, and debris, and the nurse cares for these devices when providing other hygiene measures.
- Contact lenses
- Hearing aids

CRITICAL THINKING EXERCISES

1. You have been assigned to two clients: a 75-year-old woman who is unconscious after a stroke and a 38-year-old male mechanic being treated for an ulcer. How do their hygiene needs differ?
2. You are responsible for inspecting long-term care facilities, such as nursing homes. What criteria should health care agencies meet regarding bathing facilities and hygiene policies to receive positive evaluations?
3. Explain why attending to shaving, oral hygiene, and nail care is important to families of those being cared for in long-term care facilities.
4. What strategies might a nurse use for meeting the hygiene needs of a client who refuses to bathe and perform oral care?

NEXT-GENERATION NCLEX-STYLE REVIEW QUESTIONS

1. When a home health nurse visits the home of a family being treated for pediculosis (head lice), which items should the nurse discourage?
   a. Pediculicide shampoo
   b. Fine-toothed comb
   c. Hair conditioner
   d. Warm tap water
   Test-Taking Strategy: Use the process of elimination to select the option that is unlikely to facilitate removing a lice infestation.
2. When examining the skin of a client with psoriasis, what is the nurse most likely to observe?
   a. Weeping skin lesions on the trunk of the body
   b. Red skin patches covered with silvery scales
   c. Fluid-filled blisters surrounded by crusts
   d. A red rash containing pus-filled lesions

Test-Taking Strategy: Analyze the descriptions in each option and select the one that correlates with the manifestations associated with psoriasis.

3. When a client develops pruritus (itching skin), what nursing measure is best for relieving the client's discomfort?
   a. Use a medicated bath with oatmeal or cornstarch.
   b. Apply extra wool blankets to the bed for warmth.
   c. Give frequent showers or tub baths.
   d. Rub the skin dry after bathing.
   Test-Taking Strategy: Eliminate options that are likely to aggravate itching.
4. A client experiences a shrill noise, known as *feedback*, from a hearing aid. What are some possible causes for the nurse to check? Select all that apply.
   a. Incorrect battery position
   b. Malposition within the ear
   c. Accumulation of cerumen
   d. Kinked receiver tubing
   e. Excessive volume
   f. Corroded battery
   Test-Taking Strategy: Analyze the options and select those that can cause a person who wears a hearing aid to experience shrill noise.
5. When shaving a male client's face with a safety razor, which nursing action is correct?
   a. Start at the neck working upward.
   b. Pull the razor in the direction of hair growth.
   c. Use long strokes with the razor.
   d. Replace the razor after each use.
   Test-Taking Strategy: Eliminate actions that are unlikely to produce a clean shave and promote comfort while shaving a male client.

NEXT-GENERATION NCLEX-STYLE CLINICAL SCENARIO QUESTIONS

Clinical Scenario:

After visiting his father who has been a widower for several years, it has become apparent to the son that his father is no longer attending to his physical needs such as bathing regularly, shaving, laundering, preparing meals, and maintaining the household. Arrangements are being made to admit him to a basic care nursing home.

1. From the following list, choose all of the factors that are reasons for the client to enter a basic care nursing home. Select all that apply.
   a. Client is gaining weight.
   b. Client is no longer bathing regularly.
   c. The client's household is not maintained.
   d. The client is able to make his own meals.
   e. The client's clothes are dirty and unkept.

2. From the following list, choose the most appropriate care facilities for this client.
   a. Skilled nursing facility
   b. Home health care
   c. Hospice care facility
   d. Group home for assisted living
   e. Intermediate care facilities
   f. Basic care facility
   g. Senior residential community
   h. Brushing from gum to crown of each tooth.

SKILL 17-1 Providing a Tub Bath or Shower

Suggested Action	Reason for Action
ASSESSMENT	
Check the medical record or nursing care plan for hygiene directives.	Ensures continuity of care
Assess the client's level of consciousness, orientation, strength, and mobility.	Provides data for evaluating the client's ability to carry out hygiene practices independently
Check for gauze dressings, plaster cast, or electrical or battery-operated equipment; determine whether they can be protected with waterproof material or are safe if they become wet.	Maintains the client's safety and ensures integrity of treatment devices
Determine if and when any laboratory or diagnostic procedures are scheduled.	Aids in time management
Check the occupancy, cleanliness, and safety of the tub or shower (Fig. A).	Helps organize the plan for care

Tub and shower equipped for client safety (Photo by B. Proud.)

Suggested Action	Reason for Action
PLANNING	
Clean the tub or shower if necessary.	Reduces potential for spreading microorganisms
Consult with the client about a convenient time for tending to hygiene needs.	Promotes client cooperation and participation in decision-making
Assemble supplies: floor mat, towels, face cloth, soap, clean clothes, pajamas, or gown.	Demonstrates organization and efficient time management
IMPLEMENTATION	
Escort the client to the shower or bathing room.	Shows concern for the client's safety
Demonstrate how to operate the faucet and drain.	Ensures the client's safety and comfort
Fill the tub approximately halfway with water 105°–110°F (40°–43°C) or adjust the shower to a similar temperature if the client cannot operate the faucet.	Demonstrates concern for the client's safety and comfort
Place a "Do Not Disturb" or "In Use" sign on the outer door.	Ensures privacy
Help the client into the tub or shower if they need assistance by: • Placing a chair next to the tub • Having the client swing their feet over the edge of the tub • Asking the client to lean forward, grab a support bar, and raise the buttocks and body until they can fully enter the tub	Reduces the risk of falling

SKILL 17-1 Providing a Tub Bath or Shower (*continued*)

Suggested Action	Reason for Action
Have the client sit on a stool or seat in the tub or shower if the client will have difficulty exiting the tub or may become weak while bathing (Fig. B).	Ensures safety
	Shower chair may be used for safety and comfort.

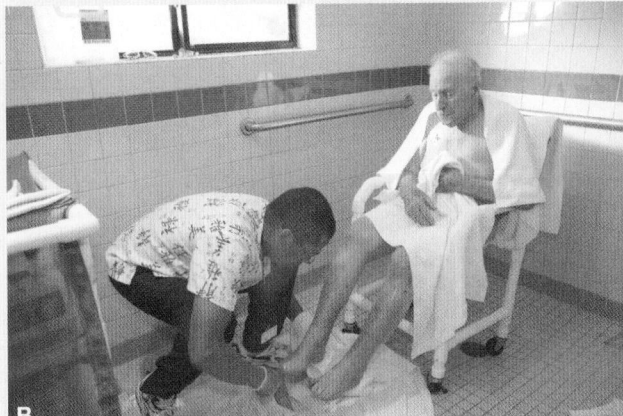

Suggested Action	Reason for Action
Show the client how to summon help.	Promotes safety
Stay close at hand.	Ensures proximity in case the client needs assistance
Check on the client frequently by knocking on the door and waiting for a response.	Shows respect for privacy yet concern for safety
Escort the client to their room after the bath or shower.	Demonstrates concern for safety and welfare
Clean the tub or shower with an antibacterial agent; dispose of soiled linen in its designated location.	Reduces the spread of microorganisms and demonstrates concern for the next person to use the tub or shower
Remove the "In Use" sign from the door.	Indicates that the bathing room is unoccupied

EVALUATION

- Client is clean.
- Client remains uninjured.

DOCUMENT

- Date and time
- Tub bath or shower

SAMPLE DOCUMENTATION[a]

Date and Time Tub bath taken independently. _____ J. Doe, LPN

[a]Generally, nurses document routine hygiene measures on a checklist, but for teaching purposes, an example of narrative charting has been provided.

SKILL 17-2 Administering Perineal Care

Suggested Action	Reason for Action
ASSESSMENT	
Inspect the client's genital and rectal areas.	Provides data for determining whether perineal care is necessary
PLANNING	
Wash hands or perform hand antisepsis with an alcohol rub (see Chapter 10).	Reduces the spread of microorganisms
Gather gloves, soap, water, and clean cloths or antiseptic wipes; a container of cleansing solution in a squeeze bottle; and several towels or absorptive pads.	Provides a means of removing debris and microorganisms

(*continued*)

SKILL 17-2 Administering Perineal Care (*continued*)

Suggested Action	Reason for Action
Explain the procedure to the client.	Reduces anxiety and promotes cooperation
Pull the privacy curtain.	Demonstrates respect for modesty
Place the client in a dorsal recumbent position and cover with a bath blanket (Fig. A).	Provides access to the perineum

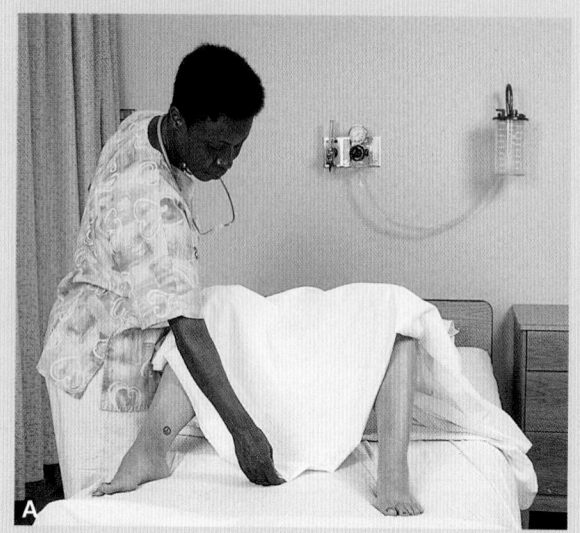

Positioning and draping the client. (Photo by B. Proud.)

Pull and fanfold the top linen to the foot of the bed while the client holds the top of the blanket.	Maintains client modesty and keeps upper linen clean and dry
For a female client, place a disposable pad beneath the buttocks or place the client on a bedpan; for a male client, place a disposable pad under the penis and beneath the buttocks.	Helps absorb liquid that may drip during cleansing

IMPLEMENTATION

Females

Bend the female client's knees and spread the legs.	Exposes area for cleansing
Put on gloves.	Prevents contact with blood, secretions, or excretions
Wash the outer folds of the labia and then separate the folds of the labia and wash from the pubic area toward the anus (Figs. B and C).	Cleanses in a direction from less soiled to more soiled; prevents reintroducing microorganisms into previously cleaned areas

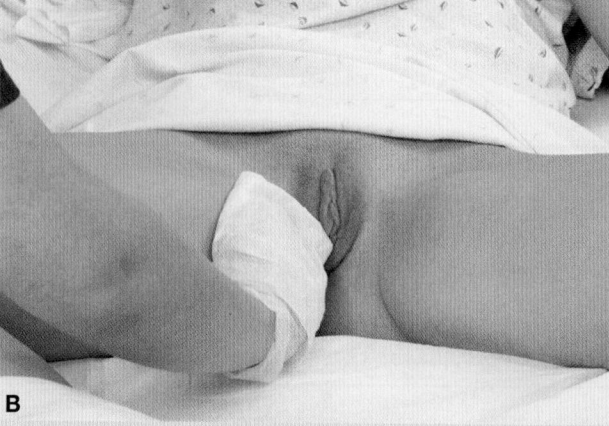

Cleansing the outer labia.

SKILL 17-2 Administering Perineal Care (*continued*)

Suggested Action	Reason for Action

C

Cleansing the inner labia toward the anus.

Suggested Action	Reason for Action
Never go back over an area that you already have cleaned. Use a clean area of the cloth or a separate antiseptic wipe for each stroke.	Avoids resoiling already clean areas
Wash debris on the outside of a urinary catheter, if one exists, especially where it is in contact with mucous membrane and genital tissue.	Reduces the number and growth of microorganisms that may ascend to the bladder
Squeeze the antiseptic solution container, if one is used, starting at the upper areas of the labia down toward the anus (Fig. D).	Ensures that the solution will drain toward more soiled body areas; prevents reintroducing microorganisms into previously cleaned areas

D

Rinsing the perineum.

Suggested Action	Reason for Action
Pat the skin dry with a towel.	Removes excess moisture
Turn the client to the side and wash from the perineum toward the anus.	Cleans in a direction toward more soiled body areas
Rinse and pat the skin dry.	Prevents skin irritation from soap residue and retained moisture; a warm, dark, moist environment contributes to fungal skin infections
Apply a clean absorbent perineal pad to clients who are menstruating or have other types of vaginal or rectal drainage.	Promotes cleanliness and reduces contact between the skin and moist drainage

(*continued*)

SKILL 17-2 Administering Perineal Care (*continued*)

Suggested Action	Reason for Action
Males	
For males, grasp the penis; if the client is uncircumcised, retract the foreskin.	Facilitates removing debris and secretions that may be trapped beneath the fold of skin
Clean the tip of the penis using circular motions (Fig. E). Never go back over an area that you have already cleaned.	Keeps the urethral opening clean

Cleansing the glans penis.

E

| Replace the foreskin. | Prevents trauma |
| Wipe the shaft of the penis toward the scrotum (Fig. F). | Keeps microorganisms and debris from the urethral opening |

Cleansing the shaft of the penis.

F

Spread the legs and wash the scrotum.	Removes debris where it may be trapped and harbor microorganisms
Pat the skin dry with a towel.	Removes excess moisture
Turn the client to the side and wash from the perineum toward the anus.	Cleans in a direction toward more soiled body areas
Rinse and pat the skin dry.	Prevents skin irritation from soap residue and retained moisture; a warm, dark, moist environment contributes to fungal skin infections.
Apply a clean absorbent pad to clients who have rectal drainage.	Promotes cleanliness and reduces contact between the skin and moist drainage
Remove damp towels and cover the client with bed linens.	Restores comfort; protects linens from soiling
Deposit wet cloths, soiled wipes, and towels in an appropriate container.	Controls the spread of microorganisms
Empty and rinse the bedpan.	Controls the spread of microorganisms

SKILL 17-2 Administering Perineal Care (*continued*)

Suggested Action	Reason for Action
Remove gloves and wash hands or perform hand antisepsis with an alcohol rub (see Chapter 10).	Reduces the spread of microorganisms
Attend to the client's comfort and safety.	Demonstrates concern for the client's welfare

EVALUATION

- Genital, perineal, and rectal areas are clean and dry.
- Cleansing has been from less to more soiled areas of the body.
- There has been no direct contact with drainage, secretions, or excretions.
- Soiled articles have been properly disposed.

DOCUMENT

- Date and time
- Care provided
- Description of drainage and tissue

SAMPLE DOCUMENTATION

Date and Time   Pericare provided to remove moderate bloody drainage coming from vagina. Perineal tissue is intact.
_____ J. Doe, LPN

SKILL 17-3 Giving a Bed Bath

Suggested Action	Reason for Action
ASSESSMENT	
Check the medical record or nursing care plan for hygiene directives.	Ensures continuity of care
Inspect the skin for signs of dryness, drainage, or secretions.	Provides data for determining whether a complete or partial bath is appropriate
PLANNING	
Consult with the client to determine a convenient time for tending to hygiene needs.	Promotes client cooperation; allows client participation in decision-making
Assemble supplies: bath blanket, towels, face cloths, soap, wash basin, clean pajamas or gown, clean bed linens, other hygiene articles such as deodorant or antiperspirant, and a razor for males.	Demonstrates organization and efficient time management
IMPLEMENTATION	
Wash hands or perform hand antisepsis with an alcohol rub (see Chapter 10).	Reduces the spread of microorganisms
Pull the privacy curtain.	Demonstrates respect for modesty
Raise the bed to an appropriate height.	Reduces muscle strain on the back when providing care
Remove extra pillows or positioning devices and place the client on their back.	Prepares the client for washing the anterior body surface
Cover the client with a bath blanket (Fig. A).	Shows respect for the client's modesty and provides warmth

Covering with a bath blanket.

(continued)

SKILL 17-3 Giving a Bed Bath (*continued*)

Suggested Action	Reason for Action
Remove the client's gown.	Facilitates washing the client
While the client holds the top of the bath blanket, pull and fanfold the top linen to the bottom of the bed or remove the linen, fold it, and lay it on a chair.	Keeps linen, which may be reused, clean
If linen is too soiled for reuse, place it in a laundry hamper.	Reduces the spread of microorganisms
Hold dirty linen away from contact with your uniform.	Reduces the spread of microorganisms
Fill a basin with 105°–110°F (40°–43°C) water; place the basin on the overbed table.	Provides comfortably warm water for bathing within easy access
Wet the washcloth and fold it to fashion a mitt (Fig. B).	Keeps water from dripping from the margins of the cloth

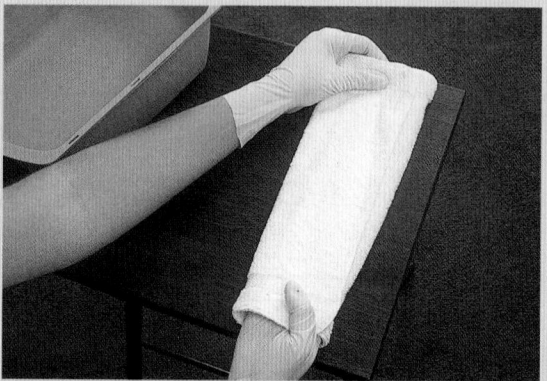
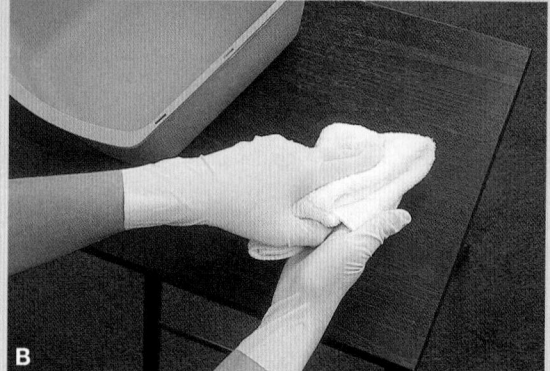

Straightening washcloth before folding info mitt.

B

Wipe each eye with a separate corner of the mitt from the nose toward the ear (Fig. C).	Prevents getting soap in the eyes

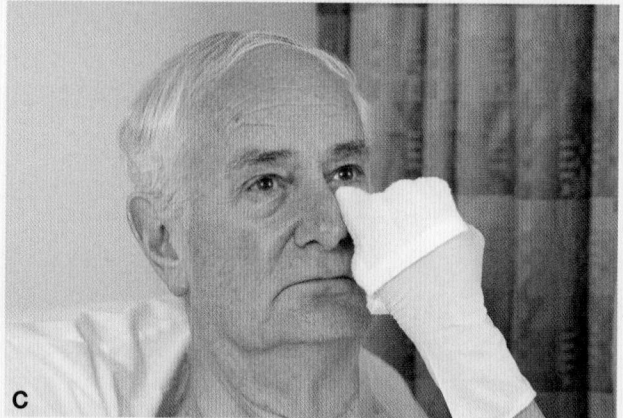

Wiping the eyes.

C

Lather the wet washcloth with soap and finish washing the face.	Removes oil, sweat, and microorganisms
Rinse the washcloth and remove soapy residue from the face, then dry well.	Prevents drying of the skin

SKILL 17-3 Giving a Bed Bath (*continued*)

Suggested Action	Reason for Action
Bathe each of the client's arms separately; the axillae may be included now or when the chest is washed (Fig. D).	Cleanses soiled material and keeps the client from becoming too chilled

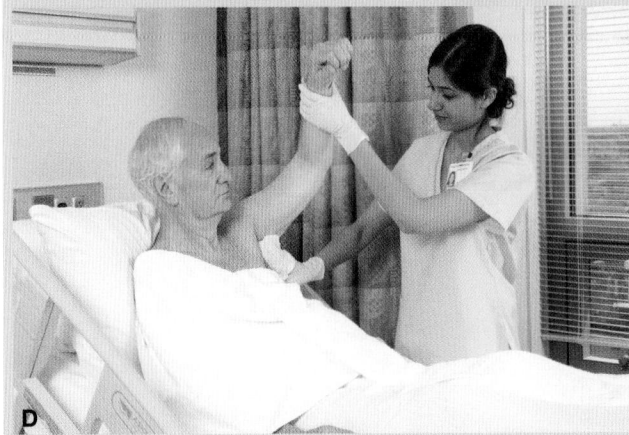

Washing the arm and axilla.

Suggested Action	Reason for Action
Offer to apply deodorant or antiperspirant after washing the axillae.	Demonstrates respect for the client's usual hygiene practices; reduces perspiration and body odor
Place each hand in the basin of water as you wash it (Fig. E).	Facilitates more thorough washing than just using the washcloth

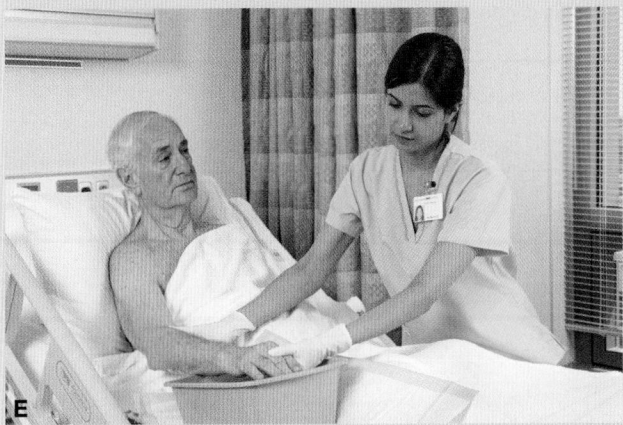

Soaking the hand in a basin.

Suggested Action	Reason for Action
Discard and replace the water in the basin; rinse the washcloth well or replace it with a clean one.	Eliminates debris, microorganisms, and soap residue and increases the warmth of the water in preparation for washing cleaner areas of the body
Wash the chest, abdomen, each leg, and then the feet following the steps described for the upper body (Fig. F).	Follows the principle of washing from cleaner to more soiled areas

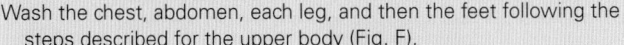
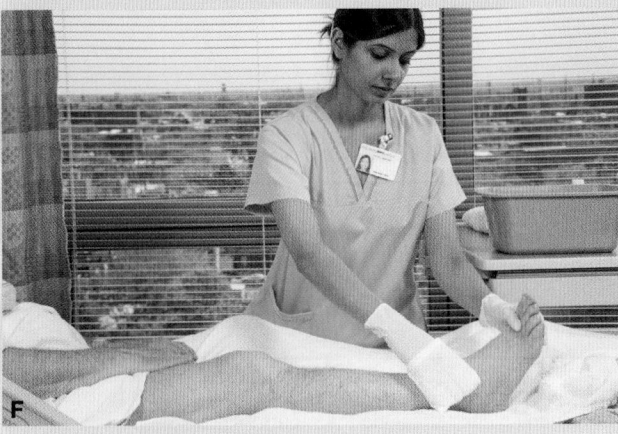

Washing a leg.

Suggested Action	Reason for Action
Help the client onto their side.	Repositions the client so you can bathe the posterior of the body
Change the water and bathe the client's back (Fig. G).	Allows washing to begin at a cleaner area on the posterior aspect of the body

(*continued*)

SKILL 17-3 Giving a Bed Bath (*continued*)

Suggested Action	Reason for Action
Offer to apply lotion and provide a backrub.	Improves circulation and relaxes the client
Put on gloves and wash the buttocks, genitals, and anus last.	Reduces the potential for contact with lesions or drainage that may contain infectious microorganisms
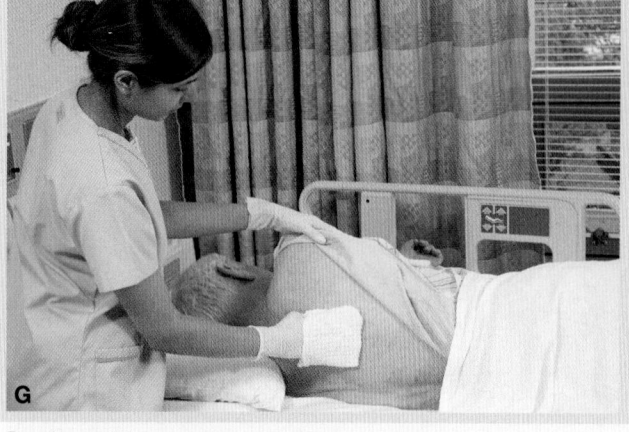 **G**	Washing the back.
Dry thoroughly.	Prevents moisture accumulation
Discard the water and wipe the basin dry.	Controls growth and spread of microorganisms
Remove gloves and help the client put on a fresh gown.	Restores comfort and modesty

EVALUATION

- Client is completely bathed.
- Client experiences no discomfort or intolerance of activity.

DOCUMENT

- Date and time
- Type and extent of hygiene
- Client response
- Assessment findings observed during bath

SAMPLE DOCUMENTATION[a]

> ***Date and Time*** Complete bed bath given. Client could wash face and genitals independently. Skin is intact. No dyspnea noted during bath. _____ J. Doe, LPN

The nurses depicted here are wearing gloves; however, gloves are not necessary when giving a bath, unless there is a risk of infectious contact.
[a]Generally, nurses document routine hygiene measures on a checklist, but for teaching purposes, an example of narrative charting has been used.

SKILL 17-4 Giving Oral Care to Unconscious Clients

Suggested Action	Reason for Action
ASSESSMENT	
Check the nursing care plan about the frequency of oral hygiene.	Maintains continuity of care
Inspect the client's mouth.	Helps to determine equipment and supplies needed
Look for oral hygiene supplies that may be at the client's bedside already.	Controls costs
PLANNING	
Arrange to brush the client's teeth once per shift and to provide additional oral care at least every 2 hours if necessary.	Promotes a schedule for removing plaque and microorganisms and moistening and refreshing the mouth

SKILL 17-4 Giving Oral Care to Unconscious Clients (*continued*)

Suggested Action	Reason for Action
Assemble the following equipment: toothbrush, toothpaste, suction catheter, water, bulb syringe, padded tongue blade, emesis basin, towel or absorbent pad, and gloves. Some agencies may stock a toothbrushing device connected directly to a suction catheter (Fig. A).	Promotes organization and efficient time management

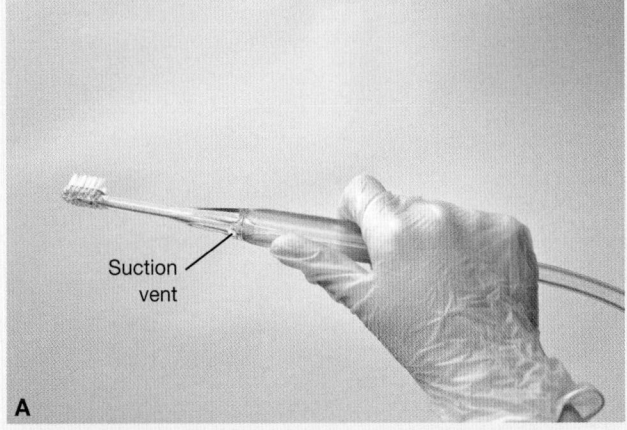

Suction vent

A

Toothbrushing device with suction catheter.

IMPLEMENTATION

Explain to the client what you are about to do.	Reduces anxiety if the client has the cognitive capacity to understand
Position the client on the side with the head slightly lowered.	Prevents liquids from draining into the airway
Place a towel beneath the head.	Absorbs liquids
Connect a suction tip or catheter to a portable or wall-mounted suction source.	Promotes safety
Spread toothpaste over a moistened toothbrush.	Prepares the toothbrush for use
Put on gloves.	Prevents direct contact with blood or microorganisms in the mouth
Use a tongue blade or lower the client's chin to open the mouth and separate the teeth.	Serves as a safe substitute for the nurse's fingers
Brush all tooth surfaces with the toothbrush (Fig. B).	Removes plaque and microorganisms

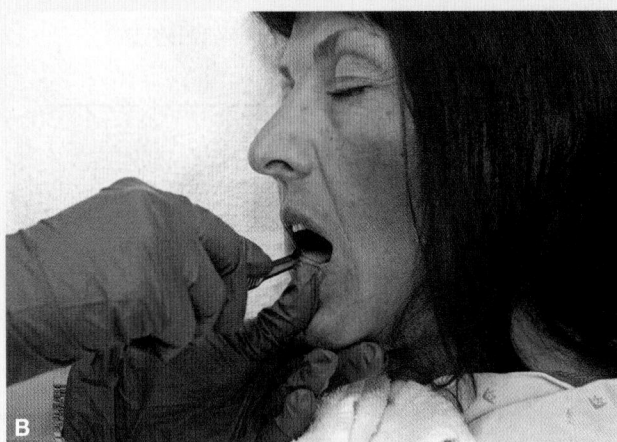

B

With the head lowered, the teeth are brushed.

(*continued*)

SKILL 17-4 Giving Oral Care to Unconscious Clients (*continued*)

Suggested Action	Reason for Action
Instill water and suction the mouth with a bulb syringe (Fig. C).	Removes loosened debris
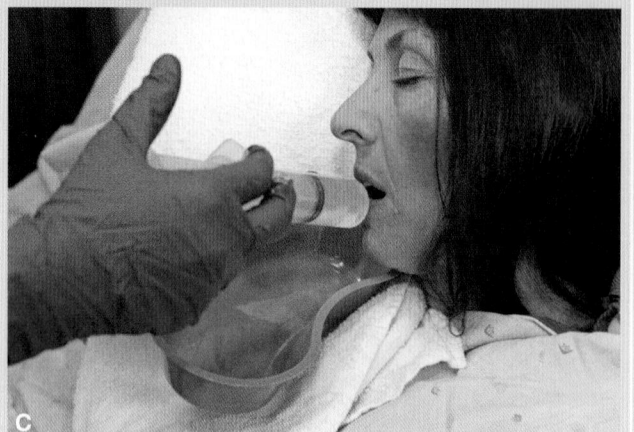	Rinsing the mouth while keeping the head lowered.
Suction the rinsing solution with a suction device (Fig. D).	Reduces the potential for aspiration
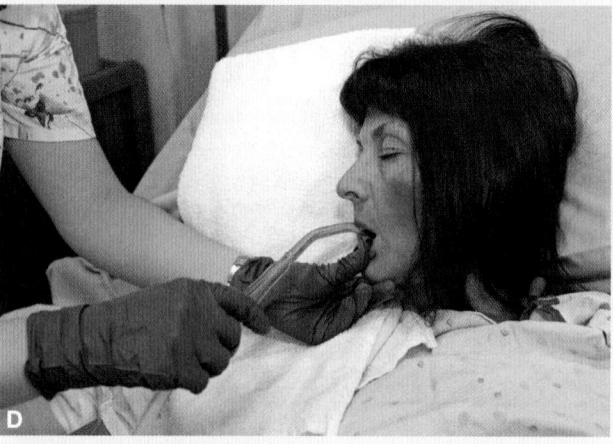	Suctioning the fluid from the mouth.
Clean and store oral hygiene supplies.	Restores cleanliness and order to the client's environment
Remove wet towel and gloves; restore client to a position of comfort and safety.	Demonstrates concern for the client's dignity and welfare

EVALUATION

- The teeth are clean.
- The oral mucosa is smooth, pink, moist, and intact.
- Safety is maintained.

DOCUMENT

- Date and time
- Assessment findings if significant
- Type of oral care
- Unusual events such as choking and nursing action that was taken
- Outcome of any nursing action

SAMPLE DOCUMENTATION

Date and Time Teeth brushed and mouth rinsed. Liquid suctioned from the mouth using a suction catheter. No choking during oral care. Lung sounds are clear bilaterally. _____ J. Doe, LPN

SKILL 17-5 Shampooing Hair

Suggested Action	Reason for Action
ASSESSMENT	
Inspect the client for oily and limp hair or signs of accumulating secretions or lesions on the scalp.	Provides data to determine the need for shampooing and what supplies may be appropriate to use
Assess for respiratory symptoms, pain, or other conditions that increase or contribute to activity intolerance.	Aids in establishing priorities for care
Determine if and when medical treatments or tests are scheduled.	Ensures that hygiene measures will not interrupt therapeutic or diagnostic procedures
Discuss the types of products available for shampooing.	Facilitates individualized care
PLANNING	
Collaborate with the client on the time of day that is best for shampooing.	Involves the client in decision-making
Assemble equipment, which may include shampoo, conditioner, hair oil treatment, towels, a water pitcher, and a shampoo basin or trough.	Promotes organization and efficient time management
IMPLEMENTATION	
Close the door to the room and pull the privacy curtain.	Reduces the potential for chilling and promotes respect for privacy
Remove the pillow and protect the upper area of the bed with towels; cover the client's chest and shoulders with a towel.	Absorbs moisture
Put on gloves if any open lesions are on or near the head.	Prevents direct contact with blood or secretions
Wet the hair thoroughly and apply shampoo (see figure).	Dilutes and distributes the shampoo

Shampooing the hair using a shampoo trough.

Suggested Action	Reason for Action
Work the shampoo into a lather.	Facilitates cleansing throughout the hair
Rinse the hair with water.	Removes oil and shampoo from the hair
Apply conditioner if requested and available.	Relaxes the hair and reduces tangles
Wrap the head with a dry towel and fluff the hair.	Absorbs water and shortens the drying time
Remove and discard gloves when there is no threat for direct contact with blood or secretions.	Facilitates hair care
Comb, braid, or style the hair according to the client's preference.	Promotes self-esteem
Clean and store shampooing supplies.	Restores cleanliness and order to the client's environment

EVALUATION

The hair is clean and dry.

DOCUMENT

- Date and time
- Assessment findings
- Type of care
- Response of the client

SAMPLE DOCUMENTATION

Date and Time Scalp and hair appear oily. Skin is intact. Bed shampoo provided. Hair dried, combed, and styled in braids. Scalp is clean and intact. No evidence of chilling, fatigue, or discomfort during shampoo. States, "I feel so much better."
_____ J. Doe, LPN

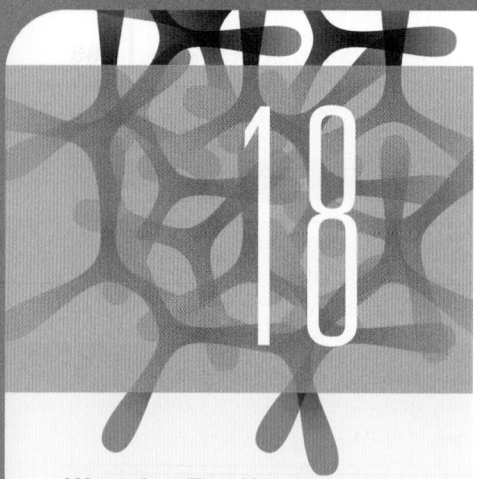

18

Comfort, Rest, and Sleep

Words To Know

apnea
automatic behavior
bruxism
cataplexy
circadian rhythm
climate control
comfort
drug tolerance
environmental psychologist
humidity
hypersomnia
hypersomnolence
hypnagogic hallucinations
hypnagogic jerks
hypnotic
hypopnea
hypoxia
insomnia
jet lag
massage
mattress overlays
melatonin
microsleep
multiple sleep latency test
narcolepsy
nocturnal enuresis
nocturnal polysomnography
occupied bed
parasomnia
photoperiod
phototherapy
progressive relaxation
relative humidity
REM rebound sleep
restless legs syndrome
sedative
sleep
sleep apnea/hypopnea syndrome
sleep diary
sleep inertia
sleep paralysis
sleep rituals
sleep–wake cycle disturbance
somnambulism
stimulants
sundown syndrome
sunrise syndrome
thermoregulation
unoccupied bed
ventilation

Learning Objectives

On completion of this chapter, the reader should be able to:

1. Differentiate between comfort, rest, and sleep.
2. Describe ways to modify the client's environment to promote comfort, rest, and sleep.
3. List standard furnishings in each client room.
4. State the functions of sleep.
5. Describe the phases of sleep and their differences.
6. Describe the general trend in sleep requirements as a person ages.
7. Identify factors that affect sleep.
8. List categories of drugs that affect sleep.
9. Name techniques for assessing sleep patterns.
10. Describe categories of sleep disorders.
11. Discuss techniques for promoting sleep.
12. Plan nursing measures that promote relaxation.
13. Discuss unique characteristics of sleep among older adults.

INTRODUCTION

Comfort (a state in which a person is relieved of distress) facilitates rest (a waking state characterized by reduced activity and mental stimulation) and **sleep** (a state of arousable unconsciousness). One factor that contributes to comfort is a safe, clean, and attractive environment.

This chapter addresses measures for ensuring that the setting for client care promotes a sense of well-being. It includes measures for maintaining the order and cleanliness of the client's bed and room and describes nursing interventions that facilitate rest and sleep.

 Gerontologic Considerations

■ Older adults may prefer warmer room temperatures because of decreased subcutaneous fat deposits. Those with cognitive impairment, however, may perceive environmental temperatures as uncomfortably warm or cool, even when the temperature is comfortable for others.

■ Older adults who reside in institutional settings, such as nursing homes or assisted living facilities, are usually more comfortable with their own bed furnishings and personal mementos and belongings.

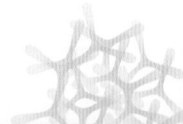

■ Older adults often experience fatigue, may report having sleep problems, and are likely to spend more time in bed without actually sleeping.

■ Short daytime naps and rest periods, usually less than 2 hours in duration, can restore energy for an older adult without interfering with nighttime sleep. However, 7 to 8 hours of sleep within a 24-hour period is the usual total amount of sleep required by older adults. Therefore, expectations for the number of sleep hours during the night must be adjusted according to the amount of daytime sleep.

■ Boredom may be a cause of daytime napping. Providing meaningful diversions may improve nighttime sleep and diminish daytime napping.

■ Older adults with limited mobility may sleep better if they participate in chair or water exercises during the day.

■ Insomnia and hypersomnia may be manifestations of depression among older adults.

■ Older adults may need an evaluation for sleep apnea if morning headaches or frequent nighttime awakenings occur.

■ Some older adults with cognitive impairment develop **sundown syndrome** (the onset of disorientation as the sun sets). Others develop **sunrise syndrome** (early-morning confusion) associated with inadequate sleep or the effects of sedative and hypnotic medications. Characteristics of sundown syndrome include:

● Alert and oriented during the day
● Onset of disorientation as the sun sets
● Disorganized thinking
● Restlessness
● Agitation
● Perseveration (ruminating over the same repetitive thought)
● Wandering

■ Any of the following relaxation techniques before bedtime can be used to improve sleep for older adults: imagery, meditation, deep breathing, soothing music, body or foot massage, chair rocking, reading nonstimulating materials, or watching light entertaining television programs.

■ Using night-lights rather than bright room lights is preferred if an older adult arises during the night. Bright lights stimulate the brain and interfere with efforts to resume sleep. Because an older adult's established pattern and circadian rhythms may not correspond to scheduled activities in institutional settings, it is important to modify the schedule to meet the needs of the older adult.

CLIENT ENVIRONMENT

The term "environment," as used here, refers to the room where the client receives nursing care. In a broader sense, however, the health care facility's location and design involve many other subtle elements that influence the client's overall impression of the institution.

Most clients are unaware of the thought and consideration that goes into their surroundings. Accessible parking, lighting inside and outside the physical building,

landscaping, barriers that reduce traffic noise, and signage that helps clients navigate the building create a positive impression among those in need of health care.

Client Rooms

Client rooms resemble bedrooms but are no longer the bare, white, sterile environments of a few decades ago. Thanks to **environmental psychologists** (specialists who study how the environment affects behavior and well-being), client rooms are now brighter, more colorful, and tastefully decorated. The wall and floor treatments, lighting, and mechanisms for maintaining climate control are practical and conducive to comfort.

Walls

Blue and colors with blue tints, such as mauve and light green, promote relaxation; these color schemes are preferred within health care settings and client rooms. If these colors are not used exclusively, they are integrated into wallpaper trim and decorative accessories, such as framed pictures. The art often depicts landscape scenes and peaceful images.

Floors

Because noise interferes with comfort, the hallways and workstations are carpeted in most agencies. The floors in client rooms have tile or linoleum surfaces to facilitate the cleaning of spills.

Lighting

Adequate lighting, both natural and artificial, is important to the comfort of clients and nursing personnel. Newer buildings have large window areas, atriums, skylights, and enclosed courtyards to facilitate exposure to sunlight as a technique for reducing stress.

Bright artificial light facilitates nursing care but is not conducive to client comfort. Therefore, most client rooms have multiple lights in various locations with adjustable intensity. Dim light and darkness promote sleep; however, injuries are more likely in dark and unfamiliar environments. Therefore, client rooms have adjustable window blinds and night-lights near the floor.

Climate Control

Climate control refers to mechanisms for maintaining temperature, humidity, and ventilation. It is a method of promoting physical comfort.

Temperature and Humidity

Most clients are comfortable when the room temperature is 68° to 74°F (20° to 23°C). Newer buildings provide thermostats in each room so that the temperature can be adjusted to suit each client.

Humidity (the amount of moisture in the air) and **relative humidity** (the ratio between the amount of moisture in the air and the greatest amount of water vapor the air can hold at a given temperature) affect comfort. At a relative humidity of 60%, the air contains 60% of its potential water capacity. A relative humidity of 30% to 60% is comfortable for most clients.

If the environmental temperature becomes greater than the skin temperature, evaporation is the only mechanism for regulating body temperature. Evaporation is reduced when humidity levels rise because air that is almost or fully saturated with water cannot absorb additional moisture. Therefore, instead of evaporating, sweat accumulates and drips from the skin. Many agencies are air conditioned. Electric fans and dehumidifiers are not always an adequate substitute but may be used if air conditioners are not available. In buildings where the air is dry, a humidifier or a cool mist machine can add moisture to the environment. Clients who have ineffective **thermoregulation** (the ability to maintain stable body temperature) may feel hot or cold even when the temperature and humidity are optimal.

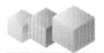 Concept Mastery Alert

Climate Control

Air conditioning is the most effective method for maintaining the humidity of the environment. If air conditioning is not available, electric fans and dehumidifiers, although less effective, can be helpful.

Ventilation

At home, methods of **ventilation** (the movement of air) include opening windows or using ceiling fans. In hospitals and nursing homes, however, open windows are a fire and safety hazard, and ceiling fans spread infectious microorganisms. Consequently, ventilation usually occurs through a system of air ducts that circulate air in and out of each client room.

Poorly ventilated rooms and buildings tend to smell bad. Removing soiled articles, emptying bedpans and urinals, and opening privacy curtains and room doors help reduce odors. An alternative is to use an air freshener or deodorizer; generally, however, scented sprays substitute one odor for another, and ill clients usually find any strong smell disagreeable. Nurses should be conscientious about their own bodies and oral hygiene, refrain from wearing overpowering fragrances, and avoid smelling of cigarette smoke.

Room Furnishings

Manufacturers of hospital furnishings attempt to design equipment that is both attractive and practical (Fig. 18-1). The bed and its components—the mattress and pillows, chairs, overbed table, and bedside stand—must be safe, durable, and comfortable.

Bed

Hospital beds are adjustable; that is, the height and position of the head and knees can be changed either electronically or manually. Adjusting the bed promotes comfort, enables self-care, and facilitates a therapeutic position (see Chapter 23). Hospital beds usually remain in their lowest position, except when clients are receiving nursing care or during a change of bed linens. Skill 18-1 describes how to

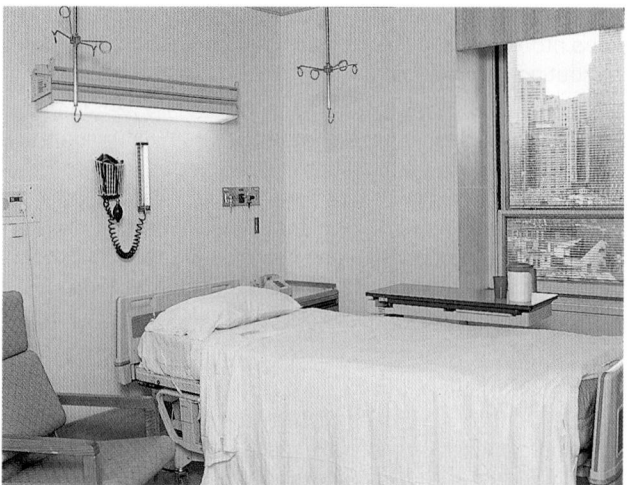

FIGURE 18-1 Typical hospital room furnishings. (Photo by B. Proud.)

make an **unoccupied bed** (changing the linens when the bed is empty).

Full or half side rails are attached to the bed frame. There is controversy as to whether raised side rails are a risk or benefit because some clients climb over them rather than seeking nursing assistance. Side rails cannot be used as a form of physical restraint in long-term care facilities, and their use for safety must be justified (Omnibus Budget Reconciliation Act of 1987; see Chapter 19).

Some beds have removable headboards (Fig. 18-2). This facilitates resuscitation efforts if the client experiences respiratory or cardiac arrest. Removing the headboard gives the code team responders better access for airway intubation. Placing the headboard under the client's upper body allows more effective cardiac compression than is possible on a mattress.

Mattress

Many people equate the comfort of a bed with the quality of the mattress. A good mattress adjusts to the shape of the body while supporting it. A mattress that is too soft alters the alignment of the spine, causing some people to awaken feeling sore from muscle and joint strain.

Hospital mattresses generally consist of tough materials that will withstand long-term use. Because mattresses are washed but not sterilized between uses, they are covered with a waterproof coating that withstands cleaning with strong antimicrobial solutions.

Occasionally, **mattress overlays** (layers of foam or other devices placed on top of the mattress; Fig. 18-3) are used to promote comfort or to keep the skin intact (see Chapter 23). Box 18-1 lists clients for whom a mattress overlay or therapeutic mattress of foam, gel, air, or water is appropriate.

Pillows

Pillows are primarily used for comfort, but they are also used to elevate a part of the body, relieve swelling, promote

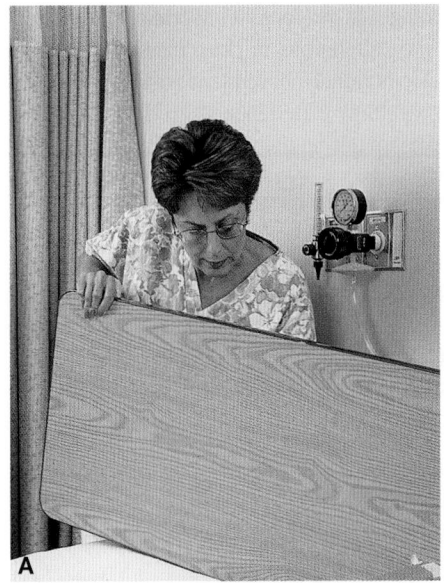
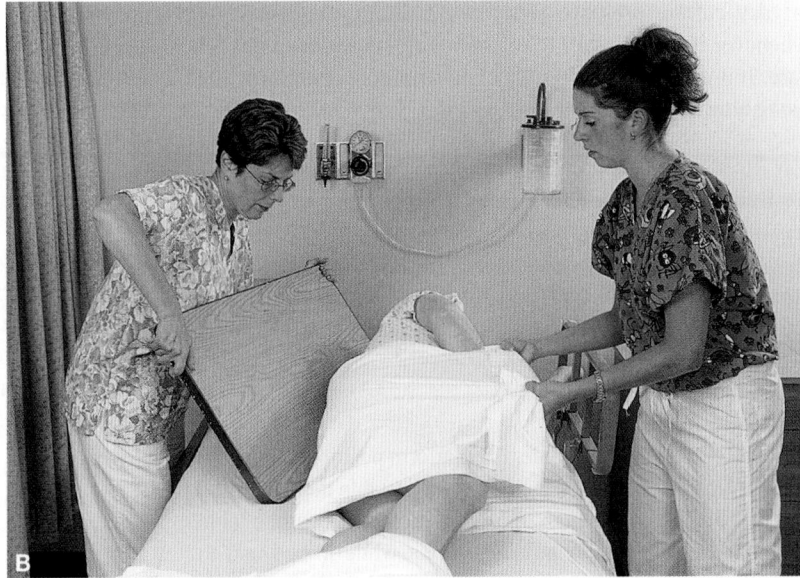

FIGURE 18-2 A. The nurse removes the headboard from a standard hospital bed. **B.** The nurse places the headboard beneath a client before resuscitation. (Photo by B. Proud.)

breathing, or help maintain a therapeutic position (see Chapter 23). In health care facilities, pillows are stuffed with foam or kapok (a mass of silky fibers) and covered with vinyl or plastic to facilitate disinfection.

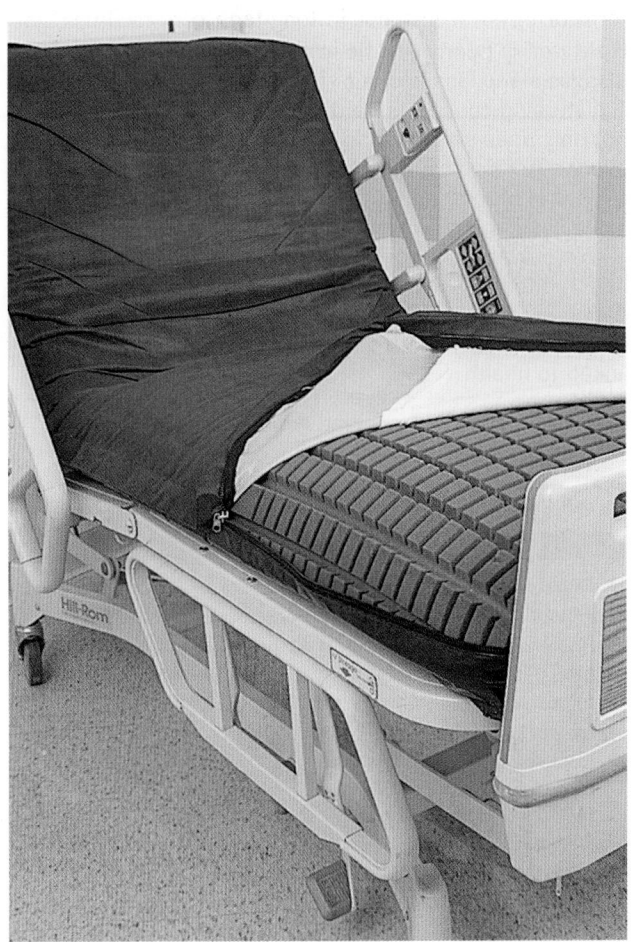

FIGURE 18-3 A waterproof mattress cover protects the mattress overlay. (Photo by B. Proud.)

Bed Linens

The linens used for most hospital beds include:

- Mattress pad
- Bottom sheet that is sometimes fitted
- Optional draw sheet that is placed beneath the client's hips
- Top sheet
- Blanket, depending on the client's preference
- Spread
- Pillowcase

Some hospitals use printed sheets to provide a more home-like atmosphere.

To control expenses, bed linens may not be changed every day, but any wet or soiled linen is changed as frequently as necessary. Sometimes, folded sheets or disposable, absorbent pads are placed between the client and the bottom sheet to avoid the need to change the entire bed when soiling occurs. Skill 18-2 explains how to make an **occupied bed** (changing the linens while the client remains in bed).

Privacy Curtain

A privacy curtain is a long fabric partition mounted from the ceiling. It can be drawn completely around the bed. The

BOX 18-1	Client Criteria for a Mattress Overlay or a Therapeutic Mattress

- Complete immobility
- Limited mobility
- Impaired skin integrity
- Inadequate nutritional status
- Incontinence of stool, urine, or both
- Altered tactile perception
- Compromised circulatory status

privacy curtain preserves the client's dignity and modesty whenever it is necessary to examine or expose the client for care. It is also used to shield a client from observation while using a urinal or bedpan.

>>> *Stop, Think, and Respond 18-1*
List situations when it would be appropriate to change some linens when providing client care and other situations in which it is more appropriate to change all linens.

Overbed Table

An overbed table is a portable, flat platform positioned over the client's lap. The height of the table is adjustable depending on whether the bed is in a high or low position. The overbed table makes it convenient for the client to eat while in bed and to perform personal hygiene or other activities requiring a flat surface. Nurses also use the overbed table to hold equipment when providing client care. Most overbed tables have a concealed compartment that may contain a mounted mirror and a place for personal items (hairbrush, comb, cosmetic bag, razor, or book).

Bedside Stand

A bedside stand is actually a small cupboard. It usually contains a drawer for personal items and two shelves. The upper shelf is used to store the client's bath basin, soap dish, soap, and a kidney-shaped basin called an *emesis basin*. The lower shelf is used to store a bedpan, urinal, and toilet paper. The elimination utensils are kept separate from the hygiene supplies to reduce the transmission of microorganisms. A carafe of water and a drinking container are placed atop the bedside stand.

Chairs

Generally, there is at least one chair in each room, but more may be available upon request. Hospital chairs are usually straight backed to facilitate good postural support. The best sitting position is when the hips, knees, and ankles are all at 90-degree angles. There may be one upholstered chair or a recliner in each client room. Although upholstered chairs are more comfortable, some clients find it difficult to rise from them. A recliner is sometimes used by a family member who stays the night with the client.

In special care areas such as orthopedic units, modified chairs called *hip chairs* may be used. Hip chairs have a higher than usual seat that makes sitting and standing less difficult.

SLEEP AND REST

No matter how comfortable the physical environment or how attractive and homelike the furnishings, failure to promote rest and sleep may sabotage or prolong recuperation. Although sleep requirements vary, alterations in sleep patterns can have serious physical and emotional consequences. Family members, especially spouses, may experience sleep disturbances if someone snores, wakes up during the night, or wanders.

Functions of Sleep

In addition to promoting emotional well-being, sleep enhances various physiologic processes. Although the exact mechanisms are not totally understood, the restorative functions of sleep can be inferred from the effects of sleep deprivation (Box 18-2). Sleep is believed to play a role in:

- Reducing fatigue
- Stabilizing mood
- Improving blood flow to the brain
- Increasing protein synthesis
- Maintaining the disease-fighting mechanisms of the immune system
- Promoting cellular growth and repair
- Improving the capacity for learning and memory storage

 Nutrition Notes

How well or poorly you sleep can affect weight gain and loss, as sleep loss is one of the risk factors for obesity A disturbing concern for individuals with obesity is that not only does sleep loss lead to weight gain, but being overweight also causes sleep issues, which may worsen biological processes that contribute to weight gain. It is a discouraging cycle, but help is available for people who are overweight or obese to improve sleep and the health effects associated with sleep loss (SleepFoundation.org, 2023a). Sleep, along with diet and exercise, is now considered to be an important lifestyle behavior linked to health.

BOX 18-2	Effects of Chronic Sleep Deprivation

- Reduced physical stamina
- Altered comfort, such as headaches and nausea
- Impaired coordination, especially of fine motor skills
- Loss of muscle mass and weight
- Increased susceptibility to infection
- Slower wound healing
- Decreased pain tolerance
- Poor concentration
- Impaired judgment
- Unstable moods
- Suspiciousness

Sleep Stages

Sleep is split into two major divisions: nonrapid eye movement (NREM) sleep and rapid eye movement (REM) sleep. These names derive from the periods during sleep when eye movements are either subdued or energetic. Sleep progresses through four stages: NREM 1 (N1), NREM 2 (N2), NREM 3 (N3), and stage 4 REM.

The combined stages of sleep provide distinct physiologic and neurologic benefits that are necessary for health and well-being. If they are disrupted, a condition known as **sleep inertia**, a feeling of incomplete awakening or grogginess as though still in a sleep state, may persist for 15 minutes or as long as 4 hours. Based on this, nurses should avoid waking a sleeping client for at least 90 to 120 minutes, the time of an average cycle of NREM sleep and REM sleep.

Nonrapid Eye Movement Sleep

NREM is quiet sleep; it is also called "slow wave sleep" because during this stage, electroencephalogram (EEG) waves appear as progressively slower oscillations. NREM 1 sleep, which occurs at the onset of sleep and lasts about 10 minutes, is characterized by drowsiness and light sleep. Sudden twitches, called **hypnagogic jerks**, are common. During this early stage of sleep, a person may be aware of sounds and conversations but avoids arousal.

During NREM 2 sleep, the response to outside stimuli is somewhat suppressed. It is believed that memory and information begin to be processed at this time.

The deepest and most restorative sleep occurs during NREM 3 sleep, during which it is difficult to awaken a person. Dreaming may occur during NREM 3 sleep, but it is not as vivid or as memorable as that which occurs during REM sleep. During the latter two stages of NREM sleep, blood pressure decreases and breathing slows. Hormones for growth and development are secreted in young persons.

Rapid Eye Movement Sleep

The REM stage of sleep follows NREM stages. It begins about 90 minutes after the onset of sleep and thereafter cyclically recurs and lengthens as the hours of sleep progress. REM sleep is also referred to as *paradoxical sleep* because the EEG waves appear similar to those produced during periods of wakefulness, indicating that the brain is quite active in concentration and thinking. However, the body is relaxed, immobile, often completely paralyzed, and unresponsive during REM sleep. It is during REM sleep that dreams take an intense and dramatic quality that can be more easily recalled than those that occur during NREM 3 sleep.

When REM sleep is interrupted, the person tends to compensate by deviating from the usual progression of NREM to REM, returns to REM earlier than usual, and stays in REM sleep longer, a phenomenon known as **REM rebound sleep**. If REM sleep is chronically shortened, the ability to learn complex tasks is impaired.

Sleep Cycles

During sleep, people alternate between NREM and REM phases (Table 18-1). NREM sleep normally precedes REM sleep, the phase during which most dreaming occurs. Although the time spent in any one phase or stage varies according to age and other variables, most people cycle between stages 2 and 3 of NREM to REM phases four to six times during the night (Fig. 18-4). The average length of an NREM–REM sleep cycle is between 90 and 110 minutes (Cherry, 2022).

Sleep Requirements

Sleep requirements vary among different age groups. The need for sleep decreases from birth to adulthood, although individuals vary (Table 18-2). Although an average of 7 to 9 hours of sleep is a requirement for young adults through older adults, many Americans report sleeping less than 6 hours a night (National Sleep Foundation, 2022).

With age, the time spent in NREM sleep decreases and REM sleep increases (Fig. 18-5). According to the National Sleep Foundation (2022), older adults sleep more on weeknights, but younger adults sleep more on weekends. Older adults nap more than younger adults, a fact that may be attributed to daytime inactivity or reduced mental stimulation.

Factors Affecting Sleep

Both the quantity and quality of sleep decrease with age. Older adults suffer disproportionately from chronic sleep deprivation (Division of Sleep and Medicine Harvard Medical School, 2024). The latter finding is not surprising because older adults awaken more frequently during the night for several reasons: pain; smaller bladder capacity, which results in an increased need to urinate; dementia-related sleep problems; side effects from medications, such as diuretics; and diminished production of neurochemicals, such as melatonin, that promote sleep. Other factors not related to age also affect the amount and quality of a person's sleep (Table 18-3).

Light

Daylight and darkness influence the sleep–wake cycle. **Circadian rhythm** (phenomena that cycle on a 24-hour basis) is a term derived from two Latin words: *circa* (about)

TABLE 18-1 Characteristics of Sleep Phases

SLEEP PHASE	LENGTH	FEATURES
NREM	90–100 minutes average	Deep, restful sleep
Stage 1	5–10 minutes in the initial cycle	Light sleep, easily aroused
		Gradual reduction in vital signs
Stage 2	10–25 minutes in the initial cycle; lengthens with each successive cycle	Deeper relaxation
		Can be awakened with effort
Stage 3	20–40 minutes in the initial cycle; shorten toward morning	Early phase of deep sleep
		Snoring
		Relaxed muscle tone
		Little or no physical movement
		Difficult to arouse
		Sleepwalking, sleep talking, and bed-wetting possible
REM	Occurs 90 minutes after the onset of sleep; 10 minutes average; lengthens up to 1 hour toward morning	Darting eye movements
		Very difficult to awaken
		Vivid, colorful, emotional dreams
		Loss of muscle tone; jaw relaxes; tongue may fall to the back of the throat.
		Vital signs fluctuate.
		Irregular respirations
		Pauses in breathing for 15–20 seconds
		Absence of snoring
		Muscle twitching
		Gastric secretions increase.
		Males may have erections.

Total: 90–110 minutes per cycle, four to five times per night
NREM, nonrapid eye movement; REM, rapid eye movement.

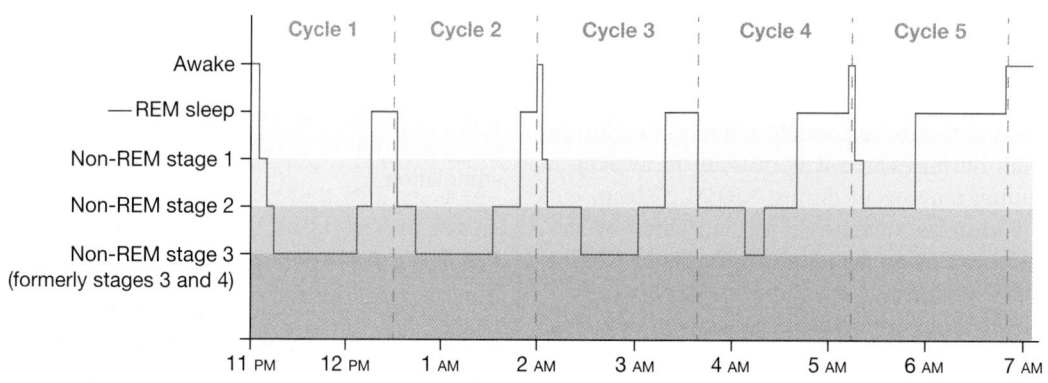

FIGURE 18-4 Example of a normal sleep pattern. REM, rapid eye movement.

TABLE 18-2 Sleep Requirements

AGE	TOTAL SLEEP TIME (HOURS)
Newborns 0–3 months	14–17
Infants 4–11 months	12–15
Toddler 1–2 years	11–14
Preschoolers 3–5 years	10–13
School-aged children 6–13 years	9–11
Teenagers 14–17 years	8–10
Young adults 18–25 years	7–9
Adults 26–64 years	7–9
Older adults >65 years	7–8

Centers for Disease Control and Prevention. (2024). *About sleep.* https://www.cdc.gov/sleep/about/index.html

and *dies* (day). Thus, drowsiness and sleep correlate with the circadian rhythm of the setting sun and night. Wakefulness corresponds with sunrise and daylight.

Researchers (Khullar, 2012) have suggested that the cycles of wakefulness followed by sleep are linked to a photosensitive system involving the eyes and the pineal gland in the brain (Fig. 18-6). As darkness develops, the pineal gland secretes **melatonin** (a hormone that induces drowsiness and sleep); light, especially daylight, triggers the suppression of melatonin secretion.

Activity

Activity, especially exercise, increases fatigue and the need for sleep. Activity appears to increase both REM and NREM

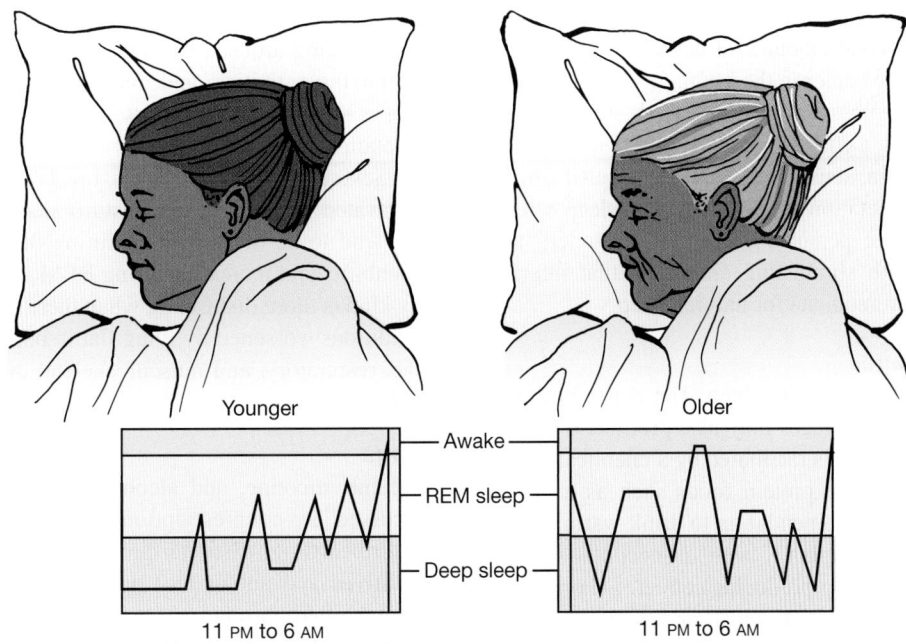

FIGURE 18-5 The time spent in rapid eye movement (REM) and non-REM sleep is different in younger adults than in older adults.

sleep, especially the deep sleep of NREM. When physical activity occurs just before bedtime, however, it has a stimulating, rather than a relaxing, effect.

Environment

Most people sleep best in their usual environments; they develop a preference for particular pillows, mattresses, and blankets. They also tend to adapt to the unique sounds where they live, such as traffic, trains, and the hum of appliance motors or furnaces. Unfamiliar sounds tend to interfere with the ability to fall or stay asleep.

In addition, **sleep rituals** (habitual activities performed before retiring) induce sleep. Examples include eating a light snack, watching television, reading, and performing hygiene. Therefore, alterations in the environment or the activities performed before bedtime—such as those occurring during vacation or when in the hospital—negatively affect a person's ability to fall and remain asleep.

Motivation

When a person has no particular reason to stay awake, sleep generally occurs easily. But if the desire to remain awake is strong, such as when a person wishes to participate in something interesting or important, the desire to sleep can be overcome.

Emotions and Moods

Depressive disorders are classically associated with an inability to sleep or the tendency to sleep more than usual. In addition, emotions such as anger, fear, anxiety, and dread

TABLE 18-3 Factors Affecting Sleep

SLEEP-PROMOTING FACTORS	SLEEP-SUPPRESSING FACTORS
Darkness, dim light	Sunlight, bright light
Consistent sleep schedule	Inconsistent sleep schedule
Secretion of melatonin	Suppression of melatonin
Familiar sleep environment	Strange sleep environment
Optimal warmth and ventilation	Cold, hot, stuffy room
Performance of sleep rituals	Disturbance of sleep rituals
Sedative, hypnotic drugs	Stimulant drugs
Depression	Depression, anxiety, worry
Relaxation	Activity
Satiation	Hunger, thirst
Proteins containing L-tryptophan	Protein-deficient diets
Excessive alcohol consumption	Metabolism of alcohol
Comfort	Pain, nausea, full bladder
Quiet	Noise
Effortless breathing	Difficulty breathing

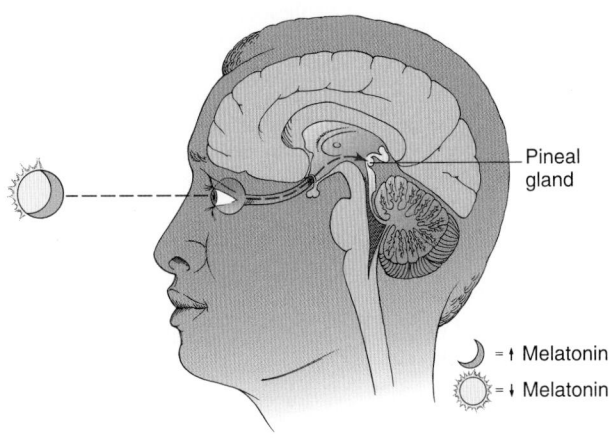

FIGURE 18-6 A photosensitive light system influences the sleep–wake cycle.

interfere with sleep. All are more than likely the result of changes in the types and amounts of neurotransmitters that affect the sleep–wake center in the brain.

Sometimes, sleeplessness is conditioned—that is, anticipating sleeplessness, a characteristic pattern of some people with chronic insomnia, actually reinforces it (a self-fulfilling prophecy). The expectation that the onset of sleep will be difficult increases the person's anxiety. The anxiety then floods the brain with stimulating chemicals that interfere with relaxation, a prerequisite for natural sleep.

Food and Beverages
Hunger or thirst interferes with sleep. The consumption of particular foods and beverages may also promote or inhibit the ability to sleep. Sleep is facilitated by a chemical known as L-tryptophan, found in protein foods such as milk and dairy products. The recommendation to drink warm milk to induce sleep may have originally been an anecdotal observation of its **hypnotic** (sleep-producing) effect. L-Tryptophan is also present in poultry, fish, eggs, and, to some extent, plant sources of protein, such as legumes.

Alcohol is a depressive drug that promotes the onset of sleep, but it tends to reduce normal REM and deep sleep stages of NREM sleep, reducing sleep's quality. As alcohol is metabolized, stimulating chemicals that were blocked by the sedative effects of the alcohol surge forth from neurons, causing early awakening. Beverages containing caffeine, a central nervous system stimulant, cause wakefulness. Caffeine is present in coffee, tea, chocolate, and most cola drinks.

Illness
Stress, anxiety, and discomfort accompany almost any illness, which can alter normal sleep patterns. In the hospital, other factors that contribute to sleep loss or fragmentation include being aroused by noise from equipment, awakened for nursing activities, and disturbed by unfamiliar sounds, such as loud talking, elevators, dietary carts, and housekeeping equipment.

Several medical disorders involve symptoms that are aggravated at night or can disturb sleep. For example, ulcers tend to be more painful during the night because hydrochloric acid increases during REM sleep. In fact, pain of any kind is more distressing when there are few distractions. Conditions worsened by lying flat in bed, such as some cardiac, respiratory, and musculoskeletal disorders, contribute to sleeplessness.

Drugs
Caffeine, nicotine, and alcohol, which have already been discussed, are nonprescription drugs that affect sleep. Some prescribed drugs also can promote or interfere with sleep. **Sedatives** and antianxiety drugs (produce a relaxing and calming effect) promote rest, a precursor to sleep. Hypnotics are drugs that induce sleep. **Stimulants** (drugs that excite structures in the brain) cause wakefulness (Table 18-4).

Some sedatives and hypnotics have a paradoxical effect when administered to older adults; they tend to produce restlessness and wakefulness instead of sleep. Many of the drug effects of hypnotics diminish after approximately 2 weeks. Therefore, hypnotic drug use is not recommended for more than 2 weeks. People who have trouble sleeping may use sleep aids (especially antihistamines) on a chronic basis. This type of drug use tends to develop **drug tolerance** (a diminished effect from the drug at its usual dosage range). Without realizing the danger, a person may increase the dose of the drug or the frequency of its administration to achieve

TABLE 18-4 Drugs That Affect Sleep

DRUG CATEGORY	DRUG FAMILY	EXAMPLE	ADVERSE REACTIONS
Drugs That Induce Sleepiness			
Sedatives/hypnotics	Benzodiazepines	Temazepam (Restoril)	Dizziness, lethargy during the day
	Nonbenzodiazepine	Zolpidem (Ambien)	Headache, nausea
	Antihistamines	Diphenhydramine (Benadryl)	Dizziness, slowed reaction time, impaired coordination
	Tricyclic antidepressants	Mirtazapine (Remeron)	Sedation is a side effect that is beneficial when the drug is given at bedtime.
	Selective serotonin reuptake inhibitor (SSRI) antidepressant	Trazodone (Oleptro)	Sedation is a side effect that is beneficial when the drug is given at bedtime.
Antianxiety	Benzodiazepines	Alprazolam (Xanax)	Dry mouth, constipation, slowed heart rate, hypotension, liver damage
Drugs That Induce Wakefulness			
Stimulants	Amphetamines	Dextroamphetamine (Dexedrine)	Insomnia, restlessness, anorexia, rapid heart rate
	Amphetamine like	Methylphenidate (Ritalin)	Nervousness, insomnia, rash, anorexia, nausea
	Caffeine		Insomnia, nervousness, restlessness, rapid heart rate
	Nicotine		Insomnia, restlessness, anorexia, rapid heart rate

the same effect first experienced at a lower dose. Increasing the dose or frequency may lead to a greater risk for falls, resulting in injury.

The abrupt discontinuation of sedatives, antianxiety agents, and hypnotics produces a disruption in sleep cycles and a period of intense stimulation that interferes with sleep. This pattern of use and discontinuation also leads to sleep disruptions, such as nightmares.

 Pharmacologic Considerations

When a diuretic (water pill) is ordered twice a day, teach the client to take the second dose before 6 PM. This will promote sleep if the client is not awakened by a full bladder.

SLEEP ASSESSMENT

Many people blame inadequate sleep for daytime fatigue, or they underestimate the actual time they sleep. Nurses can obtain a more accurate sleep pattern assessment through sleep questionnaires, sleep diaries, polysomnographic (sleep study) evaluation, and a multiple latency sleep test.

Questionnaires

Several questionnaires have been developed to help identify sleep patterns. They are either designed to obtain specific information or unstructured to give the person more freedom to respond. Nurses can gather data during interviews, or clients can answer the questions independently in the form of a self-reporting assessment.

Examples of questions for the client include:

- When you think about your sleep, what kinds of impressions come to mind?
- Does anything about your sleep bother you?
- Do you fall asleep at inappropriate times?
- Do you wake feeling rested?
- How long does it take you to fall asleep?
- Do you feel stiff and sore in the morning?
- Have you been told that you stop breathing while asleep?
- Do you fall asleep during physical activities?
- What do you do to help yourself sleep well?

Examples of questions for members of the client's household include:

- Does the client snore or gasp for air when sleeping?
- Does the client kick or thrash around while sleeping?
- Does the client sleepwalk?

Sleep Diary

A **sleep diary** is a daily account of sleeping and waking activities. The client or personnel compile the information in a sleep disorder clinic. The client notes the times they sleep, describes daily activities during each 15-minute waking period, completes a 24-hour log of consumed food and beverages, and notes when they take any medications. These self-kept diaries generally cover a 2-week period.

In addition to sleep diaries and questionnaires, sleep assessments should also include other objective diagnostic techniques for gathering data to ensure the accurate identification of sleep disorders and their etiologies.

Nocturnal Polysomnography

Nocturnal polysomnography is a diagnostic assessment technique in which a client is monitored for an entire night's sleep to obtain physiologic data. It generally takes place in a sleep disorder clinic, but it is now possible to conduct the study at the client's home; a technician monitors a computerized recording system up to 60 ft away.

Dime-sized sensors attached to the head and body (Fig. 18-7) record:

- Brain waves
- Eye movements
- Muscle tone
- Limb movement
- Body position
- Nasal and oral airflow
- Chest and abdominal respiratory effort
- Snoring sounds
- Oxygen level in the blood

The diagnostic data are compared with the patterns and characteristics of normal sleep cycles to help diagnose sleep disorders.

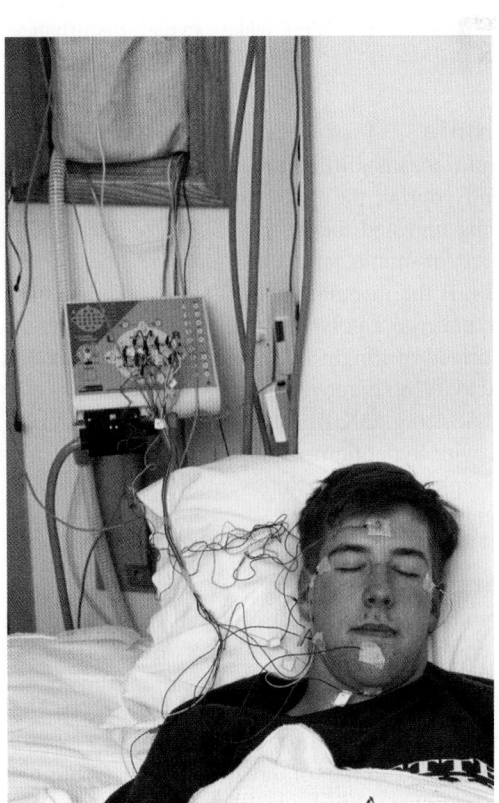

FIGURE 18-7 During a polysomnography study, electrodes are attached to the scalp, face, chest, and legs.

Multiple Sleep Latency Test

A **multiple sleep latency test** (an assessment of daytime sleepiness) is another helpful study. The person undergoing this test is asked to take a daytime nap at 2-hour intervals while being attached to sensors similar to those used in polysomnography. The client is allowed to nap for about 20 minutes. The nap periods are repeated four or five times throughout the day.

Clients who have certain sleep disorders causing daytime sleepiness have a short latency period—that is, they fall asleep in less than 5 minutes. Most well-rested persons take an average of 15 minutes before they experience the onset of daytime sleep.

Experiencing early REM sleep is also a pathologic finding that can be detected during a multiple sleep latency test. A REM period normally does not occur for at least 1 hour and after cycling through the stages of NREM. Therefore, REM should not occur during a 20-minute test nap.

SLEEP DISORDERS

According to the American Sleep Apnea Association (ASAA), 70% of American adults report occasional insufficient sleep and 11% report sleep problems on a regular basis (Sleephealth.org, 2020). The most common sleep disorder is insomnia, followed by sleep apnea. As many as one in five, or 25 million, American adults suffer from sleep apnea (Sleephealth.org, 2020). Many of those affected do not seek treatment. Most problems are short lived, but some sleep disorders are both chronic and serious.

There are four categories of sleep disorders: insomnia, hypersomnia, sleep–wake cycle disturbance, and parasomnia.

Insomnia

Insomnia means difficulty in falling asleep, awakening frequently during the night, or awakening early. It results in feeling unrested the next day. Almost everyone has experienced insomnia, and most cases resolve in less than 3 weeks. If the insomnia continues beyond 3 weeks, a client can undergo a polysomnogram, or a sleep study, which is performed overnight in a hospital and clinic, monitoring brain activity, body movement, breathing, and blood oxygen levels (ASA.org, 2020). Although chronic insomnia can be treated with hypnotic drugs, it is helpful to start treatment with nonpharmacologic interventions (Client and Family Teaching 18-1).

Hypersomnia

Hypersomnia is a sleep disorder characterized by feeling sleepy despite getting normal sleep. Two conditions of hypersomnia are sleep apnea/hypopnea syndrome and narcolepsy.

Sleep Apnea/Hypopnea Syndrome

Apnea (the cessation of breathing) and **hypopnea** (hypoventilation) are concomitant forms of hypersomnia: **sleep apnea/hypopnea syndrome**. In this disorder, the sleeper

Client and Family Teaching 18-1
Promoting Sleep

The nurse teaches the client or the family as follows:

- Resist napping during the day.
- Use the bed and bedroom just for sleeping.
- Perform sleep rituals.
- Go to bed and get up at approximately the same time, even on weekends or days off.
- If you cannot get to sleep for more than 20 to 30 minutes, get out of bed and do something else, such as reading.
- Try a bedtime relaxation tape that plays soothing music, sounds of nature, or a constant background sound (white noise).
- Exercise regularly during the day, but not late in the evening.
- Avoid alcohol, nicotine, and caffeine.
- Eat dairy products and other proteins daily.
- Modify the temperature and ventilation in the bedroom according to personal preferences.
- Use earplugs or eyeshades to reduce environmental noise or light.
- Avoid using nonprescription or prescription sleeping pills unless they have been recommended by a physician. Hypnotics should be used only on a short-term basis.
- Try drinking chamomile tea, which, some claim, improves sleep.
- Follow label directions on any medications.
- If a diuretic drug is prescribed, take it early in the morning.

stops breathing or breathing slows for 10 seconds or longer five or more times per hour. This is discussed further in Chapter 21.

During the apneic or hypopneic periods, ventilation decreases and blood oxygenation drops. The accumulation of carbon dioxide and the fall in oxygen cause brief periods of awakening throughout the night. This disturbs the normal transitions and periods of NREM and REM sleep. Consequently, clients with sleep apnea/hypopnea syndrome feel tired after having slept, or worse, their symptoms may cause a heart attack, stroke, or sudden death from **hypoxia** (decreased cellular oxygenation) of the heart, brain, and other organs.

The incidence of sleep apnea is highest among older adults, especially male adults who have excess weight and snore. Methods to reduce apneic episodes include sleeping in positions other than the supine position, losing weight, and avoiding substances that depress respirations, such as alcohol or sleeping medications. In severe cases, clients wear a continuous positive airway pressure (CPAP) mask (see Chapter 21) that keeps the alveoli inflated during sleep. Surgery on the tonsils, uvula, pharynx, tongue, or epiglottis is another treatment option when conservative measures are ineffective.

Narcolepsy

Narcolepsy is characterized by the sudden onset of daytime sleep, a short NREM period before the first REM phase, and pathologic manifestations of REM sleep. This disabling condition should not be confused with **hypersomnolence**, which is excessive sleeping for long periods.

Although the diagnosis of narcolepsy generally requires a multiple sleep latency test and polysomnography, its symptoms help distinguish it from other conditions that cause sleepiness. For example, the sleepiness of narcolepsy is accompanied by:

- **Sleep paralysis**—the person cannot move for a few minutes just before falling asleep or awakening.
- **Cataplexy**—a sudden loss of muscle tone triggered by an emotional change, such as laughing or anger
- **Hypnagogic hallucinations**—a dream-like auditory or visual experiences while dozing or falling asleep
- **Automatic behavior**—the performance of routine tasks without full awareness or later memory of having done them

If untreated, the client with narcoleptic symptoms may become involved in a motor vehicle crash or occupational accident. Prescribed stimulant drugs, such as methylphenidate (Ritalin) or amphetamine (Adderall), help improve alertness. Antidepressants reduce the symptoms associated with atypical REM sleep.

Sleep–Wake Cycle Disturbances

A **sleep–wake cycle disturbance** results from a sleep schedule that involves daytime sleeping and interferes with biologic rhythms. Changes in the intensity of light trigger sleeping. When exposure to light comes at an atypical time, the sleep–wake cycle is desynchronized. Sleep–wake cycle disorders occur among shift workers, jet travelers, and those diagnosed with seasonal affective disorder, a cyclical mood disorder believed to be linked to diminished exposure to sunlight.

Shift Work

Those who work evening or night shifts or who switch from one shift to another are especially prone to unsynchronized sleep–wake cycles. The indoor lighting to which most shift workers are exposed is not bright enough to suppress melatonin; consequently, many shift workers fight to stay awake. Some experience **microsleep**, which is unintentional sleep lasting 20 to 30 seconds. Statistics show that shift workers are more prone to errors and accidents from sleepiness (National Sleep Foundation, 2023b). Most people who work night shifts never completely adapt to the reversal of day and night activities, no matter how long the pattern is established.

Jet Travel

Jet travel causes a sudden change in the established **photoperiod** (the number of daylight hours) to which a person is accustomed. Consequently, travelers often describe having **jet lag**, or emotional and physical changes experienced when arriving in a different time zone. Many travelers have difficulty falling or staying asleep, but the disturbance caused by jet lag is more transient than that caused by shift work. Some travelers reestablish normal sleep–wake cycles, but it takes at least 1 day for each time zone that is crossed when traveling east and slightly less when traveling west.

Seasonal Affective Disorder

Seasonal affective disorder is characterized by depression, hypersomnolence, a lack of energy when awake, increased appetite accompanied by cravings for sweets, and weight gain. The symptoms begin during darker winter months and disappear as daylight hours increase in the spring. In some ways, the disorder resembles the hibernation patterns in bears and other animals.

Some suggest that seasonal affective disorder results from excessive melatonin. To counteract the symptoms, **phototherapy** (a technique for suppressing melatonin by stimulating light receptors in the eye) is prescribed. The artificial light used in phototherapy is at least 2,000 to 2,500 lux, the equivalent of the bright light measured on a sunny spring day (Fig. 18-8). Clients use the lights for 2 to 6 hours each day to simulate the number of daylight hours during sunnier months that are missing during winter months (Box 18-3). Phototherapy usually relieves symptoms within 3 to 5 days, but symptoms tend to recur in the same amount of time if a client abruptly discontinues phototherapy.

Parasomnia

Parasomnias are conditions associated with activities that cause arousal or partial arousal, usually during transitions in NREM sleep. They are not life-threatening, but they disturb others in the household—most significantly, the bed partner. Some examples of parasomnias include:

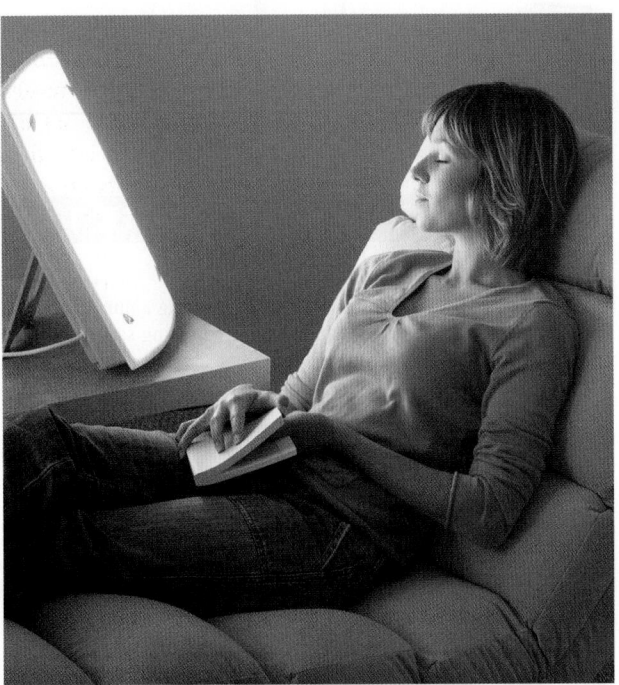

FIGURE 18-8 An example of a phototherapy device used for those with seasonal affective disorder.

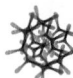

BOX 18-3 **Components of Phototherapy**

To relieve the symptoms of seasonal affective disorder, the client:
- Initiates a schedule of full-spectrum light[a] exposure beginning in October and November
- Removes eyeglasses or contact lenses that have ultraviolet filters
- Sits within 3 ft of the artificial light for approximately 2 hours soon after awakening from sleep
- Glances at the light periodically but may engage in other activities, such as reading or handiwork
- Repeats the exposure to light after sundown (to simulate extending the daylight hours) up to a cumulative time of 3 to 6 hours a day
- Continues the pattern of light exposure until spring

[a]Full-spectrum light simulates the energy of bright natural sunlight.

- **Somnambulism** (sleepwalking)
- **Nocturnal enuresis** (bed-wetting)
- Sleep talking
- Nightmares and night terrors
- **Bruxism** (grinding of the teeth)
- **Restless legs syndrome** (movement, typically in the legs but occasionally in the arms or other body parts, to relieve disturbing skin sensations)

Restless legs syndrome, also known as *nocturnal myoclonus*, may be the most disruptive parasomnia. The symptoms keep the person awake or prevent continuous sleep. Eventually, sleep deprivation affects the person's life, damaging work productivity and personal relationships. Medical etiologies, such as iron deficiency, kidney failure, and peripheral nerve pathology, can mimic the manifestations of restless legs syndrome. Once these conditions are diagnostically eliminated, the condition is confirmed with polysomnography.

Conservative treatments for parasomnias include safety measures for sleepwalkers (stair gates, security locks on doors and windows), mouth devices for bruxism, lifestyle changes, nutritional support, and good sleep hygiene. In severe cases, drug therapy is used.

NURSING IMPLICATIONS

After assessing client comfort and sleep patterns and the accompanying symptoms, nurses identify one or more nursing diagnoses that require interventions:

- Fatigue
- Sleep deprivation
- Impaired gas exchange
- Injury risk
- Insomnia

Nursing Care Plan 18-1 is an example of how the nursing process has been used to develop a plan of care for a client with insomnia. *Insomnia* is defined as either difficulty falling asleep or staying asleep that is accompanied by daytime impairments related to those sleep problems (SleepFoundation.org, 2023b).

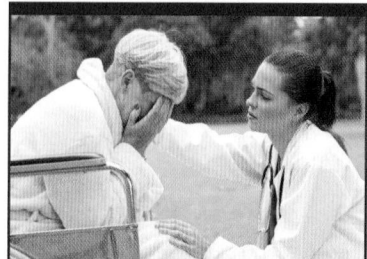

Clinical Scenario After being transferred for rehabilitation following treatment for injuries sustained in a motor vehicle accident, this client reveals that she has been getting very little sleep. The nurse adds a problem to the client's plan for care in Nursing Care Plan 18-1.

NURSING CARE PLAN 18-1 Insomnia

Assessment
- Ask the client to rate their quality of sleep using a numeric scale of 10 indicating severe disturbance to 0 indicating satisfactory.
- Identify sleep aids including medications, alcohol, and sleep rituals and lifestyle practices, such as excessive consumption of caffeine, that may interfere with sleep.
- Inquire about the client's usual time for retiring and awakening without an alarm clock.
- Have the client keep a diary for several days for:
- Bedtime
- Approximate time for onset of sleep
- Number of times awakened during sleep and reason for awakening
- Time of awakening in the morning
- Number and length of daytime naps
- Compare collected data with age-related norms.
- Determine the client's level of stress, emotional stability, attention, and exercise endurance.

Nursing Diagnosis. Insomnia related to excessive neurostimulation secondary to anxiety over slow recovery from rehabilitation as evidenced by the statement, "I'd rate the quality of my sleep at 5. It seems that it takes forever to fall asleep. It's been 2 weeks since I've gotten more than 4 hours of sleep. I worry constantly that I'll never go home again," and need for barbiturate hypnotic that is repeated each night

Expected Outcome. The client will sleep within 30 minutes of going to bed and remain asleep for a minimum of 7 hours within 5 days (by 3/15).

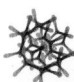

NURSING CARE PLAN 18-1   Insomnia (*continued*)

Interventions	Rationales
Have the client retire at 2100 each evening and arise at 0730 each morning, regardless of the duration or quality of sleep.	Retiring and arising at a consistent time helps develop a consistent sleep–wake pattern.
Allow naps only in the early morning.	More rapid eye movement (REM) sleep occurs during early morning than afternoon naps. Increasing REM will improve a feeling of rest and well-being.
Limit naps to less than 90 minutes.	Short naps promote longer sleep cycles during the night, which, in turn, contributes to additional REM periods of sleep.
Avoid disturbing the client at night within 90- to 120-minute blocks of sleep.	The duration of a complete cycle of nonrapid eye movement (NREM) and REM sleep is approximately 90 minutes during the early period of sleep and 120 minutes during later periods. Sleep cycles occur four or five times a night.
Reduce or eliminate the client's intake of caffeine.	Caffeine is a central nervous system stimulant that interferes with relaxation and sleep.
Encourage moderate exercise for at least 20 minutes three times a day, but no later than 1930.	Regular exercise promotes sleep but may overstimulate a person if performed too close to bedtime.
Provide milk, yogurt, vanilla pudding, custard, or some other dairy product at approximately 2030.	Dairy products are a good source of L-tryptophan, which promotes sleep.
Delay administering sleeping medication and give a back massage at bedtime.	Massage promotes relaxation, which is a precursor to sleep. Sleep medications can interfere with REM sleep and may cause daytime drowsiness.

Evaluation of Expected Outcome

- The client was observed to fall asleep in 30–45 minutes.
- The client experienced uninterrupted sleep for 3 hours.
- The client's total duration of sleep was 6–7 hours.

Several sleep-promoting nursing measures, such as maintaining sleep rituals, reducing the intake of stimulating chemicals, promoting daytime exercise, and adhering to a regular schedule for retiring and awakening, have already been discussed. Two additional beneficial methods are assisting the client with progressive relaxation exercises and providing a back massage.

Progressive Relaxation

Progressive relaxation is a therapeutic exercise in which a person actively contracts and then relaxes muscle groups to break the worry–tension cycle that interferes with relaxation (see Nursing Guidelines 18-1).

NURSING GUIDELINES 18-1

Facilitating Progressive Relaxation

- Select a room that is quiet, private, and dimly lit. *Such a setting reduces stimulation of the arousal center in the brain, which responds to noise, bright lights, and activity.*
- Encourage the client to assume a comfortable position; this usually involves lying down or sitting. *Sitting or lying down provides external support for the body, which facilitates muscle relaxation.*
- Advise the client to avoid talking and instead listen to the suggestions that will follow. *Advising the client to take a passive role reduces performance anxiety (a worry about appearing incompetent or foolish).*
- Instruct the client to close the eyes and consciously focus on breathing. *Closing the eyes blocks visual stimuli; focusing on breathing helps turn the client's attention away from distracting thoughts and feelings.*
- Tell the client to inhale deeply through the nose and exhale slowly out the mouth. Repeat the activity several times. *This breathing oxygenates the blood and brain and reduces the heart rate.*

- Tell the client to tighten the muscles in an area of the body, such as the foot, and hold the position for at least 5 seconds. *Tightening a muscle depletes the level of stimulating neurotransmitters.*
- Direct the client to relax the tensed muscles and focus on the pleasant feeling. *Focusing on the pleasant feeling directs the cortex's attention to the desired outcome and raises the client's awareness.*
- Proceed with sequence after sequence of muscle contraction followed by relaxation until all muscle groups in the body have been exercised. *Continued tensing and relaxation lead to higher planes of relaxation.*
- Continue suggesting throughout that the client focuses on how relaxed or weightless they feel. *These verbal cues reinforce relaxation.*
- Tell the client that as you reach 0 after counting backward from 10, they can begin to move. *This provides a gradual end to the relaxation period.*

Clients can learn to perform progressive relaxation exercises independently using self-suggestion. Some clients eventually omit the muscle contraction phase and go directly to progressive relaxation of muscle groups.

Back Massage

Massage (stroking the skin) promotes two desired outcomes; it relaxes tense muscles and improves circulation (Skill 18-3). Nurses perform massage using various stroking techniques (Table 18-5). Stimulating strokes are omitted if the purpose is to relax the client.

>>> *Stop, Think, and Respond 18-2*

Describe techniques for maximizing the positive effects of a back massage.

TABLE 18-5 Massage Techniques

TECHNIQUE	DESCRIPTION	METHOD
Effleurage	To skim the surface	The hands are used to make a circular pattern using long strokes over the massaged area.
Pétrissage	To knead	The skin is lifted and compressed or pulled in opposing directions.
Frôlement	To brush	The skin is lightly touched with the fingertips.
Tapotement	To tap	The skin is lightly struck with the sides of the hands.
Vibration	To set in motion	The skin is moved rhythmically with open or cupped palms, causing the tissue to quiver.
Friction	To rub	The skin is pulled from opposite directions using the thumbs and fingers.

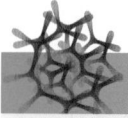

KEY POINTS

- Client environment
  - Client rooms
  - Walls
  - Floors
  - Lighting
  - Climate control
    - Ventilation
    - Humidity
  - Room furnishings
    - Bed: Hospital or regular
    - Side rails
    - Mattress
    - Mattress overlay
    - Pillow
    - Linens
    - Privacy curtain
    - Overbed stand
    - Side table
    - Chairs
- Functions of sleep
  - Reducing fatigue
  - Stabilizing mood
  - Improving blood flow to the brain
  - Increasing protein synthesis
  - Maintaining the disease-fighting mechanisms of the immune system
  - Promoting cellular growth and repair
  - Improving the capacity for learning and memory storage
- Sleep stages
  - NREM: Quiet sleep
  - REM: The body is relaxed, immobile, often completely paralyzed, and unresponsive during REM sleep.
- Sleep requirements are different for all age groups.
- Factors affecting sleep
  - Light
  - Activity
  - Environment
  - Motivation
  - Emotion and moods
  - Food and beverages
  - Illness
  - Drugs
- Sleep assessments: Gathering data during interviews, or clients can answer the questions independently in the form of a self-reporting assessment.
- Sleep disorders
  - Insomnia: Difficulty in falling asleep, awakening frequently during the night, or awakening early
  - Hypersomnia: A sleep disorder characterized by feeling sleepy despite getting normal sleep
  - Sleep apnea/hypopnea syndrome: The sleeper stops breathing or breathing slows for 10 seconds or longer five or more times per hour.
  - Narcolepsy: Characterized by the sudden onset of daytime sleep
  - Sleep–wake cycle disturbances: Results from a sleep schedule that involves daytime sleeping and interferes with biologic rhythms
  - Parasomnia: Sleepwalking, restless legs syndrome, bed-wetting, night terrors, sleep talking, grinding of the teeth (bruxism)
- Progressive relaxation: Facilitates relaxation by tightening and relaxing muscle groups to break the worry–tension cycle
- Back massages: Relaxes tense muscles and improves circulation

CRITICAL THINKING EXERCISES

1. What items in the health care environment would you find important in supporting your comfort, rest, and sleep?

2. What actions could a nurse take to promote sleep among clients in a hospital or other types of health care facility such as a nursing home?

3. Discuss possible effects of suffering from or living with a person who has a sleep disorder.

4. Explain why nursing interventions that promote sleep may be preferable to administering a medication that promotes sleep.

NEXT-GENERATION NCLEX-STYLE REVIEW QUESTIONS

1. When observing an unlicensed nursing assistant make an occupied bed, which action indicates a need for further learning?
   a. The assistant loosens all the linen under the client.
   b. The assistant wears gloves to remove soiled linen.
   c. The assistant keeps the bed in a low position.
   d. The assistant rolls the client to the far side of the bed.
   Test-Taking Strategy: Eliminate actions that are appropriate when making an unoccupied bed leaving an option that describes an action that warrants reteaching.

2. To help a client suffering from insomnia, which plan for nursing care is best?
   a. Administer a prescribed hypnotic drug each night.
   b. Try to duplicate the client's pattern of sleep rituals.
   c. Have the client exercise for 30 minutes at bedtime.
   d. Suggest the client go to bed earlier than the usual time.

Test-Taking Strategy: Note the key word, "best." Eliminate options that may be inappropriate or plausible, and select the option that is better than any of the others.

3. Which are aseptic practices that are appropriate when making an unoccupied bed? Select all that apply.
   a. Raise the bed to a high position.
   b. Loosen the bed linens from the mattress.
   c. Place clean linens on a chair.
   d. Hold soiled linens away from the uniform.
   e. Place soiled linens directly into a hamper.
   Test-Taking Strategy: Note the key words, "aseptic practices." Analyze the choices and select options that reduce the transmission of microorganisms.

4. What interval of time should the nurse allow to avoid interrupting a sleeping client's full cycle of NREM and REM sleep?
   a. 30 to 60 minutes
   b. 60 to 90 minutes
   c. 90 to 120 minutes
   d. 120 to 150 minutes
   Test-Taking Strategy: Note the key words, "full cycle." Select the option that most closely resembles the combined time of NREM and REM.

5. When assessing a sleeping client, which nursing observations suggest the client is in REM sleep? Select all that apply.
   a. Muscle twitching
   b. Snoring
   c. Little physical movement
   d. Darting movement beneath the eyelids
   e. Talking while asleep
   Test-Taking Strategy: Use the process of elimination to select options that differentiate REM from NREM sleep.

SKILL 18-1 Making an Unoccupied Bed

Suggested Action	Reason for Action
ASSESSMENT	
Check the medical record or nursing care plan to determine the client's activity level.	Determines whether the client can be out of bed during bed-making
Inspect the linen for moisture or evidence of soiling.	Indicates what and how much linen must be changed and if gloves are appropriate when removing soiled linen
PLANNING	
Plan to change the linen after the client's hygiene needs have been met.	Reduces the potential for wetting or soiling the clean linen
Wash hands or perform hand antisepsis with an alcohol rub (see Chapter 10). Use gloves if there is a potential for direct contact with blood, stool, or other body fluids.	Reduces the transmission of microorganisms
Bring necessary bed linen to the room.	Demonstrates organization and efficient time management
Place the clean linen on a clean, dry surface such as the seat or back of a chair (Fig. A).	Reduces transmission of microorganisms to clean supplies

Arranging clean bed linens (Photo by B. Proud.)

Assist the client from the bed.	Facilitates bed-making
IMPLEMENTATION	
Raise the bed to a high position and lower the side rails.	Prevents postural and muscular strain
Remove equipment attached to the bed linens such as the signal cord and drainage tubes and check for personal items.	Avoids breakage, spills, or loss of personal items
Loosen the bed linen from where it has been tucked under the mattress.	Facilitates removal or retightening
Fold any linen that may be reused and place it on a clean surface.	Promotes efficiency, orderliness, and asepsis
Put on gloves, if necessary, and roll linen that will be replaced so that the soiled surface is enclosed (Fig. B).	Gloves are a standard precaution to provide a barrier between the nurse and the blood or other body fluids; gloves are unnecessary if linen does not contain blood or body fluid. Rolling linen with the soiled side inward reduces contact with sources of microorganisms.

SKILL 18-1 Making an Unoccupied Bed (*continued*)

Suggested Action	Reason for Action
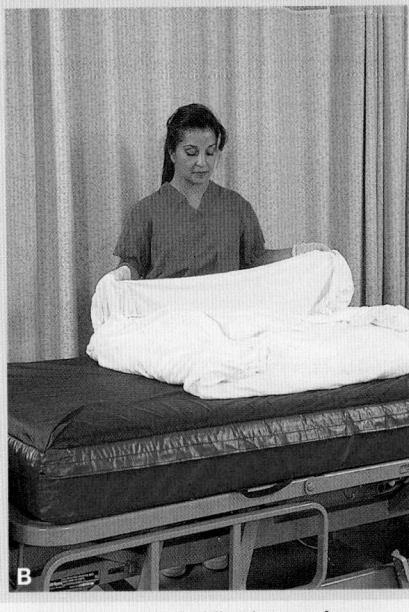	Enclosing soiled side of linens. (Photo by B. Proud.)
Remove the soiled linen while holding it away from your uniform (Fig. C).	Prevents transferring microorganisms to your uniform and then to other clients
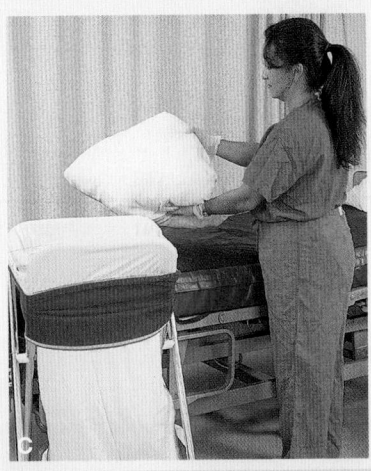	Avoiding contact with uniform. (Photo by B. Proud.)
Place the soiled linen directly into a pillowcase, laundry hamper, or self-made pouch from one of the removed sheets (Fig. D). *Do not place the soiled linen on the floor.*	Keeps the soiled linen from being further contaminated
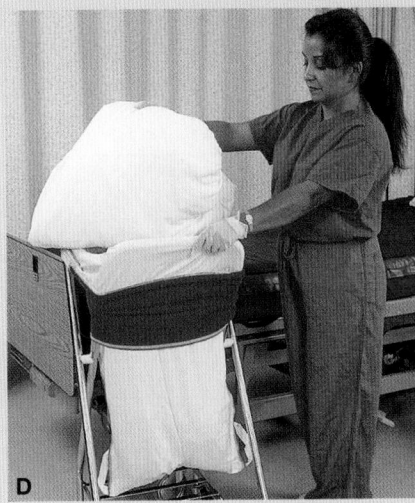	Placing soiled linens in hamper. (Photo by B. Proud.)

(*continued*)

Suggested Action	Reason for Action
Remove gloves and wash hands or perform hand antisepsis with an alcohol rub (see Chapter 10) once contact with body secretions is no longer likely.	Facilitates use of the hands and promotes asepsis
Reposition the mattress so it is flush with the headboard.	Provides maximum foot room
Tighten any linen that will be reused.	Removes wrinkles, which promotes client comfort
If the bottom sheet needs changing, center the longitudinal fold and open the layers of folded linen to one side of the bed.	Reduces postural strain
If using a flat sheet, make sure the flat edge of the hem is flush with the edge of the mattress at the foot end.	Prevents skin pressure and irritation
If using a flat sheet, tuck the upper portion under the mattress. Make a mitered or square corner at the top of the bed.	Anchors the bottom sheet
If using a fitted sheet, position the upper and lower corners of the mattress within the contoured corners of the sheet (Fig. E).	Anchors the fitted sheet

Stretching the fitted sheet taut. (Photo by B. Proud.)

If the client is apt to soil the linen with urine or stool, fold a flat sheet horizontally with the smooth edge of the hem toward the foot of the bed and tuck it in place approximately where the buttocks will be. Do the same if a draw sheet is available (Fig. F).	Reduces the need to change all the bottom linens

Smoothing the draw sheet before securing it snugly under the mattress. (Photo by B. Proud.)

Position the top linen on one half of the bed at this time. Move to the other side of the bed, pull the linen taut, and tuck the free edges beneath the mattress.	Saves time by reducing the number of moves around the bed
Alternatively, wait until you have secured all the bottom linen to position the top sheet.	Secures and smooths the bottom linen
Center the top sheet and unfold it to one side, leaving sufficient length at the top to make a fold over the spread.	Provides a smooth edge next to the client's neck
Add blankets if the client wishes.	Demonstrates concern for the client's comfort
Cover the top sheet with the spread if desired. Tuck the excess linen at the foot of the bed under the bottom of the mattress and finish the sides with a mitered or square corner (Fig. G).	Secures the top linen

SKILL 18-1 Making an Unoccupied Bed (*continued*)

Suggested Action	Reason for Action

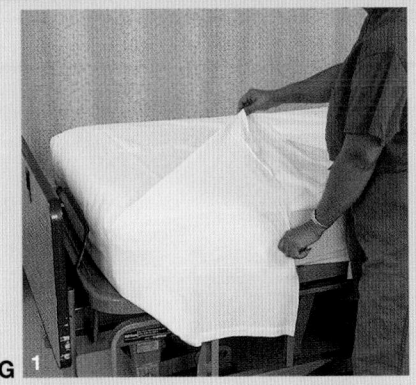 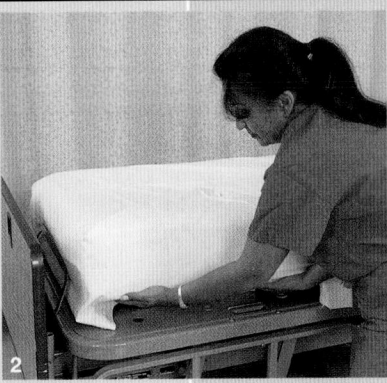 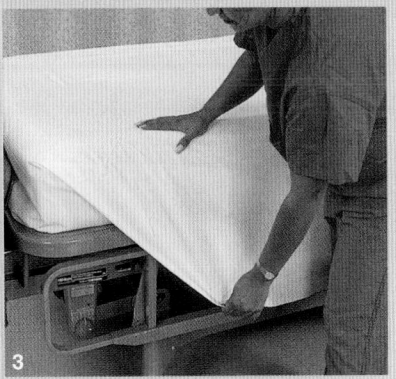

(1) Folding the edge of the top sheet back onto itself. (2) Tucking the edge hanging from the bed under the mattress. (3) Pulling the top sheet taut. (Photo by B. Proud.)

Smooth the top sheet (Fig. H).	Creates comfort and tidiness

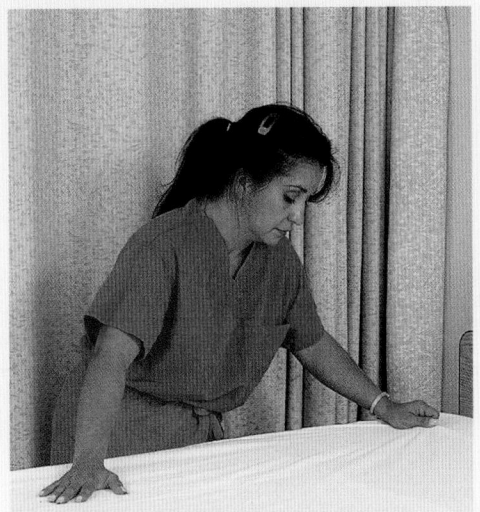

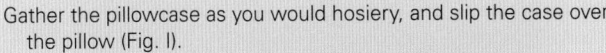

Smoothing the top sheet. (Photo by B. Proud.)

Gather the pillowcase as you would hosiery, and slip the case over the pillow (Fig. I).	Prevents contact between the pillow and your uniform

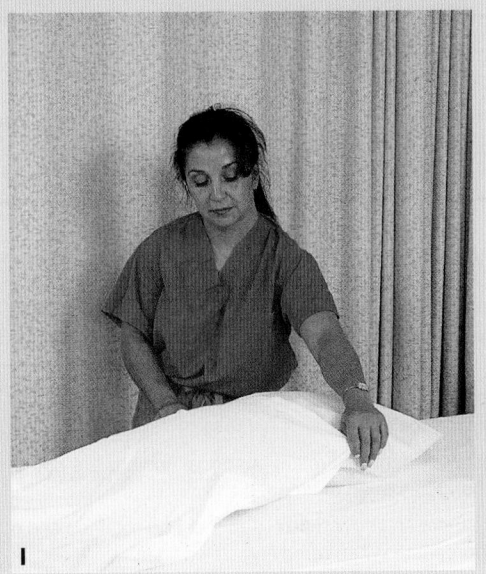

Covering the pillow. (Photo by B. Proud.)

(*continued*)

SKILL 18-1 Making an Unoccupied Bed (*continued*)

Suggested Action	Reason for Action
Place the pillow at the head of the bed with the open end away from the door and the seam of the pillowcase toward the headboard.	Presents a tidy view of the room from the hallway; prevents pressure on the skin around the head and neck
Fanfold or pie-fold the top linen toward the foot of the bed (Fig. J).	Facilitates returning to bed

Prefolding the linen. (Photo by B. Proud.)

Suggested Action	Reason for Action
Secure the signal device on or to the bed.	Ensures that the client can receive nursing assistance
Adjust the bed to a low position.	Enables the client to return to bed
Wash hands or perform hand antisepsis with an alcohol rub (see Chapter 10).	Reduces the transmission of microorganisms

EVALUATION

- The bed is clean and dry.
- The linen is free of wrinkles.
- The environment is orderly.
- The client feels comfortable.

DOCUMENT

- Date and time
- Characteristics of drainage, if present
- Any unique measures taken to ensure client comfort

SAMPLE DOCUMENTATION

Date and Time Menses established. Bed linen changed while shower taken. Given a supply of sanitary napkins. Absorbent pad placed over bottom sheet. _____ J. Doe, LPN

SKILL 18-2 Making an Occupied Bed

Suggested Action	Reason for Action
ASSESSMENT	
Check the medical record or nursing care plan to confirm that the client must remain in bed.	Demonstrates compliance with the care plan
Assess the client's level of consciousness, physical strength, breathing pattern, heart rate, and blood pressure.	Indicates a need for bed rest if abnormal findings are noted, whether it has been prescribed
Inspect the linen for moisture or evidence of soiling.	Indicates what and how much linen must be changed and if gloves are appropriate when removing soiled linen

SKILL 18-2 Making an Occupied Bed (*continued*)

Suggested Action	Reason for Action
Determine who might be available to assist if the client is too weak or unable to cooperate.	Avoids postural or muscular injury and ensures the client's comfort and safety

PLANNING

Suggested Action	Reason for Action
Plan to change the linen after the client's hygiene needs have been met.	Reduces the potential for wetting or soiling the clean linen
Wash hands or perform hand antisepsis with an alcohol rub (see Chapter 10). Use gloves if there is a potential for direct contact with blood, stool, or other body fluids.	Reduces the transmission of microorganisms
Bring necessary bed linens to the room.	Demonstrates organization and efficient time management
Place the clean linen on a clean, dry surface, such as the back of a chair.	Reduces the transmission of microorganisms to clean supplies

IMPLEMENTATION

Suggested Action	Reason for Action
Explain what you plan to do.	Informs the client and promotes cooperation
Raise the bed to a high position.	Prevents postural and muscular strain
Cover the client with a bath blanket or leave the top sheet loosened but in place.	Maintains warmth and demonstrates respect for modesty
Fold the top sheet or spread if it will be reused and place it on a clean surface.	Promotes efficiency, orderliness, and asepsis
Unfasten equipment attached to the bottom linen and check for personal items.	Avoids breakage, spills, or loss of personal items
Loosen the bed linen from where it has been tucked under the mattress.	Facilitates removal or retightening
Lower the rail on the side of the bed where you are standing, and roll the client toward the opposite side rail.	Provides room for making the bed while ensuring the client's safety
Roll the soiled bottom sheets as close to the client as possible.	Facilitates removal
Proceed to unfold and tuck the bottom sheet and draw sheet on the vacant side of the bed, as described in Skill 18-1 (Fig. A).	Remakes half of the bed with clean linen

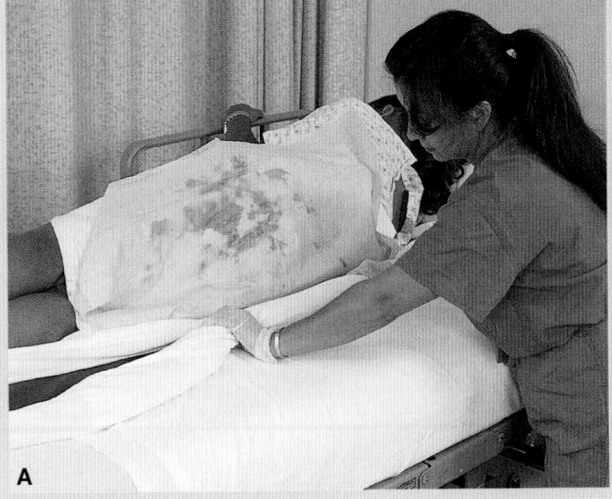

A

Changing linen on half of the bed. (Photo by B. Proud.)

Suggested Action	Reason for Action
Fold the free edges of the sheet under the folded portion of the soiled sheets.	Keeps the clean sheet from becoming soiled; facilitates pulling the sheets from under the client
Raise the side rail and move to the opposite side of the bed.	Prevents postural and muscular strain
Lower the side rail, in your new position, and help the client to roll over the mound of sheets.	Helps reposition the client on the clean side of the bed
Pull the soiled laundry close to the edge of the bed and the clean linen close beside it.	Reduces the mound of linen in the center of the bed
Remove the soiled linen and place it into a pillowcase or pouch that is off the floor.	Keeps the soiled linen from becoming further contaminated

(*continued*)

SKILL 18-2 Making an Occupied Bed (continued)

Suggested Action	Reason for Action
Pull the clean bottom sheet until it is unfolded from beneath the client (Fig. B).	Ensures the client is in contact with clean sheets

B

Pulling the clean linen through. (Photo by B. Proud.)

Suggested Action	Reason for Action
Miter or square the upper corner of the sheet; pull and tuck the free edges under the mattress.	Secures the clean sheets
Assist the client to the middle of the bed.	Ensures comfort and safety
Straighten or replace the top sheet, blankets, and spread; remove and replace the pillowcase if necessary.	Restores comfort and orderliness to the environment
Reposition the client according to the therapeutic regimen or comfort.	Demonstrates adherence to the care plan; shows concern for client comfort
Lower the height of the bed and raise the remaining side rail if appropriate.	Reduces the potential for injury
Dispose of the soiled linens in a laundry hamper outside the room.	Restores order to the room and ensures that the linens will be collected for laundering
Wash hands or perform hand antisepsis with an alcohol rub (see Chapter 10).	Reduces the transmission of microorganisms

EVALUATION

- The bed is clean and dry.
- The linen is free of wrinkles.
- The environment is orderly.
- The client feels comfortable.

DOCUMENT

- Date and time
- Characteristics of drainage, if present
- Measures taken to ensure client comfort

SAMPLE DOCUMENTATION

Date and Time Unresponsive even to painful stimuli. Complete bed bath given followed by linen change. Repositioned on L. side with head at a 45-degree elevation. Full side rails raised. Bed in low position. _____ J. Doe, LPN

SKILL 18-3 Giving a Back Massage

Suggested Action	Reason for Action
ASSESSMENT	
Observe if the client is still awake 30 minutes after retiring for sleep.	Indicates a delay in the usual onset of sleep
Determine whether the client is experiencing pain, has a need for bladder or bowel elimination, is hungry, is too warm or cold, or has any other physical or environmental problem that may be easily overcome.	Eliminates all but psychophysiological etiologies as the cause for sleeplessness
Check the medical record to determine whether the client has any condition that would contraindicate a backrub, such as fractured ribs or a back injury.	Demonstrates concern for the client's safety and comfort
Ask the client if they would like a back massage.	Allows the client an opportunity to participate in decision-making
PLANNING	
Obtain lotion or an alternative substance such as alcohol or powder if the client's skin is oily.	Demonstrates organization and efficient time management
Put on gloves if there are any open, draining lesions on the skin.	Provides a barrier against blood-borne microorganisms
Reduce environmental stimuli, such as bright lights and loud noise.	Decreases stimulation of the wake center in the brain
IMPLEMENTATION	
Pull the privacy curtain around the client's bed.	Demonstrates respect for modesty
Raise the bed to an appropriate height to avoid bending at the waist.	Reduces back strain
Wash hands or perform hand antisepsis with an alcohol rub (see Chapter 10); put on gloves if appropriate.	Reduces the spread of microorganisms
Help the client lie on the abdomen or side and untie the hospital gown or remove it completely.	Provides access to the back
Instruct the client to breathe slowly and deeply in and out through an open mouth.	Promotes ventilation and relaxation
Squirt a generous amount of lotion into your hands and rub them together.	Warms the lotion
Place the entire surface of the hands on either side of the lower spine and move them upward over the shoulders and back again using long, continuous strokes. Repeat the stroke pattern several times (Fig. A).	Uses effleurage to promote relaxation

A
Effleurage (example 1).

Effleurage (example 2).

Apply firmer pressure with the upstroke and lighter pressure during the downstroke.	Enhances relaxation by alternating pressure and rhythm
Make smaller circular strokes up and down the length of the back with the thumbs.	Improves blood flow and removes chemicals that accumulate in contracted muscles

(continued)

SKILL 18-3 Giving a Back Massage (*continued*)

Suggested Action	Reason for Action
Lift and gently compress tissue with the fingers, starting at the base of the spine and ending at the neck and shoulder areas (Fig. B).	Uses pétrissage to increase blood circulation

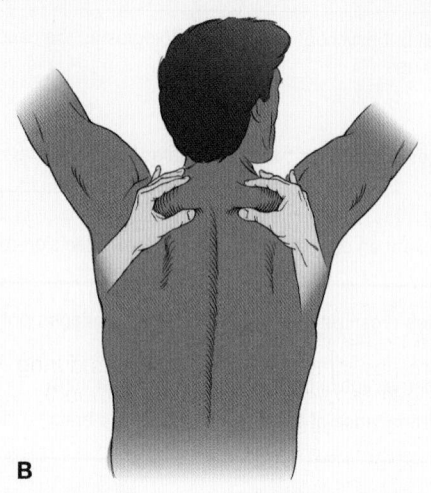

B

Pétrissage (example 1).

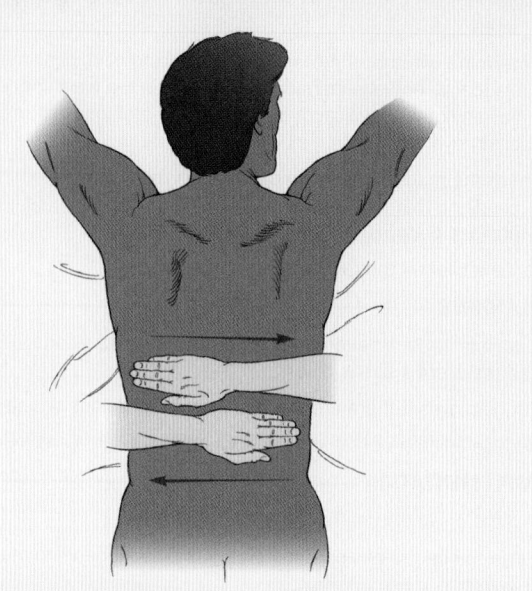

Pétrissage (example 2).

Suggested Action	Reason for Action
Pull the skin in opposite directions in a kneading manner to lift and stretch it from the base of the spine to the shoulder areas.	Uses another pétrissage technique to reduce tension in muscles and improve circulation
End the backrub by lightly stroking the length of the back, gradually lightening the pressure as you move the fingers downward (Fig. C).	Uses frôlement to prolong the sensation of relaxation

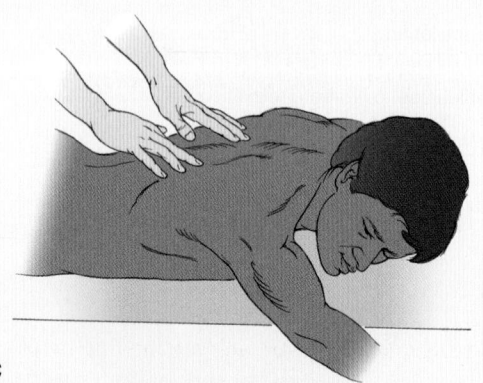

C

Frôlement.

Suggested Action	Reason for Action
Lightly cover the client and lower the bed.	Extends the period of relaxation by reducing activity and may induce nonrapid eye movement (NREM) sleep

EVALUATION

- Client feels relaxed.
- Sleep is promoted.

DOCUMENT

- Date and time of back massage
- Response of client

SAMPLE DOCUMENTATION

Date and Time   Unable to sleep. Assisted to bathroom to void. Light snack of graham crackers and milk provided. Back massaged for 10 minutes. Observed to be sleeping 20 minutes later. _____ J. Doe, LPN

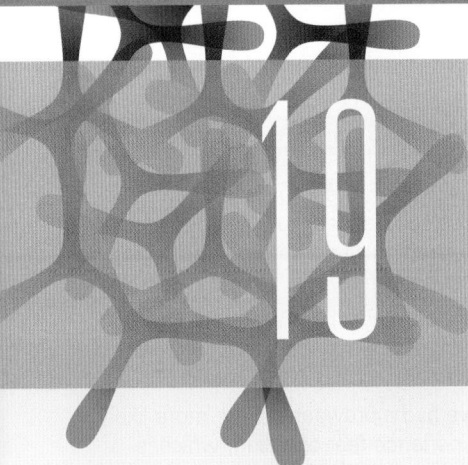

19

Safety

Learning Objectives

On completion of this chapter, the reader should be able to:

1. Discuss the purpose of the National Patient Safety Goals (NPSGs) and methods for implementing them.
2. Give an example of a common injury that predominates during each developmental stage (infancy through older adulthood).
3. Name injuries that result from environmental hazards.
4. Identify methods for reducing latex sensitization.
5. Discuss measures for preventing burns.
6. List areas of responsibility incorporated into most fire plans.
7. Describe the indications for using each class of fire extinguishers.
8. Name common causes of asphyxiation.
9. Discuss methods for preventing drowning.
10. Explain why humans are susceptible to electrical shock.
11. Discuss methods for preventing electrical shock.
12. Name common substances associated with poisonings.
13. Discuss methods for preventing poisonings.
14. Explain why older adults are prone to falling.
15. Discuss the benefits and risks of using physical restraints.
16. Explain the basis for enacting restraint legislation and The Joint Commission's accreditation standards.
17. Identify criteria for applying a physical restraint.
18. Differentiate between a restraint and a restraint alternative.
19. Describe areas of concern during an accident.

INTRODUCTION

Safety (measures that prevent accidents or unintentional injuries) remains a primary focus in health care since many hospital deaths and injuries are attributed to medication errors and adverse medication effects, infections, and surgical errors. Medical errors are a serious public health problem and a leading cause of death in the United States (Medical Error Reduction and Prevention, 2022). Such findings validate the conclusion that receiving health care is an extreme risk to a person's safety. This chapter examines factors that place people at risk for injuries, environmental hazards in homes and health care facilities, and nursing measures that keep clients safe. The Joint Commission (TJC), or other health care regulating agencies, began considering safety a priority when caring for clients and began establishing the **National Patient Safety Goals (NPSGs)** in 2003. Since that time, there have been subsequent updates, the most recent being in 2023. The purpose of these goals is to help health care organizations obtain and retain their accreditation by demonstrating safe and effective care of the highest quality by reducing the risk of adverse client outcomes. The goals are revised regularly based on the recommendations of the Patient Safety Advisory Group, which comprises nurses, physicians, pharmacists, and others to reduce the incidences of deaths and injuries among those being cared for in health care agencies (Table 19-1). Methods of implementing the goals are integrated within the nursing skills that appear in this text.

TABLE 19-1 Summary of Hospital NPSGs

GOAL	IMPLEMENTATION
Identify patients correctly.	Use at least two ways to identify patients. For example, use the patient's name and date of birth. This is done to make sure that each patient gets the correct medicine and treatment.
Improve staff communication.	Get important test results to the right staff person on time.
Use medicines safely.	Before a procedure, label medicines that are not labeled. For example, medicines in syringes, cups, and basins. Do this in the area where medicines and supplies are set up. Take extra care with patients who take medicines to thin their blood. Record and pass along correct information about a patient's medicines. Find out what medicines the patient is taking. Compare those medicines to new medicines given to the patient. Give the patient written information about the medicines they need to take. Tell the patient it is important to bring their up-to-date list of medicines every time they visit a doctor.
Use alarms safely.	Make improvements to ensure that alarms on medical equipment are heard and responded to on time.
Prevent infection.	Use the hand cleaning guidelines from the Centers for Disease Control and Prevention or the World Health Organization. Set goals for improving hand cleaning. Use the goals to improve hand cleaning.
Identify patient safety risks.	Reduce the risk for suicide.
Improve health care equity	Improving health care equity is a quality and patient safety priority. For example, health care disparities in the patient population are identified and a written plan describes ways to improve health care equity.
Prevent mistakes in surgery.	Make sure that the correct surgery is done on the correct patient and at the correct place on the patient's body. Mark the correct place on the patient's body where the surgery is to be done. Pause before the surgery to make sure that a mistake is not being made.

Adapted from The Joint Commission. (2024). *Hospital: 2024 National Patient Safety Goals.* https://www.jointcommission.org/standards/national-patient-safety-goals/hospital-national-patient-safety-goals/

 Gerontologic Considerations

■ Protect older adults with cognitive impairments from accidental ingestion of toxic substances, such as medications and cleaning agents, by keeping all potentially harmful substances in a secure, locked location.

■ Osteoporosis (loss of bone mass) increases the risk of fractures. Osteoporotic fractures may occur with little or no trauma and even without a fall.

■ Older adults who have had a previous fall are more likely to fall again and may experience fear of falling, which is characterized by gait changes and being overly cautious. Fear of falling can significantly limit mobility, which may actually increase the risk for falls.

■ Practical methods such as assessing risk factors for falls and teaching fall management should be initiated. Placing beds at low heights may diminish risks from falls.

■ Wandering is not a justification for restraining clients. Older adults who are confused or otherwise cognitively impaired without an awareness or appreciation for personal safety may need alternative precautions to prevent wandering.

■ Helpful devices include placing a specially designed net with a stop sign across the exit doorway with Velcro, using bells over doors to alert caregivers, or disguising an exit door by covering it with a curtain or wallpaper that blends in with the surrounding environment. Several different types of monitors, identification bracelets (that include a phone number), and alert/alarm devices are available to reduce the risk for wandering.

■ Special environments may be designed so that the hallways form a circle around the nursing stations, allowing the older adult to walk, yet remain in view of the nursing staff.

■ Caregivers should be aware that early identification is necessary so that proper precautions can be initiated. Daily documentation of what a person is wearing is helpful should the client wander and need to be identified.

■ The Alzheimer's Association sponsors a program called "Safe Return," which facilitates the reporting and return of people with cognitive impairments who become lost. Local police departments may provide a service of digital photography of the older adult and coded identification bracelets. The photos and identification codes are stored in the computers maintained by the police department for identification of an adult found wandering. Clients with dementia may also be fitted with a global positioning satellite (GPS) device to facilitate locating a missing person.

AGE-RELATED SAFETY FACTORS

No age group is immune to accidental injury. Distinct differences among age groups exist, however, because of varying levels of cognitive function and judgment, activity and mobility, and degree of supervision, as well as the design of and safety devices within physical surroundings.

Infants and Toddlers

Infants rely on the safety consciousness of their adult care-givers. They are especially vulnerable to injuries resulting from falling off changing tables or being unrestrained in automobiles. Toddlers are naturally inquisitive and more mobile than infants and fail to understand the dangers that accompany climbing. Consequently, they are often the victims of accidental poisoning, falls down the stairs or from high chairs, burns, electrocution from exploring outlets or manipulating electric cords, and drowning.

School-Aged Children and Adolescents

School-aged children are physically active, which makes them prone to play-related injuries. Many adolescents suffer sports-related injuries because they participate in physically challenging activities—sometimes without adequate protective equipment—before their musculoskeletal systems can withstand the stress. Adolescents also tend to be impulsive and take risks as a result of poor judgment and peer pressure.

Adults

Adults are at risk for injuries from ignoring safety issues, such as driving while texting or talking on a cell phone, failing to use seat belts, fatigue, sensory changes, and the effects of disease. The types of injuries that young, middle aged, and older adults incur depend on their social, developmental, and physical differences (Table 19-2).

ENVIRONMENTAL HAZARDS

Environmental hazards are potentially dangerous conditions in the physical surroundings. Examples in the home and health care environment include latex sensitization, thermal burns, asphyxiation, electrical shock, poisoning, and falls.

BOX 19-1	Common Items Containing Latex
Medical gloves	Intravenous injection ports
Bandages	Nondisposable sheet protectors
Bulb syringes	Stethoscope tubing
Medication vial stoppers	Tourniquets
Urinary catheters	Elastic stockings/elastic in clothing
Condoms/diaphragms	Foam mattresses and pillows/ mattress covers
Wound drains	Dental bands and products
Endoscopes	Blood pressure cuffs and tubing

Latex Sensitization

Increasing numbers of people are developing **latex sensitivity** (allergic response to the proteins in latex). Latex, a natural rubber sap that originates from a species of tree indigenous to Brazil, is a component of many household items, such as balloons, envelope glue, erasers, and carpet backing, as well as health care products. Health-related sensitization is partly the result of repeated exposure to latex in medical gloves and other equipment (Box 19-1). Clients predisposed to latex sensitivity include those with a history of asthma and allergies to other substances, multiple surgeries, and recurring medical procedures.

Types of Latex Reactions

Sensitization follows latex exposure through the skin, mucous membranes, inhalation, ingestion, injection, or wound management. The two forms of allergic reactions to latex or the chemicals used in its manufacture are as follows:

- **Contact dermatitis,** a delayed localized skin reaction that occurs within 6 to 48 hours and lasts for several days (Fig. 19-1)

TABLE 19-2 Age-Related Factors Affecting Adult Safety

ADULT GROUP	CONTRIBUTING FACTORS	COMMON TYPES OF INJURIES
Young adults	Alcohol and drug misuse Emancipation from parental supervision Naiveté about workplace hazards	Motor vehicle collisions Boating accidents Head and spinal cord injuries Eye injuries, chemical burns, traumatic amputations, and soft tissue and back injuries
Middle-aged adults	Failure to use safety devices Overexertion and fatigue Disregard for use of seat belts and car safety harnesses Lack of expertise in performing home maintenance or repairs	Physical trauma (see previous) Burns and asphyxiation related to nonfunctioning smoke, heat, and carbon monoxide detectors
Older adults	Visual impairment Urinary urgency Postural hypotension Reduced coordination Impaired mobility Inadequate home maintenance Mental confusion Impaired temperature regulation	Falls Poisoning/medication errors Hypothermia and hyperthermia Scalds and burns

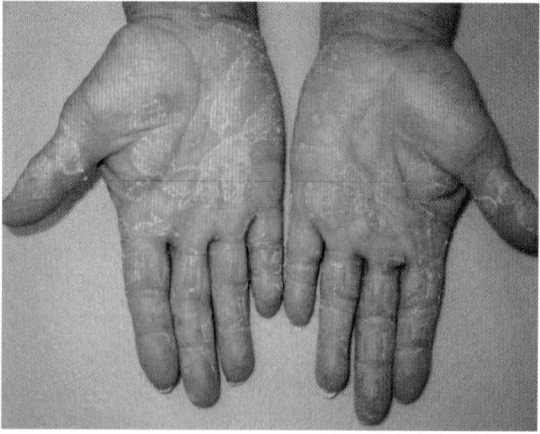

FIGURE 19-1 Contact dermatitis from exposure to latex in gloves. (Image provided by Stedman's.)

- **Acute hypersensitivity**, an instantaneous or fairly prompt systemic reaction manifested by a variety of signs and symptoms such as swelling, itching, respiratory distress, hypotension, and death in severe cases (Fig. 19-2)

Sensitized people can also develop a cross-reaction to fruits and vegetables, such as avocados, bananas, almonds, peaches, kiwi, tomatoes, and others, because the molecular structure of latex and other plant substances is similar.

Safeguarding Clients and Health Care Providers

One of the best techniques for preventing latex sensitization and allergic reactions is to minimize or eliminate latex exposure. Health care agencies now provide health care providers with more than one type of glove (Table 19-3). If they use latex gloves, nurses should:

- Use powder-free gloves.
- Avoid "snapping" the gloves when donning or removing to avoid air dispersal of powder and latex proteins.

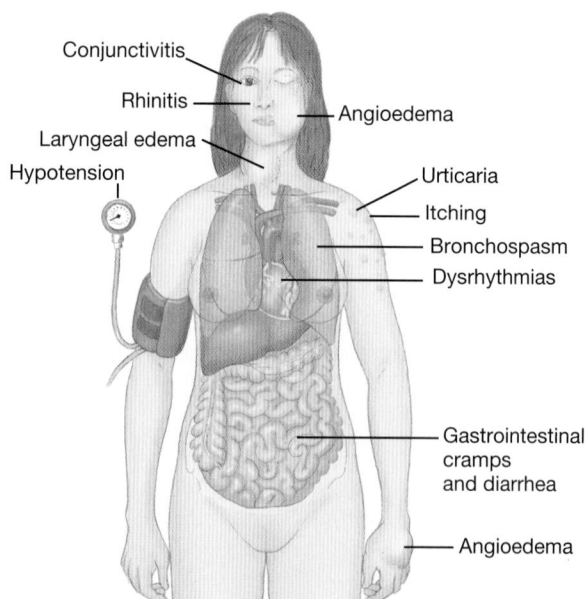

FIGURE 19-2 Manifestations that accompany an acute hypersensitivity reaction. (From Donnelly-Moreno, L., & Moseley, B. [2021]. *Introductory medical-surgical nursing* [12th ed.]. Lippincott Williams & Wilkins.)

- Reduce the time the gloves are worn.
- Wash hands thoroughly with a pH-balanced soap after removing the gloves.
- Avoid using oil-based hand creams or lotions.

Other measures to protect clients and health care providers include:

- Obtain an allergy history, and ask about sensitivity to latex in particular.
- Flag the chart and room door (Fig. 19-3), and attach an allergy alert identification bracelet to latex-sensitive clients.
- Assign clients with latex allergies to private rooms or a **latex-safe environment** (room stocked with latex-free equipment and wiped clean of glove powder).
- Stock a latex-safe cart containing synthetic gloves and latex-free client care and resuscitation equipment in the room of a client sensitive to latex.
- Communicate with personnel in other departments so that they use nonlatex equipment and supplies during diagnostic or treatment procedures.
- Report allergic events and their possible causes promptly to the agency's administration; administrators are required to report injuries, serious illnesses, or deaths from unsafe equipment to the U.S. Food and Drug Administration (FDA).
- Refer sensitized clients to latex allergy support groups.
- Recommend that latex-sensitive clients wear a MedicAlert bracelet at all times.
- Advise latex-sensitive clients to notify their employer's health officer about the allergy in case of a future claim for worker's compensation or a legal case concerning discrimination in the workplace.

Burns

A **thermal burn** is a skin injury caused by flames, hot liquids, or steam and is the most common form of burn. U.S. fire departments respond to an estimated average of 5,750 structure fires in health care properties each year (www.nfpa.org). The number of those fires varies according to the type of health facility (Fig. 19-4). Cooking equipment was the leading cause of these fires at 66% (www.nfpa.org) (Fig. 19-5).

Burn Prevention

Because many adults become complacent about safety hazards, the nurse should review burn prevention measures with clients being treated for thermal-related accidents (Client and Family Teaching 19-1).

Exits must be identified, lit, and unlocked. Most fire codes require that public buildings, including hospitals and nursing homes, have a functioning sprinkler system. Sprinkler systems help control fires and limit structural damage.

Fire Plans

To prevent or limit burn injuries in a health care setting, all employees must know and follow the agency's **fire plan** (procedure followed for a possible or actual fire). Compliance with the fire plan is a major component of TJC's inspection. Every accredited health care agency must demonstrate

TABLE 19-3 Types of Medical Gloves

TYPE	ADVANTAGES	DISADVANTAGES
Latex		
Powdered latex	Inexpensive Elastic Adequate barrier against blood-borne pathogens	Releases latex protein allergen into the air via powder
Low-powder latex	Less potential for airborne distribution of latex and chemical proteins	Unproven ability to prevent sensitization
Powder-free latex	Reduced sensitization of nonallergic individuals from lack of airborne distribution of latex allergen	Deposits latex protein on surface environment, causing symptoms in sensitized individuals Slightly more expensive than powdered latex gloves
Low-protein latex	Less latex protein	No significant evidence that use eliminates sensitization
Nonlatex		
Vinyl powder and powder free	Similar strength of latex gloves Costs approximately the same as powdered latex gloves	Less durable and more likely to leak than latex Recommend changing after 30 minutes to maintain barrier protection
Nitrile	Better resistance to tears, punctures, and chemical disintegration than latex or vinyl gloves	Possible contact dermatitis from chemicals contained in nitrile More expensive than latex or vinyl
Neoprene	Fit, strength, and barrier protection similar to latex	Contains potentially allergic chemicals More expensive than nitrile gloves
Thermoplastic elastomer	Strength and protection similar or superior to latex	Free of latex or chemical allergens Most expensive of all gloves

and document that all new and current staff members have been trained in the following five areas:

- Specific roles and responsibilities at and away from the fire's point of origin
- Use of the fire alarm system
- Roles in preparing for building evacuation
- Location and proper use of equipment for evacuation or transporting clients to areas of refuge
- Building compartmentalization procedures for containing smoke and fire. To obtain TJC's accreditation, staff members

on each shift must also participate in fire drills, the frequency of which must be identified in the agency's fire plan.

Fire Management

The National Fire Protection Association, whose Life Safety Code is the basis for TJC's management standards, recommends using the acronym "RACE" to identify the basic steps to take when managing a fire:

R—Rescue
A—Alarm
C—Confine the fire
E—Extinguish

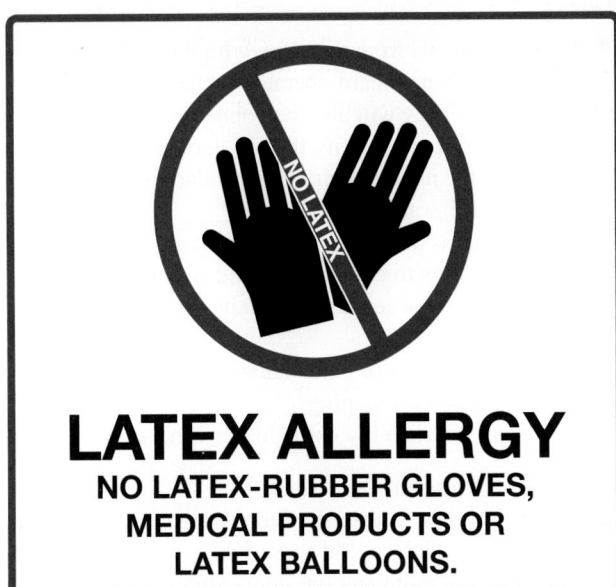

FIGURE 19-3 Example of a sign posted to alert health care providers and others that the client has an allergy to latex.

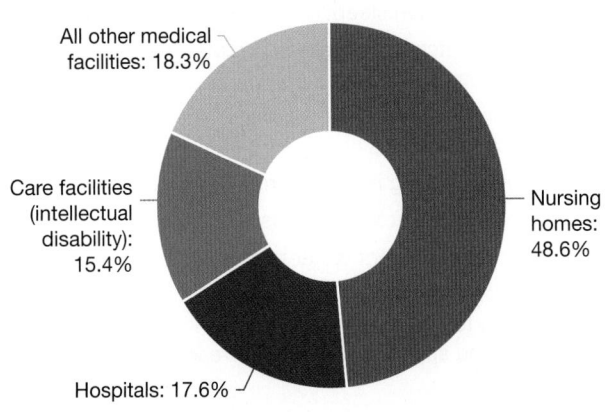

FIGURE 19-4 Data Snapshot: Medical Facility Fires (2014-2016). (FEMA & U.S. Fire Administration. [2022]. https://www.usfa.fema.gov/statistics/reports/where-fires-occur/snapshot-medical-facility.html.)

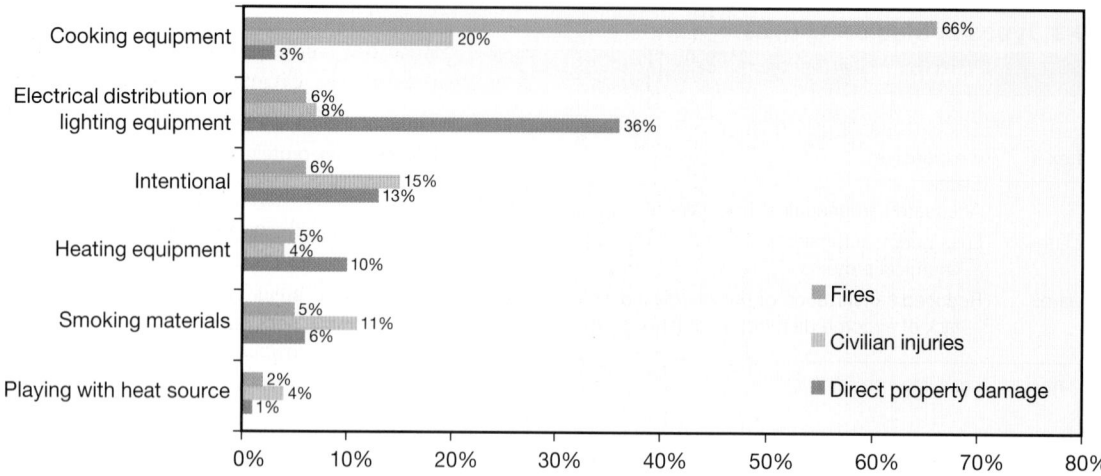

FIGURE 19-5 Fire loss in the United States 2023. (FEMA & U.S. Fire Administration. [2022]. Medical facility fires [2014-2016]. https://www.usfa.fema.gov/downloads/pdf/statistics/snapshot_medical_facility.pdf.)

Client and Family Teaching 19-1
Burn Prevention

The nurse teaches the client or the family the following:

- Change the batteries in smoke, heat, and carbon monoxide detectors at least every year.
- Equip the home with at least one fire extinguisher.
- Develop an evacuation plan (and an alternate escape route) and a place for family members to meet after exiting a burning home.
- Practice the evacuation plan periodically.
- Keep all windows and doors barrier free.
- Identify the location of exits when staying in a hotel.
- Dispose of rags that have been saturated with solvents.
- Keep items away from the pilot lights on the furnace, water heater, or clothes dryer.
- Avoid storing gasoline, kerosene, turpentine, or other solvents.
- Go to public firework displays rather than igniting them at home.
- Never smoke when sleepy or around oxygen equipment.
- Use safety matches rather than a lighter; children are less capable of using matches.
- Buy clothing, especially sleepwear, made from natural or flame-resistant fabrics.
- Never run if clothing is on fire; instead stop, drop, and roll.
- Do not overload electrical outlets or circuits.
- Set thermostats on hot water heaters to less than 120°F (48.8°C).
- Keep cords to coffee pots, electric frying pans, or other small cooking appliances above the reach of young children.
- Follow label directions about the use of gloves when using chemicals.
- Flush chemicals with copious amounts of water if they come in contact with skin.
- Go inside if the weather is threatening or you see lightning.
- If you are inside a burning building:
  - Feel if the surface of a door is hot before opening it.
  - Close doors behind you.
  - Crawl on the floor if the room is smoke filled.
  - Use stairs rather than elevators.
  - Never go back inside, regardless of whom or what has been left there.
- Go to a neighbor's home to call the fire department or 911 operator.

Most health care agencies incorporate these concepts by including the following sequence of actions in their fire plans:

1. Evacuate clients from the room with the fire.
2. Inform the switchboard operator of the fire's location (Fig. 19-6). They will alert personnel over the public address system and notify the fire department.
3. Return to the nursing unit when an alarm sounds; do not use the elevator.
4. Clear the halls of visitors and equipment.
5. Close the doors to client rooms and stairwells as well as fire doors between adjacent units. Wait for further directions.
6. Place moist towels or bath blankets at the threshold of doors if smoke is escaping.
7. Use an appropriate fire extinguisher if necessary.

Rescue and Evacuation

The first priority is to rescue clients in the immediate vicinity of the fire. Nurses lead those who can walk to a safe area and close the room and fire doors after exiting. Using a variety of techniques, nursing personnel evacuate those who cannot walk (Fig. 19-7).

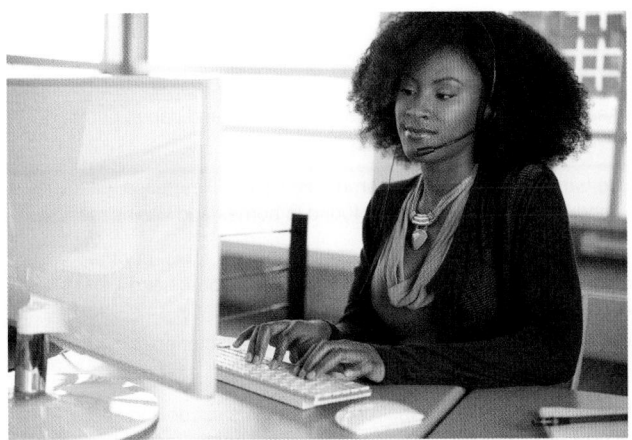

FIGURE 19-6 The nurse notifies the switchboard operator who will announce and initiate the fire plan and notify the fire department. (ESB Basic/Shutterstock.)

Fire Extinguishers

There are various types of fire extinguishers (Table 19-4). Each type is labeled. Nurses must know the type of extinguisher that is appropriate for the burning substance and how to use it (Nursing Guidelines 19-1). The U.S. Fire Administration (2022) recommends remembering the mnemonic "PASS":

- *P*ull the pin with the extinguisher in a downward position and release the locking mechanism.
- *A*im the nozzle of the extinguisher at the base of the fire.
- *S*queeze the lever slowly and evenly.
- *S*weep the nozzle from side to side.

Asphyxiation

Asphyxiation (an inability to breathe) can result from airway obstruction (see Chapter 37), drowning, or inhalation of noxious gases such as smoke or carbon monoxide (CO).

Smoke Inhalation

Smoke can be more deadly than fire. It consists of incinerated particles, chemicals, and gases. The effects range from asphyxiation to chemical irritation and thermal damage. Health care facilities have banned cigarette smoking; consequently, smoke inhalation in those locations now accounts for far fewer deaths. However, when a fire occurs, regardless of its location or cause, smoke inhalation rather than burn injuries results.

Symptoms from smoke inhalation range from coughing to impaired judgment, unconsciousness, and respiratory arrest. If superheated gases are inhaled, they can burn the respiratory tract and form **carboxyhemoglobin** (compound of CO with hemoglobin) in the bloodstream, thereby depriving oxygen to the brain and other vital organs (Fig. 19-8).

Despite efforts to ban smoking, there continues to be a risk for fires from smoking in health care facilities and other nonresidential locations. Home fires may occur when people who smoke fall asleep with a burning cigarette or when children play with matches or lighters.

Many homes and apartment buildings are equipped with smoke detectors. However, some people dismantle their smoke detector when it begins to emit an audible alarm signaling low battery power, and they fail to replace the batteries twice a year when going from and into daylight, saving time as recommended.

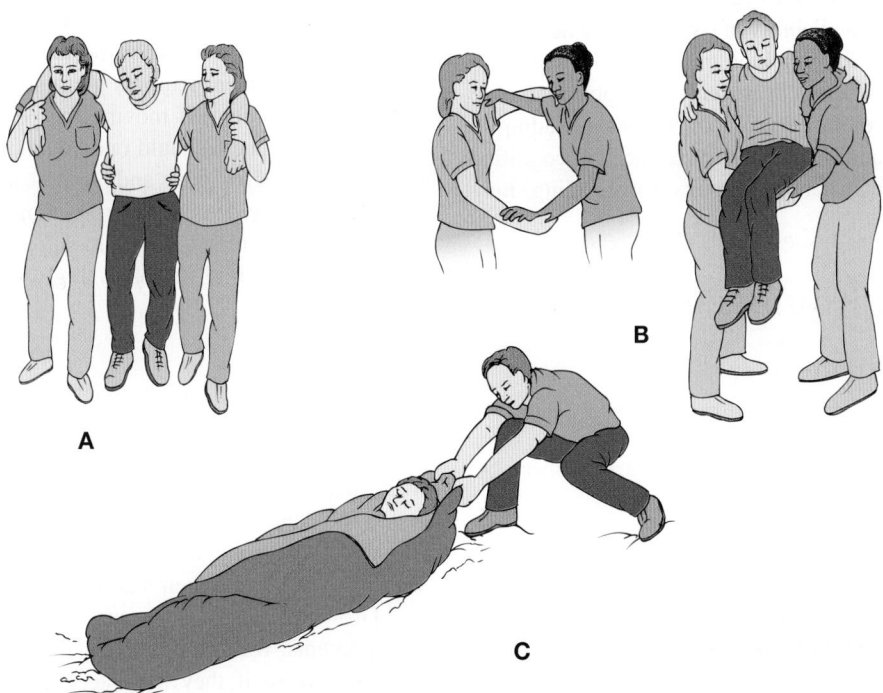

FIGURE 19-7 Evacuation of clients. **A.** Human crutches—rescuers secure a weak but ambulatory client's arm and waist. **B.** Seat carry—rescuers interlock arms and carry a nonambulatory client. **C.** Body drag—rescuer drags an unconscious victim or one who cannot assist on a blanket or sheet.

TABLE 19-4 Types of Fire Extinguishers and Uses

TYPE	SYMBOL	CONTENTS	USE
Class A	A	Water under pressure	For use with ordinary materials like cloth, wood, and paper. Often found in homes and businesses.
Class B	B	Carbon dioxide	For use with combustible and flammable liquids like grease, gasoline, oil, and oil-based paints. Often found in homes and businesses.
Class C	C	Dry chemicals	For use with electrical equipment like appliances, tools, or other equipment that is plugged in. Often found in homes and businesses.
Class D	D	Dry powder agent	For use with flammable metals. Often found in factories.
Class K	K	Wet chemical agent composed of potassium	For use with vegetable oils, animal oils, and fats in cooking appliances. Often found in commercial kitchens (restaurants, cafeterias, catering businesses).

U.S. Fire Administration. (n.d.). *Choosing and using fire extinguishers.* https://www.usfa.fema.gov/prevention/home-fires/prepare-for-fire/fire-extinguishers/index.html

Carbon Monoxide Poisoning

CO is extremely lethal because it is colorless, odorless, and tasteless, making poisoning with it an "invisible death." CO is released during the incomplete combustion of carbon products, such as fossil fuels; some examples in which CO poisoning can occur include when unvented kerosene or space heaters are used, when a chimney is blocked or partially obstructed, when a motor vehicle attached to a garage is allowed to stand idling, and when using a hibachi or charcoal grill indoors.

When inhaled, CO binds with hemoglobin in preference to oxygen; consequently, there is little oxygen available to cells and tissues. In addition, CO binds to myoglobin, the protein that carries and stores oxygen in muscle cells like the heart. With a reduced availability of oxygen to the heart, cardiac output is decreased and blood pressure falls, depriving the brain of oxygen. When cells suffer from hypoxia, aerobic metabolism is replaced by anaerobic metabolism, leading to metabolic acidosis and death. If survival occurs, cognitive defects, such as impairment in memory and learning, may persist (Fig. 19-9).

 NURSING GUIDELINES 19-1

Using a Fire Extinguisher

- Know the location of each type of fire extinguisher. *Doing so minimizes response time.*
- Free the extinguisher from its enclosure. *The extinguisher must be removed for use.*
- Remove the pin that locks the handle. *The pin must be removed for use.*
- Aim the nozzle near the edge, not the center, of the fire. *The chemical will contain the fire.*
- Move the nozzle from side to side. *Doing so increases the effectiveness of fire control.*
- Avoid skin contact with the contents of the fire extinguisher. *The chemicals in the extinguisher can cause injury.*
- Return the extinguisher to the maintenance department. *The extinguisher will be replaced or refilled for future use.*

The average level of CO in homes is 5 to 15 parts per million (ppm). Prolonged exposure to levels above 70 ppm produces flu-like symptoms, such as headache, nausea, vomiting, weakness, and confusion. When CO gases accumulate above 150 to 200 ppm, disorientation, unconsciousness, and death are possible. One of the classic signs of CO poisoning is a bright cherry red skin color that may persist even after death occurs (Fig. 19-10).

Prevention and Treatment

Because CO can be present even without smoke, the nurse recommends that CO detectors should be installed in all homes and the fire department should be summoned to investigate alarms. Without detectors, victims may be unaware that their symptoms are due to the accumulating level of CO (Box 19-2). If a person is suspected of being poisoned by CO, initial treatment requires getting the victim out of the present environment. If moving the person out of doors is impossible, rescuers should open windows and doors to reduce the level of toxic gas and promote adequate ventilation. Once emergency personnel arrive, they administer oxygen. In the case of extremely high blood levels of CO, the victim may be treated with hyperbaric (high-pressure) oxygen (see Chapter 21).

Drowning

Drowning is when fluid occupies the airway and interferes with ventilation. It can happen to swimmers and nonswimmers alike. Accidental drownings occur during water activities, such as fishing, boating, swimming, and water skiing. Some incidents are linked to alcohol misuse, which tends to interfere with judgment and promotes risk-taking. Other victims overestimate their stamina.

Drownings can also occur at home or in health care environments. Young children can drown if left momentarily in a bathtub or if they have access to a swimming pool. Swimming pools should be fenced and locked, and children should never be left unattended in a bathtub or pool.

Although the potential for drowning in a health care institution is statistically remote, it can happen. Therefore,

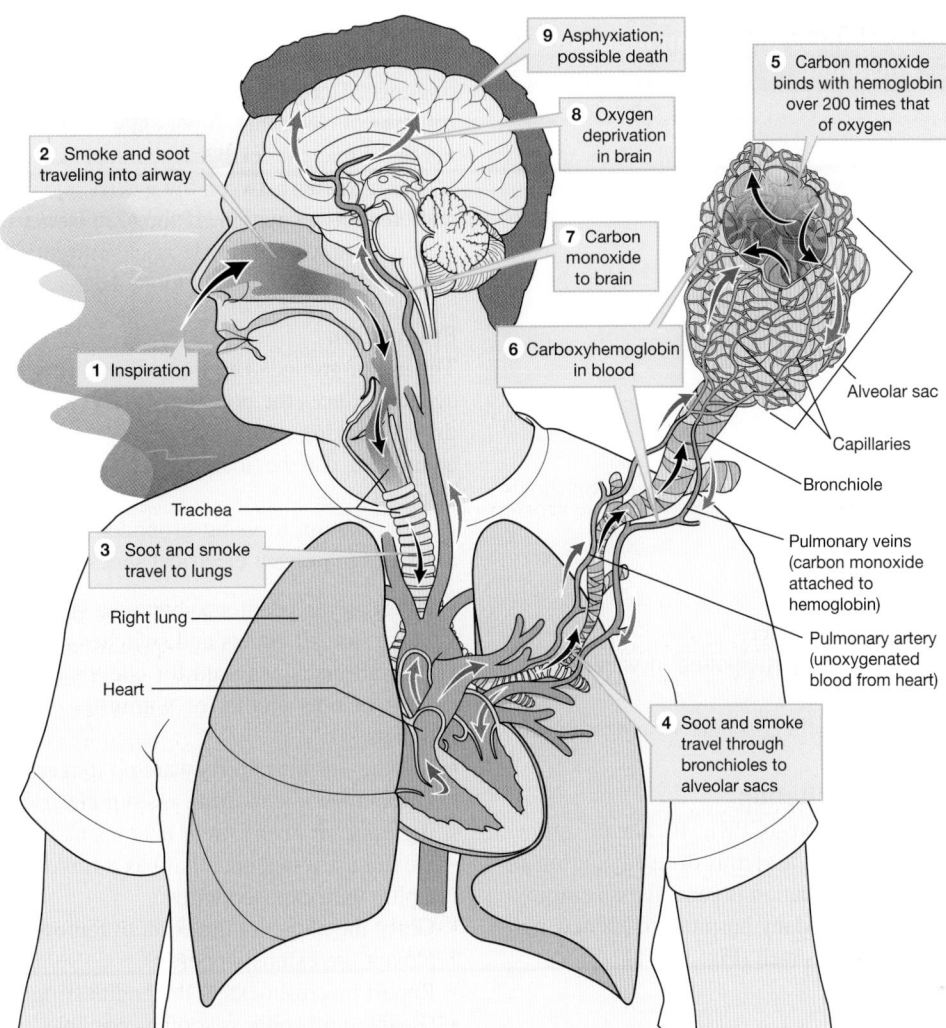

FIGURE 19-8 Effects produced by smoke inhalation.

nurses should never leave any helpless or cognitively impaired client, young or old, alone in a tub of water, regardless of its depth.

Prevention

Victims of cold water drownings are more likely to be resuscitated because the cold temperature lowers metabolism,

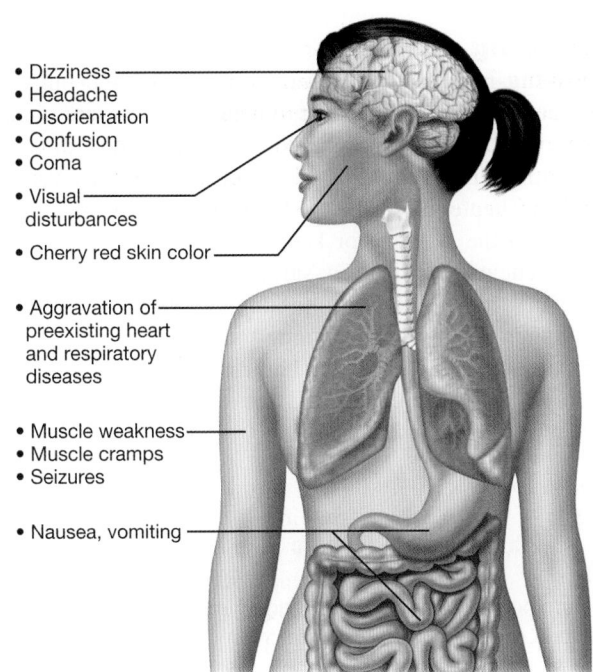

FIGURE 19-9 Symptoms associated with carbon monoxide poisoning.

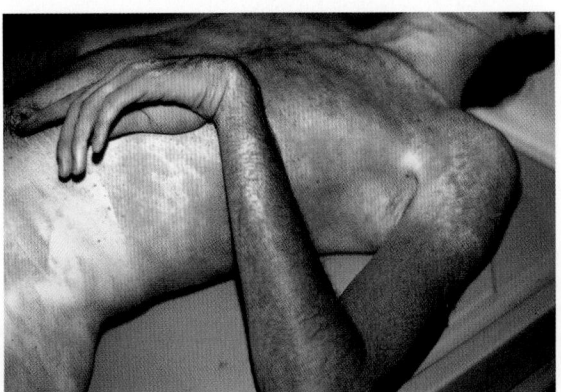

FIGURE 19-10 Bright cherry red skin color in a victim of carbon monoxide poisoning. (From Preston, R. R., & Wilson, T. [2019]. *Lippincott illustrated reviews: Physiology* [2nd ed.]. Lippincott Williams & Wilkins.)

BOX 19-2	Symptoms of Carbon Monoxide Poisoning

Nausea

Vomiting

Headache

Dizziness

Muscle weakness

Confusion

Shortness of breath

Cherry red skin color

Loss of consciousness

thus conserving oxygen (see Chapter 12). Prevention, however, is far better:

- Learn to swim.
- Never swim alone.
- Wear an approved flotation device.
- Do not drink alcohol when participating in water-related sports.
- Notify a law enforcement officer if boaters appear unsafe.

Cardiopulmonary Resuscitation

Cardiopulmonary resuscitation (CPR), if begun immediately, may be lifesaving for a victim of asphyxiation or drowning. Current CPR certification is generally an employment requirement for nurses. Many hospitals teach new parents how to administer CPR as well (Fig. 19-11).

Electrical Shock

Electrical shock (the discharge of electricity through the body) is a potential hazard wherever there are machines and electrical equipment. The body is susceptible to electrical shock because it is composed of water and electrolytes, both of which are good conductors of electricity. A **conductor** is a substance that facilitates the flow of electrical current; an **insulator** is a substance that contains electrical currents so they do not scatter. Electric cords are covered with rubber or some other insulating substance.

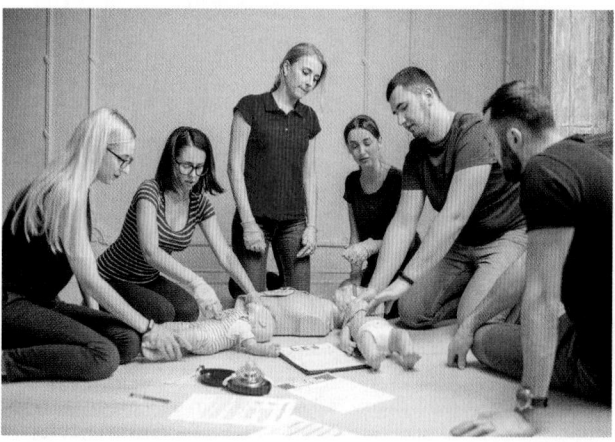

FIGURE 19-11 Parents being taught cardiopulmonary resuscitation as part of discharge planning. (RossHelen/Shutterstock.)

Macroshock is a harmless distribution of low-amperage electricity over a large area of the body. It feels like a slight tingling. **Microshock** is low-voltage but high-amperage distribution of electricity. A person with intact skin usually does not feel a microshock because intact skin offers resistance or acts as a barrier between the electrical current and the water and electrolytes within. If the skin is wet or its integrity is impaired, however, the electrical current can be fatal, especially if delivered directly to the heart.

Prevention

The use of grounded equipment in the home and health care agency reduces the potential for electrical shock. A **ground** diverts leaking electrical energy to the earth. Grounded equipment can be identified by the presence of a three-pronged plug.

In addition to using grounded equipment, other safety measures to prevent electrical shock include:

- Never use an adaptor to bypass a grounded outlet.
- Make sure all outlets and switches have cover plates.
- Plug all machines used for client care into outlets within 12 ft of one another or within the same cluster of wall outlets.
- Unplug machines if they are no longer necessary.
- Discourage clients from resting electric hair dryers, curling irons, or razors on or near a sink that contains water.
- Do not use a machine that has a frayed or cracked cord or a plug with exposed wires.
- Grasp the plug, not the cord, to remove it from an outlet.
- Do not use extension cords.
- Report macroshocks to the engineering department.
- Clean liquid spills as soon as possible.
- Stand clear of the client and bed during cardiac defibrillation.

Poisoning

Poisoning is an injury caused by the ingestion, inhalation, or absorption of a toxic substance. These are more common in homes than in health care institutions, though medication errors could be considered a form of poisoning (see Chapter 32). Preventing medication errors is addressed in the NPSGs for keeping people safe in health care agencies. Medication safety is discussed in more depth in Unit 9, Medication Administration. Accidental poisonings usually occur among toddlers and commonly involve substances located in bathrooms or kitchens (Box 19-3). Many children treated for accidental poisoning have repeat episodes.

 P h a r m a c o l o g i c   C o n s i d e r a t i o n s

Acetaminophen overdose is a leading cause of acute liver failure in children. Individuals are often unaware they have exceeded the daily recommended dose of 3 g when fever and pain relief drugs are coupled with over-the-counter cough and cold remedies that also contain acetaminophen.

<table>
</table>

BOX 19-3 — Common Substances Associated with Childhood Poisonings

Drugs: Particularly over-the-counter remedies, such as aspirin, acetaminophen, and other pain pills, topical medicines, vitamins, antihistamines, antacids, antibiotics, dietary supplements, herbals, and homeopathic remedies
Cleaning agents: Bleach, toilet bowl or tank disks, detergent pods, and drain cleaners
Paint solvents: Turpentine, kerosene, and gasoline
Heavy metals: Lead paint chips
Chemical products: Glue, shoe polish, antifreeze, and insecticides
Cosmetics: Hair dye, shampoo, and nail polish remover
Plants: Mistletoe berries, rhubarb leaves, foxglove, and castor beans

Poison Control National Capital Poison Center. (2020). *Poison statistics national data 2020*. https://www.poison.org/poison-statistics-national

Health care facilities have fewer poisonings because they secure medications. By law, they must keep chemicals such as liquid antiseptics, which are intended for external use, separate from other drugs. Nevertheless, medication errors persist (see Chapter 32) in which the wrong medication or dose at an incorrect time is administered or given to the wrong client.

Prevention

Children should be educated about the hazards of poisons. The American Association of Poison Control Centers promotes awareness for assistance with accidental poisoning with a "poison help" logo (Fig. 19-12). The logo provides a nationwide toll-free number that, when dialed, automatically connects the caller to the closest poison control center. Nurses and pharmacists who are certified specialists in poison information answer emergency calls around the clock. All nurses can teach parents and others how to reduce the risk of poisoning in the home (Client and Family Teaching 19-2). Adults who have trouble remembering or who cannot administer their own medications safely can use containers prefilled by a responsible person (Fig. 19-13).

Treatment

Initial treatment for a victim of suspected poisoning involves maintaining breathing and cardiac function. After that, rescuers attempt to identify what was ingested, how much, and when. Definitive treatment depends on the substance, the

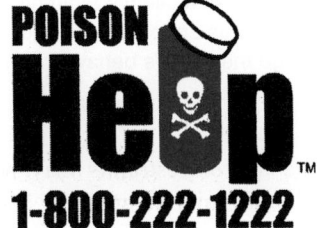

FIGURE 19-12 The toll-free number provides immediate access to an expert at a poison control center with answers to questions about poisons and poisonings.

Client and Family Teaching 19-2 Preventing Childhood Poisoning

The nurse teaches the parents or the caregivers the following:
* Install child-resistant latches on cupboard doors.
* Request childproof caps on all prescription medications.
* Buy chemicals and nonprescription drugs with tamper-proof lids.
* Never transfer a toxic substance to a container usually used for storing food.
* Do not refer to medications as "candy," and do not tell children they taste "yummy."
* Do not keep drugs in your purse.
* Remind grandparents or babysitters to "childproof" their homes.
* Remove toxic houseplants from the home.
* Keep the home well ventilated when using an aerosol or another substance that leaves lingering fumes in the air.

client's condition, and if the substance is still in the stomach. For ingestions of commercial products containing multiple ingredients, the poison control center is consulted. Otherwise, treatment follows the decision tree in Figure 19-14.

Falls

More than any other injury discussed thus far, falls are the most common accident experienced by older adults and have the most serious consequences for this age group. According to the Centers for Disease Control and Prevention (CDC), each year, 3 million older people are treated in emergency departments for fall injuries, and at least 300,000 older people are hospitalized for hip fractures (2023b).

Most falls among older adults occur at home. Common injuries include those to the head, wrist, spine, and hip.

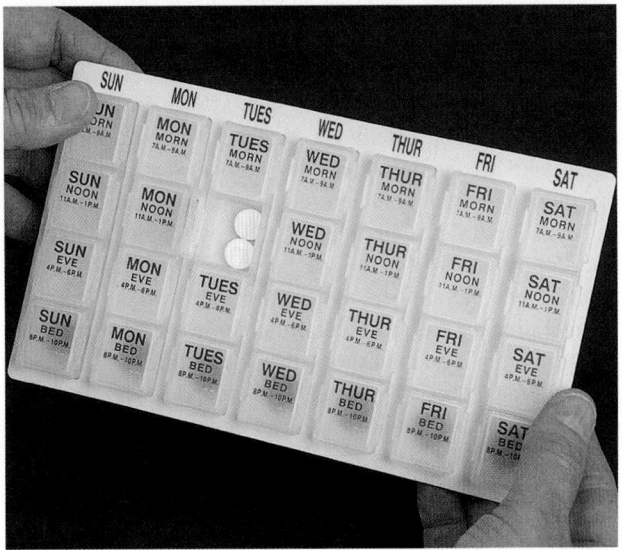

FIGURE 19-13 A pill organizer may help reduce the incidence of medication overdoses. (Photo by B. Proud.)

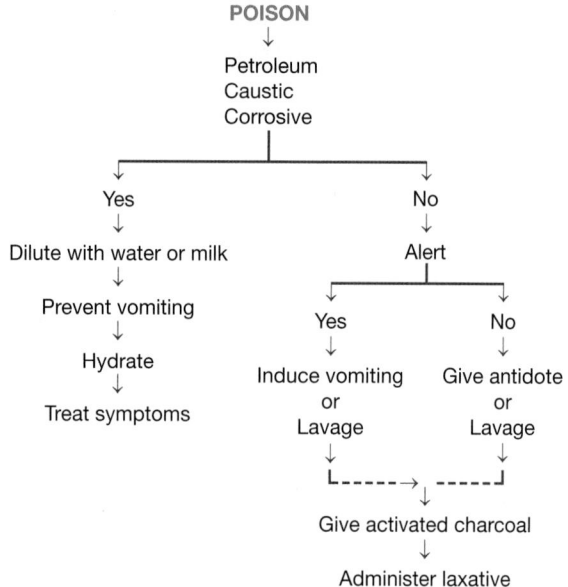

POISON
↓
Petroleum
Caustic
Corrosive

Yes → Dilute with water or milk → Prevent vomiting → Hydrate → Treat symptoms

No → Alert

Yes → Induce vomiting or Lavage

No → Give antidote or Lavage

Give activated charcoal
↓
Administer laxative

FIGURE 19-14 Decision tree for treating ingested poisons.

Many who survive a fall suffer years of disability, impaired mobility, and pain.

The incidence of falls in general as well as in hospitals must be reduced not only for the associated pain and suffering but also for financial reasons. In 2020, the total medical costs for falls were more than $50 billion, and Medicare and Medicaid paid for 75% of these expenses (CDC, 2023a). As an incentive to control costs, the Centers for Medicare & Medicaid Services (CMS) has classified falls as one of several **hospital-acquired conditions** (HACs). An HAC is a complication of hospitalization that is reasonably preventable. As such, CMS will no longer cover the cost of care that was incurred by a fall. Several major private insurers are adopting similar reimbursement practices in cases of preventable medical errors (National Conference of State Legislatures, 2020).

Contributing Factors

Older adults are more prone to falls for several reasons. Many have age-related changes such as visual impairments and disorders that affect gait, balance, and coordination. Some take medications that lower blood pressure, causing dizziness upon rising. Others have urinary urgency and rush to reach the toilet. Other social and environmental factors also contribute to the risk of falling. For example, older adults may wear slippers to accommodate swollen feet. Although slippers are more comfortable, less expensive, and less tiring to put on than shoes, they might offer less support or traction. Clutter may accumulate around the house if the older adult lacks the energy to clean or does not want to discard old items.

For hospitalized older adults, the risk for falls increases. They are in an unfamiliar environment. They must rely on nursing assistance for mobility, and such assistance may not be prompt. Medications and altered health status may cause temporary confusion and poor judgment.

Assessment

Determining which clients are at higher risk can prevent some falls. Identifying at-risk clients and preventing falls are also the NPSGs (see Table 19-1). Accredited hospitals and long-term care (LTC) agencies use assessment tools to determine which clients need fall prevention protocols (Fig. 19-15).

Prevention

Different fall prevention approaches are used in the home and health care facilities. Measures for preventing falls are modified based on the client's circumstances (Client and Family Teaching 19-3).

Older adults should keep a list of emergency numbers posted by the phone. Those who live alone may want to become part of a daily phone tree in which someone investigates if an older adult does not call in or answer a call. Personal response services are also available in which the subscriber wears a wireless, waterproof pendant with a button that they can use to summon help in an emergency. Activating the button places a call to the manufacturer's emergency response center; once connected, the user can carry on a two-way hands-free conversation. The center directs calls for assistance to predetermined people, such as family, neighbors, the physician, or emergency personnel. If the user cannot communicate, the center dispatches emergency personnel to the user's location.

RESTRAINTS

In health care agencies, fall prevention measures are necessary for identified clients. The use of restraints, however, is closely regulated. **Physical restraints** are methods that immobilize or reduce the ability of a client to freely move their arms, legs, body, or head. **Chemical restraints** are medications that are not a standard treatment or dosage for the client's condition but rather are used to manage a client's behavior or freedom of movement. These are generally warranted to manage violent or self-destructive behavior that jeopardizes the immediate physical safety of the client, staff, or others. The goal is to use the least restrictive type of restraint possible and only as a last resort when the risk of injury to the client or others is too high.

 Concept Mastery Alert

Chemical Restraints

Remember, chemical restraints are not medications commonly included as part of a client's regimen. Rather, they are medications, such as antipsychotic agents, given to specifically manage the client's behavior or freedom of movement.

Although the use of restraints may be intended to prevent falls and other injuries, in many cases, their risks outweigh their benefits. Restrained clients become increasingly confused; suffer chronic constipation, incontinence, and infections such as pneumonia and pressure injuries; and experience a progressive decline in their

Hendrich II Fall Risk Model

RISK FACTOR	RISK POINTS	SCORE
Confusion/Disorientation/Impulsivity	4	
Symptomatic Depression	2	
Altered Elimination	1	
Dizziness/Vertigo	1	
Gender (Male)	1	
Any Administered Antiepileptics (Anticonvulsants): (Carbamazepine, Divalproex Sodium, Ethotoin, Ethosuximide, Felbamate, Fosphenytoin, Gabapentin, Lamotrigine, Mephenytoin, Methsuximide, Phenobarbital, Phenytoin, Primidone, Topiramate, Trimethadione, Valproic Acid)[1]	2	
Any Administered Benzodiazepines:[2] (Alprazolam, Chlordiazepoxide, Clonazepam, Clorazepate Dipotassium, Diazepam, Flurazepam, Halazepam,[3] Lorazepam, Midazolam, Oxazepam, Temazepam, Triazolam)	1	
Get-Up-and-Go Test: "Rising from a Chair" If unable to assess, monitor for change in activity level, assess other risk factors, document both on patient chart with date and time.		
Ability to Rise in Single Movement—No Loss of Balance with Steps	0	
Pushes Up, Successful in One Attempt	1	
Multiple Attempts Successful	3	
Unable to Rise without Assistance During Test If unable to assess, document this on the patient chart with the date and time.	4	
(A Score of 5 or Greater = High Risk)	**TOTAL SCORE**	

© 2012 AHI of Indiana, Inc. All rights reserved. U.S. Patent No. 7,282,031 and U.S. Patent No. 7,682,308. Reproduction of copyright and patented materials without authorization is a violation of federal law.

Ongoing Medication Review Updates:

[1] Levetiracetam (Keppra) was not assessed during the original research conducted to create the Hendrich Fall Risk Model. As an antiepileptic, levetiracetam does have a side effect of somnolence and dizziness, which contributes to its fall risk and should be scored (effective June 2010).

[2] The study did not include the effect of benzodiazepine-like drugs since they were not on the market at the time. However, due to their similarity in drug structure, mechanism of action, and drug effects, they should also be scored (effective January 2010).

[3] Halazepam was included in the study but is no longer available in the United States (effective June 2010).

FIGURE 19-15 The Hendrich II Fall Risk Model, a fall risk assessment tool recommended by the Hartford Institute for Geriatric Nursing. (Used with permission of Ann Hendrich, Inc.)

Client and Family Teaching 19-3 Preventing Falls

The nurse teaches the client or the family as follows:

- Keep the environment well lit.
- Install and use handrails on stairs inside and outside the home.
- Place a strip of light-colored adhesive tape on the edge of each stair for visibility.
- Remove scatter rugs.
- Keep extension cords next to the wall.
- Do not wax floors.
- Wear well-fitting shoes that enclose the heel and toe of the foot and have nonskid soles.
- Keep pathways clutter free.
- Wear short robes without cloth belts that may loosen and trip the client.
- Use a cane or walker if prescribed.
- Replace the tip on a cane as it wears down.
- Stay indoors when the weather is icy or snowy.
- Sit down when using public transportation, even if it means asking someone for their seat.
- Install and use grab bars in the shower and near the toilet.
- Place a nonskid mat or decals on the floor of the tub or shower.
- Use soap-on-a-rope or a suspended container of liquid soap to prevent slipping on a loose soap bar.
- Use a flashlight or nightlight when it is dark.
- Make sure pets are not underfoot.
- Mop up spills immediately.
- Use long-handled tongs rather than climbing on a chair to reach high objects.

ability to perform activities of daily living. Restrained clients are more likely to die during their hospital stay than those who are not restrained.

It is unethical and a violation of TJC's standards to use physical or chemical restraints for disciplinary reasons or to compensate for limited personnel. Restraints must be the last intervention after trying all other measures to solve the problem. Nurses must take measures to protect the restrained client's autonomy, health, safety, dignity, rights, and well-being.

Legislation

After research studies revealed the widespread use of physical restraints in LTC facilities, federal legislation known as the *Nursing Home Reform Law* was incorporated in the Omnibus Budget Reconciliation Act (OBRA) in 1987 (Box 19-4). Compliance with the law has been mandatory since 1990.

Accreditation Standards

TJC followed the lead of the OBRA legislation by developing restraint and seclusion standards in 1991. They continue to revise these standards, which differ for nonpsychiatric and psychiatric institutions; the most recent revision occurred in 2022. The standards address three areas: agency restraint protocol, medical orders, and client monitoring and documentation of nursing care.

Agency Restraint Protocol

A **protocol** is a plan or set of steps to follow when implementing an intervention. During TJC inspection, the accrediting team examines an agency's protocol for restraint use that the medical staff has approved. The protocol must identify the criteria that justify the application and discontinuation of restraints. Nonphysical interventions, such as reorienting a person to place and circumstances, or "time-out," which involves removing the client from the immediate environment to a quiet room, is preferred. In the case of a

---

BOX 19-4	**OBRA Legislation Addressing Restraints**

The Omnibus Budget Reconciliation Act of 1987 specifies that:

The resident (patient) has the right to be free from any physical restraints imposed or psychoactive drug administered for purposes of discipline or convenience, and not required to treat the resident's (patient's) medical symptoms. ... Restraints may only be imposed to ensure the physical safety of the resident or other residents and only upon the written order of a physician that specifies the duration and the circumstances under which the restraints are to be used (except in emergency situations which must be addressed in the facility's restraint policy).

---

client attempting to remove an endotracheal tube that facilitates mechanical ventilation, personnel must first attempt less restrictive measures, such as having someone sit with the client.

Medical Orders

A physician must write a restraint order, or a nurse must obtain one from a physician by telephone within 1 hour after the restraint is initiated. If a physician is unavailable, a registered nurse who has knowledge, training, and experience in the techniques that necessitate the use of restraints may initiate restraint use based on appropriate assessment of the client. If need for a restraint used to protect the physical safety of a nonviolent or nondestructive client is ongoing, the physician must renew the medical order according to the agency's protocol.

Monitoring and Documentation

The client's chart must contain documented evidence of frequent and regular nursing assessments of the restrained client's vital signs, circulation, skin conditions or signs of injury, psychological status and comfort, and readiness for discontinuing restraint. In addition, the nurse must record nursing care concerning toileting, nutrition, hydration, and range of motion while the client is restrained. The documented care must reflect the agency's established protocol. The nurse also promptly communicates with the client's family regarding the need for restraints and notes the time in the documentation. When the assessment findings indicate that the client has improved, the nurse must legally and ethically remove the restraint.

Restraint Alternatives

Agencies are being challenged to implement interventions that protect clients from injury while ensuring their freedom, mobility, and dignity. The intent of both the OBRA legislation and TJC standards is to promote **restraint alternatives** (protective or adaptive devices that promote client safety and postural support but that the client can release independently) and, eventually, restraint-free client care.

Restraint alternatives are generally appropriate for clients who tend to need repositioning to maintain their body alignment or improve their independence and functional status. Some examples include seat inserts or gripping materials that prevent sliding, support pillows, seat belts or harnesses with front-releasing Velcro or buckle closures, and commercial or homemade tilt wedges (Fig. 19-16). If the client is unaware of or cannot release the restraint alternative, it is considered a restraint.

Other supplementary measures may also reduce the need for restraints. Health care providers are encouraged to improve gait training, provide physical exercise, reorient clients, encourage assistive ambulatory devices such as walkers and hall rails, and use electronic seat and bed

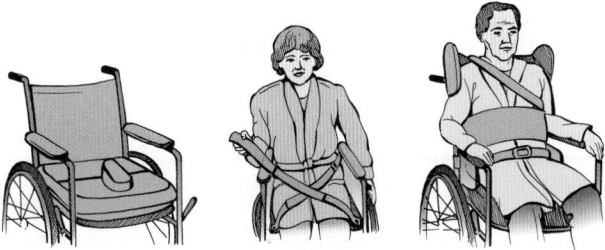

FIGURE 19-16 Examples of restraint alternatives.

>>> *Stop, Think, and Respond 19-1*
List some methods for avoiding a lawsuit when restraints are necessary.

monitors that sound an alarm when clients get up without assistance (Fig. 19-17). Before considering the use of physical restraints, the nurse observes and documents the client's response to other alternatives. When clients are in a wheelchair, nurses must position them correctly.

Use of Restraints

When the use of restraints is justified, nurses and the health care providers they supervise must demonstrate continued competency in their safe application. Skill 19-1 explains how to apply restraints and use them appropriately.

NURSING IMPLICATIONS

Nurses must recognize safety hazards and identify clients at greatest risk for injury. Once they gather and analyze the data, they may identify several nursing diagnoses:

- Latex allergy reaction
- Injury risk
- Acute confusion
- Chronic confusion

Nursing Care Plan 19-1 gives sample interventions for a client like the one described in the Clinical Scenario with a nursing diagnosis of injury risk. *Injury risk* is defined as the state in which a person is at risk for injury as a result of environmental conditions interacting with the individual's adaptive and protective resources.

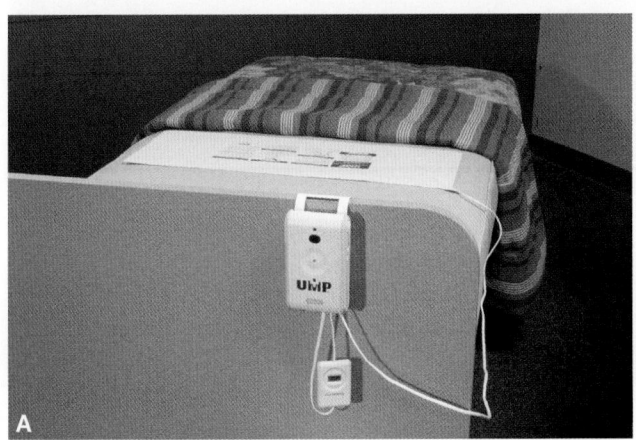
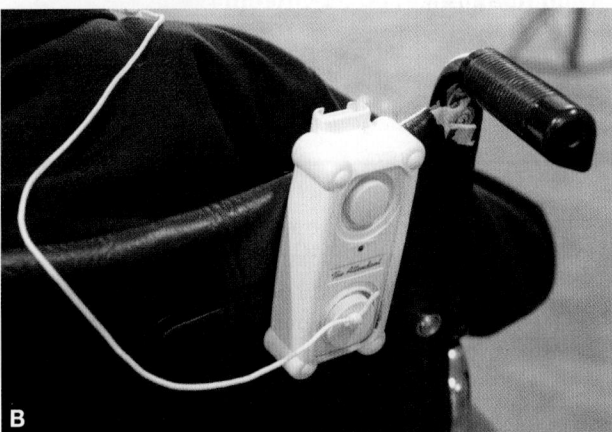

FIGURE 19-17 Alarm devices used in lieu of a restraint to alert nursing staff of a client who is wandering. **A.** Bed alarm. **B.** Wheelchair alarm.

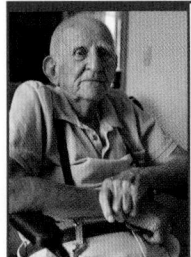

Clinical Scenario   A nurse makes a home visit to an 80-year-old male client who depends on a wheelchair and walker for mobility. The nurse discovers that the client postpones using the toilet until it becomes absolutely necessary due to the effort involved in navigating to the bathroom. The nurse believes that the client is not drinking sufficient fluids to maintain a stable blood pressure. The nurse consults the client, his family, and physician about transferring him to an extended care facility for a period of time to obtain physical therapy to improve his muscle strength and ambulation skills to avoid further injuries.

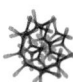

NURSING CARE PLAN 19-1 | Injury Risk

Assessment
- Note evidence of altered mental status.
- Determine signs of impaired mobility, balance, and coordination.
- Take vital signs and document postural changes in blood pressure.

- Consult drug references for medications that cause sensory or motor effects or deficits.
- Check the client's use of an ambulatory aid, such as crutches, canes, or a walker.
- Communicate with the client regarding self-assessment of functional status.

Nursing Diagnosis. **Injury risk** related to impaired mobility and postural hypotension as evidenced by a difference of 20 mm Hg in systolic pressure when lying and standing (135/85 lying; 115/80 standing), previous fall that resulted in a fractured hip, inconsistent use of walker, and client's statement, "I've had some near-falls at home since my surgery. I get dizzy when I hurry, and my feet get all tangled up."

Expected Outcome. The client will remain free of injury throughout the duration of care.

Interventions	Rationales
Assess blood pressure (BP) lying and standing daily at 0800.	Determines the effects of postural changes on BP regulation
Keep the bed in a low position.	Facilitates safety when relocating from the bed to a wheelchair, chair, or walker to ambulate
Reinforce the need to use the call signal.	Obtaining assistance with ambulation reduces the potential for falling.
Assist the client into a sitting position until dizziness passes before standing.	Given time, baroreceptors for regulating BP can adjust to accommodate for venous pooling.
Keep the walker within reach at all times.	Enhances the possibility that the client will use the ambulatory aid
Help client put on nonskid shoes or slippers and glasses for ambulation.	Footwear with traction and support and maximizing vision help reduce the risk for falling.

Evaluation of Expected Outcomes

- Ambulation is delayed briefly until dizziness has passed.
- Client is assisted with putting on nonskid slippers and glasses before ambulating.
- Client ambulates with assistance and the use of a walker.
- No falls occur.

Despite appropriate assessments and plans for preventing injuries, accidents still occur. When they do, the nurse's first concerns are the safety of the client and the potential for allegations of malpractice. Therefore, if an accident occurs, the nurse takes the following actions:

- Checks the client's condition immediately
- Calls for help if the client is in danger

- Begins resuscitation measures if necessary
- Comforts and reassures the client
- Avoids moving the client until safe to do so
- Reports the accident and assessment findings to the physician
- Completes an incident report as soon as the client is stabilized (see Chapter 3)

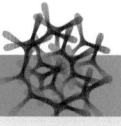

KEY POINTS

- NPSGs: The purpose of the NPSGs is to improve patient safety. The goals address problems in the following areas:
  - Patient identification
  - Staff communication
  - Medication safety
  - Alarm safety
  - Infection prevention
  - Identifying patient safety risks
  - Preventing mistakes in surgery
- Age-related safety factors
  - Infants and toddlers

- School-aged children and adolescents
- Adults
- Environmental hazards
  - Latex allergies: Minimize or eliminate latex exposure
  - Burns: Burn prevention, fire plans, safety management, fire extinguishers
  - Asphyxiation: Smoke inhalation, carbon monoxide poisoning
  - Drowning: Prevention and CPR
  - Electrical shock: Prevention and grounded cords
  - Poisoning: Prevention and poison control centers
  - Falls: Age, medications, clutter; fall prevention

- Restraints
  - Physical: Methods that immobilize or reduce the ability of a client to freely move their arms, legs, body, or head
  - Chemical: Medications that are not a standard treatment or dosage for the client's condition but rather are used to manage a client's behavior or freedom of movement

- Agency restraint protocol: A plan or set of steps to follow when implementing an intervention
- Restraint alternatives: Protective or adaptive devices that promote client safety and postural support but that the client can release independently for, eventually, restraint-free client care

CRITICAL THINKING EXERCISES

1. What rationale would you give as the reason TJC identified NPSG as a criterion for compliance with accreditation?
2. If someone you know is contemplating a career in nursing but is hesitant because of a latex allergy, what information would you offer?
3. When discharging an older adult to the care of a family member, what safety measures are appropriate to include in the discharge instructions?
4. Without resorting to the use of restraints, how can you prevent falls in a client with an unsteady gait?

NEXT-GENERATION NCLEX-STYLE REVIEW QUESTIONS

1. When examining an unconscious client, which nursing assessment finding is most indicative of CO poisoning?
   a. Bilaterally dilated pupils
   b. Cherry red skin color
   c. Smoky odor to clothing
   d. Rapid, irregular pulse rate
   Test-Taking Strategy: Note the key word and modifier, "most indicative." Eliminate any options that are incorrect; narrow the selection to the one option that is better than any of the others.

2. Place the following nursing actions in the order they should be performed when a fire is discovered.
   a. Clear the halls of visitors and equipment.
   b. Locate and use a fire extinguisher.
   c. Notify the switchboard operator.
   d. Shut doors to rooms and stairwells.
   e. Rescue persons near the fire.
   Test-Taking Strategy: Analyze the options and place them in a sequence that is consistent with health care agency fire plans.

3. When providing health teaching to caregivers, which should be the priority focus for preventing injuries to older adults?
   a. Chemical poisoning
   b. Thermal burns
   c. Electrical shock
   d. Accidental falls
   Test-Taking Strategy: Note the key word and modifier, "priority focus." Analyze the choices and select the hazard that most commonly affects older adults.

4. Which nursing action is best to recommend initially when someone reports that an alert person has just ingested multiple medications in a suicide attempt?
   a. Induce vomiting.
   b. Administer an antacid.
   c. Transport the person to the emergency department.
   d. Call the person's personal physician immediately.
   Test-Taking Strategy: Note the key words, "best," "initially," and "just ingested." Analyze the options and select the most immediate priority before proceeding with any of the other actions.

5. If a nurse determines that a physical restraint is necessary to maintain a client's safety, which action is essential?
   a. Obtaining a medical order for its use
   b. Notifying the nursing supervisor
   c. Administering a mild sedative
   d. Relocating the client near the nursing station.
   Test-Taking Strategy: Note the key word, "essential." Analyze the options to select one nursing action that must be implemented.

NEXT-GENERATION NCLEX-STYLE CLINICAL SCENARIO QUESTIONS

Clinical Scenario:

A nurse makes a home visit to an 80-year-old male client who depends on a wheelchair and walker for mobility. The nurse discovers that the client postpones using the toilet until it becomes absolutely necessary due to the effort involved in navigating to the bathroom. The nurse believes that the client is not drinking sufficient fluids to maintain a stable blood pressure. The nurse consults the client, his family, and physician about transferring him to an extended care facility for a period of time to obtain physical therapy to improve his muscle strength and ambulation skills to avoid further injuries.

Place an "x" under "effective" identifying behaviors that would promote the client's health. Place an "x" under "ineffective" identifying poor behavioral health choices.

BEHAVIOR	EFFECTIVE	INEFFECTIVE
Postponing toilet use		
Using the wheelchair and walker		
Not drinking enough fluids		
Transfer to LTC facility		
Physical therapy program		
Poorly placed throw rugs in the home's hallways, between the bedroom and bathroom		

SKILL 19-1 Using Physical Restraints

Suggested Action	Reason for Action
ASSESSMENT	
Assess the client's physical and mental status for signs suggesting the need for safety.	Provides data for determining the need for physical protective restraints
Consult with staff and the family on options other than restraints.	Supports the principle of using less restrictive approaches initially
Observe the client's response to alternative measures.	Determines the need to revise the current plan for care
Contact the physician for an order for the use of restraints.	Complies with The Joint Commission (TJC) requirements
Review the agency's restraint policy or procedure if unable to contact the physician.	Follows the standards for care
Assess the client's skin and circulation.	Provides a baseline of information for future comparisons
Inspect the restraint that will be used and avoid any that are in poor condition.	Ensures safety
PLANNING	
Choose a restraint compatible with the client's size.	Prevents injury
Approach the client slowly and calmly. Speak in a soft, controlled voice.	Reduces agitation
Use the client's name and make eye contact.	Helps secure the client's attention
Explain why a restraint is necessary.	Promotes understanding and cooperation
Reassure the client that the restraints will be discontinued when the possibility for injury no longer exists.	Indicates the criteria for releasing restraints
Plan to remove or loosen the restraints at times established by agency policy to assess circulation, provide joint mobility, provide skin care, assist with elimination, offer food and fluids, and evaluate whether restraints are still needed.	Demonstrates attention to basic physiologic and safety needs; supports the principle that restraints are not applied longer than necessary
IMPLEMENTATION	
Place the client in a position of comfort with proper body alignment.	Maintains functional position and reduces discomfort
Protect any bony prominences or fragile skin that a restraint may injure.	Reduces or prevents injury
Upper Extremity Restraints	
Apply mitts rather than wrist restraints if possible (Fig. A).	Maintains freedom to move elbows and shoulders

A netted hand mitt. (Photo by B. Proud.)

A

SKILL 19-1 Using Physical Restraints (*continued*)

Suggested Action	Reason for Action
Use soft cloth restraints instead of stiff leather (Fig. B).	Promotes skin integrity

B

	Soft wrist restraints are applied over padded bony prominences. Ensure that two fingers can be inserted between the restraint and the wrist. (Photo by B. Proud.)
Provide as much length as possible without allowing the client to pull at tubes or other treatment devices.	Facilitates movement

Wheelchair Restraints

Avoid back cushions if possible.	Creates the potential for slack if they become dislodged
Make sure the client's hips are flush with the back of the chair.	Promotes good posture and skeletal alignment
Apply belts snugly over the thighs with at least a 45-degree angle between the belt and the knees (Fig. C).	Minimizes sliding up toward the ribs and compromising breathing

45°

C

	With the lap strap at a 45-degree angle to the knees, the hips are held toward the back of the chair.
Apply vests with Velcro or zipper closures at the back (Fig. D); use crisscrossing vests with front closures only on docile clients.	Keeps fasteners out of reach; prevents strangulation

(*continued*)

SKILL 19-1 Using Physical Restraints (*continued*)

Suggested Action	Reason for Action
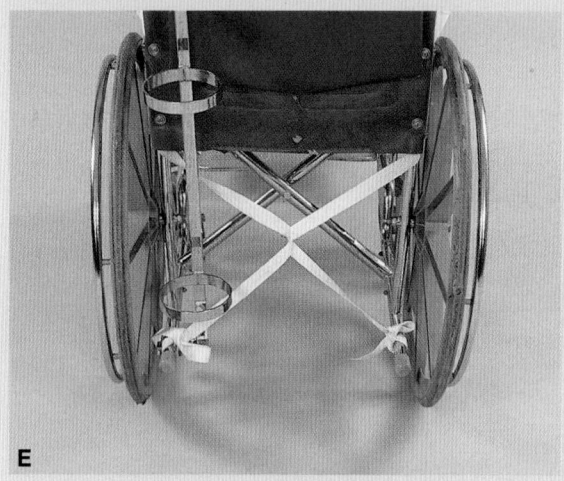	Example of a vest restraint that fastens in the back. (Carter, P. J., & Goldschmidt, W. M. [2009]. *Lippincott's textbook for long-term care nursing assistants.* Wolters Kluwer.)
Support the feet on footrests.	Reduces pressure behind the knees and promotes blood circulation
Tie restraints under the chair, not behind the back (Fig. E).	Prevents suffocation if the client should slide downward
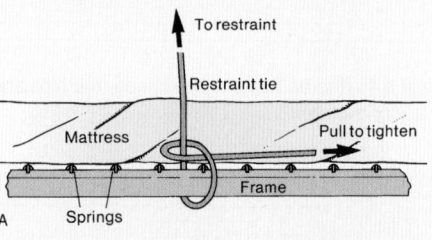	Restraint ties are secured beneath the chair. (Photo by B. Proud.)
Use a quick-release knot when tying any type of restraint (Fig. F).	Facilitates removal should the client's safety become compromised
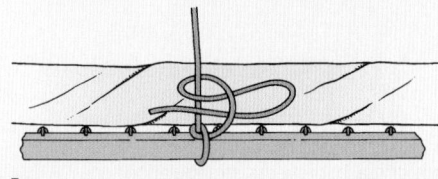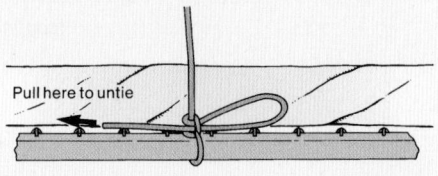	Follow the sequence in steps A, B, and C to tie a quick-release knot.

SKILL 19-1 Using Physical Restraints (*continued*)

Suggested Action	Reason for Action
Keep the client in sight whenever restraints are used.	Aids in monitoring the client's safety
Never restrain a client to a toilet.	Prevents drowning or falls
Bed Restraints	
Position the client in the center of the mattress.	Allows maximum movement and proper body alignment
Use full side rails and maintain them in an "up" position while the client is restrained.	Prevents injury from slipping between or below half rails
Apply side rail covers or pad the rails with soft bath blankets if the client is extremely restless.	Reduces the potential for becoming caught or injured within the open spaces of the rails
Apply jacket restraints snugly enough to prevent harm but not so tight as to constrict the chest and interfere with breathing.	Ensures ventilation
Secure the straps to the moveable part of the bed frame, not the side rails or stationary frame (Fig. G).	Prevents sliding and chest compression

G

Monitor aggressive, agitated, or restless clients frequently.	Promotes client safety

EVALUATION

- Restraints are applied correctly.
- Client remains free of injury.
- Restraints are released according to policy.
- Basic needs are met.
- Restraints are discontinued when no longer needed.

DOCUMENT

- Assessment findings that indicate a need for restraint
- Types of restraint alternatives and the client's response
- Condition of skin, circulation, sensation, and joint mobility before restraint application
- Type of restraint applied
- Communication with physician and responsible family member
- Frequency of release and assessment findings
- Nursing measures used to promote skin integrity and joint flexibility and to meet nutritional and elimination needs
- Assessments indicating an ongoing need for restraints

SAMPLE DOCUMENTATION

Date and Time Pulling on urinary catheter. Reminded to leave catheter alone. Placed close to nursing station to allow quick intervention. Given a skein of yarn to wrap as a ball to distract client from catheter. Continues to tug at catheter. Catheter is patent, but urine now appears bloody. Order obtained for soft cloth wrist restraints. Skin over wrists is intact, no edema, full mobility, fingers are warm and pink, can differentiate sharp from dull sensation. Restraints secured to arms of wheelchair. Daughter notified of need to use restraints at this time and concurs with treatment plan. _____ J. Doe, LPN

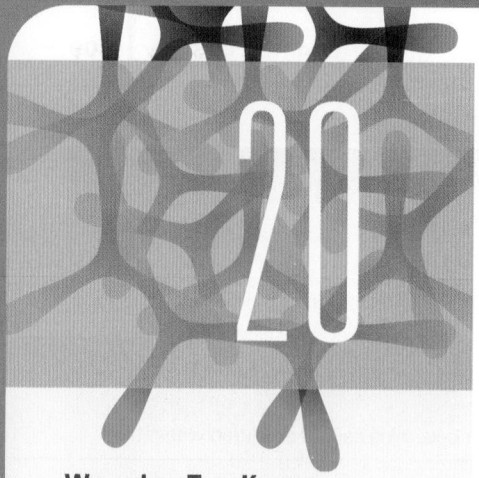

Pain Management

Words To Know

acupressure
acupuncture
acute pain
adjuvants
analgesic
biofeedback
bolus
chronic pain
complementary and alternative
    medical (CAM) therapy
controlled substances
cordotomy
cutaneous pain
distraction
endogenous opioids
equianalgesic dose
fifth vital sign
hypnosis
imagery
intractable pain
intraspinal analgesia
loading dose
lockout
malingerer
meditation
modulation
neuropathic pain
neuropeptides
nociceptors
nonopioids
opioids
pain
pain management
pain threshold
pain tolerance
patient-controlled analgesia (PCA)
perception
percutaneous electrical nerve
    stimulation (PENS)
placebo
referred pain
relaxation
rhizotomy
somatic pain
suffering
transcutaneous electrical nerve
    stimulation (TENS)
transduction
transmission
visceral pain

Learning Objectives

On completion of this chapter, the reader should be able to:

1. Give a general definition of pain.
2. List phases in the pain process.
3. Explain the differences among pain perception, pain threshold, and pain tolerance.
4. List pain theories.
5. Describe the gate control theory and how it applies to methods for reducing the perception and intensity of pain.
6. Explain how endogenous opioids reduce pain transmission.
7. Name types of pain.
8. Differentiate the characteristics of acute pain from those of chronic pain.
9. List components of a basic pain assessment.
10. Identify occasions when it is essential to perform a pain assessment and document assessment findings.
11. Name common pain intensity assessment tools used by nurses.
12. Name physiologic mechanisms for managing pain.
13. Give categories of drugs used either alone or in combination to manage pain.
14. Identify surgical procedures used when other methods of pain management are ineffective.
15. List complementary and alternative medical (CAM) therapies for managing pain.
16. Define addiction.
17. Discuss how fear of addiction affects pain management.
18. Discuss the most common reason why clients request frequent administrations of pain-relieving drugs.
19. Define placebo and explain the basis for its positive effect.

INTRODUCTION

Pain is a predominant cause of physical distress among clients. Clients have a right to expect access to the most effective pain relief that can safely be provided. This chapter provides information about pain, nursing, and multidisciplinary techniques for pain relief.

 Gerontologic Considerations

■ Research on pain in older adults lags behind other areas of pain research, but much evidence points toward the conclusion that pain is underdetected and poorly managed among older adults.

■ A guiding principle with regard to pain in older adults is to consider the person's age as one of the many variables that can influence assessment and management.

- Older adults may not report pain for several reasons, such as not wanting to be perceived as a nuisance or a complainer, believing that pain is expected with aging or is an indicator of weakness, fearing addiction to pain medication, or misperceiving that nothing can be done to alleviate the pain.

- Chronic illnesses (e.g., peripheral vascular disease, diabetic neuropathies, orthopedic problems, cancer) can increase the risk of pain in older adults.

- Pain is one of the most commonly reported symptoms by older people, who are more likely to have atypical presentations of pain.

- Older adults with cognitive impairment may not be able to report pain or discomfort. Changes in mental status or behavior can be primary manifestations of pain in people with dementia. When assessing pain in older adults, attention should be focused on how the pain or discomfort interferes with activities of daily living and quality of life.

- Astute assessment of physiologic indicators and behavioral changes such as increased pulse, respiration, restlessness, agitation, and wandering may provide the primary clues to pain in older adults with cognitive impairments.

- Adverse effects of analgesics, even over-the-counter products, are often more pronounced in older adults. Common adverse effects include confusion, disorientation, gastritis, constipation, urinary retention, blurred vision, and gastrointestinal bleeding.

- Physiologic changes in older adults such as decreased gastric acid production, decreased gastrointestinal motility, and changes in liver and kidney function can affect drug absorption, metabolism, and excretion. These age-related changes can result in increased variability in the response of older adults and an increased risk of adverse effects and toxicity, even when the dose is in the therapeutic range. Older adults have increased sensitivity to opioids. Initial dosing should be at the lower levels (begin with half of the recommended dose) and titrated to the most effective dose. "Start low, go slow" is a rule of thumb for analgesic administration.

- Death rates from drug overdoses among people aged 65 years and older have more than tripled over the past two decades (2.4 deaths per 100,000 people aged 65 years and older in 2000 vs. 8.8 in 2020), with faster rates of increase for men than women in the recent period (CDC, 2022).

- Although the administration of low doses of antidepressants, anticonvulsants, or stimulants may enhance the effectiveness of analgesics for older adults, these agents also increase the risk for adverse effects and drug interactions.

- To ensure safety, it is important to assess the condition of the skin and cognitive level of older adults prior to using topical application of heat or cold.

PAIN

Pain is an unpleasant sensation usually associated with disease or injury. It causes physical discomfort and is accompanied by **suffering**, which is the emotional component of pain. Understanding how pain is produced and perceived is essential to finding mechanisms for pain relief. Extensive research is ongoing to discover more about pain transmission, types of pain, and the management of pain.

The Process of Pain
The process by which people experience pain occurs in four phases: transduction, transmission, perception, and modulation (Fig. 20-1).

Transduction
Transduction refers to the conversion of chemical information at the cellular level into electrical impulses that move toward the spinal cord. Transduction begins when injured cells release chemicals, such as substance P, prostaglandins, bradykinin, histamine, and glutamate. These chemicals excite **nociceptors**, sensory nerve receptors activated by around 20 **neuropeptides**, noxious chemicals released from damaged tissue, such as substance P, serotonin, histamine, and arachidonic acid, which is metabolized into prostaglandin, acetylcholine, and others (Kendroud et al., 2024). Nociceptors are located throughout the skin, bones, joints, muscles, and internal organs (Fig. 20-2).

Transmission
Transmission is the phase during which stimuli move from the peripheral nervous system toward the brain. Transmission occurs when peripheral nociceptors form synapses with neurons within the spinal cord that carry pain impulses and other sensory information such as pressure and temperature changes via fast and slow nerve fibers. Impulses through the fast pain pathway, *A-delta fibers*, result in sharp, acute initial sensations like those felt when touching a hot iron. The result is that the person almost immediately withdraws from the pain-provoking stimulus. Following the fast transmission, impulses from small unmyelinated fibers known as *C-fibers* carry impulses at a slower rate of 0.5 to 2 m/sec. They are responsible for the throbbing, aching, or burning sensation that persists after the initial discomfort.

With the help of substance P, pain impulses move to sequentially higher levels in the brain, such as the reticular activating system, thalamus, cerebral cortex, and limbic system. Prostaglandin, a chemical released from the injured cells, speeds up the transmission. As the pain impulses are transmitted, pain receptors become increasingly sensitized. This finding helps explain the clinical observation that established pain is more difficult to suppress.

When pain impulses reach the thalamus within the brain, two responses occur. First, the thalamus transmits the message to the cortex, where the location and severity of the injury are identified. Second, it notifies the nociceptors that the message has been received and that continued transmission is no longer necessary. A malfunction in this secondary process may be one reason why chronic pain lingers.

Perception
Perception (the conscious experience of discomfort) occurs when the **pain threshold** (the point at which sufficient pain-transmitting stimuli reach the brain) is reached. Once pain is perceived, structures within the brain determine its intensity, attach meaningfulness to the event, and provoke emotional responses.

Pain thresholds tend to be the same among healthy people, but each person tolerates or bears the sensation of pain differently. **Pain tolerance** (the amount of pain a person

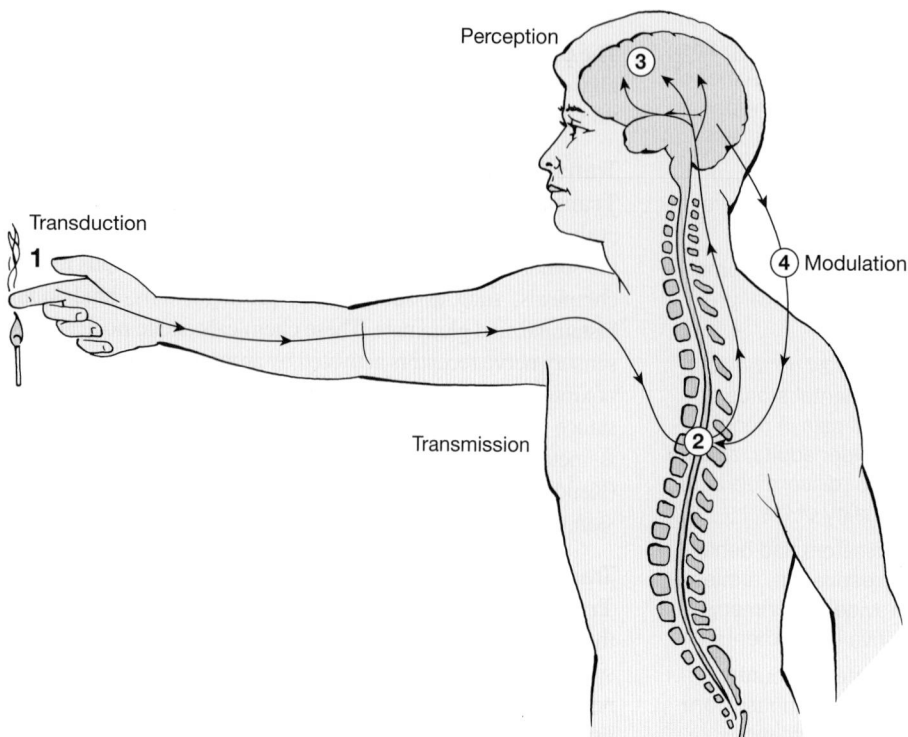

Perception

Transduction

1

Transmission

4 Modulation

FIGURE 20-1 The phases of pain.

endures) is influenced by genetics; learned behaviors specific to gender, age, and culture (see Chapter 6); and other biopsychosocially unique factors such as current anxiety level, past pain experiences, and overall emotional disposition (The Emotional Impact of the Pain Experience, 2022).

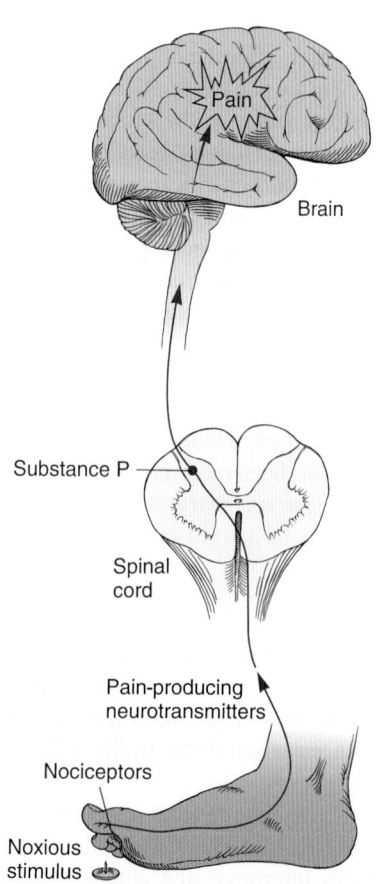

Pain

Brain

Substance P

Spinal cord

Pain-producing neurotransmitters

Nociceptors

Noxious stimulus

FIGURE 20-2 Pain transmission pathway.

Modulation

Modulation is the last phase of pain impulse transmission during which the brain interacts with the spinal nerves in a downward manner to subsequently alter the pain experience. At this point, the release of pain-inhibiting neurochemicals reduces the painful sensation. Examples of such neurochemicals include endogenous opioids (discussed later in this chapter), gamma-aminobutyric acid (GABA), and others.

Research into developing new types of pain-modulating drugs is ongoing. Current efforts are being directed at medications that (1) occupy cell receptors for neurotransmitters, such as acetylcholine and serotonin; (2) block glutamate receptors and peptides (protein compounds), such as tachykinin—neurokinin and substance P; and (3) reduce cytokines (a type of immune system protein) that trigger pain by promoting inflammation.

Theories of Pain

Several theories attempt to explain how pain is transmitted and reduced. No one theory is all encompassing.

Specificity Theory

The specificity theory was one of the earliest explanations for how pain is transmitted. Its hypothesis, which originated in the 1800s, proposed that one type of sensory nerve was continuous from the periphery to the brain and functioned specifically to transmit pain signals. This theory has been discounted because the transmission and perception of pain and other sensations involve sensory nerves in the periphery and structures in the spinal cord before eventually reaching the brain.

Pattern Theory

The pattern theory proposed that sensory stimuli such as touch, heat, cold, and pain produce various patterns. Once a pattern develops, it is transmitted to the brain where the pattern is perceived as either damaging or nondamaging.

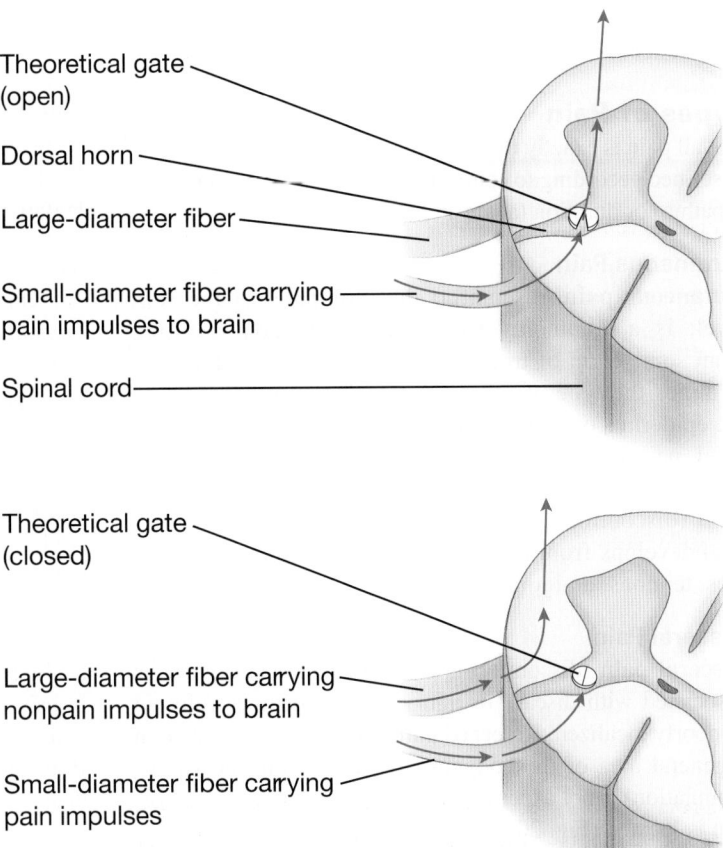

FIGURE 20-3 Pain impulse transmission and blocking according to the gate control theory. (From Taylor, C., Lynn, P., & Bartlett, J. [2022]. *Fundamentals of nursing: The art and science of nursing care* [10th ed.]. Lippincott Williams & Wilkins.)

Gate Control Theory

In the mid-1960s, Ronald Melzack, a Canadian psychologist, and his physiologist colleague, Patrick Wall, revolutionized the thinking of the scientific community with their gate control theory. Together, they proposed that sensory information travels over slow, small fibers as well as fast, large fibers. Slow fibers, through which pain stimuli travel, open gates within the spinal cord, allowing its transmission toward the brain. Fast fibers that are responsible for transmitting other types of sensory information can close the gates through which pain stimuli travel (Fig. 20-3). The gating mechanism may help explain pain relief via direct simple mechanical stimulation of receptors in the skin, muscles, and joints, such as that from massage, joint mobilization, traction, compression, thermal stimulation, transcutaneous electrical nerve stimulation (TENS), and other electrical stimulation of muscles (www.physiotherapy-treatment.com, 2020).

Neuromatrix Theory

In 1999, Melzack offered another dimension to the pain experience when he introduced the neuromatrix theory. The neuromatrix theory incorporates biopsychosocial variables. Melzack indicated that the perception and modulation of the pain experience are affected by each person's unique psychological and cognitive thought processes. For example, past memories, current stressors, and anxiety can either exacerbate or inhibit the experience of pain.

Endogenous Opioid Theory

The endogenous opioid theory is based on the fact that nociceptors contain receptors that can bind with neurotransmitters called **endogenous opioids**—endorphins, dynorphins, and enkephalins (or exogenous opioids such as morphine)—that modulate pain. When endogenous opioids are released, they are thought to attach to sites on the nerve cell's membrane, blocking the transmission of pain-conducting chemicals, such as substance P and prostaglandin (Fig. 20-4). If endogenous opioid production

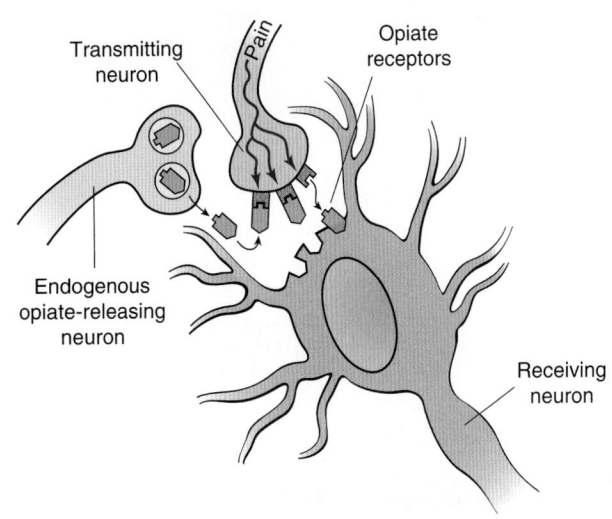

FIGURE 20-4 Mechanism of pain transmission and interference.

or storage is suppressed, pain of varying degrees will be experienced.

Types of Pain

Not all pain is exactly the same. Five types of pain have been described according to source (cutaneous, visceral, and neuropathic) or duration (acute and chronic).

Cutaneous Pain

Cutaneous pain, discomfort that originates at the skin level, is a commonly experienced sensation resulting from some form of trauma. The depth of the trauma determines the type of sensation felt. Damage confined to the epidermis produces a burning sensation. At the dermis level, pain is localized and superficial. Subcutaneous tissue injuries produce an aching, throbbing pain. **Somatic pain** (discomfort generated from deeper connective tissue) develops from injury to structures such as the muscles, tendons, and joints.

Visceral Pain

Visceral pain (discomfort arising from internal organs) is associated with disease or injury. It is sometimes referred or poorly localized. **Referred pain** (discomfort perceived in a general area of the body, usually away from the site of stimulation) is not experienced in the exact site where an organ is located (Fig. 20-5). Other autonomic nervous system symptoms such as nausea, vomiting, pallor, hypotension, and sweating may accompany visceral pain.

Neuropathic Pain

Neuropathic pain is often described as a shooting or burning pain. It may go away on its own but is often chronic. It is frequently the result of nerve damage or a malfunctioning nervous system. It may affect both the site of the injury and the areas around it.

One example of neuropathic pain is *phantom limb pain* or *phantom limb sensation*, when a person with an amputated limb perceives that the limb still exists and feels burning, itching, and deep pain in tissues that have been surgically removed. The nerves are now misfiring and causing sensation, though the limb has been removed.

Acute Pain

Acute pain (discomfort that has a short duration) lasts for a few seconds to less than 6 months. It is associated with tissue trauma, including surgery or some other recent identifiable etiology. Although severe initially, acute pain eases with healing and eventually disappears. The gradual reduction in pain promotes coping with the discomfort because there is a reinforcing belief that the pain will disappear in time. Both acute and chronic pain result in physical and emotional distress and can be intermittent (incorporating periods of relief), but that is where the similarities end.

REFERRED PAIN

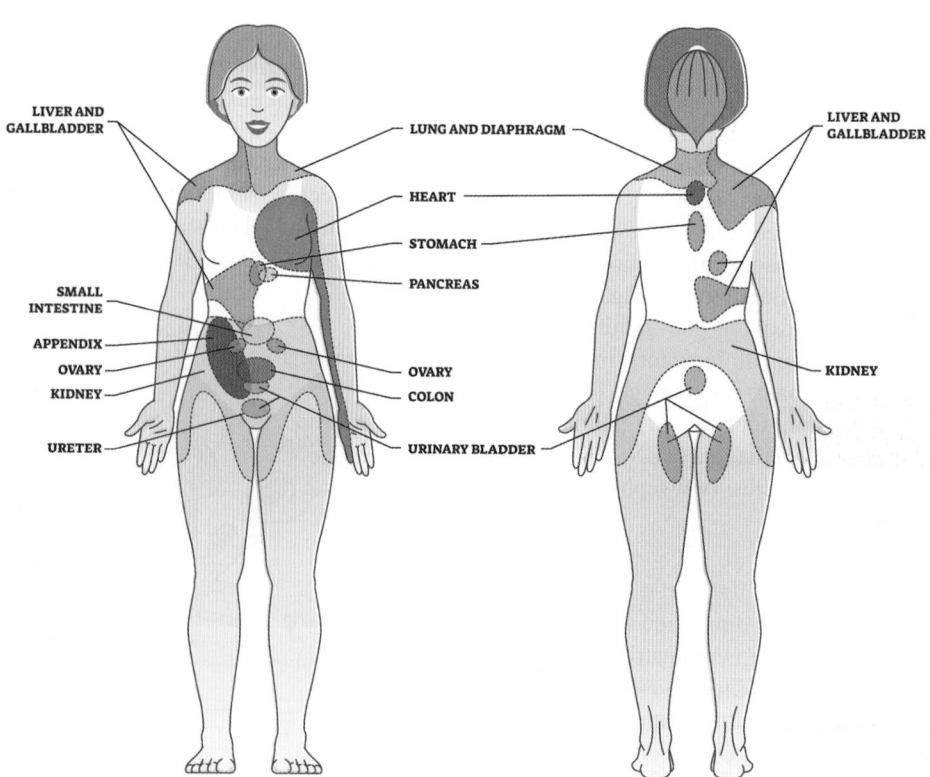

FIGURE 20-5 Areas of referred pain. (Vectormine/Shutterstock.)

TABLE 20-1 Characteristics of Acute and Chronic Pain

ACUTE PAIN	CHRONIC PAIN
Recent onset	Remote onset
Symptomatic of primary injury or disease	Uncharacteristic of primary injury or disease
Specific and localized	Nonspecific and generalized
Severity associated with the acuity of the injury or disease process	Severity out of proportion to the stage of the injury or disease
Favorable response to drug therapy	Poor response to drug therapy
Requires less and less drug therapy	Requires more and more drug therapy
Diminishes with healing	Persists beyond the healing stage
Suffering is decreased.	Suffering is intensified.
Associated with sympathetic nervous system responses such as hypertension, tachycardia, restlessness, and anxiety	Absence of autonomic nervous system responses; depression and irritability are manifested.

Chronic Pain

The characteristics of **chronic pain** (discomfort that lasts longer than 6 months) are almost totally opposite from those of acute pain (Table 20-1). The longer the pain exists, the more far-reaching its effects on the sufferer (Box 20-1). Family members in a relationship with a person who has chronic pain may begin to show negative reactions. Some of the following are common:

- Anger for thinking the person in pain is not trying hard enough to resolve it
- Anger with the medical system for not having answers
- Anger at insurance companies for denying or delaying approvals for procedures
- Guilt for being angry
- Guilt for wanting to leave the relationship
- Feelings of being trapped
- Loneliness from social isolation
- Resentment for having to assume extra burdens
- Questioning if the person in pain is exaggerating to shirk responsibilities
- Becoming less attentive and withdrawing from intimacy

STANDARDS OF PAIN ASSESSMENT

The American Pain Society has called pain the **fifth vital sign**. In other words, the nurse should check and document the client's pain every time they assess the client's other vital signs, temperature, pulse, respirations, and blood pressure. The Joint Commission established a Pain Assessment and Management Standards scale, which was updated in 2023.

BOX 20-1   Quality-of-Life Activities Affected by Chronic Pain

- Exercising
- Working around the house
- Sleeping
- Enjoying hobbies and leisure time
- Socializing
- Walking
- Concentrating
- Having sex
- Maintaining relationships with family and friends
- Working a full day
- Caring for children

It includes how all accredited health care organizations must comply with pain assessments and management. Aspects incorporated in The Joint Commission standards include:

- Everyone cared for in an accredited hospital, long-term care facility, home health care agency, outpatient clinic, or managed care organization has the right to an assessment and management of pain.
- Pain is assessed using a tool appropriate for the person's age, developmental level, health condition, and cultural identity. Refer to Table 20-2 for pain-related information that is included in an initial comprehensive pain assessment.

TABLE 20-2 Components of a Comprehensive Pain Assessment

COMPONENT	FOCUS OF ASSESSMENT
Intensity	Rating for present pain, worst pain, and least pain using a consistent scale
Location	Site of pain or identifying mark on a diagram
Quality	Description in client's own words
Onset	Time the pain began
Duration	Period that pain has existed
Variations	Pain characteristics that change
Patterns	Repetitiveness or lack thereof
Alleviating factors	Techniques or circumstances that reduce or relieve the pain
Aggravating factors	Techniques or circumstances that cause the pain to return or escalate in intensity
Present pain management regimen	Approaches used to control the pain and results and effectiveness
Pain management history	Past medications or interventions and response; manner of expressing pain; personal, cultural, spiritual, or ethnic beliefs that affect pain management
Effects of pain	Alterations in self-care, sleep, dietary intake, thought processes, lifestyle, and relationships
Person's goal for pain control	Expectations for level of pain relief, tolerance, or restoration of functional abilities
Physical examination of pain	Assessment of structures that relate to the site of pain

If clients have pain in more than one area, assessment data are collected for each.

- Pain is assessed regularly throughout health care delivery.
- Pain is treated in the health care agency, or the client is referred elsewhere.
- Health care providers are educated regarding pain assessment and management.
- Clients and their families are educated about effective pain management as an important part of care.
- The client's choices regarding pain management are respected.

In pain assessment and management, The Joint Commission states there are key concepts organizations need to understand regarding the pain management requirements in the Leadership and Provision of Care, Treatment, and Services. The key concepts are standards that must be adhered to and are as follows:

- Providing staff and licensed practitioners (LPs) with educational programs and resources regarding pain management and safe use of opioid medication
- Leadership responsibilities for developing and monitoring performance improvement activities specific to pain management and safe opioid prescribing
- Providing information to staff and LPs on available services for consultation and referral of patients with complex pain management needs
- Acceptable nonpharmacologic pain treatment modalities

To comply with the established standards of care, the nurse assesses pain whenever they consider it appropriate and routinely in the following circumstances:

- When the client is admitted
- Whenever the nurse takes vital signs
- At least once per shift when pain is problem focused or a risk
- When the client is at rest and when involved in a nursing activity
- After each potentially painful procedure or treatment
- Before implementing a pain management intervention, such as administering an **analgesic** (a pain-relieving drug), and again 30 minutes later

PAIN ASSESSMENT DATA

A basic or brief pain assessment includes the client's description of the *onset*, *quality*, *intensity*, *location*, and *duration* of the pain (Table 20-3). Nurses also ask about symptoms that accompany the pain and what, if anything, makes it better or worse. During an admission assessment, the nurse also asks questions such as:

- What activities are you unable to do because of pain?
- Do you ever take pain medication? If so, when?
- What are the names and dosages of pain medicine you take?
- What nondrug methods, such as rest, do you use to relieve your pain?
- How does your pain change with self-treatment?
- What are your preferences for managing your pain?
- What pain level is an acceptable goal for you if total pain relief is not possible?

TABLE 20-3 Basic Components of Pain Assessment

CHARACTERISTIC	DESCRIPTION	EXAMPLES
Onset	Time or circumstances under which the pain became apparent	After eating, while shoveling snow, during the night
Quality	Sensory experiences and degree of suffering	Throbbing, crushing, agonizing, annoying
Intensity	Magnitude of pain	None, slight, mild, moderate, severe; or numeric scale from 0 to 10
Location	Anatomic site	Chest, abdomen, jaw
Duration	Time span of pain	Continuous, intermittent, hours, weeks, months

When caring for clients, especially those who are often underassessed and undertreated (Box 20-2), the nurse observes for behavioral signs that are common nonverbal indicators of pain, such as moaning, crying, grimacing, guarded position, increased vital signs, reduced social interactions, irritability, difficulty concentrating, and changes in eating and sleeping. Autonomic nervous system responses such as tachycardia, hypertension, dilated pupils, perspiration, pallor, rapid and shallow breathing, urinary retention, reduced bowel motility, and elevated blood glucose levels may be apparent. Clients with chronic pain are not as likely to manifest autonomic nervous system responses.

PAIN INTENSITY ASSESSMENT TOOLS

There is no perfect way for externally determining whether someone's pain exists and how severe it is. Because no machines or laboratory tests can measure pain, nurses are limited to the subjective information that only clients can provide. Individual characteristics, family, culture, and ethnicity influence tolerance and expression of pain.

Nurses generally use one of four simple assessment tools to quantify a client's pain intensity: a numeric scale, a word scale, a linear scale (Fig. 20-6), and a visual analog (picture) scale. Clients identify how their pain compares with the choices on the scale.

BOX 20-2 Underassessed and Undertreated Pain Populations

- Infants
- Children younger than 7 years
- Clients from historically marginalized backgrounds
- Clients who are cognitively impaired
- Clients with dementia (diminished brain function)
- Clients who are hearing—or speech impaired
- Clients who are psychologically disturbed

Pain intensity scales

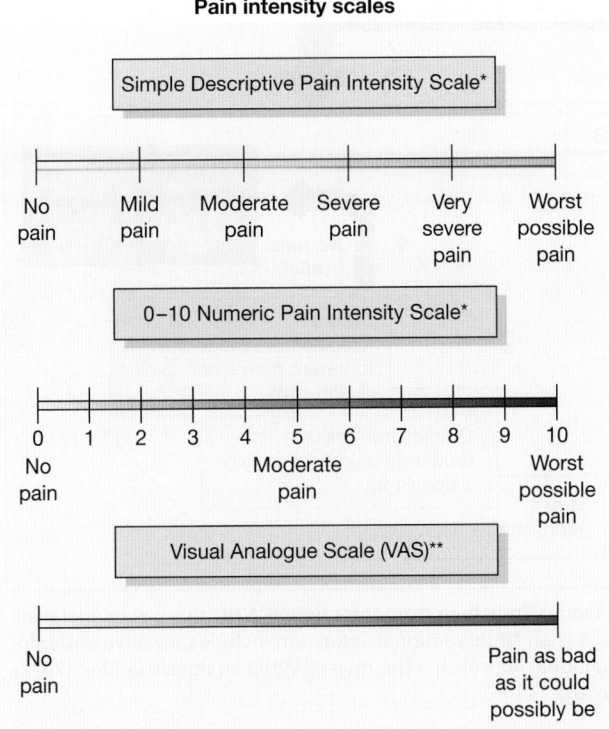

* If used as a graphic rating scale, a 10-cm baseline is recommended.
** A 10-cm baseline is recommended for VAS.

FIGURE 20-6 Pain assessment tools: word scale (top), numeric scale (middle), and linear scale (bottom).

One scale is not better than another. A numeric scale is the most commonly used tool when assessing adults. A picture scale like the Wong–Baker FACES pain rating scale is best for children or clients who have language barriers or are cognitively impaired. Children as young as 3 years can use the FACES scale. Regardless of the assessment tool used, many clients may underrate or minimize their pain intensity.

PAIN MANAGEMENT

Because of the wide variety of the types of pain and effects on lifestyle and personal relationships, management of the client's pain is a priority. Despite the fact that the client is the only reliable source for quantifying pain, nurses are not consistent in responding to different clients' reports of pain because of personal biases.

In 2018, the American Nurses Association (ANA) published a position statement regarding the nurse's responsibility in pain management. The ANA believes the relief of pain and suffering is an ethical responsibility of nurses and that it is best relieved by a multidisciplinary approach (ANA, 2018).

Treatment Biases

McCaffery and Ferrell (1999) were the first to note that nurses sometimes delay pain-relieving measures because "[they] expect someone in severe pain to *look* as if he hurts." Because of the recent opioid epidemic in the United States, nurses have become constrained in pain management.

"Recognizing biases, preventing moral disengagement, creating ethical practice environments, and addressing financial inequities are tactics for minimizing constraints and approaching better relief of pain and suffering" (ANA, 2018).

Neither behaviors nor physiologic data, however, are irrefutable indicators of pain. Responses to pain and coping techniques are learned, and clients may express them in a variety of ways. If a client's expressions of pain are incongruent with the nurse's expectations, pain management may not be readily forthcoming. Consequently, the client's pain may be undertreated.

Pain Management Techniques

Pain management (techniques for preventing, reducing, or relieving pain) is a major focus for quality improvement programs in health care agencies. The objective of a collaborative effort is to improve how pain is assessed and controlled. The effort has been expanded to include the assessment and treatment of pain in all client populations.

Most techniques for managing pain fall into one of the four general physiologic categories (Table 20-4).

Drug Therapy

Drug therapy, either alone or in combination with other therapeutic measures, is the cornerstone of pain management. The World Health Organization (WHO, 2022a, 2022b) recommends following a four-tiered drug approach based on the pain intensity and the client's response to therapy. The fourth tier was added in 2022 to address clients who have not had pain relief with medication. The fourth tier adds invasive and minimally invasive interventions (Yang et al., 2020; Fig. 20-7). The original target of the WHO's analgesic ladder in 1996 was to address methods for relieving pain from cancer. Nevertheless, the principles continue to be applicable for managing pain from cancer as well as other causes of pain.

Using a tiered approach, physicians prescribe one or more of the following classes of drugs: **nonopioids, opioids,**

TABLE 20-4 Approaches to Pain Management

APPROACH	INTERVENTION	EXAMPLES
Interrupting pain-transmitting chemicals at the site of injury	Local anesthetics, antiinflammatory drugs	Procaine, lidocaine, aspirin, ibuprofen, acetaminophen, naproxen, indomethacin
Altering transmission at the spinal cord	Intraspinal anesthesia and analgesia, neurosurgery	Epidural, caudal, rhizotomy, cordotomy, sympathectomy
Substituting sensory stimuli for pain-producing stimuli	Cutaneous stimuli	Massage, acupuncture, acupressure, heat, cold, therapeutic touch, electrical stimulation
Blocking brain perception	Opioids, nondrug techniques	Morphine, codeine, hypnosis, imagery, distraction

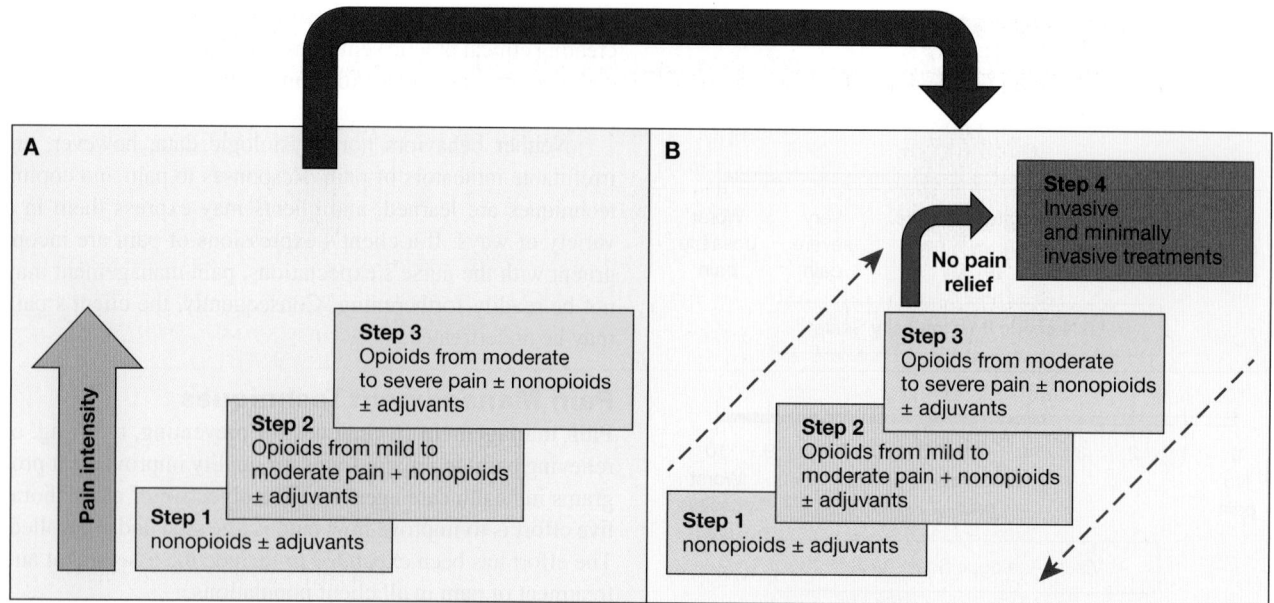

FIGURE 20-7 The revised World Health Organization (WHO) analgesic ladder. Transition from the original WHO three-step analgesic ladder **(A)** to the revised WHO fourth-step form **(B)**. The additional step 4 is an "interventional" step and includes invasive and minimally invasive techniques. This updated WHO ladder provides a bidirectional approach. (The revised WHO analgesic ladder. [2022]. https://www.ncbi.nlm.nih.gov/books/NBK554435/figure/article-31358.image.f1/)

and **adjuvants** (drugs that assist in accomplishing the desired effect of a primary drug). The choice of drug, its dose, and the timing of medication administration are critical in achieving optimal pain relief. When medications do not provide relief, invasive or minimally invasive interventions are recommended.

Pharmacologic Considerations

Although the terms "opioid" and "narcotic" were once interchangeable, law enforcement agencies have generalized the term "narcotic" to mean a drug that is addictive and misused or used illegally. Health care providers use the term "opioid" to describe drugs used in pain relief.

Nonopioid Drugs

Nonopioid drugs include aspirin, acetaminophen (Tylenol), and nonsteroidal antiinflammatory drugs (NSAIDs), such as ibuprofen (Motrin, Advil, Nuprin), ketoprofen (Orudis KT), and naproxen sodium (Naprosyn, Aleve). These drugs relieve pain by altering neurotransmission peripherally at the site of injury.

Another category of nonopioid drugs is the cyclooxygenase-2 (COX-2) inhibitors. COX is an enzyme with two subtypes: COX-1 protects the gastrointestinal tract and urinary system, and COX-2 promotes the production of pain-transmitting and inflammatory chemicals, such as prostaglandins. The inhibition of just COX-2 is believed to relieve pain better with fewer gastric side effects than older NSAIDs, which suppress both COX-1 and COX-2 enzymes. Currently, celecoxib (Celebrex) is the only COX-2 inhibitor available. Evidence of a greater risk for heart attack and stroke forced the removal of other COX-2 inhibitors from

the market. This warning of heart attack and stroke is being recommended for all NSAIDs. Therefore, assessing the patient for cardiovascular disease before administering any NSAIDs is recommended.

Most nonopioids are effective at relieving pain caused by inflammation. The exception is acetaminophen, which has limited antiinflammatory activity; however, it is still an effective analgesic. Almost all of the NSAIDs cause gastrointestinal irritation and bleeding, so they should be taken with food.

Opioid Drugs

When pain is no longer controlled with a nonopioid, the nonopioid is combined with an opioid, for example, aspirin with codeine or acetaminophen with codeine or an adjuvant drug, which is discussed later. Opioids and opiate analgesics are **controlled substances** (drugs that have prescription and dispensing that are regulated by federal law because they have the potential for being misused). Examples include:

- Morphine sulfate
- Codeine sulfate
- Meperidine (Demerol)
- Fentanyl (Duragesic, Sublimaze)

Opioids interfere with central pain perception (at the brain) and are generally reserved for treating moderate and severe pain. They are administered primarily by the oral, rectal, transdermal, or parenteral (injected) route. Opioids cause sedation, nausea, constipation, and respiratory depression.

Treating and prescribing medications with opioids have been reduced in recent years due to the addictive properties of the drug. According to the National Institute on Drug Abuse (NIDA), 130 Americans died daily from opioid overdose in 2020 (2022). See Figure 20-8.

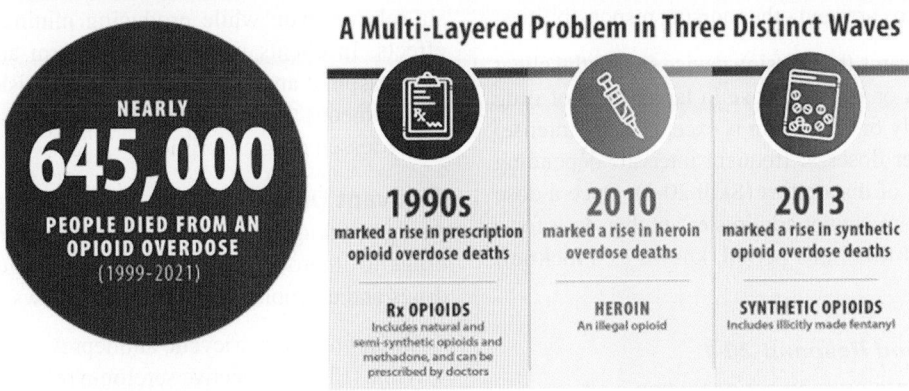

RISE IN OPIOID OVERDOSE DEATHS IN AMERICA

A Multi-Layered Problem in Three Distinct Waves

NEARLY
645,000
PEOPLE DIED FROM AN
OPIOID OVERDOSE
(1999-2021)

1990s
marked a rise in prescription
opioid overdose deaths

Rx OPIOIDS
Includes natural and
semi-synthetic opioids and
methadone, and can be
prescribed by doctors

2010
marked a rise in heroin
overdose deaths

HEROIN
An illegal opioid

2013
marked a rise in synthetic
opioid overdose deaths

SYNTHETIC OPIOIDS
Includes illicitly made fentanyl

www.cdc.gov

Learn more about the evolving opioid overdose crisis: **www.cdc.gov/drugoverdose**

FIGURE 20-8 The rates of overdose deaths associated with three categories of opioids, as well as opioids overall, according to the Centers for Disease Control and Prevention. (Opioid Data Analysis and Resources. [2023]. https://www.cdc.gov/overdose-prevention/data-research/facts-stats/index.html

 Pharmacologic Considerations

Morphine is considered the "gold standard" for opioid pain management; all other drugs are compared to this drug for equal analgesic conversions. Fentanyl is an opioid 100 times more potent than morphine and used for intractable pain associated with causes such as the large tumor burden of certain cancers. Transdermal patches or lozenges of fentanyl make administration of the medication easier when clients are unable to take the drug orally.

Because of the increased rates of addiction and overdose in recent years, opioids tend to be underprescribed even if clients can benefit from their use. NIDA and the National Institutes of Health (NIH) have taken steps to decrease opioid use and misuse and recommend alternative, nonaddictive treatments. They are also working on finding new ways to treat opioid use disorders. The use of evidence-based treatments, including medication-assisted therapy (MAT), is a comprehensive way to address the needs of individuals that combines the use of medication (methadone, buprenorphine, or naltrexone) with counseling and behavioral therapies (CDC, 2023). Beginning January 2020, the Centers for Medicare & Medicaid Services (CMS) started paying Opioid Treatment Programs for opioid use disorder treatment services provided to people with Medicare Part B (NIDA, 2024).

Patient-Controlled Analgesia

Patient-controlled analgesia (PCA) is an intervention that allows clients to self-administer opioid pain medication through the use of an infusion device (Fig. 20-9). PCA is used primarily to relieve acute pain after surgery, but this technology is finding its way into the home health arena where nonhospitalized clients with cancer are using it.

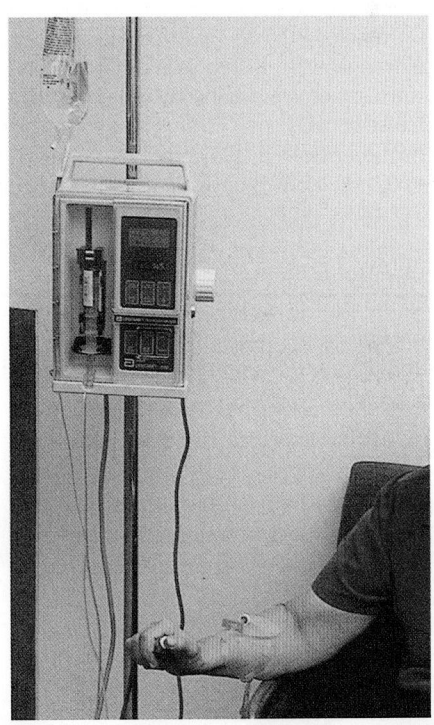

FIGURE 20-9 Patient-controlled analgesia. (From Acosta, W. R. [2020]. *Pharmacology for health professionals* [2nd ed.]. Lippincott Williams & Wilkins.)

PCA has several advantages to both clients and nurses:

- Pain relief is rapid because the drug is delivered intravenously.
- Pain is kept within a constant tolerable level.
- Less of the drug is used because small doses continuously control the pain.
- Clients are spared the discomfort of repeated injections.
- Anxiety is reduced because the client does not have to wait for the nurse to prepare and administer an injection.
- Side effects are reduced with smaller individual dosages and lower total dosages.

- Clients tend to ambulate and move more, reducing the potential for complications from immobility.
- Clients take an active role in their pain management.
- The nurse is free to carry out other nursing responsibilities.

The nurse programs the infusion device so that the client can receive a **bolus** or **loading dose** (a larger dose of drug administered initially or when pain is exceptionally intense) and additional lower doses at frequent intervals depending on the client's level of discomfort (Skill 20-1). Once a dose is delivered, the client cannot administer another dose for a specified amount of time; this period, known as a **lockout**, prevents overdoses.

 Stop, Think, and Respond 20-1

Discuss appropriate nursing actions when a client uses the maximum doses of drug with a patient-controlled analgesia infuser.

Pharmacologic Considerations

Meperidine (Demerol) is occasionally used rather than morphine for acute pain management, such as in a PCA machine. Some physicians are less apt to prescribe the drug because it can potentially cause convulsions. The drug meperidine is metabolized into "normeperidine" by the body. When this metabolite is not excreted quickly, it builds up and can cause seizures.

Intraspinal Analgesia

Intraspinal analgesia is a method of relieving pain by instilling an opioid or local anesthetic through a catheter into the subarachnoid or epidural space of the spinal cord (Fig. 20-10). It is another technique for managing pain. The intraspinal analgesic is administered several times per day or as a continuous low-dose infusion. Intraspinal analgesia relieves pain while producing minimal systemic drug effects. In clients who need long-term analgesia, the use of intraspinal analgesia diminishes the risk for injuring the subcutaneous tissue with repeated injections that may eventually lessen drug absorption.

Adjuvant Drugs

Analgesic drugs are combined with a wide range of adjuvant drugs to improve pain control. The categories of adjuvant drugs and examples of each are as follows:

- *Antidepressants*: tricyclic antidepressants such as amitriptyline (Elavil), selective serotonin reuptake inhibitors such as fluoxetine (Prozac) and paroxetine (Paxil), and serotonin–norepinephrine reuptake inhibitors such as duloxetine (Cymbalta)
- *Anticonvulsants*: carbamazepine (Tegretol), gabapentin (Neurontin)
- *N-methyl-D-aspartate (NMDA) receptor antagonists*: dextromethorphan, ketamine (Ketalar)
- Nutritional supplements such as glucosamine

Each category of adjuvant drugs acts by different mechanisms. The antidepressants may produce their analgesic-enhancing effect by increasing norepinephrine and serotonin levels, augmenting the release of endorphins. Anticonvulsants are believed to inhibit the transmission of pain by regulating and potentiating the inhibitory neurotransmitter GABA (see Chapter 5). NMDA drugs interfere with the function of nociceptive nerve fibers, perhaps blocking the release of substance P, its nerve-sensitizing properties, and

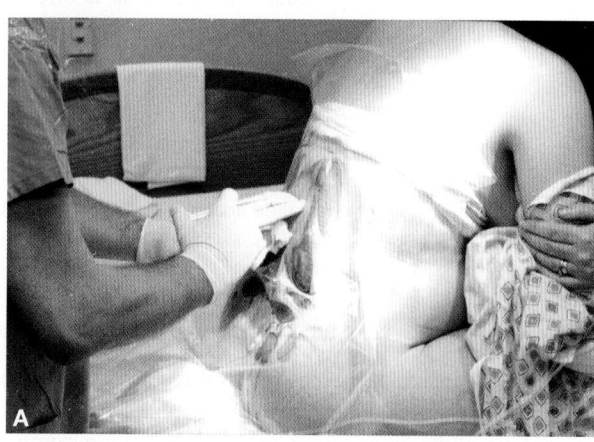

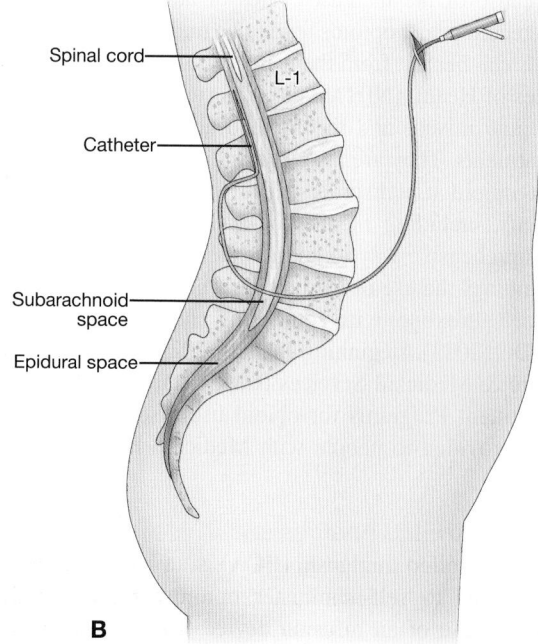

FIGURE 20-10 Intraspinal anesthesia. **A.** Inserting the catheter into the subarachnoid or epidural space. **B.** Catheter location for epidural anesthesia. (**A**, From Ricci, S. S. [2020]. *Essentials of maternity, newborn, and women's health nursing* [5th ed.]. Lippincott Williams & Wilkins; **B**, from *Lippincott's nursing procedures and skills*. [2022]. [9th ed.] Lippincott Williams & Wilkins.)

other inflammatory chemicals. Those who favor **complementary and alternative medical (CAM) therapy** (methods used in addition to conventional medical treatment, known as *integrative medicine*) contend that glucosamine slows the breakdown of joint cartilage and promotes its regeneration, relieving pain associated with joint diseases. However, in a recent study on glucosamine use, participants showed no significant improvement in knee pain or function, although there was an improvement in a small subset group that took glucosamine and chondroitin together (NCCIH. NIH.gov, 2023).

Adjuvant drugs are never used as a first-line treatment for pain. When they are used as combination drug therapy, however, the dose of the primary drug can often be decreased. With a lowered opioid dosage, for instance, the client will have less sedation and fewer undesirable side effects.

Botulinum Toxin Therapy

Botulinum toxin, one of the most poisonous biologic substances known, is a neurotoxin produced by the bacterium *Clostridium botulinum*, which is found in soil and water. In 2002, the U.S. Food and Drug Administration (FDA) approved the use of Botox (botulinum toxin A, or BTX-A) for the cosmetic purpose of temporarily reducing forehead frown lines. Of the seven types of neurotoxins it produces, BTX-A, which was approved in 1989, was found useful for treating painful musculoskeletal conditions and various types of headaches.

When injected directly into a muscle, the toxin blocks the action of acetylcholine. Research shows pain relief may occur due to muscle paralysis, increased blood flow, decompressing nerve fibers, and the effects of the toxin on nociceptive neurons (Di Maio et al., 2023). Injections must be repeated to continue the therapeutic effect. The duration of each injection's effect tends to become shorter over time. Clinical resistance may result from the development of neutralizing BTX-A antibodies.

Those who are candidates for BTX-A therapy may experience local pain, bruising, or infection at the injection site. The muscle weakness may be somewhat disturbing to some; a few develop new patterns of pain. Since the treatment with BTX-A has a short duration, some may discontinue the treatment.

Surgical Approaches

Intractable pain (pain unresponsive to other methods of pain management) can be relieved with surgery. Rhizotomy and cordotomy are neurosurgical procedures that provide pain relief.

Rhizotomy

Rhizotomy refers to the surgical sectioning of a nerve root close to the spinal cord (Fig. 20-11). This prevents sensory impulses from entering the spinal cord and traveling to the brain. Generally, more than one nerve needs to be sectioned to achieve the desired result. Chemical rhizotomy, which uses alcohol or phenol, and percutaneous rhizotomy, which uses radiofrequency waves, are nonsurgical alternatives for destroying nerve fibers. The latter can be performed on an outpatient basis. However, affected nerves regenerate in

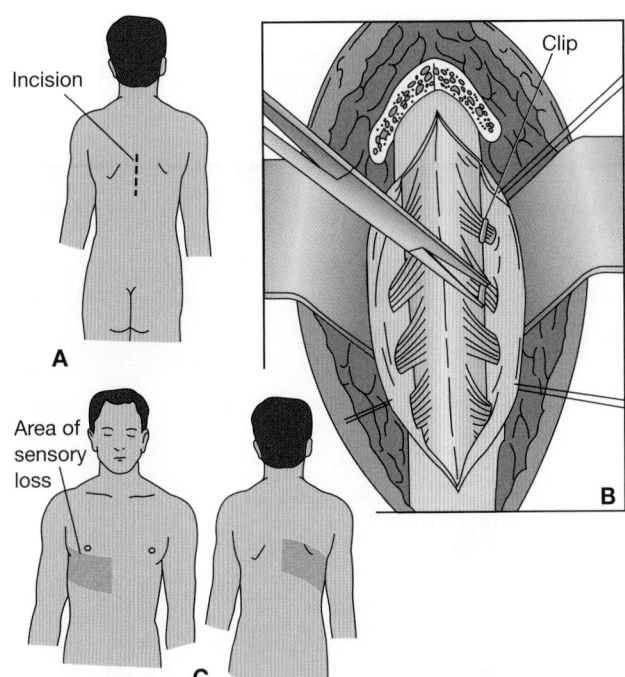

FIGURE 20-11 A. Incision site for a rhizotomy. **B.** Nerve roots are divided, banded, and clipped. **C.** Areas where there is a loss of sensation. (From Hinkle, J. L., Cheever, K. H., & Overbaugh, K., [2021]. *Brunner and Suddarth's textbook of medical-surgical nursing* [15th ed.]. Lippincott Williams & Wilkins; adapted with permission from Ballantyne, J., Fishman, S., & Rathmell, J. [2018]. *Bonica's management of pain* [5th ed.]. Lippincott Williams & Wilkins.)

approximately 5 to 8 months, and the client will experience pain again, requiring repeated treatment.

Cordotomy

Cordotomy refers to the interruption of pain pathways in the spinal cord. The surgical procedure in which bundles of nerves are severed has all but been replaced by a percutaneous approach in the area of cervical vertebrae (Fig. 20-12). In the percutaneous approach, an electrode is directed into a section of the spinal cord under fluoroscopy or computed tomography (CT). The electrode then creates a lesion using radiofrequency. Although both procedures interrupt the sensation of pain, they also inhibit the perception of pressure and temperature in the area supplied by the nerves. Consequently, there is a risk for undesirable secondary effects.

Complementary and Alternative Medical Interventions

Several CAM interventions can be used to help manage pain. Some independent nursing measures include education, imagery, distraction, relaxation techniques, and applications of heat or cold. Interventions, such as TENS, acupuncture and acupressure, percutaneous electrical nerve stimulation (PENS), biofeedback, and hypnosis, require collaboration with people who have specialized training and expertise. CAM interventions are more likely to be used for clients with chronic pain or those for whom acute pain management techniques have been unsuccessful or are contraindicated (Fig. 20-13).

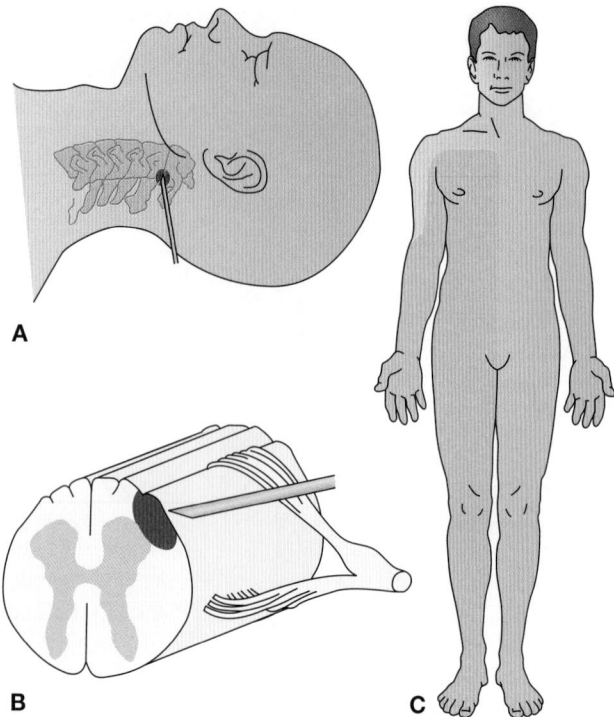

FIGURE 20-12 A percutaneous cordotomy performed at the level of cervical vertebrae 1 and 2 produces a lesion that produces analgesia. **A.** An electrode is directed into a section of the spinal cord using fluoroscopy or computed tomography. **B.** The electrode then creates a lesion using radiofrequency. **C.** Area where the perception of pressure and temperature is inhibited. (From Hinkle, J. L., Cheever, K. H., & Overbaugh, K. [2021]. *Brunner and Suddarth's textbook of medical-surgical nursing* [15th ed.]. Lippincott Williams & Wilkins.)

Client Education

Educating clients about pain and methods of pain management supports the principle that clients who assume an active role in their treatment achieve positive outcomes sooner than others (Client and Family Teaching 20-1). It may be

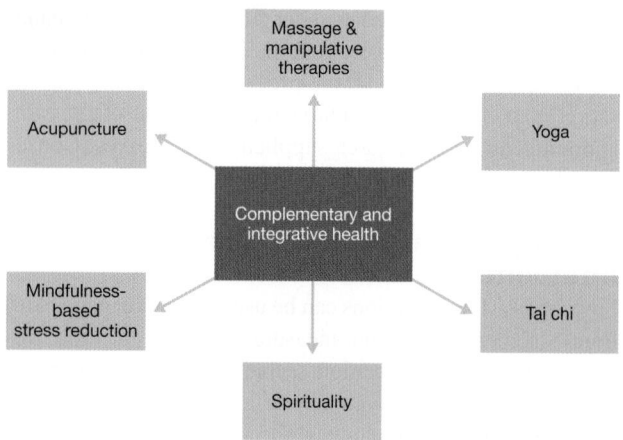

This list is nonexhaustive

FIGURE 20-13 Complementary and integrative health approaches for the treatment or management of pain conditions consist of a variety of interventions. (From U.S. Department of Health and Human Services. [2019]. *Pain management best practices inter-agency task force report.* https://www.hhs.gov/sites/default/files/pmtf-final-report-2019-05-23.pdf)

 Client and Family Teaching 20-1
Pain and Its Management

The nurse teaches the client and the family as follows:

- Ask the doctor what to expect from the disorder and its treatment.
- Discuss pain control methods that have worked well or not as well previously.
- Talk with the doctor and nurses about any concerns you have about pain medicine.
- Identify any drug allergies you have.
- Inform the doctor and nurses about other medicines you take in case they may interact with pain medications.
- Help the doctor and nurses measure your pain on a pain scale by stating the number or word that best describes the pain.
- Ask for or take pain-relieving drugs when pain begins or before an activity that causes pain.
- Set a pain control goal such as having no pain worse than 4 on a scale of 0 to 10.
- Inform the doctor and nurses if the pain medication is not working.
- Perform simple techniques such as abdominal breathing and jaw relaxation to increase comfort.
- Consult with the doctor or nurses about using cold or hot packs or other nondrug techniques to enhance pain control.

unrealistic for clients to expect to be totally pain free, but they should not have to endure severe pain.

Imagery

Imagery means using the mind to visualize an experience and sometimes is referred to as *intentional daydreaming*. The person chooses images based on pleasant memories. In *guided imagery*, the nurse or another person suggests the image to use, such as a walk in the woods, and describes the sensory experiences in great detail. Audio recordings for guided imagery and relaxation (discussed later) are also available, but the subject matter and descriptions can become boring when played repeatedly. Some prefer to use recorded sounds of nature, making it easy to conjure different images each time.

Physiologically, the process of imagery produces an alteration in consciousness that allows the client to forget uncomfortable sensory experiences, such as pain. Some believe imagery stimulates the visual portion of the brain's cortex, located in the right hemisphere, where abstract concepts and creative activities occur. While the person is experiencing imagery, neurotransmitters are released that calm the body physically and promote emotional well-being.

Meditation

Meditation involves concentrating on a word or idea that promotes tranquility or often the breath. Those who use this technique tend to successfully experience a relaxed state with lowered blood pressure and pulse rates, and research supports many health benefits from regular meditation.

Distraction

Distraction is the intentional diversion of attention to switch the person's focus from an unpleasant sensory experience to one that is neutral or more pleasant. The distraction occurs in the "here and now;" it is not imagined. Examples include talking with someone, watching television, participating in a hobby, and listening to music. The mind can attend to only one stimulus at a time; while the person is occupied with the diversional activity, consciousness is blocked from perceiving painful stimuli.

Relaxation

Relaxation is a technique for releasing muscle tension and quieting the mind, which helps reduce pain, relieve anxiety, and promote a sense of well-being. Consciously relaxing breaks the circuit among neurons that are overloading the brain with distressing thoughts and painful stimuli. Client and Family Teaching 20-2 outlines a procedure clients can learn for relaxation.

Heat and Cold

Applications of heat or cold (thermal therapy) are well-established techniques for relieving pain. In some areas of practice, nurses must obtain permission from the physician before applying heat or cold.

Pain caused by an injury is best treated initially with cold applications (ice bag or chemical pack). The cold reduces localized swelling and promotes vasoconstriction, decreasing the circulation of pain-producing chemicals. Many believe that cold applications relieve pain faster and sustain pain relief longer. Heat applications (hot water bottle, rice bag [cloth bag containing uncooked rice that is heated in the

Client and Family Teaching 20-2
Relaxation

The nurse teaches the client and family as follows:

- Assume a comfortable position, either sitting or lying down.
- Close your eyes and clear your mind.
- Let the chair or bed effortlessly support your body.
- Become aware of how your body feels.
- Take deep abdominal breaths.
- Focus on the rhythm of your breathing.
- Relax with each breath in and out.
- Tighten and then release muscles in sequential parts of your body, such as the toes, feet, lower legs, thighs, and buttocks. Progress toward the face and scalp.
- Visualize healing energy flowing from your feet through your head. Release your worries and discomfort as it passes through.
- Let yourself sleep if possible.
- At the end of the session, wake up or begin to move gradually.

microwave], or moist packs) are placed over a painful area 24 to 48 hours after the injury.

Thermal applications, whether hot or cold, are never used longer than 20 minutes at any one time (see Chapter 28). The skin is always protected with an insulating layer, such as a cloth or a towel. The client should never go to sleep while a hot or cold pack is in place, and hot and cold applications are contraindicated in areas of the body where circulation or sensation is impaired.

Menthol (Icy Hot, BenGay) and capsaicin (Zostrix), a compound found in red pepper, are over-the-counter products that are applied topically. They increase blood flow in the area of application, creating a warm or cool feeling that lasts for several hours.

Transcutaneous Electrical Nerve Stimulation

Transcutaneous electrical nerve stimulation (TENS), a medically prescribed pain management technique that delivers bursts of electricity to the skin and underlying nerves, is an intervention nurses can implement (Skill 20-2). The client perceives the electrical stimulus, generated by a battery-powered stimulator, as a pleasant tapping, tingling, vibrating, or buzzing sensation. TENS is used intermittently for 15 to 30 minutes or longer whenever the client feels a need for it. TENS-like devices can be purchased on the internet without a physician's prescription.

For some time, clients with chronic pain have used TENS, but surgical clients are now using it as well. Reports of its effectiveness range from "useless" to "fantastic." It is unclear exactly how TENS works. It is possible the transmission of electrical stimuli over larger myelinated nerves takes precedence over the transmission of pain-producing stimuli to the brain. Others believe that TENS stimulates the body to release endogenous opioids, and still others posit TENS is an application of the gate control theory.

TENS is a nonopioid, noninvasive method without harmful side effects. It is contraindicated in pregnant patients because its effect on the unborn fetus has not been determined. Clients with cardiac pacemakers (especially the demand type), clients prone to an irregular heartbeat, and clients with previous heart attacks are not candidates for TENS.

≫ Stop, Think, and Respond 20-2
Give some reasons that a person may object to using a transcutaneous electrical nerve stimulation unit for pain management.

Acupuncture and Acupressure

Acupuncture is a pain management technique in which long, thin needles are inserted into the skin (Fig. 20-14) at precise points. **Acupressure** is a technique that involves tissue compression rather than needles to reduce pain. Both are based on ancient traditions of Chinese medicine and have been demonstrated to prevent or relieve pain.

Their exact analgesic mechanisms, however, are not completely understood. Some speculate that these techniques stimulate the body's production of endogenous opioids or

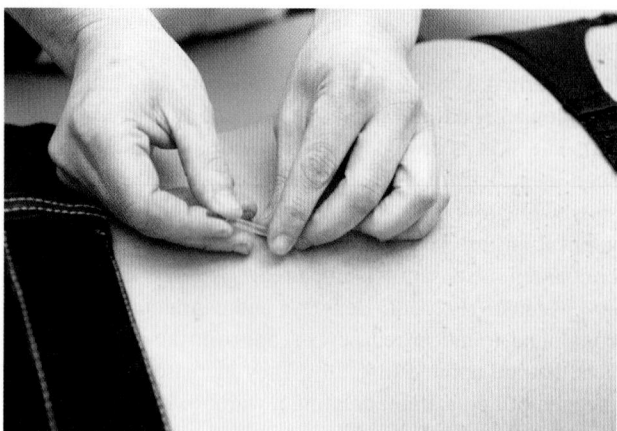

FIGURE 20-14 Acupuncture needles are inserted in meridians based on Chinese healing practices. (From DeLaet, R. [2020]. *Introduction to health care & careers.* Lippincott Williams & Wilkins.)

that the twisting and vibration of the needles and the pressure applied are forms of cutaneous stimuli that interfere with pain-transmitting neurochemicals. Others believe that the pain relief is a result of a placebo effect (see later discussion); however, combining acupuncture with conventional treatment has shown better results for some than with conventional treatment alone. Acupuncture and acupressure are becoming increasingly accepted as effective forms of pain therapy in the United States.

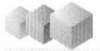 Concept Mastery Alert

Acupressure and Biofeedback

Acupressure involves the process of cutaneous stimulation, as pressure is applied to various points of the body to prevent or relieve pain. It is not to be confused with biofeedback, which involves a conscious effort to relax.

Percutaneous Electrical Nerve Stimulation

Another technique for acute and chronic pain management is **percutaneous electrical nerve stimulation (PENS)**, a pain management technique involving a combination of acupuncture needles and TENS. Acupuncture needles are inserted into the soft tissue at the site of pain, and an electrical stimulus is conducted through the needles (Fig. 20-15). Percutaneous neuromodulation therapy is an investigational variation of PENS, the difference being that the needle-like filaments are of different lengths and are placed in anatomic landmarks rather than at the sites of pain.

PENS is considered superior to TENS in providing pain relief because the needles are located closer to nerve endings. PENS therapy is administered three times a week for 30 minutes for 4 weeks or more. Sustained analgesia for a period of time can be obtained by performing PENS for at least 8 weeks. The technique has been successful in research trials on clients with low back pain, pain caused by the spread of cancer to bones, shingles (acute herpes zoster viral infection), diabetic neuropathy, and migraine headaches.

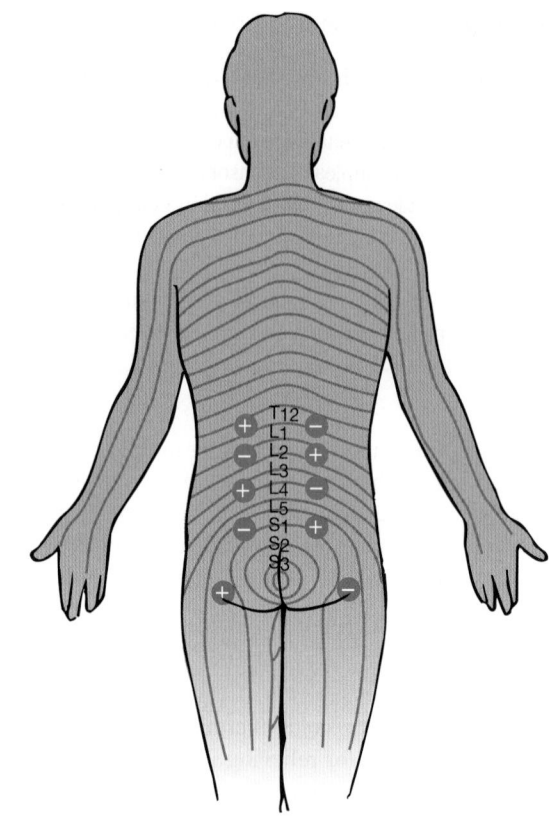

FIGURE 20-15 With percutaneous electrical nerve stimulation therapy, five pairs of electrical stimulating leads (alternating positive and negative current) are connected to needles inserted into the lumbar and sacral regions of the spine.

Biofeedback

With **biofeedback**, a client learns to control or alter a physiologic phenomenon (e.g., pain, blood pressure, headache, heart rate and rhythm, seizures) as an adjunct to traditional pain management. Initially, the client is connected to a physiologic sensing instrument, such as a pulse oximeter or an electromyography machine. The instrument produces a visual or audible signal that correlates with the person's heart rate, skin temperature, or muscle tension. The client is encouraged to reduce or extinguish the signal using whatever mechanism they can—generally by physically relaxing. The feedback from the machine demonstrates to the client how well they are accomplishing the goal. Eventually, clients can learn to control their symptoms without the assistance of the equipment, using self-suggestion alone.

Hypnosis

Hypnosis is a therapeutic technique in which a person enters a trance-like state, resulting in an alteration in perception and memory. During hypnosis, the suggestion is made that the person's pain will be eliminated or that the client will experience the sensation in a more pleasant way.

Although self-hypnosis is possible, more often, hypnosis is induced with the help of a hypnotherapist. Hypnotherapists receive special clinical training; their professional organizations include the American Society of Clinical Hypnosis and the International Society for Medical and Psychological Hypnosis.

NURSING IMPLICATIONS

Nurses must increase their knowledge about pain, take every client's pain seriously, and implement measures for treating pain effectively. Whenever a client's pain is not controlled to their satisfaction, the nurse pursues better goal achievement by collaborating with pain experts (Nursing Guidelines 20-1).

 NURSING GUIDELINES 20-1

Managing Pain

- Never doubt the client's description of pain or need for relief. *Bias on the nurse's part may lead to withholding prescribed medication or undertreating the symptoms.*
- Follow the written medical orders for administering pain medications. *This practice demonstrates compliance with nurse practice acts.*
- Administer pain-relieving drugs as soon as the need becomes evident. *Prompt administration of drugs reduces the client's suffering.*
- Consult the physician if the current drug therapy is not controlling the client's pain. *Consulting with the physician demonstrates client advocacy.*
- Collaborate with the physician to develop several pain management options involving combinations of drugs, alternative routes of administration, and different dosing schedules. *Developing options individualizes pain management.*
- Support the formation of an interdisciplinary pain management team (physicians, surgeons, nurses, pharmacists, anesthesiologists, physical therapists, massage therapists, and so forth) who can be consulted on hard-to-manage pain problems. *Such a group makes the expertise of a variety of health care providers available.*
- Administer pain medication before an activity that produces or intensifies pain. *This timing prevents pain, which is much easier than treating it.*
- When the client's pain is continuous, administer analgesic drugs on a scheduled basis rather than irregularly. *Administering the drugs regularly controls pain when it is at a lower intensity.*
- Monitor for drug side effects, such as respiratory depression, decreased levels of consciousness, nausea, vomiting, and constipation. *Careful monitoring demonstrates concern for the client's safety and comfort.*
- Consult the professional literature or experts on the **equianalgesic dose** (an oral dose that provides the same level of pain relief as a parenteral dose). *This prevents undertreatment of pain because of changes in drug absorption or drug metabolism.*
- Change the client's position, elevate a swollen limb to reduce swelling, loosen a tight dressing, and assist the client with bowel or bladder elimination. *These measures reduce factors that intensify the pain experience.*
- Implement independent and prescribed nondrug interventions, such as client teaching, imagery, meditation, distraction, and transcutaneous electrical nerve stimulation (TENS), as additional techniques for pain management. *These techniques reduce mild-to-moderate pain when used alone or potentiate pain management when combined with drug therapy.*
- Allow rest periods between activities. *Exhaustion reduces the client's ability to cope with pain.*

Clients with pain are likely to have various nursing diagnoses, including the following:

- Acute pain
- Chronic pain
- Impaired comfort
- Acute anxiety
- Chronic anxiety
- Fear
- Coping impairment
- Knowledge deficiency

Nursing Care Plan 20-1 is an example of how a nurse can follow the steps in the nursing process when planning the care of any client with acute pain, a nursing diagnosis defined as pain occurring suddenly, beginning as sharp or intense, and that serves as a warning sign of disease or threat to the body.

Addiction

One of the leading factors interfering with adequate pain management is the fear of addiction. The American Society for Pain Management Nursing describes addiction as "a chronic, relapsing, treatable disease" characterized by:

- Craving
- Dysfunctional behaviors
- Inability to control impulses regarding consumption of a substance
- Compulsive use despite harmful consequences

Fears of addiction, especially in light of the recent U.S. opioid epidemic, may interfere with clients receiving pain relief, often needlessly. Nurses often assume that a client's desire to experience the drug's pleasant effects motivates their desire for frequent doses of opioids. What may be happening is that the prescribed dose or frequency of administration is not controlling the pain, a phenomenon that occurs as clients develop drug tolerance. Nurses may undertreat the pain or may convince the physician to prescribe a placebo.

Placebos

A **placebo** is an inactive substance or treatment used as a substitute for an analgesic drug or conventional therapeutic measure. Placebos can relieve pain, especially when clients have confidence in their health care providers. The trust a client has in the nurse or physician probably has more to do with the efficacy of placebos than any other factor. Consequently, it is wrong to assume that a client whose pain is relieved with placebos is addicted or is a **malingerer** (someone who pretends to be sick or in pain). Using deception and withholding pain medication are considered unethical.

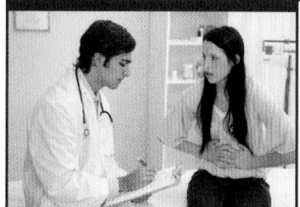

Clinical Scenario A young college student has come to the campus health center because of sudden abdominal discomfort that began the previous night. She is interviewed by the triage nurse prior to being seen by the physician. She is subsequently admitted to a local hospital for diagnostic and treatment purposes.

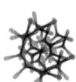

NURSING CARE PLAN 20-1 Acute Pain

Assessment

- Determine the source of the client's pain; when it began; its intensity, location, and characteristics; and related factors such as what makes the pain better or worse.
- Ask how the client's pain interferes with life such as diminishing the person's ability to meet their own needs for hygiene, eating, sleeping, activity, social interactions, emotional stability, and concentration.
- Identify at what level the client can tolerate pain.

- Measure the client's vital signs.
- Note pain-related behaviors, such as grimacing, crying, moaning, and assuming a guarded position.
- Perform a physical assessment, taking care to gently support and assist the client to turn as various structures are examined. Use light palpation in areas that are tender. Show concern when assessment techniques increase the client's pain. Postpone nonpriority assessments until the client's pain is reduced.

Nursing Diagnosis. Acute pain related to cellular injury or disease as manifested by the statement, "I'm in severe pain," rating pain at a 10 using a numeric scale, describing the pain as being "continuous and stabbing that started the previous night" without any known cause

Expected Outcomes. The client will rate the pain intensity at their tolerable level of 5 within 30 minutes of implementing a pain management technique.

Interventions	Rationales
Assess the client's pain and its characteristics at least every 2 hours while awake and 30 minutes after implementing a pain management technique.	Prompt interventions prevent or minimize pain.
Modify or eliminate factors that contribute to pain such as a full bladder, uncomfortable position, pain-aggravating activity, excessively warm or cool environment, noise, and social isolation.	Multiple stressors decrease tolerance of pain.
Determine the client's choice for pain relief techniques from among those available.	Doing so encourages and respects the client's participation in decision-making.
Administer prescribed analgesics or alternative pain management techniques promptly.	Suffering contributes to the pain experience; eliminating delays in nursing responses can reduce suffering.
Advocate on the client's behalf for doses of prescribed analgesics or the addition of adjuvant drug therapy if pain is not satisfactorily relieved.	The Joint Commission standards mandate nurses and other health care workers facilitate pain relief for all clients.
Administer a prescribed analgesic before a procedure or activity that is likely to result in pain or intensify pain that already exists.	Prophylactic interventions facilitate keeping pain within a manageable level.
Plan for periods of rest between activities.	Fatigue and exhaustion interfere with pain tolerance.
Reassure the client that there are many ways to moderate the pain experience.	Suggesting that there are additional options not yet tried reduces frustration or despair that there is no hope for pain relief.
Assist the client with visualizing a pleasant experience.	Visualization interrupts pain perception.
Help the client focus on deep breathing, relaxing muscles, watching television, putting a puzzle together, or talking to someone on the telephone.	Diverting attention to something other than pain reduces pain perception.
Apply warm or cool compresses to a painful site.	Flooding the brain with alternative sensory stimuli interrupts impulses that transmit pain.
Gently massage a painful area or the same area on the opposite side of the body (contralateral massage).	Massage promotes the release of endorphins and enkephalins that moderate the sensation of pain.
Promote laughter by suggesting that the client relate a humorous story or watch a video or comedy program of their choice.	Laughter releases endorphins and enkephalins that promote a feeling of well-being.

Evaluation of Expected Outcomes

- The client reports that pain is gone or at a tolerable level.
- The client perceives the pain experience realistically and copes effectively.
- The client can participate in self-care activities without undue pain.

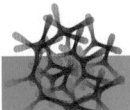

KEY POINTS

- Pain occurs in four phases.
  - Transduction: Begins when the injured cells release chemicals that are changed into electrical impulses that move toward the spinal cord
  - Transmission: The stimuli move from the peripheral nervous system toward the brain.
  - Perception: The conscious experience of discomfort; the pain threshold is reached, and pain is perceived.
  - Modulation: The last phase of pain; the brain interacts with the spinal nerves in a downward manner to subsequently alter the pain experience.
- Five types of pain
  - Cutaneous
    - Discomfort that originates at the skin level (e.g., trauma)
    - Somatic pain: Discomfort that generates from deeper connective tissue, such as the muscles or joints
  - Visceral
    - Discomfort arising from internal organs, associated with disease or injury (e.g., nausea, vomiting)
    - Referred pain: Pain that is not experienced at the site where the organ is located (e.g., cardiac pain)
  - Neuropathic (functional pain): Occurs days, weeks, or months after the pain has been treated and resolved (e.g., phantom limb pain)

- Acute pain: Discomfort that has a short duration, lasts for a few seconds to less than 6 months
- Chronic pain: Discomfort that lasts longer than 6 months
- Pain is considered the fifth vital sign after temperature, pulse, respirations, and blood pressure.
- Pain assessment data: Includes the client's description of the *onset*, *quality*, *intensity*, *location*, duration, symptoms that accompany the pain, and what makes the pain better or worse
- Pain intensity tool: Numerical scale, word scale, linear scale, picture scale (e.g., Wong–Baker FACES scale)
- Drug therapy for pain
  - Nonopioids (e.g., aspirin, acetaminophen)
  - Opioids (e.g., morphine sulfate, codeine sulfate, fentanyl; used cautiously due to high addiction rate)
  - Adjuvants: Drugs like antidepressants that improve pain when combined with analgesics
  - Placebo: Inactive substance or treatment used as a substitute for an analgesic drug or conventional therapeutic measure
- Other treatments for pain
  - Neurosurgical procedures for pain control: Rhizotomy, cordotomy
  - Complementary and alternative medicine: Imagery, meditation, distraction, relaxation, heat and cold, TENS unit, acupuncture, acupressure, PENS, biofeedback, and hypnosis

CRITICAL THINKING EXERCISES

1. Describe factors that can intensify pain.
2. How would you respond to a coworker who believes a client is "faking" pain to receive medication?

NEXT-GENERATION NCLEX-STYLE REVIEW QUESTIONS

1. When a nurse observes that a client is curled in a fetal position and rocking back and forth, which action would help most to determine whether these findings are due to pain?
   a. Determine whether the client can stop moving.
   b. Ask the client to rate pain from 0 to 10.
   c. Observe whether the client is perspiring heavily.
   d. Monitor the client's response to a pain-relieving drug.
   Test-Taking Strategy: Note the key word, "help most." Analyze the options and select one that provides the best criteria for determining whether the client is experiencing pain.

2. Which are essential components of a basic pain assessment? Select all that apply.
   a. Nonverbal indicators of pain
   b. Time of pain onset
   c. History of analgesic use
   d. Location of pain
   e. Characteristics of pain
   f. Intensity of pain
   Test-Taking Strategy: Note the key word and modifier, "essential components." Analyze the options and select those that are the core elements of a pain assessment.

3. When assessing a client, which finding is likely in a client experiencing acute pain?
   a. The temperature may be elevated.
   b. The pulse rate may be rapid.
   c. The respiratory rate may be slow.
   d. The blood pressure may fall.
   Test-Taking Strategy: Use the process of elimination to select the most likely effect pain has on vital signs.

4. Which is the best nursing action for sustaining maximum pain relief when caring for a client with a terminal illness?
   a. Give analgesic medication whenever the client requests it.
   b. Administer pain medication every 3 hours as prescribed.
   c. Ask the physician to prescribe a high dose of pain medication.
   d. Give pain medication when the client's pain is severe.

   Test-Taking Strategy: Note the key words, "best" and "sustaining." Analyze the options and select the action that is better than any of the others for safely providing a consistent level of pain relief.

5. Which categories of medications are adjuvant drugs that enhance a client's prescribed analgesic? Select all that apply.
   a. NSAIDs
   b. Botulinum toxin
   c. Antidepressants
   d. Anticonvulsants
   e. Opioids

   Test-Taking Strategy: Use the process of elimination to select categories of drugs that may be co-prescribed to enhance the pain-relieving quality of an analgesic.

SKILL 20-1 Preparing a Patient-Controlled Analgesia Infuser

Suggested Action	Reason for Action
ASSESSMENT	
Check the written medical order for the use of a patient-controlled analgesia (PCA) infusion device, the prescribed drug, the initial loading dose, the dose per self-administration, and the lockout interval.	Provides data for programming the infusion device
Check the client's wristband.	Prevents medication errors
Obtain two forms of identification such as asking the client's name and date of birth.	Supports The Joint Commission's National Patient Safety Goal for identifying clients correctly
Assess what the client understands about PCA.	Indicates the type and amount of teaching that must be provided
Check that the currently infusing intravenous (IV) solution is compatible with the prescribed analgesic.	Avoids incompatibility reactions
PLANNING	
Obtain the following equipment: the infuser, the PCA tubing, and the prefilled medication container.	Promotes organization and efficient time management
Plug the power cord into the electrical wall outlet.	Prolongs the life of the battery
Explain the equipment and how it functions.	Reduces anxiety and promotes independence
IMPLEMENTATION	
Wash hands or perform hand antisepsis with an alcohol rub (see Chapter 10).	Reduces the transmission of microorganisms
Attach the PCA tubing to the assembled syringe (Fig. A).	Provides a pathway for delivering the medication

Connecting the tubing. (Photo by B. Proud.)

Suggested Action	Reason for Action
Open the cover or door of the infuser and load the syringe into its cradle (Fig. B).	Stabilizes the syringe within the infuser

Loading the syringe within the PCA machine. (Photo by B. Proud.)

Suggested Action	Reason for Action
Fill the PCA tubing with fluid.	Displaces air from the tubing
Connect the PCA tubing to the IV tubing.	Facilitates intermittent administration of medication

(*continued*)

SKILL 20-1 Preparing a Patient-Controlled Analgesia Infuser (*continued*)

Suggested Action	Reason for Action
Assess the client's pain.	Provides data from which to evaluate the drug's effectiveness
Set the volume for the prescribed loading dose (Fig. C).	Administers a slightly larger dose of the drug to establish a reduced level of pain rather quickly

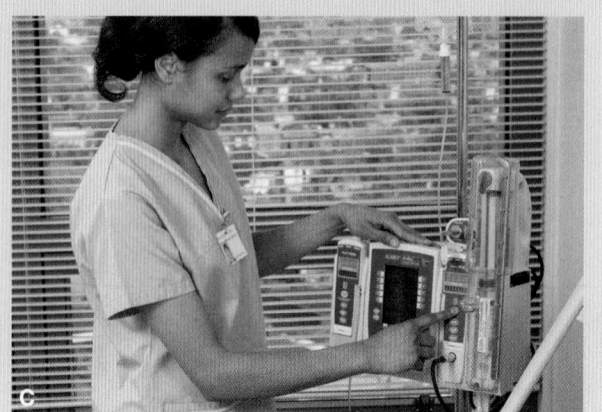

Setting the loading dose. (Photo by B. Proud.)

Suggested Action	Reason for Action
Program the infuser according to the individual dose and lockout period.	Prevents overdosing
Close the security door and lock it with a key (Fig. D).	Prevents tampering

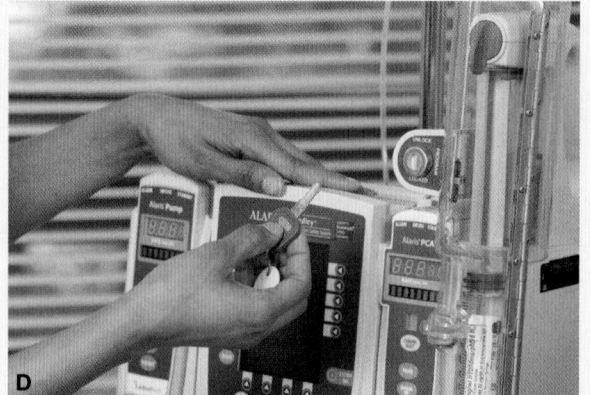

Locking the infuser within the PCA machine. (Photo by B. Proud.)

Suggested Action	Reason for Action
Instruct the client to press and release the control button each time pain relief is needed (Fig. E).	Educates the client on how to operate the equipment

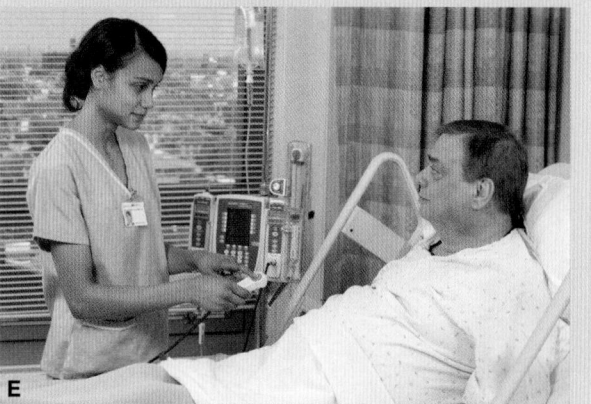

Explaining the use of the PCA infuser. (Photo by B. Proud.)

Suggested Action	Reason for Action
Explain that a bell will sound when the infuser delivers medication.	Provides sensory reinforcement that the machine is working
Assess the client's pain at least every 2 hours.	Complies with standards of care
Replace the medication syringe when it becomes empty.	Maintains continuous pain management
Change the primary IV solution container every 24 hours.	Complies with infection control policies

SKILL 20-1 Preparing a Patient-Controlled Analgesia Infuser (*continued*)

Suggested Action	Reason for Action

EVALUATION

- The client self-administers pain medication.
- The client's pain is controlled within a tolerable level.

DOCUMENT

- Date and time
- Volume and type of analgesic solution
- Name of analgesic drug
- Initial pain assessment
- Loading dose
- Individual dose and time schedule
- Reassessments of pain
- Total volume self-administered per shift

SAMPLE DOCUMENTATION

Date and Time A 30-mL syringe of saline with 30 mg of morphine sulfate inserted into a PCA pump. Describes pain around abdominal incision as continuous and stabbing. Rates the pain at a level of 7 on a scale of 0–10. Loading dose of 2 mg administered. Infuser programmed to deliver 0.1 mL—the equivalent of 0.1 mg—at no more than 10-minute intervals. Rates pain at a level of 5 within 10 minutes after loading dose. Instructed and observed to self-administer a subsequent dose.
_____ J. Doe, LPN

SKILL 20-2 Operating a Transcutaneous Electrical Nerve Stimulation Unit

Suggested Action	Reason for Action
ASSESSMENT	
Check the written medical order for providing the client with a transcutaneous electrical nerve stimulation (TENS) unit.	Demonstrates collaboration with the medical management of client care
Ask the physician or physical therapist about the best location for electrode placement. Some possible variations are: • On or near the painful site • On either side of an incision • Over cutaneous nerves • Over a joint	Optimizes pain management by individualizing electrode placement
Read the client's history to determine whether there are any conditions for which the use of a TENS unit is contraindicated.	Ensures client safety
Check the client's wristband, ask the client to identify themselves, and state their date of birth.	Prevents errors and ensures proper client identification
Assess what the client understands about TENS.	Indicates the type and amount of teaching that the nurse must provide
PLANNING	
Obtain the TENS unit and two to four self-adhesive electrodes (Fig. A).	Promotes organization and efficient time management

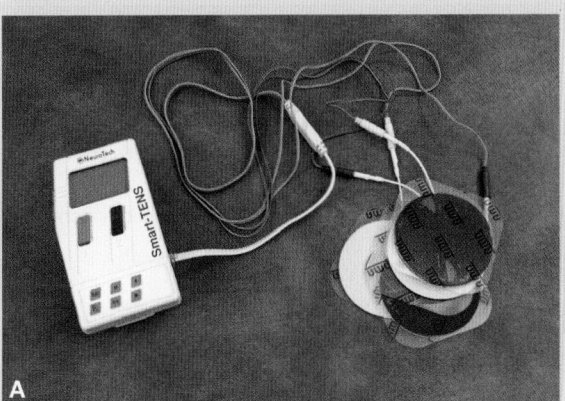

A

TENS unit.

(*continued*)

SKILL 20-2 Operating a Transcutaneous Electrical Nerve Stimulation Unit (*continued*)

Suggested Action	Reason for Action
Explain the equipment and how it functions.	Reduces anxiety and promotes independence
Establish a goal with the client for the level of pain management desired.	Aids in evaluating the effectiveness of the intervention

IMPLEMENTATION

Wash hands or perform hand antisepsis with an alcohol rub (see Chapter 10).	Reduces the transmission of microorganisms
Peel the backing from the adhesive side of the electrodes.	Facilitates skin contact
Position each electrode flat against the skin (Fig. B).	Enhances contact with the skin for maximum effectiveness

Applying electrodes.

Space the electrodes at least the width of one from the other.	Prevents the potential for burning caused by close proximity of the electrodes
Make sure the settings on the TENS unit are off.	Prevents premature stimulation to the skin
Attach the cords from the electrodes to the outlet jacks on the TENS unit, much like a headset connects with a radio.	Completes the circuitry from the electrodes to the battery-operated power unit
Turn the amplitude (intensity) knob onto the lowest setting and assess whether the client can feel a tingling, buzzing, or vibrating sensation.	Helps acquaint the client with the sensation that the TENS unit produces
Gradually increase the intensity to the point at which the client experiences a mild or moderately pleasant sensation (Fig. C).	Adjusts intensity according to the client's response—a high intensity does not always provide the most pain relief; in fact, it may cause discomfort, muscle contractions, or itching

Adjusting the TENS settings.

Set the rate (pulses per second) at low and increase upward; a rate of 80–125 pulses per second is a conventional setting.	Adjusts the frequency of stimuli according to the client's comfort and tolerance
Set the pulse width (the duration of each pulsation); a pulse width of 60–100 µsec usually is used for acute pain, but 220–250 µsec at higher amplitudes may be necessary for chronic or intense pain.	Provides wider and deeper stimulation as the pulse width increases
Turn the unit off when a sufficient level of pain relief occurs and turn it back on when pain reappears.	Tests whether the TENS unit may be sufficient for intermittent rather than continuous use

SKILL 20-2 Operating a Transcutaneous Electrical Nerve Stimulation Unit (*continued*)

Suggested Action	Reason for Action
Turn the unit off and remove the cord from the outlet jacks before bathing the client.	Reduces hazards from potential contact of electrical equipment with water
Remove the electrode patches periodically to inspect the skin; re-apply electrodes if they become loose.	Aids in skin assessment
Slightly change the position of the electrodes if skin irritation develops.	Promotes skin integrity
Replace or recharge the batteries as needed.	Maintains function of the unit

EVALUATION

- Pain is managed at the goal set by the client.
- Activity is increased.
- Less pain medication is required.
- Emotional outlook is improved.

DOCUMENT

- Date and time
- Initial pain assessments
- Location of electrodes
- Power settings
- Length of time TENS unit is in use
- Reassessments of pain 30 minutes after application of unit and at least once per shift
- Time when TENS is stopped or discontinued

SAMPLE DOCUMENTATION

Date and Time Rates pain intensity as 10 on a scale from 0 to 10. Pain is described as "piercing" and continuous. Points to lower spine when asked to identify location of pain. Electrodes placed to the immediate R and L of the lumbosacral vertebrae. TENS unit initially set at a rate of 80 pulses per second and a pulse width of 60 μsec. Used for 30 minutes, at which time rated pain at "moderate." Rate increased to 100 pulses per second with a pulse width of 150. _____ J. Doe, LPN

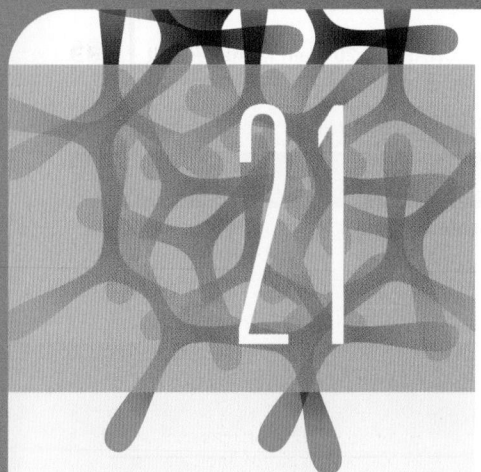

Oxygenation

Learning Objectives

On completion of this chapter, the reader should be able to:

1. Explain the difference between ventilation and respiration.
2. Differentiate between external and internal respiration.
3. Name methods for assessing the oxygenation status of clients at the bedside.
4. List signs of inadequate oxygenation.
5. Name nursing interventions that can be used to improve ventilation and oxygenation.
6. Name sources for supplemental oxygen.
7. Identify items that may be needed when providing oxygen therapy.
8. List common oxygen delivery devices.
9. Discuss hazards related to the administration of oxygen.
10. Describe additional therapeutic techniques that relate to oxygenation.
11. Discuss facts concerning oxygenation that affect the care of older adults.

INTRODUCTION

Oxygen, which measures approximately 21% in the Earth's atmosphere, is essential for sustaining life. Each cell of the human body uses oxygen to metabolize nutrients and produce energy. Without oxygen, cell death occurs rapidly.

This chapter describes the anatomic and physiologic aspects of breathing, techniques for assessing and monitoring oxygenation, types of equipment used in oxygen therapy, and skills needed to maintain respiratory function. Techniques for airway management, such as suctioning and other methods for maintaining a patent airway, are presented in Chapter 36.

 Gerontologic Considerations

■ Reduced gas exchange and efficiency in ventilation are age-related changes that can affect respiratory function, even in healthy older adults.

■ Functional changes to the respiratory system include diminished coughing and gag reflexes, increased use of accessory muscles for breathing, diminished efficiency of gas exchange in the lungs, and increased mouth breathing and snoring.

■ Some changes in lung volumes occur, resulting in a slight decrease in overall efficiency and increased energy expenditure by older adults.

■ Careful assessment of older adults who demonstrate restlessness or confusion is imperative for differentiating signs of inadequate oxygenation accurately from signs of delirium or dementia.

■ Older adults who require home oxygen need encouragement to continue socializing with others outside the home to prevent feelings of isolation and depression. It is important to teach older adults and their caregivers about portable oxygen equipment.

■ The skin behind the ears of older adults as well as others should be assessed for breakdown if oxygen administration equipment is secured by tubing or elastic.

■ Older adults who have lost weight and subcutaneous fat in their cheeks or who are not wearing their dentures may not receive the prescribed amounts of oxygen by mask because of an inadequate facial seal.

■ Advise older adults to receive annual influenza immunizations and a pneumonia immunization after 65 years of age or earlier if there is a history of chronic illness. Current guidelines recommend a booster dose for older adults who received their initial pneumonia immunization 5 or more years ago.

ANATOMY AND PHYSIOLOGY OF BREATHING

The elasticity of lung tissue allows the lungs to stretch and fill with air during **inspiration** (breathing in) and return to a resting position after **expiration** (breathing out). **Ventilation** (the movement of air in and out of the lungs) facilitates **respiration** (the exchange of oxygen and carbon dioxide). **External respiration** takes place at the most distal point in the airway between the alveolar and capillary membranes

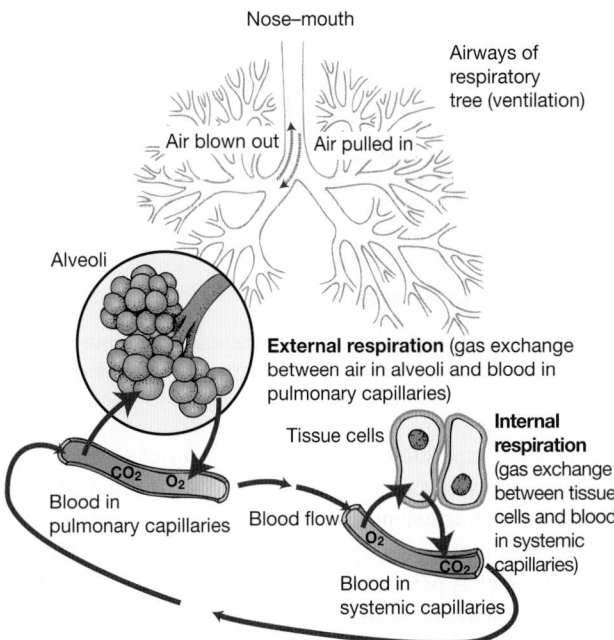

FIGURE 21-1 External and internal respiration.

(Fig. 21-1). **Internal respiration** occurs at the cellular level by means of hemoglobin and body cells. For people without respiratory disease, increased blood levels of carbon dioxide and hydrogen ions trigger the stimulus to breathe, both chemically and neurologically.

Ventilation results from pressure changes within the thoracic cavity produced by the contraction and relaxation of respiratory muscles (Fig. 21-2). During inspiration, the dome-shaped diaphragm contracts and moves downward in the thorax. The intercostal muscles move the chest outward by elevating the ribs and sternum. This combination expands the thoracic cavity. Expansion creates more chest space, causing the pressure within the lungs to fall below that in

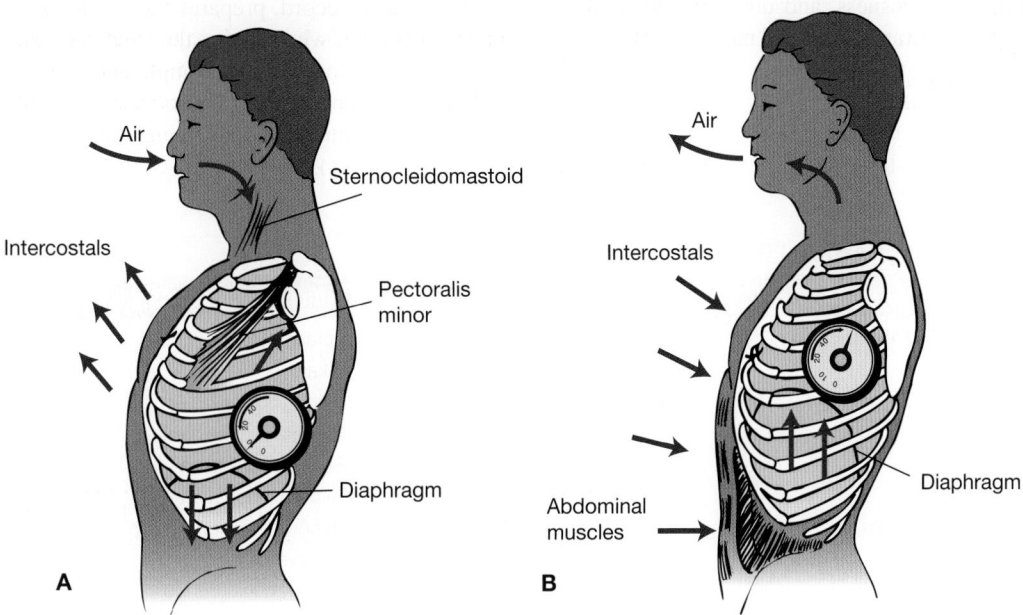

FIGURE 21-2 Ventilation and thoracic pressure changes. **A.** Inspiration. **B.** Expiration.

the atmosphere. Because air flows from an area of higher pressure to one of lower pressure, air is pulled in through the nose, filling the lungs. When there is an acute need for oxygen, additional muscles known as *accessory* muscles of respiration (the pectoralis minor and sternocleidomastoid) contract to assist with even greater chest expansion.

 Concept Mastery Alert

Inspiration and Chest Pressure

During inspiration, the chest cavity increases, but the chest pressure decreases, allowing air to move into the lungs.

During expiration, the respiratory muscles relax, the thoracic cavity decreases, the stretched elastic lung tissue recoils, intrathoracic pressure increases as a result of the compressed pulmonary space, and air moves out of the respiratory tract. A person can forcibly exhale additional air by contracting abdominal muscles, such as the rectus abdominis, transverse abdominis, and external and internal obliques.

ASSESSING OXYGENATION

The nurse can determine the quality of a client's oxygenation by collecting physical assessment data, monitoring arterial blood gases (ABGs), and using pulse oximetry. A combination of these measures helps identify signs of **hypoxemia** (insufficient oxygen within arterial blood) and **hypoxia** (inadequate oxygen at the cellular level).

Physical Assessment

The nurse physically assesses oxygenation by monitoring the client's respiratory rate, observing the breathing pattern and effort, checking chest symmetry, and auscultating lung sounds (see Chapter 13). Additional assessments include recording the heart rate and blood pressure, determining the client's level of consciousness, and observing the color of the skin, mucous membranes, lips, and nail beds (Box 21-1).

Arterial Blood Gases

An **arterial blood gas** (ABG) assessment is a laboratory test using arterial blood to evaluate or assess oxygenation,

BOX 21-1	Common Signs of Inadequate Oxygenation

- Decreased energy
- Restlessness
- Rapid, shallow breathing
- Rapid heart rate
- Sitting up to breathe
- Nasal flaring
- Use of accessory muscles
- Hypertension
- Sleepiness, confusion, stupor, coma

 Pharmacologic Considerations

All clients under 5 years of age, over 65 years, or anyone with a compromising chronic health condition should be assessed for and offered Prevnar 13, a pneumococcal vaccine. This vaccine is effective in reducing infection with 13 strains of *Streptococcus pneumoniae*.

ventilation, and acid–base balance. It measures the partial pressure of oxygen dissolved in plasma (PaO_2), the percentage of hemoglobin saturated with oxygen (SaO_2), the partial pressure of carbon dioxide in plasma ($PaCO_2$), the pH of blood, and the level of bicarbonate (HCO_3) ions (Table 21-1). Arterial blood is preferred for sampling because arteries have greater oxygen content than veins and are responsible for carrying oxygen to all cells. Initial and subsequent ABGs are ordered to assess the client in acute respiratory distress or to monitor the progress of a client receiving medical treatment.

In most situations, a laboratory technician and the nurse collaboratively collect arterial blood. The nurse notifies the laboratory of the need for the blood test, records pertinent assessments on the laboratory request form and in the client's medical record, prepares the client, assists the laboratory technician who obtains the specimen, and implements measures for preventing complications after the arterial puncture. In emergencies, a nurse who is trained in performing arterial punctures may obtain the specimen (Nursing Guidelines 21-1).

TABLE 21-1 Values for Arterial Blood Gases

COMPONENT	NORMAL RANGE	ABNORMAL FINDINGS	INDICATION OF ABNORMAL FINDINGS
pH	7.35–7.45	<7.35	Acidosis
		>7.45	Alkalosis
PaO_2	80–100 mm Hg	60–80 mm Hg	Mild hypoxemia
		40–60 mm Hg	Moderate hypoxemia
		<40 mm Hg	Severe hypoxemia
		>100 mm Hg	Hyperoxygenation
$PaCO_2$	35–45 mm Hg	<35 mm Hg	Hyperventilation
		>45 mm Hg	Hypoventilation
SaO_2	95%–100%	<95%	Hypoventilation
			Anemia
HCO_3	22–26 mEq	<22 or >26 mEq	Compensation for acid–base imbalance

NURSING GUIDELINES 21-1

Assisting with an arterial blood gas (ABG)

- Perform the Allen test before the arterial puncture by doing the following:
- Flex the client's elbow and elevate the forearm where the arterial puncture will be made.
- Compress the radial and ulnar arteries simultaneously (Fig. A).
- Instruct the client to open and close the fist until the palm of the hand appears blanched.
- Release pressure from the ulnar artery while maintaining pressure on the radial artery (Fig. B).
- Observe whether the skin flushes or remains blanched.
- Release pressure on the radial artery.

The Allen test determines whether the hand has an adequate ulnar arterial blood supply should the radial artery become damaged or occluded. The radial artery should not be punctured if the Allen test shows absent or poor collateral arterial blood flow as evidenced by continued blanching after pressure on the ulnar artery has been released. Alternative sites include the brachial, femoral, or dorsalis pedis arteries.

- Keep the client at rest for at least 30 minutes before obtaining the specimen unless the procedure is an emergency. *Because an ABG reflects the client's status at the moment of blood sampling, activity can transiently lower oxygen levels in the blood and lead to an incorrect interpretation of the test results.*
- Record the client's current temperature, respiratory rate, and level of activity if other than resting. *Increased metabolism and activity affect cellular oxygen demands. Therefore, the data help in interpreting the results of laboratory findings.*
- Record the amount of oxygen the client is receiving at the time of the test (either room air or prescribed amount) and ventilator settings. *This information helps determine whether oxygen therapy is necessary or aids in evaluating its current effectiveness.*

- Hyperextend the wrist over a rolled towel. *Hyperextension brings the radial artery nearer the skin surface to facilitate penetration.*
- Comfort the client during the puncture. *An arterial puncture tends to be painful unless a local anesthetic is used.*
- After obtaining the specimen, expel all air bubbles from it. *Doing so ensures that the only gas in the specimen is that contained in the blood.*
- Rotate the collected specimen. *Rotation mixes the blood with the anticoagulant in the specimen tube, ensuring that the blood sample will not clot before it can be examined.*
- Place the specimen on ice immediately. *Blood cells deteriorate outside the body, causing changes in the oxygen content of the sample. Cooling the sample slows cellular metabolism and ensures more accurate test results.*
- Apply direct manual pressure to the arterial puncture site for 5 to 10 minutes. *Arterial blood flows under higher pressure than venous blood. Therefore, prolonged manual pressure is necessary to control bleeding.*
- Cover the puncture site with a pressure dressing composed of several 4 × 4 in gauze squares and tape. *Tight mechanical compression provides continued pressure to reduce the potential for arterial bleeding.*
- Assess the puncture site periodically for bleeding or formation of a hematoma (collection of trapped blood) beneath the skin. *Periodic inspection aids in the early identification of arterial bleeding, which can lead to substantial blood loss and discomfort.*
- Report the laboratory findings to the prescribing physician as soon as they are available. *Collaboration with the physician assists in making changes in the treatment plan to improve the client's condition.*

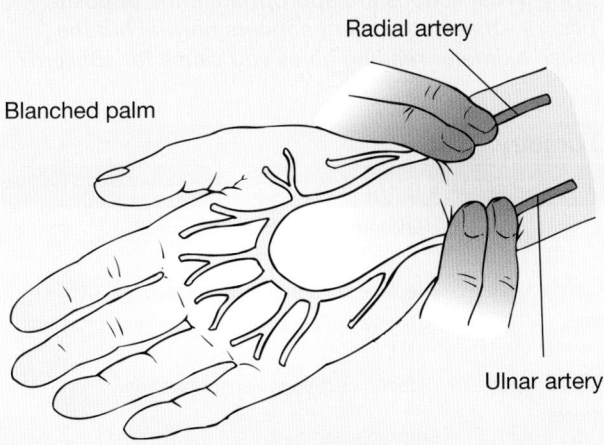

A

Simultaneous compression of radial and ulnar arteries.

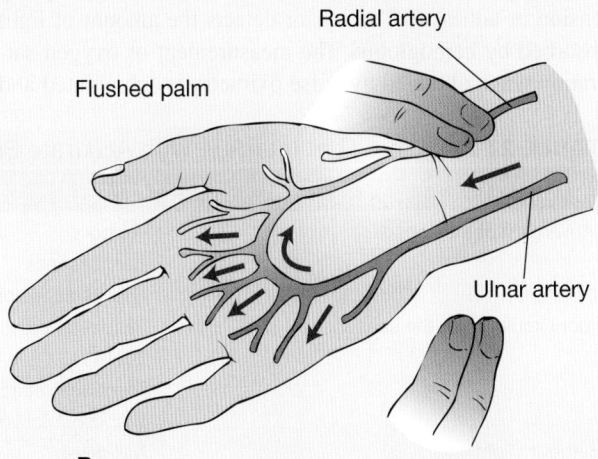

B

Pressure on the ulnar artery is released.

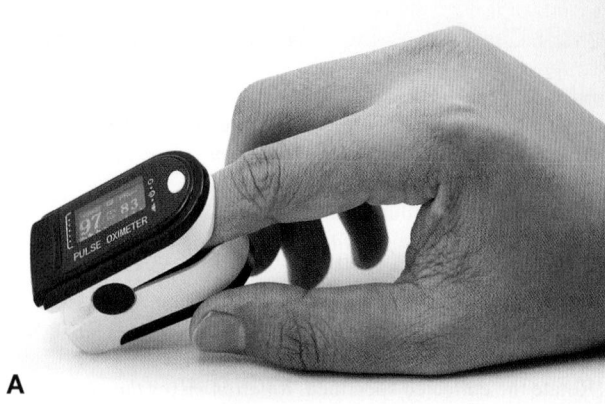

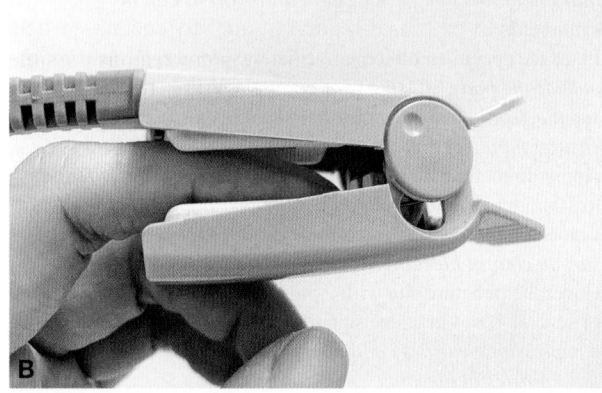

FIGURE 21-3 A. Pulse oximetry (TomoTaro/Shutterstock). **B.** Close-up of pulse oximeter showing infrared light emitter (DaViDa S/Shutterstock).

Pulse Oximetry

Pulse oximetry is a noninvasive, transcutaneous technique for periodically or continuously monitoring the oxygen saturation of blood. A pulse oximeter is composed of a photodetector sensor, a red and infrared light emitter, and a microprocessor (Fig. 21-3). The sensor is attached to a finger, toe, earlobe, or the bridge of the nose using spring tension or adhesive. The sensor detects the amount of light absorbed by hemoglobin. The measurement of oxygen saturation when obtained by pulse oximetry is abbreviated and

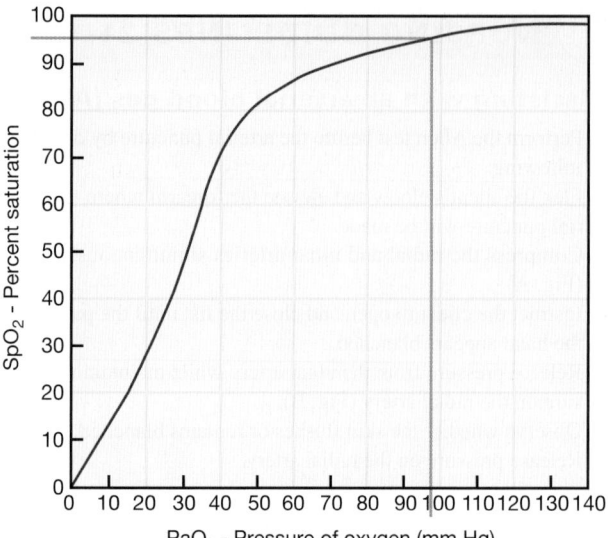

FIGURE 21-4 Draw a line from the SpO_2 in the left column across the graph to the point at which it intersects the curve. Use the numeric scale at the bottom to calculate the PaO_2. In this example, with an SpO_2 of 95%, the PaO_2 is approximately 98 mm Hg.

recorded as SpO_2 to distinguish it from the SaO_2 measurement obtained from arterial blood.

Based on the oxygen–hemoglobin dissociation curve (Fig. 21-4), it is possible to infer the PaO_2 from the pulse oximetry measurement. The normal SpO_2 is 95% to 100%. A sustained level of less than 90% is cause for concern. If the SpO_2 remains low, the client needs oxygen therapy. Various factors, however, affect the accuracy of the displayed information (Table 21-2). Troubleshooting the equipment, performing current physical assessments, and obtaining an ABG help confirm the significance of the displayed findings.

»» *Stop, Think, and Respond 21-1*

What actions are appropriate if a client appears to be hypoxemic but the pulse oximeter indicates a normal SpO_2? What actions are appropriate if the opposite occurs—that is, the client appears normal but the pulse oximeter reading gives you cause for concern?

TABLE 21-2 Factors That Interfere with Accurate Pulse Oximetry

FACTOR	CAUSE	REMEDY
Movement of the sensor	Tremor	Relocate sensor to another site.
	Restlessness	
	Loss of adhesion	Replace sensor or tape in place.
Poor circulation at the sensor site	Peripheral vascular disease	Change the sensor location or type of sensor.
	Edema	
	Tourniquet effect from taped sensor	Loosen or change sensor location.
	Vasoconstrictive drug effects	
Barrier to light	Nail polish	Discontinue use temporarily.
	Thick toenails	Remove polish.
	Acrylic nails	Relocate sensor.
		Remove acrylic nails.
Extraneous light	Direct sunlight	Cover sensor with a towel.
	Treatment lights	
Hemoglobin saturation with other substances	Carbon monoxide poisoning	Discontinue use temporarily.

PROMOTING OXYGENATION

Many factors affect ventilation and subsequently respiration (Table 21-3). Positioning and teaching breathing techniques are two nursing interventions frequently used to promote oxygenation. Adhesive nasal strips can be used to improve oxygenation by reducing nasal airway resistance and improving ventilation.

Positioning

Unless contraindicated by a condition, clients with hypoxia are placed in high **Fowler position** (an upright seated position; see Chapter 23). This position eases breathing by allowing the abdominal organs to descend away from the diaphragm. As a result, the lungs have the potential to fill with a greater volume of air.

As an alternative, clients who find breathing difficult may benefit from variations of Fowler position. An option is a **tripod position** in which the client is in a seated position with the arms supported on pillows or the armrests of a chair, or leaning over while allowing the hands to push on their thighs. The tripod position increases a client's breathing capacity by using the arms to lift the chest upward (Fig. 21-5A). Another option is an **orthopneic position** in bed. In the orthopneic position, the client leans forward over the bedside table or a chair back (Fig. 21-5B). The orthopneic position allows room for maximum vertical and lateral chest expansion and provides comfort while resting or sleeping.

Breathing Techniques

Breathing techniques such as deep breathing with or without an incentive spirometer, pursed-lip breathing, and diaphragmatic breathing help clients breathe more efficiently.

Deep Breathing

Deep breathing is a technique for maximizing ventilation. Taking in a large volume of air fills alveoli to a greater capacity, thus improving gas exchange. Deep breathing is therapeutic for clients who tend to breathe shallowly, such as those who are inactive or in pain. To encourage deep breathing, the client learns to take in as much air as possible, hold the breath briefly, and exhale slowly. In some cases, it is helpful to use an incentive spirometer; however, deep breathing alone is sufficiently beneficial when performed effectively.

Incentive Spirometry

Incentive spirometry, a technique for deep breathing using a calibrated device, encourages clients to reach a goal-directed volume of inspired air. Although spirometers

TABLE 21-3 Factors Affecting Oxygenation

FACT	NURSING IMPLICATION
Adequate respiration depends on a minimum of 21% oxygen in the environment and normal function of the cardiopulmonary system.	Clients with cardiopulmonary disorders require > 21% oxygen to maintain adequate oxygenation of blood and cells.
Breathing can be voluntarily controlled.	Assist clients who are hyperventilating to slow the rate of breathing; teach clients to perform pursed-lip breathing to exhale more completely.
Clients with chronic lung diseases are stimulated to breathe by low blood levels of oxygen, called the "hypoxic drive to breathe."	Giving high percentages of oxygen can depress breathing in clients with chronic lung disease. No > 2–3 L oxygen is safe unless the client is mechanically ventilated.
Smoking causes increased amounts of inhaled carbon monoxide that compete and bond more easily than oxygen to the hemoglobin.	Clients who smoke have a greater potential for compromised gas exchange and acquiring chronic pulmonary and cardiac diseases.
Nicotine increases the heart rate and constricts arteries.	Teach people who do not smoke never to start.
	Identify products that are available, such as nicotine skin patches and gum, which can help with smoking cessation.
Pregnant people who smoke have a risk for low-birth-weight infants because low blood oxygenation affects fetal metabolism and growth.	Promote smoking cessation for pregnant people who are addicted to nicotine.
Pulmonary secretions within the airway and fluid within the interstitial space between the alveoli and the capillaries interfere with gas exchange.	Encourage coughing, deep breathing, turning, and ambulating to keep the alveoli inflated and the airway clear.
	Antibiotics, diuretics, and drugs that improve heart contraction reduce fluid within the lungs.
Gas exchange is increased by maximum lung expansion and compromised by any condition that compresses the diaphragm, such as obesity, intestinal gas, pregnancy, and an enlarged liver.	Assist clients to sit up to lower abdominal organs away from the diaphragm.
	Encourage weight loss, expulsion of gas via ambulation and bowel elimination, and assist with removing abdominal fluid by paracentesis (see Chapter 14) to improve breathing.
Activity and emotional stress increase the metabolic need for greater amounts of oxygen.	Provide rest periods and teach stress reduction techniques such as muscle relaxation to promote maintenance of blood oxygen levels.
Pain associated with muscle movement around abdominal and flank surgical incisions decreases the incentive to breathe deeply and cough forcefully.	Teach and supervise deep breathing before surgery. Support the incision with a pillow and administer drugs that relieve pain to facilitate ventilation.

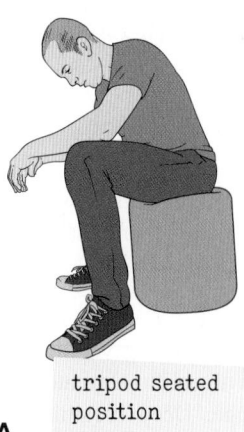 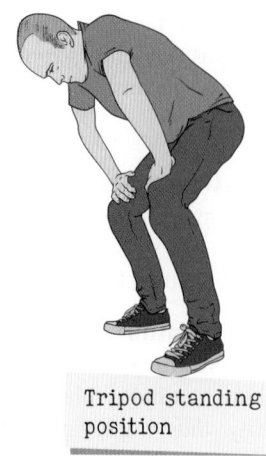

A

tripod seated position

Tripod standing position

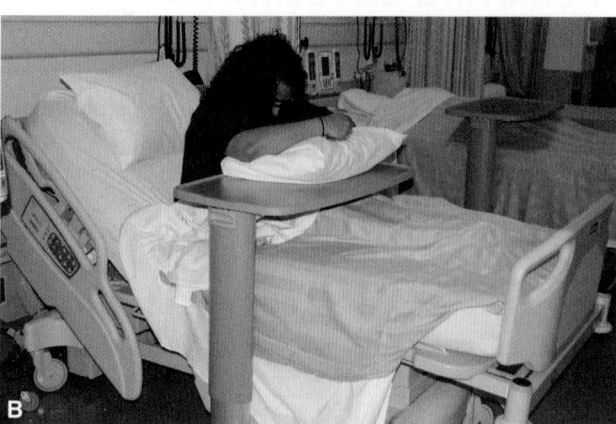

B

FIGURE 21-5 A. Different tripod positions used to reduce shortness of breath (EreborMountain/Shutterstock). **B.** The orthopneic position.

are constructed in different ways, all are marked in at least 100-mL increments and include some visual cues, such as elevation of lightweight balls, to show how much air the client has inhaled (Fig. 21-6). The calibrated measurement also helps the nurse evaluate the effectiveness of the client's breathing efforts (Client and Family Teaching 21-1).

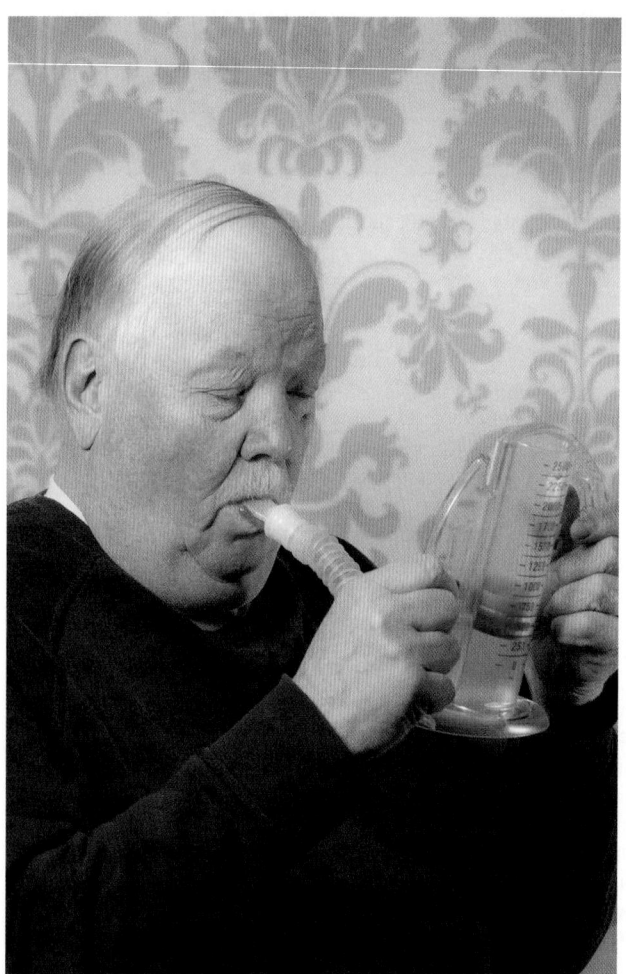

FIGURE 21-6 Incentive spirometry. During deep inhalation, a ball rises in an incentive spirometer (Debra Anderson/Shutterstock).

**Client and Family Teaching 21-1
Using an Incentive Spirometer**

The nurse teaches the client and the family as follows:
- Sit upright unless contraindicated.
- Identify the mark indicating the goal for inhalation.
- Exhale normally.
- Insert the mouthpiece, sealing it between the lips.
- Inhale slowly and deeply until the predetermined volume has been reached.
- Hold the breath for 3 to 6 seconds.
- Remove the mouthpiece and exhale normally.
- Relax and breathe normally before the next breath with the spirometer.
- Repeat the exercise 10 to 20 times/hour while awake or as prescribed by the physician.

Pursed-Lip Breathing
Pursed-lip breathing is a form of controlled ventilation in which the client consciously prolongs the expiration phase of breathing. This is another technique for improving gas exchange, which helps clients eliminate more than the usual amount of carbon dioxide from the lungs when done correctly. Pursed-lip breathing and diaphragmatic breathing are especially helpful for clients who have chronic obstructive pulmonary disorders (COPDs), such as emphysema, which are characterized by chronic hypoxemia and **hypercarbia** (excessive levels of carbon dioxide in the blood). The client performs pursed-lip breathing as follows:

- Inhale slowly through the nose while counting to three.
- Purse the lips as though to whistle.
- Contract the abdominal muscles.
- Exhale through pursed lips for a count of six or more.

Expiration should be two to three times longer than inspiration. Not all clients can achieve this goal initially, but with practice, the length of expiration can increase.

Diaphragmatic Breathing

Diaphragmatic breathing is breathing that promotes the use of the diaphragm rather than the upper chest muscles. It is used to increase the volume of air exchanged during inspiration and expiration. With practice, diaphragmatic breathing reduces respiratory effort and relieves rapid, ineffective breathing (Client and Family Teaching 21-2).

Nasal Strips

Adhesive nasal strips, commercially available in drugstores, are used to reduce airflow resistance by widening the breathing passageways of the nose. Increasing the nasal diameter promotes easier breathing. Common users of nasal strips are people with ineffective breathing as well as athletes, whose oxygen requirements increase during sustained exercise. Another use for nasal strips is to reduce or eliminate snoring.

OXYGEN THERAPY

When positioning and breathing techniques are inadequate for keeping the blood adequately saturated with oxygen, oxygen therapy is necessary. **Oxygen therapy** is an intervention for administering more oxygen than is present in the atmosphere to prevent or relieve hypoxemia. It requires an oxygen source, a flowmeter, in some cases an oxygen analyzer or humidifier, and an oxygen delivery device.

Oxygen Sources

Oxygen is supplied from any one of four sources: wall outlet, portable tank, liquid oxygen unit, or oxygen concentrator.

Wall Outlet

Most modern health care facilities supply oxygen through a wall outlet in the client's room. The outlet is connected to a large central reservoir filled with oxygen on a routine basis.

Client and Family Teaching 21-2
Diaphragmatic Breathing

The nurse teaches the client and the family as follows:

- Lie down with knees slightly bent.
- Place one hand on the abdomen and the other on the chest.
- Inhale slowly and deeply through the nose while letting the abdomen rise more than the chest.
- Purse the lips.
- Contract the abdominal muscles and begin to exhale.
- Press inward and upward with the hand on the abdomen while continuing to exhale.
- Repeat the exercise for 1 full minute; rest for at least 2 minutes.
- Practice the breathing exercises at least twice a day for a period of 5 to 10 minutes.
- Progress to diaphragmatic breathing while upright and active.

Portable Tanks

When oxygen is not piped into individual rooms or if the client needs to leave the room temporarily, oxygen is provided in portable tanks (Fig. 21-7) that hold various volumes under extreme pressure. A large tank of oxygen contains 2,000 lb of pressure per square inch. Therefore, tanks are delivered with a protective cap to prevent accidental force against the tank outlet. Any accidental force applied to a partially opened outlet could cause the tank to take flight like a rocket with disastrous results. Therefore, oxygen tanks are transported and stored while strapped to a wheeled carrier.

Before oxygen is administered from a portable tank, the tank is "cracked," a technique for clearing the outlet of dust and debris. Cracking is done by turning the tank valve slightly with a wrench to allow a brief release of pressurized oxygen (Fig. 21-8). The force causes a loud hissing noise, which may be frightening. Therefore, it is best to crack the tank away from the client's bedside.

Liquid Oxygen Unit

A **liquid oxygen unit** is a device that converts cooled liquid oxygen into gas by passing it through heated coils (Fig. 21-9). Ambulatory clients at home primarily use these small, lightweight, portable units because they allow greater mobility inside and outside the home. Each unit holds approximately 4 to 8 hours' worth of oxygen. Potential problems include that liquid oxygen is more expensive, the unit may leak during warm weather, and frozen moisture may occlude the outlet.

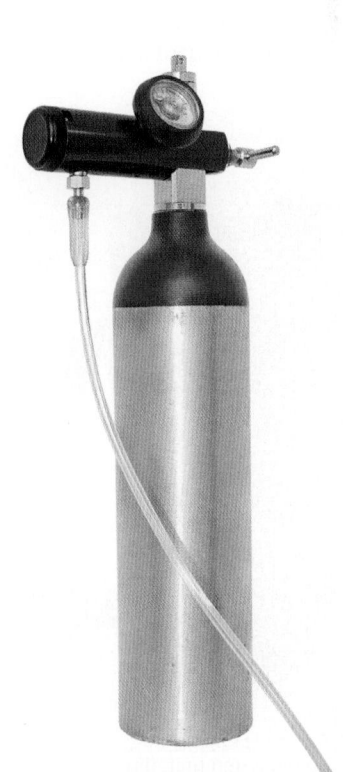

FIGURE 21-7 Portable oxygen tank (rCarner/Shutterstock).

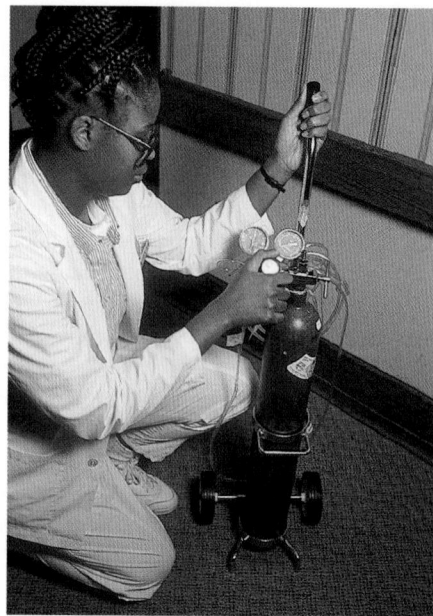

FIGURE 21-8 A nurse opens a portable oxygen tank with a wrench.

Liquid Oxygen Concentrator

An **oxygen concentrator** is a machine that collects and concentrates oxygen from room air and stores it for client use. The oxygen concentrator works on electricity; it takes in room air, removes nitrogen from it, and provides up to 95% pure oxygen (Fig. 21-10). Oxygen concentrators typically provide oxygen flows of 1 to 10 L/minute. When concentrators were first introduced, they were large, heavy pieces of equipment. Now, portable oxygen concentrators (POCs) are lighter in weight; some weigh as little as 5 lb, and they can be powered by both standard household AC 110 currents

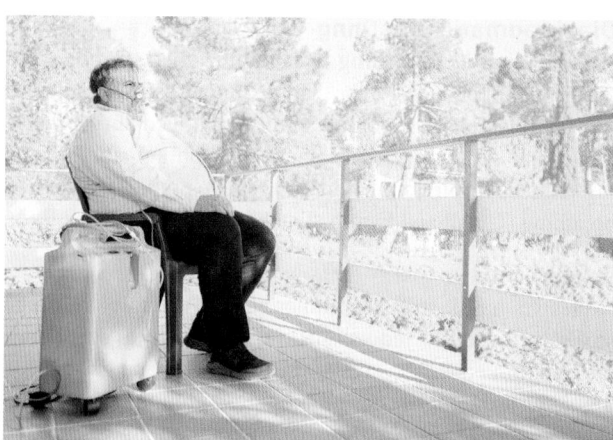

FIGURE 21-10 A portable oxygen concentrator extracts nitrogen and concentrates oxygen to enable clients who require oxygen therapy to travel about or maintain their lifestyles without the need for multiple tanks of oxygen (Itxu/Shutterstock).

and the DC outlet found in motor vehicles and rechargeable batteries (webmd, 2023).

An oxygen concentrator eliminates the need for a central reservoir of piped oxygen or the use of bulky tanks that must be constantly replaced. This type of oxygen source is used in home health care and long-term care facilities, primarily because of its convenience and economy. It is essential that clients have a secondary source of oxygen available in case of a power failure.

Equipment Used in Oxygen Administration

In addition to an oxygen source, other pieces of equipment used during the administration of oxygen are a flowmeter, oxygen analyzer, and humidifier.

Flowmeter

The flow of oxygen is measured in liters per minute (L/minute). A **flowmeter** is a gauge used to regulate the amount of oxygen delivered to the client and is attached to the oxygen source (Fig. 21-11). To adjust the rate of flow, the nurse turns the dial until the indicator is directly beside the prescribed amount.

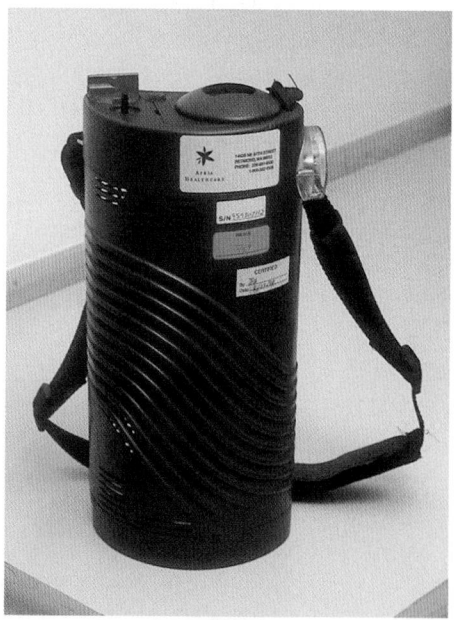

FIGURE 21-9 A liquid oxygen unit. (From Craven, R. F., Hirnle, C. J., & Henshaw, C. [2020]. *Fundamentals of nursing* [9th ed.]. Wolters Kluwer.)

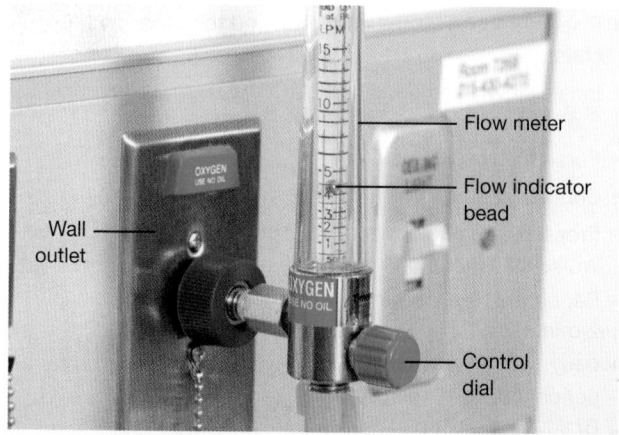

FIGURE 21-11 A flowmeter attached to a wall outlet for oxygen administration.

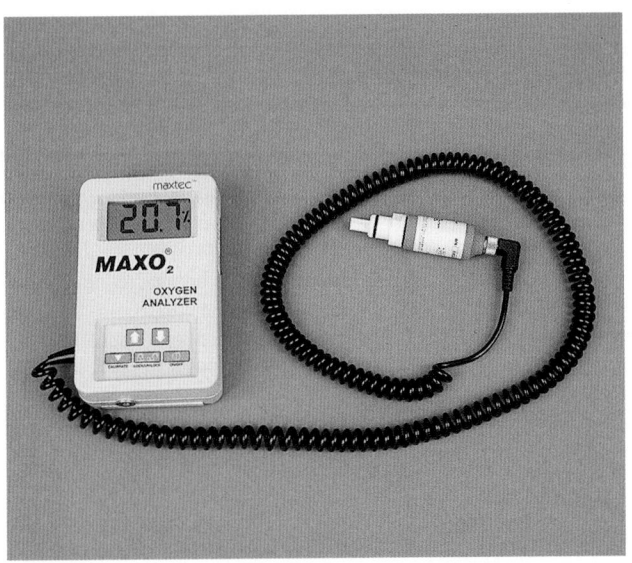

FIGURE 21-12 An oxygen analyzer. (Photo by B. Proud.)

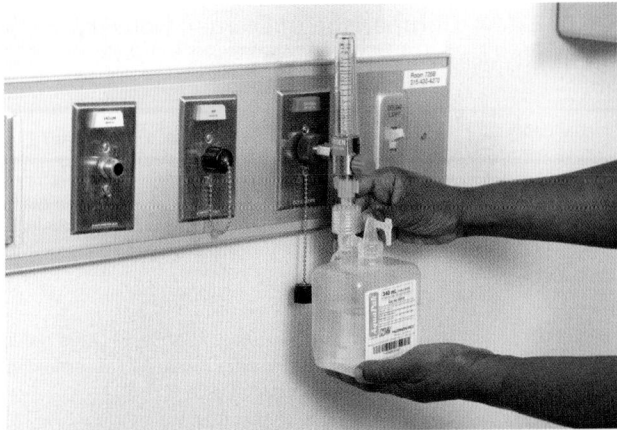

FIGURE 21-13 An oxygen humidifier attached to a flowmeter.

The physician prescribes the concentration of oxygen, also called the **fraction of inspired oxygen** (FIO_2; the portion of oxygen in relation to total inspired gas), as a percentage or as a decimal (e.g., 40% or 0.40). The prescription is based on the client's condition. The Joint Commission recommends that oxygen be prescribed as a percentage rather than in liters per minute because, depending on the oxygen delivery device, liters per minute may provide different percentages of oxygen.

Oxygen Analyzer

An **oxygen analyzer** is a device that measures the percentage of delivered oxygen to determine whether the client is receiving the amount prescribed by the physician (Fig. 21-12). The nurse or respiratory therapist first checks the percentage of oxygen in the room air with the analyzer. If there is a normal mixture of oxygen and other gases in the environment, the analyzer indicates 0.21 (21%). When the analyzer is positioned near or within the device used to deliver oxygen, the reading should register at the prescribed amount (over 0.21). If there is a discrepancy, the nurse adjusts the flowmeter to reach the desired amount. Oxygen analyzers are used most often when caring for newborns in isolettes, children in croup tents, and clients who are mechanically ventilated.

Humidifier

A **humidifier** is a device that produces small water droplets and may be used during oxygen administration because oxygen is drying to the mucous membranes. In most cases, oxygen is humidified only when more than 4 L/minute is administered for an extended period. When humidification is desired, a bottle is filled with distilled water and attached to the flowmeter (Fig. 21-13). A respiratory therapist or nurse checks the water level daily and refills the bottle as needed.

Common Delivery Devices

Common oxygen delivery devices include a nasal cannula, masks, a face tent, a tracheostomy collar, and a T-piece

(Table 21-4). The device prescribed depends on the client's oxygenation status, physical condition, and amount of oxygen needed. Skill 21-1 describes how to administer oxygen by common delivery methods.

Nasal Cannula

A **nasal cannula**, the most common oxygen delivery device, is a hollow tube with 1/2-in prongs placed into the client's nostrils. It is held in place by wrapping the tubing around the ears and adjusting the fit beneath the chin (Fig. 21-14). The skin around the ears and cheeks should be assessed for pressure. Padding the area around the ears may be required to keep the skin intact. Frequent mouth and nasal care are indicated.

A nasal cannula provides a means of administering low concentrations of oxygen. Therefore, it is ideal for clients who are not extremely hypoxic or who have chronic lung diseases. High percentages of oxygen are contraindicated for clients with chronic lung disease because they have adapted to excessive levels of retained carbon dioxide and low blood oxygen levels to stimulate the drive to breathe. Consequently, if clients with chronic lung disease receive more than 2 to 3 L of oxygen over a sustained period, the respiratory rate slows or even stops.

Traditional nasal cannulas can effectively provide up to 4 to 6 L/minute of supplemental oxygen; however, newer high-flow nasal cannula therapy is an oxygen supply system that is capable of delivering up to 100% humidified and heated oxygen at a flow rate of up to 60 L/minute. The high-flow nasal therapy must be monitored closely by respiratory therapists, nurses, and the medical provider (Sharma et al., 2022).

>>> *Stop, Think, and Respond 21-2*

Explain the difference between a flowmeter and an oxygen analyzer.

Masks

Oxygen can be delivered using a simple mask, a partial rebreather mask, a nonrebreather mask, or a venturi mask.

Simple Mask

A **simple mask** fits over the nose and mouth and allows atmospheric air to enter and exit through side ports (Fig. 21-15).

TABLE 21-4 Comparison of Oxygen Delivery Devices

DEVICE	COMMON RANGE OF ADMINISTRATION	ADVANTAGES	DISADVANTAGES
Nasal cannula	2–6 L/minute	Is easy to apply; promotes comfort	Dries nasal mucosa at higher flows
	FIO_2 24%–40%[a]	Does not interfere with eating or talking	May irritate the skin on the cheeks, nose, and behind ears
		Is less likely to create a feeling of suffocation	Is less effective in some clients who tend to mouth breathe
			Does not facilitate administering high FIO_2 to hypoxic clients
High-flow nasal cannula	Capable of delivering up to 100% humidified and heated oxygen at a flow rate of up to 60 L/minute	Does not interfere with eating or smoking	Is a newer treatment and education for use of the equipment is necessary
	FIO_2 from 21% to 100% irrespective of flow rates	Creates a positive pressure environment that increases oxygenation potential	
Masks			
Simple	5–8 L/minute	Provides higher concentrations than possible with a cannula	Requires humidification
	FIO_2 35%–50%[a]	Is effective for mouth breathers or clients with nasal disorders	Interferes with eating and talking
	Allows a client to inhale a mixture of 75% room air and 25% oxygen	Can cause anxiety among those who are claustrophobic	Creates a risk for rebreathing CO_2 retained within mask when <6 L/minute is administered
Partial rebreather	6–10 L/minute	Increases the amount of oxygen with lower liter flows	Requires a minimum of 6 L/minute
	FIO_2 35%–60%[a]		Creates a risk for suffocation
			Requires monitoring to verify that the reservoir bag remains inflated at all times
Nonrebreather	6–10 L/minute	Delivers highest FIO_2 possible with a mask	See partial rebreather mask
	FIO_2 60%–90%[a]	Prevents breathing room air	Creates a risk for oxygen toxicity
			Exhaled air is not rebreathed.
Venturi	4–8 L/min	Delivers FIO_2 precisely through adjustable ports	Permits condensation to form in tubing, which diminishes the flow of oxygen
	FIO_2 24%–40%[a]		
		Buildup of carbon dioxide is minimal.	
Face tent	8–12 L/min	Provides a comfortable fit	Interferes with eating
	FIO_2 30%–55%[a]	Is useful for clients with facial trauma, facial burns, or who are claustrophobic when an oxygen mask is applied	May result in inconsistent FIO_2, depending on environmental loss
		Facilitates humidification	
Tracheostomy collar	4–10 L/minute	Facilitates humidifying and warming oxygen	Allows water vapor to collect in tubing, which may drain into airway
	FIO_2 24%–100%[a]		
T-piece	4–10 L/minute	Delivers any desired FIO_2 with high humidity	May pull on tracheostomy tube
	FIO_2 24%–100%[a]		Allows humidity to collect and moisten gauze dressing

[a]American Association for Respiratory Care (AARC).

An elastic strap holds it in place. The simple mask, like other types of masks, allows for the administration of higher levels of oxygen than are possible with a cannula. A simple mask is sometimes substituted for a cannula when a client has nasal trauma or breathes through the mouth. When a simple mask is used, oxygen is delivered at no less than 5 L/minute.

The efficiency of any mask is affected by how well it fits the face. Without a good seal, the oxygen leaks from the mask, thus diminishing its concentration. Other problems are associated with masks as well. All oxygen masks interfere with eating and make verbal communication difficult to understand. Also, some clients become anxious when the nose and mouth are covered because it creates a feeling of being suffocated. Skin care also becomes a priority because masks create pressure and trap moisture.

Partial Rebreather Mask

A **partial rebreather mask** is an oxygen delivery device through which a client inhales a mixture of atmospheric air, oxygen from its source, and oxygen contained within a

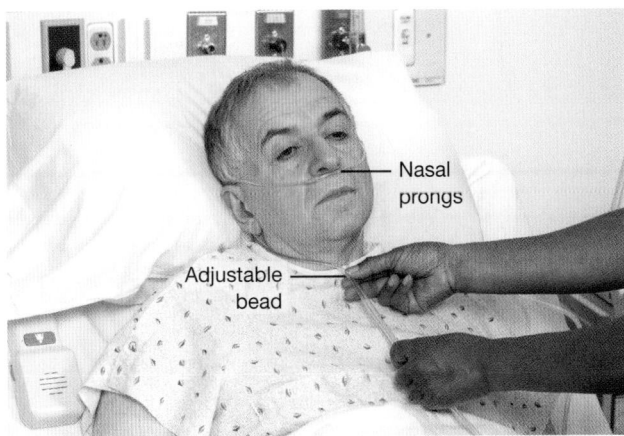

FIGURE 21-14 Oxygen delivered with a nasal cannula.

reservoir bag (Fig. 21-16). It provides a means for recycling oxygen and venting all the carbon dioxide during expiration from the mask. During expiration, the first third of exhaled air enters the reservoir bag. The portion of exhaled air in the reservoir bag contains a high proportion of oxygen because it comes directly from the upper airways; the gas in this area has not been involved in gas exchange at the alveolar level. Once the reservoir bag is filled, the remainder of exhaled air is forced from the mask through small ports. With a simple mask, some carbon dioxide always remains within the mask and is reinhaled.

Nonrebreather Mask

A **nonrebreather mask** is an oxygen delivery device in which all the exhaled air leaves the mask rather than partially entering the reservoir bag (Fig. 21-17). It is designed to deliver an F_{IO_2} of 90% to 100%. This type of mask contains one-way valves that allow only oxygen from its source, as well as the oxygen in the reservoir bag, to be

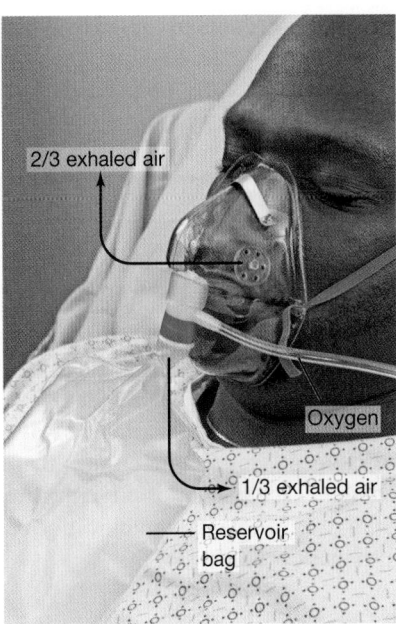

FIGURE 21-16 A partial rebreather mask delivers a higher percentage of oxygen than a simple mask.

inhaled. No air from the atmosphere is inhaled. All the air that is exhaled is vented from the mask. None enters the reservoir bag. Obviously, clients for whom nonrebreather masks are used are those who require high concentrations of oxygen. They are usually critically ill and may eventually need mechanical ventilation. Despite the high concentration of oxygen, humidification is not employed when a mask with a reservoir bag is used. Also, clients with partial and nonrebreather masks are monitored closely to ensure that the reservoir bag remains partially inflated at all times.

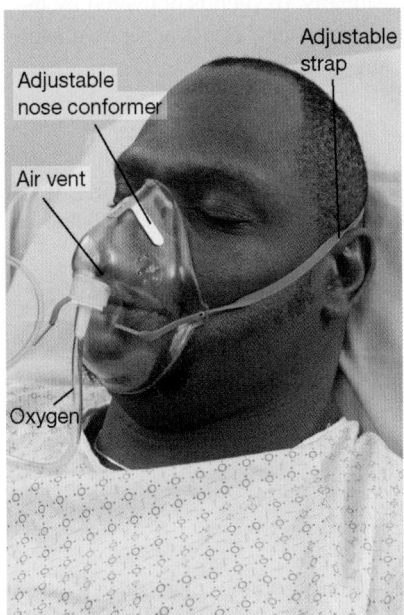

FIGURE 21-15 A simple mask is used to administer oxygen.

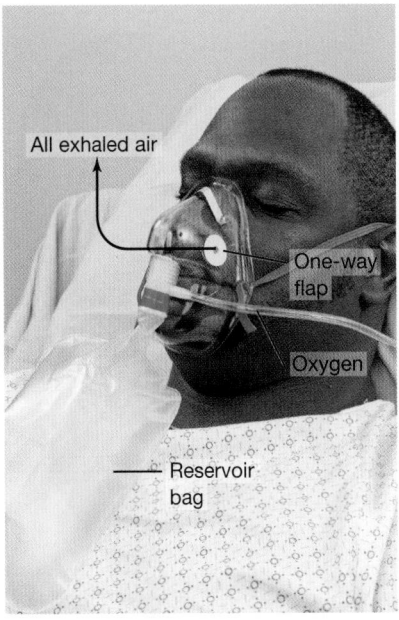

FIGURE 21-17 A nonrebreather mask can deliver the highest amount of oxygen without the use of a mechanical ventilator.

Oxygen toxicity, a condition caused by breathing a high concentration of oxygen, can develop among clients who require the prolonged use of a nonrebreather mask and is discussed later in this chapter. Oxygen toxicity can result in irreversible pulmonary damage as well as decreases the stimulus to breathe that naturally occurs when carbon dioxide levels rise.

Venturi Mask

A **venturi mask** mixes a precise amount of oxygen and atmospheric air. Sometimes called a *venti mask*, this mask has a large ringed tube extending from it (Fig. 21-18). Adapters within the tube, which are color coded or regulated by a dial system, permit only specific amounts of room air to mix with the oxygen. This feature ensures that the venturi mask delivers the exact amount of prescribed oxygen. Unlike masks with reservoir bags, humidification can be added when a venturi mask is used.

Face Tent

A **face tent** provides oxygen to the nose and mouth without the discomfort of a mask (Fig. 21-19). Because the face tent is open and loose around the face, clients are less likely to feel claustrophobic. An added advantage is that a face mask can be used for clients with facial trauma or burns. A disadvantage is that the amount of oxygen clients actually receive may be inconsistent with what is prescribed because of environmental losses.

Tracheostomy Collar

A **tracheostomy collar** delivers oxygen near an artificial opening in the neck (Fig. 21-20). It is applied over a tracheostomy—an opening into the trachea through which a client breathes (see Chapter 36). Because it bypasses the warming and moisturizing functions of the nose, a tracheostomy collar provides a means for both oxygenation and

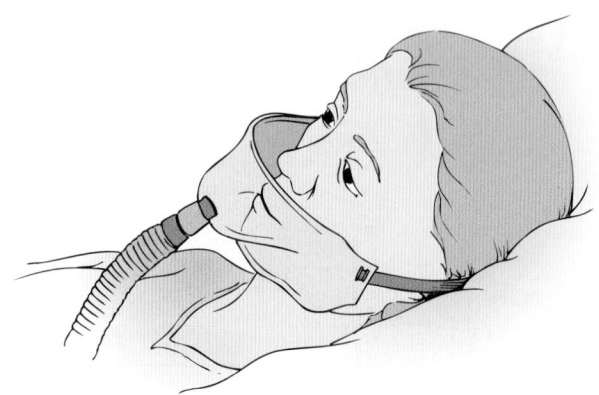

FIGURE 21-19 A face tent supplies oxygen toward the nose and mouth of a client.

humidification. The moisture that collects, however, tends to saturate the gauze dressing around the tracheostomy, making it necessary to change it frequently.

T-Piece

A **T-piece** fits securely onto a tracheostomy tube or endotracheal tube (Fig. 21-21). It is similar to a tracheostomy collar but is attached directly to the artificial airway. Although the gauze around the tracheostomy usually remains dry, the moisture that collects within the tubing tends to condense and may enter the airway during position changes if it is not drained periodically. Another disadvantage is that the weight of the T-piece, or its manipulation, may pull on the tracheostomy tube, causing the client to cough or experience discomfort. To avoid displacing the tracheostomy tube, the T-piece may need to be supported with a rolled towel.

Additional Delivery Devices

Other methods for delivering oxygen are used less commonly. Occasionally, oxygen is delivered by means of a nasal catheter, oxygen tent, transtracheal catheter, or positive airway pressure machines.

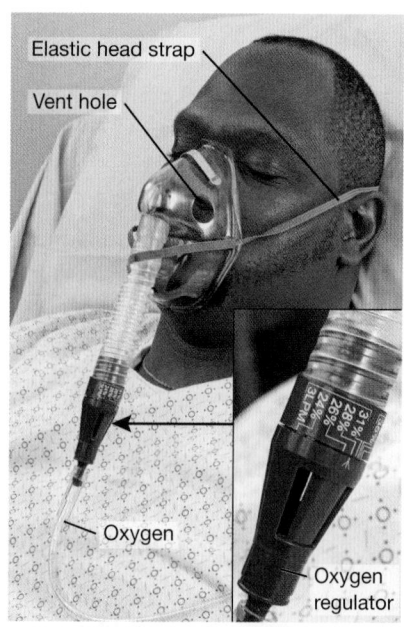

FIGURE 21-18 A venturi mask can be adjusted to deliver a variety of oxygen percentages.

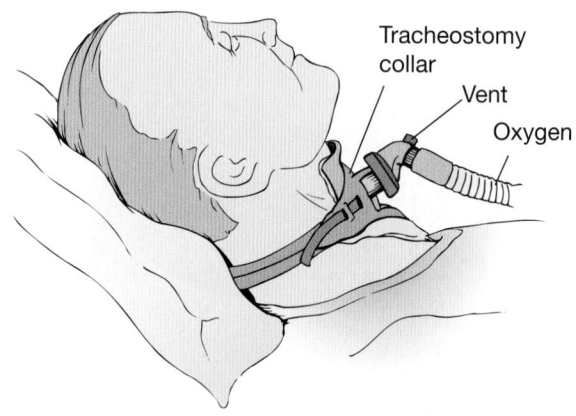

FIGURE 21-20 A tracheostomy collar is used to deliver oxygen via an artificial airway when the client does not breathe through the nose or mouth.

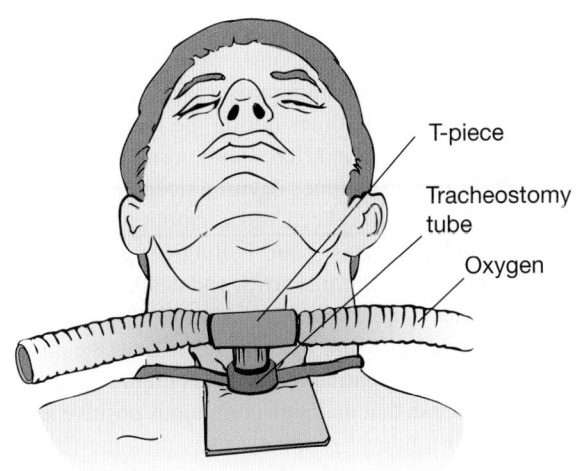

FIGURE 21-21 A T-piece attached to an airway.

Nasal Catheter

A **nasal catheter** is a method for delivering oxygen with a tube inserted through the nose into the posterior nasal pharynx (Fig. 21-22). It is used for clients who tend to breathe through the mouth or experience claustrophobia when a mask covers the face. The catheter tends to irritate the nasopharynx; therefore, some clients find it uncomfortable. If a catheter is prescribed, the nurse secures it to the nose to avoid displacement and regularly cleans the nostril with a cotton applicator to remove the dried mucus.

Transtracheal Oxygen

Some clients who require long-term oxygen therapy may prefer its administration through a **transtracheal catheter** (a hollow tube inserted within the trachea to deliver oxygen; Fig. 21-23). This device is less noticeable than a nasal cannula. The client is adequately oxygenated with lower flows, decreasing the costs of replenishing the oxygen source.

Before transtracheal oxygen is used, a **stent** (tube that keeps a channel open) is inserted into a surgically created opening and remains there until the wound heals. Thereafter, the stent is removed, and the catheter is inserted and held in place with a necklace-type chain. Clients learn how to clean

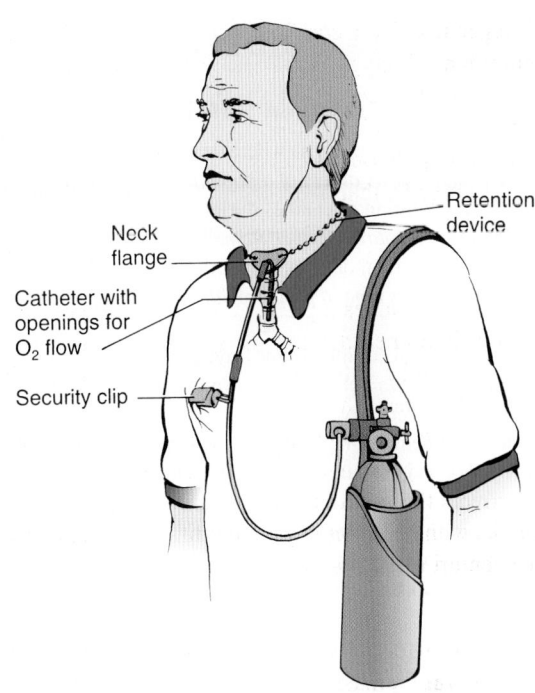

FIGURE 21-23 Transtracheal oxygen administration.

the tracheal opening and catheter, a procedure performed several times a day. During cleaning, clients administer oxygen with a nasal cannula.

Oxygen Tent

An **oxygen tent** is a clear plastic enclosure that provides cooled, humidified oxygen. It is most often used in the care of active toddlers. Children at this age are less likely to keep a mask or cannula in place but may require oxygenation and humidification for respiratory conditions, such as croup or bronchitis. A face hood may be used for less active infants.

Oxygen concentrations are difficult to control when an oxygen tent is used. Therefore, when caring for a child in an oxygen tent, the edges of the tent must be tucked securely beneath the mattress; limit opening the zippered access ports so that oxygen does not escape too freely. Oxygen levels must be monitored with an oxygen analyzer.

>>> **Stop, Think, and Respond 21-3**
What evidence indicates that a client is well oxygenated?

Oxygen Hazards

Regardless of which device is used, oxygen administration involves potential hazards: first and foremost, oxygen's capacity to support fires, and second, the potential for oxygen toxicity.

Fire Potential

Oxygen itself does not burn, but it does support combustion; in other words, it contributes to the burning process. Therefore, it is necessary to control all possible sources of open flames or ungrounded electricity (Nursing Guidelines 21-2).

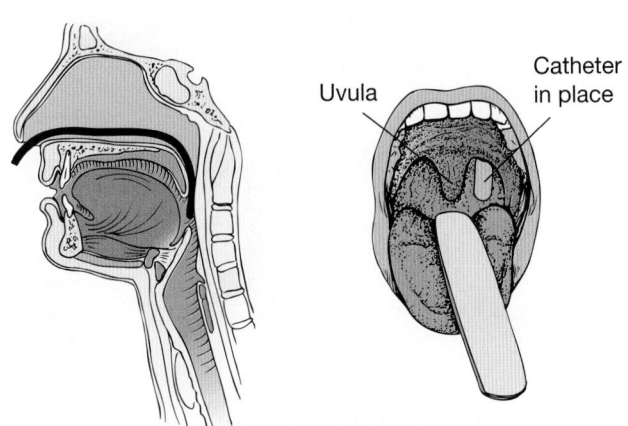

FIGURE 21-22 Nasal catheter placement.

NURSING GUIDELINES 21-2

Administering Oxygen Safely

- Post "Oxygen in Use" signs wherever oxygen is stored or in use. *The sign warns others of a potential fire hazard.*
- Prohibit the burning of candles during religious rites. *Doing so eliminates a source of open flames.*
- Check that electrical devices have a three-pronged plug (see Chapter 19). *This type of plug provides a ground for leaking electricity.*
- Inspect electrical equipment for frayed wires or loose connections. *Inspection helps prevent sparks or an uncontrolled pathway for electricity.*
- Avoid using petroleum products, aerosol products (such as hair spray), and products containing acetone (such as nail polish remover) where oxygen is used. *This measure prevents ignition of flammable substances.*
- Secure portable oxygen cylinders to rigid stands. *Doing so prevents the tank from rupturing.*

Oxygen Toxicity

Oxygen toxicity refers to lung damage that develops when oxygen concentrations of more than 50% are administered for longer than 48 to 72 hours. The exact mechanism by which hyperoxygenation damages the lungs is not definitely known. One theory is that it reduces **surfactant**, which is a lipoprotein produced by cells in the alveoli that promotes elasticity of the lungs and enhances gas diffusion. Once oxygen toxicity develops, it is difficult to reverse. Unfortunately, early symptoms are quite subtle (Box 21-2). The best prevention is to administer the lowest F_{IO_2} possible for the shortest amount of time.

RELATED OXYGENATION TECHNIQUES

Additional techniques that relate to oxygenation include positive airway pressure machines, water-seal chest tube drainage systems, and hyperbaric oxygen therapy (HBOT).

Positive Airway Pressure Machines

Positive airway pressure machines are devices that help relieve impaired oxygen levels caused by apnea or hypopnea during sleep. The underlying cause of sleep apnea/hypopnea is a temporary relaxation of muscles that should support

BOX 21-2	Signs and Symptoms of Oxygen Toxicity

- Nonproductive cough
- Substernal chest pain
- Nasal stuffiness
- Nausea and vomiting
- Fatigue
- Headache
- Sore throat
- Hypoventilation

structures in the soft palate and tongue. As a result of the muscle relaxation, the airway becomes obstructed and breathing becomes difficult or temporarily ceases. Those affected awaken briefly multiple times during the night in an effort to restore breathing that interferes with normal sleep cycles. Consequently, they experience daytime sleepiness, difficulty concentrating on work-related tasks, emotional irritability, headaches, and even chest pain. Falling oxygen saturation levels may precipitate cardiac arrest and death.

Sleep apnea can be relieved with one of several types of positive airway pressure machines that keep the airways open with controlled ventilation. Some examples include full face or nasal masks that maintain continuous positive airway pressure (CPAP), bilevel positive airway pressure (BiPAP), and other variations or mode adjustments of the two.

Continuous Positive Airway Pressure Mask

A **CPAP mask** attached to a portable ventilator maintains CPAP keeping the alveoli partially inflated even during periods of expiration (Fig. 21-24). The positive pressure prevents the airway from collapsing, allowing inflated alveoli to diffuse oxygen into the blood during apneic episodes that may last 10 seconds or more as frequently as 10 to 15 times an hour.

However, some find it difficult to adjust to wearing the mask during the night as well as overcoming an effort to exhale against a continuous fixed level of pressure. Some abandon treatment due to their discomfort. An alternative is to switch to a BiPAP mask.

Bilevel Positive Airway Pressure Mask

A **BiPAP mask**, which looks similar to a CPAP device, provides two different levels of airway pressure: *inspiratory positive airway pressure*, which is higher during inhalation, and *expiratory positive airway pressure*, which is lower during expiration. The variation promotes better tolerance among those requiring positive airway pressure therapy.

Further modifications are available. They include systems known as *automatically adjusting positive airway pressure* (APAP) and *variable positive airway pressure* (VPAP) machines. The APAP machine adjusts the pressure

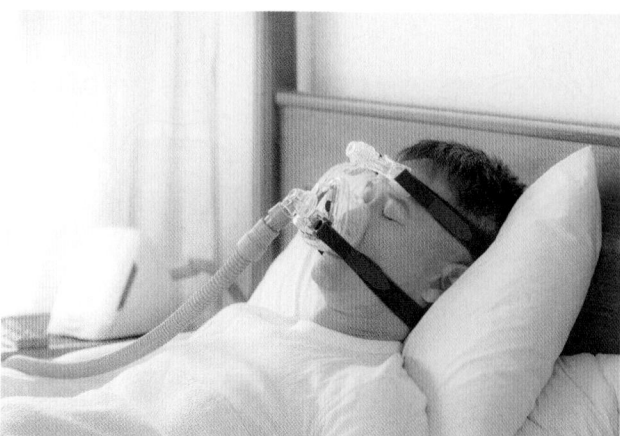

FIGURE 21-24 A continuous positive airway pressure mask (sbw18/Shutterstock).

according to the sleeper's position in bed and stages of sleep. A VPAP device normalizes breathing on a breath-by-breath basis, thus suppressing apnea and promoting the time spent in rapid eye movement (REM) sleep (see Chapter 18).

Water-Seal Chest Tube Drainage

Water-seal chest tube drainage is a technique for evacuating air or blood from the pleural cavity, which helps restore negative intrapleural pressure and reinflate the lung. Clients who require water-seal drainage have one or two chest tubes connected to the drainage system.

Several companies provide equipment for water-seal drainage. All of these products consist of a three-chamber system (Fig. 21-25):

- One chamber collects blood or acts as an exit route for pleural air.
- A second compartment holds water that prevents atmospheric air from reentering the pleural space (hence the term "water seal").
- A third chamber, if used, facilitates the use of suction, which may speed the evacuation of blood or air.

One of the most important principles when caring for clients with water-seal drainage is that the chest tube must never be separated from the drainage system unless it is clamped. Even then, the tube is clamped for only a brief time. Additional nursing responsibilities are included in Skill 21-2.

⟫⟫ Stop, Think, and Respond 21-4

Discuss how a collapsed lung affects oxygenation.

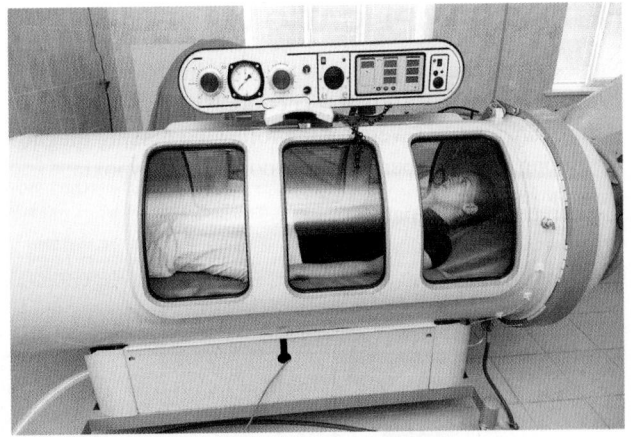

FIGURE 21-26 A hyperbaric oxygen chamber (Viktoriia Novokhatska/Shutterstock).

Hyperbaric Oxygen Therapy

Hyperbaric oxygen therapy (HBOT) consists of the delivery of 100% oxygen at three times the normal atmospheric pressure within an airtight chamber (Fig. 21-26). Treatments, which last approximately 90 minutes, are repeated over days, weeks, or months of therapy. Providing pressurized oxygen can deliver 15 times as much oxygen to tissues as can be obtained by breathing room air. Providing clients with brief periods of breathing room air helps prevent oxygen toxicity.

HBOT helps regenerate new tissue at a faster rate; thus, its most popular use is for promoting wound healing. It is also used to treat carbon monoxide poisoning, gangrene associated with diabetes or other conditions of vascular insufficiency, decompression sickness experienced by deep sea divers, anaerobic infections (especially in clients with burn), and several other medical conditions.

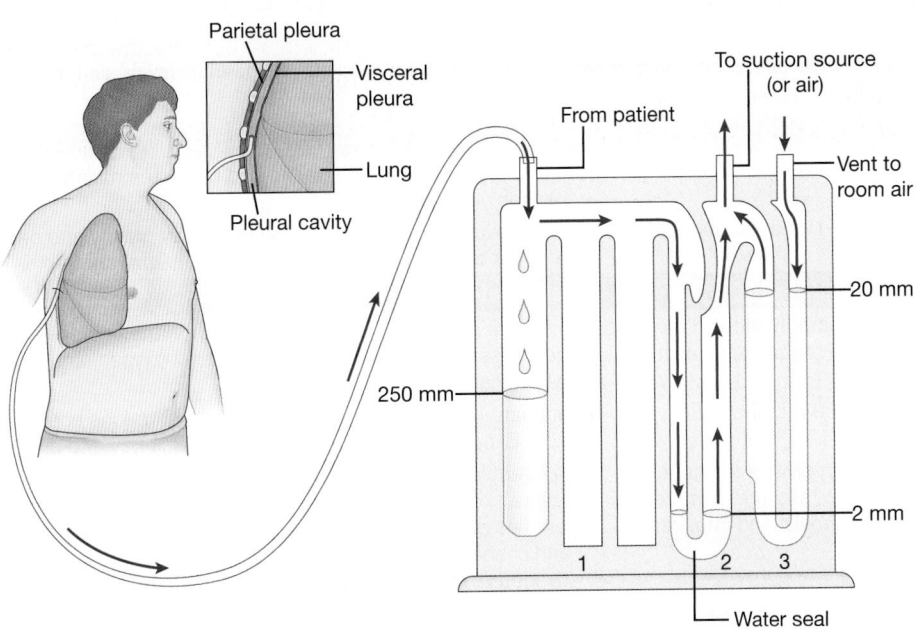

FIGURE 21-25 The three-chambered water-seal drainage system: (1) drainage collection chamber from the client, (2) the water-seal chamber, and (3) the suction control chamber attached to a source of suction and vented to room air.

NURSING IMPLICATIONS

Nurses assess the oxygenation status of clients on a day-by-day and a shift-by-shift basis. Therefore, it is not unusual to identify any one or several of the following nursing diagnoses among clients experiencing hypoxemia or hypoxia:

- Altered breathing pattern
- Impaired gas exchange
- Activity intolerance

- Chronic/acute anxiety
- Risk for ineffective airway clearance

Abnormal assessment findings often lead to collaboration with the physician and the prescription for oxygen therapy.

Nursing Care Plan 21-1 is one example of how the nursing process applies to a client with the nursing diagnosis of impaired gas exchange. This diagnostic nursing problem is defined as an alteration in the balance of oxygen and carbon dioxide.

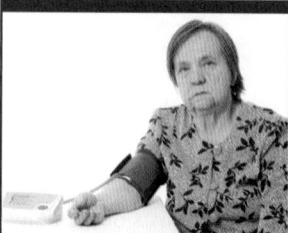

Clinical Scenario An older adult client is assessed by her physician because she has developed a frequent productive cough. She has a history of smoking one to two packs of cigarettes daily for 30 years. She tells her physician, "It seems so hard for me to get my breath. I cannot work in my flower garden because I get winded when I try to do any gardening. I cannot sleep lying down because I cannot breathe so I sleep in a chair." Her physical examination reveals a barrel chest and diminished lung sounds bilaterally. The physician arranges a hospital admission.

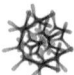

NURSING CARE PLAN 21-1   Impaired Gas Exchange

Assessment

- Determine the client's respiratory rate and effort.
- Check the radial or apical pulse rate.
- Measure the client's blood pressure.
- Note the client's level of consciousness and mental status.
- Assess for the evidence of a cough and its characteristics.
- Observe the use of accessory thoracic and abdominal muscles for breathing.
- Observe the client's chest contour.
- Inspect the skin, oral mucous membranes, and nail beds for signs of cyanosis.
- Palpate the client's abdomen for evidence of distention that could crowd the diaphragm.

- Note the client's body position, which may or may not facilitate breathing.
- Measure the client's SpO_2 with a pulse oximeter.
- Review the results of arterial blood gas (ABG) measurements.
- Auscultate anterior, posterior, and lateral lung sounds.
- Ask the client to describe their current status of oxygenation.
- Perform a pain assessment.
- Inquire as to the client's medical history of respiratory disorders or other conditions that can affect ventilation.
- Identify the client's smoking history.
- Review the client's current medication history for drugs that can impair oxygenation.

Nursing Diagnosis. Impaired gas exchange related to the retention of carbon dioxide secondary to chronic pulmonary damage from long-term cigarette smoking as manifested by rapid, shallow breathing at 40 breaths/minute accompanied by the use of accessory muscles to breathe.

Expected Outcome. The client's respiratory assessments will show improvement over baseline levels, and the client will show signs of improved gas exchange.

Interventions	Rationales
Provide periods of rest between activities.	Rest decreases oxygen demand and facilitates maintenance or restoration of oxygen within blood.
Elevate the head of the bed up to 90 degrees.	Head elevation lowers abdominal organs by gravity and provides an increased area for chest expansion when the diaphragm contracts.

Interventions	Rationales
Teach how to perform diaphragmatic and pursed-lip breathing and practice the same at least twice daily (bid).	Pursed-lip breathing decreases respiratory rate, increases tidal volume, decreases arterial CO_2, increases arterial oxygen, and improves exercise performance.
Provide a minimum of 2,000 mL of oral fluid per 24 hours.	Adequate hydration liquefies respiratory secretions and facilitates expectoration. Expectoration of sputum clears the airway and promotes ventilation.
Monitor for signs and symptoms of respiratory acidosis, including anxiety, shortness of breath, wheezing, insomnia, cyanosis, and impaired coordination.	Hypoventilation and associated hypoxemia lead to respiratory distress or failure.
	Identifies areas of decreased ventilation (atelectasis) or airway obstruction and changes as the patient deteriorates or improves, reflecting the effectiveness of treatment, dictating therapy needs
Monitor arterial blood gas levels, as ordered.	Evaluates therapy need and effectiveness
Monitor pulse oximetry, as ordered	Bedside pulse oximetry monitoring is used to show early changes in oxygenation before other signs or symptoms are observed.

Administer oxygen per nasal cannula at 2 L/minute as prescribed by the physician if SpO₂ falls below 90% and is sustained there.	Supplemental oxygen relieves hypoxemia. Administering 2–3 L/minute prevents suppressing the hypoxic drive to breathe, experienced by clients with chronic respiratory diseases.
Explore nicotine cessation therapy with transdermal skin patches.	Transdermal nicotine skin patches reduce symptoms associated with nicotine withdrawal. The dose of nicotine can be reduced gradually to promote nicotine cessation.

Evaluation of Expected Outcomes

- Respiratory rate decreases from 34 to 26 when placed in high Fowler position.
- SpO₂ increases from 86% to 90% with 2 L of oxygen per minute.
- The client demonstrates and performs pursed-lip breathing.
- Fluid intake for 24 hours is between 1,800 and 2,200 mL.
- The client demonstrates improved ventilation and adequate oxygenation of tissues as evidenced by ABGs within client's acceptable limits and the absence of symptoms of respiratory distress.
- The client verbalizes understanding of causative factors and appropriate interventions.
- The client participates in the treatment regimen within the level of ability/situation.

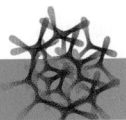

KEY POINTS

- Assessing oxygenation
  - Monitoring ABGs
  - Pulse oximeter
- Symptoms of decreased oxygenation
  - Decreased energy
  - Restlessness
  - Rapid, shallow breathing
  - Rapid heart rate
  - Sitting up to breathe
  - Nasal flaring
  - Use of accessory muscles
  - Hypertension
  - Sleepiness, confusion, stupor, coma
- Normal range for pH in arterial blood = 7.35–7.45
- Allen test: Determines whether the hand has an adequate ulnar arterial blood supply should the radial artery become damaged or occluded while performing the blood gas analysis
- Ways to promote effective oxygenation in clients
  - Positioning
  - Breathing techniques
    - Deep breathing
    - Incentive spirometry
    - Pursed-lip breathing
    - Diaphragmatic breathing
    - Nasal strips

- Oxygen therapy sources
  - Wall outlet
  - Portable tanks
  - Liquid oxygen unit
  - Oxygen concentrator
- Oxygen delivery devices
  - Nasal cannula
  - Masks: Simple, partial rebreather, nonrebreather, venturi
  - Face tent
  - Tracheostomy collar
  - T-piece
- Additional O₂ devices
  - Nasal catheter
  - Transtracheal oxygen
  - Oxygen tent
- Oxygen hazards
  - Fire potential: Oxygen's capacity to support fires
  - Oxygen toxicity: Long-term use of greater than 50% oxygen concentration for longer than 72 hours
- Related oxygen techniques
  - Positive airway pressure devices: CPAP, BiPAP
  - Water-seal chest tube drainage
  - HBOT

CRITICAL THINKING EXERCISES

1. What levels of oxygen saturation and pulse rates are a cause for nursing concern and indicate a need for further assessment?
2. Discuss some differences between oxygen therapy in a health care setting and that in a home environment.
3. What health teaching would you provide to reduce potential problems with oxygenation?
4. What nursing actions may be appropriate if the alarm on a pulse oximeter sounds frequently because the sensor does not stay on a client's finger?

NEXT-GENERATION NCLEX-STYLE REVIEW QUESTIONS

1. When a nurse assesses a client returning from surgery, which sign is an early indication that the client's oxygenation status is compromised?
   a. The client's dressing is bloody.
   b. The client becomes restless.
   c. The client's heart rate is irregular.
   d. The client reports being thirsty.
   Test-Taking Strategy: Note the key words, "early indication." Select a sign that correlates with hypoxemia.

2. When the nurse uses a pulse oximeter, what range in the Spo₂ measurement indicates the client is adequately oxygenated?
   a. 80 to 100 mm Hg
   b. 95 to 100 mm Hg
   c. 80% to 100%
   d. 95% to 100%
   Test-Taking Strategy: Use the process of elimination to select the measurement and range for normal Spo₂.

3. When administering oxygen with a partial rebreather mask, which observation is most important for the nurse to report to the respiratory therapy department?
   a. Moisture accumulates inside the mask.
   b. The reservoir bag collapses during inspiration.
   c. The mask covers the mouth and nose.
   d. The strap around the head is snug.
   Test-Taking Strategy: Note the key word and modifier, "most important." Select the option that requires immediate action more so than any of the others.

4. When the physician orders oxygen by nasal cannula at 5 L/minute for a client with chronic pulmonary disease, what is the most appropriate initial nursing action?
   a. Add an oxygen humidifier to the flowmeter.
   b. Apply a pulse oximeter sensor to a finger.
   c. Question the prescribed oxygen flow rate.
   d. Substitute a mask for the nasal cannula.
   Test-Taking Strategy: Note the key words and modifier, "most appropriate" and "initial." Analyze the options and select the one that promotes the safety of the client.

5. When the nurse assesses a client with a chest tube connected to a water-seal drainage system, what are indications that the nurse should take corrective action? Select all that apply.
   a. Fluid in the water-seal chamber rises and falls with respirations.
   b. The fluid in the water seal is at the 2-cm mark.
   c. There is dark red blood in the drainage compartment.

d. Fluid vigorously bubbles in the suction chamber.
e. There is 10 cm of water in the suction chamber.
Test-Taking Strategy: Use the process of elimination to select options that do not correlate with the safe use of water-seal drainage system.

NEXT-GENERATION NCLEX-STYLE CLINICAL SCENARIO QUESTIONS

Clinical Scenario:

An older adult client is assessed by her physician because she has developed a frequent productive cough. She has a history of smoking one to two packs of cigarettes daily for 30 years. She tells her physician, "It seems so hard for me to get my breath. I cannot work in my flower garden because I get winded when I try to do any gardening. I cannot sleep lying down because I cannot breathe so I sleep in a chair." Her physical examination reveals a barrel chest and diminished lung sounds bilaterally. The physician arranges a hospital admission.

1. Select all of the indicators that may suggest impaired gas exchange and risk for ineffective airway clearance.
   a. Productive cough
   b. Kneeling in the garden
   c. Smoking one to two packs of cigarettes for 30 years
   d. Not being able to sleep lying flat
   e. Clear breath sounds
   f. Diminished breath sounds
   g. Barrel chest

2. Choose the most likely options for the information missing from the statement below by selecting from the list of options provided.

   The client's _____1_____ is contributing to her physical examination findings of _____2_____.

OPTION 1	OPTION 2
gardening	barrel chest
sleeping with one pillow	healthy skin tone
30-year history of smoking	slow pulse

SKILL 21-1 Administering Oxygen

Suggested Action	Reason for Action
ASSESSMENT	
Perform physical assessment techniques that focus on oxygenation.	Provides a baseline for future comparisons
Monitor the Spo$_2$ level with a pulse oximeter.	Provides a baseline for future comparisons
Check the medical order for the type of oxygen delivery device, liter flow or prescribed percentage, and whether the oxygen is to be administered continuously or only as needed.	Ensures adherence to the plan for medical treatment because oxygen therapy is medically prescribed (except in emergencies)
Note whether a wall outlet is available or if another type of oxygen source must be obtained.	Promotes organization and efficient time management
Determine how much the client understands about oxygen therapy.	Indicates the need for and the type of teaching that must be done
PLANNING	
Obtain equipment, which usually includes a flowmeter, delivery device, and, in some cases, a humidifier.	Promotes organization and efficient time management
Contact the respiratory therapy department for equipment if that is agency policy.	Follows interdepartmental guidelines; ensures nursing collaboration with various health care providers to provide client care
"Crack" the portable oxygen tank if that is the type of oxygen source being used.	Prevents alarming the client
Explain the procedure to the client.	Decreases anxiety and promotes cooperation
Eliminate safety hazards that may support a fire or explosion.	Demonstrates concern for safety because open flames, electrical sparks, smoking, and petroleum products are contraindicated when oxygen is in use
IMPLEMENTATION	
Wash hands or perform hand antisepsis with an alcohol rub (see Chapter 10).	Reduces the transmission of microorganisms
Assist the client into a Fowler or alternate position.	Promotes optimal ventilation
Attach the flowmeter to the oxygen source (Fig. A).	Provides a means for regulating the prescribed amount of oxygen

Attaching the flowmeter. (Photo by B. Proud.)

Fill a humidifier bottle with distilled water to the appropriate level if administering 4 L/minute or more.	Provides moisture because oxygen dries mucous membranes; potential increases with the percentage being administered

(continued)

SKILL 21-1 Administering Oxygen (*continued*)

Suggested Action	Reason for Action
Connect the humidifier bottle to the flowmeter (Fig. B).	Provides a pathway through which moisture is added to the oxygen

Connecting the humidification bottle. (Photo by B. Proud.)

Suggested Action	Reason for Action
Insert the appropriate color-coded valve or dial the prescribed percentage if a venturi mask is being used.	Regulates the F_{IO_2}
Attach the distal end of the tubing from the oxygen delivery device to the flowmeter or humidifier bottle (Fig. C).	Provides a pathway for oxygen from its source to the client

Attaching tubing from the delivery device. (Photo by B. Proud.)

Suggested Action	Reason for Action
Turn on the oxygen by adjusting the flowmeter to the prescribed volume.	Fills the delivery device with oxygen-rich air
Note bubbles that appear in the humidifier bottle if one is used or that air is felt at the proximal end of the delivery device.	Indicates oxygen is being released
Make sure that if a reservoir bag is used, it is partially filled and remains that way throughout oxygen therapy.	Prevents asphyxiation and promotes high oxygenation; a reservoir bag must never become totally deflated during inhalation
Attach the delivery device to the client.	Provides oxygen therapy
Drain any tubing that collects condensation.	Maintains a clear pathway for oxygen and prevents accidental aspiration when turning a client
Remove the oxygen delivery device and provide skin, oral, and nasal hygiene at least every 4–8 hours.	Maintains intact skin and mucous membranes; reduces the growth of microorganisms
Reassess the client's oxygenation status every 2–4 hours.	Indicates how well the client is responding to oxygen therapy
Notify the physician if the client manifests signs of hypoxemia or hypoxia despite oxygen therapy.	Demonstrates concern for the client's safety and well-being

SKILL 21-1 Administering Oxygen (*continued*)

Suggested Action	Reason for Action

EVALUATION

- Respiratory rate is 12–24 breaths/minute at rest.
- Breathing is effortless.
- Heart rate is less than 100 bpm.
- Client is alert and oriented.
- Skin and mucous membranes are normal in color.
- Spo2 is greater than or equal to 90%.
- Fio2 and delivery device correspond to medical order.

DOCUMENT

- Assessment data
- Percentage or liter flow of oxygen administration
- Type of delivery device
- Length of time in use
- Client's response to oxygen therapy

SAMPLE DOCUMENTATION

Date and Time Restless, pulse rate 120, respiratory rate 32 with nasal flaring. Placed in high Fowler position. Spo$_2$ at 85%–88%. Simple mask applied with administration of oxygen at 6 L/minute. After 15 minutes of oxygen therapy, is less agitated, pulse rate 100, respiratory rate 28, no nasal flaring noted. Spo$_2$ at 90%–92%. Oxygen continues to be administered.
_____ J. Doe, LPN

SKILL 21-2 Maintaining a Water-Seal Chest Tube Drainage System

Suggested Action	Reason for Action

ASSESSMENT

Review the client's medical record to determine the condition that necessitated inserting a chest tube.	Indicates whether to expect air, bloody drainage, or both; any condition that causes an opening between the atmosphere and pleural space results in a loss of intrapleural negative pressure and subsequent lung deflation
Determine whether the physician has inserted one or two chest tubes (Fig. A).	Helps direct assessment; the usual sites for chest tubes are at the second intercostal space in the midclavicular line and in the fifth to eighth intercostal spaces in the midaxillary line
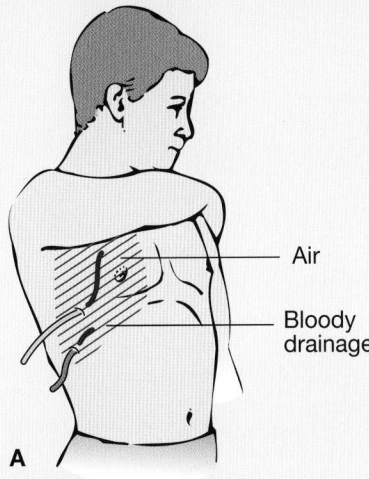 Air Bloody drainage **A**	Determining whether the physician has inserted one or two chest tubes.

(*continued*)

SKILL 21-2 Maintaining a Water-Seal Chest Tube Drainage System (*continued*)

Suggested Action	Reason for Action
Note the date of chest tube(s) insertion.	Provides a point of reference for analyzing assessment data
Check the medical orders to determine whether the drainage is being collected by gravity or with the addition of suction.	Provides guidelines for carrying out medical treatment; mechanical suction is used when there is a large air leak or potential for a large accumulation of drainage

PLANNING ⎯⎯⎯⎯⎯⎯⎯⎯⎯⎯⎯⎯⎯⎯⎯⎯⎯⎯⎯⎯⎯⎯⎯⎯⎯⎯⎯⎯⎯

Arrange to perform a physical assessment of the client and equipment as soon as possible after receiving the report.	Establishes a baseline and early opportunity for troubleshooting abnormal findings
Locate a roll of tape and a container of sterile distilled water.	Facilitates efficient time management for general maintenance of the drainage system

IMPLEMENTATION ⎯⎯⎯⎯⎯⎯⎯⎯⎯⎯⎯⎯⎯⎯⎯⎯⎯⎯⎯⎯⎯⎯⎯⎯⎯⎯⎯

Introduce yourself to the client and explain the purpose for the interaction.	Reduces anxiety and promotes cooperation
Wash hands or perform hand antisepsis with an alcohol rub (see Chapter 10).	Reduces the transmission of microorganisms; conscientious hand hygiene is one of the most effective methods for preventing infection
Check to see that a pair of hemostats (instruments for clamping) is at the bedside.	Facilitates checking for air leaks in the tubing or clamping the chest tube in the event the drainage system must be replaced to prevent the reentry of atmospheric air within the pleural space, thus maintaining lung expansion
Turn off the suction regulator if one is used before assessing the client.	Eliminates noise that may interfere with chest auscultation
Assess the client's lung sounds.	Provides a baseline for future comparison; because lung sounds cannot be heard in uninflated areas, lung sounds in previously silent areas indicate reexpansion
Inspect the dressing for signs that it has become loose or saturated with drainage (Fig. B).	Indicates a need for changing the dressing

Palpate around the chest tube insertion site to assess for signs of drainage. Inspecting the dressing for signs that it has become loose or saturated with drainage. (Photo by B. Proud.)

B

SKILL 21-2 Maintaining a Water-Seal Chest Tube Drainage System (*continued*)

Suggested Action	Reason for Action
Palpate the skin around the chest tube insertion site to feel and listen for air crackling in the tissues (Fig. C).	Indicates a subcutaneous air leak and an internal displacement of the drainage tube

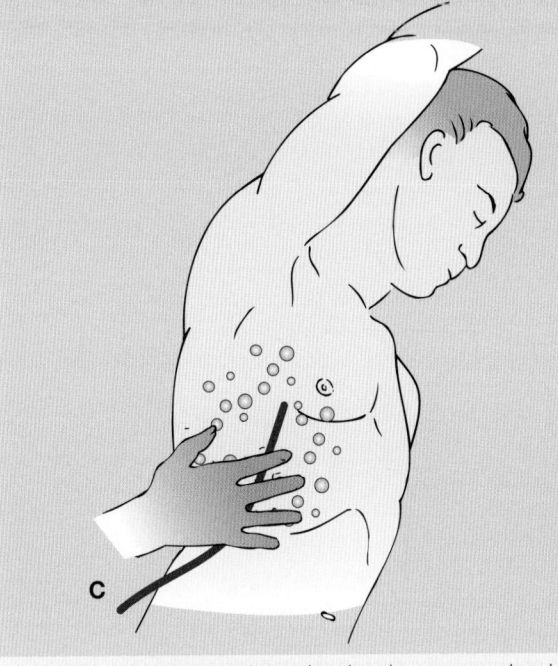

Palpating the skin around the chest tube insertion site to feel and listen for air crackling in the tissue.

Suggested Action	Reason for Action
Inspect all connections to determine that they are taped and secure.	Indicates appropriate care has been taken and ensures that the drainage system will not become accidentally separated
Reinforce connections where the tape may be loose.	Prevents accidental separation
Check that all tubing is unkinked and hangs freely into the drainage system (Fig. D).	Ensures the evacuation of air and bloody drainage because fluid cannot drain upward against gravity; neither air nor fluid can pass through a physical obstruction

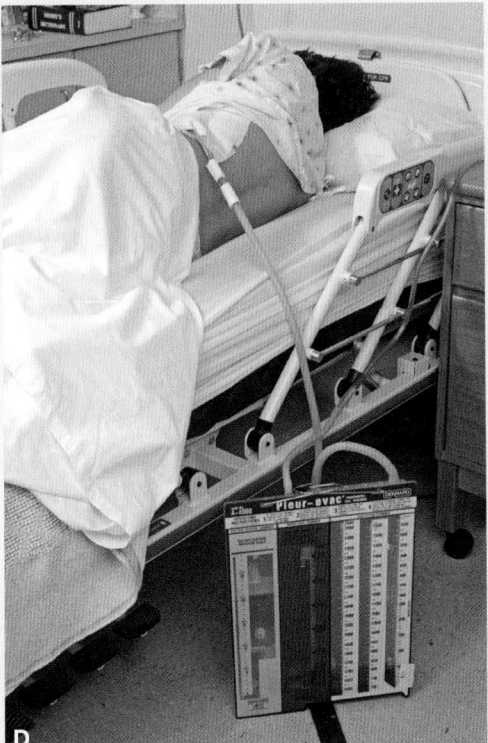

Keeping chest tubes unobstructed from the client to the drainage chamber.

(*continued*)

SKILL 21-2 Maintaining a Water-Seal Chest Tube Drainage System (*continued*)

Suggested Action	Reason for Action
Observe the fluid level in the water-seal chamber to see if it is at the 2-cm level and that the water in the suction chamber is at the 20-cm mark or the pressure prescribed by the physician (Fig. E).	Maintains the water seal, preventing the passage of atmospheric air into the pleural space and provides the usual water level for suction

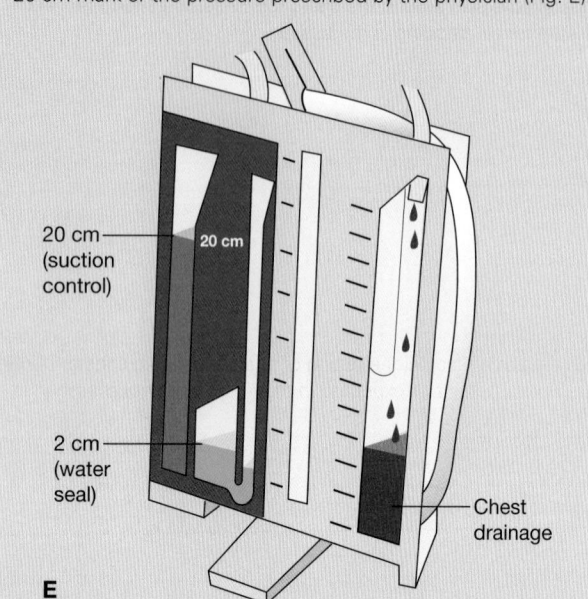

20 cm (suction control)

20 cm

2 cm (water seal)

Chest drainage

E

Noting water levels.

| Add sterile distilled water to the 2-cm mark in the water-seal chamber or 20-cm mark to the suction control chamber if the fluid is below standard (Fig. F). | Two centimeters of water maintains the water seal; the 20-cm depth of water in the suction chamber determines the amount of negative pressure, *not* the pressure setting on the suction source. |

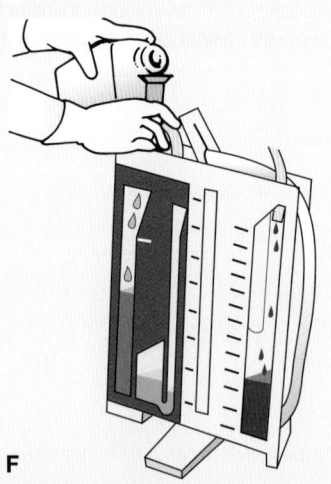

F

Adding water to the suction control chamber.

| Note if the water is **tidaling** (the rise and fall of water in the water-seal chamber that coincides with respiration) (Fig. G). | Indicates that the tubing is unobstructed and the lung has not completely inflated; intrathoracic pressure changes during breathing cause the fluid to rise and fall |

SKILL 21-2 Maintaining a Water-Seal Chest Tube Drainage System (*continued*)

Suggested Action	Reason for Action
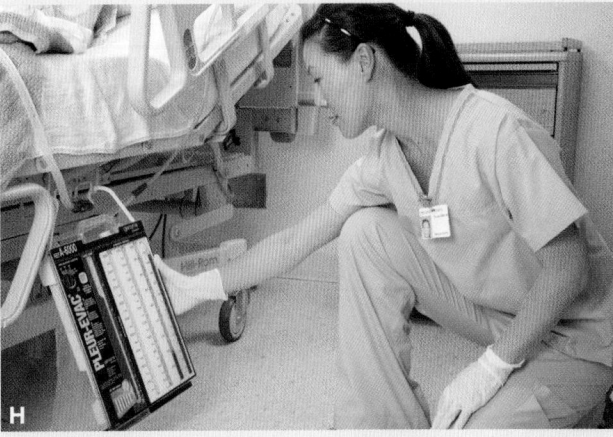	Watching for tidaling—movement of water up and down in the water-seal chamber.
Observe for continuous bubbling *in the water-seal chamber*.	Indicates an air leak in the tubing or at a connection; constant bubbling is normal and expected *in the suction control chamber* as long as it is used
If constant bubbling is observed, clamp hemostats at the chest within a few inches away; observe if the bubbling stops; continue releasing and reapplying the hemostats toward the drainage system until the bubbling stops.	Provides a means for determining the location of an air leak within the tubing because gas escapes through the path of least resistance
Apply tape around the tube above where the last clamp was applied when the bubbling stopped.	Seals the origin of the air leak
Regulate the wall suction so that it produces gentle bubbling.	Prevents rapid evaporation and unnecessary noise
Observe the nature and amount of drainage in the collection chamber (Fig. H).	Provides comparative data; more than 100 mL/hour or bright red drainage is reported immediately
	Observing drainage characteristics.
Keep the drainage system below chest level.	Maintains gravity flow of drainage
Position the client to avoid compressing the tubing.	Facilitates drainage
Curl and secure excess tubing on the bed.	Avoids dependent loops to facilitate drainage
Milk the tubing, a process of compressing and stripping the tubing to move stationary clots, but only if necessary.	Creates extremely high negative intrapleural pressure; milking is never done routinely
Encourage coughing and deep breathing at least every 2 hours while awake.	Promotes lung reexpansion because the mechanics of breathing and forceful coughing help evacuate air and fluid

(*continued*)

SKILL 21-2 Maintaining a Water-Seal Chest Tube Drainage System (*continued*)

Suggested Action	Reason for Action
Instruct the client to move around in bed, ambulate while carrying the drainage system, and exercise the shoulder on the side of the drainage tube(s).	Prevents hazards of immobility and maintains joint flexibility with no danger to the client while the tube to the suction source is disconnected as long as the water seal remains intact
Never clamp the chest tube for an extended period.	Predisposes client to developing a **tension pneumothorax** (extreme air pressure within the lung when there is no avenue for its escape); clamping a chest tube *briefly* is safe, for example, when changing the entire drainage system
If the tube and drainage system become separated, insert a separated chest tube within sterile water until it can be reattached and secured to the drainage system.	Provides a temporary water seal to prevent the entrance of atmospheric air, which can recollapse the lung
Prevent air from entering the tube insertion site by covering it with a gloved hand or woven fabric if the tube is accidentally pulled out.	Reduces the amount of lung collapse
Mark the drainage level on the collection chamber at the end of each shift (Fig. I).	Provides data about fluid loss without the risk of recollapsing the lung; *never* empty the drainage container

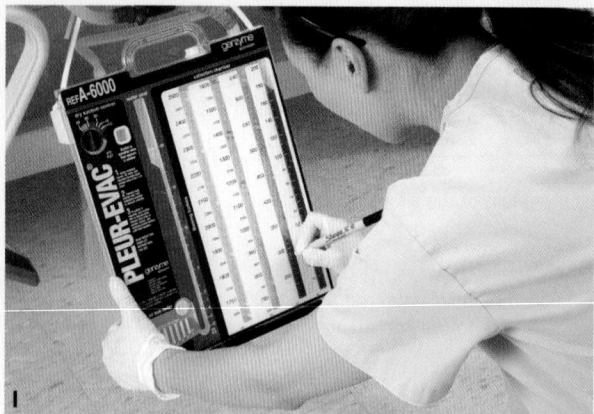

I

Marking the drainage level.

EVALUATION

- Client exhibits no evidence of respiratory distress.
- Dressing is dry and intact.
- No subcutaneous air is detected around the site of the tube insertion.
- Equipment is functioning appropriately.
- Water is at recommended levels.

DOCUMENT

- Assessment findings
- Care provided
- Amount of drainage during period of care

SAMPLE DOCUMENTATION

Date and Time Upper and lower chest tubes connected to water-seal drainage system. Normal lung sounds heard throughout chest, except in apex and base of left lung, where chest tubes are inserted. Tidaling still observed in water-seal chamber. 20 cm of suction maintained. Dark red chest tube drainage measures a scant 50 mL. Ambulated in hall while disconnected from suction. Performed full range of motion with left shoulder. _____ J. Doe, LPN

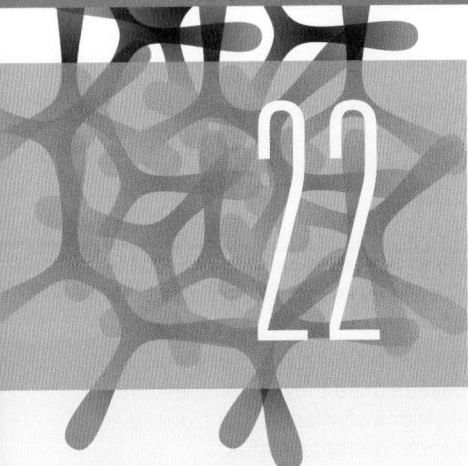

Infection Control

Learning Objectives

On completion of this chapter, the reader should be able to:

1. Define infectious diseases.
2. Differentiate between infection and colonization.
3. List the stages in the course of an infectious disease.
4. Define infection control measures.
5. Name two major techniques for infection control.
6. Identify the elements of standard precautions.
7. Discuss situations in which nurses use standard precautions and transmission-based precautions.
8. Describe the rationale for using airborne, droplet, and contact precautions.
9. Explain the purpose of personal protective equipment (PPE).
10. Discuss the rationale for removing PPE in a specific sequence.
11. Explain how nurses perform double bagging.
12. List psychological problems common among clients with infectious diseases.
13. Provide teaching suggestions for preventing infections.
14. Discuss unique characteristics of older adults in relation to infectious diseases.

INTRODUCTION

Infectious diseases are spread by pathogens or toxins among susceptible individuals. Infectious diseases can be classified as **communicable diseases** when they are transmitted from one source to another by infectious bacteria or viral organisms. An example of *noncommunicable* disease is a disease caused by toxins from food poisoning or infection caused by toxins in the environment, such as tetanus. **Contagious diseases** are communicable diseases that can spread rapidly among individuals in close proximity to each other. Another distinction is to classify infections as **community-acquired infections**, those that are not present or incubating prior to care provided by health care providers, and **health care–associated infections** (HCAIs) that are acquired within a health care facility.

HCAIs are the most common adverse event in hospitals. Infections increase morbidity and mortality among those affected. The nation and world experienced unprecedented challenges due to the COVID-19 pandemic, which impacted surveillance for and incidence of HCAIs. Hospitals across the nation experienced higher than usual hospitalizations, as well as shortages in health care personnel and equipment, which may have resulted in decreased surveillance activities and reporting. The Centers for Medicare & Medicaid (CMS) implemented the extraordinary circumstance exception (ECE) policy that excused facilities from HCAI surveillance and reporting for the 2019Q4 through 2020Q2 reporting quarters. During this time, facilities were not required to report HAI data to CMS's reporting programs. Reporting levels during the second half of 2020 were close to prepandemic time periods for most HCAIs (CDC, 2021).

Despite vaccines, aggressive public health measures, and advances in drug therapy, infectious diseases have not disappeared. In fact, the microorganisms that cause tuberculosis (TB), gonorrhea, and some forms of wound and respiratory infections have developed drug-resistant strains (see Chapter 10). HIV/AIDS (Box 22-1), severe acute respiratory syndrome (SARS), and bird flu (avian influenza) continue to pose threats. Mosquito-transmitted infections such as the West Nile virus, Zika virus, and Heartland virus and the 2014 to 2016 Ebola and coronavirus 2019 (COVID-19) outbreaks proved hard to contain. It is clear that humans have not won the war against pathogens.

BOX 22-1 | **Facts and Myths about the Transmission of HIV**

Facts

HIV is transmitted by:

- Having unprotected vaginal, anal, or oral sexual contact with an infected person
- Sharing needles or syringes with an infected person
- Acquiring a needlestick injury with the blood of an infected person (see Chapter 34)
- Receiving transfusions of infected blood or blood products
- Being born to or breast-fed by an HIV-infected mother
- Having contact with the blood of an infected person through unsterilized equipment for ear piercing, tattooing, acupuncture, dental procedures, safety razors, or toothbrushes
- Contacting blood of an infected person through an open cut or splashes into the mucous membranes, such as the eyes or inside of the nose
- Artificial insemination with infected semen
- Organ transplant from an HIV-infected donor

Myths

HIV is *not* transmitted by:

- Donating blood
- Being bitten by insects
- Sharing cups and eating utensils
- Inhaling droplets from sneezes or coughs
- Hugging, touching, or closed-mouth kissing of an infected person
- Sharing telephones or computer keyboards
- Going to any public place with people infected with HIV
- Using public drinking fountains or toilet seats
- Swimming in pools

From HIV.gov. (2023). *How Do You Get or Transmit HIV?* https://www.hiv.gov/hiv-basics/overview/about-hivd-an-aids/how-is-hivtransmitted

---

 Gerontologic Considerations

■ Many long-term care residents, older hospitalized clients, and health care personnel are colonized with antibiotic-resistant bacteria, possibly with few or no symptoms.

■ Older adults are more susceptible to infections because of an age-related decrease in immune system functioning. Additional risk factors common in older adults are inadequate nutrition and fluid intake.

■ Symptoms of infections tend to be subtle among older adults. Because older adults tend to have a lower baseline temperature, a temperature in the normal range may actually be elevated for an older adult.

■ Infections are more likely to have a rapid course and life-threatening consequences once they become established. Common manifestations of infections in older adults include changes in behavior and mental status.

■ Age-related changes, such as thinning, drying, and diminished blood supply to the skin, predispose the older person to skin infections. Maintaining intact skin is an excellent first-line defense against acquiring infections.

■ Infections are often transmitted to vulnerable older adults and others through equipment reservoirs, such as indwelling urinary catheters, humidifiers, and oxygen equipment, or through incisional sites, such as those for intravenous tubing, parenteral nutrition, or tube feedings. The use of proper aseptic techniques is essential for preventing the introduction of microorganisms. A daily assessment for any signs of infection is imperative.

■ Older adults, family caregivers and members in close contact with older people, and all personnel in health care settings should obtain annual immunizations against influenza. Those who are 65 years and older and younger people with chronic diseases should receive the pneumococcal vaccine, doses of which vary depending on the type administered.

■ Visitors with respiratory infections need to wear masks or avoid contact with older adults in their home or long-term care settings until their symptoms have subsided. In addition to a mask, frequent and thorough hand hygiene can help prevent the transfer of organisms.

■ Health care providers who are ill should avoid exposing susceptible clients to infectious organisms.

■ Older adults with cognitive impairment may need more assistance with adhering to infection control measures.

■ The incidence of TB in community-living older adults has been decreasing steadily across all age groups in recent years, but rates for people aged 65 years and older are higher than for any other age group. All long-term care facilities are required to test each resident on admission and each new employee for TB.

 Nutrition Notes

■ Microorganisms that cause foodborne illness are found widely in nature and are transmitted to people from within the food (e.g., eggs), from on the food (e.g., raw vegetables), from unsafe water, and from human and animal feces.

■ Foods most often associated with foodborne illness are raw or undercooked animal products, such as meat, poultry, eggs, and unpasteurized milk; raw fruits and vegetables; raw sprouts; unpasteurized fruit juice; and any uncooked food that was handled by someone who is ill.

This chapter discusses precautions that confine the reservoir of infectious agents and block their transmission from one host to another. To understand the concepts of infection control, it is important to understand the chain of infection (see Chapter 10) and the course of an infection.

P h a r m a c o l o g i c   C o n s i d e r a t i o n s

Fear of vaccines prevents individuals from immunizing their children and themselves. Always ask about the client's immunization status during an initial and ongoing assessments. Early diagnosis, treatment, and isolation of a person with a communicable disease will reduce transmission.

INFECTION

Infection is a condition that results when microorganisms cause injury to a host. Infection differs from **colonization**, a condition in which microorganisms are present, but the host does not manifest any signs or symptoms of infection. Regardless of whether the host is infected or colonized, the host can transmit pathogens and infectious diseases to others.

Infections progress through distinct stages (Table 22-1). The characteristics and length of each stage may differ depending on the infectious agent. For example, the incubation period for the common cold is approximately 2 to 4 days before symptoms appear, but it may take months or years before a person infected with HIV demonstrates symptoms of AIDS.

INFECTION CONTROL PRECAUTIONS

Infection control precautions are physical measures designed to curtail the spread of infectious diseases. They are essential when caring for clients in any health care facility. Infection control precautions require knowledge of the mechanisms by which an infectious disease is transmitted and the methods that will interfere with the chain of infection. Infection control practices include:

- Hand hygiene and hand antisepsis measures (see Chapter 10)
- Using standard precautions
- Following transmission-based precautions
- Wearing personal protective equipment (PPE)
- Cleaning, disinfecting, or sterilizing equipment used by more than one client (see Chapter 10)
- Keeping the client's environment clean (see Chapter 10)

P h a r m a c o l o g i c   C o n s i d e r a t i o n s

It is recommended that health care providers and those who volunteer in facilities obtain annual influenza immunizations.

In 2022, the Centers for Disease Control and Prevention (CDC) updated guidelines for major categories of infection control precautions, including standard precautions, isolation precautions, and transmission-based precautions.

Standard Precautions

Standard precautions are measures for reducing the risk of microorganism transmission from both recognized and unrecognized sources of infection. Health care providers follow standard precautions when caring for all clients, regardless of the suspected or confirmed infection status (Box 22-2). This precautionary system combines methods previously known as *universal precautions* and body *substance isolation*. The use of standard precautions reduces the potential for transmitting infectious agents in blood, body fluids, secretions, excretions (except sweat), nonintact skin, mucous membranes, and equipment or items in the client's environment that may contain transmissible infectious agents whether they contain visible blood. Health care providers follow standard precautions when caring for all clients in all settings in which health care is delivered. Standard precautions include hand hygiene; using **personal protective equipment** (PPE) like garments that block the transfer of pathogens from one person, place, or object to oneself or others; and safe injection practices (see Chapter 34). PPE use, such as that with gloves, gowns, masks, eye protection, and face shields, is determined by the nature of the client interaction and the extent of anticipated blood, body fluid, or pathogen exposure. A sign that alerts health care providers of the appropriate PPE to use may be posted in various areas of the health care agency (Fig. 22-1).

Respiratory Hygiene/Cough Etiquette
Respiratory hygiene/cough etiquette (Fig. 22-2) refers to infection control measures used at the first point of an encounter with clients, family, or friends of persons with signs of illness suggesting an undiagnosed transmissible respiratory infection. It includes:

- Covering the mouth and nose with a tissue when coughing (coughing or sneezing into an upper sleeve or elbow is another alternative when a tissue is unavailable)

TABLE 22-1 Course of Infectious Diseases

STAGE	CHARACTERISTIC
Incubation period	Infectious agent reproduces, but there are no recognizable symptoms. The infectious agent may, however, exit the host at this time and infect others.
Prodromal stage	Initial symptoms appear, which may be vague and nonspecific. They may include mild fever, headache, and loss of usual energy.
Acute stage	Symptoms become severe and specific to the tissue or organ that is affected. For example, tuberculosis is manifested by respiratory symptoms.
Convalescent stage	The symptoms subside as the host overcomes the infectious agent.
Resolution	The pathogen is destroyed. Health improves or is restored.

BOX 22-2 Standard Precautions

Hand Hygiene
- Use an alcohol-based product or plain (nonantimicrobial) soap for routine hand hygiene.
- Perform hand hygiene after touching blood, body fluids, secretions, excretions, and contaminated items, whether gloves are worn.
- Perform hand hygiene immediately after gloves are removed, between client contacts, and when otherwise indicated; perform hand hygiene between tasks and procedures on the same client to prevent cross-contamination of different body sites.
- Use an antimicrobial agent or a waterless antiseptic agent to control outbreaks or **hyperendemic infections** (infections that are highly infectious in all age groups).

Gloves
- Wear clean, nonsterile gloves that fit snugly around the wrist when touching blood, body fluids, secretions, excretions, and contaminated items; latex or nitrile gloves are preferred for clinical procedures that require manual dexterity or involve more than brief client contact.
- Change gloves between tasks on the same client after contact with material that may contain a high concentration of microorganisms and before touching portable computer keyboards or other mobile equipment that is transported from room to room.
- Remove gloves and perform hand hygiene immediately before caring for another client.

Mask, Eye Protection, Face Shield
- Wear a mask and eye protection (goggles) or face shield to protect the eyes, nose, and mouth when there is a likelihood that splashes or sprays of blood, body fluids, secretions, or excretions will occur; eyeglasses and contact lenses are not adequate for eye protection.
- Obtain a user-seal check (also called a "fit check") to minimize air leakage around the facepiece of a respirator; reuse of a particulate respirator by the same person is acceptable as long as the respirator is not damaged or soiled, the fit is not compromised by change in shape, and the respirator has not been contaminated with blood or body fluids.

Gown
- Wear a clean, nonsterile gown that covers the arms and body from neck to midthigh or below when there is a likelihood that

splashes or sprays of blood, body fluids, secretions, or excretions will occur.
- Remove a soiled gown promptly and perform hand hygiene.

Client Care Equipment
- Locate containers for used disposable or reusable personal protective equipment (PPE) at a site that is convenient for the removal and disposal of contaminated materials.
- Handle equipment soiled with blood, body fluids, secretions, and excretions so as to prevent the transfer of microorganisms to oneself, others, or the environment.
- Ensure that soiled reusable equipment is cleaned and disinfected or sterilized before another subsequent use.
- Discard soiled single-use equipment properly.

Environmental Control
- Ensure that procedures for the routine cleaning and disinfection of environmental surfaces, beds, bedrails, bedside equipment, and other frequently touched surfaces are carried out.

Linens
- Handle, transport, and process soiled linen in such a way as to prevent exposure to oneself, others, and the environment.

Occupational Health and Blood-Borne Pathogens
- Prevent injuries when using needles, scalpels, and other sharp devices.
- Never recap used needles.
- Use either a one-handed "scoop" method or a mechanical device for covering a needle.
- Place all disposable sharp items in a puncture-resistant container as close to the location of use as possible; transport reusable syringes and needles in a puncture-resistant container for reprocessing.
- Use mouthpieces, resuscitation bags, or other ventilation devices as an alternative to mouth-to-mouth resuscitation methods in areas where the need for resuscitation is predictable.

Client Placement
- Place potentially infectious clients in a private room whenever possible.
- Consult with an infection control professional concerning alternatives if a private room is not available.
- Place a client who contaminates the environment, who does not—or cannot be expected to—assist in maintaining appropriate hygiene or environmental control in a private room.

Adapted from Centers for Disease Control and Prevention. (2024). *Standard precautions for all patient care.* https://www.cdc.gov/infectioncontrol/basics/standard-precautions.html

- Disposing of used tissues promptly
- Performing hand hygiene after contact with respiratory secretions
- Using a surgical mask on a coughing client who can tolerate this measure
- Distancing the person with respiratory symptoms at least 3 to 6 ft from others in common waiting areas

Safe Injection Practices
Safe injection practices are infection control measures that prevent the transmission of viral hepatitis B virus (HBV) and hepatitis C virus (HCV) to the health care

worker by using aseptic techniques involving the preparation and administration of parenteral medications (see Chapter 34). Health care providers are advised to (1) use a sterile, single-use, disposable syringe for each injection; (2) prevent the contamination of injection equipment and medication; and (3) use single-dose vials rather than multiple dose vials when administering medications to multiple clients. Measures to handle needles and other sharp devices ("sharps") in a manner that avoids injury to the user and others who may encounter the device during or after a procedure continue to be a standard practice (see Chapters 34 and 35).

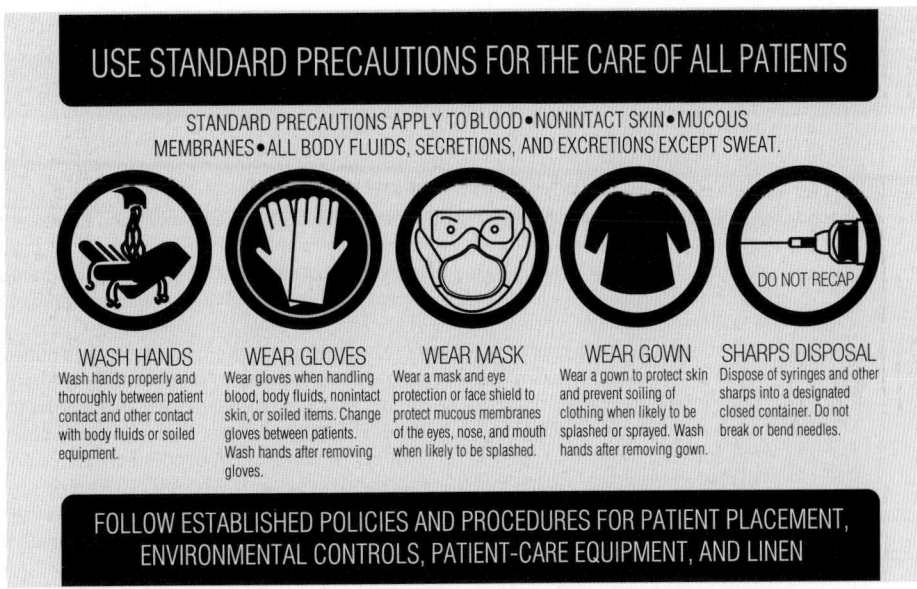

USE STANDARD PRECAUTIONS FOR THE CARE OF ALL PATIENTS

STANDARD PRECAUTIONS APPLY TO BLOOD•NONINTACT SKIN•MUCOUS
MEMBRANES•ALL BODY FLUIDS, SECRETIONS, AND EXCRETIONS EXCEPT SWEAT.

WASH HANDS
Wash hands properly and thoroughly between patient contact and other contact with body fluids or soiled equipment.

WEAR GLOVES
Wear gloves when handling blood, body fluids, nonintact skin, or soiled items. Change gloves between patients. Wash hands after removing gloves.

WEAR MASK
Wear a mask and eye protection or face shield to protect mucous membranes of the eyes, nose, and mouth when likely to be splashed.

WEAR GOWN
Wear a gown to protect skin and prevent soiling of clothing when likely to be splashed or sprayed. Wash hands after removing gown.

SHARPS DISPOSAL
Dispose of syringes and other sharps into a designated closed container. Do not break or bend needles.

DO NOT RECAP

FOLLOW ESTABLISHED POLICIES AND PROCEDURES FOR PATIENT PLACEMENT,
ENVIRONMENTAL CONTROLS, PATIENT-CARE EQUIPMENT, AND LINEN

FIGURE 22-1 A sign that identifies standard precautions.

Infection Control Practices for Special Lumbar Puncture Procedures

Lumbar puncture procedures are performed for a number of reasons, such as performing a myelogram, administering spinal and epidural anesthesia, placement of spinal catheters, and injecting medications within the spinal canal. Because there has been an increase in the incidence of bacterial meningitis, most likely from respiratory droplet transmission at the time these procedures were performed, it is now recommended that the person performing the procedure wear a mask in addition to the usual protective equipment that is used.

Transmission-Based Precautions

Transmission-based precautions, also called *isolation* precautions, are measures for controlling the spread of highly transmissible or epidemiologically important infectious agents from clients when the known or suspected routes of transmission are not completely interrupted using standard precautions alone. The three types of transmission-based precautions are airborne precautions, droplet precautions, and contact precautions (Table 22-2). These three types replace the earlier categories of strict isolation, contact isolation, respiratory isolation, TB (acid–fast bacilli, or AFB) isolation, enteric precautions, and drainage/secretion

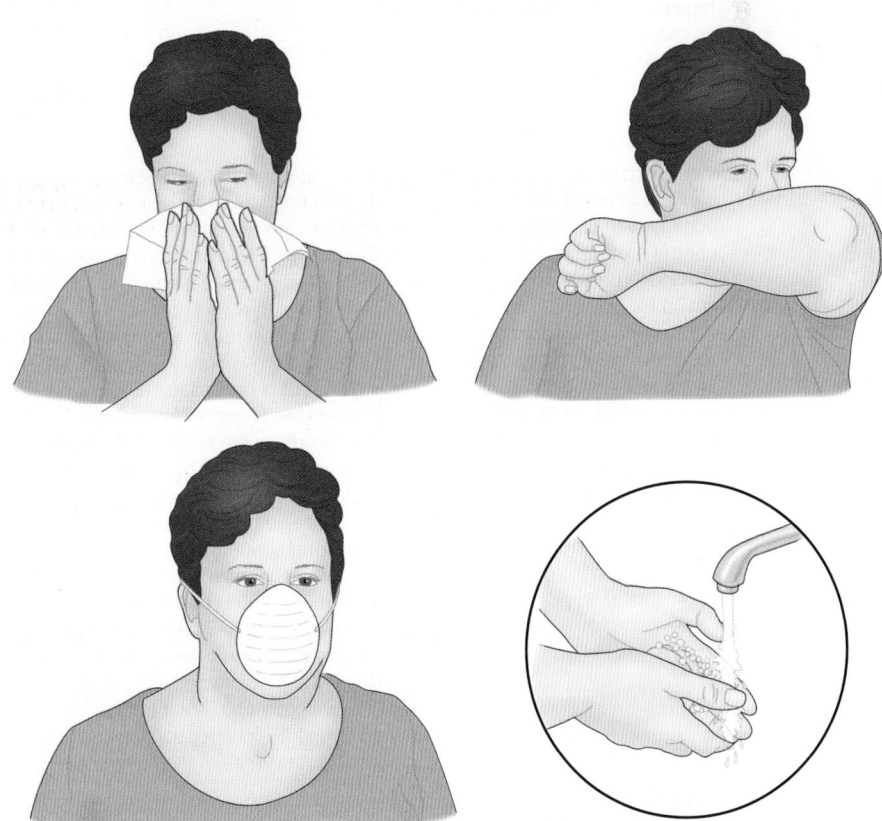

FIGURE 22-2 Techniques for preventing or reducing the spread of respiratory pathogens.

TABLE 22-2 Transmission-Based Precautions

TYPE OF PRECAUTION	CLIENT PLACEMENT	PROTECTION	EXAMPLES OF DISEASES
Airborne	Private room or in a room with a similarly infected client Negative air pressure[a] Six to 12 air changes per hour Discharge of room air to environment or filtered before being circulated Precautions: in settings where airborne precautions cannot be implemented due to limited engineering resources, masking the patient and placing the patient in a private room with the door closed will reduce the likelihood of airborne transmission until the patient is either transferred to a facility with an AIIR or returned home.	Source control: put a mask on the patient. Restrict susceptible health care personnel from entering the room of the patients known or suspected to have measles, chickenpox, disseminated zoster, or smallpox if other immune health care personnel are available. Use personal protective equipment (PPE) appropriately, including a fit-tested NIOSH-approved N95 or higher level respirator for health care personnel. Limit transport and movement of patients outside the room to medically necessary purposes. If transport or movement outside an AIIR is necessary, instruct the patients to wear a surgical mask, if possible, and observe respiratory hygiene/cough etiquette. Health care personnel transporting patients who are on airborne precautions do not need to wear a mask or respirator during transport if the patient is wearing a mask and infectious skin lesions are covered. Immunize susceptible persons as soon as possible following unprotected contact with vaccine-preventable infections (e.g., measles, varicella, or smallpox).	Pulmonary TB Measles (rubeola) Chickenpox (varicella) SARS Influenza A: avian H7N9, Asian H5N1
Droplet	Private room or in a room with a similarly infected client or one in which there are at least 3 ft between other clients and visitors In long-term care and other residential settings, make decisions regarding patient placement on a case-by-case basis considering infection risks to other patients in the room and available alternatives. In ambulatory settings, place patients who require droplet precautions in an examination room or cubicle as soon as possible and instruct the patients to follow respiratory hygiene/cough etiquette recommendations.	Source control: put a mask on the patient. Use PPE appropriately. Don mask upon entry into the patient room or patient space. Limit transport and movement of patients outside the room to medically necessary purposes. If transport or movement outside the room is necessary, instruct the patient to wear a mask and follow respiratory hygiene/cough etiquette.	Influenza Rubella Streptococcal pneumonia Meningococcal meningitis Whooping cough Coronavirus disease 2019 (COVID-19)
Contact	Private room or in a room with similarly infected client or consult with an infection control professional if the previous options are not available Ensure appropriate patient placement in a single patient space or room if available in acute care hospitals. In long-term and other residential settings, make room placement decisions balancing risks to other patients. In ambulatory settings, place patients requiring contact precautions in an exam room or cubicle as soon as possible.	Use PPE appropriately, including gloves and gown. Wear a gown and gloves for all interactions that may involve contact with the patient or the patient's environment. Donning PPE upon room entry and properly discarding before exiting the patient room are done to contain pathogens. Limit transport and movement of patients outside the room to medically necessary purposes. When transport or movement is necessary, cover or contain the infected or colonized areas of the patient's body. Remove and dispose of contaminated PPE and perform hand hygiene prior to transporting patients on contact precautions. Don clean PPE to handle the patient at the transport location. Use disposable or dedicated patient care equipment (e.g., blood pressure cuffs). If common use of equipment for multiple patients is unavoidable, clean and disinfect such equipment before use on another patient. Prioritize cleaning and disinfection of the rooms of patients on contact precautions ensuring rooms are frequently cleaned and disinfected (e.g., at least daily or prior to use by another patient if outpatient setting) focusing on frequently touched surfaces and equipment in the immediate vicinity of the patient.	Gastrointestinal, respiratory, skin, or wound infections that are drug resistant Gas gangrene Acute diarrhea Acute viral conjunctivitis Draining abscess Hepatitis type A and E virus: diapered or incontinent persons

AIIR, airborne infection isolation room; NIOSH, U.S. National Institute for Occupational Safety and Health; SARS, severe acute respiratory syndrome; TB, tuberculosis.
[a]Negative air pressure pulls air from the hall into the room when the door is opened, as opposed to positive air pressure, which pulls room air into the hall.
Centers for Disease Control and Prevention. (2023). *Transmission-based precautions.* https://www.cdc.gov/infectioncontrol/basics/transmission-based-precautions.html

precautions. Health care providers base the decision to use one or a combination of precautions on the mechanism of transmission of the pathogen. They use one or more categories of transmission-based precautions concurrently when diseases have multiple routes of transmission. For instance, during the COVID-19 outbreak, both contact and droplet precautions were initiated (CDC, 2020).

Transmission-based precautions are required for various lengths of time, depending on how long the risk of transmission of the infectious agent persists or for the duration of the illness. Health care providers discontinue some precautions, with the exception of standard precautions, when culture or other laboratory findings document that the disease has been resolved, when a wound or lesion stops draining, after the initiation of effective therapy, or when state laws and regulations dictate discontinuation. Sometimes, health care providers employ them throughout a client's treatment.

Airborne Precautions

Airborne precautions are measures that reduce the risk for transmitting pathogens that remain infectious over long distances when suspended in the air (see Table 22-2). They block pathogens, 0.3 microns or smaller, that are present in the residue of evaporated droplets that remain suspended in the air as well as those attached to dust particles.

TB is an example of a disease transmitted through the air. Caregivers must wear a specific type of mask when caring for clients with TB. An **N95 respirator**, which is individually fitted for each caregiver, can filter particles 1 micron (smaller than a millimeter) with an efficiency of 95% or more, provided the device fits the face snugly (Fig. 22-3A). A **powered air-purifying respirator** (PAPR) is an alternative if a caregiver has not been fitted with an N95 respirator or has facial hair or a facial deformity that prevents a tight

seal with an N95 respirator (Fig. 22-3B). A PAPR blows atmospheric air through belt-mounted air-purifying canisters to the facepiece through a flexible tube. A PAPR can also be used when rescuing victims exposed to hazardous chemicals or bioterrorist substances.

Concept Mastery Alert

Mask Choices

If a nurse has abundant facial hair, such as a beard, a PAPR is the better choice over the N95 mask when caring for clients with TB. The N95 mask must fit tightly around the mouth, which is not possible with facial hair.

Droplet Precautions

Droplet precautions are measures that block infectious pathogens within moist droplets larger than 5 microns. They are used to reduce pathogen transmission from close contact (usually 3 ft or less) with respiratory secretions or mucous membranes between infected persons or a person who is a carrier of a droplet-spread microorganism and others. Microorganisms carried on droplets commonly exit the body during coughing, sneezing, talking, and procedures such as airway suctioning (see Chapter 36) and bronchoscopy. Airborne precautions are not used because droplets do not remain suspended in the air.

Contact Precautions

Contact precautions are measures used to block the transmission of pathogens by direct or indirect contact. This is the final category of transmission-based precautions. Direct contact involves skin-to-skin contact with an infected or colonized person. Indirect contact occurs by touching a contaminated intermediate object in the client's environment.

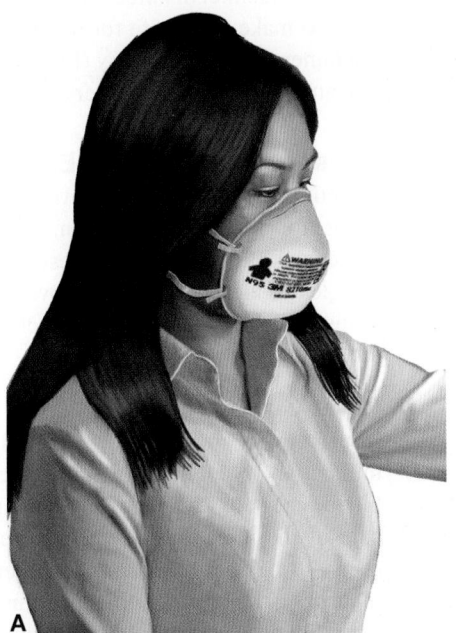
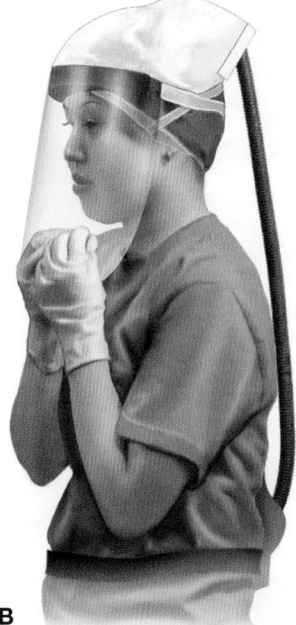

A   B

FIGURE 22-3 A. An N95 respirator must fit tightly around the mouth and nose with straps that attach it to the head. A secure seal is evidenced by a slight bulging on exhalation and slight collapse upon inhalation. **B.** A powered air-purifying respirator uses a blower to remove contaminated air through a filter and supplies purified air to a facepiece.

Additional precautions are necessary if the microorganism is resistant to antibiotics.

>>> **Stop, Think, and Respond 22-1**
Which type of transmission precautions do health care personnel follow when caring for clients with the following medical diagnoses: (1) pulmonary TB, (2) streptococcal pneumonia, (3) an infected wound, (4) acute diarrhea, and (5) meningococcal meningitis?

Some infectious diseases such as chickenpox (varicella), smallpox (variola), COVID-19, and SARS require both airborne and contact precautions.

INFECTION CONTROL MEASURES

Infection control measures involve the use of PPE and techniques that serve as barriers to transmission (Fig. 22-4). Depending on the type of precautions used, nurses implement all or some of the following measures:

• Locating a client and equipping a room so as to confine pathogens to one area
• Using PPE such as cover gowns, face shields or goggles, cloth or paper masks or respirators (see Chapter 10), and gloves to prevent spreading microorganisms through direct and indirect contact
• Disposing of contaminated linen, equipment, and supplies in such a way that nurses do not transfer pathogens to others
• Using infection control measures to prevent pathogens from spreading when transporting laboratory specimens or clients

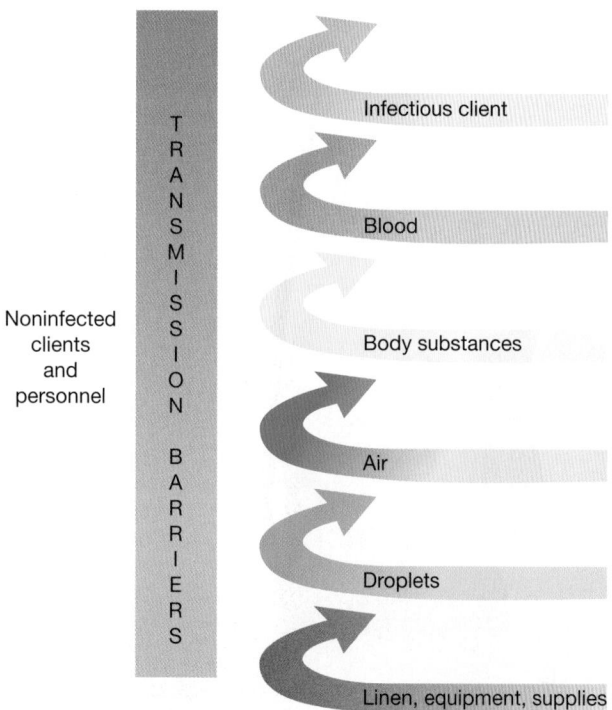

FIGURE 22-4 Blocking sources of infectious disease transmission.

Client Environment

The client environment includes the room designated for the care of a client with an infectious disease and the equipment and supplies essential for controlling transmission of the pathogens.

Infection Control Room

Except when using standard precautions, most health care agencies assign infectious or potentially infectious clients to private rooms. Infection control personnel can offer alternatives if a private room is not available (see Table 22-2). They keep the door to the room closed to control air currents and the circulation of dust particles.

The room has a private bathroom so that personnel can flush contaminated liquids and biodegradable solids. A sink is also located in the room for hand hygiene.

Health care providers in the nursing unit post an instruction card on the door or nearby at eye level stating that isolation precautions are required (Fig. 22-5). Nurses are responsible for teaching visitors how to adhere to the infection control measures.

In accordance with the principles of medical asepsis, housekeeping personnel clean the infectious client's room last to avoid transferring organisms on the wet mop to other client areas. They deposit the mop head, if not disposable, with the soiled linen and wipe the mop handle with a disinfectant. They flush solutions used for cleaning down the toilet.

Equipment and Supplies

The infection control room contains the same equipment and supplies as any other hospital room with a few modifications. A dedicated stethoscope and sphygmomanometer remain in the client's room whenever possible. This prevents the need to clean and disinfect these items each time they need to be removed.

For the same reason, disposable thermometers are preferred. Personnel disinfect electronic or tympanic thermometers to make them safe for the next client. Items such as a container for soiled laundry (Fig. 22-6), lined waste containers, and liquid soap dispensers are also placed in the room.

Personal Protective Equipment

Infection control measures involve the use of one or more items for personal protection. PPE, also called "barrier garments" (Fig. 22-7), includes gowns, masks, respirators, goggles or face shields, and gloves (see Chapter 10). These items are located just outside the client's room or in an anteroom (Fig. 22-8).

Cover Gowns

Cover gowns are worn for two reasons: they prevent contamination of clothing and protect the skin from contact with blood and body fluids. When they are removed after direct care of the infectious client, they reduce the possibility of transmitting pathogens from the client, the client's environment, or contaminated objects. Many types of cover gowns exist, but all have the following common characteristics:

• They open in the back to reduce inadvertent contact with the client and objects.

> # Visitors—Report to Nurses' Station Before Entering Room
>
> 1. Masks are indicated for all persons entering room.
> 2. Gowns are indicated for all persons entering room.
> 3. Gloves are indicated for all persons entering room.
> 4. HANDS MUST BE WASHED AFTER TOUCHING THE PATIENT OR POTENTIALLY CONTAMINATED ARTICLES AND BEFORE TAKING CARE OF ANOTHER PATIENT.
> 5. Articles contaminated with infective material should be discarded or bagged and labeled before being sent for decontamination and reprocessing.

FIGURE 22-5 A door instructional card.

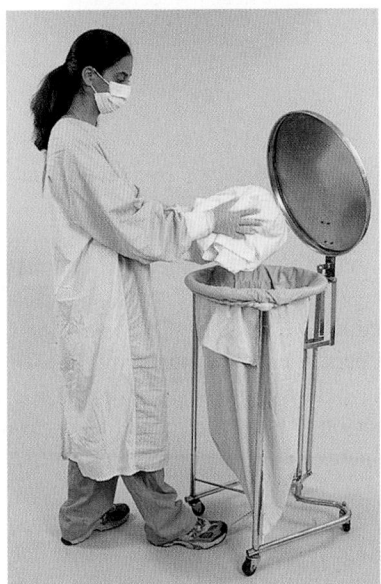

FIGURE 22-6 Containing soiled laundry. (Photo by B. Proud.)

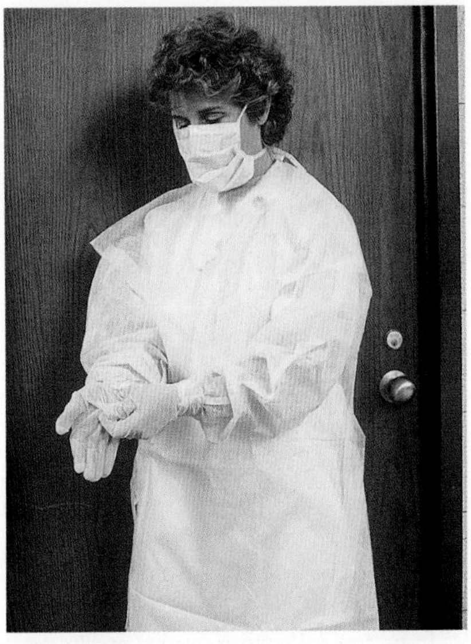

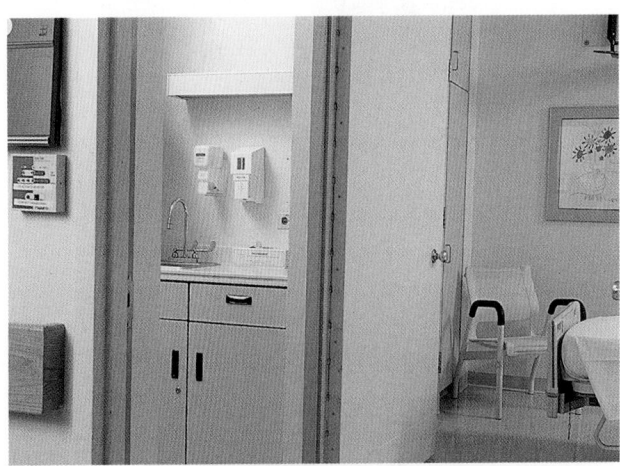

FIGURE 22-7 Putting on personal protective equipment helps prevent the transmission of infectious microorganisms. (Photo by B. Proud.)

- They have close-fitting wristbands to help avoid contaminating the forearms.
- They fasten at the neck and waist to keep the gown securely closed, thus covering all the wearer's clothing.

Nurses wear a cover gown only once and then discard it. They place discarded cloth gowns in the client's laundry hamper and remove them with the soiled linen. Cloth cover gowns are laundered before being used again. Disposable paper gowns are placed in a waste container and incinerated.

Face Protection Devices

Depending on the mode of transmission of the pathogen, health care providers wear a mask or respirator (see Chapter 10), goggles, or a face shield. They always put on these items before entering the client's room.

Gloves

Gloves are required when an infectious disease is transmitted by direct contact or contact with blood and body fluid substances. Health care providers always put on gloves before or immediately upon entering the client's room. After one use, they are discarded.

FIGURE 22-8 An anteroom outside the infection control room. (Photo by B. Proud.)

Gloves are not a total and complete barrier to microorganisms. They are easily punctured and can leak; the potential for leakage increases with the stress of use. Wearing gloves does not replace the need for hand antisepsis (see Chapter 10) after removal. Hands can be contaminated during glove removal, and microorganisms that were present on the hands before gloving grow and multiply rapidly in the warm, moist environment beneath the gloves.

>>> **Stop, Think, and Respond 22-2**
Which personal protective items would you expect to wear when managing the care of a client with a draining wound abscess?

Removing Personal Protective Equipment

Regardless of which garments they wear, nurses follow an orderly sequence for removing them (Skill 22-1). The goal is to leave the client's room without contaminating oneself or one's uniform. The procedure involves making contact between two contaminated surfaces or two clean surfaces. Nurses remove the garments that are most contaminated first, preserving the clean uniform underneath (Fig. 22-9).

Nurses can modify the technique to accommodate the removal of any combination of equipment. The most important nursing action is to perform thorough hand hygiene before leaving the client's room and before touching any other client, health care provider, environmental surface, or client care items.

Disposing of Contaminated Linens, Equipment, and Supplies

Receptacles in the client's room are used to collect contaminated items. Soiled waste containers are emptied at the end of each shift or more often if their contents accumulate (Fig. 22-10). To avoid spreading pathogens, some items are double bagged.

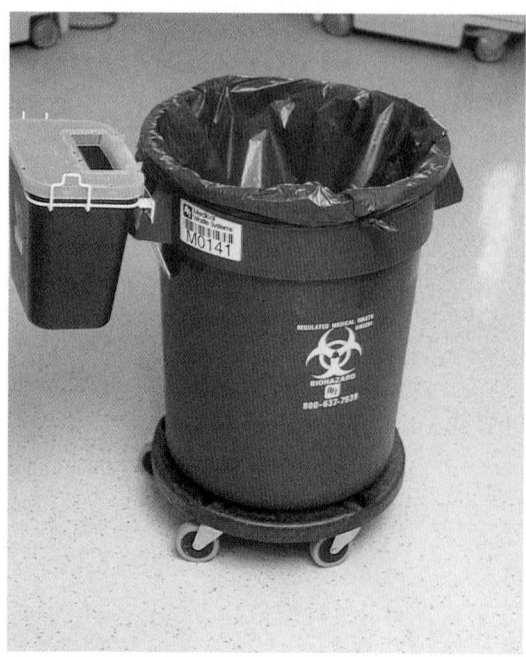

FIGURE 22-10 A waste container used for infectious waste. (Photo by B. Proud.)

Double bagging is an infection control measure in which one bag of contaminated items, such as trash or laundry, is placed within another. This measure requires two people. One person bags the items and deposits the bag in a second bag held by another person outside the client's room. The person holding the second bag prevents contamination by manipulating the bag underneath a folded cuff (Fig. 22-11).

The CDC has relaxed its recommendations concerning double bagging. Its revised position is that one bag is adequate if the bag is sturdy and the articles are placed in the bag without contaminating the outside of the bag. Otherwise, double bagging is used.

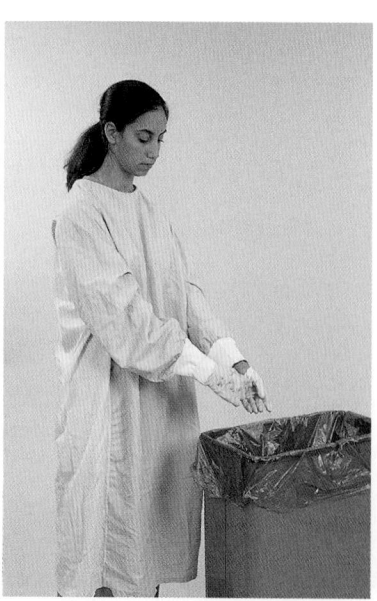

FIGURE 22-9 Removing and disposing the most contaminated garments first. (Photo by B. Proud.)

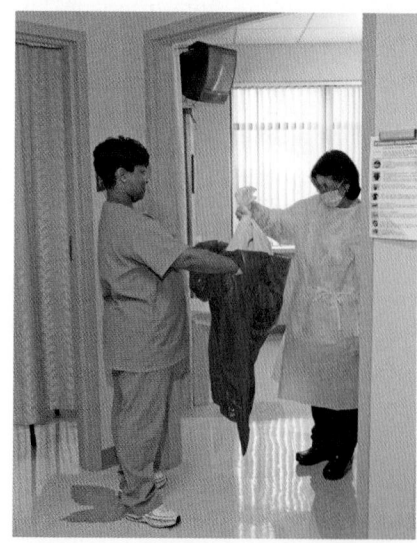

FIGURE 22-11 Double bagging technique. (From Carter, P. J. [2019]. *Lippincott's textbook for nursing assistants* [5th ed.]. Lippincott Williams & Wilkins.)

Following the termination of transmission-based precautions, equipment that will be used again for other client care must first be thoroughly cleaned and disinfected.

Discarding Biodegradable Trash

Biodegradable trash is refuse that will decompose naturally into less complex compounds. It includes items such as unconsumed beverages, paper tissues, the contents of drainage collectors, urine, and stool. All these items can be flushed down the toilet in the client's room. Chemicals and filtration methods in sewage treatment centers are sufficient for destroying pathogens in human wastes.

Nurses place bulkier items in a lined trash container and remove them from the room by single or double bagging. They wrap moist items such as soiled dressings so that during their containment, flying or crawling insects cannot transfer pathogens. Eventually, the bag and its contents are destroyed by incineration, or they are autoclaved. Autoclaved items can be safely disposed of in landfills.

Removing Reusable Items

To reduce the need for disinfection of reusable items, disposable equipment and supplies such as plastic bedpans, basins, eating utensils, and paper plates and cups are used as much as possible. Following the termination of transmission-based precautions, equipment that will be used again for other client care must first be thoroughly cleaned, disinfected, and sterilized (see Chapter 10).

Delivering Laboratory Specimens

Specimens are delivered to the laboratory in sealed containers in plastic biohazard bags. When the testing is complete, most specimens are flushed, incinerated, or sterilized.

Transporting Clients

Clients with infectious diseases may need to be transported to other areas such as the X-ray department. During transport, nurses use methods to prevent the spread of pathogens either directly or indirectly from the client. For example, to prevent the exit of pathogens from the client onto transport equipment, nurses line the surface of the wheelchair or stretcher with a clean sheet or bath blanket to protect the surface from direct client contact. They use a second sheet or blanket to cover as much of the client's body as possible during transport. The client wears a mask or particulate air filter respirator if the pathogen is transmitted by the airborne or droplet route. Any hospital health care providers who have direct contact with the client use PPE similar to that used in client care.

Interdepartmental coordination is important. The department to which the client is transported is made aware that the client has an infectious disease. This facilitates the expeditious care of the client and avoids unnecessary waiting in areas with other clients.

When the client returns, the nurse deposits the soiled linen in the linen hamper in the client's room, touching only the outside surface of the protective covers. Some agencies also spray or wash the transport vehicle with a disinfectant before reuse.

PSYCHOLOGICAL IMPLICATIONS

Although infection control measures are necessary, they often leave clients feeling shunned or abandoned. Clients with infectious diseases continue to need human contact and interaction, both of which are often minimal because of the elaborate precautions taken upon entering and leaving the room. Fearful family and friends may avoid visiting, and clients are restricted from leaving their rooms. Measures are needed to relieve the client's feelings of isolation by providing social interaction and sensory stimulation.

Promoting Social Interaction

When transmission-based precautions are in effect, it is important to plan frequent contact with the client. Nurses encourage visitors to come as often as the agency's policies and the client's condition permit. They use every opportunity to emphasize that as long as visitors follow the infection control precautions, they are not likely to acquire the disease.

Combating Sensory Deprivation

Sensory deprivation results when a person experiences insufficient sensory stimulation or is exposed to sensory stimulation that is continuous and monotonous. The goal is to provide a variety of sensory experiences at intervals (Nursing Guidelines 22-1).

 NURSING GUIDELINES 22-1

Providing Sensory Stimulation

- Move the bed to various places in the room or periodically rearrange the furnishings in the room. *Such a change provides a new perspective for the client.*
- Position the client so that they can look out the window. *Having something different to look at reduces boredom.*
- Encourage the client to use the telephone. *Telephone calls allow social interaction.*
- Communicate using the intercom system if entering the room is inconvenient. *This shows that the nurse is paying attention to the client.*
- Converse with the client about current world events. *Conversation stimulates the client's thought processes.*
- Help the client select television or radio programs. *Watching television or listening to the radio engages the client's attention.*
- Change the location of equipment that produces monotonous sounds. *Changing the location will vary the volume or pitch of the noise.*
- Encourage the client to be active within the confines of the room. *Activity provides a means of stimulation.*
- Encourage activities that the client can do independently, such as reading, working crossword puzzles, playing solitaire, and putting picture puzzles together. *Such activities are diverting.*
- Offer a wide choice of foods with different flavors, temperatures, and textures. *Eating a variety of foods stimulates oral and olfactory sensations.*
- Use touch appropriately by giving a backrub or changing the client's position. *Touch produces tactile stimulation.*

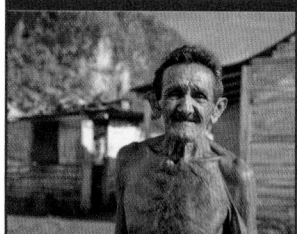

Clinical Scenario A 76-year-old male has come to a public health clinic. He admits that he has not seen a physician in many years, but he tells the nurse that he has been increasingly concerned about having a chronic productive cough that sometimes contains blood. He has been losing weight and admits to having night sweats. The nurse who examines him and takes his vital signs notes that he has a fever. The attending physician sends the man to the hospital where he is admitted for a diagnostic sputum test and chest X-ray. The physician suspects the man has TB.

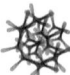

NURSING CARE PLAN 22-1   Infection Risk Transmission

Assessment

- Monitor laboratory test findings for evidence of infection such as an elevated white blood cell count or the results of a culture indicating the growth of a pathogen.
- Check the client's temperature regularly and note if there is a persistent elevation.
- Inspect the skin, mucous membranes, wounds, sputum, urine, and stool for signs of purulent or unusual drainage.
- Listen for abnormal lung sounds, especially if the client has a cough.

- Inspect the area around invasive devices such as an intravenous catheter, wound drain, and abdominal feeding tube.
- Ask whether the client has a decreased appetite, has lost weight, or feels weak and tired.
- Inquire about recent travel in a country or area where there has been an incidence of infectious disease or contact with others who have been ill lately.
- Ask about the client's immunization history.
- Read the results of a current skin test for tuberculosis (TB) or refer to a person who is certified to do so.

Nursing Diagnosis. Infection risk through transmission related to the airborne spread of the pathogen causing TB (positive TB test and suspicious chest X-ray)

Expected Outcome. The client will adhere to infection control measures and accurately describe postdischarge drug therapy and medical follow-up by the time of discharge.

Interventions	Rationales
Follow airborne transmission precautions until sputum culture is negative; follow standard precautions throughout the length of stay.	Airborne transmission precautions are the specified infection control measures for preventing the spread of TB to susceptible individuals. Nurses implement standard precautions during the care of all clients. Once sputum specimens are free of infectious microorganisms, the client will no longer require airborne transmission precautions.

Interventions	Rationales
Postinfection control measures on the room door, but do not identify the name of the disease.	Posting instructions on the client's door informs personnel, family, and friends how to protect themselves from contact with organisms that can cause infectious disease. Privacy regulations require that the client's health problem be kept confidential.
Wear a particulate air filter respirator during client care.	A particulate air filter respirator is more efficient than a cloth or paper mask because it can filter particles 0.3 microns in size with a minimum efficiency of 95%.
Teach the client to cover their nose and mouth with a paper tissue when coughing, sneezing, or laughing and dispose of tissue in a paper bag.	A paper tissue collects moist respiratory secretions and decreases airborne transmission. Paper is disposable and is incinerated to destroy microorganisms present in secretions.

Interventions	Rationales
Directly observe the client taking prescribed drug therapy.	A combination of various medications can eliminate the infectious organism that causes TB when a client is compliant with drug therapy.
Explain the purpose of combination drug therapy and the need to continue its uninterrupted administration to avoid treatment failure and the development of a drug-resistant strain.	An informed and knowledgeable client promotes adherence.
Direct the client to provide a sputum specimen at the public health department within 2–3 weeks following discharge.	Continued monitoring of the client's sputum provides a means for evaluating whether the client is noninfectious and responding to treatment.
Recommend TB skin testing for close family members or friends.	TB is usually spread among those who have close contact with the infected person. Any person who previously had a negative skin test and now tests positive is placed on prophylactic drug therapy.

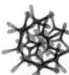

NURSING CARE PLAN 22-1 — Infection Risk Transmission (*continued*)

Evaluation of Expected Outcome

- The client remained in a private infection control room.
- The client used a paper tissue when coughing, sneezing, and talking.
- The client took all prescribed medications.
- The client's family and friends followed posted infection control instructions.
- The client's spouse and children have received TB skin tests with negative results.
- The client verbalized how to self-administer his medications and the importance for remaining compliant.
- The client identified the date for a follow-up appointment with the Public Health Department for a repeat of sputum analysis.

NURSING IMPLICATIONS

Caring for clients with infectious diseases involves meeting their physical and emotional needs. Some frequently identified nursing diagnoses include:

- Infection risk
- Acute anxiety
- Grief
- Fear

Nursing Care Plan 22-1 demonstrates how nurses apply the nursing process when caring for a client with the nursing diagnosis of infection risk. Through implementation and planning of this nursing diagnosis, the nurse must address the concern of infection transmission.

Nurses also play a pivotal role by teaching measures to prevent infection (Client and Family Teaching 22-1).

Client and Family Teaching 22-1
Preventing Infections

The nurse teaches the client and the family as follows:

- Bathe daily and perform other forms of personal hygiene such as oral care.
- Keep the home environment clean and uncluttered.
- Use diluted household bleach (1:10 or 1:100) as a disinfectant.
- Obtain appropriate adult immunizations.
  - Tetanus vaccine at 10-year intervals
  - Influenza vaccine yearly
  - Tdap booster to prevent tetanus, diphtheria, and pertussis (whooping cough)
- A zoster vaccine is recommended for adults aged 60 years or older to prevent shingles if they had chickenpox as children.
- A pneumococcal pneumonia immunization lasts a lifetime or revaccination is required every 5 years for extremely high-risk people.
- Investigate necessary vaccines, water purification techniques, and foods to avoid when traveling outside the United States.
- Practice a healthy lifestyle such as eating the recommended number of servings from the MyPlate nutrition guidelines (see Chapter 15).
- Perform frequent handwashing, especially before eating, after contact with nasal secretions, and after using the toilet.
- Use disposable tissues rather than a cloth handkerchief for nasal and oral secretions.
- Avoid sharing personal care items, such as washcloths and towels, razors, and cups.
- Stay home from work or school when ill rather than exposing others to infectious pathogens.
- Assume the task of cooking if the family member who usually cooks is ill.
- Keep food refrigerated until used.
- Cook food thoroughly.
- Avoid crowds and public places during outbreaks of influenza.
- Follow infection control instructions when visiting hospitalized family members and friends.
- Adhere to drug therapy when prescribed.

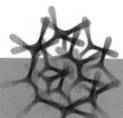

KEY POINTS

- Infectious diseases: Spread by pathogens or toxins among susceptible individuals
- Communicable diseases: Transmitted from one source to another by infectious bacteria or viral organisms
- Contagious diseases: Communicable diseases that can spread rapidly among individuals in close proximity to each other
- Community-acquired infections: Those that are not present or incubating prior to care provided by health care providers
- HCAIs: Acquired within health care facilities
- Stages of infection
  - Incubation period: No symptoms but infectious
  - Prodromal stage: Vague, nonspecific symptoms
  - Acute stage: Severe, specific symptoms related to tissue or organ affected
  - Convalescent stage: Symptoms subside
  - Resolution: Pathogen destroyed, health improves
- Hand hygiene is the best method of infection control.
- Standard precautions: The minimum infection prevention practices that apply to all patient care regardless of suspected or confirmed infection status of the patient in any setting where health care is delivered
- Transmission-based precautions: Also called isolation precautions, measures for controlling the spread of highly transmissible infectious agents from clients when the known

or suspected routes of transmission are not completely interrupted using standard precautions alone
- Airborne precautions: Measures that reduce the risk for transmitting pathogens that remain infectious over long distances when suspended in the air
- Droplet precautions: Measures that block infectious pathogens within moist droplets larger than 5 microns
- Contact precautions: Measures used to block the transmission of pathogens by direct or indirect contact
- Infection control measures
  - Client environment
  - Infection control room
  - Equipment and supplies
  - PPE
  - Cover gowns
  - Face protection devices
  - Gloves
- Disposing of contaminated linens, equipment, and supplies
  - Double bagging
- Disposing biodegradable trash
- Psychological implications of infection control with isolation
  - Promote social interactions
  - Provide sensory stimulation

CRITICAL THINKING EXERCISES

1. Explain why controlling the spread of infectious diseases is difficult among children cared for in day care centers.
2. Discuss some reasons why new cases of AIDS occur despite the fact that its mode of transmission is known.
3. What actions are appropriate to take if there are several residents in a long-term care facility who acquire an infection with a transmittable pathogen and there are not enough private rooms to relocate them?
4. A recent influenza vaccine has been found to be less effective because one of the viruses (type A, H3N2) used in the vaccine mutated. If there is an outbreak in the community of H3N2, what measures might a long-term health care facility take to protect clients?

NEXT-GENERATION NCLEX-STYLE REVIEW QUESTIONS

1. When a nurse empties the secretions from a wound suction container, which personal protective measure is most important at this time?
   a. Wear a mask.
   b. Wear a gown.
   c. Wear goggles.
   d. Wear gloves.

Test-Taking Strategy: Note the key word and modifier, "most important." Analyze the choices and select the option that identifies a primary barrier from body fluid that may contain a pathogen.

2. When a person comes to the emergency department with respiratory symptoms, which infection control measure is appropriate to use initially?
   a. Contact precautions
   b. Airborne precautions
   c. Respiratory hygiene/cough etiquette
   d. Droplet precautions

Test-Taking Strategy: Note the key word, "initially." Analyze the choices and select the option that is appropriate to use at the first point of encounter with a client with a possible infectious respiratory condition.

3. When exiting the room of a client being cared for with contact precautions, arrange the steps in the order in which personal protection items are removed.
   a. Take off the mask or particulate air respirator.
   b. Untie and remove the gown.
   c. Remove gloves one at a time.
   d. Remove goggles, if worn.

Test-Taking Strategy: Analyze the choices and select the personal protection items from most contaminated to least contaminated.

4. What is the best advice the nurse can give to someone who is allergic to latex, yet must wear gloves for standard precautions?
   a. Rinse the latex gloves with running tap water before donning them.
   b. Apply a petroleum ointment to both hands before donning latex gloves.
   c. Eliminate wearing gloves, but wash both hands vigorously with alcohol afterward.
   d. Wear two pairs of vinyl gloves if there is a potential for contact with blood or body fluid.

   Test-Taking Strategy: Analyze the choices and select the option that offers protection from contact with a pathogen and allergen.

5. Other than obtaining an immunization against influenza, what is the best advice the nurse can give to high-risk people to avoid acquiring this infection?
   a. Consume adequate vitamin C.
   b. Avoid going to crowded places.
   c. Dress warmly in cold weather.
   d. Reduce daily stress and anxiety.

   Test-Taking Strategy: Note the key word and modifier, "best advice." Analyze the choices and select the one that is better than any of the others at preventing the potential for acquiring a respiratory infection like influenza.

NEXT-GENERATION NCLEX-STYLE CLINICAL SCENARIO QUESTIONS

Clinical Scenario:

A 76-year-old male has come to a public health clinic. He admits that he has not seen a physician in many years, but he tells the nurse that he has been increasingly concerned about having a chronic productive cough that sometimes contains blood. He has been losing weight and admits to having night sweats. The nurse who examines him and takes his vital signs notes that he has a fever. The attending physician sends the man to the hospital where he is admitted for a diagnostic sputum test and chest X-ray. The physician suspects the man has TB.

1. Select all of the indicators that may suggest a cause for concern regarding an infection risk.
   a. Chronic productive cough
   b. Weight gain
   c. Losing weight
   d. Increased appetite
   e. Night sweats
   f. Fever
   g. Swelling in the ankles
   h. Blood streaked sputum

2. Place an x under "effective" to identify methods that will help with infection control measures. Place an x under "ineffective" to identify methods that are not likely to help with infection control.

METHODS	EFFECTIVE	INEFFECTIVE
Follow airborne transmission precautions until sputum culture is negative.		
Take vitamin and herbal supplements.		
Postinfection control measures on the room door.		
Verify the client's diet and nutrition.		
Teach the client to cover their nose and mouth with a paper tissue when coughing, sneezing, or laughing and dispose of tissue in a paper bag.		
Wear a particulate air filter respirator during client care.		

SKILL 22-1 Removing Personal Protective Equipment

Suggested Action	Reason for Action
ASSESSMENT	
Determine which type of infection control precautions is being used.	Indicates whether garments must be removed and discarded within the room
Note whether there are sufficient hand hygiene supplies, paper towels, a laundry hamper, and a lined waste receptacle within the room.	Provides a means for hand antisepsis and confining soiled garments and materials
PLANNING	
Make sure that all direct care of the client has been completed.	Avoids having to put on barrier garments a second time
IMPLEMENTATION	
Proceed with removing gloves.	Gloves are the most contaminated personal protection item
Remove one glove by grasping at the wrist and pulling the glove inside out with a gloved hand. Insert the fingers of the ungloved hand under the wrist of the remaining glove. Pull the remaining glove inside out while holding the first removed glove (Fig. A).	Contains the contaminated surface inside the glove

Removing gloves. (Ursula Page/Shutterstock.)
Reduces contact with the most contaminated surface of the gloves
Enfolds the contaminated surface inside the glove

A

SKILL 22-1 Removing Personal Protective Equipment (*continued*)

Suggested Action	Reason for Action
Untie or unfasten the neck and then the back closure of the cover gown (Fig. B).	The back of the gown is considered less contaminated than the front and can be touched with the bare hands.

Untying the back closures on the cover gown. (From LifeART.2023 Philadelphia, PA: Lippincott Williams & Wilkins. All rights reserved.)

B

Suggested Action	Reason for Action
Remove the gown by inserting your fingers at the shoulder and pulling the gown forward to turn the gown inside out (Fig. C).	Prevents gross contamination of the hands with contaminated areas of the gown

Removing a cover gown. (From LifeART. 2023 Philadelphia, PA: Lippincott Williams & Wilkins. All rights reserved.)

C

(*continued*)

SKILL 22-1 Removing Personal Protective Equipment (*continued*)

Suggested Action	Reason for Action
Fold the soiled side of the gown to the inside while holding it away from your uniform.	Prevents contamination of the hands and uniform
Roll up the gown with the inner surface exposed and discard it in the waste container if it is made of paper. If the gown is made of cloth, discard it in the laundry hamper in the room (Fig. D).	Confines contaminated garments

D

Enclosing the contaminated surface of the gown to the inside before discarding it. (From LifeART. 2023 Philadelphia, PA: Lippincott Williams & Wilkins. All rights reserved.)

| Remove mask (see Chapter 10) or other disposable face protection items by touching only the ties or elastic bands and discard them in the waste container (Fig. E). | The ties or other materials used to attach the mask or other face protection items are considered "clean" and can be touched with the bare hands; the surface covering the eyes and face is considered contaminated. |

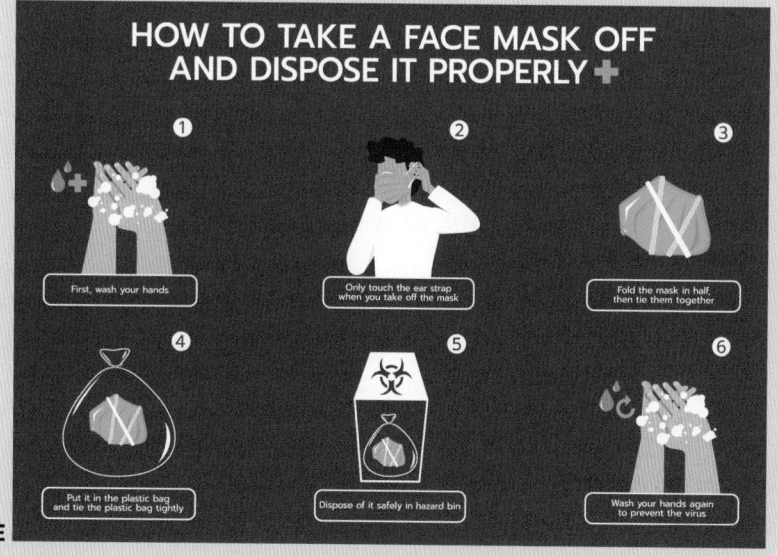

HOW TO TAKE A FACE MASK OFF AND DISPOSE IT PROPERLY

① First, wash your hands
② Only touch the ear strap when you take off the mask
③ Fold the mask in half, then tie them together
④ Put it in the plastic bag and tie the plastic bag tightly
⑤ Dispose of it safely in hazard bin
⑥ Wash your hands again to prevent the virus

E

Removal of mask. (Health Care Vector Life/Shutterstock.)

SKILL 22-1 Removing Personal Protective Equipment (*continued*)

Suggested Action	Reason for Action
Wash hands or use an alcohol-based hand rub.	Removes microorganisms that may have been inadvertently transferred during face protection items and gown removal
Use a clean paper towel to open the room door.	Protects clean hands from recontamination
Discard the paper towel in the waste container in the client's room.	Confines contaminated material
Leave the room, taking care not to touch anything.	Prevents recontamination
Go directly to the utility room and perform hand antisepsis one final time.	Removes microorganisms; it is always safer to overdo than underdo any practice that controls the spread of pathogens

EVALUATION

- Appropriate personal protective equipment (PPE) was worn.
- Garments were removed with the least contamination possible.
- Handwashing was performed appropriately.

DOCUMENT

- Type of transmission-based precautions being followed
- Care provided
- Response of client

SAMPLE DOCUMENTATION

Date and Time   Contact precautions followed. Assisted with bath. States, "I wish the door to my room could be left opened. It gets rather boring in here." Reinforced the purpose for keeping the door closed. _____ J. Doe, LPN

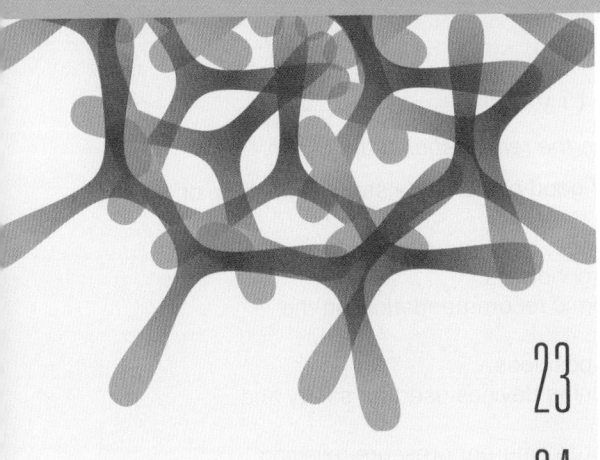

UNIT 6 | Assisting the Inactive Client

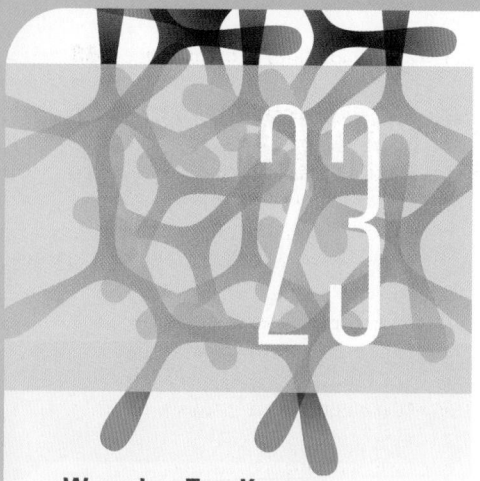

Body Mechanics, Positioning, and Moving

Words To Know

alignment
anatomic position
balance
bariatric client
base of support
bed board
body mechanics
center of gravity
contractures
disuse syndrome
energy
ergonomics
foot drop
Fowler position
functional mobility
functional position
gravity
lateral oblique position
lateral position
line of gravity
muscle spasms
neutral position
posture
prone position
repetitive strain injuries
shearing
Sims position
supine position
transfer

Learning Objectives

On completion of this chapter, the reader should be able to:

1. Identify characteristics of good posture in a standing, sitting, or lying position.
2. Describe principles of correct body mechanics.
3. Explain the purpose of ergonomics.
4. Give examples of ergonomic recommendations in the workplace.
5. Describe common client positions.
6. Describe different positioning devices used for safety and comfort.
7. Discuss advantages of three different pressure-relieving devices.
8. Identify types of transfer devices.
9. Outline general guidelines that apply to transferring clients.
10. Describe signs and symptoms associated with the disuse syndrome.

INTRODUCTION

Inactivity leads to a deterioration of health. Multiple complications can occur among people with limited activity and movement (Table 23-1).

The consequences of inactivity are collectively referred to as **disuse syndrome** (signs and symptoms that result from inactivity). Nursing care activities such as positioning and moving clients reduce the potential for disuse syndrome. Nurses can become injured, however, if they fail to use good posture and body mechanics while performing these activities.

This chapter describes how to position and move clients to prevent complications associated with inactivity. It also discusses methods for protecting nurses from work-related injuries. Basic terms are defined in Box 23-1.

 Gerontologic Considerations

■ By the seventh or eighth decade of life, muscle strength, endurance, and coordination decline. Engaging in physical activity is an important health promotion intervention for preventing mobility limitations. The risk for social isolation among older adults increases as mobility is limited.

■ Skeletal changes such as kyphosis, lordosis, or scoliosis change the older person's center of gravity.

■ Kyphotic changes can cause pressure on cervical vertebrae when someone is in a supine position. The effects of this can be minimized by placing a small towel or cervical pillow under the neck.

■ Teach older adults to use appropriate body mechanics, such as sitting in a chair when lifting an object. Also, teach about the importance of positioning oneself directly in front of objects when lifting to prevent pulling of lateral back muscles or vertebral disk compression.

■ Elevated toilet seats with handrails may help older adults use their arm muscles during transfers.

■ Older adults require extra time and assistance during positioning, transferring, and ambulating. Positions should be modified to address pain or functional limitations.

■ Allow extra time when older adults are changing their positions, such as from supine to sitting or standing, to prevent orthostatic hypotension. Teach the client to wait until any dizziness has resolved before moving, thus decreasing the risk for falls.

■ Older adults may limit their mobility due to fear of falling. Handrails may be strategically placed to promote confidence in ambulation. In addition, placing chairs along usual walking pathways will provide a "rest stop," thus increasing confidence in ambulation.

■ Older adults with cognitive impairment may have difficulty following directions regarding positioning and transferring. Instructions should be given using clear, simple words to make one request at a time. Demonstrations and illustrations can be used to help convey the message.

TABLE 23-1 Dangers of Inactivity

SYSTEMS	EFFECTS
Muscular	Weakness Decreased tone/strength Decreased size (atrophy)
Skeletal	Poor posture Contractures Foot drop
Cardiovascular	Impaired circulation Thrombus (clot) formation Dependent edema
Respiratory	Pooling of secretions Shallow respirations Atelectasis (collapsed alveoli)
Urinary	Oliguria (scanty urine) Urinary tract infections Calculi (stone) formation Incontinence (inability to control elimination)
Gastrointestinal	Anorexia (loss of appetite) Constipation Fecal impaction
Integumentary	Pressure sores
Endocrine	Decreased metabolic rate Decreased hormonal secretions
Central nervous	Sleep pattern disturbances Psychosocial changes

---

BOX 23-1 | **Basic Terminology Used in Body Mechanics**

Gravity: Force that pulls objects toward the center of the earth. The pull of gravity causes objects, such as an item dropped from the hand, to fall to the ground. It causes water to drain to its lowest level.

Energy: Capacity to do work. Energy is used to move the body from place to place. Energy is required to overcome the force of gravity.

Balance: Steady position with weight. A person falls when off balance.

Center of gravity: Point at which the mass of an object is centered. The center of gravity for a standing position is the center of the pelvis and about halfway between the umbilicus and the pubic bone.

Line of gravity: Imaginary vertical line that passes through the center of gravity. The line of gravity in a standing person is a straight line from the head to the feet through the center of the body.

Base of support: Area on which an object rests. The feet are the base of support when a person is in a standing position.

Alignment: Parts of an object being in proper relationship to one another. The body is in good alignment in a position of good posture.

Neutral position: The position of a limb that is turned neither toward nor away from the body's midline.

Anatomic position: Frontal and back views with arms at the sides and palms forward.

Functional position: Position in which an activity is performed properly and normally. In the hand, the wrists are slightly dorsiflexed between 20 and 35 degrees and the proximal finger joints are flexed between 45 and 60 degrees, with the thumb in opposition and in alignment with the pads of the fingers.

MAINTAINING GOOD POSTURE

Posture (the position of the body, or the way in which it is held) affects a person's appearance, stamina, and ability to use the musculoskeletal system efficiently. Good posture, whether in a standing, sitting, or lying position, distributes gravity through the center of the body over a wide base of support (Fig. 23-1). Good posture is important for both clients and nurses.

 Pharmacologic Considerations

Female older adults may be prescribed bisphosphonate drugs (bone resorption inhibitors), such as alendronate (Fosamax), to maintain bone density and prevent bone fractures. Specific administration guidelines must be followed for best results and to prevent gastrointestinal side effects.

When a person performs work while using poor posture, **muscle spasms** (sudden, forceful, and involuntary muscle contractions) may result. They occur more often when muscles are strained and forced to work beyond their capacity.

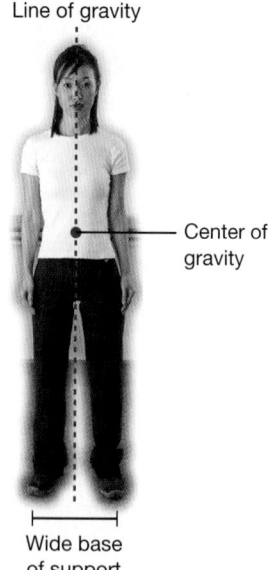

Line of gravity

Center of gravity

Wide base of support

FIGURE 23-1 Good posture helps align gravity through the center of the body. A wide stance provides a stable base for support.

Standing

To maintain good posture in a standing position (Fig. 23-2):

- Keep the feet parallel, at right angles to the lower legs, about 4 to 8 in (10 to 20 cm) apart.
- Distribute weight equally on both feet to provide a broad base of support.
- Bend the knees slightly to avoid straining the joints.
- Maintain the hips at an even level.

- Pull in the buttocks and hold the abdomen up and in to keep the spine properly aligned. This position supports the abdominal organs and reduces strain on both the back and abdominal muscles.
- Hold the chest up and slightly forward and extend or stretch the waist to give internal organs more space and maintain good alignment of the spine.
- Keep the shoulders even and centered above the hips.
- Hold the head erect with the face forward and the chin slightly tucked.

Sitting

In a good sitting position (Fig. 23-3), the buttocks and upper thighs become the base of support. Both feet rest on the floor. The knees are bent, with the posterior of the knee free from the edge of the chair to avoid interfering with distal circulation.

Lying Down

Good posture in a lying position looks the same as in a standing position, except the person is horizontal (Fig. 23-4). The head and neck muscles are in a neutral position, centered between the shoulders. The shoulders are level, and the arms, hips, and knees are slightly flexed, with no compression of the arms or legs under the body. The trunk is straight, and the hips are level. The legs are parallel to each other with the feet at the right angles to the leg.

BODY MECHANICS

The use of proper **body mechanics** (the efficient use of the musculoskeletal system) increases muscle effectiveness, reduces fatigue, and helps avoid **repetitive strain injuries**

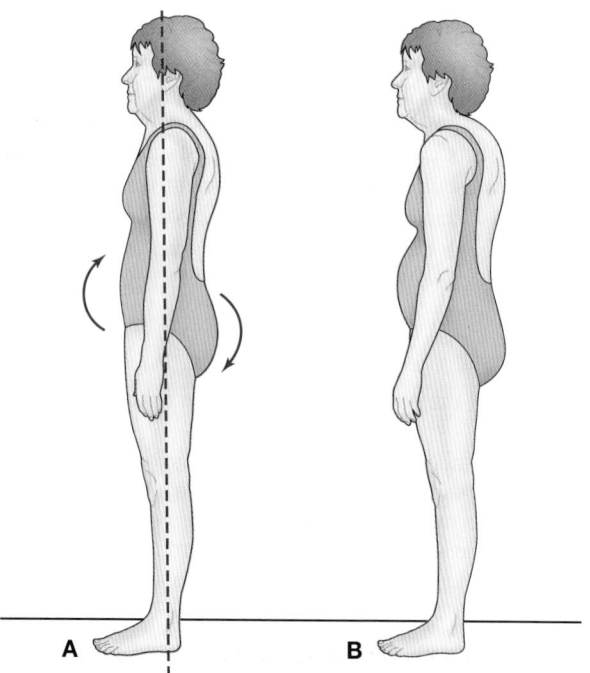

FIGURE 23-2 A. A good standing posture results when abdominal and gluteal muscles are contracted. **B.** A poor standing posture results when abdominal muscles are relaxed, causing altered body alignment.

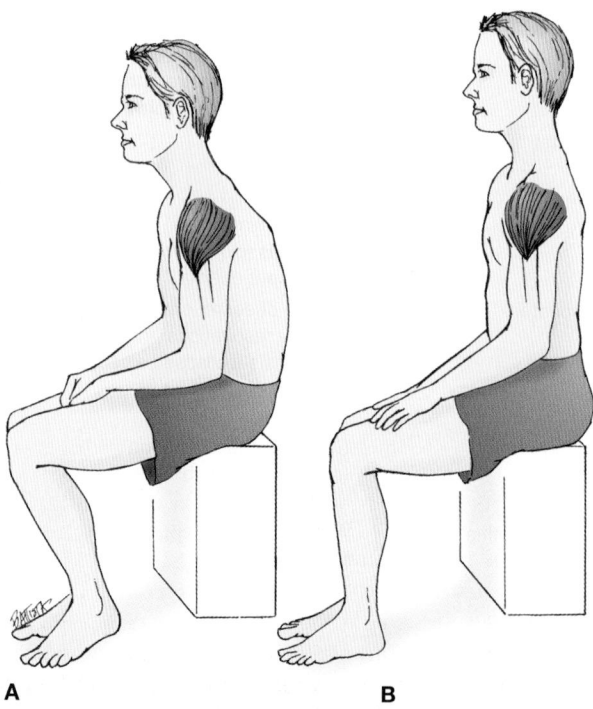

FIGURE 23-3 A. An incorrect sitting posture. **B.** A correct sitting posture. (From Hendrickson, T. [2020]. *Massage and manual therapy for orthopedic conditions* [2nd ed.]. Jones & Bartlett Learning.)

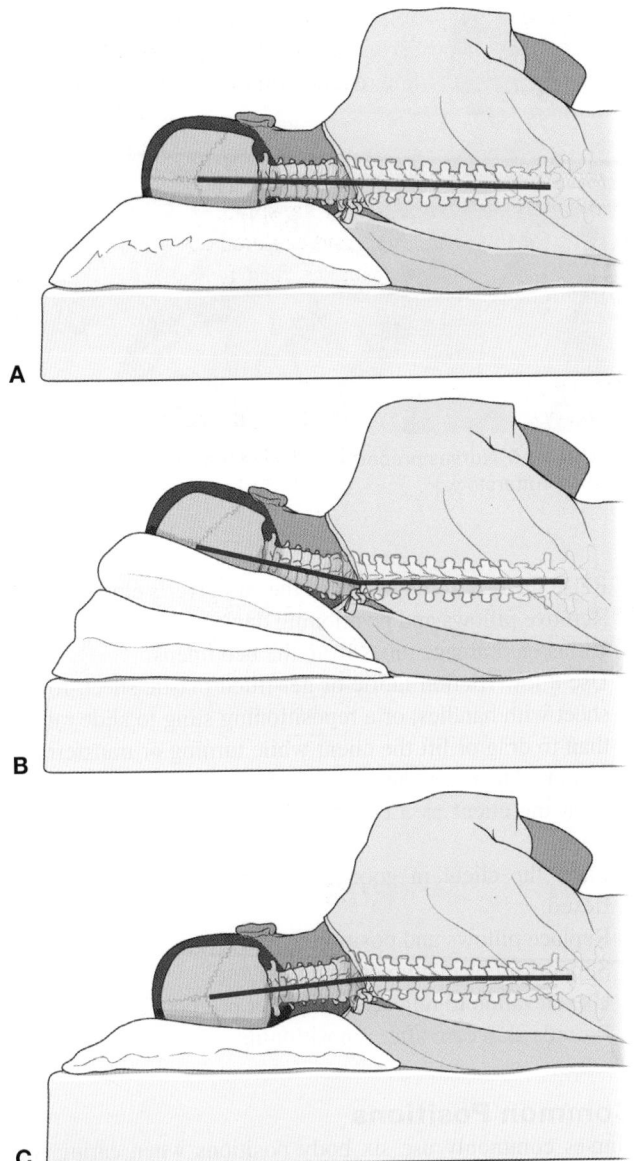

FIGURE 23-4 A. Maintaining the spine in neutral position facilitates the best lying posture. Positions that create neck flexion **(B)** or **(C)** hyperextension are undesirable.

(disorders that result from cumulative trauma to musculoskeletal structures). Basic principles of body mechanics are important regardless of a person's occupation or daily activities, but body mechanics alone will not necessarily reduce musculoskeletal injuries (Nursing Guidelines 23-1).

ERGONOMICS

Using proper body mechanics is one component of preserving the integrity of the body. Another component is applying and implementing **ergonomics** (a specialty field of engineering science devoted to promoting comfort, performance, and health in the workplace). Ergonomics is used to improve the design of the work environment and equipment. The National Institute for Occupational Safety and Health (NIOSH), a division of the Centers for Disease Control and Prevention (CDC), requires employers to comply with many ergonomic recommendations. Examples include:

NURSING GUIDELINES 23-1

Using Good Body Mechanics

- Use the longest and strongest muscles of the arms and legs. *Use of these muscles provides the greatest strength and potential for performing work.*
- When lifting a heavy load, center it over the feet. *Such positioning creates a base of support.*
- Hold objects close to the body. *Doing so increases balance.*
- Bend the knees. *Bending the knees prepares the spine to accept the weight of the load.*
- Contract the abdominal muscles and make a long midriff. *Doing so protects the muscles of the abdomen and pelvis and prevents strain and injury to the abdominal wall.*
- Push, pull, or roll objects whenever possible rather than lifting them. *Lifting requires more effort.*
- Use body weight as a lever to assist with pushing or pulling an object. *This reduces muscle strain.*
- Keep feet apart for a broad base of support. *This stance lowers the center of gravity, which promotes stability.*
- Bend the knees and keep the back straight when lifting an object, rather than bending over from the waist with straight knees. *This stance makes the best use of the longest and strongest body muscles and improves balance by keeping the weight of the object close to the center of gravity.*
- Avoid twisting and stretching muscles during work. *Twisting can strain muscles because the line of gravity is outside the body's base of support.*
- Rest between periods of exertion. *Resting promotes work endurance.*

- Using assistive devices to lift or transport heavy items or clients
- Using alternative equipment for tasks that require repetitive motion—for instance, telephone headsets or automatic staplers
- Positioning equipment no more than 20 to 30 degrees away—about an arm's length—to avoid reaching or twisting the trunk or neck
- Using a chair with good back support. A chair should be high enough so the user can place their feet firmly on the floor. There should be room for two fingers between the edge of the seat and the back of the knees. Armrests should allow a relaxed shoulder position.
- Keeping the elbows flexed no more than 100 to 110 degrees, or resting the wrists in a neutral position when working at a computer
- Working under lighting without glare

Despite being taught principles of good body mechanics, health care providers, particularly nurses, are vulnerable to ergonomic hazards in the workplace as a direct consequence of (1) lifting heavy loads (i.e., clients), (2) reaching and lifting with loads far from the body, (3) twisting while lifting, (4) unexpected changes in load demand during the lift, (5) reaching low or high to begin a lift, and (6) moving or carrying a load a significant distance. In 2018, the CDC introduced a musculoskeletal health council to review and suggest preventative measures for workplace musculo-skeletal injuries. Health care workers occupy the first and second places for most musculoskeletal injuries in the workplace (CDC, 2022). Because of the pervasiveness of the problem and its direct link to a shortage of employed nurses, the American Nurses Association (ANA) established the 2003 *Handle with Care Campaign* to reduce injuries to nurses and their clients. More recently, along with the CDC, the ANA introduced a guide to reducing musculoskeletal injuries called *Safe Patient Handling and Mobility: Interprofessional National Standards*. The goal is to reduce injuries through the use of assistive equipment and devices, which would result in many advantages (Box 23-2). In 2015, these principles were incorporated in a U.S. Congressional bill (H.R. 4266) known as the *Nurse and Health Care Worker Protection Act* (www.govtrack.us). The bill mandates health care employers create and put in place a safe patient handling, mobility, and injury prevention program; train workers on safe patient handling, mobility, and injury prevention; and post a notice that explains the standard procedures to report patient handling–related injuries and workers' rights.

POSITIONING CLIENTS

Good posture and body mechanics and ergonomically designed assistive devices are necessary when inactive clients require positioning and moving. An inactive client's position is changed to relieve pressure on bony areas of the body, promote **functional mobility** (an alignment that maintains the potential for movement and ambulation), and provide for therapeutic needs. General principles for positioning are as follows:

- Change the inactive client's position at least every 2 hours.
- Enlist the assistance of at least one other caregiver.

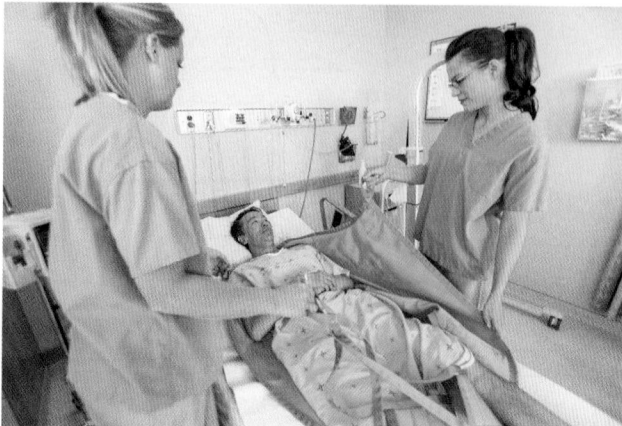

FIGURE 23-5 Nurses preparing to transfer a client. (Tyler Olson/Shutterstock.)

- Raise the bed to the height of the caregiver's elbow.
- Remove pillows and positioning devices.
- Unfasten drainage tubes from the bed linens.
- Use a low-friction fabric or gel-filled plastic sheet, roller sheet with handles, or a repositioning sling to slide rather than to drag or lift the client while turning or transferring from bed to a stretcher (Fig. 23-5).
- Turn the client as a complete unit to avoid twisting the spine.
- Place the client in good alignment with joints slightly flexed.
- Replace pillows and positioning devices.
- Support limbs in a functional position.
- Use elevation to relieve swelling or promote comfort.
- Provide skin care after repositioning.

Common Positions

Nurses commonly use six body positions when caring for bedridden clients: supine, lateral, lateral oblique, prone, Sims, and Fowler.

Supine Position

In the **supine position**, the person lies on their back (Fig. 23-6).

BOX 23-2	Advantages of Assistive Devices

Nurses
- Lessens physical exertion during positioning, moving, and transferring clients
- Reduces musculoskeletal injuries
- Decreases sick or absentee time
- Lowers medical costs, pain, and suffering
- Decreases workers' compensation claims
- Maintains workforce of employed nurses

Clients
- Provides more security during repositioning and transfers from bed, chairs, toilets, stretchers
- Results in fewer handling mishaps and secondary injuries
- Relieves anxiety concerning safety
- Promotes comfort by reducing awkward or forceful manual handling
- Maintains dignity and self-esteem
- Promotes faster recovery

Adapted from American Nurses Association. (n.d.). *Handle with care campaign.* http://www.nursingworld.org/handlewithcare

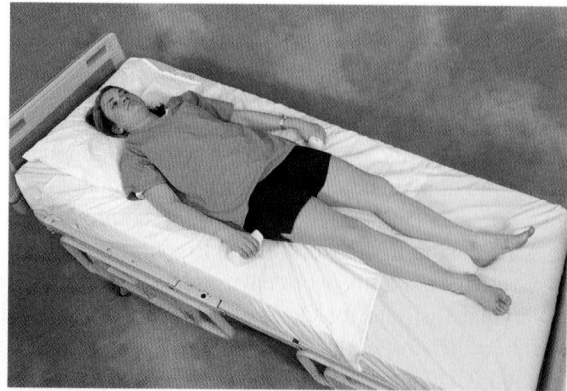

FIGURE 23-6 Supine position.

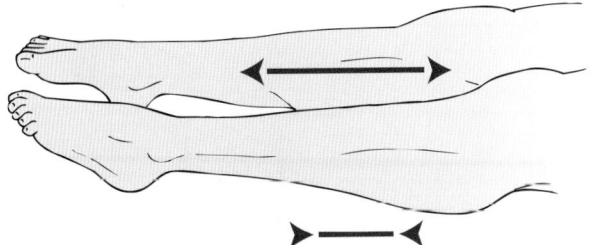

FIGURE 23-7 Foot drop is a consequence of weakened muscles for dorsiflexion, resulting in permanent plantar flexion.

There are two primary concerns associated with the supine position: prolonged pressure, especially at the end of the spine, leads to skin breakdown; and gravity, combined with pressure on the toes from bed linen, creates a potential for **foot drop** (a permanent dysfunctional position caused by a shortening of the calf muscles and a lengthening of the opposing muscles on the anterior leg; Fig. 23-7). Foot drop hinders ambulation because it interferes with a person's ability to place the heel on the floor.

Lateral Position
With the **lateral position** (a side-lying position), foot drop is of less concern because gravity does not pull the feet down as happens when clients are supine (Fig. 23-8). Nevertheless, unless the upper shoulder and arm are supported, they may rotate forward and interfere with breathing.

Lateral Oblique Position
In the **lateral oblique position** (a variation of the side-lying position), the client lies on the side with the top leg placed at 30 degrees of hip flexion and 35 degrees of knee flexion (Fig. 23-9). The calf of the top leg is placed behind the midline of the body on a support such as a pillow. The back is supported, and the bottom leg is in a neutral position. This position produces less pressure on the hip than a strictly lateral position and reduces the potential for skin breakdown.

Prone Position
The **prone position** (one in which the client lies on the abdomen, Fig. 23-10) is an alternative position for the person with skin breakdown from pressure ulcers (see Chapter 28). The prone position also provides good drainage from bronchioles, stretches the trunk and extremities, and keeps the

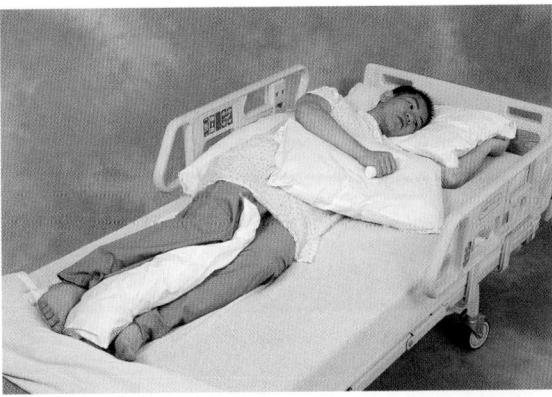

FIGURE 23-9 Lateral oblique position.

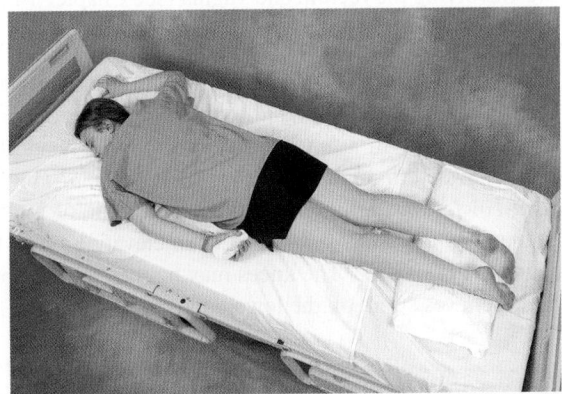

FIGURE 23-10 Prone position.

hips in an extended position. The prone position has been found to improve arterial oxygenation in critically ill clients with acute respiratory distress syndrome who are mechanically ventilated, it was shown to improve oxygenation and decrease dyspnea (Venus et al., 2020). The prone position poses a nursing challenge for assessing and communicating with clients, however, and it is uncomfortable for clients with recent abdominal surgery or back pain and interferes with eating.

Sims Position
In **Sims position** (a semiprone position), the client lies on the left side, with the right knee drawn up toward the chest (Fig. 23-11). An arm is positioned along the client's back, and the chest and abdomen are allowed to lean forward. The

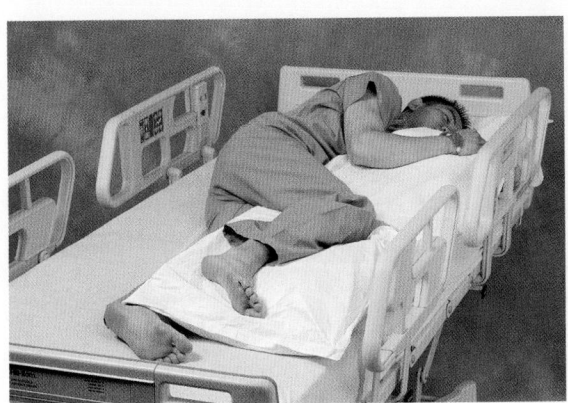

FIGURE 23-8 Lateral position.

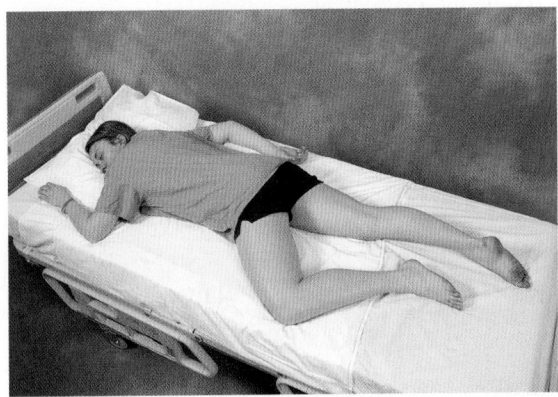

FIGURE 23-11 Sims position.

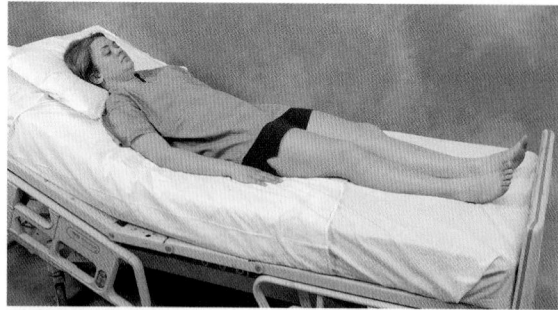

FIGURE 23-12 Low Fowler position.

Sims position is also used for the examination of and procedures involving the rectum and vagina (see Chapter 14).

Fowler Position

The **Fowler position** (a semi-sitting position) makes it easier for the client to eat, talk, and look around. Three variations are common. In a *low Fowler position*, the head and torso are elevated to 30 degrees (Fig. 23-12). A *mid-Fowler* or *semi-Fowler position* refers to an elevation of up to 45 degrees. A *high Fowler position* is an elevation of 60 to 90 degrees (Fig. 23-13). The knees may not be elevated, but doing so relieves strain on the lower spine.

> ### ⟫ *Stop, Think, and Respond 23-1*
> *Give one advantage and one disadvantage each for the supine, lateral, lateral oblique, prone, Sims, and Fowler positions.*

The Fowler position is especially helpful for clients with dyspnea because it causes the abdominal organs to drop away from the diaphragm. Relieving pressure on the diaphragm allows the exchange of a greater volume of air. Sitting for a prolonged period, however, decreases blood flow to tissues in the coccyx area and increases the risk for pressure ulcers in that area.

Positioning Devices

Many devices are available to help maintain good body alignment in bed and to prevent discomfort or pressure. Any position, no matter how comfortable or anatomically correct, must be changed frequently.

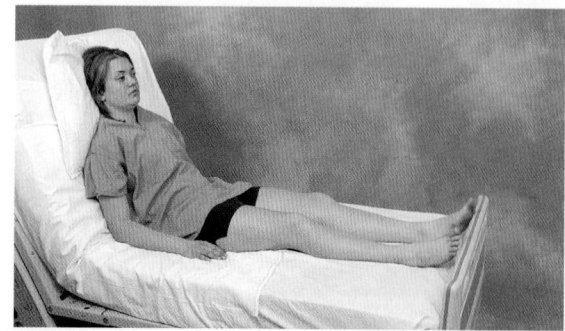

FIGURE 23-13 High Fowler position.

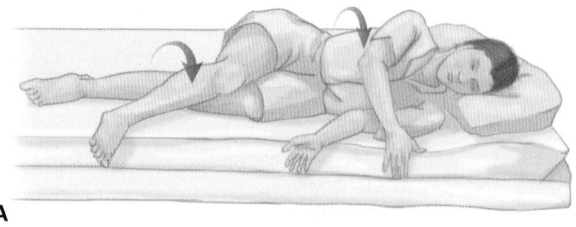

A

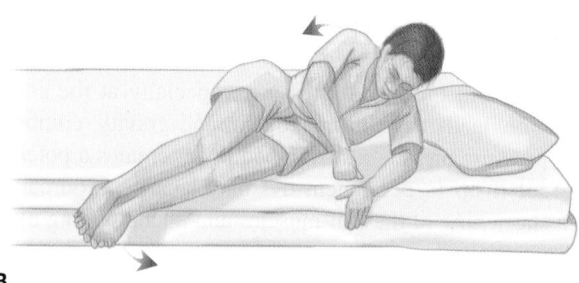

B

FIGURE 23-14 A. Place the bed in the lowest position. Grasping the mattress and pushing down with the other hand is an independent technique for sitting on the edge of the bed. **B.** Preparing the client to safely get out of bed for ambulation. (From Craven, R. F., Hirnle, C. J., & Henshaw, C. [2019]. *Fundamentals of nursing* [9th ed.]. Wolters Kluwer Health.)

Adjustable Bed

The adjustable bed (see Chapter 18) can be raised or lowered and allows the position of the head and knees to be changed. The high position facilitates the performance of nursing care. Raising the head of the bed helps the client look around without twisting and bending. It also promotes drainage of the upper lobes of the lungs and prepares the client for eventually standing and walking. The low position enables an independent client to get in and out of the bed safely (Fig. 23-14). Placing a bed in a slight Trendelenburg position may help keep the client from sliding down toward the foot of the bed (Fig. 23-15).

Mattress

A comfortable, supportive mattress is firm but flexible enough to permit good body alignment. An unsupportive mattress promotes an unnatural curvature of the spine.

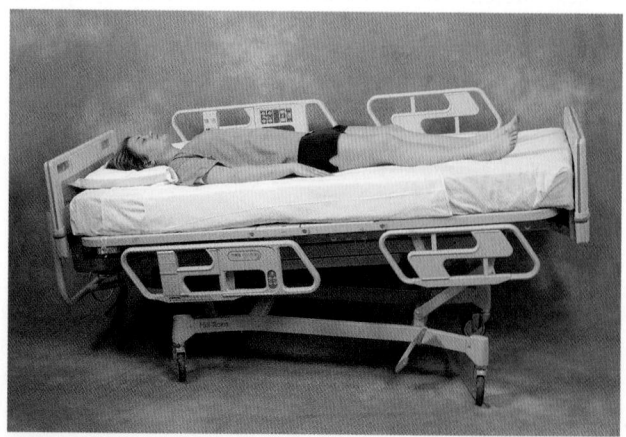

FIGURE 23-15 In the Trendelenburg position, the head is lower than the feet.

Bed Board

A **bed board** (a rigid structure placed under a mattress) provides additional skeletal support. Bed boards are usually made of plywood or some other firm material. The size varies with the situation. If sections of the bed (the head and foot) can be raised, the board must be divided into hinged sections. For home use, full bed boards can be purchased or made from sheets of plywood.

Pillows

Pillows are used to support and elevate a body part. Small pillows, such as contour pillows, triangular wedges, and bolsters, are ideal for supporting and elevating the head, extremities, and shoulders. For home use, oversized pillows are useful for elevating the upper part of the body if an adjustable bed is not available.

Roller Sheet

A roller sheet (also known as a *slider* sheet) that extends from the upper back to the midthigh is a helpful positioning device. Some are designed with handles on either side. When made of substances that reduce friction, the roller sheets diminish the work of turning a client and avoid the potential for skin injuries. They are used to slide and roll rather than to lift the client. They help clients move up in bed from a supine position in the center of the bed to the side of the bed, to turn clients to a lateral position, or to transfer clients from bed to a stretcher. Working as a team, nurses use the roller sheet to change the client to an alternate position while avoiding any stooping, reaching, or twisting. The sheet is removed after being used or kept dry and free of wrinkles to prevent skin

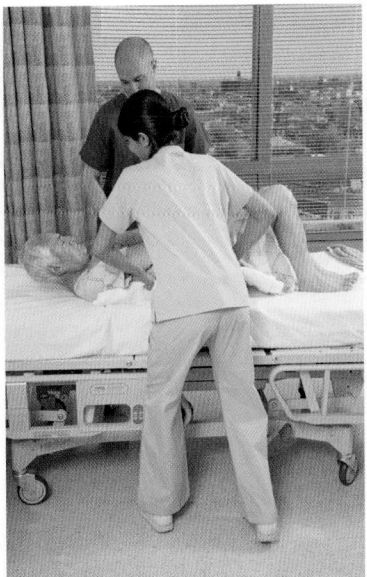

FIGURE 23-16 A roller sheet is used for turning, moving, and repositioning.

breakdown. A mechanical lift, which is discussed later, or a repositioning sling is recommended when major repositioning is required. The roller sheet is placed close to the sides of the client's body during repositioning (Fig. 23-16).

Turning and Moving Clients

In some cases, the client may be fully capable of assisting with turning or moving. The amount of client assistance depends on factors such as size, weight, mental status, and strength (Fig. 23-17).

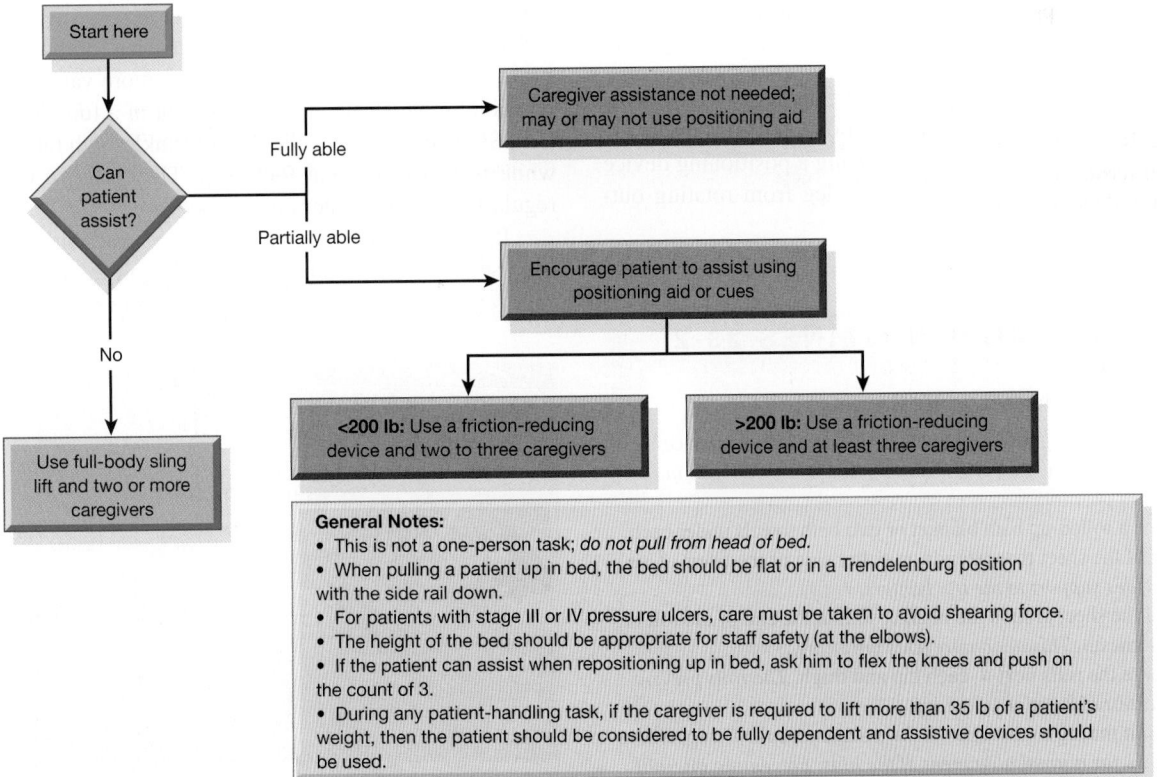

FIGURE 23-17 Repositioning algorithm for reposition in bed, from side to side or up. (VISN 8 Patient Safety Center. [2005]. *Safe patient handling and movement algorithms.* https://www.lmcins.com/uploads/3/2/0/7/3207324/safe_patient_handling.pdf) Up to date 2023.

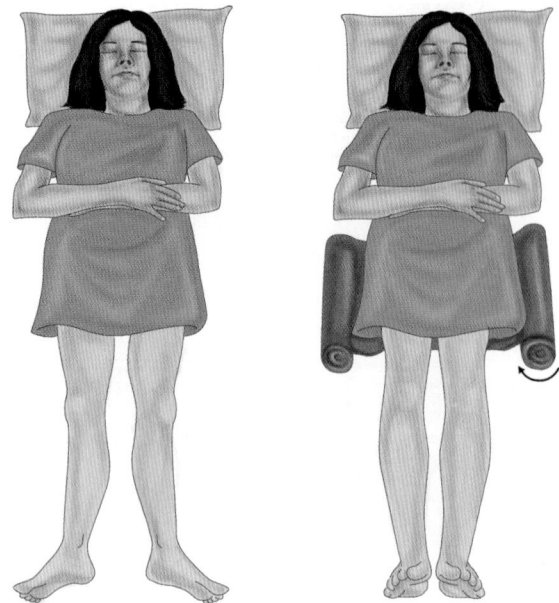

FIGURE 23-18 Placement of trochanter rolls. (From Taylor, L. P., & Bartlett, J. [2023]. *Fundamentals of nursing* [10th ed.]. Wolters Kluwer Health.)

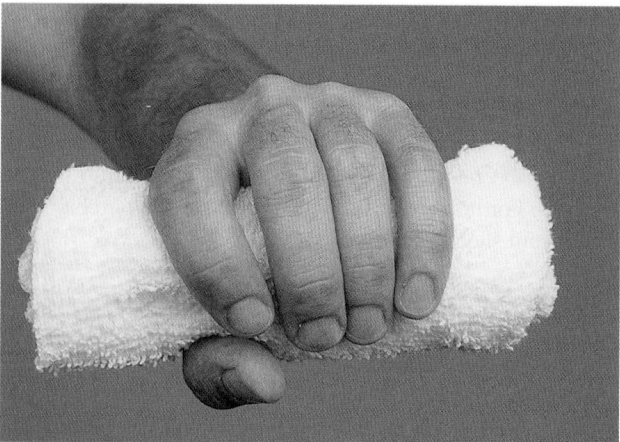

FIGURE 23-19 A hand roll. (Photo by B. Proud.)

If all criteria suggest that the nurse and client can accomplish the task at hand, the nurse enlists the client's cooperation by explaining the plan and how the client can help. Assistive devices and additional caregivers are needed when turning or moving a client who cannot change from one position to another independently or who needs help doing so. Good turning and moving skills are important to prevent injury to the nurse and the client. Skill 23-1 describes the process of repositioning and moving clients.

Trochanter Rolls

Trochanter rolls (Fig. 23-18) prevent the legs from turning outward. The trochanters are the bony protrusions at the head of the femur near the hip. Placing a positioning device at the trochanters helps prevent the leg from rotating outward (Nursing Guidelines 23-2).

NURSING GUIDELINES 23-2

Using a Trochanter Roll

- Fold a sheet lengthwise in half or in one-thirds and place it under the client's hips. *The sheet will anchor the body in the correct position.*
- Place a rolled-up bath blanket or two bath towels under each end of the sheet that extends on either side of the client. *This provides support to the trochanters.*
- Roll the sheet around the blanket so that the end of the roll is underneath. *This action prevents unrolling.*
- Secure the rolls next to each hip and thigh. *The rolls prevent an external rotation of the hip.*
- Permit the leg to rest against the trochanter roll. *This position allows for normal alignment of the hips, preventing internal or external rotation.*

Hand Rolls

Hand rolls (Fig. 23-19) are devices that preserve the client's functional ability to grasp and pick up objects. Hand rolls prevent **contractures** (permanently shortened muscles that resist stretching) of the fingers. They keep the thumb positioned slightly away from the hand and at a moderate angle to the fingers. The fingers are kept in a slightly neutral position rather than a tight fist. A rolled-up washcloth or a ball can be used as an alternative to commercial hand rolls. Hand rolls are removed regularly to facilitate movement and exercise.

Footboards, Boots, and Foot Splints

Footboards, boots, and splints are devices that prevent foot drop by keeping the feet in a functional position (Fig. 23-20). Some commercial footboards have supports that prevent the outward rotation of the foot and lower leg.

If the client is short and cannot reach a footboard, a foot splint is used. A foot splint allows for more variety in body positioning while maintaining the foot in a functional position. Some nurses have clients wear ankle-high tennis shoes while in bed to prevent foot drop. They remove the shoes regularly and administer proper foot care.

If a foot splint or footboard is not available, the nurse can use a pillow and large sheet. They roll the pillow in the sheet and twist the ends of the sheet before tucking it under

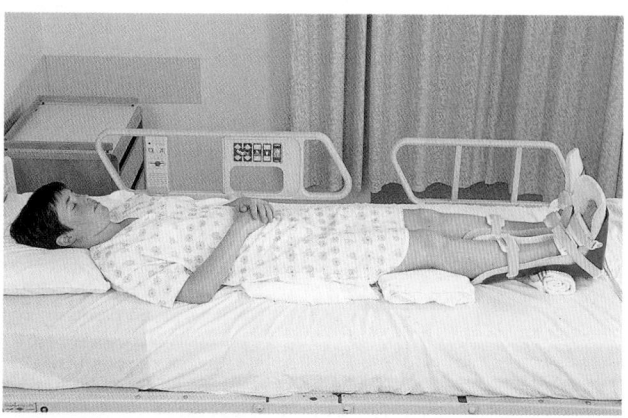

FIGURE 23-20 Protective boots to avoid foot drop. (Photo by B. Proud.)

the foot of the mattress. A pillow support does not provide the firmness of a board or splint, and the nurse replaces it as soon as possible with a sturdier device.

Trapeze

A trapeze is a triangular piece of metal hung by a chain over the head of the bed (Fig. 23-21). The client grasps the trapeze to lift the body and move about in bed. Unless arm movement or lifting is undesirable, a trapeze is an excellent device for helping a bedridden client increase activity.

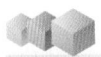
Concept Mastery Alert

Client Independence

Promoting client independence with movement and activity is an important intervention for clients with musculoskeletal problems. Unlike log rolling and pull sheets that are nurse-initiated methods, the overhead trapeze is used by the client.

PROTECTIVE DEVICES

Items such as side rails, mattress overlays, cradles, and specialty beds protect inactive clients from harm or complications.

Side Rails

Side rails (Fig. 23-22) are a valuable device to aid clients in changing their position and moving while in bed. With side rails in place, the client can safely turn from side to side and sit up in bed. These activities help clients maintain or regain muscle strength and joint flexibility.

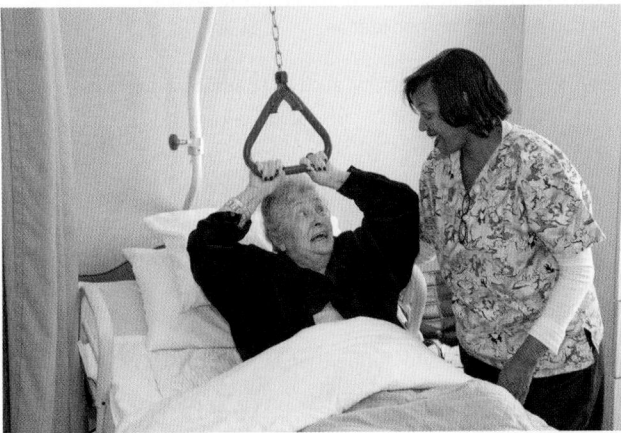

FIGURE 23-21 Using a trapeze to facilitate movement. (From Taylor, C., Lynn, P., & Bartlett, J. [2023]. *Fundamentals of nursing* [10th ed.]. Wolters Kluwer Health.)

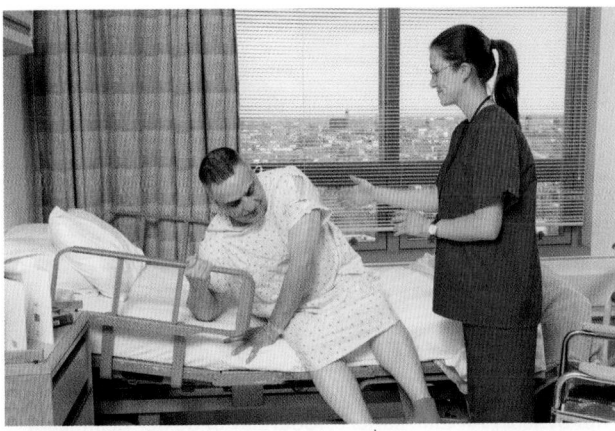

FIGURE 23-22 Using side rails to prepare for ambulation and to change position.

Mattress Overlays

Mattress overlays are accessory items made of foam or containing gel, air, or water that nurses place over a standard hospital mattress. Nurses use mattress overlays to reduce pressure and restore skin integrity (see Chapter 28).

Foam and Gel Mattresses

Several types of foam mattresses, made of latex or polyethylene, are available. Foam acts like a layer of subcutaneous tissue because it conforms to the client's body and acts like a cushion. Consequently, it redistributes pressure over a greater area, reducing the compressive effect on skin and tissue. Foam also contains channels and cells filled with air that allow for the evaporation of moisture and the escape of heat.

Some foam mattresses are convoluted or made with a series of elevations and depressions, resembling an egg crate (see Chapter 18) or waffle. The density of the foam and the manner in which the foam is formed determine the degree of pressure reduction. Egg-crate foam mattresses provide minimal pressure reduction and are recommended for comfort only. Thicker, waffle-shaped foam mattresses offer greater pressure reduction; nurses can use them to prevent skin breakdown.

Gel is an alternative substance used to fill cushions and mattresses. It differs from foam in that it suspends and supports the body part. Nurses place gel and foam cushions in wheelchairs to prevent the "hammock effect"—the posterior and lateral compression that occurs when sitting in a sling-like seat.

Static Air Mattress

A static air pressure mattress is filled with a fixed volume of air. It is similar in appearance to those used for recreational purposes. It suspends the client on a buoyant surface, distributing the pressure on the underlying tissue. If the mattress becomes underinflated, however, it loses its effectiveness as a pressure-relieving device. Because plastic is nonabsorbent, air mattresses permit less evaporation of moisture than foam. Also, sharp objects can damage the integrity of the mattress.

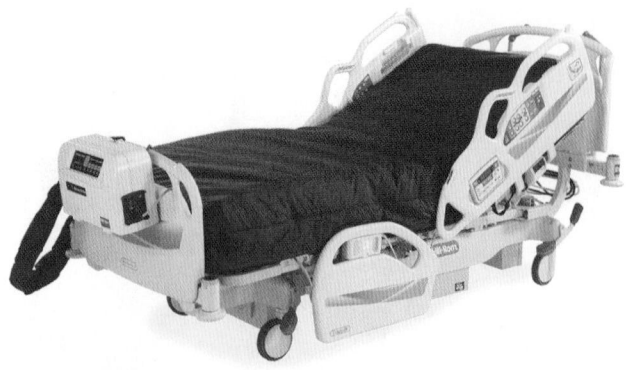

FIGURE 23-23 Synergy Air Elite surface of Advanta 2 bed with Synergy Air Elite surface. (Courtesy of Baxter Healthcare Corporation.)

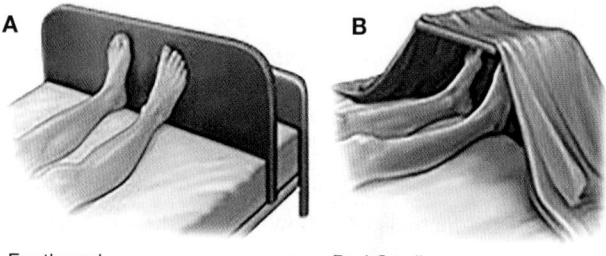

Footboard   Bed Cradle

FIGURE 23-24 **A.** A footboard can help keep your feet in proper position. **B.** A bed cradle beneath the top sheet. (https://www.drugs.com/cg/how-to-use-bed-cradles-and-footboards.html)

Alternating Air Mattress
An alternating air mattress (Fig. 23-23) is similar to a static one with one exception: every other channel inflates as the next one deflates. The process is then reversed. The wave-like redistribution of air cyclically relieves pressure over bony prominences. This repetitive process promotes blood flow and keeps the tissues supplied with oxygen. The tubing connecting the mattress to its motor-driven compressor must not become kinked. The noise may disturb some clients.

Water Mattress
A water mattress supports the body and equalizes the pressure per square inch over its surface. The pressure-relieving effect is maintained regardless of any shift in the client's position. Many claim that sleeping on a waterbed produces a feeling of tranquility, which may provide beneficial emotional effects. Water mattresses are heavy; therefore, the floor and the bed frame must be able to support the weight. Puncturing leads to damage. Filling and emptying, though done infrequently, are time-consuming.

Cradle
A cradle is a metal frame secured to or placed on top of the mattress. It forms a shell over the client's lower legs to keep bed linen off the feet or legs (Fig. 23-24). A cradle is often used for clients with burns, painful joint disease, and fractures of the leg. Footboards will also keep your feet in proper position while you are in bed.

Specialty Beds
Specialty beds such as low–air-loss beds, air-fluidized beds, oscillating support beds, and circular beds offer more functions than standard hospital beds. Like mattress overlays, they are used to relieve pressure and to prevent other problems associated with inactivity and immobility (Table 23-2).

TABLE 23-2 Pressure-Relieving Devices

DEVICE	EXAMPLES	INDICATIONS FOR USE
Foam mattress or gel cushion	Egg crate / Geo-Mat	Intact skin and minimal risk for breakdown / Changes in position occur spontaneously or require minimal assistance.
Static air, alternating air, or water mattress	TENDER Cloud / Sof-Care / Pulsair / Lotus	At some risk for skin breakdown / A superficial or single deep break in skin but pressure easily relieved / Need for prolonged bed rest with immobilization
Oscillating support bed	Roto Rest / Tilt and Turn / Paragon 9000	At high risk for systemic effects of immobility, such as pneumonia and skin breakdown
Low–air-loss bed	KinAir / FLEXICAIR / Mediscus	Combination of the following: • Impaired skin • Continued existence of risk factors for further skin breakdown • Alternative positions limited, less than adequate, or impossible • Assistance required for frequent transfers from bed
Air-fluidized bed	Clinitron / FluidAir	Combination of the following: • Impaired skin • Continued existence of risk factors for further skin breakdown • Alternative positions limited, less than adequate, or impossible • Seldom transferred from bed
Circular bed	CircOlectric	Current or high risk for skin breakdown because of multiple traumas, especially if it involves the head, neck, or spine / Burns that require frequent dressing changes or topical applications

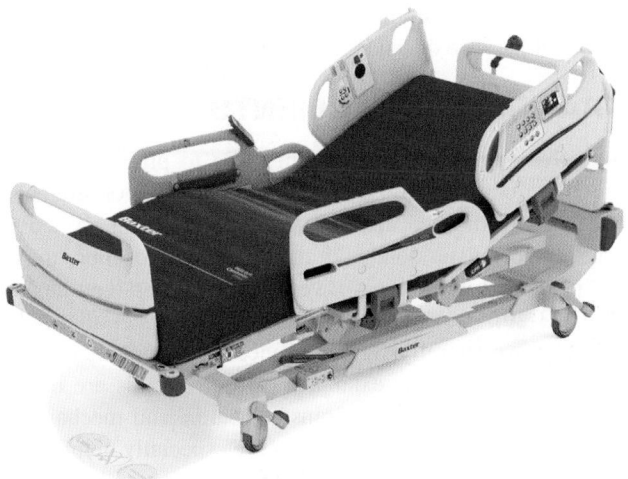

FIGURE 23-25 Centrella bed with max surface. (Courtesy of Baxter Healthcare Corporation.)

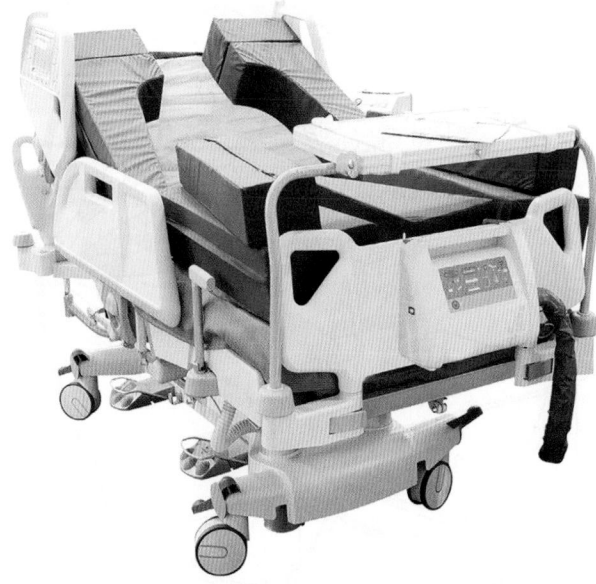

FIGURE 23-27 An oscillating bed. (Vereshchagin Dmitry/Shutterstock.)

Low–Air-Loss Bed

A low–air-loss bed (Fig. 23-25) contains inflated air sacs within the mattress. It maintains capillary pressure well below that which can interfere with blood flow. Regardless of changes in body position, the mattress selectively responds by redistributing the air to maintain low pressure to all skin areas.

Air-Fluidized Bed

An air-fluidized bed (Fig. 23-26) contains a collection of tiny beads within a mattress cover. The beads are blown upward on warm air. When suspended, the dry beads take on the characteristics of fluid, allowing the client to float on the lifted beads. Excretions and secretions drain away from the body and through the beads, thereby preventing skin irritation and maceration from moisture. The pressure-relieving effects of this type of bed have been shown to speed the healing of severely impaired tissue.

An air-fluidized bed is better used for a client who is likely to remain in bed for long periods. Fluid balance may become a problem because of the accelerated evaporation

caused by the warm, blowing air. Puncturing or tearing of the mattress is also a potential problem.

Oscillating Support Bed

An oscillating bed (Fig. 23-27) slowly and continuously rocks the client from side to side in a 124-degree arc. Oscillation relieves skin pressure and helps mobilize respiratory secretions. Foam-covered supports applied to the head, arms, and legs prevent sliding and skin **shearing** (the force exerted against the surface and layers of the skin as tissues slide in opposite but parallel directions). Compartments within the bed are removed temporarily to facilitate assessment and care of the posterior body.

Circular Bed

A circular bed supports the client on a 6- or 7-ft anterior or posterior platform suspended across the diameter of the frame (Fig. 23-28). This type of bed allows the client to remain passively immobilized during a position change.

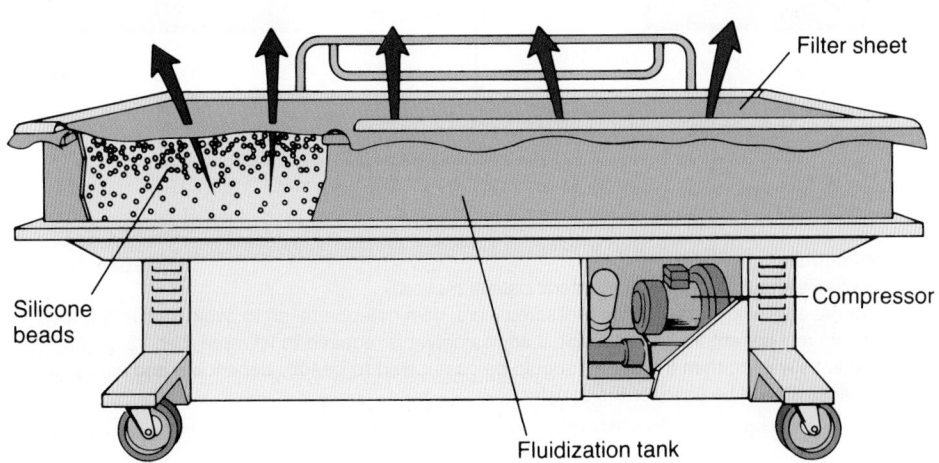

Filter sheet
Silicone beads
Compressor
Fluidization tank

FIGURE 23-26 An air-fluidized bed.

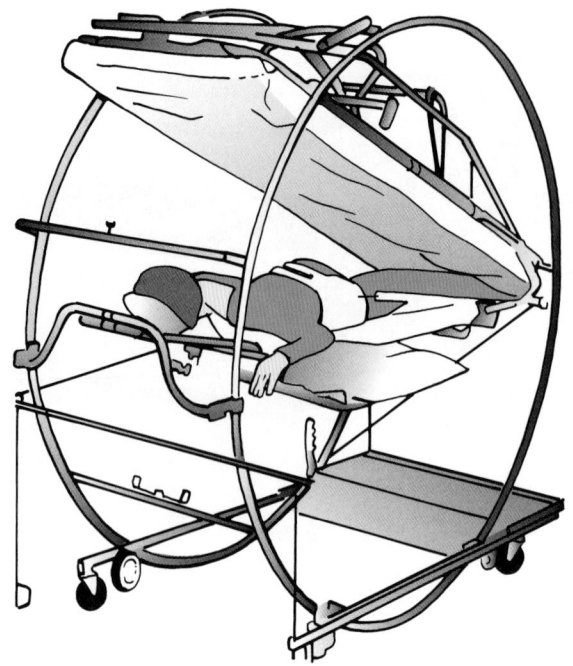

FIGURE 23-28 A circular bed.

The bed has the capacity to rotate the client, who is sandwiched between the anterior and posterior frames in a 180-degree arc. Turning permits access to the client for nursing care. Clients learn how to operate the bed to make minor

adjustments in position. This promotes a sense of control among otherwise dependent clients.

TRANSFERRING CLIENTS

Transfer (moving a client from place to place) refers to moving a client from the bed to a chair, toilet, or stretcher and back to the bed again. The client assists in an active transfer. A transfer done with the help of one or more nursing personnel with an assistive device is a passive transfer (Fig. 23-29). Transfer aids are assistive devices that help clients move laterally. Several devices are available to help transfer clients. Some examples of transfer aids are transfer handles, transfer belts, transfer boards, and mechanical or electrical lifts. Transfer devices are especially helpful for decreasing the potential for injury to caregivers and clients or, for times, when caring for clients who fear falling or who lack confidence in the ability of personnel to transfer them safely and comfortably.

Transfer Handle

Some clients with disabilities find that a transfer handle helps them remain active and independent (Fig. 23-30). A transfer handle fits between the mattress and the bed frame or box spring and serves as a combination grab bar and handrail to support the client's weight while exiting and returning to bed. A transfer handle is not considered a restrictive device like side rails because the client is free to move around. It promotes activity and mobility for many who are physically challenged.

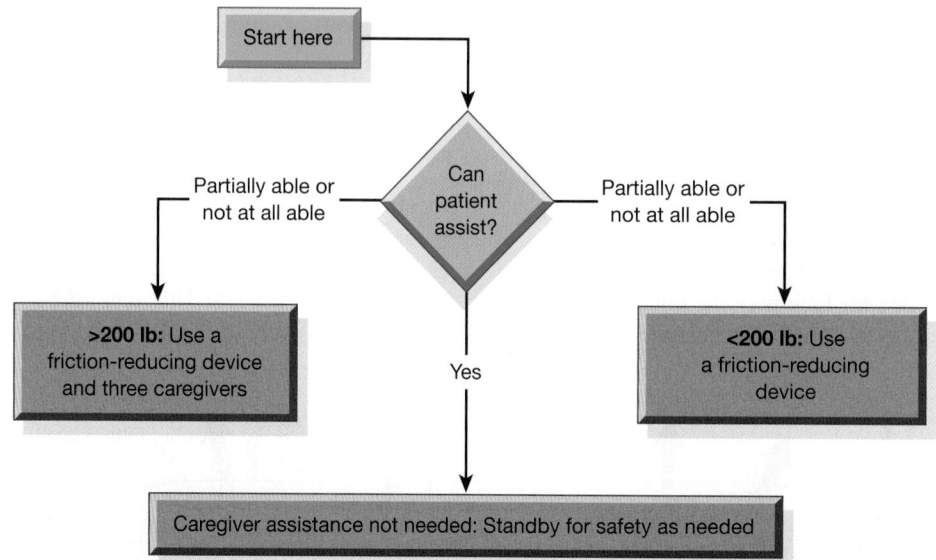

FIGURE 23-29 Algorithm for lateral transfer options to and from bed. (VISN 8 Patient Safety Center. [2005]. *Safe patient handling and movement algorithms.* https://www.lmcins.com/uploads/3/2/0/7/3207324/safe_patient_handling.pdf) Up to date 2023.

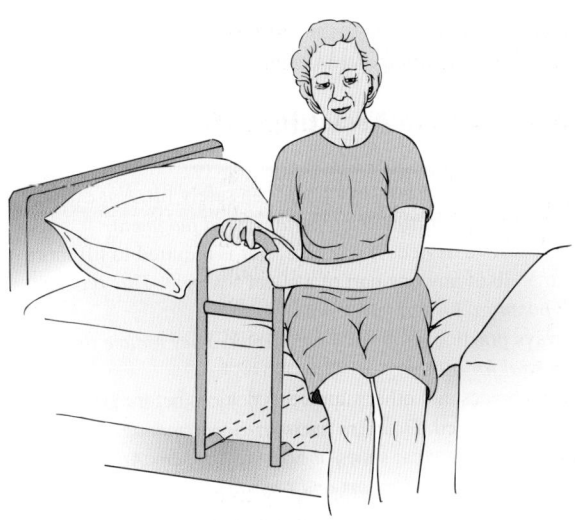

FIGURE 23-30 A transfer handle.

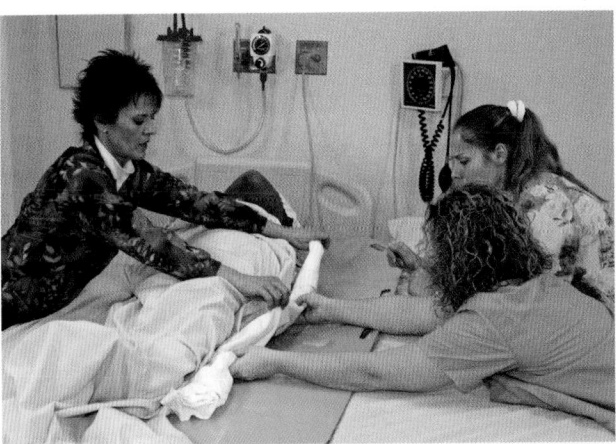

FIGURE 23-32 A transfer board is used to move a client from the bed to a stretcher.

Transfer Belt

A transfer belt is a padded device secured around the client's waist. Its handles provide a means of gripping and supporting the client (Fig. 23-31). This device is designed for clients who can bear weight and help with the transfer but are unsteady. It may also be used as a walking belt to provide safety and security while assisting a client with ambulation (see Chapter 26).

Transfer Boards

A transfer board serves as a supportive bridge between two surfaces, such as the bed and a wheelchair, the bed and a stretcher, the wheelchair and a car seat, or the wheelchair and the toilet. Transfer boards come in a variety of widths and lengths. Some are curved to facilitate transferring around fixed armrests; others may have wheels underneath. Transfer boards are positioned in such a way that the client's buttocks or body can slide across what would otherwise be an open space or a gap in height between two surfaces (Fig. 23-32).

Some clients with strong arm and upper body muscles can use a transfer board independently. For clients who need assistance, the nurse uses a transfer belt in conjunction with a transfer board. Full-body transfer boards also are available for moving supine clients to a stretcher or an X-ray table. A low-friction roller sheet may be used in conjunction with a transfer board.

Mechanical Lift

A mechanical lift (Fig. 23-33) helps move heavy clients or those with limited ability to assist from the bed to a chair, toilet, or tub and back again. Both electric and hydraulic models are available with a lifting capacity of 350 to 600 lb. Using a mechanical lift enables a caregiver to raise and lower clients secured in a canvas sling and move them around on a wheeled frame. The wheels are locked when a stationary position is desired, such as when lowering a client into place. Standing assist lifts are an alternative for use when clients have some ability to bear weight (Fig. 23-34).

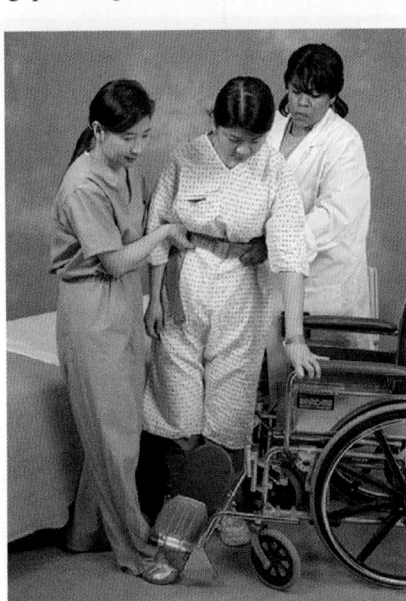

FIGURE 23-31 A belt is used to assist with transferring a client from the bed to a wheelchair and back to the bed.

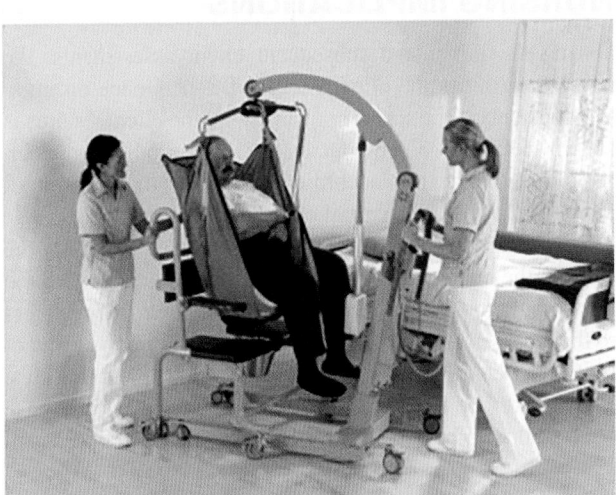

FIGURE 23-33 A hydraulic mechanical lift is used to raise and transfer a client who is obese or helpless to some other location and return the client to bed. (From U.S. Department of Veteran Affairs. [2021]. *Safe patient handling and mobility design criteria.* https://www.cfm.va.gov/til/etc/dcSPHM.pdf)

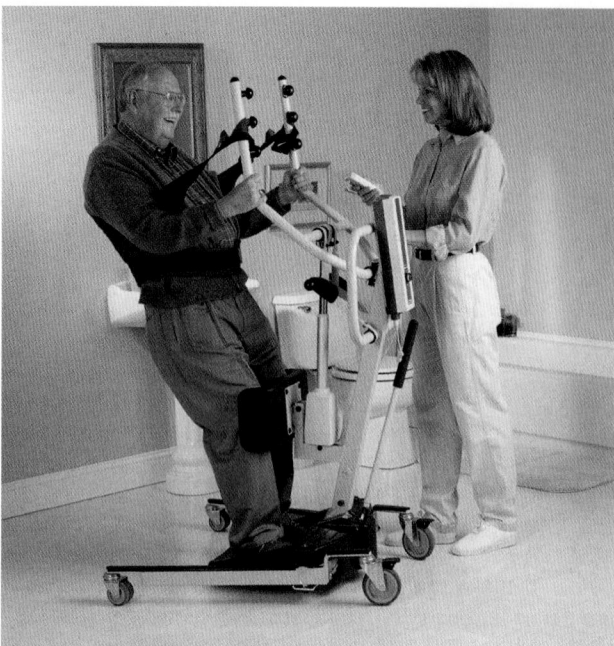

FIGURE 23-34 A standing lift supports a client who can bear some body weight. It also facilitates lowering the client to a sitting position on a chair or toilet.

>>> *Stop, Think, and Respond 23-3*

List the various devices for transferring clients in a sequence from the one that requires the least work on the part of the nurse to the one that may require the most.

It is best to use assistive devices when they are needed, observe the guidelines in Nursing Guidelines 23-3, and use the recommendations in Skill 23-2 when transferring clients.

NURSING IMPLICATIONS

During the initial and subsequent client assessments, the nurse determines the client's level of dependence on nursing assistance. One scale for quantifying the client's status is shown in Box 23-3. The nurse selects positioning, transfer, and protective devices according to whether the client is independent or requires partial or total assistance.

Nursing Care Plan 23-1 illustrates how nurses apply the steps in the nursing process when caring for a client with the nursing diagnosis of deconditioning. *Deconditioning* refers to the changes in the body that occur during a period of inactivity. The changes happen in the heart, lungs, and muscles. They make one feel tired and weak (fatigued) and decrease one's ability to be active. It can result in functional losses in

 NURSING GUIDELINES 23-3

Managing Pain Assisting with Client Transfer

- Be realistic about how much you can safely lift. *Not exceeding one's capabilities demonstrates good judgment.*
- Use assistive devices if any caregiver is required to lift more than 35 lb of any one part of a client's weight. *This reduces the potential for caregiver injuries.*
- Always practice good body mechanics. *They reduce the potential for injury.*
- Put on braces and other supportive devices before getting a client out of bed. *Doing so maximizes time management.*
- Have the client wear shoes or nonskid slippers. *Appropriate footwear provides support and prevents foot injuries.*
- Plan to transfer clients across the shortest distance. *A short transfer reduces the potential for injury.*
- Make sure the client's stronger leg, if there is one, is nearest the chair to which the client is transferring. *This action ensures safety.*
- Stand on the side of the bed to which the client will be moving. *This position helps the nurse assist the client.*
- Explain to the client what will be done, step by step, and solicit the client's help as much as possible. *These actions inform the client, encourage self-help, and reduce the workload.*

areas such as mental status, the degree of continence, and the ability to accomplish activities of daily living (ADLs).

While providing nursing care, there may be opportunities to teach clients and their caregivers about techniques that promote activity or reduce the potential for complications from inactivity. See Client and Family Teaching 23-1.

BOX 23-3	Levels of Functional Status

0 = Completely independent
1 = Requires the use of an assistive device
2 = Needs minimal help
3 = Needs assistance and/or some supervision
4 = Needs total supervision
5 = Needs total assistance or unable to assist
Various nursing diagnoses may apply to inactive clients:
- Risk for altered skin integrity
- Activity of daily living (ADL) deficit
- Deconditioning
- Injury risk
- Safety
- Fall risk
- Pressure injury risk

Client and Family Teaching 23-1
Promoting Activity and Mobility

The nurse teaches the client and the family as follows:

- Balance periods of activity with periods of rest.
- Become aware of the dangers of inactivity.
- Allow adequate time for performing activities.
- Join a club that involves social activities.
- Develop hobbies or recreational interests.
- Become a volunteer at the hospital, your church, or a municipal group.
- Join a local group—a coffee club, a book club, or card game.

- Remove objects that might pose safety hazards, such as throw rugs or electrical cords. Make sure chair legs are not in the way. Promptly mop up any water spilled on the floor.
- Rent or purchase hospital equipment from a medical supply company.
- Investigate the loan of equipment for homebound terminal clients from national organizations, such as the American Cancer Society.
- Ask about community services that encourage independent living, such as homemaker services, trained assistance dogs, Meals on Wheels, social services, and church organizations.

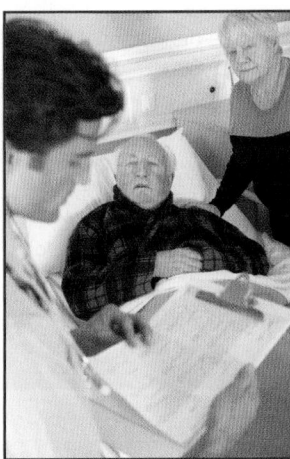

Clinical Scenario A 77-year-old male client is recovering after surgery to remove a tumor from his colon. He is depressed and has refused to ambulate as well as perform bed exercises. He lies in bed and is not motivated to assist with his hygiene. It has been 3 days since his last bowel movement. The nurse explains his potential for developing complications due to his inactivity.

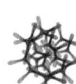

NURSING CARE PLAN 23-1   Deconditioning

Assessment
- Assess the client's independent movement and activity status.
- Inspect the integrity of the skin.
- Inquire as to the client's bowel elimination pattern and characteristics of stool.
- Observe the client's depth of respirations and the ability to raise pulmonary secretions.
- Check skin color, capillary refill of nail beds, and urinary output for evidence of circulatory perfusion.
- Palpate distal peripheral pulses for rate and quality.

- Determine whether there is a potential for infection of any type, such as an indwelling urinary or venous catheter, artificial airway, and wound.
- Observe if the client has sufficient muscle strength and coordination to protect themself from a potential injury.
- Assess if there is any impairment of vision, hearing, and tactile sensation.
- Note the client's mental status for signs of dementia, depression, or apathy.

Nursing Diagnosis. Deconditioning

Expected Outcome. The client will have no evidence of complications associated with deconditioning as evidenced by intact skin/tissue integrity, full range of joint motion, clear lung sounds, capillary refill in less than 3 seconds, strong peripheral pulses, regular bowel movements of soft stool, and urinary output greater than 1,500 mL/day throughout length of care.

Interventions	Rationales
Assess the patient's ability to perform activities of daily living (ADLs).	Emphasizes functional capacity and evaluates ADLs, hearing, fecal and urinary continence, balance, and cognition
Reposition the client every 2 hours around the clock.	Position changes relieve pressure and maintain sufficient capillary circulation to ensure cellular and tissue integrity.
Provide clean, dry, and wrinkle-free bedding at all times.	Clean dry linen prevents the maceration of skin from prolonged contact with moisture. Keeping the linen wrinkle-free prevents compromised circulation from increased pressure per square inch (PSI) of skin.

(continued)

NURSING CARE PLAN 23-1 — Deconditioning (*continued*)

Interventions	Rationales
Use and check incontinence pads on bed every 2 hours; change immediately when soiled.	Incontinence pads wick moisture away from the client and keep the bed linen dry. Changing soiled incontinence pads prevents skin maceration from contact with moisture and waste products of elimination.
Assist the client to the bedside commode every 4 hours when awake.	Transferring from bed to a commode promotes the use of the musculoskeletal system, increases circulation and breathing, and relieves pressure on skin from lying positions in bed. Use of the commode promotes continence and dignity.
Use a foam mattress on the bed.	Foam acts like a layer of subcutaneous tissue and redistributes pressure over a greater area, reducing the potential for skin breakdown.
Use trochanter rolls for supine positioning.	Trochanter rolls prevent external rotation of the hips and legs. Maintaining a neutral position facilitates the potential for ambulation and independence.
Apply a footboard to the bed or foot splints to both legs.	These devices prevent foot drop and help ensure the potential for normal ambulation.
Collaborate with physical therapy, as appropriate, to implement an individualized therapy program to increase strength and endurance.	Activity reduces the potential for complications associated with deconditioning.
Vary the daily routine when possible.	Variety in the routine stimulates the mind and cognitive processes.
Include the client in planning the daily routine.	Giving the client a locus of control maintains dignity and self-esteem.
Teach the family how to turn and position the client.	Involving the client's family provides a sense of personal satisfaction for being involved in the care of a loved one. Teaching helps prepare them to assist the client when eventually discharged or transferred to another level of care.

Evaluation of Expected Outcome

- The client's skin is pink, dry, and intact in all areas.
- The client has full range of motion in all joints.
- The client's lungs are clear to auscultation anteriorly, posteriorly, and laterally.
- The pedal pulses are present and strong bilaterally.
- The capillary refill in nail beds of great toes is 2–3 seconds.
- The client has a daily bowel movement without straining.
- The client's urine is clear yellow with a daily volume between 2,000 and 2,200 mL.
- No foot drop or external rotation of hips and legs is noted when footboard and trochanter rolls are in use.

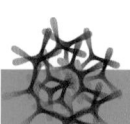

KEY POINTS

- Body mechanics: The efficient use of the musculoskeletal system; the way we move during daily activities; proper body mechanics can help avoid injury and muscle fatigue, increase muscle effectiveness, reduce fatigue, and avoid repetitive strain injuries (disorders that result from cumulative trauma to musculoskeletal structures)
- Advantages of assistive devices:
  - Nurses: Lessens physical exertion during positioning, moving, and transferring clients
  - Clients: Helps with maintaining a degree of independence despite sensory, physical, or cognitive problems
- Positioning clients
  - Good posture and body mechanics and ergonomically designed assistive devices are necessary when inactive clients require positioning and moving.
  - Functional mobility: Alignment that maintains the potential for movement and ambulation, providing for therapeutic needs

- Common positions for clients (remember to change and chart position changes every 2 hours):
  - Supine: The client lies on the back.
  - Lateral position: A side-lying position
  - Lateral oblique position: A variation of the side-lying position
  - Prone position: The client lies on the abdomen.
  - Sims position: A semiprone position
  - Fowler position: A semi-sitting position
  - High Fowler position: Sitting straight up
- Positioning devices: Adjustable bed, mattress, bed board, pillows, roller sheet
- Protective devices: Side rails, mattress overlays, foam and gel mattresses, static air mattresses, alternating air mattress, water mattress, cradle, specialty beds, low–air-loss mattress, air-fluidized bed, oscillating support bed, circular bed
- Transferring clients: Transfer handle, transfer belt, transfer board, mechanical lift

CRITICAL THINKING EXERCISES

1. You observe a coworker using incorrect body mechanics while administering care to a client. How would you approach this coworker? What suggestions would you give?
2. List nursing activities that predispose one to work-related injuries. How can the nurse reduce the risk for injury during each activity?
3. What precautions would you advocate for repositioning or moving a **bariatric client**, one who is defined by the Obesity Action Coalition (2015) as severely obese with a body mass index of 40 or more than 100 lb over their ideal body weight?
4. What factors pose unique challenges in positioning and moving geriatric clients?

NEXT-GENERATION NCLEX-STYLE REVIEW QUESTIONS

1. When the nurse instructs a nursing assistant to place a client in a Sims position, which description indicates the nursing assistant has performed the task correctly?
   a. The client is in a side-lying position.
   b. The client is lying on their back.
   c. The client is in a semi-sitting position.
   d. The client is in a semiprone position.
   Test-Taking Strategy: Use the process of elimination to select a position that correlates with the definition of a Sims position.
2. Which nursing measure is best to keep a client from sliding down in bed?
   a. Place trochanter rolls at the client's hips.
   b. Place the client in a slight Trendelenburg position.
   c. Place a roller sheet from the client's back to midthigh.
   d. Place a trapeze at the head of the bed.
   Test-Taking Strategy: Note the key word, "best." Analyze the choices and select the option that is better than any of the others for preventing the client from sliding toward the foot of the bed.
3. To avoid a nurse-related injury as well as promote safe handling of a client before repositioning from a supine to a lateral position, which nursing assessment question is most important?
   a. Is the client cooperative?
   b. Is the client able to assist?
   c. What does the client weigh?
   d. When was the position last changed?
   Test-Taking Strategy: Analyze the choices and select the option that identifies information that is better than any other for avoiding potential injuries.
4. Which items are appropriate for the nurse to prevent pressure sores when caring for an inactive client? Select all that apply.
   a. Footboard
   b. Alternating air mattress
   c. Trochanter roll
   d. Foam mattress overlay
   e. Bed cradle
   f. Air-fluidized bed
   Test-Taking Strategy: Note the key phrase, "prevent pressure sores." Analyze the choices and pick options that are primarily used to avoid the breakdown of skin that is presently intact.
5. A client who works in a warehouse and must lift heavy objects asks the nurse how to avoid musculoskeletal injuries. Which information would the nurse include? Select all that apply.
   a. Stand with your feet close together.
   b. Bend from the knees.
   c. Stoop over when lifting.
   d. Carry objects close to your body.
   e. Push rather than lift heavy objects.
   Test-Taking Strategy: Analyze the choices and select the options that are characteristics of good body mechanics and ergonomics.

NEXT-GENERATION NCLEX-STYLE CLINICAL SCENARIO QUESTIONS

Clinical Scenario:

A 77-year-old male client is recovering after surgery to remove a tumor from his colon. He is depressed and has refused to ambulate as well as perform bed exercises. He lies in bed and is not motivated to assist with his hygiene. It has been 3 days since his last bowel movement. The nurse explains his potential for developing complications due to his inactivity.

1. From the following list, select the factors that may contribute to the client developing complications, postsurgery.
   a. Depression
   b. Refusing to ambulate
   c. Eating a well-balanced meal
   d. Rehabilitation therapy twice a day
   e. Unwilling to perform ADLs
   f. Lying in bed
2. Place an "x" under "effective" for activities that can help the client recuperate from surgery. Place an "x" under "ineffective" for that issues may contribute to the client's potential complications.

ACTIVITIES/ISSUES	EFFECTIVE	INEFFECTIVE
Eating a well-balanced meal		
Refusing to participate in physical therapy		
Repositioning in bed		
Performing bed exercises		
Not showering during the hospital stay		

SKILL 23-1 Turning and Moving a Client

Suggested Action	Reason for Action
ASSESSMENT	
Assess for risk factors that may contribute to inactivity.	Indicates a need to reposition more frequently
Determine the time of the last position change.	Ensures following the plan for care
Assess the physical, mental, and emotional ability to assist in turning, positioning, or moving.	Determines whether additional help or assistive devices are needed
Inspect for drainage tubes and equipment.	Ensures that they will not be displaced or cause discomfort to the client
PLANNING	
Explain the procedure to the client.	Increases cooperation and decreases anxiety
Remove all pillows and current positioning devices, such as trochanter rolls.	Reduces interference during repositioning
Raise the bed to elbow height, which is a suitable working height.	Prevents back strain by maintaining the center of gravity
Secure two or three additional caregivers, positioning and moving devices (e.g., roller sheets, repositioning sling, mechanical lift), or both if the client cannot assist.	Ensures safety and reduces the potential for musculoskeletal injuries
Close the door or draw the bedside curtain.	Demonstrates respect for privacy
IMPLEMENTATION	
Turning the Client from Supine to Lateral or Prone Position	
Wash hands or use an alcohol-based hand rub when appropriate (see Chapter 10).	Reduces the transmission of microorganisms
Secure two or three additional caregivers, positioning and moving devices (e.g., roller sheets, repositioning sling, mechanical lift), or both if the client cannot assist.	Ensures safety and reduces the potential for musculoskeletal injuries
Help or have the client slide to one side of the bed.	Provides room when repositioning
Raise the side rail.	Ensures safety
Flex the client's knee over the other with the arms across the chest.	Aids in turning and protects the client's arms
Spread your feet, flex your knees, and place one foot behind the other.	Provides a broad base of support
Place one hand on the client's shoulder and one on the hip.	Facilitates turning
Roll the client toward the side rail (Fig. A).	Reduces effort

A

Directing the client to turn.

SKILL 23-1 Turning and Moving a Client (*continued*)

Suggested Action	Reason for Action
Place pillows behind the back, between the legs, and under the upper arm (Fig. B).	Aids in maintaining position and provides comfort
 B	Supporting arms and legs with pillows.
Raise the side rails and lower the height of the bed.	Ensures safety
Wash hands or use an alcohol-based hand rub when appropriate (see Chapter 10).	Reduces the transmission of microorganisms
For a Prone Position	
Begin as described earlier for the lateral position.	Follows the same principles
Secure two or three additional caregivers, positioning and moving devices (e.g., roller sheets, repositioning sling, mechanical lift), or both if the client cannot assist.	Ensures safety and reduces the potential for musculoskeletal injuries
Have the client turn their head opposite to the direction for rolling and leave the arms extended at each side (Fig. C).	Prevents pressure on the face and arms during and after repositioning
 C	Preparing for prone positioning.

(*continued*)

SKILL 23-1 Turning and Moving a Client (*continued*)

Suggested Action	Reason for Action
Shift your hands from the posterior of the shoulder and hip to the anterior as the client rolls independently onto their abdomen (Fig. D).	Controls the speed with which the client is repositioned
D	Assist the client as they roll from the supine to the prone position.
Center the client in bed.	Prevents pressure on arms
Arrange pillows.	Provides for comfort and support
Raise the side rails and lower the height of the bed.	Ensures safety
Wash hands or use an alcohol-based hand rub when appropriate (see Chapter 10).	Reduces the transmission of microorganisms
Moving the Mobile Client Up in Bed (One-Nurse and Client Technique)	
Wash hands or use an alcohol-based hand rub when appropriate (see Chapter 10).	Reduces the transmission of microorganisms
Remove the pillow from under the client's head.	Prevents strain on the neck and head during moving
Place the pillow against the headboard.	Cushions the head from contact with the headboard
Position the client on their back or in a slight Trendelenburg position with the side rails down.	Facilitates use of gravity
Raise the bed to elbow height.	Reduces back strain
Place a roller/slider sheet beneath the buttocks to facilitate movement if needed if the client is weak or unable to fully assist.	Promotes gliding and reduces friction
Instruct the client to bend both knees and grasp a trapeze if one is available.	Aids in assisting by using the stronger muscles of the arms and legs
Ask the client to push down on the count of 3 with their feet, causing the legs to straighten (Fig. E). Repeat again if necessary.	Creates momentum to facilitate moving
E	Moving up in bed.

SKILL 23-1 Turning and Moving a Client (*continued*)

Suggested Action	Reason for Action
Rearrange pillows and remove the roller sheet unless it will be needed again in the near future.	Restores comfort
Place the client in a slight Trendelenburg position if sliding downward is a persistent problem.	Gravity keeps the client from sliding downward.
Wash hands or use an alcohol-based hand rub when appropriate (see Chapter 10).	Reduces the transmission of microorganisms

Two-Nurse and Roller Sheet Technique

Secure an additional caregiver, positioning and moving devices (e.g., roller sheets, repositioning sling, mechanical lift), or both if the client cannot assist.	Ensures safety and reduces the potential for musculoskeletal injuries
Wash hands or use an alcohol-based hand rub when appropriate (see Chapter 10).	Reduces the transmission of microorganisms
Protect the headboard with a pillow.	Ensures client safety
Raise the bed to elbow height.	Reduces back strain
Place a roller/slider sheet beneath the client's shoulders and buttocks.	Facilitates gliding the client rather than lifting
Stand facing each other on opposite sides of the bed between the client's hips and shoulders.	Aids in coordinating movement between nurses
Roll the slider sheet to the sides of the client.	A palms-up grip provides more strength by keeping the elbows close to the body, thus reducing the workload.
Grasp the rolled sheet with the palms up and the knuckles in contact with the bed sheet.	Keeping the knuckles in contact with the bed sheet ensures a sliding, rather than a lifting, motion.
Bend hips and knees; spread feet.	Follows principles of good body mechanics and provides momentum to facilitate sliding
Slide the client up on reaching a previously agreed signal (Fig. F), such as the count of 3.	Promotes coordination of effort

Moving the client up in bed with a rolled sheet and the assistance of two people.

Avoid shrugging the shoulders while moving the client.	Shrugging the shoulders indicates the client is being lifted.
Rearrange pillows; remove the roller sheet unless it will be needed again in the near future.	Restores comfort
Place the client in a slight Trendelenburg position if sliding downward is a persistent problem.	Gravity keeps the client from sliding downward.
Wash hands or use an alcohol-based hand rub when appropriate (see Chapter 10).	Reduces the transmission of microorganisms

(continued)

SKILL 23-1 Turning and Moving a Client (*continued*)

Suggested Action	Reason for Action

EVALUATION

- Movement is achieved.
- Client is comfortable.
- Pressure is relieved.
- Joints and limbs are supported.

DOCUMENT

- Frequency of turning and moving
- Positions used
- Use of positioning devices
- Assistance required
- Client's response

SAMPLE DOCUMENTATION

Date and Time   Position changed q2h from supine to R and L lateral positions with assistance of client. Pillows used to support limbs and maintain positions. Footboard in place. No shortness of breath noted. No evidence of discomfort during repositioning.
_____ J. Doe, LPN

SKILL 23-2 Transferring Clients

Suggested Action	Reason for Action
ASSESSMENT	
Check the health record, nursing care plan, and medical orders for activity level.	Complies with the plan for care
Assess the client's strength and mobility as well as their mental and emotional status.	Determines the need for additional personnel or a mechanical lifting device
Secure additional caregivers, positioning and moving devices (e.g., roller sheets, repositioning sling, mechanical lift), or both if the client cannot assist.	Ensures safety and reduces the potential for musculoskeletal injuries
PLANNING	
Consult with the client on the preferred time for getting out of bed.	Helps client participate in decision-making
Locate a straight-backed chair, wheelchair, or stretcher to which the client will be transferred.	Facilitates efficient time management
Arrange the chair or stretcher next to or close to the bed on the client's stronger side, if there is one.	Ensures safety
Lock the wheels of the bed, wheelchair, or stretcher.	Prevents rolling and ensures safety
Explain how the transfer will be accomplished.	Reduces anxiety and promotes cooperation
IMPLEMENTATION	
From Bed to Chair	
Wash hands or use an alcohol-based hand rub when appropriate (see Chapter 10).	Reduces the transmission of microorganisms
Assist the client into a sitting position on the side of the bed.	Reduces dizziness; enables the client to stand
Help the client put on a bathrobe and nonskid slippers.	Ensures warmth, modesty, and safety
Place the chair parallel to the bed on the client's stronger side; raise the footrests if using a wheelchair.	Provides for easy access

SKILL 23-2 Transferring Clients (*continued*)

Suggested Action	Reason for Action
Apply a transfer belt or other assistive device if needed (Fig. A). 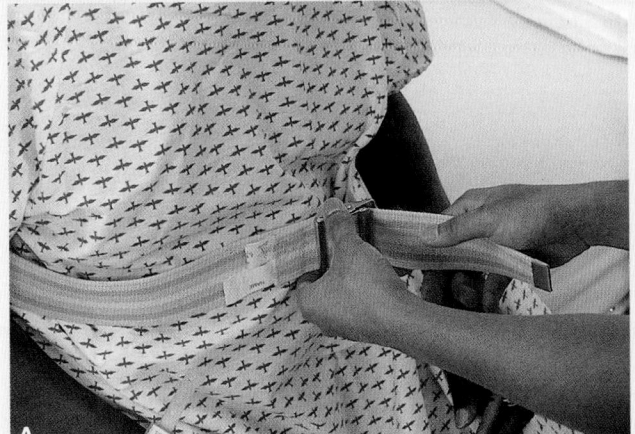 **A**	Reduces the risk for falling Applying a transfer belt.
Grasp the transfer belt or reach under the client's arms.	Helps support the upper body
Instruct the client to grasp your shoulders.	Gives the client leverage for rising
Bend the hips and knees; brace the client's knees (Fig. B). 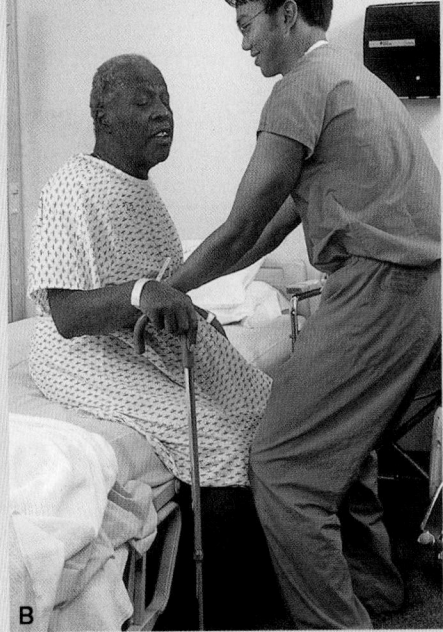 **B**	Stabilizes the client and follows principles of good body mechanics Bracing the client's knees.
Rock the client to a standing position at an agreed signal while encouraging the client to straighten their knees and hips.	Provides momentum and reduces the need to lift the client
Pivot the client with their back toward the chair.	Positions the client for sitting
Tell the client to step back until they feel the chair at the back of the legs.	Places the client in close proximity with the chair

(*continued*)

SKILL 23-2 Transferring Clients (*continued*)

Suggested Action	Reason for Action
Instruct the client to grasp the arms of the chair while you stabilize their knees and lower the client into the chair (Fig. C).	Promotes safety

Backing into a wheelchair.

Suggested Action	Reason for Action
Support the feet on the footrests.	Facilitates good posture
Using a Transfer Board	
Wash hands or use an alcohol-based hand rub when appropriate (see Chapter 10).	Reduces the transmission of microorganisms
Remove an arm from the wheelchair.	Reduces interference with transfer
Lock the brakes on the bed and wheelchair.	Prevents rolling and ensures safety
Slide the client to the edge of the bed.	Maintains the shortest distance for transfer
Angle the transfer board from the client's buttocks and hips down toward the seat of the chair.	Places the board where there is maximum weight
Position the transfer board beneath the client.	Supports upper body
Support and brace the client's knee with your knees while maintaining proper body mechanics.	Prevents injury
Slide the client down the transfer board into the seat of the chair at an agreed-upon signal (Fig. D).	Reduces the need to lift the client

Using a transfer board. (Photo by B. Proud.)

Suggested Action	Reason for Action
Wash hands or use an alcohol-based hand rub if appropriate (see Chapter 10).	Reduces the transmission of microorganisms

SKILL 23-2 Transferring Clients (*continued*)

Suggested Action	Reason for Action
Using a Mechanical Lift	
Secure an additional caregiver and a mechanical lift.	Prevents musculoskeletal injuries when a client is fully dependent
Wash hands or use an alcohol-based hand rub if appropriate (see Chapter 10).	Reduces the transmission of microorganisms
Raise the bed to a height that places the client near the nurse's center of gravity.	Reduces the risk for back injury
Lock the brakes on the bed.	Prevents the bed from moving and causing injury
Place the canvas sling under the client from the shoulders to midthigh (Fig. E).	Positions the sling where it will support the greatest mass of the client

Applying the lift's sling.

Move the lift device on the same side of the bed as the chair or stretcher to which the client will be transferred.	Facilitates safety when the client and equipment are within close proximity
Position the boom on the lift over the client's torso.	Enables the attachment of lifting chains to the canvas sling
Lock the wheels on the lift.	Stabilizes the lift in place
Attach the hooks on the lifting chain or straps to the holes in the canvas sling (Fig. F).	Connects the lift to the client

Positioning the lift and the client.

Position the client's arms across their chest.	Protects the client's arms and hands from being injured

(*continued*)

SKILL 23-2 Transferring Clients (*continued*)

Suggested Action	Reason for Action
Pump the jack handle to elevate the client to about 6 in above the mattress (Fig. G).	Aids in assessing whether the client is properly and safely within the sling

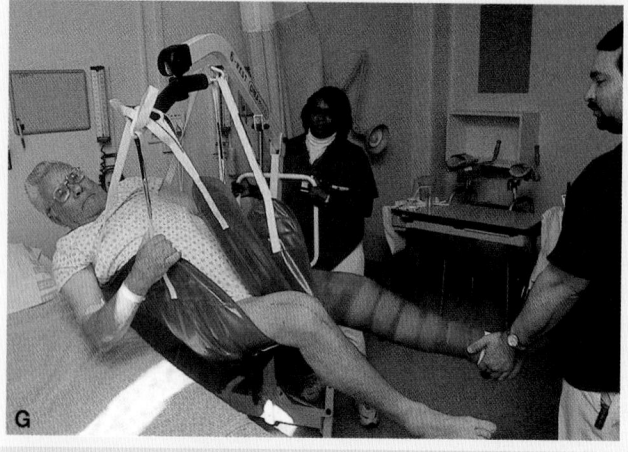

G

	Raising the client.
Unlock the wheels on the lift and move the lifted client directly over the chair or stretcher.	Relocates the client to the desired location
Relock the wheels of the lift.	Ensures the client's safety
Release the jack handle slowly.	Lowers the client from the suspended position
Remove the lifting chains, but leave the canvas sling in place beneath the client.	Facilitates returning the client to bed
Wash hands or perform an alcohol-based hand rub if appropriate (see Chapter 10).	Reduces the transmission of microorganisms

EVALUATION

- Client is relocated.
- No injury occurs to client or health care providers.

DOCUMENT

- Method of transfer
- Response of client

SAMPLE DOCUMENTATION

Date and Time Transferred from bed to wheelchair by standing and pivoting with weight bearing on right leg. Transient pain rated at 1 on a scale of 0 to 10 experienced in left hip during transfer. Declined offer for pain medication. Up in chair approximately 1 hour.
_____ J. Doe, LPN

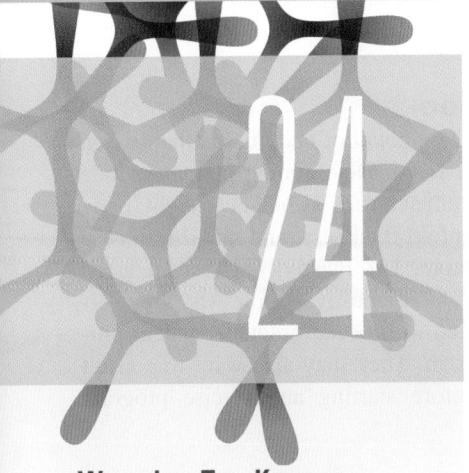

24

Fitness and Therapeutic Exercise

Learning Objectives

On completion of this chapter, the reader should be able to:

1. List benefits of regular exercise.
2. Define fitness.
3. Identify factors that interfere with fitness.
4. Name methods of fitness testing.
5. Describe how to calculate a person's target heart rate.
6. Define metabolic energy equivalent.
7. Differentiate fitness exercise from therapeutic exercise.
8. Differentiate isotonic exercise from isometric exercise.
9. Give examples of isotonic, isometric, and isokinetic exercises.
10. Differentiate between active exercise and passive exercise.
11. Discuss how and why range of motion exercises are performed.
12. Provide suggestions for helping older adults become or stay physically active.

INTRODUCTION

Exercise (purposeful physical activity) is beneficial to people of all age groups (Box 24-1), and the health risks of a sedentary lifestyle are well documented. This chapter addresses techniques for improving health and maintaining or restoring muscle and joint function by promoting exercise. Because exercise must be individualized, nurses are responsible for assessing each person's fitness level before initiating an exercise program with a client.

 Gerontologic Considerations

■ Older adults, especially those who are disabled, need to balance periods of physical activity with periods of rest. Shortness of breath or an increased heart rate indicates that the level of activity is beyond the client's tolerance.

■ Older adults need to eliminate their intake of caffeinated and alcoholic beverages before and during physical activity to avoid depleting fluid volume. Water is the preferred drink for fluid replacement.

■ Encourage families and caregivers of older adults with cognitive impairment to help older persons participate in physical activities, such as walking and ball throwing. If the older person has difficulty with balance, exercises may be done while sitting or lying down. Active range of motion (ROM) exercises should be scheduled daily and may be divided into short sessions. If the older adult cannot participate actively in an exercise program, caregivers can perform passive ROM exercises at least daily to prevent muscle atrophy and disuse syndrome.

■ Many shopping malls permit and even encourage people to walk through the mall before stores open for business.

■ Swimming or exercising in water puts less stress on joints and is beneficial for older adults.

■ Many physically challenging sports, such as bowling, golfing, walking in marathons, and weight lifting, have competition categories for older adults.

■ Precautions, such as wearing safe shoes with nonskid soles, are necessary to prevent falls when older adults exercise. Complications from falls contribute to morbidity and mortality among older people.

FITNESS ASSESSMENT

Fitness means the capacity to exercise. Factors such as a sedentary lifestyle, health problems, compromised muscle and skeletal function, obesity, advanced age, smoking, and high blood pressure can impair a client's fitness and stamina. They could even result in injury during exercise. Therefore, before a client begins an exercise program, assessment of their fitness level is necessary. Some assessment techniques include measuring body composition, evaluating trends in vital signs, and performing fitness tests.

BOX 24-1 **Benefits of Physical Exercise**

• Lower risk of all-cause mortality
• Lower risk of cardiovascular disease mortality
• Lower risk of cardiovascular disease (including heart disease and stroke)
• Lower risk of hypertension
• Lower risk of type 2 diabetes
• Lower risk of adverse blood lipid profile
• Lower risk of cancers of the bladder, breast, colon, endometrium, esophagus, kidney, lung, and stomach
• Improved cognition[a]
• Reduced risk of dementia (including Alzheimer disease)
• Improved quality of life
• Reduced anxiety
• Reduced risk of depression
• Improved sleep
• Slowed or reduced weight gain
• Weight loss, particularly when combined with reduced calorie intake
• Prevention of weight regain following initial weight loss
• Improved bone health
• Improved physical function
• Lower risk of falls (older adults)
• Lower risk of fall-related injuries (older adults)

[a]Reduced risk of dementia, including Alzheimer disease, and improved cognition: executive function, attention, memory, crystallized intelligence, and processing speed.

U.S. Department of Health and Human Services. (2023). *Physical activity guidelines for Americans.* 2nd ed. https://health.gov/sites/default/files/2019-09/Physical_Activity_Guidelines_2nd_edition.pdf

Body Composition

Body composition is the amount of body tissue that is lean versus the amount that is fat. Determining factors include anthropometric measurements such as height, weight, body mass index (BMI), skinfold thickness, and midarm muscle circumference (see Chapter 13). Inactivity without reduced food intake tends to promote obesity. People who are overweight and inactive need to proceed gradually when initiating an exercise program. They may also want to consult a medical provider before starting an exercise program (Flack e al., 2023).

Vital Signs

Vital signs—temperature, pulse rate, respiratory rate, and blood pressure—reflect a person's physical status (see Chapter 12). Elevated pulse rate, respiratory rate, and blood pressure while resting are signs that the person may have life-threatening cardiovascular symptoms during exercise. After a period of modified exercise, vital signs may decrease, thus reducing the potential for heart-related complications.

Fitness Tests

Fitness tests provide an objective measure of a person's current fitness level and their potential for safe exercise. They also help establish safe parameters for the level and duration of exercise. Two methods of fitness testing are a stress electrocardiogram (ECG) and an ambulatory ECG. Another is a **submaximal fitness test**, which is an exercise test that does not stress a person to exhaustion. Examples of submaximal fitness tests include a step test and a walk-a-mile test. Because submaximal tests are less demanding, the validity of their results is less reliable than the results obtained through ECG testing.

Stress Electrocardiogram

A **stress electrocardiogram** tests electrical conduction through the heart during maximal activity and is performed in an acute care facility or an outpatient clinic (Fig. 24-1). The client first walks slowly on a flat treadmill. As the test progresses, the speed and incline of the treadmill are increased. The examiner notes the client's heart rate and rhythm, blood pressure, breathing, and symptoms such as dizziness and chest pain. A pulse oximeter (see Chapter 21) is used to measure peripheral oxygenation. The examiner stops the test if the client develops an abnormal heart rhythm, **cardiac ischemia** (impaired blood flow to the heart), elevated blood pressure, or exhaustion.

Ambulatory Electrocardiogram

An **ambulatory electrocardiogram** is a continuous recording of heart rate and rhythm during normal activity. It requires the client to wear a device called a *Holter monitor* for 24 hours. This less taxing version of a stress ECG is used when the person has had prior cardiac-related symptoms, such as chest pain, or has major health risks that contraindicate a stress ECG.

An ambulatory ECG helps assess the heart's response to normal activity rather than activity imposed during a stress

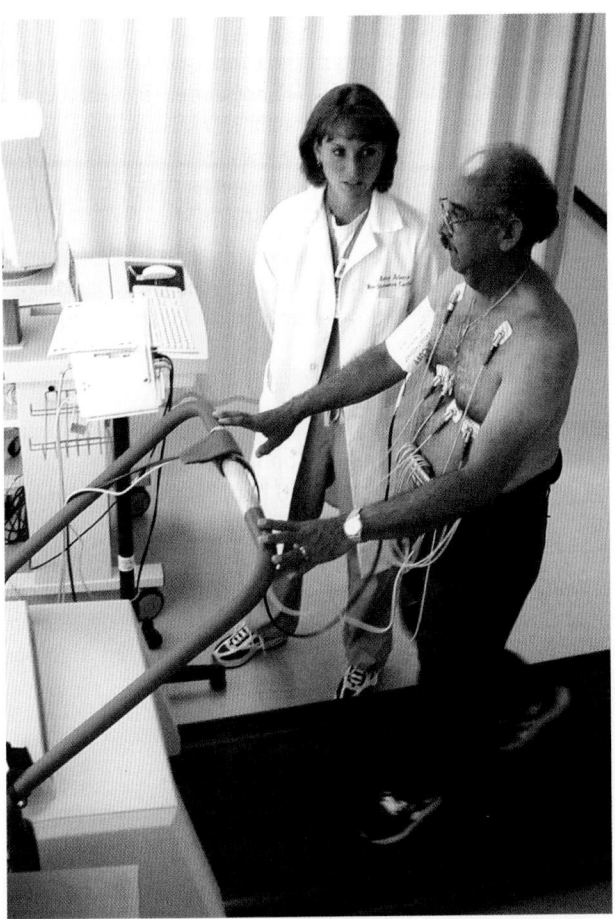

FIGURE 24-1 A stress electrocardiogram test. (Image Texas Heart Institute, www.texasheart.org.)

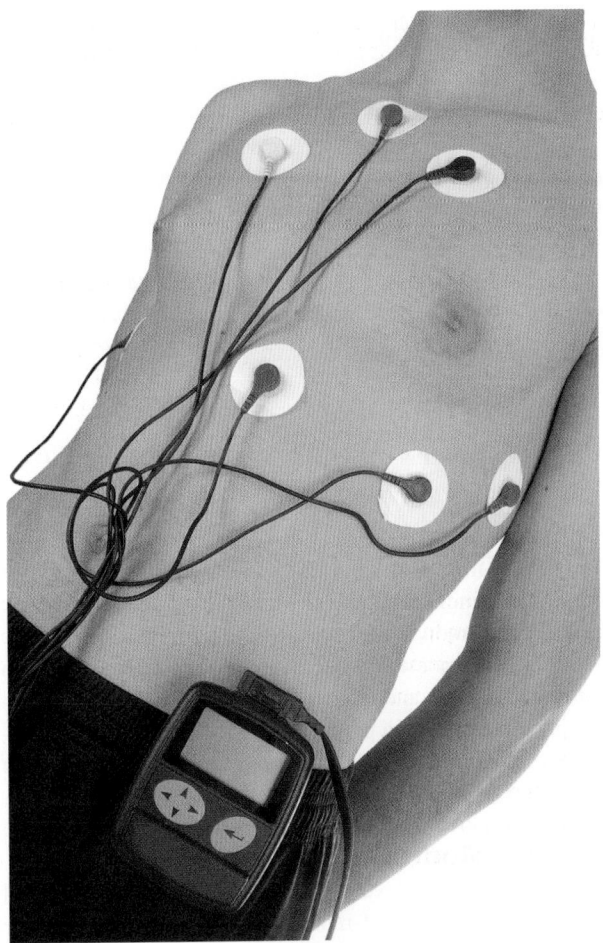

FIGURE 24-2 Ambulatory electrocardiography.

ECG. It also helps evaluate how a person is responding to cardiac rehabilitation and medical therapy.

The Holter monitor, which is connected to chest leads, is attached to a belt or shoulder strap or carried in a pocket (Fig. 24-2). During an ambulatory ECG, the client should not shower or swim; a sponge bath is permitted as long as the monitor does not get wet. The client should also avoid magnets, metal detectors, electric blankets, and high-voltage areas that may cause **artifacts** (abnormal appearance due to external distortion) on the recordings that interfere with an accurate interpretation of the test results.

The client keeps a diary of the time and type of activities performed, when they took medications, and when symptoms, if any, were experienced. After the test period, the client returns the monitor and then a computer and the physician check the electrically recorded information. The physician compares the client's diary with the ECG. The assessment results help determine whether oxygenation to the heart muscle was temporarily impaired during an activity or if an abnormal heart rhythm developed. Either finding indicates that exercise should be delayed until further treatment or started at a very low intensity and for a short duration.

Step Test

A **step test** is a submaximal fitness test involving a timed stepping activity. Several variations include the Harvard

Step Test, the Queens College Step Test, and the Chester Step Test. A person undergoing this type of fitness analysis will step up and down on a platform of a prescribed height (20 in for men, 16 in for women) for 3 to 5 minutes at a rate of at least 76 steps/minute. A step up or down is considered one step. The time is shortened when the client can no longer sustain the prescribed rate or develops discomfort. The examiner uses a metronome and a stopwatch to keep track of the rate and the time.

Examiners calculate the client's **recovery index** (a guide for determining a person's fitness level) by taking a 30-second pulse rate at 1, 2, and 3 minutes after the test using the following formula:

$$\frac{\text{Recovery}}{\text{index}} = \frac{(100 \times \text{test deration in seconds})}{2 \times \text{total of the 30} - \text{seconds pulse assessments}}$$

The examiner compares results with standardized fitness levels (Table 24-1). A fit person has a smaller decline in heart rate at each assessment. Another fitness indicator is how close the pulse rate at the end of recovery compares with the pretest pulse rate. The more similar the pretest and posttest pulse rates, the fitter the person is.

The step test must be used with caution. Personnel certified in cardiopulmonary resuscitation and use of an

TABLE 24-1 Cardiovascular Endurance Fitness Levels

SCORE	FITNESS CLASSIFICATION
≥96	Excellent
83–96	Good
68–82	Average
54–67	Low average
≤54	Poor

Data from Fox, E. L., Billings, C. E. Jr., Bartels, R. L., & Mathews, D. (1973). Fitness standards for male college students. *Internationale Zeitschrift fur angewandte Physiologie, 31*(3), 231–236. https://doi.org/10.1007/BF00697601

TABLE 24-3 Pedometer Assessment

NUMBER OF STEPS	ACTIVITY LEVEL
0–4,999	Sedentary
5,000–7,499	Low active
7,500–9,999	Somewhat active
10,000–12,499	Active
≥12,500	Highly active

Data from 10,000 Steps. (2023). *Counting your steps.* https://www.10000steps .org.au/articles/counting-steps/

automated electronic defibrillator should be available to assist if there is an adverse cardiac event (see Chapter 37).

Walk-a-Mile Test

The **walk-a-mile test**, devised by the American College of Sports Medicine, measures the time it takes a person to walk 1 mile. The person is instructed to walk 1 mile on a flat surface as fast as possible. The examiner calculates the time from start to finish and interprets the results using the guidelines in Table 24-2. If a person walks at a brisk pace, approximately 3 to 4 mph, it will take approximately 30 minutes to complete 1 to 2 miles.

Activity Monitoring

A person's activity level can be monitored and evaluated with a **pedometer**, a self-monitoring motion-sensing device that tracks total steps and distance walked. Another option is a wristband monitor, such as a Fitbit. A common daily goal is 10,000 steps/day or approximately 5 miles. An individual's activity level can be compared with the levels in Table 24-3.

EXERCISE PRESCRIPTIONS

The prescription for an exercise program involves determining the person's target heart rate and the metabolic energy equivalents (METs) of particular activities based on the person's fitness level.

Target Heart Rate

Target heart rate refers to the goal for heart rate during exercise. It is determined by first calculating the person's **maximum heart rate** (the highest limit for heart rate during exercise). Maximum heart rate is determined by subtracting

a person's age from 220. Thus, a 20-year-old has a maximum heart rate of 200 beats/minute (bpm), whereas a 50-year-old has a maximum heart rate of 170 bpm. The target heart rate for moderate intensity is 64% to 76% of the maximum heart rate (Centers for Disease Control and Prevention, 2020). Beginners should not exceed 50%, intermediate athletes can exercise up to 70%, and competitive athletes may tolerate 70% to 85% of their maximum heart rate during vigorous intensive activity.

> **》》 Stop, Think, and Respond 24-1**
> What is the maximum heart rate and minimum target heart rate for a person who is 25 years old and a competitive athlete who is 32 years old?

Exercising at the target rate for 15 minutes (excluding the warmup and cool-down periods) three or more times per week strengthens the heart muscle and promotes the use of fat reserves for energy. Exercising beyond the target heart rate reduces endurance by increasing fatigue.

Metabolic Energy Equivalent

Because fitness levels vary, different types of exercise are prescribed according to their **metabolic energy equivalent** (the measure of energy and oxygen consumption during exercise). This is the prescribed amount that a person's cardiovascular system can safely support. Low-to-vigorous physical activities and their approximate METs are listed in Table 24-4.

TYPES OF EXERCISE

Exercise is performed to promote fitness or to achieve therapeutic outcomes. The two major types of exercise are fitness exercise and therapeutic exercise.

Fitness Exercise

Fitness exercise means physical activity performed by healthy adults. Fitness exercise develops and maintains cardiorespiratory function, muscular strength, and endurance (Fig. 24-3). The three categories of fitness exercise are isotonic, isometric, and isokinetic.

Isotonic exercise is an activity that involves movement and work. The muscles being exercised change length; they shorten and lengthen during contraction (Fig. 24-4).

TABLE 24-2 Evaluation Criteria for the Walk-a-Mile Test

PERFORMANCE TIME FOR MEN (MINUTES)	PERFORMANCE TIME FOR WOMEN (MINUTES)	FITNESS LEVEL[a]
≥15:3	≥17:3	Poor
14:01–14:42	15:07–16:06	Average
12:54–14:00	14:12–15:06	Good
<12:54	<14:12	Excellent

[a]Based on adults aged 40 to 49 years.

TABLE 24-4 Levels of Physical Activity

PHYSICAL ACTIVITY INTENSITY	
Light-intensity activity: <2 METs	Nonsedentary waking behavior Examples include walking at a slow or leisurely pace (≤2 mph), cooking activities, or light household chores.
Moderate-intensity activity: 3–<6 METs	Examples include walking briskly (2.5–4 mph), playing doubles tennis, or raking the yard.
Vigorous-intensity activity: ≥6.0 METs	Examples include jogging, running, carrying heavy groceries or other loads upstairs, shoveling snow, or participating in a strenuous fitness class. Many adults do no vigorous-intensity physical activity.

U.S. Department of Health and Human Services. (2023). *Physical activity guidelines for Americans* (2nd ed.). https://health.gov/sites/default/files/2019-09/Physical_Activity_Guidelines_2nd_edition.pdf

METABOLIC ENERGY EQUIVALENT (MET)	EXAMPLES OF ACTIVITIES
1	Sewing Watching television Dressing
1–2	Walking 1 mph on level ground Bowling
2–3	Golfing with a cart Mowing lawn with a power mower
3–4	Playing badminton (doubles) Raking leaves
4–5	Slow swimming Lifting 50 lb
5–6	Square dancing Shoveling snow
6–7	Water skiing Moving heavy furniture
7–8	Playing basketball Playing noncompetitive handball
8–9	Cross country skiing Playing contact football
≥10	Running 6 mph or faster

Aerobic exercise is an example of isotonic exercise. It involves rhythmically moving all parts of the body at a moderate to slow speed without hindering the ability to breathe (Fig. 24-5). In other words, the person can talk comfortably if the exercise is within their level of fitness. To promote cardiorespiratory conditioning and increase lean muscle mass, a person should perform isotonic exercise at their target heart rate.

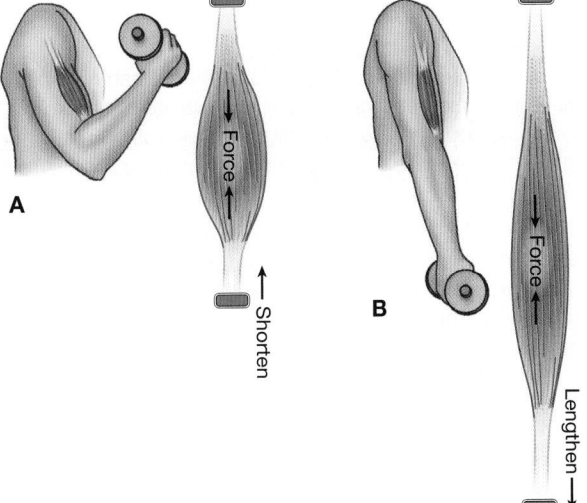

FIGURE 24-4 Example of an isotonic exercise with shortening (**A**) and lengthening (**B**) of muscles. (**A**, *Left* from McArdle, W. D., Katch, F. I., & Katch, V. L. [2022]. *Essentials of exercise physiology* [9th ed.]. Lippincott Williams & Wilkins; *Right*, from Kraemer, W. J., Fleck, S. J., & Deschenes, M. R. [2020]. *Exercise physiology* [3rd ed.]. Lippincott Williams & Wilkins; **B,** *Left* from McArdle, W. D., Katch, F. I., & Katch, V. L. [2022]. *Essentials of exercise physiology* [9th ed.]. Lippincott Williams & Wilkins; *Right*, from Kraemer, W. J., Fleck, S. J., & Deschenes, M. R. [2020]. *Exercise physiology* [3rd ed.]. Lippincott Williams & Wilkins.)

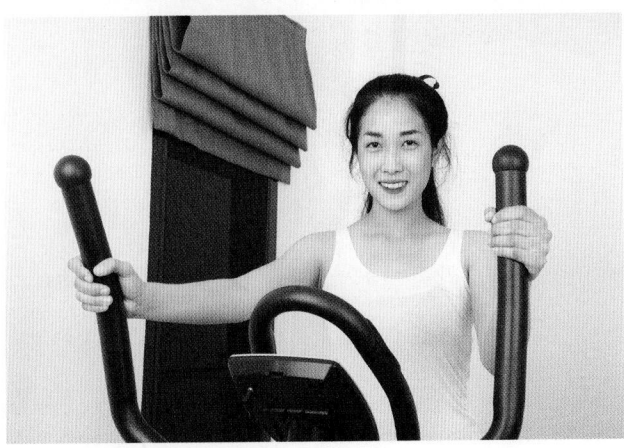

FIGURE 24-3 Fitness exercise.

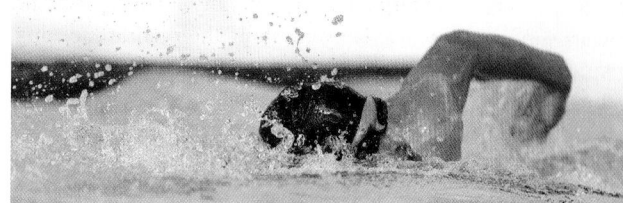

FIGURE 24-5 Example of aerobic exercise.

Isometric exercise consists of stationary exercises during which there is no change in the length of the contracting muscle. The concept involves working to hold a position still. Examples include holding weights in a steady position, using an elastic band or stationary ball to achieve a static position and holding the position, or less intense activities such as simply contracting and relaxing muscle groups while sitting or standing (Fig. 24-6). Isometric exercises increase muscle mass and strength and tone and define muscle groups. Although they improve blood circulation, they do *not* promote cardiorespiratory function. In fact, strenuous isometric exercises elevate blood pressure temporarily.

Isokinetic exercise combines movement at a constant speed with a form of resistance. The speed and resistance are preprogrammed and controlled with a machine. For example, a stationary bicycle like those in therapeutic settings or fitness centers (Fig. 24-7) can be set at a level that allows a certain number of revolutions per minute. Isokinetic exercises are often used for the purpose of rehabilitation after an athlete experiences an injury (Fig. 24-8) or to strengthen the weakened muscles when a person is recovering from a stroke or accident.

 Nutrition Notes

■ Because muscle is composed of protein, many people believe that it is necessary to eat more protein to build muscle. Although protein is vital to the process, the amount needed to stimulate exercise-related muscle growth is relatively small.

■ Nutritionally, the most important factor for increasing muscle mass is calories. If calorie intake is adequate, muscle growth can occur over a range of protein intakes. Protein and amino acid supplements are not more effective than protein in food for increasing muscle mass.

Before beginning any exercise program, the nurse can offer information about how to promote safety and prevent injuries (Client and Family Teaching 24-1).

Therapeutic Exercise

Therapeutic exercise is an activity performed by people with health risks or those being treated for an existing health problem, such as following cardiac surgery. Clients perform therapeutic exercise to prevent health-related complications or to restore lost functions (see "Performing Leg Exercises" in Chapter 27 and "Strengthening Pelvic Floor Muscles" in

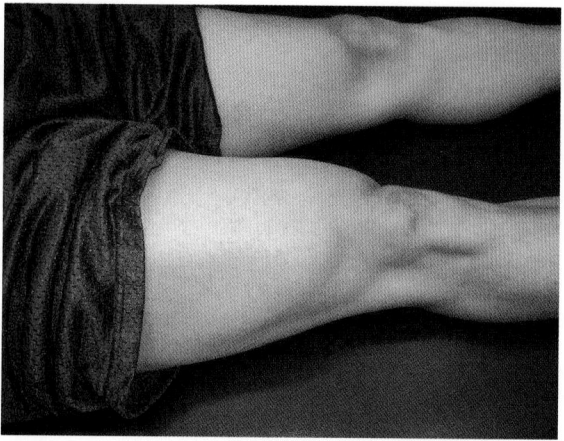

FIGURE 24-6 Isometric exercise occurs by repeatedly tensing and relaxing muscles, such as the quadriceps, with little or no movement of the exercised body part. (From Lotke, P. A., Abboud, J. A., & Ende, J. [2013]. *Lippincott's primary care orthopaedics* [2nd ed.]. Lippincott Williams & Wilkins.)

Chapter 30). Therapeutic exercise may be isotonic or isometric; isotonic exercises are performed actively or passively.

Active Exercise

Active exercise is therapeutic activity that the client performs independently after proper instruction. For example,

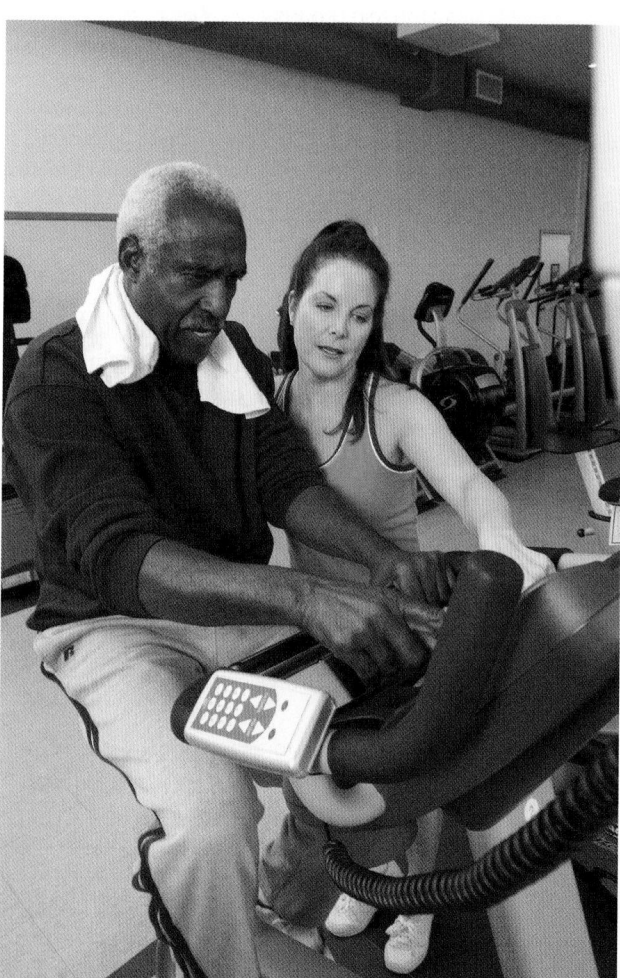

FIGURE 24-7 Isokinetic exercise using a stationary bike.

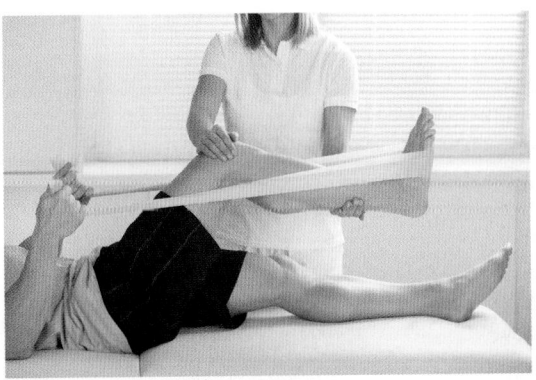

FIGURE 24-8 Isokinetic exercise to recover strength following an injury.

Client and Family Teaching 24-1
A Safe Exercise Program

The nurse teaches the client and the family about safe exercise as follows:

- Seek a preliminary exercise fitness evaluation from a health care provider or a certified sports trainer.
- Determine the target heart rate according to fitness level.
- Determine the appropriate level of METs
- Choose a form of exercise that seems pleasurable and involves as many muscle groups as possible.
- Increase physical activity gradually over time to meet key guidelines or health goals. Inactive people should "start low and go slow" by starting with lower intensity activities and gradually increasing how often and how long activities are done.
- Exercise with a partner for safety and motivation.
- Avoid exercising in extreme weather conditions (high humidity, smog).
- Dress in layers according to the temperature and weather conditions.
- Wear supportive shoes.
- Wear reflective clothing after dark.
- Walk or jog against traffic; cycle in the same direction as traffic.
- Eat complex carbohydrates (pasta, rice, cooked cereal) rather than fasting or eating simple sugars (cookies, chocolate, sweetened drinks) before exercising.
- Avoid drinking alcohol, which dilates the blood vessels, promotes heat loss, and interferes with good judgment.
- Warm up for 5 minutes by stretching muscle groups or doing light calisthenics.
- Measure the heart rate two or three times while exercising.
- Slow down if the heart rate exceeds the preestablished target.
- Try to sustain the target heart rate for at least 12 to 15 minutes.
- Never stop exercising abruptly.
- Cool down for at least 5 minutes in a manner similar to the warmup.

clients who have undergone a mastectomy learn to exercise the arm on the surgical side by combing their hair, squeezing a soft ball, finger climbing the vertical surface of a wall, and swinging a rope attached to a doorknob.

Active therapeutic exercise is often limited to a particular part of the body that is in a weakened condition. It is assumed that clients will use their unaffected muscle groups while performing activities of daily living (ADLs), such as bathing and dressing.

Passive Exercise

Passive exercise is therapeutic activity that the client performs with assistance and is provided when a client cannot move one or more parts of the body. For example, for clients who are comatose or paralyzed from a stroke or spinal injury, nurses perform exercises that maintain muscle tone and flexible joints. One form of frequently provided passive therapeutic exercise is ROM exercise. Another form is delivered with a continuous passive motion (CPM) machine, which is discussed later.

Range of Motion Exercises

Range of motion (ROM) exercises are therapeutic activities that move the joints. They are performed for the following reasons:

- To assess joint flexibility before initiating an exercise program
- To maintain joint mobility and flexibility in inactive clients
- To prevent **ankylosis** (the permanent loss of joint movement)
- To stretch joints before performing more strenuous activities
- To evaluate the client's response to a therapeutic exercise program

During ROM exercises, the client moves or is assisted with moving joints in the positions that the joint normally permits (Table 24-5). Whenever possible, the client actively exercises as many joints as possible while the nurse assists with those who are compromised (see Nursing Guidelines 24-1).

 Concept Mastery Alert

Passive Range of Motion Exercises

When performing passive ROM exercises, the nurse evaluates the client's tolerance for the exercises, noting any verbal and nonverbal expressions of discomfort or pain. Extra caution is needed when performing passive ROM exercises with nonresponsive clients because of their inability to communicate discomfort or pain.

>> *Stop, Think, and Respond 24-2*
Why would a nurse promote active ROM exercises in the upper body for a client who is paralyzed below the waist after a motor vehicle collision?

Nurses perform ROM exercises whenever they care for inactive clients (Skill 24-1).

TABLE 24-5 Joint Positions

POSITION	DESCRIPTION
Flexion	Bending so as to decrease the angle between two adjoining bones
Extension	Straightening so as to increase the angle between two adjoining bones up to 180 degrees
Hyperextension	Increasing the angle between two adjoining bones >180 degrees
Abduction	Moving away from the midline
Adduction	Moving toward the midline
Rotation	Turning from side to side as in an arc
External rotation	Turning outward, away from the midline of the body
Internal rotation	Turning inward, toward the midline of the body
Circumduction	Forming a circle
Pronation	Turning downward
Supination	Turning upward
Plantar flexion	Bending toward the sole of the foot
Dorsiflexion	Bending the foot toward the dorsum or anterior side
Inversion	Turning the sole of the foot toward the midline
Eversion	Turning the sole of the foot away from the midline

Data from TeachMeAnatomy. (n.d.). *Anatomical terms of movement.* https://teachmeanatomy.info/the-basics/anatomical-terminology/terms-of-movement/

Continuous Passive Motion Machine

A **continuous passive motion (CPM) machine** is a mechanical device powered electrically as a supplement or substitute for manual ROM exercise. A machine-assisted

NURSING GUIDELINES 24-1

Performing Range of Motion Exercises

- Use good body mechanics (see Chapter 23). *Doing so conserves energy and avoids muscle strain and injury.*
- Remove pillows and other positioning devices. *Such items can interfere with the exercises.*
- Position the client to facilitate movement of the joint through all its usual positions. *This positioning makes it easier to perform a comprehensive exercise program.*
- Follow a systematic, repetitive pattern, such as beginning at the head and moving down. *A routine prevents overlooking a joint.*
- Perform similar movements with each extremity. *Doing so exercises the joints bilaterally.*
- Support the joint being exercised. *Support reduces discomfort.*
- Move each joint until there is resistance but not pain. *This method exercises each joint to its point of limitation.*
- Watch for nonverbal communication. *Nonverbal signs may indicate the client's response.*
- Avoid exercising a painful joint. *Doing so can contribute to injury.*
- Stop if spasticity develops as manifested by a sudden, continuous muscle contraction. *Taking a break gives muscles time to relax and recover.*
- Apply gentle pressure to the muscle or move the spastic limb more slowly. *These actions relieve spasticity.*
- Expect the client's respiratory and heart rates to increase during exercise but to return to a resting rate later. *This is a normal cardiopulmonary response to activity.*
- Teach the family to perform ROM exercises. *A regular exercise program improves the potential for regaining function.*

⟩⟩ **Stop, Think, and Respond 24-3**

List examples of assessment findings that indicate a positive response to the use of a CPM machine.

ROM is sometimes preferred during the rehabilitation of clients who have experienced burns or have had knee or hip replacement surgery because the machine precisely controls the degree of joint movement and can increase it in specific increments throughout recovery.

NURSING IMPLICATIONS

Few people exercise sufficiently to promote optimal health. With this in mind, the Department of Health and Human Services has established *Physical Activity Guidelines for Americans* for improving the health of U.S. citizens (Table 24-6). Nurses can set an example for others in the community by improving their own physical fitness and encouraging others to do so.

For people with medical disorders, nurses may identify one or more of the following nursing diagnoses that are treated with activity or an exercise regimen:

- Activity intolerance
- Deconditioning
- ADL deficit

Nursing Care Plan 24-1 illustrates how a nurse can incorporate exercise into the care of a client with a stroke using the nursing diagnosis of ADL deficit. *ADL deficit* is defined as a decline in the ability to accomplish one or more basic activities independently, such as bathing, dressing, grooming, eating, toileting, and mobility/transferring.

TABLE 24-6 Physical Activity Guidelines for Americans

Moderate-intensity activities	• Walking briskly (2.5 mph or faster) • Recreational swimming • Bicycling slower than 10 mph on level terrain • Tennis (doubles) • Active forms of yoga (e.g., vinyasa or power yoga) • Ballroom or line dancing • General yard work and home repair work • Exercise classes like water aerobics
Vigorous-intensity activities	• Jogging or running • Swimming laps • Tennis (singles) • Vigorous dancing • Bicycling faster than 10 miles per hour • Jumping rope • Heavy yard work (digging or shoveling, with heart rate increases) • Hiking uphill or with a heavy backpack • High-intensity interval training • Exercise classes like vigorous step aerobics or kickboxing

GOAL	RECOMMENDATION	STRATEGIES	EXAMPLES
Increase aerobic physical activities.	Do at least 2½ hours of moderate-level activities or 1¼ hours of vigorous activities per week.	Build up time slowly. Do at least 10 minutes at a time. Combine moderate and vigorous activities.	*Moderate* (can talk, but not sing during performance): • Walking briskly • Ballroom and line dancing • Biking on level ground or with few hills
Increase muscle strengthening activities.	Do at least 2 days/week.	Include all the major muscle groups (legs, hips, back, chest, stomach, shoulders, and arms). Repeat 8–12 times for each muscle group per session.	General gardening (raking, trimming shrubs) Sports in which you catch and throw (baseball, softball, volleyball) Water aerobics *Vigorous* (can say a few words without stopping for a breath): • Jogging • Fast or aerobic dancing • Biking faster than 10 mph • Heavy gardening (digging, hoeing) • Jumping rope • Swimming fast or swimming laps • Sports with a lot of running (basketball, soccer, hockey)

From U.S. Department of Health and Human Services. (2023). *Physical activity guidelines for Americans* (2nd ed.). https://health.gov/sites/default/files/2019-09/Physical_Activity_Guidelines_2nd_edition.pdf

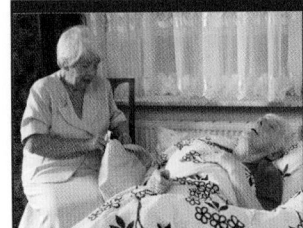

Clinical Scenario An 88-year-old female is a resident in a nursing home following a stroke. She has lost motor skills including ROM on the right side of her body. She does not notice people or objects on her affected side. Her muscle mass and strength on the right side have diminished due to neglect of her arm and leg as well as its position. She depends on others for turning, positioning, and ADLs.

NURSING CARE PLAN 24-1   ADL Deficit

Assessment
• Observe the client's movement or lack of movement.
• Note whether the client is able to complete ADLs in an integrated and coordinated manner.

• Determine whether the client omits, ignores, or favors activities or objects consistently.
• Check the client's vision and sensation bilaterally.

(continued)

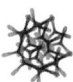

NURSING CARE PLAN 24-1 **ADL Deficit (*continued*)**

Nursing Diagnosis. **ADL deficit** related to the inability to perform her ADLs due to her recent stroke

Expected Outcome. The client will identify the cause of decline in ADL functions and difficulties to recovery of function and to increase the ability for independent functioning.

Interventions	Rationales
Assess the client's strength to complete ADLs efficiently and carefully on a daily basis using a proper assessment tool.	The client may only need help with some self-care measures.
Evaluate the client's need for assistive devices.	Assistive devices improve confidence in performance of ADLs.
Recognize choice for food, personal care items, and other things.	The client will be eager to submit to the treatment schedule that supports their specific preferences.
Present positive support for all activities attempted, note any partial achievements.	External resources of positive support may promote ongoing efforts. Clients often have trouble seeing progress.
Apply routines and allow sufficient time for the patient to complete a task.	An established routine becomes habit and requires less effort. This helps the client organize and perform self-care skills.
Corroborate with health care staff the need for home health care after discharge.	Shortened hospital stays have resulted in clients being more debilitated on discharge and, as a result, are requiring more assistance at home.
Educate family to promote autonomy and to intercede if the patient becomes tired, not capable of carrying out task, or become aggravated.	This shows caring and concern but does not deter client's efforts to achieve independence.

Evaluation of Expected Outcomes

- The client is able to accomplish their ADLs sufficiently.
- The client is able to be discharged with Home Health to assist them at home.
- The client's family is willing to continue support for independent ADLs.

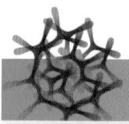

KEY POINTS

- Exercise: Purposeful physical activity
- Fitness: The capacity to exercise
- Fitness assessment
  - Body composition analysis
  - Vital signs
  - Fitness test
    - Stress ECG
    - Ambulatory ECG
    - Step test
  - Walk-a-mile test
  - Activity monitoring
- Exercise prescriptions
  - Target heart rate
  - Metabolic energy equivalent
- Fitness exercise: Physical activity performed by healthy adults; develops and maintains cardiorespiratory function, muscular strength, and endurance

- Isotonic: Activity that involves movement and work; muscles being exercised change length, shortening and lengthening during contraction
- Isometric: Stationary exercises during which there is no change in the length of the contracting muscle; involves working to hold a position still
- Isokinetic: Combines movement at a constant speed with a form of resistance
- Therapeutic exercise: Activity performed by people with health risks or those being treated for an existing health problem
  - Active: Therapeutic activity that the client performs independently
  - Passive: Therapeutic activity that the client performs with assistance
  - ROM: Therapeutic activities that move the joints

CRITICAL THINKING EXERCISES

1. List excuses people give for not exercising and offer counterarguments for each.
2. A client with paralysis of the lower extremities is depressed and questions the purpose of performing passive ROM exercises on the lower body. Assuming paralysis is permanent and the client will never walk again, how would you respond?
3. What advantages would you offer to a friend who is physically inactive and could benefit from exercise?
4. What are some reasons the federal government sets goals and objectives for physical activity and fitness in its *Healthy People* campaigns?

NEXT-GENERATION NCLEX-STYLE REVIEW QUESTIONS

1. When the nurse teaches a client how to perform isometric exercises of the quadriceps muscles, which instruction is correct?
   a. Move your toes toward and away from your head.
   b. Tighten and relax the muscles on the front of your thigh.
   c. Lift your lower leg up and down from the bed.
   d. Bend your knee, and pull your lower leg upward.
   Test-Taking Strategy: Analyze the choices and select the option that describes keeping the exercised limb stationary.

2. When the nursing team develops a plan of care for a client with a stroke, which area of nursing management is most important to the client's rehabilitation?
   a. Regulating bowel and bladder elimination
   b. Dealing with problems of disturbed body image
   c. Preventing contractures and joint deformities
   d. Facilitating positive outcomes from grieving
   Test-Taking Strategy: Note the key word and modifier, "most important." Analyze the choices and select one that promotes restoration of the client's future mobility and self-care.

3. When a client asks of what benefit a stress ECG will be, what is the most accurate answer from the nurse?
   a. A stress ECG shows how the heart performs during progressive exercise.
   b. A stress ECG helps determine the client's potential target heart rate.
   c. A stress ECG verifies how much exercise is needed to improve fitness.
   d. A stress ECG can predict whether the client will have a heart attack soon.
   Test-Taking Strategy: Note the key word and modifier, "most accurate." Analyze the choices and select the option that describes the primary purpose of a stress ECG better than any of the others.

4. When the nurse performs ROM exercises on a sedentary client, which indicates the exercise should be stopped immediately? Select all that apply.
   a. The joint movement is accompanied by pain.
   b. The joint movement causes a sudden muscle spasm.
   c. The joint movement meets with slight resistance.
   d. The joint movement increases the client's respirations.
   e. The joint movement results in a grimaced expression.
   Test-Taking Strategy: Note the key word, "immediately." Analyze the choices and select options that indicate the exercise may be too excessive at the present time.

5. What information is essential for the nurse to document when caring for a client for whom the physician has ordered the use of a CPM machine? Select all that apply.
   a. Condition of the sutures around the incision
   b. Degree of joint flexion
   c. Amount of time the client used the machine
   d. Characteristics of drainage from the wound
   e. Number of cycles per minute
   f. Presence and quality of arterial pulses
   Test-Taking Strategy: Note the key word, "essential." Analyze the choices and select options that provide information to team members about the current therapy using a CPM machine.

NEXT-GENERATION NCLEX-STYLE CLINICAL SCENARIO QUESTIONS

Clinical Scenario:
An 88-year-old female is a resident in a nursing home following a stroke. She has lost motor skills including ROM on the right side of her body. She does not notice people or objects on her affected side. Her muscle mass and strength on the right side have diminished due to neglect of her arm and leg as well as its position. She depends on others for turning, positioning, and ADLs.

1. Select all of the indicators that may suggest a cause for concern regarding an inability to perform ADLs.
   a. Lost motor skills
   b. Recent stroke
   c. Increased appetite
   d. Increased muscle mass
   e. Diminished strength
   f. Unable to reposition herself

2. From the following list, identify self-care measures that may assist the client with her ADLs.
   a. Implement measures to promote independence.
   b. Apply regular routines, and allow adequate time for the patient to complete the task.
   c. Allow the patient to feed herself as soon as possible.
   d. Use a cane to assist the client in ambulating.
   e. Allow the client to toilet on her own.
   f. Consider using energy conservation techniques.

SKILL 24-1 Performing Range of Motion Exercises

Suggested Action	Reason for Action
ASSESSMENT	
Review the medical record and nursing plan for care.	Determines whether activity problems have been identified
Assess the client's level of activity and joint mobility.	Indicates whether, and the extent to which, joints should be passively exercised
Assess the client's understanding of the hazards of inactivity and purposes for exercise.	Determines the type and amount of health teaching needed
PLANNING	
Explain the procedure for performing ROM exercises.	Reduces anxiety and promotes cooperation
Consult with the client on when ROM exercises may be best performed.	Shows respect for independent decision-making
Suggest performing ROM exercises during a time that requires general activity, such as bathing.	Demonstrates efficient time management
Perform ROM exercises at least twice a day.	Promotes recovery or maintains functional use
Exercise each joint at least two to five times during each exercise period.	Increases exercise benefits
IMPLEMENTATION	
Wash your hands or use an alcohol-based hand rub (see Chapter 10).	Reduces the potential for transferring microorganisms
Help the client into a sitting or lying position.	Promotes relaxation and access to the body
Pull the privacy curtains.	Demonstrates respect for modesty
Drape the client loosely or suggest loose-fitting underwear or shorts.	Avoids exposing the client
Begin at the head.	Facilitates organization
Support the client's neck and bring the chin toward the chest and then as far back in the opposite position as possible (Fig. A).	Flexes and hyperextends the neck

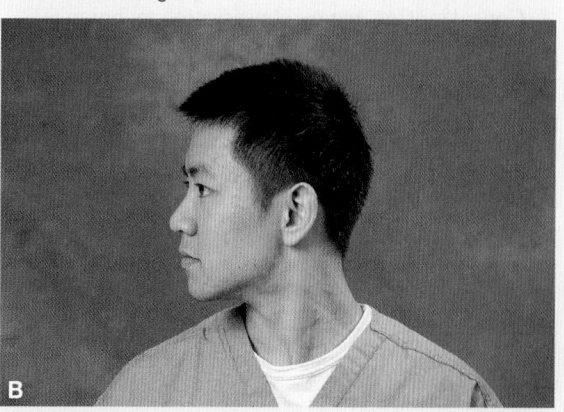

Neck hyperextension.

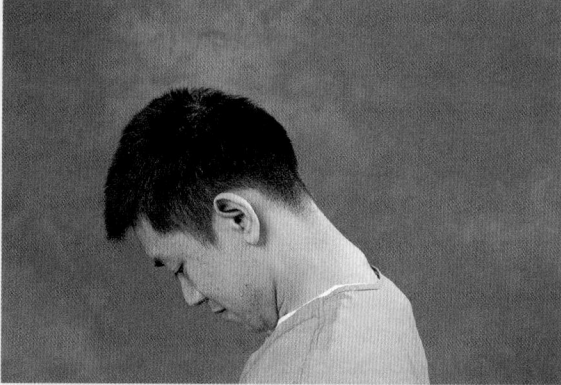

Neck flexion.

Place a hand on either side of the head and move the neck from side to side (Fig. B).

Rotates the neck

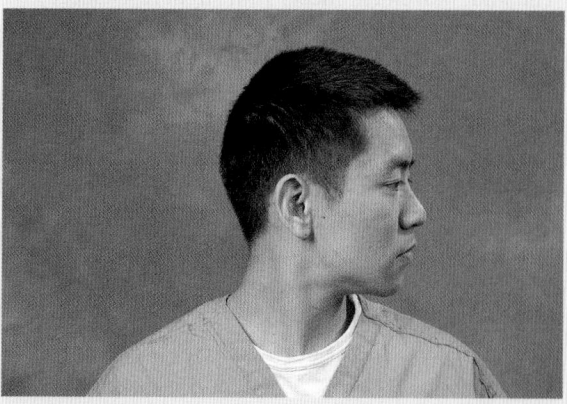

SKILL 24-1 Performing Range of Motion Exercises (*continued*)

Suggested Action	Reason for Action
Neck rotation.	
Turn the head in a circular manner (Fig. C).	Puts the head and neck through circumduction

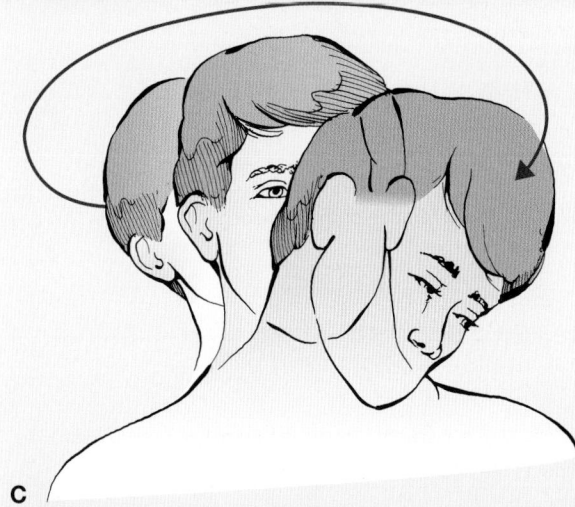

Circumduction of the neck.

C

Support the elbow and wrist while moving the straightened arm above the head and behind the body (Fig. D).	Flexes, extends, and then hyperextends the shoulder

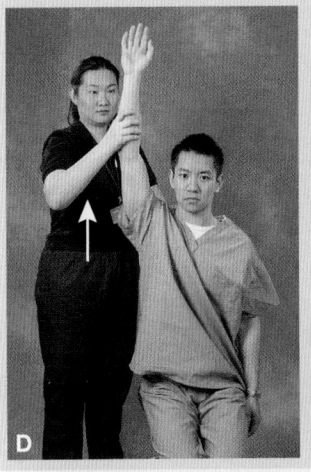 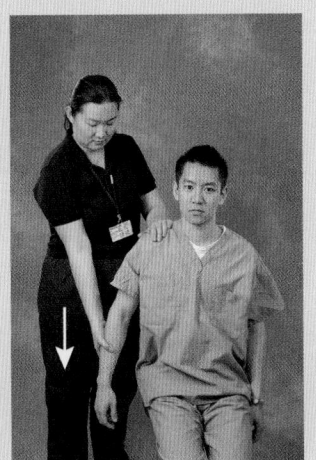

Flexion and extension of the shoulder.

D

Move the straightened arm away from the body and then toward the midline (Fig. E).	Abducts and adducts the shoulder

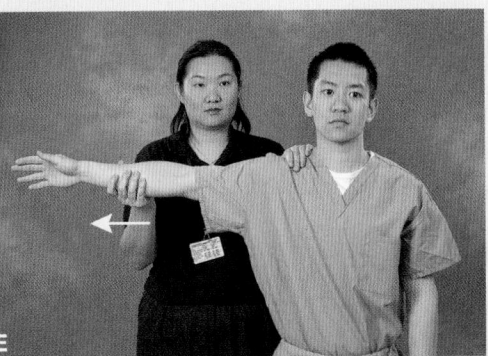 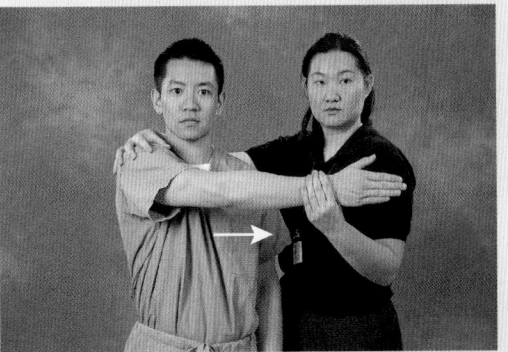

E

Abduction and adduction of the shoulder.

(*continued*)

SKILL 24-1 Performing Range of Motion Exercises (*continued*)

Suggested Action	Reason for Action
Bend the elbow and move the arm so that the palm is upward and then downward (Fig. F).	Produces internal and external rotation of the shoulder
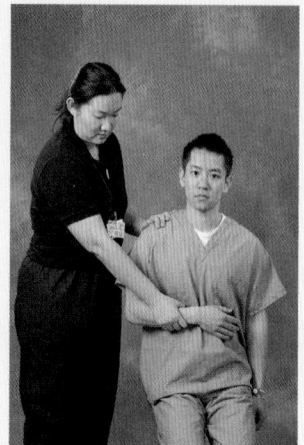 Internal and external rotation of the shoulder.	
Move the arm in a full circle (Fig. G).	Circumducts the shoulder
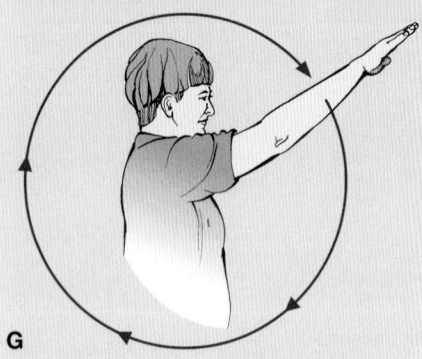 Circumduction of the shoulder.	
Place the arm at the client's side and bend the forearm toward the shoulder and then straighten it again (Fig. H).	Flexes and extends the elbow
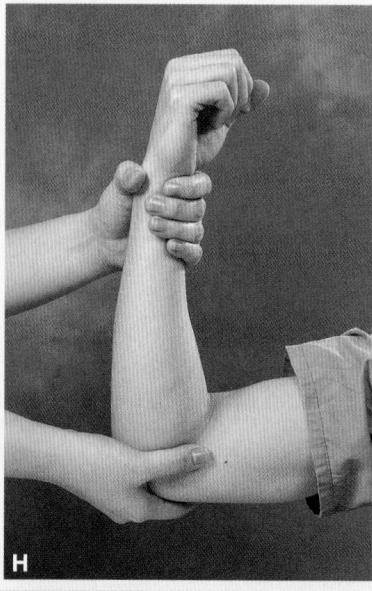 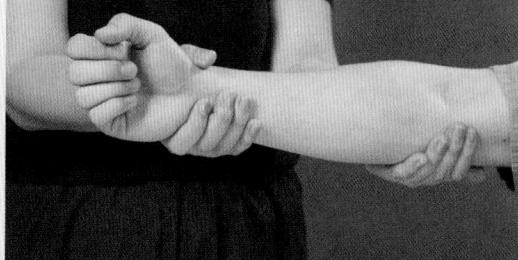 Flexion and extension of the elbow.	

SKILL 24-1 Performing Range of Motion Exercises (*continued*)

Suggested Action	Reason for Action
Bend the wrist forward and then backward (Fig. I).	Moves the wrist from flexion to extension and then hyperextension Flexion and extension of the wrist.
Twist the wrist to the right and then left (Fig. J).	Rotates the wrist joint Rotation of the wrist.
Bend the thumb side of the hand away from the wrist and then in the opposite direction (Fig. K).	Provides adduction and then abduction of the wrist Abduction and adduction of the wrist.

(*continued*)

SKILL 24-1 Performing Range of Motion Exercises (*continued*)

Suggested Action	Reason for Action
Turn the palm downward and then upward (Fig. L).	Pronates and supinates the wrist

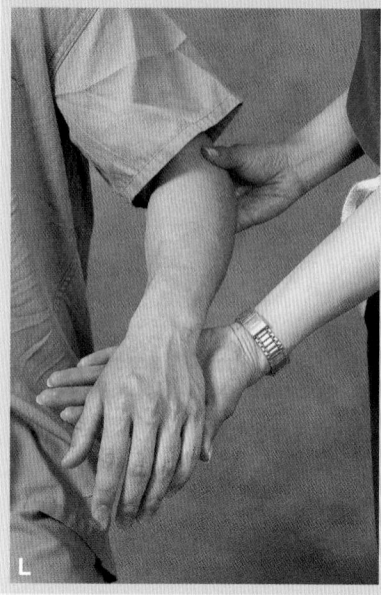 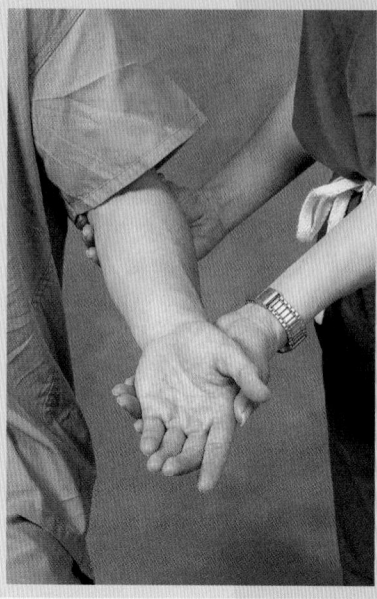

Pronation and supination of the wrist.

Suggested Action	Reason for Action
Open and close the fingers as though making a fist (Fig. M).	Extends and flexes the fingers

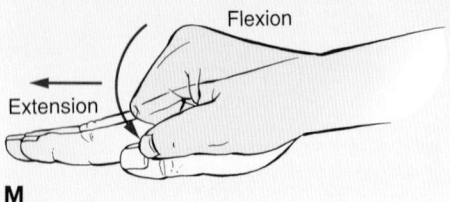

Flexion

Extension

M

Flexion and extension of the fingers.

Suggested Action	Reason for Action
Bend the thumb toward the center of the palm and then back to its original position (Fig. N).	Flexes and extends the thumb

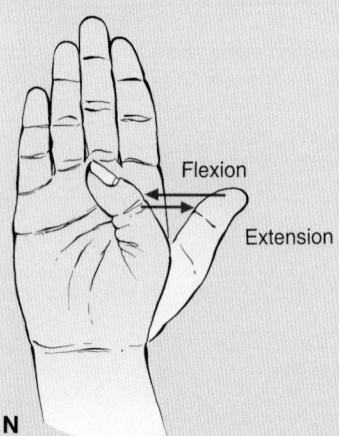

Flexion

Extension

N

Flexion and extension of the thumb.

SKILL 24-1 Performing Range of Motion Exercises (*continued*)

Suggested Action	Reason for Action
Spread the fingers and thumb as widely as possible and then bring them back together again (Fig. O).	Abducts and adducts the fingers and thumb

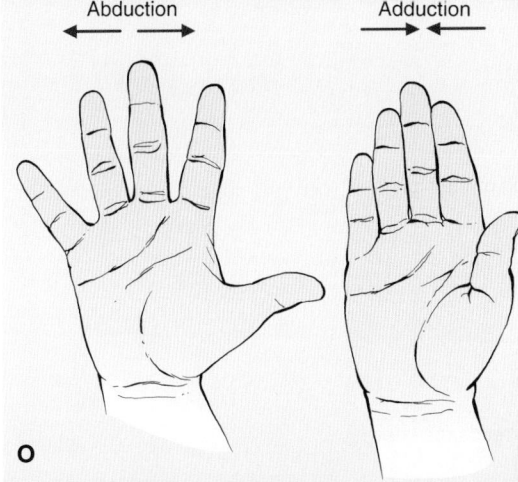

Abduction and adduction of the fingers and thumb.

| Bring the straightened leg forward and backward from the body in a standing position (Fig. P). | Flexes, extends, and hyperextends the hip |

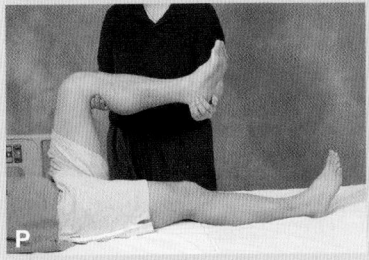 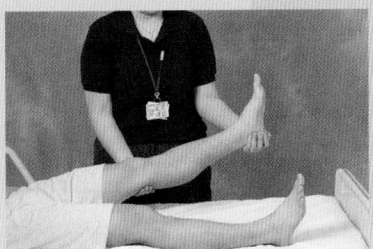

Flexion and extension of the hip in a lying position.

| Move the straightened leg away from the body and back beyond the midline (Fig. Q). | Abducts and then adducts the hip |

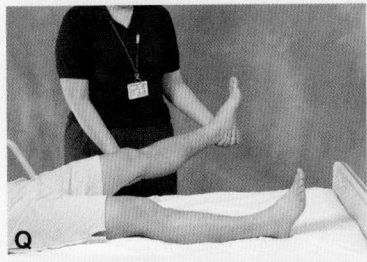 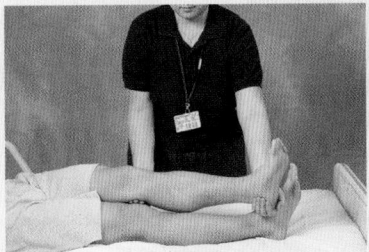

Abduction and adduction of the hip.

| Turn the leg away from the other leg and then toward it (Fig. R). | Rotates the hip externally and then internally |

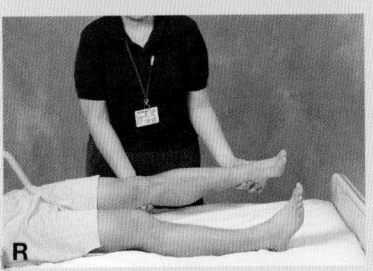 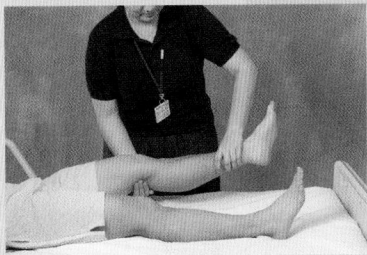

Internal and external rotation of the hip.

(*continued*)

SKILL 24-1 Performing Range of Motion Exercises (*continued*)

Suggested Action	Reason for Action
Turn the leg in a circle (Fig. S).	Circumducts the hip

S

Circumduction of the hip.

Bend the knee and then straighten it again (Fig. T).	Flexes and extends the knee

Extension   Flexion

T

Flexion and extension of the knee.

Bend the foot toward the ankle and then away from the ankle (Fig. U).	Causes dorsiflexion and plantar flexion

U

Dorsiflexion and plantar flexion of the foot.

SKILL 24-1 Performing Range of Motion Exercises (*continued*)

Suggested Action	Reason for Action
Bend the sole of the foot toward the midline and then away from midline (Fig. V).	Inverts and everts the ankle

Inversion

Eversion

V

Inversion and eversion of the ankle.

| Bend and then straighten the toes (Fig. W). | Flexes and extends the toes |

W

Flexion and extension of the toes.

EVALUATION

All joints are exercised to the extent possible.

DOCUMENT

- Performance of exercise regimen
- Response of the client

SAMPLE DOCUMENTATION

Date and Time Assisted in performing ROM exercises during bath. Actively moves all joints on the right side of the body. Joints on the left side passively exercised through full ranges. No resistance or pain experienced. _____ J. Doe, LPN

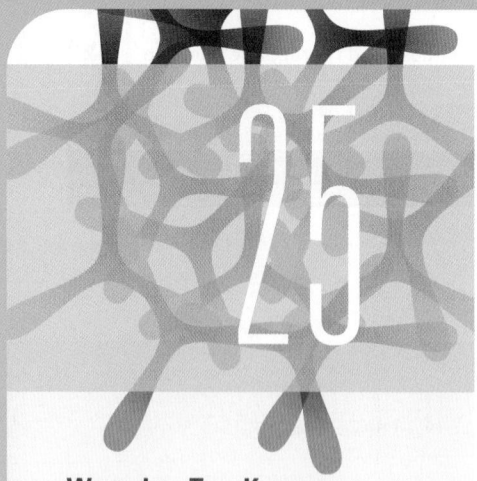

Mechanical Immobilization

Words To Know

bivalved cast
body cast
braces
cast
cervical collar
compartment syndrome
controlled ankle movement
(CAM)
cylinder cast
external fixator
functional braces
immobilizers
inflatable splints
manual traction
molded splints
orthopedic boot/walking boot
orthoses
petals
pin site
pneumatic splints
prophylactic braces
rehabilitative braces
skeletal traction
skin traction
sling
spica cast
splint
traction
traction splints
window

Learning Objectives

On completion of this chapter, the reader should be able to:

1. List purposes of mechanical immobilization.
2. Name types of splints.
3. Discuss why slings and braces are used.
4. Explain the purpose of a cast.
5. Name types of casts.
6. Describe nursing actions that are appropriate when caring for clients with casts.
7. Discuss how casts are removed.
8. Explain what traction implies.
9. List types of traction.
10. Explain principles that apply to maintaining effective traction.
11. Describe the purpose of an external fixator.
12. Identify the rationale for performing pin site care.

INTRODUCTION

Some clients are inactive and physically immobile as a result of an overall debilitating condition. For others, impaired mobility results from trauma or its treatment. Such is the case for clients with **orthoses**, which are orthopedic devices that support or align a body part and prevent or correct deformities. Examples of orthoses include splints, immobilizers, and braces. Other clients have limited mobility when the use of slings, casts, traction, and external fixators is necessary. Caring for clients who are mechanically immobilized with orthopedic devices requires specialized nursing skills described in this chapter.

 Gerontologic Considerations

■ As adults live longer, many are dealing with the pain and loss of function associated with arthritis. Treatment options include rehabilitation with various types of mechanical devices in the home or rehabilitation setting.

■ Some fractures in older adults are treated nonsurgically by limiting movement of the bone or joint. Occupational and physical therapists are helpful in assisting older adults to regain function and range of motion following any period of immobilization to prevent a decrease or a permanent loss of function.

■ Because of diminished tactile sensation, older adults may be unaware of skin pressure from a splint, cast, traction, or other mechanical device. Assess the skin of an older person daily for redness or other signs of pressure. If the older person cannot change positions, the caregiver is responsible for ensuring that pressure is relieved at least every 2 hours.

Concept Mastery Alert

Crutches and Orthoses

Crutches are not considered orthoses. Orthoses support or align a body part. Crutches are aids to promote ambulation.

PURPOSES OF MECHANICAL IMMOBILIZATION

Most clients who require mechanical immobilization have suffered trauma to the musculoskeletal system. Such injuries are painful and heal less rapidly than injuries to the skin or soft tissue. They require a period of inactivity to allow new cells to restore integrity to the damaged structures.

Mechanical immobilization of a body part accomplishes the following:

- Relieves pain and muscle spasm
- Supports and aligns skeletal injuries
- Restricts movement while injuries heal
- Maintains a functional position until healing is complete
- Allows activity while restricting movement of an injured area
- Prevents further structural damage and deformity

MECHANICAL IMMOBILIZING DEVICES

The use of various immobilizing devices can achieve therapeutic benefits. Examples of such devices include splints, slings, braces, casts, and traction.

Splints

Some conditions are treated with a **splint**, which is a device that immobilizes and protects an injured body part. Splints are used before or instead of casts or traction.

Emergency Splints

Splints often are applied as a first aid measure for suspected sprains or fractures (Fig. 25-1; Nursing Guidelines 25-1).

Commercial Splints

Commercial splints are more effective than improvised splints. They are available in various designs depending on the injury. Examples include inflatable splints, traction splints, immobilizers, molded splints, and cervical collars. Inflatable and traction splints are intended for short-term use; they are

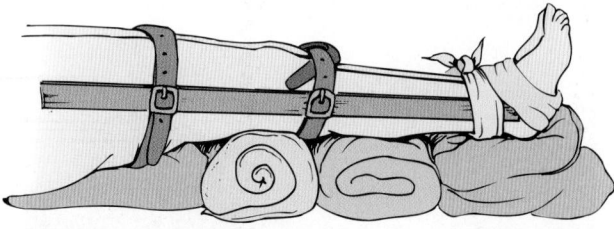

FIGURE 25-1 Emergency first aid splinting immobilizes the injured leg to the uninjured leg with a makeshift splint, such as a board, broom handle, or golf club. Neckties, belts, or scarves keep the splint in place.

 NURSING GUIDELINES 25-1

Applying an Emergency Splint

- Avoid changing the position of the injured part even if it appears grossly deformed. *Keeping the injured part in place prevents additional injuries.*
- Leave a high-top shoe or a ski boot in place if the injury involves an ankle. *The shoe or boot limits movement and reduces pain and swelling.*
- Cover any open wounds with clean material. *The covering absorbs blood and prevents dirt and additional pathogens from entering.*
- Select a rigid splinting material such as a flat board, broom handle, or rolled-up newspaper. *Rigid material provides support while restricting movement.*
- Pad bony prominences with soft material. *Padding reduces pressure and prevents friction on the skin.*
- Apply the splinting device so that it spans the injured area from the joint above to the joint below the injury. *Such placement immobilizes the injured tissue.*
- Use an uninjured area of the body adjacent to the injured part as a splint, if no other sturdy material is available. *The uninjured part can serve as a substitute for an external splint.*
- Use wide tape or wide strips of fabric to confine the injured part to the splint. *Securing the body part prevents displacement and reduces the risk for compromising circulation.*
- Loosen the splint or the material used to attach it if the fingers or toes are pale, blue, or cold. *Loosening the splint facilitates circulation.*
- Elevate the immobilized part if possible so that the lowest point is higher than the heart. *Elevation reduces swelling and enhances venous return to the heart.*
- Keep the client warm and safe. *Shock is a risk.*
- Seek assistance in transporting the client to a health care agency. *The client requires more sophisticated treatment.*

usually applied just after the injury and are removed shortly after a more thorough assessment of the injury. Immobilizers and molded splints are used for longer periods.

Inflatable Splints

Inflatable splints, also called "**pneumatic splints,**" are immobilizing devices that become rigid when filled with air (Fig. 25-2). In addition to limiting motion, they control

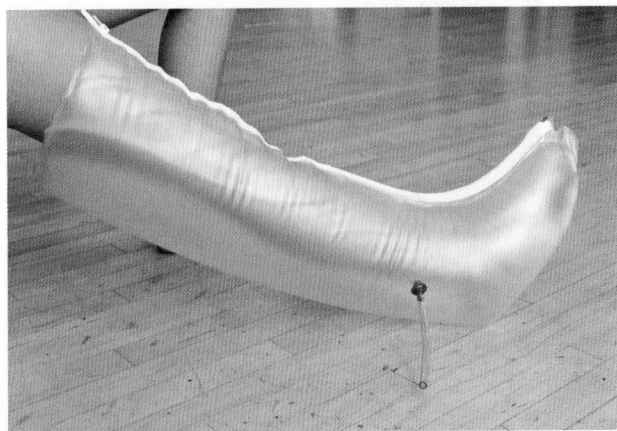

FIGURE 25-2 An inflatable splint.

bleeding and swelling. The injured body part is inserted into the deflated splint. When air is infused, the splint molds to the contour of the injured part, preventing movement. The splint is filled with air to the point at which it can be indented 0.5 in (1.3 cm) with the fingertips. Inflatable splints are most often used in emergency first aid. The injury should be examined and treated soon after application of the splint; otherwise, circulation may be affected. If an inflatable splint is to remain in place for some time, a stockinette (a stretchable cotton fabric) is loosely applied over the extremity and the splint is inflated just enough to immobilize the part.

Traction Splints

Traction splints are metal devices that immobilize and pull on contracted muscles. They are not as easy to apply as inflatable splints. One example is a *Thomas splint*, which requires special training for its application to prevent additional injuries (Fig. 25-3). A Thomas splint may also be used to suspend a leg in traction.

Immobilizers

Immobilizers are commercial splints made from cloth and foam and held in place by adjustable hook and loop tape (such as Velcro) straps (Fig. 25-4). As the name implies, immobilizers limit motion in the area of a painful but healing injury, such as that of the knee. They are removed for brief periods during hygiene and dressing.

Molded Splints

Molded splints are orthotic devices made of rigid materials and are used for chronic injuries accompanied by inflammation. They may be appropriate for clients with repetitive motion disorders such as carpal tunnel syndrome, or *plantar fasciitis* (inflammation of the plantar fascia that supports the arch of the foot causing heel pain), and *Achilles tendonitis* (inflammation of a tendon in the calf where it attaches to the heel). Molded splints provide support and limit movement

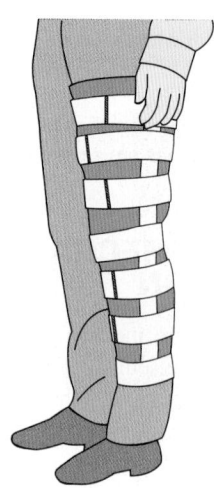

FIGURE 25-4 A leg immobilizer.

to prevent further injury and pain (Fig. 25-5). They maintain the body part in a functional position to prevent contractures and muscle atrophy during immobility.

Orthopedic Boots

An **orthopedic boot/walking boot** is used to help clients recover from an injured foot or ankle or postsurgery. Other terms often used are CAM walker, fracture boot, or orthopedic boot. CAM stands for **controlled ankle movement**. It is used as a cast alternative and a transition from the walking cast after a client experiences a foot or ankle injury (Fig. 25-6). A walking boot/orthopedic boot can help keep the foot stable so it can heal. It can keep weight off an area, such as the toe, as it heals. Most boots have between two and five adjustable straps and go mid-way up the calf (drugs.com, 2023).

Cervical Collars

A **cervical collar** is a foam or rigid splint placed around the neck. It is used to treat athletic neck injuries and other trauma that results in a neck sprain or strain. Neck strain is sometimes referred to as *whiplash* or a *whiplash injury*. The incidence of whiplash injuries has decreased primarily for two reasons: improved athletic protective equipment and the use of shoulder harnesses and neck supports in automobiles. When a neck injury—which is generally more painful the day after trauma—is mild or moderate,

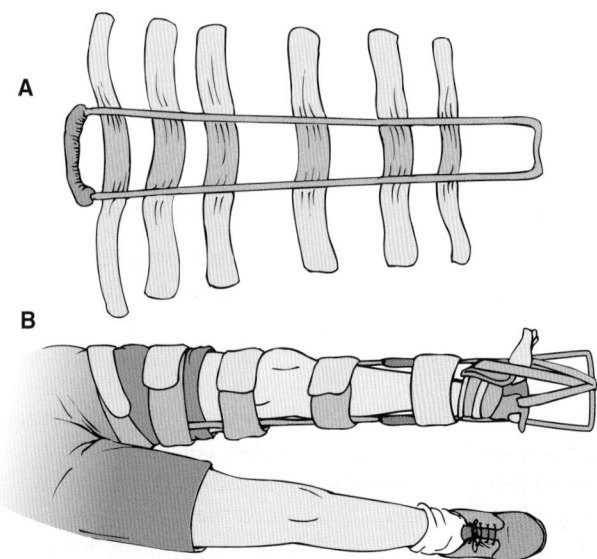

FIGURE 25-3 A. A Thomas splint. **B.** A Thomas splint applied to the lower extremity.

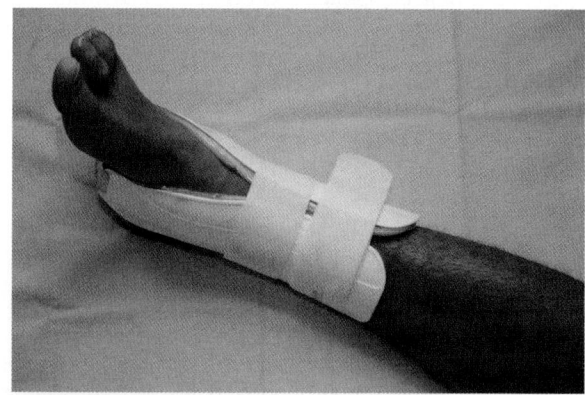

FIGURE 25-5 A molded splint.

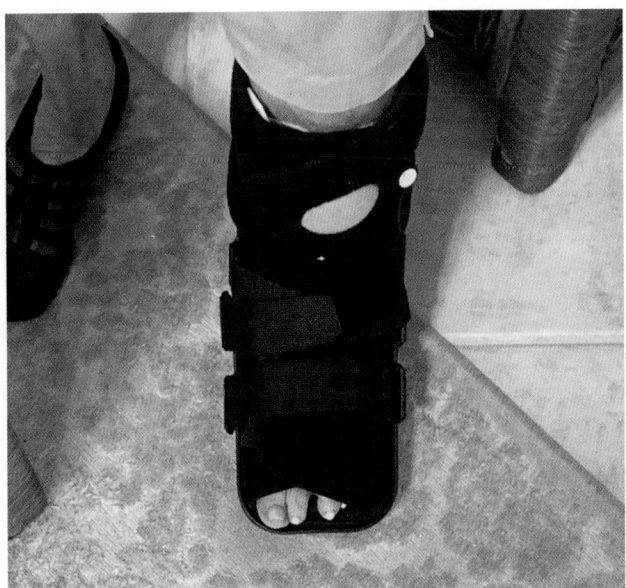

FIGURE 25-6 Orthopedic boot/walking boot, used after a foot injury to allow the client to ambulate, while securing the foot/ankle. (Photo by L. Moreno.)

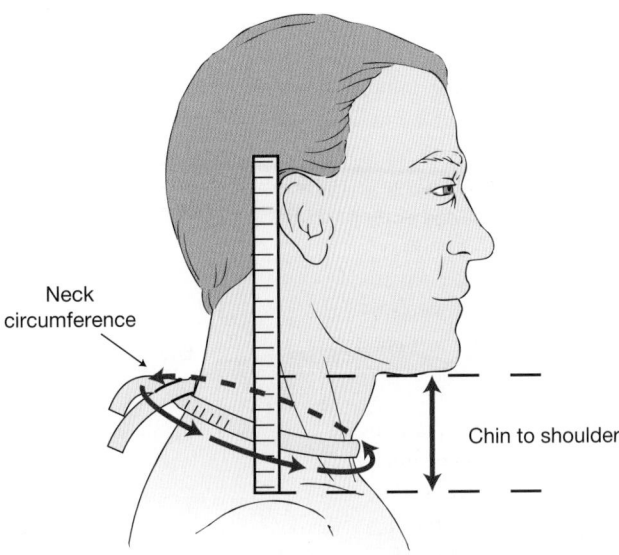

FIGURE 25-8 Vertical and circumferential measurements for cervical collar size.

a foam collar covered with a stockinette is used. When the client wears it, it is a reminder to limit neck and head movements. For more serious injuries, a rigid splint made from polyurethane is used to control neck motion and support the head, reducing its load-bearing force on the cervical spine (Fig. 25-7).

To determine the proper collar size, the nurse measures the neck circumference and the distance between the shoulder and the chin (Fig. 25-8). The nurse then compares measurements with the size guide suggested by the collar manufacturer. For example, a person with a neck size of 15 to 20 in and a shoulder-to-chin height of 3 in probably would require a regular adult size. Adult sizes also come in short, tall, and extra tall. Pediatric collars are also available.

When applying a cervical collar, the head is placed in a neutral position (see Chapter 23). The front of the collar is

positioned well beneath the chin and slid upward until the chin is well supported. The opening of the collar is centered at the back of the neck. Straps made of Velcro or other materials are used to secure the collar in the desired position. When applied appropriately, the client can breathe and swallow effortlessly while wearing the collar.

Clients wear cervical collars almost continuously, even while sleeping, for 10 days to 2 weeks. They remove them to do gentle range-of-motion neck exercises (see Chapter 24). The sooner a client performs exercise (within their pain tolerance), the faster revascularization and recovery occur. Prolonged dependence on the collar for comfort can lead to permanent stiffness in the neck.

During recovery, the nurse assesses the client's neuromuscular status by having the client perform movements that correlate with muscular functions controlled by cervical spine and peripheral nerve roots. If neuromuscular function is intact, the client can:

- Elevate both shoulders.
- Flex and extend the elbows and the wrists.
- Generate a strong handgrip.
- Spread the fingers.
- Touch the thumb to the little finger on each hand.

The nurse documents and communicates to the physician any difference in strength or movement on one side or the other.

Slings

A **sling** is a cloth device used to elevate, cradle, and support parts of the body. Slings are applied commonly to the arm, leg, or pelvis after immobilization and examination of the injury. Most ambulatory clients use a commercially made arm sling; a triangular piece of muslin cloth occasionally may be used to fashion a sling (Fig. 25-9). To be effective, slings require proper application (Skill 25-1).

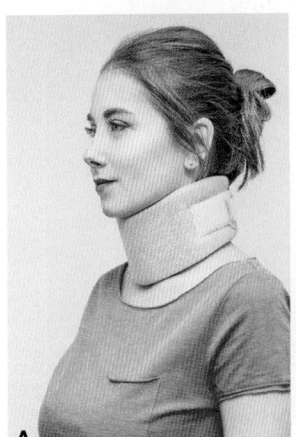
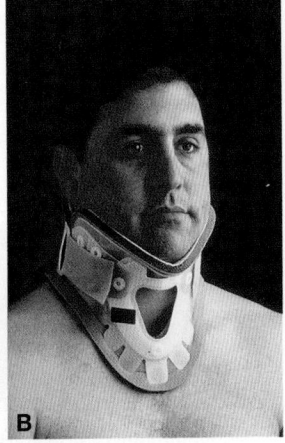

FIGURE 25-7 **A.** A foam cervical collar. **B.** A rigid cervical collar. (Okrasiuk/Shutterstock.)

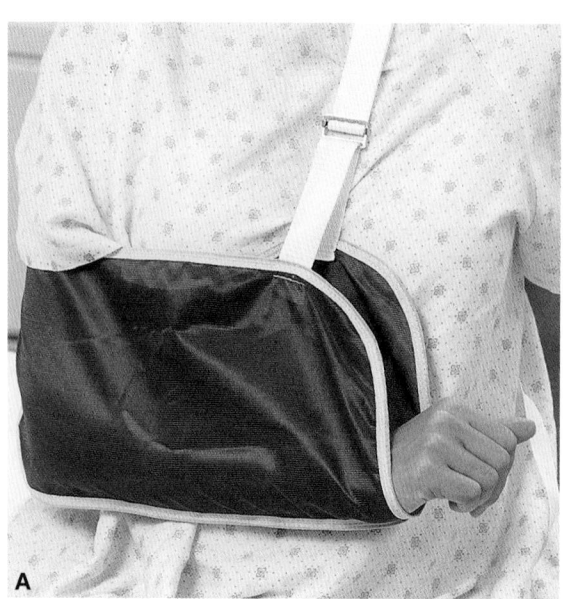
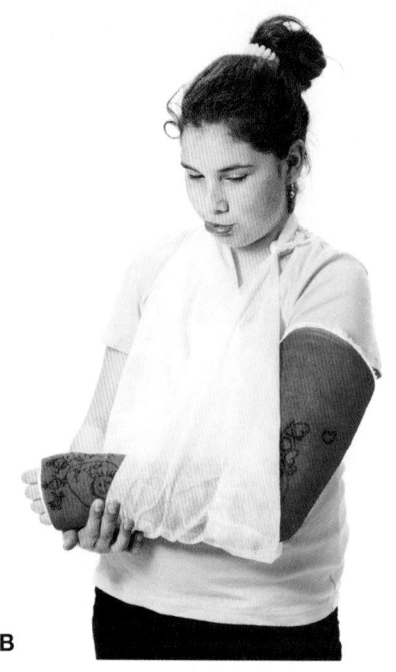

FIGURE 25-9 Examples of slings. **A.** A commercial sling used for arm suspension. (Photo by B. Proud.) **B.** Cloth triangular sling.

⟫ *Stop, Think, and Respond 25-1*

List the advantages and disadvantages of using a commercially made canvas sling and a triangular cloth sling.

Braces

Braces are custom-made or custom-fitted devices designed to support weakened structures. The three categories of braces are (1) **prophylactic braces** that are used to prevent or reduce the severity of a joint injury, (2) **functional braces** that provide stability for an unstable joint, and (3) **rehabilitative braces** that allow protected motion of an injured joint that has been treated operatively (Fig. 25-10).

Because clients generally wear braces during active periods, braces are made of sturdy materials such as metal or leather. Leg braces may be incorporated into a shoe. Some back braces are made of cloth with metal staves, or strips, sewn within the fabric of the brace. An improperly applied or ill-fitting brace can cause discomfort, deformity, and skin ulcerations from friction or prolonged pressure.

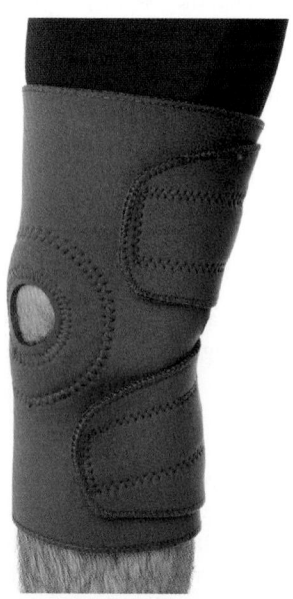
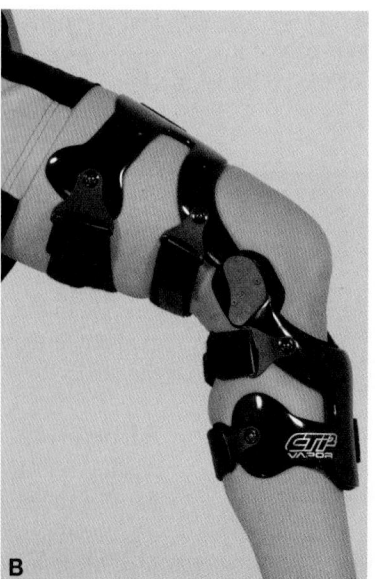
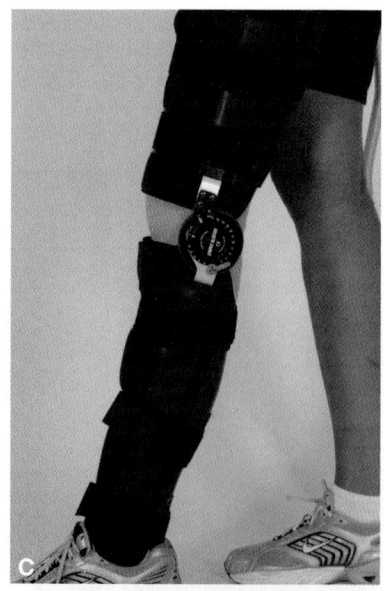

FIGURE 25-10 Types of braces. **A.** Prophylactic brace. **B.** Functional brace. **C.** Rehabilitative brace. (**A**, copyright Julian Rovagnati; **B** and **C** from Anderson, M. K., & Barnum, M. [2021]. *Foundations of athletic training: Prevention, assessment, and management* [7th ed.]. Lippincott Williams & Wilkins.)

TABLE 25-1 Cast Materials

SUBSTANCE	ADVANTAGES	DISADVANTAGES
Plaster of Paris	Inexpensive Easy to apply Low incidence of allergic reactions	Takes 24–48 hours to dry; large casts may take up to 72 hours to dry. Weight-bearing must be delayed until thoroughly dried. Heavy Prone to cracking or crumbling, especially at the edges Softens when wet
Fiberglass	Lightweight Porous Dries in 5–15 minutes Allows immediate weight-bearing Durable Unaffected by water	Expensive Not recommended for severe injuries or those accompanied by excessive swelling Macerates skin if padding becomes wetCast edges may be sharp and cause skin abrasions.

Casts

A **cast** is a rigid mold placed around an injured body part after it has been restored to correct the anatomic alignment. The purpose of the cast is to continuously immobilize the injured structure. Casts usually are applied to fractured (broken) bones. They are formed using either wetted rolls of plaster of Paris or premoistened rolls of fiberglass (Table 25-1).

Types of Casts

There are basically three types of casts: cylinder, body, and spica. Cylinder and body casts may be bivalved.

Cylinder Cast

A **cylinder cast**, the most common type of cast, encircles an arm or leg and leaves the toes or fingers exposed. The cast extends from the joints above and below the affected bone. This prevents movement in the injured area, thereby maintaining correct alignment during healing. As healing progresses, the cast may be trimmed or shortened.

Body Cast

A **body cast** is a larger form of a cylinder cast and encircles the trunk of the body instead of an extremity (Fig. 25-11). It generally extends from the nipple line to the hips. For some clients with spinal problems, the body cast extends from the back of the head and chin areas to the hips, with modifications for exposing the arms.

Bivalved Cast

The physician may create a **bivalved cast** (one that is cut into two pieces lengthwise) from either a body or a cylinder cast. A bivalved cast on an extremity (Fig. 25-12) is created when:

- Swelling compresses tissue and interferes with circulation.
- The client is being weaned from the cast.
- A sharper X-ray image is needed.
- Painful joints need to be immobilized temporarily for a client with arthritis.

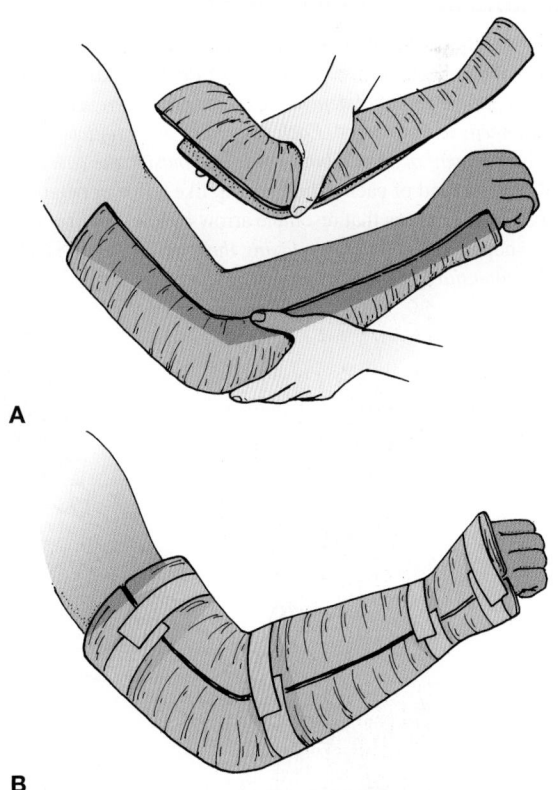

A

B

FIGURE 25-12 A. A bivalved cast. **B**. The two halves are rejoined. (From Donnelly-Moreno, L. A., & Moseley, B. [2021]. *Introductory medical-surgical nursing* [13th ed.]. Wolters Kluwer.)

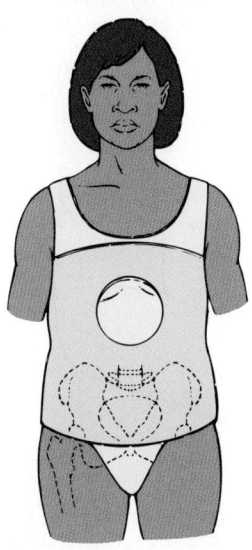

FIGURE 25-11 Example of a body cast. (From LifeART, copyright 2016, Lippincott Williams & Wilkins. All rights reserved.)

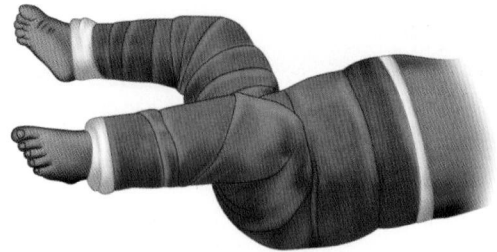

FIGURE 25-13 Hip spica cast. (From Eltorai, A., George, P., & Rougas, S. [2022]. *The pre-clerkship guide: Procedures and skills for clinical rotations.* Wolters Kluwer.)

Creating a front and a back for a body cast facilitates bathing and skin care. If the physician approves, half of the shell is removed temporarily for hygiene while the other half remains in place. The process is repeated when caring for the opposite body area. Once care has been completed, the removed piece is replaced and the two halves are held in place by wrapping them together with an elastic bandage.

Spica Cast

A **spica cast** encircles one or both arms or legs and the chest or trunk. It may have an abduction bar to help maintain the position of the repaired injury. When applied to the upper body, the cast is referred to as a *shoulder spica*; one applied to the lower extremities is called a *hip spica* (Fig. 25-13). Spica casts, especially those on the lower extremities, are heavy, hot, and frustrating because they severely restrict movement and activity.

When applied to a lower extremity, the cast is trimmed in the anal and genital areas to allow for the elimination of urine and stool. Clients with hip spicas cannot sit during elimination, so the nurse protects the cast from soiling using plastic wrap and positions the client on a small bedpan known as a fracture pan (see Chapter 30).

Cast Application

Cast application generally requires more than one person. The nurse prepares the client, assembles the cast supplies, and helps the physician during the cast application (Skill 25-2). A light-cured fiberglass cast requires exposure to ultraviolet light to harden.

Basic Cast Care

Some clients need extended care after surgery that has included the application of a cast. The nurse is responsible for caring for the cast and making appropriate assessments to prevent complications (Skill 25-3). See Nursing

---

 NURSING GUIDELINES 25-2

Making and Applying Petals

- Cut multiple strips of adhesive tape approximately 2 in wide by 2 to 3 in in length or use precut ovals from moleskin. *The width of the tape is optional depending on the circumference of the cast that needs to be covered. Each petal must be of sufficient length for placement of an end both inside and outside the cast edges.*
- Round the end of each adhesive strip like a flower petal or trim to create chevrons that resemble arrows; moleskin may already be shaped into an oval. *Modifying the ends of the tape reduces the potential for wrinkles.*

- Tuck one end of the tape or moleskin inside the cast edge, taking care to avoid wrinkles. *Wrinkles can cause friction on the skin and may lead to abrasions.*
- Overlap the strips of tape or moleskin around the rough cast edge (see figure). *Overlapping ensures there are no gaps that expose a rough area that will continue to irritate the skin.*
- Continue to monitor the skin for signs of impairment. *If petals do not relieve skin irritation, the physician may need to smooth the edge with additional strips of plaster.*

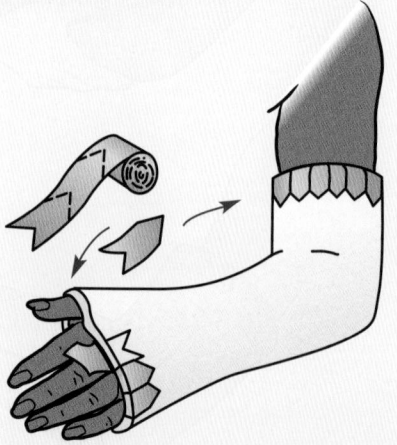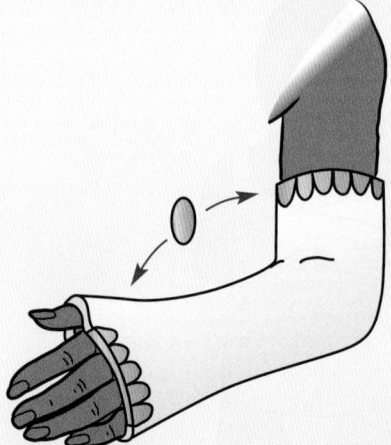

Petals are overlapped and applied around the edge circumference of a cast.

Guidelines 25-2 for instructions on making and applying **petals**, strips of adhesive tape or moleskin for the purpose of reducing skin irritation from the rough edges of a cast.

Cast Removal

In most cases, casts are removed when they need to be changed and reapplied, or when the injury has healed sufficiently that the cast is no longer necessary. A cast is removed prematurely if complications develop.

Most casts are removed with an electric cast cutter, an instrument that looks like a circular saw (Fig. 25-14). The cast cutter is noisy and may frighten clients. There is a natural expectation that an instrument sharp enough to cut a cast is sharp enough to cut skin and tissue. Proper use of an electric cast cutter, however, leaves the skin intact. While a physician should know proper cast saw techniques, many cast technicians, physician assistants, and medical assistants are also qualified to use the cast cutter.

When the cast is removed, the unexercised muscle is usually smaller and weaker. The joints may have a limited range of motion. The skin usually appears pale and waxy and may contain scales or patches of dead skin. The skin is washed as usual with soapy warm water, but the semi-attached areas of skin are left in place; they are not forcibly removed. Applying lotion to the skin adds moisture and tends to prevent the rough skin edges from catching on clothing. Eventually, the dead skin fragments will shed.

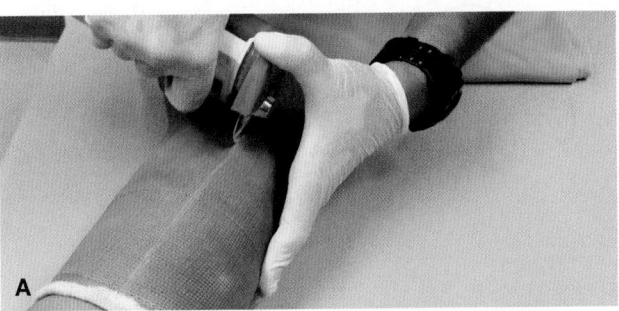
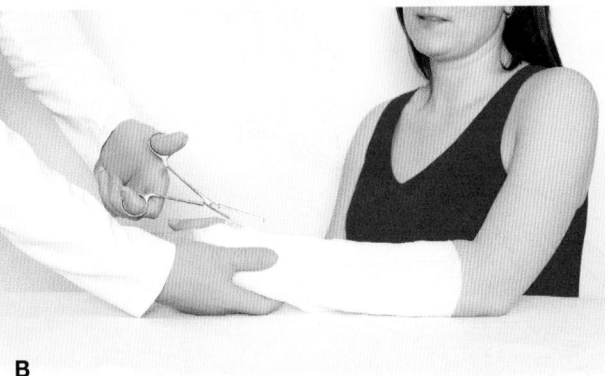

FIGURE 25-14 Cast removal. **A.** The cast is bivalved with an electric cast cutter. (porjai kittawornrat/Shutterstock) **B.** The padding is manually cut. (HenadziPechan/Shutterstock).

›› Stop, Think, and Respond 25-2

Discuss the discharge teaching for a client who has had a cast applied.

Traction

Traction is a pulling effect exerted on a part of the skeletal system. It is a treatment measure for musculoskeletal trauma and disorders. Traction is used to accomplish the following:

- Reduce muscle spasms
- Realign bones
- Relieve pain
- Prevent deformities

The pull of the traction generally is offset by the counterpull from the client's own body weight. Except for traction exerted with the hands, application of traction involves the use of weights connected to the client through a system of ropes, pulleys, slings, and other equipment.

Types of Traction

The three basic types of traction are manual, skin, and skeletal. The categories reflect the manner in which traction is applied.

Manual Traction

Manual traction means pulling on the body using a person's hands and muscular strength (Fig. 25-15). It is most often used briefly to realign (set) a broken bone. It is also used to replace a dislocated bone into its original position within a joint.

Skin Traction

Skin traction means a pulling effect on the skeletal system by applying devices to the skin, such as a pelvic belt and a cervical halter (Fig. 25-16). Other names for commonly applied forms of skin traction are Buck traction and Russell traction (Fig. 25-17).

Skeletal Traction

Skeletal traction means pull exerted directly on the skeletal system by attaching wires, pins, or tongs into or through a bone (Fig. 25-18). Skeletal traction is applied continuously for an extended period to the skull, humerus, and femur, for example.

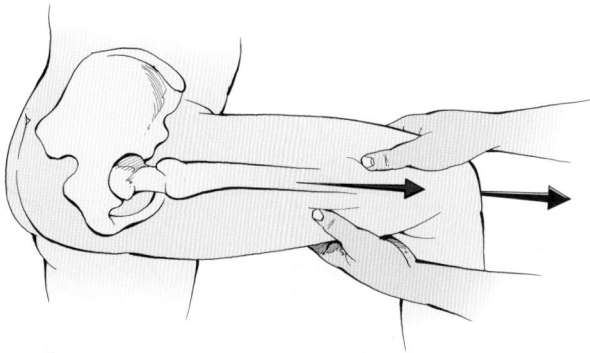

FIGURE 25-15 Manual traction.

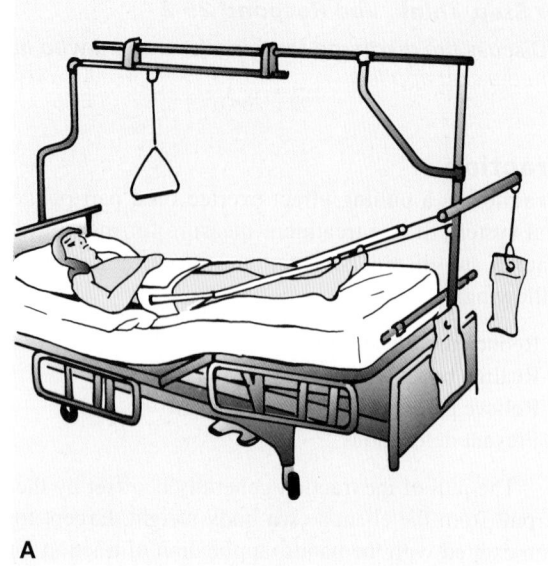

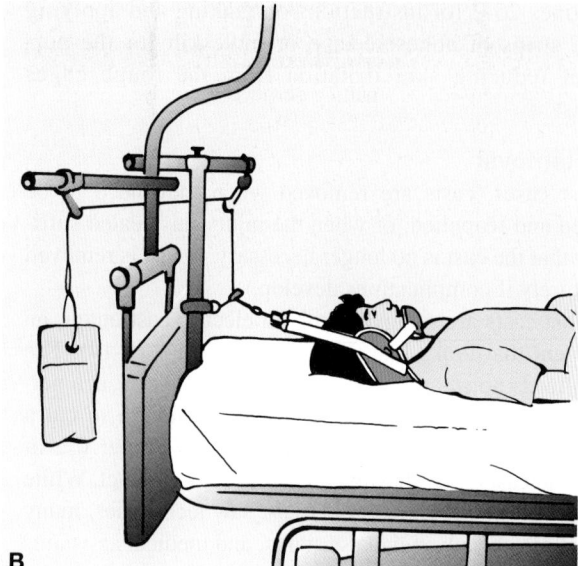

FIGURE 25-16 A. A pelvic belt. **B.** A cervical halter.

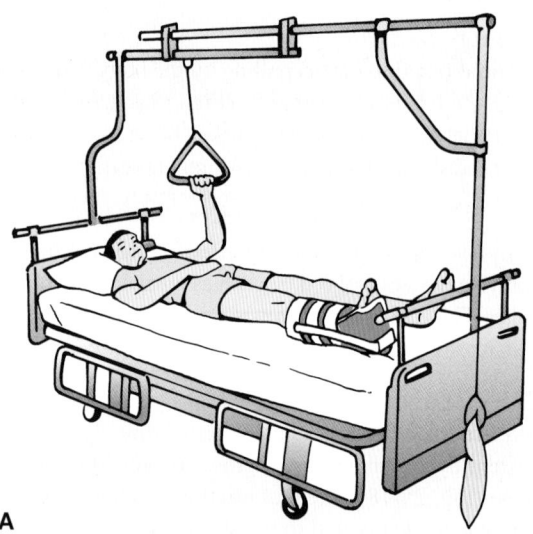

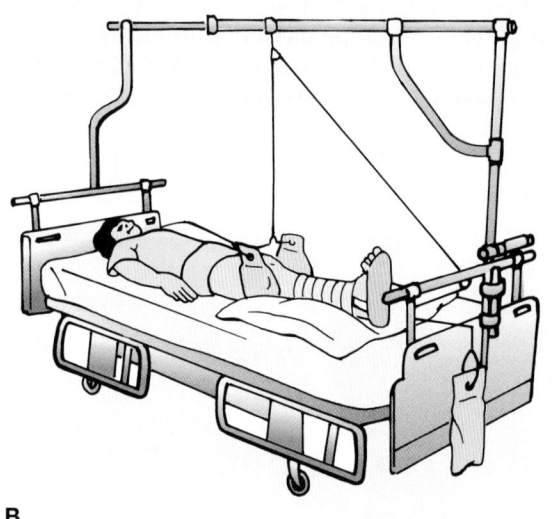

FIGURE 25-17 A. Buck traction. **B.** Russell traction.

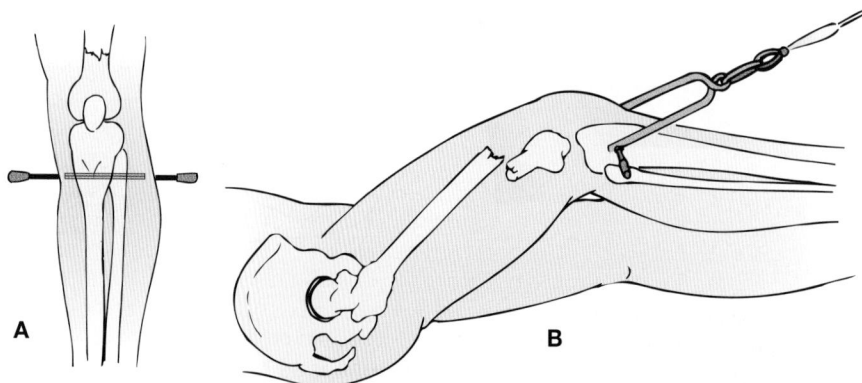

FIGURE 25-18 The application of skeletal traction. **A.** A pin transects the bone. **B.** Traction is applied.

BOX 25-1 Principles for Maintaining Effective Traction

- Traction must produce a pulling effect on the body.
- Countertraction (counterpull) must be maintained.
- The pull of traction and the counterpull must be in exactly opposite directions.
- Splints and slings must be suspended without interference.
- Ropes must move freely through each pulley.
- The prescribed amount of weight must be applied.
- The weights must hang free.

Traction Care

Regardless of the type of traction used, its effectiveness depends on the application of certain principles during the client's care (Box 25-1, Skill 25-4).

External Fixators

An **external fixator** is a metal device inserted into and through one or more broken bones to stabilize fragments during healing (Fig. 25-19). Although the external fixator immobilizes the area of injury, the client is encouraged to be active and mobile (see Chapter 26 for information about ambulatory aids).

During recovery, the nurse provides care for the **pin site** (the location where pins, wires, or tongs enter or exit the skin). In conjunction with an external fixator and skeletal traction, pin site care is essential to prevent infection. Insertion of pins impairs skin integrity and provides a port of entry for pathogens. Caring for a pin site is described in Skill 25-5.

⟫ Stop, Think, and Respond 25-3

A culture from a specimen taken at a pin site reveals that the pin site is infected with Staphylococcus aureus. What nursing actions are required for contact precautions to control transmission of the pathogen? (Use information in Chapter 22 as a resource or to review.)

NURSING IMPLICATIONS

Clients with immobilizing devices such as casts and traction may have one or more of the following nursing diagnoses:

- Acute pain
- Altered skin integrity risk

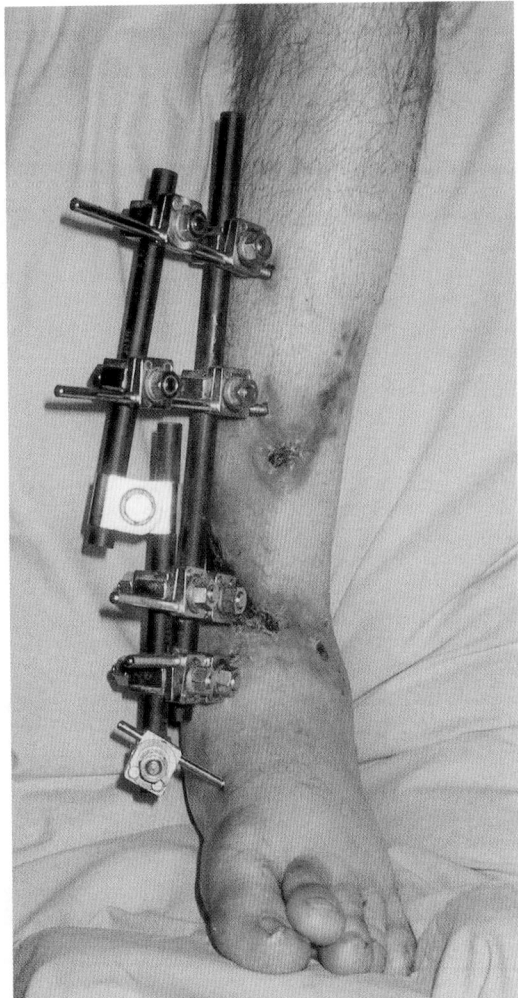

FIGURE 25-19 An external fixator. Metal rods exert traction between two sets of skeletal pins.

- Altered tissue integrity risk
- Altered tissue perfusion
- Bathing/hygiene ADL deficit
- Venous thromboembolism risk

Nursing Care Plan 25-1 describes the nursing process as it applies to a client with a nursing diagnosis of altered tissue perfusion, defined as the lack of oxygenated blood flow to areas of the body.

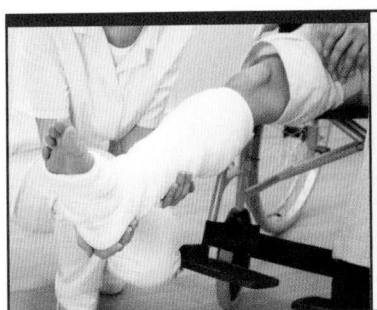

Clinical Scenario A 28-year-old male has returned to the emergency department within 24 hours following his discharge after having surgery on a leg fracture with the application of a cast. The client reports pain in the casted extremity that he rates as a "10" despite self-administering prescribed pain medication, which followed discharge instructions to keep the limb elevated and intermittently apply an ice bag. The nurse collects data and suspects the client may have a condition known as *compartment syndrome*. **Compartment syndrome** occurs when there is swelling within fascia that does not expand. The pressure from the swelling interferes with blood flow to tissues and nerves.

NURSING CARE PLAN 25-1 | Altered Tissue Perfusion

Assessment

- Monitor peripheral circulation:
  - Check for the presence and quality of peripheral pulses in affected and unaffected extremities.
  - Feel the temperature of exposed toes or fingers and compare findings with the opposite extremity.
  - Compress the nail beds and measure the time for the color to return following blanching.
  - Observe for swelling in the affected extremity in comparison to the unaffected extremity.

- Look at the skin color and compare differences in the extremities.
- Assess the client's neurologic status in both extremities:
  - Ask the client to move the toes or fingers in the extremities.
  - Touch the client's extremities with objects that are sharp, dull, warm, or cold to determine whether the client can differentiate the stimuli without actually seeing the source of stimulation.
  - Quantify the client's level of pain, its location, characteristics, and whether it decreases or increases with usual pain-relieving measures.

Nursing Diagnosis. Altered tissue perfusion related to tissue swelling and compression of blood vessels and nerves secondary to injury and recent cast application to the injured leg

Expected Outcome. The client's neurovascular status will be normal as evidenced by a report of pain relief from present rate of 10 to 7 or less. Pedal pulses will be equally strong. Movement and sensation will be equal in both extremities. Capillary refill will be 3 seconds or less bilaterally within 3 hours today (8/20).

Interventions	Rationales
Elevate the casted leg so that toes are higher than the client's heart.	Use of gravity facilitates the venous return of blood from distal areas to the heart.
Have client exercise toes of the foot in the cast every 15 minutes while awake.	Contraction of skeletal muscles compresses capillaries and veins, which propels venous blood toward the heart.
Apply an ice bag on the cast over the area of injury; empty and refill ice bag every 20 minutes.	Application of cold causes blood vessels to constrict and reduces tissue swelling.
Monitor circulatory status, sensation including tactile and pain, and mobility of toes in affected extremity every 30 minutes.	Lack of improvement or escalation of signs suggesting neurovascular impairment indicates a medical emergency.
Report worsening of symptoms to the charge nurse and physician immediately.	Failure to report and implement additional interventions can cause the client to permanently lose function in the limb or require surgical amputation.

Evaluation of Expected Outcomes

- The pedal pulse is diminished in extremity in cast; pulse is strong and regular in unaffected foot despite the elevation of casted leg on three pillows.
- The client performs active exercises with toes every 15 minutes.
- Client rates pain at 10 after receiving Demerol 75 mg IM.
- Capillary refill is 2 seconds in toes on both feet. Pedal pulses are palpable and equal bilaterally. The client moves and detects sensation equally bilaterally and rates pain at 5 after cast is bivalved.
- Affected leg remains elevated with ice bag applied. Client does exercises as directed.

KEY POINTS

- Purposes of mechanical immobilization
  - Relieves pain and muscle spasms
  - Supports and aligns skeletal injuries
  - Restricts movement while injuries heal
  - Maintains a functional position until healing is complete
  - Allows activity while restricting movement of an injured area
  - Prevents further structural damage and deformity
- Splints: Some conditions are treated with a splint, which is a device that immobilizes and protects an injured body part. Splints are used before or instead of casts or traction.
  - Emergency splint
  - Inflatable splint
  - Traction splint
  - Immunizers
  - Molded splints
  - Cervical collar
  - Slings
  - Braces

- Casts: A rigid mold placed around an injured body part after it has been restored to correct the anatomic alignment. The purpose of the cast is to continuously immobilize the injured structure.
  - Material used for casts
    - Plaster of Paris
    - Fiberglass
  - Types of casts
    - Cylinder cast
    - Body cast
    - Spica cast
  - Cast care
    - Monitor peripheral circulation
    - Assess neurologic status in both extremities
- Traction: A pulling effect exerted on a part of the skeletal system; a treatment measure for musculoskeletal trauma and disorders
  - Manual
  - Skin
  - Skeletal

CRITICAL THINKING EXERCISES

1. Although slings are applied most often to support injured extremities, discuss possible reasons for applying a sling on an arm paralyzed by stroke.
2. Discuss the differences and similarities between caring for clients with casts and caring for clients in traction.
3. Discuss ways to provide diversions for clients with a cast or in traction who are confined to bed while their injuries heal.
4. A nursing assistant reports that a client with a cast is experiencing pain that is being rated at higher and higher levels since the cast was applied this morning. What actions should the nurse take? What complication could be the cause of the client's discomfort?

NEXT-GENERATION NCLEX-STYLE REVIEW QUESTIONS

1. As the physician wraps the arm of a client with rolls of wet plaster, what is the most appropriate method the nurse should use for supporting the wet cast?
   a. Support the wet cast on a soft mattress.
   b. Support the wet cast on a firm surface.
   c. Support the wet cast with the tips of the fingers.
   d. Support the wet cast with the palms of the hands.
   Test-Taking Strategy: Note the key words and modifier, "most appropriate method." Review the choices and select the option that is better than any of the others when handling a wet cast.

2. When a client asks the nurse to explain the advantage of a fiberglass cast over one made of plaster, which is an accurate response?
   a. Fiberglass casts are generally less expensive.
   b. Fiberglass casts are generally more lightweight.
   c. Fiberglass casts are generally more flexible.
   d. Fiberglass casts are generally less restrictive.
   Test-Taking Strategy: Note the key word, "accurate." Analyze the choices and select the option that is a correct description.

3. Which technique is best for assessing circulation in the casted extremity of a client with a long leg plaster cast?
   a. Ask the client whether the cast feels exceptionally heavy.
   b. Feel the cast to determine whether it is unusually cold.
   c. Depress the nail bed and time the return of color.
   d. See whether there is room to insert a finger within the cast.
   Test-Taking Strategy: Note the key word, "best." Analyze the choices and select the option that is better than any of the others for assessing the quality of distal circulation.

4. Which nursing assessments suggest a client with a cylinder cast on a leg is developing compartment syndrome? Select all that apply.
   a. There is a foul odor from under the cast.
   b. The client has intense unrelieved pain.
   c. The client reports severe itching under the cast.
   d. The distal peripheral pulse in the casted leg is weak.
   e. The toes of the casted leg are colder than the uncasted leg.
   f. The toes on the casted foot are red and swollen.
   Test-Taking Strategy: Use the process of elimination to select only the options that correspond with signs and symptoms associated with compartment syndrome.

5. While providing nursing care for a client in Buck skin traction, which finding indicates a need for immediate action?
   a. The traction weights are hanging above the floor.
   b. The leg is in line with the pull of the traction.
   c. The client's foot is touching the end of the bed.
   d. The rope is in the groove of the traction pulley.
   Test-Taking Strategy: Note the key words, "immediate action." Analyze the choices and select the option that if left unmanaged interferes with the client's treatment.

NEXT-GENERATION NCLEX-STYLE CLINICAL SCENARIO QUESTIONS

Clinical Scenario:

A 28-year-old male has returned to the emergency department within 24 hours following his discharge after having surgery on a leg fracture with the application of a cast. The client reports pain in the casted extremity that he rates as a "10" despite self-administering prescribed pain medication, which followed discharge instructions to keep the limb elevated and intermittently apply an ice bag. The nurse collects data and suspects the client may have a condition known as compartment syndrome. Compartment syndrome occurs when there is swelling within fascia that does not expand. The pressure from the swelling interferes with blood flow to tissues and nerves.

1. Select all of the indicators that may suggest a cause for concern regarding an altered tissue perfusion.
   a. Leg fracture and application of a cast
   b. Pain at a "10"
   c. Applying a hot pack
   d. Noted swelling at the toes
   e. Cyanosis noted on toes
   f. Walking a half a mile

2. Choose the most likely options for the information missing from the statement below by selecting from the list of options provided.
   a. The _____1_____ is contributing to the pain and the compartment syndrome is a result of the _____2_____.

OPTION 1	OPTION 2
cold compress	non-expanding fascia
limb elevation	pain medicine
swelling	cyanosis

SKILL 25-1 Applying an Arm Sling

Suggested Action	Reason for Action
ASSESSMENT	
Check the medical orders.	Integrates nursing activities with medical treatment
Assess the skin color and temperature, capillary refill time, and amount of edema; verify the presence of peripheral pulses in the injured arm (don gloves if there is a potential for contact with blood or nonintact skin).	Provides baseline objective data for future comparisons
Ask the client to describe how the fingers and arm feel and to rate any pain on a scale of 0–10.	Provides baseline subjective data for future comparisons
Determine whether the client required an arm sling in the past.	Indicates the level and type of health teaching needed
PLANNING	
Explain the purpose of the sling.	Adds to the client's understanding
Obtain a canvas or triangular sling, depending on what is available or prescribed for use.	Complies with medical practice
IMPLEMENTATION	
Wash your hands or use an alcohol-based hand rub (see Chapter 10).	Reduces the potential for transferring microorganisms
Position forearm across the client's chest with the thumb pointing upward.	Flexes the elbow
Avoid more than 90 degrees of flexion, especially if the elbow has been injured.	Facilitates circulation
CANVAS SLING	
Slip the flexed arm into the canvas sling so that the elbow fits flush with the corner of the sling (Fig. A).	Encloses the forearm and wrist

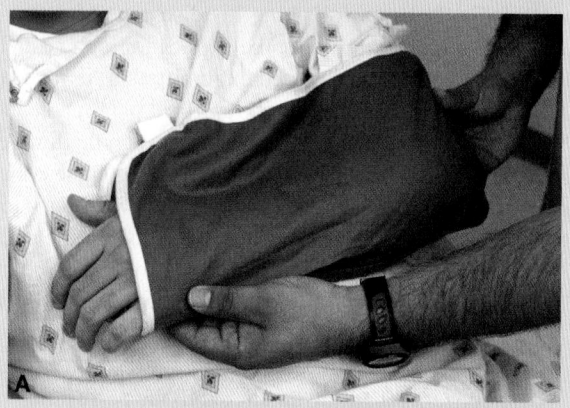

Positioning a commercial arm sling.

Bring the strap around the opposing shoulder and fasten it to the sling (Fig. B).	Provides the means for support

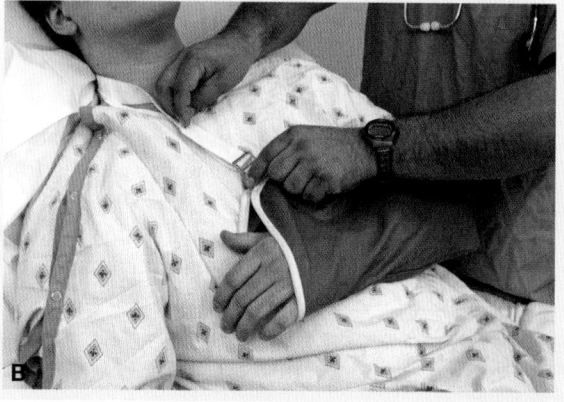

Placing the strap around the neck

SKILL 25-1 Applying an Arm Sling (*continued*)

Suggested Action	Reason for Action
Pad and tighten the strap sufficiently (Fig. C).	Reduces friction and pressure to preserve skin integrity
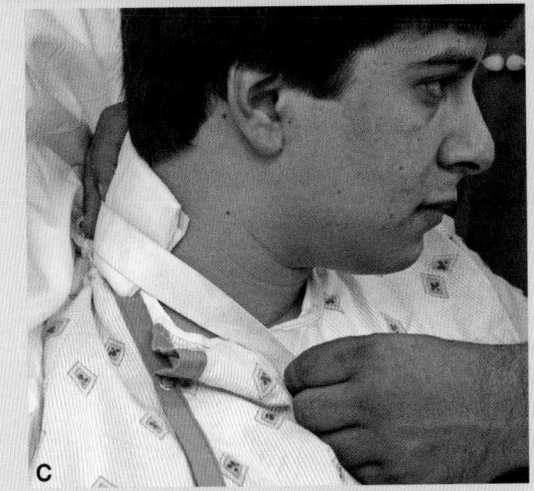	Placing padding between the strap and neck
Keep the elbow flexed and the wrist elevated (Fig. D).	Promotes circulation
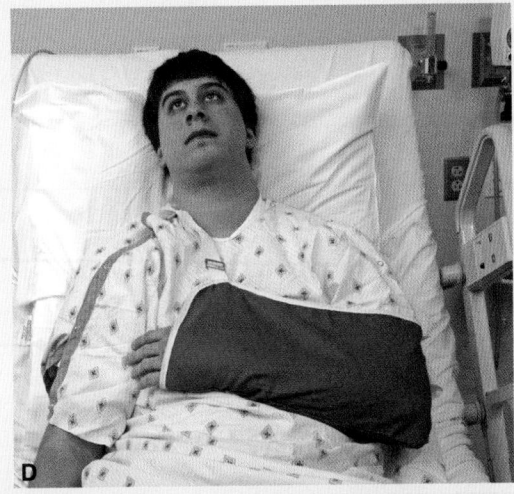	The sling in place

TRIANGULAR SLING

Place the longer side of the sling from the shoulder opposite the injured arm to the waist.	Positions the sling where length is needed
Position the apex or point of the triangle under the elbow (Fig. E).	Facilitates making a hammock for the arm
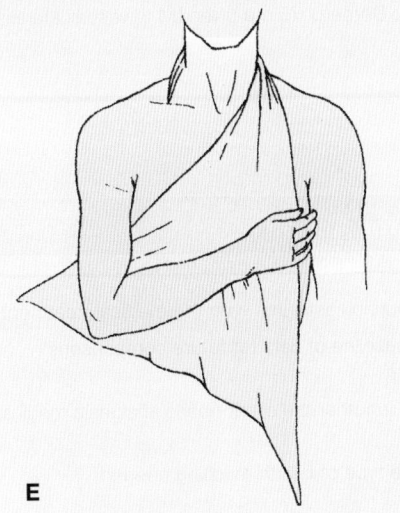	Positioning a triangular sling

(continued)

SKILL 25-1 Applying an Arm Sling (*continued*)

Suggested Action	Reason for Action
Bring the point at the waist up to join the point at the neck and tie them.	Encloses the injured arm
Position the knot to the side of the neck.	Avoids pressure on the vertebrae
Fold in and secure excess fabric at the elbow; a safety pin may be necessary (Fig. F).	Keeps the elbow enclosed
	A completed sling
Inspect the condition of the skin at the neck and the circulation, mobility, and sensation of the fingers at least once per shift.	Provides comparative data
Pad the skin at the neck with soft gauze or towel material if the skin becomes irritated.	Reduces pressure and friction
Tell the client to report any changes in sensation, especially pain with limited movement or pressure.	Indicates developing complications

F

EVALUATION

- Forearm is supported.
- Wrist is elevated.
- Pain and swelling are reduced.
- Circulation, mobility, and sensation are maintained.

DOCUMENT

- Baseline and comparative assessment data
- Type of sling applied or used
- To whom significant abnormal assessments were reported
- Outcomes of the verbal report

SAMPLE DOCUMENTATION

Date and Time   Fingers on R hand are pale, cool, and swollen. Capillary refill is sluggish, taking 4 seconds for color to return. Can move all fingers. Can discriminate sharp and dull stimuli. No tingling identified. Pain rated at 8 on a scale of 0–10. All above data reported to Dr. Stuckey. Orders received for pain medication and canvas sling. Demerol 75 mg given IM in vastus lateralis. Sling applied. _____ J. Doe, LPN

SKILL 25-2 Assisting with a Cast Application

Suggested Action	Reason for Action
ASSESSMENT	
Check the medical orders.	Integrates nursing activities with the medical treatment
Assess the appearance of the skin that the cast will cover; also check circulation, mobility, and sensation.	Provides a baseline of data for future comparisons
Ask the client to describe the location, type, and intensity of any pain.	Determines whether the client needs analgesic medication
Determine what the client understands about the application of a cast.	Indicates the type of health teaching needed

SKILL 25-2 Assisting with a Cast Application (*continued*)

Suggested Action	Reason for Action
Check with the physician as to whether a plaster of Paris or fiber-glass cast will be applied.	Facilitates assembling appropriate supplies

PLANNING

Suggested Action	Reason for Action
Obtain a signature on a treatment consent form if required.	Ensures legal protection
Administer pain medication if prescribed.	Relieves discomfort
Remove the client's clothing that may not stretch over the cast once it is applied.	Avoids having to cut and destroy clothing
Provide a gown or drape.	Preserves dignity and protects clothing
Assemble materials, which may include stockinette, felt padding, cotton batting, rolls of cast material, gloves, and apron.	Facilitates organization and efficient time management
Anticipate that if the cast is being applied to a lower extremity, the client will need crutches and instructions on their use (see Chapter 26).	Shows awareness of discharge planning
Have an arm sling available if applying the cast to an upper extremity.	Shows awareness of discharge planning

IMPLEMENTATION

Suggested Action	Reason for Action
Explain how the cast will be applied. If using plaster of Paris, be sure to tell the client that it will feel warm as it dries.	Reduces anxiety and promotes cooperation
Wash your hands or use an alcohol-based hand rub (see Chapter 10).	Reduces the potential for transferring microorganisms
Wash the client's skin with soap and water and dry well.	Removes dirt, body oil, and some microorganisms
Cover the skin with a stockinette and protective padding as directed (Fig. A).	Protects the skin from direct contact with the cast material and provides a fabric cushion that protects the skin

A

Stockinette in place

Suggested Action	Reason for Action
If applying a plaster cast, open rolls and strips of plaster gauze material. Briefly dip them one at a time in water and wring out the excess moisture.	Prepares the cast material for application
If using fiberglass material, open the foil packets one at a time.	Reduces the risk of rapidly drying and becoming unfit for use

(*continued*)

SKILL 12-2 Assisting with a Cast Application (*continued*)

Suggested Action	Reason for Action
Support the extremity while the physician wraps the cast material around the arm or leg (Fig. B).	Facilitates going around the injured area; ensures proper alignment because fiberglass is harder to mold

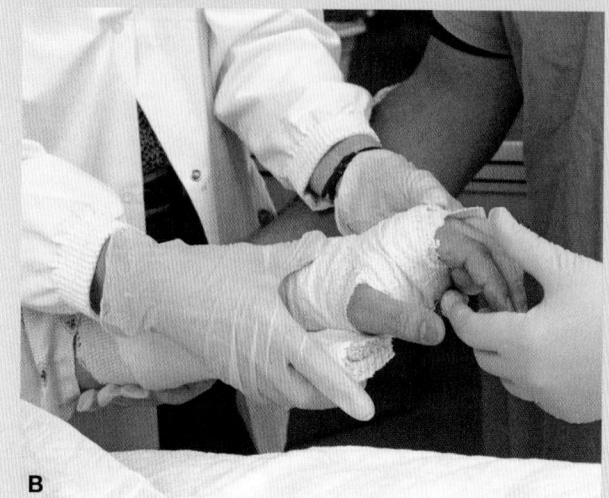

B

	Casting material being applied
For a fiberglass cast, hold the extremity in this position until the cast is dry (approximately 15 minutes).	Maintains desired position
Help fold back the edges of the stockinette at each end of the cast just before the final layer of cast material is applied (Fig. C).	Forms a smooth, soft edge at the margins of the cast, which may protect the skin from becoming irritated

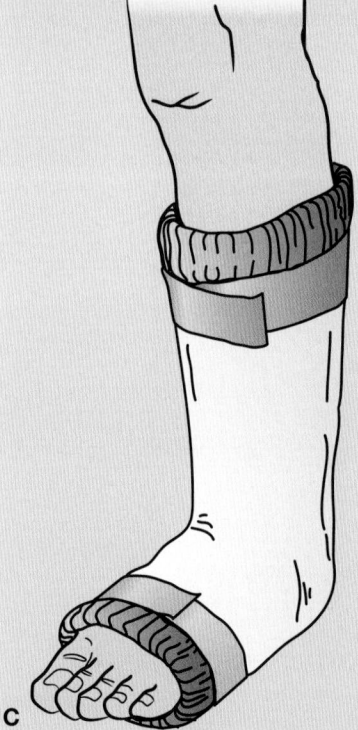

C

	The folded stockinette beneath the cast protects the skin from the sharp edges of the cast.
Elevate the cast on pillows or other support.	Helps reduce swelling and pain
If a plaster cast was applied, use a special sink with a plaster trap to dispose of the water in which plaster rolls were soaked.	Prevents clogging of plumbing
Provide verbal and written instructions on cast care.	Facilitates independence and safe self-care

SKILL 25-2 Assisting with a Cast Application (*continued*)

Suggested Action	Reason for Action

EVALUATION

- Skin has been cleaned and protected.
- Cast has been applied and is drying or dried.
- Circulation and sensation are within acceptable parameters.
- Client can repeat discharge instructions.

DOCUMENT

- Assessment data
- Type of cast
- Cast material
- Name of physician who applied the cast
- Discharge instructions

SAMPLE DOCUMENTATION

Date and Time Wrist appears swollen but skin is warm, dry, and intact. Capillary refill <3 seconds. X-ray department reports a fracture of the wrist. Dr. Roberts notified. Dr. Roberts applied cylinder fiberglass cast from middle of hand to above elbow. Assessment findings remain unchanged after cast application. Casted arm supported in a canvas sling. Standard instructions for cast care provided (see copy attached). Instructed to call Dr. Roberts if pain or swelling increases and make an office appointment in 2 weeks.
_____ J. Doe, LPN

SKILL 25-3 Providing Basic Care of a Client with a Cast

Suggested Action	Reason for Action
ASSESSMENT	
Determine the type of cast, the body location, and when the cast was initially applied.	Plaster casts do not completely dry for 24–72 hours or longer depending on the size and type of cast; fiberglass casts dry within 30 minutes.
Check whether there is a trapeze on the client's bed.	A trapeze helps a client change position or move up or down in bed.
PLANNING	
Plan to check the condition of the cast, the neurovascular status, and the condition of the skin on the limb enclosed by the cast every 30 minutes initially and twice per shift once it has dried.	A plaster cast is vulnerable to changing shape until it has dried; neurovascular complications are more likely to occur in the early hours after the initial cast application; and the risk for impaired skin integrity and infection is ongoing.
Explain the purpose and methods for assessment to the client.	Adds to the client's understanding
IMPLEMENTATION	
Place the bed at a comfortable height.	Prevents back strain
Wash your hands or use an alcohol-based hand rub (see Chapter 10).	Removes transient microorganisms and reduces the transmission of pathogens
Observe and feel the condition of the cast on the anterior as well as posterior surfaces. Position a fresh plaster cast on pillows without plastic covers.	A dry cast is white, shiny, and odorless; a damp cast is gray, dull, and musty-smelling. The buoyancy of the pillow reduces the direct force of the hard mattress against the cast that may alter its shape. Plastic-covered pillows trap heat and moisture, which slows drying.
Use the palms of the hands, not the fingers, to move or reposition the cast before it is thoroughly dry.	Use of the fingers can cause indentations, which can cause pressure sores to develop under the cast.
Leave a freshly applied plaster cast uncovered until it is dry; turn the client periodically to expose all the surfaces of the cast to air.	Aids in the evaporation of water from the plaster, which is necessary for drying the cast
Avoid using the abduction bar in a hip spica cast when turning a client.	Pulling on the abduction bar is likely to break it free from its attachment to the cast.
Observe the color, temperature, and size of the fingers or toes on the extremity with the cast; compare with those on the opposite extremity.	Digits that are pink, warm, and of a similar size bilaterally suggest that there is an adequate distal blood supply.

(*continued*)

SKILL 25-3 Providing Basic Care of a Client with a Cast (*continued*)

Suggested Action	Reason for Action
Assess capillary refill in exposed fingers or toes (Fig. A); compare with the uncasted digits.	Color should reappear in 2–3 seconds as the capillaries refill following blanching; checking the opposite nail beds provides comparative data.

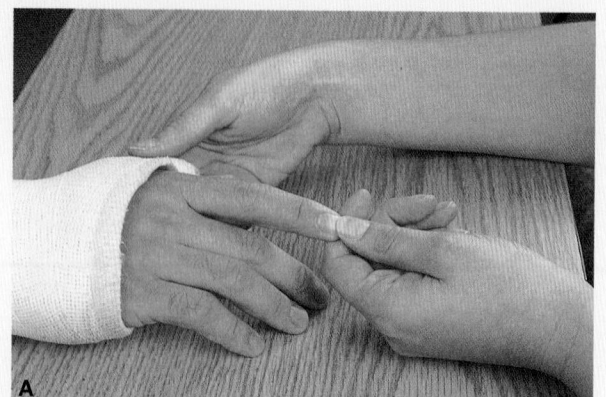

Assessing capillary refill (Photo by B. Proud.)

Suggested Action	Reason for Action
Elevate an extremity that appears swollen.	Elevation promotes the return of venous blood to the heart that may be trapped distally by a swelling extremity
Circle areas where blood has seeped through the cast; note the time on the cast. Recircle any expanding blood seepage and identify the time.	Helps in evaluating the significance of blood loss
Apply ice packs to the cast at the level of injury or where surgery has been performed if swelling is evident (Fig. B).	Cold is conducted through the skin causing vasoconstriction, which helps control swelling and bleeding.

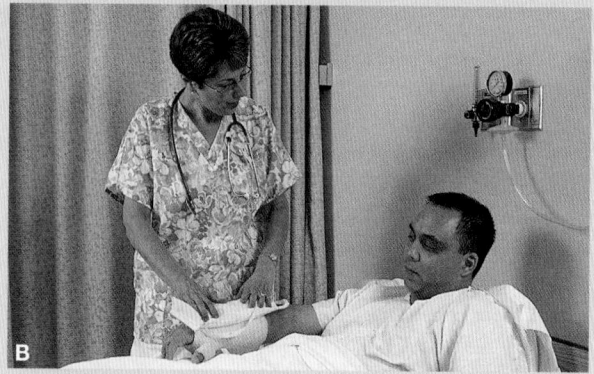

Applying an ice pack (Photo by B. Proud.)

Suggested Action	Reason for Action
Monitor the mobility of the fingers or toes (Fig. C).	The ability to move the fingers or toes upon request reflects intact neuromuscular status.

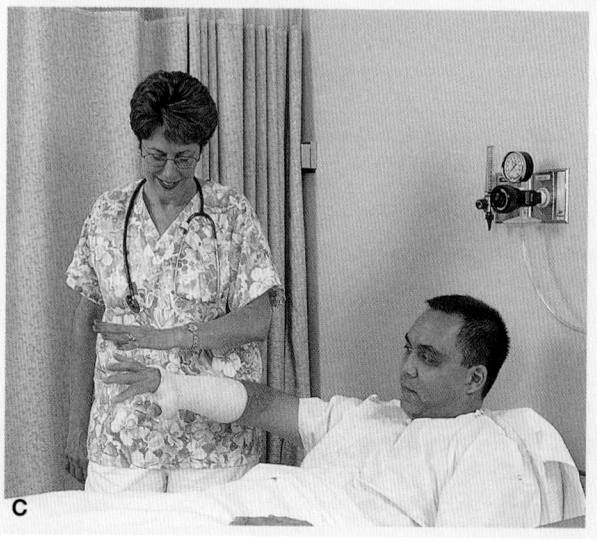

Checking mobility (Photo by B. Proud.)

SKILL 25-3 Providing Basic Care of a Client with a Cast (*continued*)

Suggested Action	Reason for Action
Assess sensation in exposed fingers or toes (Fig. D).	Ability to feel sensation indicates intact neurologic status

Assessing sensation in exposed fingers (Photo by B. Proud.)

Suggested Action	Reason for Action
Assess the presence and quality of pain in the area covered by the cast, especially if it is unrelieved by elevation, cold applications, and analgesic medication.	Unrelieved pain of increasing intensity suggests compartment syndrome, which is caused by pressure due to swelling within the inelastic fascia that surrounds muscles.
Report pain that escalates and does not respond to pain-relieving measures.	The pressure from compartment syndrome, if unrelieved, disrupts circulation and damages nerves, which may cause permanent disability.
Be aware of any foul odor or purulent drainage coming from within the cast.	Suggests possible infection
Encourage the client to exercise fingers or toes frequently.	Exercise helps increase circulation, decrease swelling, and prevent stiffness.
Swab remnants of plaster from the skin with a damp cloth; remove fiberglass resin from the skin with alcohol or acetone.	Water moistens plaster, allowing it to be removed; alcohol and acetone are chemical solvents.
Avoid getting a cast wet. If it becomes wet, dry the area using a blow dryer on a cool setting.	Water softens plaster and may saturate the padding next to the skin of both plaster and fiberglass casts. Prolonged dampness weakens plaster; damp padding can macerate the skin.
Ensure the edges of the cast are smooth and padded (Fig. E). Rough edges can be reinforced with petals made of tape or moleskin (see Nursing Guidelines 25-2).	Reduces the risk for skin irritation and breakdown

Soft cast edges minimize the risk for skin impairment. (Photo by B. Proud.)

Suggested Action	Reason for Action
Caution clients not to insert objects (e.g., straws, combs, utensils) within the cast.	Can impair skin integrity by causing abrasions or prolonged pressure if retained within the cast
Report itching, which may be treated with oral medication or by blowing cool air from a hair dryer down the cast.	Antipruritic medications relieve itching but may cause drowsiness. Cool blown air is not harmful and does not cause side effects.
Advise clients not to paint a fiberglass cast, but friends may write or draw on either type of cast.	Painting fiberglass interferes with its porosity.
Replace a **window**, a small square cut from a cast for the purpose of inspecting the skin or incision beneath a cast, by taping it back in place.	Prevents the skin from bulging into the open space, causing impaired skin and circulation in the area
Ambulate clients as soon as possible or have them exercise in bed.	Prevents complications from immobility

(continued)

SKILL 25-3 Providing Basic Care of a Client with a Cast (*continued*)

Suggested Action	Reason for Action

EVALUATION

- The cast is dry without any evidence of dents or cracks.
- The skin is warm and of appropriate color without evidence of swelling.
- Pain is absent or reduced using pain-relieving measures.
- The client is able to move fingers or toes and has normal sensory perception.
- The exposed skin at the cast edges is intact.
- There is no evidence of purulent drainage.

DOCUMENT

- Date, time, and results of assessments
- Measures used to relieve swelling or itching, if any occurred
- Level of pain, pain-relieving techniques, and outcomes following their use
- Skin care provided
- To whom abnormal findings were communicated, the content of the reported information, and the response of the caregiver receiving the information

SAMPLE DOCUMENTATION

Date and Time Long leg cast on left leg is dry and shiny, and elevated on two pillows. No evidence of dents or cracks in cast. Toes are pink, warm, and similar in size to those on the right. Capillary refill of toes on left is 2 seconds. Can move all toes and perceives being touched. Rates pain at a level 3 and refuses any pain-relieving measures. _____ J. Doe, LPN

SKILL 25-4 Caring for Clients in Traction

Suggested Action	Reason for Action
ASSESSMENT	
Check the medical orders to determine the type of traction and amount of weight that has been prescribed.	Integrates nursing activities with medical treatment
Note whether there is a trapeze attached to the overbed frame.	Facilitates mobility and self-care
Inspect the mechanical equipment used to apply traction.	Determines the status of the equipment
Check whether traction ropes move freely through the pulleys.	Fraying or knots in the traction ropes may interfere with the pull of traction.
Determine whether the weights are hanging free of the bed or floor.	Unobstructed and unsupported weights ensure the effectiveness of traction.
Observe the client's body position.	Effective traction occurs when the body part is positioned in an opposite line with the pull of the traction equipment.
Wash your hands or use an alcohol-based hand rub (see Chapter 10).	Removes transient microorganisms and reduces the transmission of pathogens
Inspect the skin and pin sites.	Pressure from traction equipment, immobility, and tissue compromised by skeletal pins predispose a client to impaired skin integrity and the risk of infection.
Assess the client's circulation and sensation in the area to which traction has been applied.	Neurovascular complications can occur when a part of the body is immobilized.
Determine the client's last date of bowel elimination.	Immobility and use of a bedpan predispose the client to constipation and fecal impaction.
Note the frequency, volume, and color of urine.	Certain traction positions interfere with the complete emptying of the bladder; urinary stasis predisposes the client to stone formation and bladder infection.
Auscultate the client's lungs.	Immobilized clients tend to breathe shallowly, creating a risk for pneumonia.
Review the trend in the client's temperature.	Elevation in body temperature suggestive of infection
Assess the client's level of pain or discomfort.	Determines need for pain relief measures
Observe the client's emotional state.	Prolonged confinement, immobilization, and decreased sensory stimulation place the client at risk for boredom, depression, and loneliness.

SKILL 25-4 Caring for Clients in Traction (*continued*)

Suggested Action	Reason for Action
PLANNING	
Explain the purpose of the traction and the care that will follow.	Adds to the client's understanding
IMPLEMENTATION	
Keep the traction applied continuously unless there are medical orders to the contrary.	Fosters the achievement of desired outcomes
Raise the height of the bed to ensure the weights hang above the floor.	Provides the musculoskeletal pull in traction
Limit the client's positions to those indicated in the medical orders or standards for care.	Positions that alter the pull and counterpull of traction interfere with therapy.
Provide for the client's hygiene and oral needs, encouraging as much self-care as possible.	Promotes client independence
Bathe the backs of clients who must remain in a supine or other back-lying position by depressing the mattress enough to insert a hand.	Facilitates skin care and hygiene
Remove and apply bottom bed linen from the foot of the bed rather than turning the client from side to side.	Maintains body alignment
Avoid tucking top sheets, blankets, or bedspread beneath the mattress.	Can interfere with the pull of traction equipment
Do not use a pillow if the client's head or neck is in traction unless medical orders indicate otherwise.	Can disturb the line of pull and counterpull
Use pressure-relieving devices (see Chapters 23 and 28) and a regimen of frequent conscientious skin care if the client is confined to bed for a prolonged time.	Prevents impaired skin integrity
Insert padding within slings if they tend to wrinkle.	Helps cushion and distribute pressure, prevents interference with circulation, and reduces the risk for skin breakdown
Cleanse the skin around a skeletal pin insertion using an antimicrobial agent (see Skill 25-5).	Reduces the risk of infection
Cover the tips of protruding metal pins or other sharp traction devices with corks or other protective material.	Prevents accidental injury
Use a small bedpan, called a "fracture pan," if elevating the hips alters the line of pull.	Ensures alignment and maintains the effectiveness of traction
Encourage isometric, isotonic, and active range-of-motion exercises.	Maintains the tone, strength, and flexibility of the musculoskeletal system
Provide diversional activities as often as possible.	Relieves boredom and sensory deprivation

EVALUATION

- The type of traction and amount of traction weight correlate with the medical orders.
- The weights hang freely above the floor.
- There are no knots in the traction rope close to the pulleys.
- The traction ropes are intact and move freely through the pulleys.
- The client lies in the center of the bed in proper alignment with the pull of the traction.
- There is a trapeze within reach of the client.
- Physical assessment data are normal.
- Hygiene is accomplished on a regular basis.

DOCUMENT

- Date and time of care
- Type of traction and location of application
- Amount of weight currently applied
- Results of physical assessment
- To whom abnormal findings were reported and changes recommended as a result of the report

SAMPLE DOCUMENTATION

Date and Time Buck skin traction applied to left leg with 5 lb of weight attached. Ropes move freely through pulleys and weights hang freely off the floor. Client in supine position with left leg aligned with pull of traction. Peripheral pulses are present and strong in both extremities; capillary refill is less than 2–3 seconds in toes on the left, the toes on the left are warm and move when instructed to do so, sensation in left foot is normal. Skin remains intact and free of redness. Eliminating stool and urine regularly. Lung sounds are clear upon auscultation. Pain rated at 2 which is within a tolerable range. Mood is appropriate for situation. _____ J. Doe, LPN

SKILL 25-5 Providing Pin Site Care

Suggested Action	Reason for Action
ASSESSMENT	
Check the medical orders or standards for care regarding the frequency of pin site care and the preferred cleansing agent.	Demonstrates collaboration with the medical treatment
Review the medical record for trends in the client's temperature, white blood cell count, reports of pain, and frequency for treating pain.	Uses data that reflect indications of infection
Inspect the area around the pin insertion site for redness, swelling, increased tenderness, and drainage.	Provides data for current and future comparisons
Examine the pin for signs of bending or shifting.	Identifies potential problems with maintaining traction and desired position
PLANNING	
Explain the purpose and technique for pin site care to the client.	Adds to the client's understanding
Assemble gloves, the prescribed cleansing agent (usually sterile normal saline, hydrogen peroxide, or povidone iodine), and sterile cotton-tipped applicators. Sometimes presaturated swabs are used.	Contributes to organization and efficient time management
Place the bed at a comfortable height.	Prevents back strain
IMPLEMENTATION	
Wash your hands or use an alcohol-based hand rub (see Chapter 10).	Removes transient microorganisms and reduces the transmission of pathogens
Put on gloves; clean gloves can be used to hold the stick end of the applicator.	Prevents skin contact with blood or body fluid
Open the package containing cotton-tipped applicators without touching the applicator tips.	Avoids contaminating the point of contact between the applicator tip and the client's skin
Pour enough cleansing agent to saturate the dry applicators while holding them over a basin or wastebasket.	Prepares applicators for use while maintaining the sterility of the applicator tip
Cleanse the skin at the pin site moving outward in a circular manner (see figure).	Prevents moving microorganisms toward the area of open skin

Providing pin site care

Gently remove crusted secretions.	Removes debris that supports the growth of microorganisms
Use a separate applicator for each pin site or if the site needs more than one circular swipe for additional cleansing.	Prevents reintroducing microorganisms into cleaned areas
Avoid applying ointment to pin sites unless prescribed.	Reduces retained moisture at the site and occludes drainage, both of which increase the risk for microbial growth
Check with the physician or infection control policy about obtaining a wound culture if *purulent drainage* (that which contains pus) is present.	Aids in determining the identity of pathogenic microorganisms and the need to institute infection control measures, such as contact precautions (see Chapter 22)
Teach the client to not touch the pin sites.	Prevents introducing transient and resident microorganisms into the wound

SKILL 25-5 Providing Pin Site Care (*continued*)

Suggested Action	Reason for Action
Discard soiled supplies in an enclosed, lined container; remove gloves; and wash hands or use an alcohol-based hand rub.	Demonstrates the principles of medical asepsis (see Chapter 10)

EVALUATION

- The skin and tissue around the pin site are free of redness, swelling, or pain.
- There is no evidence of purulent drainage.
- The client's temperature and white blood cell count are within normal ranges.

DOCUMENT

- Date, time, and location of pin site care
- Type of cleansing agent
- Appearance of the pin site and the client's subjective remarks regarding the presence of tenderness or pain
- Collection of a wound specimen for a culture test, if ordered, and time of its delivery to the laboratory
- Person to whom abnormal findings were communicated, the content of the reported information, and the response of the caregiver receiving the information

SAMPLE DOCUMENTATION

Date and Time Pin sites on medial and lateral sides of L thigh cleansed with povidone iodine. Sites appear dry and without evidence of inflammation. No complaints of pain or discomfort. _____ J. Doe, LPN

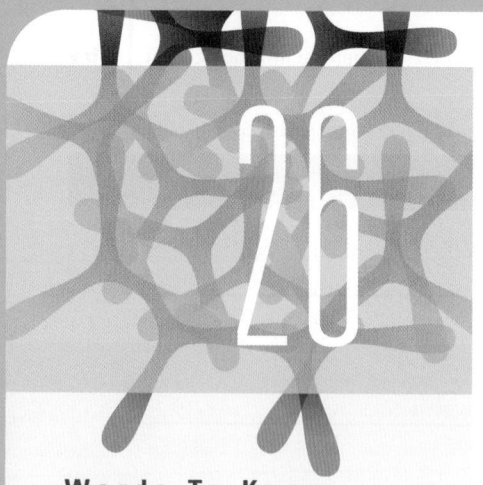

Ambulatory Aids

Learning Objectives

On completion of this chapter, the reader should be able to:

1. Name activities that prepare clients for ambulation.
2. Give examples of isometric exercises that tone and strengthen lower extremities.
3. Identify techniques for building upper arm strength.
4. Explain the reason for dangling clients or using a tilt table.
5. Name devices used to assist clients with ambulation.
6. Give examples of ambulatory aids.
7. Identify the most stable type of ambulatory aid.
8. Describe characteristics of appropriately fitted crutches.
9. Name types of crutch-walking gaits.
10. Explain the purpose of a temporary prosthetic limb.
11. Name four components of above-the-knee and below-the-knee prosthetic limbs.
12. Describe how a prosthetic limb is applied.
13. Discuss age-related changes that affect the gait and ambulation of older adults.

INTRODUCTION

Clients with disorders of or injuries to the musculoskeletal system and those who are weak or unsteady because of age-related or neurologic problems may have difficulty walking. This chapter provides information on nursing activities and devices used to promote or enhance mobility.

 Gerontologic Considerations

■ Maintaining independence is important to the older person. Mobility facilitates staying active and independent.

■ An older adult's self-perception is often linked to functional ability. Functional ability involves both mobility and making adaptations to compensate for changes that are associated with aging or disease processes. Older people may need encouragement and support to integrate adaptations for mobility to maintain their activities of daily living.

■ An elevated toilet seat and grab bars may be needed to improve an older adult's ability to transfer safely and to maintain independence.

■ A walking or gait belt can be used to assist an older person with transferring, even if the client is not ambulatory. Instruct the older client to balance on their stronger extremity while being supported with the gait belt. The client should never be forced to walk if unable.

■ Limited or unsteady mobility may be a problem for some older adults as a result of pathologic conditions or age-related postural changes. It may lead to the development of a swaying or shuffling gait.

- As a person ages, they may develop flexion of the spine, which can alter the center of gravity and may result in an increased risk for falls.

- If a client appears to have an unusual gait, assess the feet for corns, calluses, bunions, and ingrown or long toenails. If any of these conditions are found, a podiatry referral may be indicated. Vascular changes may lead to numbness and a decreased sensory ability to perceive contact with the ground, which can also change a person's gait.

- Older adults sometimes use a "step–stop" pattern when using an ambulatory aid; that is, they take one step, then stop, and repeat again. If that is the case, encourage a smooth, progressive cadence.

- Some older adults develop the habit of picking up and carrying a walker rather than having it make contact with the floor. In these situations, the person may benefit from another type of walker such as a walker with wheels or a three-wheeled walker. A physical therapist can assess the situation and recommend an appropriate walker.

- Rubber tips and handgrips on ambulatory aids should be kept clean and replaced when they are worn. Worn or dirty tips and handgrips contribute to falls and unsafe mobility.

- Before discharging an older person who will be using a mobility device, advise the family to make the home safer by removing scatter rugs and ensuring that lighting is adequate and that no electric cords are in passageways. Furniture may have to be rearranged and railings or grab bars may need to be added to bathrooms and outside entrances.

- A ramp with a handrail helps older adults enter and leave their residence more conveniently and safely when they are using an ambulatory aid.

- Older adults who have difficulty going up and down stairs may consider rearranging their homes so all necessary furnishings are on one level. A bedside commode decreases the number of trips up and down stairs if the bathroom is not on the same level as the bedroom or living area.

PREPARING FOR AMBULATION

Debilitated clients (those who are frail or weak from prolonged inactivity) require physical conditioning before they can ambulate again. Some techniques for increasing muscular strength and the ability to bear weight include performing isometric exercises with the lower limbs, performing isotonic exercises with the upper arms, dangling at the bedside, and using a device called a tilt table.

Isometric Exercises

Isometric exercises (see Chapter 24) are used to promote muscle tone and strength. **Tone** means the ability of muscles to respond when stimulated; **strength** means the power to perform. Both tone and strength are inherent in maintaining mobility. Frequent contraction of muscle fibers retains or improves muscle tone and strength. Active people maintain these two qualities through everyday activities, but inactive people and those who have been immobilized in casts or traction may require focused periods of exercise to reestablish their previous ability to walk.

Client and Family Teaching 26-1
Quadriceps and Gluteal Setting Exercises

The nurse teaches the client and the family as follows:

- Tighten (contract) the quadriceps muscles by flattening the backs of the knees into the mattress. If that is not possible, place a rolled towel under the knee or heel before attempting to tighten the quadriceps muscles.
- Check to see that the kneecaps move upward. This is an indication that the client is performing the exercise correctly.
- Hold the contracted position for a count of five.
- Relax and repeat two or three times each hour.
- Tighten (contract) the gluteal muscles by clenching the cheeks of the buttocks together.
- Hold the contracted position for a count of five.
- Relax and repeat two or three times each hour.

Quadriceps setting and gluteal setting exercises are two types of isometric exercises that promote tone and strength in weight-bearing muscles. Both types are easily performed in bed or in a chair. They are initiated long before the anticipated time when ambulation will start. Most clients can perform these exercises independently once they have been instructed (Client and Family Teaching 26-1).

Quadriceps Setting
Quadriceps setting is an isometric exercise in which the client alternately tenses and relaxes the quadriceps muscles. This type of exercise is sometimes referred to as "quad setting." The quadriceps muscles (rectus femoris, vastus intermedius, vastus medialis, and vastus lateralis) cover the front and side of the thigh. Together they aid in extending the leg. Exercising the quadriceps muscles, therefore, enables clients to stand and support their body weight.

Gluteal Setting
Gluteal setting is the contraction and relaxation of the gluteal muscles (gluteus maximus, gluteus medius, and gluteus minimus) to improve their strength and tone. As a group, the muscles in the buttocks aid in extending, abducting, and rotating the leg—functions that are essential to walking.

Upper Arm Strengthening
Clients who will use a walker, cane, or crutches also need upper arm strength. An exercise regimen to strengthen the upper arms typically includes flexion and extension of the arms and wrists, raising and lowering weights with the hands, squeezing a ball or spring grip, and performing modified hand push-ups in bed.

Clients perform modified push-ups (exercises that support the upper body on the hands and arms) in several ways, depending on age and condition. While sitting in bed, a client may lift the hips off the bed by pushing down on the mattress with the hands (Fig. 26-1). If the mattress is soft, the nurse places a block or books on the bed under the client's

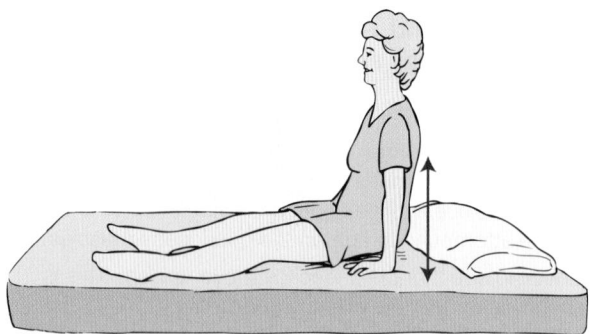

FIGURE 26-1 Modified hand push-ups are performed by extending the elbows and flexing the wrists to lift the buttocks slightly off the mattress.

hands. If a sturdy armchair is available, the client can raise their body from the seat while pushing on the armrests.

If the client can lie on the abdomen, they perform push-ups in the following sequence:

1. Flex the elbows.
2. Place the hands palms down at approximately shoulder level.
3. Straighten the elbows to lift the head and chest off the bed (Fig. 26-2).

For effectiveness, clients must perform push-ups three or four times a day.

Dangling

Dangling (sitting on the edge of the bed; Fig. 26-3) helps normalize blood pressure, which may drop when the client rises from a reclining position (see the section on postural hypotension in Chapter 12; see Nursing Guidelines 26-1).

Using a Tilt Table

A **tilt table** is a device that raises the client from a supine to a standing position (Fig. 26-4). It helps clients adjust to being upright and bearing weight on their feet. Although the tilt table is usually located in the physical therapy department, nurses often prepare the client for this type of preambulation therapy and communicate with the therapists about the client's response.

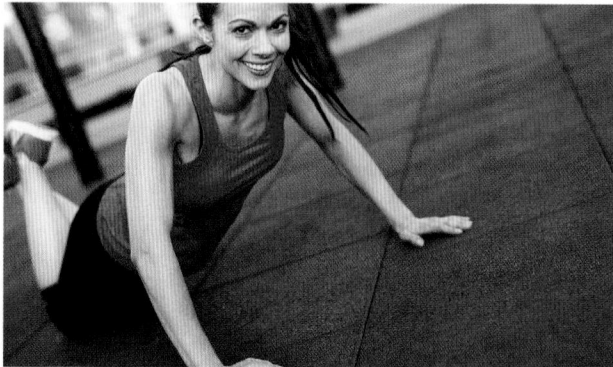

FIGURE 26-2 Push-ups in a prone position. (Ground Picture/Shutterstock.)

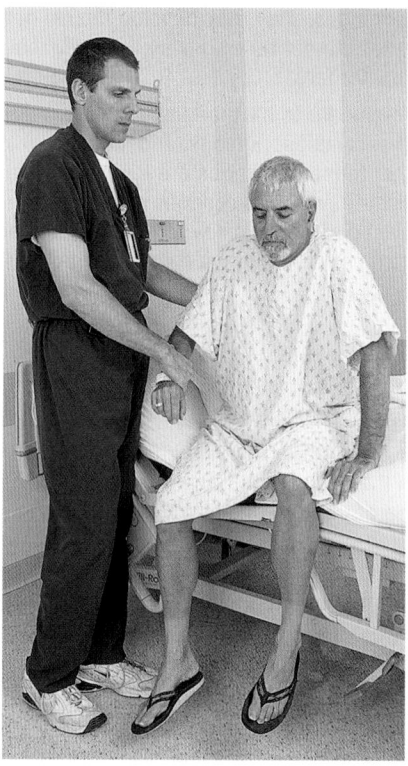

FIGURE 26-3 Dangling. (Photo by B. Proud.)

Just before using a tilt table, the nurse applies elastic stockings (see the section on antiembolism stockings in Chapter 27). These stockings help compress vein walls, thus preventing the pooling of blood in the extremities, which may trigger fainting. After being transferred from the bed or stretcher to the horizontal tilt table, the client is strapped securely to prevent a fall. The feet are positioned against the foot rest. The entire table is then tilted in increments of 15 to 30 degrees until the client is in a vertical position.

 NURSING GUIDELINES 26-1

Assisting Clients to Dangle

- Perform dangling before ambulating whenever a client has been inactive for an extended period. *Performing dangling before ambulating demonstrates concern for the client's safety.*
- Place the client in a Fowler position for a few minutes. *This position maintains safety should the client become dizzy or faint.*
- Lower the height of the bed. *With a lowered bed, the client can use the floor for support.*
- Provide a foot stool if the client's feet do not reach the floor. *A foot stool is an alternative for supporting the feet.*
- Fold back the top linen. *Linen can interfere with movement.*
- Provide the client with a robe and slippers. *Doing so maintains warmth and shows respect for the client's modesty.*
- Help the client pivot a quarter of a turn to swing the legs over the side and sit on the edge of the bed. *This position helps the client adjust to the sitting position.*
- Stay with the client until they no longer feel dizzy or lightheaded. *The nurse can provide immediate assistance.*

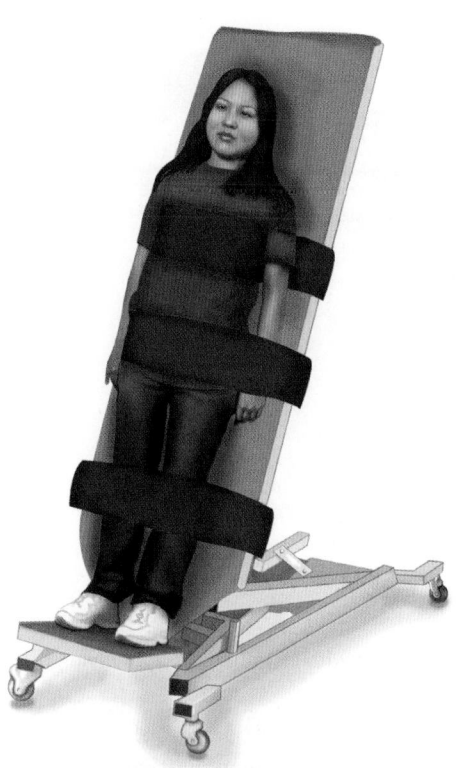

FIGURE 26-4 A tilt table.

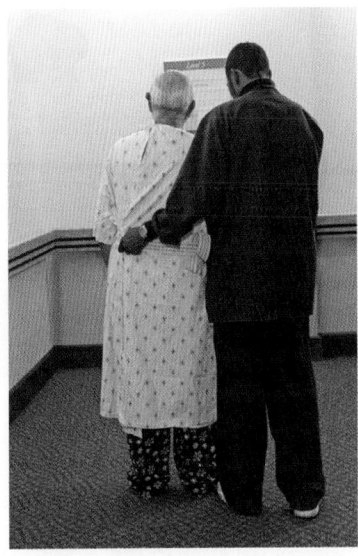

FIGURE 26-5 Supporting the client with a walking belt. (From Lynn, P. [2022]. *Taylor's Handbook of clinical nursing skills* [6th ed.]. Lippincott Williams & Wilkins.)

If symptoms such as dizziness and hypotension develop, the table is lowered or returned to the horizontal position.

AMBULATORY ASSISTIVE DEVICES

Some clients still need assistance in ambulating independently even after performing strengthening exercises. Two devices used to provide support and assistance with walking are a walking belt, which is also known as a gait belt, and parallel bars.

A **walking belt** is applied around the client's waist. If the client loses balance, the nurse can support them and prevent injuries. When assisting a client with ambulating, the nurse walks slightly behind the client, holding the walking belt or the client's own belt and supporting the client's arm (Fig. 26-5).

Clients use **parallel bars** (a double row of stationary bars) as handrails to gain practice in ambulating. Sometimes a tilt table is positioned just in front of the parallel bars so that the client can progress from being upright to actually walking again (Fig. 26-6).

The nurse observes the ambulating client for pallor, weakness, or dizziness. If fainting seems likely, the nurse supports the client by sliding an arm under the axilla and placing a foot to the side, forming a wide base of support.

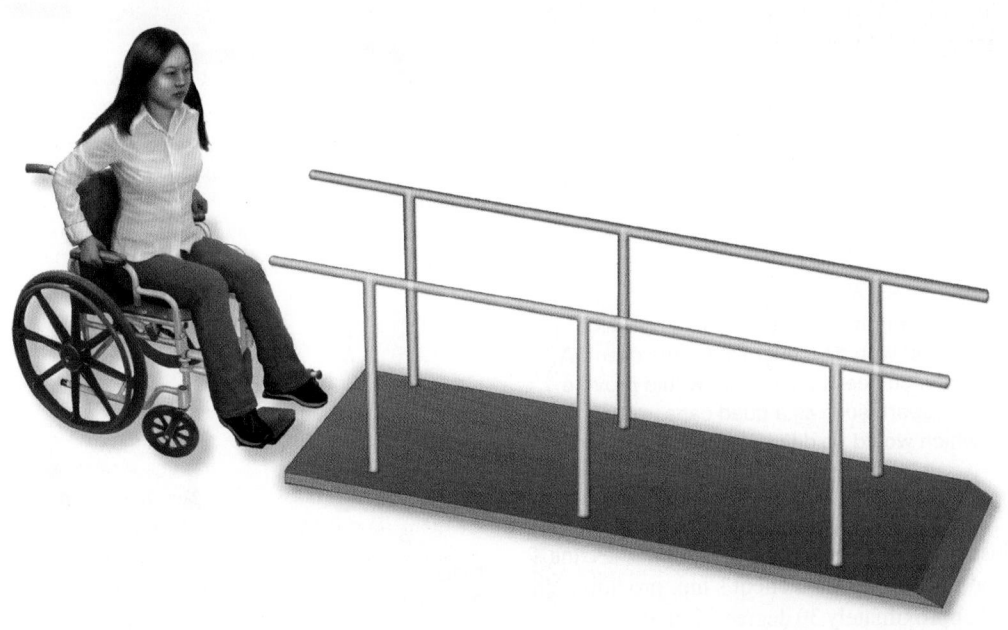

FIGURE 26-6 Parallel bars.

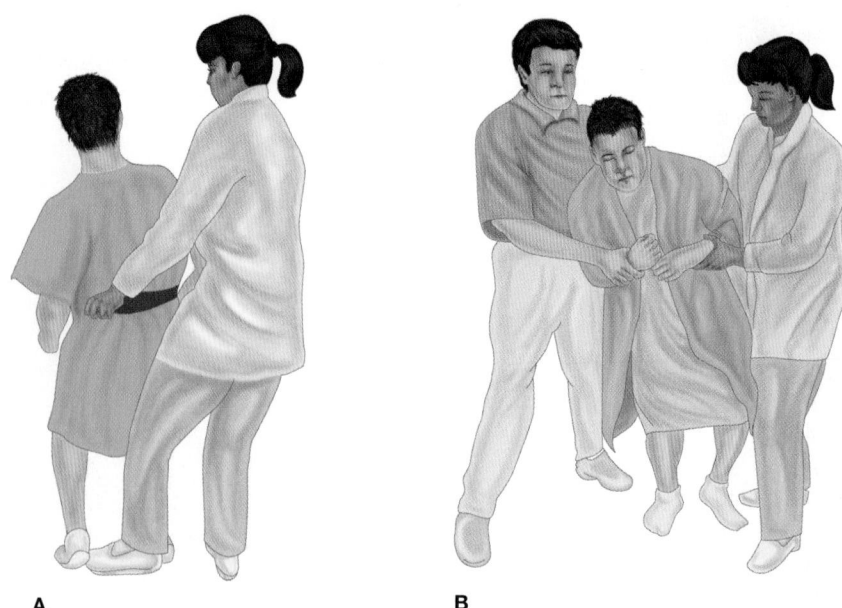

FIGURE 26-7 A. One nurse guides a client to the floor. **B.** A client is lowered to the floor with two nurses. (From Taylor, C., Lynn, P., & Bartlett, J. [2018]. *Fundamentals of nursing* [9th ed.]. Lippincott Williams & Wilkins.)

With the client's weight braced, the nurse balances the client on a hip until help arrives or slides the client down the length of the nurse's leg to the floor (Fig. 26-7).

AMBULATORY AIDS

Three aids are used to help with ambulation: canes, walkers, and crutches.

Canes

A client who has weakness on one side of the body uses a **cane**, a handheld ambulation device made of wood or aluminum. Aluminum canes are more common. Canes have rubber tips to reduce the potential for slipping.

Clients may use different types of canes depending on their physical deficits. For clients who need minimal support, a cane with a half-circle handle is appropriate. A T-handle cane has a handgrip with a slightly bent shaft, offering the user more stability. A quad cane has four supports at the base and provides even more stability than the other types (Fig. 26-8).

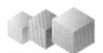 Concept Mastery Alert

Choosing an Ambulatory Aid
Consider the client's condition when determining which type of ambulatory aid would be the best for the client. A client with poor balance needs an aid that would provide a strong base of support, such as a quad cane, rather than crutches, which would be difficult to maneuver and control.

A cane must be the right height for the client. The cane's handle should be parallel with the client's hip, providing an elbow flexion of approximately 30 degrees. Removing a portion of the lower end can shorten wooden canes. Depressing

metal buttons in the telescoping shaft can shorten or lengthen aluminum canes (Client and Family Teaching 26-2).

When clients begin to use a cane, the nurse assists by applying a walking belt and standing toward the back of the client's stronger side (Fig. 26-9).

Walkers

Clients who require considerable support and assistance with balance use a **walker**, the most stable form of ambulatory aid. Examples of clients who commonly use walkers are those beginning to ambulate after prolonged bed rest or after hip surgery.

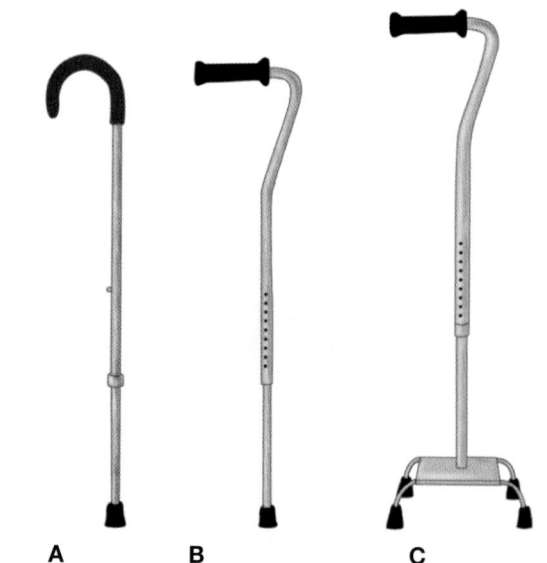

FIGURE 26-8 Three types of canes. **A.** Standard cane. **B.** Functional cane. **C.** Quad cane. (From Kronenberger, J., & Woodson, D. [2016]. *Lippincott Williams & Wilkins' clinical medical assisting* [5th ed.]. Lippincott Williams & Wilkins.)

Client and Family Teaching 26-2
Using a Cane

The nurse teaches the client and the family as follows:

- Place the cane on the stronger side of the body.
- Stand upright with the cane 4 to 6 in (10 to 15 cm) to the side of the toes (Fig. A).
- Move the cane forward at the same time as the weaker extremity.
- Take the next step with the stronger extremity.
- When using stairs:
  - Use a stair rail rather than the cane when going up or down stairs if possible (Fig. B).
  - Take each step up with the stronger leg followed by the weaker one. Reverse the pattern for descending the stairs.
  - If there is no stair rail, advance the cane just before rising or descending with the weaker leg.
- When sitting:
  - Back up to the chair until the seat is against the back of the legs (Fig. C).
  - Rest the cane close by.
  - Grip the armrests with both hands.
  - Sit down.
- When getting up from a chair:
  - Grip the armrest while holding the cane in the stronger hand.
  - Advance the stronger leg.

- Lean forward.
- Push with both arms against the armrests.
- Stand until balanced and any symptoms of dizziness pass.

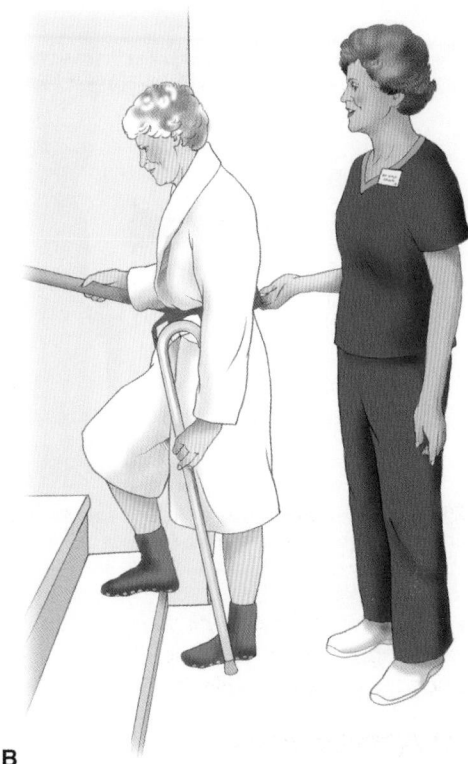

B

(From *Lippincott's procedures.* [2022]. Lippincott Williams & Wilkins.)

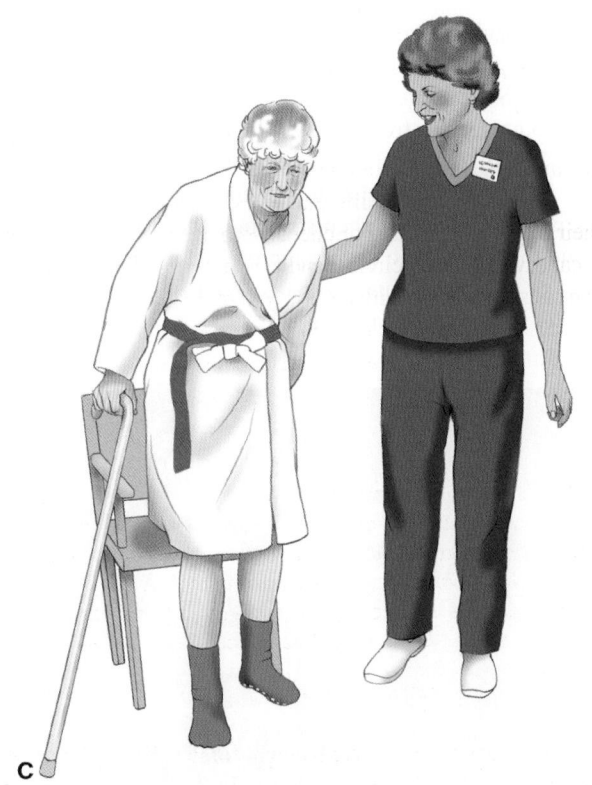

C

(From *Lippincott's nursing procedures and skills.* [2022]. Lippincott Williams & Wilkins.)

A

(Roman Samborskyi/Shutterstock)

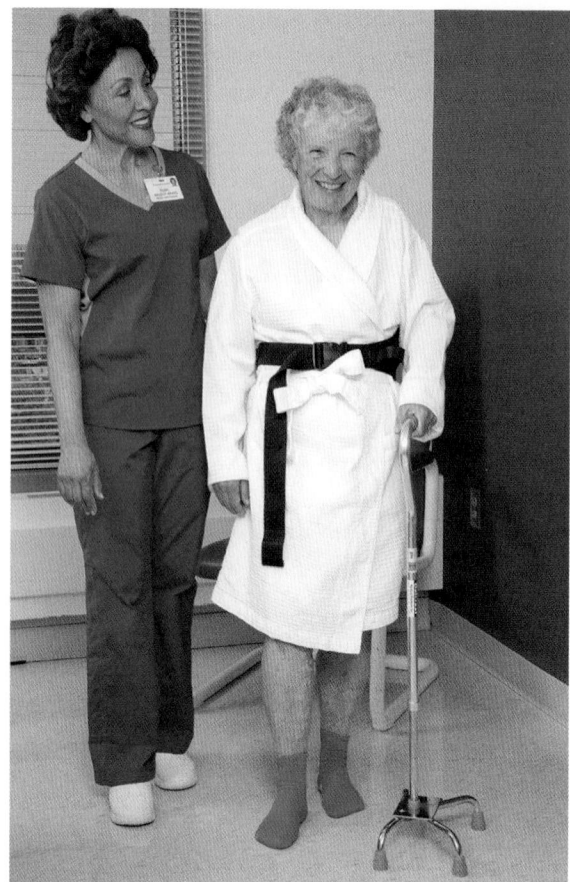

FIGURE 26-9 Assisting a client with a cane. (From *Lippincott procedures* [9th ed.]. [2022]. Lippincott Williams & Wilkins.)

Standard walkers are constructed of curved aluminum bars that form a three-sided enclosure with four legs for support. Some have legs that must be advanced with each step; others have front wheels and may also have a seat (Fig. 26-10). Optional attachments for walkers include baskets and hanging pouches that clients can use when carrying personal items or when shopping. Other adaptations are made for clients who have compromised use of one or both arms or those who must use stairs. The height of a walker as well as a cane is adjustable.

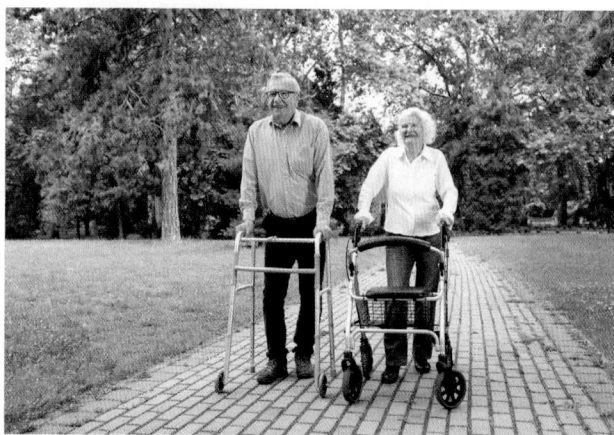

FIGURE 26-10 Two types of walkers, left to right: pick-up walker; rolling walker on wheels. (didesign021/Shutterstock.)

Nurses instruct clients who use a walker without wheels to:

- Stand within the walker.
- Hold on to the walker at the padded handgrips.
- Pick up the walker and advance it 6 to 8 in (15 to 20 cm).
- Take a step forward.
- Support the body weight on the handgrips when moving the weaker leg (for clients with partial or non–weight-bearing on one leg).

When the client with a walker wants to sit down, the technique is similar to that with a cane, with one exception. When the legs are at the front of the chair seat, the client grips an armrest with one arm while placing the other hand on the walker and using the stronger leg for support. The client releases the grip on the walker while using the free hand to grasp the opposite armrest and lowers themselves into the chair. To rise, the client moves to the edge of the chair and repositions the walker. After pushing up on the armrests with both arms until the body weight is centered, the client uses one hand, then the other to grasp the walker.

Crutches

Crutches, an ambulatory aid generally used in pairs, are constructed of wood or aluminum. Because the use of crutches requires a great deal of upper arm strength and balance, older adults or weak clients do not commonly use them.

The three basic types of crutches are axillary, forearm, and platform (Fig. 26-11). The most familiar type is **axillary crutches** (the standard type of crutches) that have a bar which, when used, allows a two-finger space beneath the axilla (Fig. 26-12).

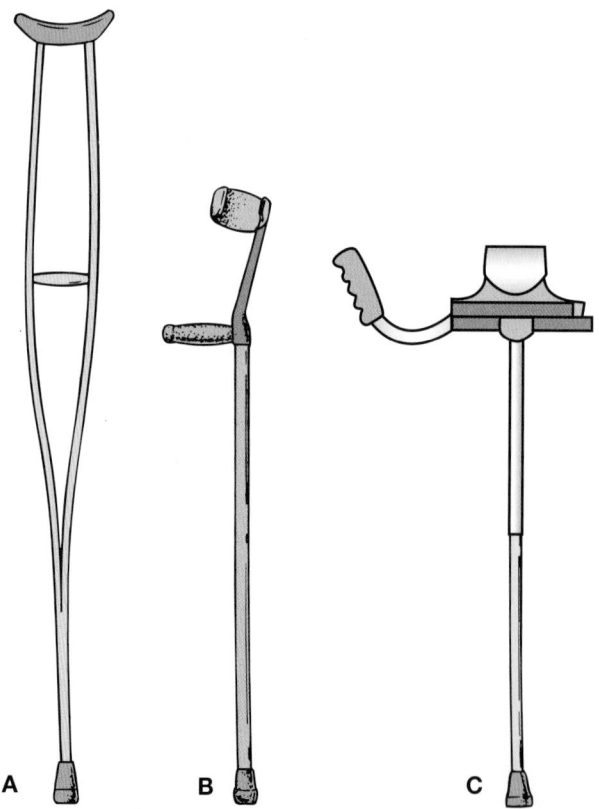

A   B   C

FIGURE 26-11 Three types of crutches: axillary (**A**), forearm (**B**), and platform (**C**).

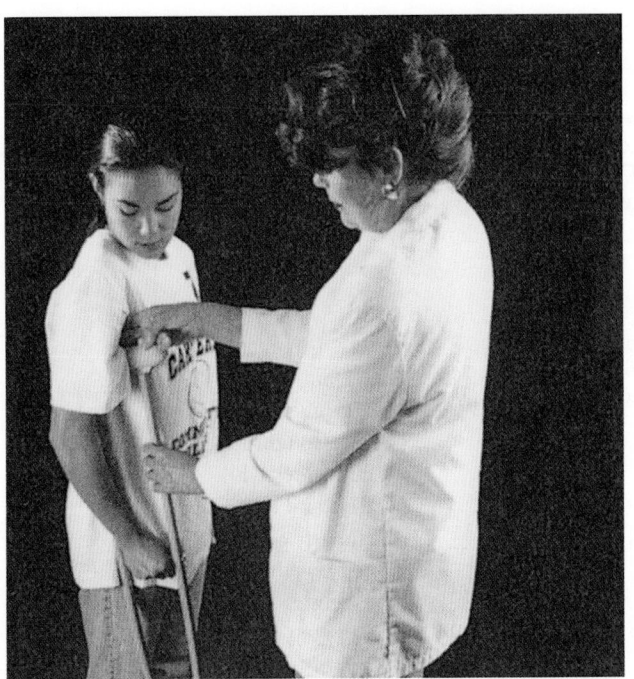

FIGURE 26-12 There must be room for two fingers between the axilla and the crutch bar to prevent nerve damage. (Hinkle, J. L., & Cheever, J. H. [2014]. *Brunner & Suddarth's textbook of medical-surgical nursing* [13th ed.]. Lippincott Williams & Wilkins.)

Clients who need brief, temporary assistance with ambulation are likely to use axillary crutches. Lofstrand and Canadian crutches are examples of **forearm crutches**; they have an arm cuff but no axillary bar. Forearm crutches are generally used by experienced clients who need permanent assistance with walking. **Platform crutches** (crutches that support the forearm) are used by clients who cannot bear weight with their hands and wrists. Many clients with arthritis use them. Sometimes a client uses one axillary crutch and one platform crutch—for example, when one arm is broken.

Once the type of ambulatory aid is medically prescribed, the client is measured (Skill 26-1).

Crutch-Walking Gaits

The term *gait* refers to one's manner of walking. A crutch-walking gait is the walking pattern used when ambulating with crutches; clients use some of the same gaits with walkers or canes.

The four types of crutch-walking gaits are the four-point gait, the three-point gait (non–weight-bearing or partial weight-bearing), the two-point gait, and the swing-through gait (Table 26-1). The word *point* refers to the sum of the crutches and legs used when performing the gait. Nurses are responsible for assisting clients who are learning to walk with crutches (Skill 26-2).

TABLE 26-1 Crutch-Walking Gaits

GAIT	INDICATIONS FOR USE	GAIT PATTERN	ILLUSTRATION
Four point	Bilateral weakness or disability such as arthritis or cerebral palsy	One crutch, opposite foot, other crutch, remaining foot	
Two point	Same as for four point, but clients have more strength, coordination, and balance	One crutch and opposite foot moved in unison followed by the remaining pair	
Three-point non–weight-bearing	One amputated, injured, or disabled extremity (fractured leg or severe ankle sprain)	Both crutches move forward followed by the weight-bearing leg	

(continued)

TABLE 26-1 Crutch-Walking Gaits (*continued*)

GAIT	INDICATIONS FOR USE	GAIT PATTERN	ILLUSTRATION
Three-point partial weight-bearing	Client with an amputation learning to use prosthesis, minor injury to one leg, or previous injury showing signs of healing	Both crutches are advanced with the weaker leg; the stronger leg is placed parallel to the weaker leg	
Swing-through	Injury or disorder affecting one or both legs, such as a paralyzed client with leg braces or an client with an amputation before being fitted with a prosthesis	Both crutches are moved forward; one or both legs are advanced beyond the crutches	

>>> Stop, Think, and Respond 26-1

What negative consequences can occur when a client uses ambulatory aids?

PROSTHETIC LIMBS

Some clients with leg amputations ambulate using a **prosthetic limb** (a substitute for an arm or leg) without the assistance of crutches or other ambulatory aids. The design of a prosthetic limb varies depending on whether the lower extremity is amputated at the foot (Syme amputation), a below-the-knee (BK) amputation, a disarticulation at the knee, an above-the-knee (AK) amputation, or the entire leg and a portion of the hip (hemipelvectomy) are removed.

There are currently a few different options for prosthetics, for use in either upper or lower body limbs.

- Passive prosthetic: designed to look like the natural limb, these prostheses are lightweight and while they do not have active movement, they may improve a person's function
- Body-powered prosthesis: operated by a system of cables, harnesses, and sometimes manual control
- Electrically powered prosthetic: includes motors and batteries that provide movement and power to the prosthesis
- Hybrid prosthesis: combines body-powered and electrically powered components in one prosthesis
- Activity-specific prosthesis: designed for an activity in which a residual limb with no prosthesis, or passive, body-powered, or electrically powered prostheses, could be damaged or simply won't work as needed for the specific activities (Arm Dynamics, 2024)

Temporary Prosthetic Limb

In many cases, clients return from surgery with an immediate postoperative prosthesis (IPOP), which is a temporary artificial limb. It consists of a walking pylon, a lightweight tube, attached to a shell made of plaster or plastic on the residual limb, and a rigid foot (Fig. 26-13). A belt with garters keeps the temporary prosthesis in place. The belt is loosened while the client is in bed and is tightened during ambulation. Some IPOPs are attached to the residual limb with a pneumatic air bag or with a clamshell design, which permits removal when the client is not ambulating. An IPOP facilitates early ambulation and promotes an intact body image immediately after surgery. It also helps control residual limb swelling.

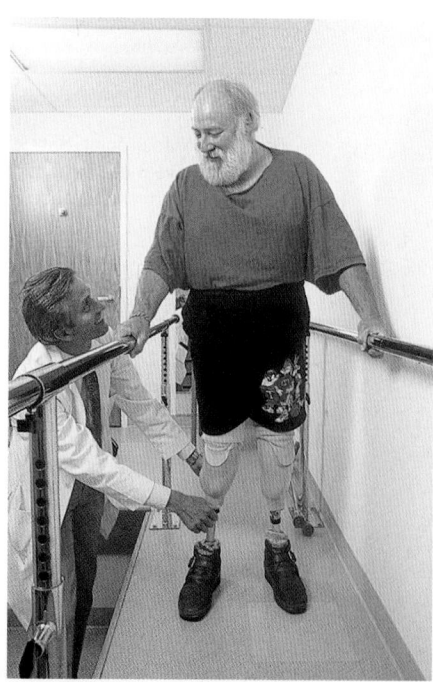

FIGURE 26-13 Many people with amputations receive prostheses soon after surgery and begin learning to use them with the support of the rehabilitation team.

The nurse is responsible for ensuring that the incision heals and that no complications, such as joint contractures or infection, develop. Complications delay rehabilitation. Contractures interfere with limb and prosthetic alignment, which ultimately affects the client's ability to walk.

Permanent Prosthetic Components

Construction of a permanent prosthesis is delayed for several weeks or months until the wound heals and the residual limb size is relatively stable. The permanent prosthesis is custom-made to conform to the residual limb and to meet the client's needs.

Permanent prostheses for clients with BK amputations include a socket, a shank, and an ankle/foot system. AK prostheses also include a knee system to replace the knee joint. The socket, a molded cone, holds the residual limb and enables the amputee to move the prosthesis. It is held in place by suction or by a leather belt, also referred to as a sling. Many clients wear one or more socks over the residual limb as a layer between the skin and the socket. Residual limb socks, made of wool or cotton, come in a variety of thicknesses to accommodate slight changes in residual limb size. Tube socks are not an appropriate substitute. Despite the expense, residual limb socks must be replaced whenever holes develop, or they become worn; a darned residual limb sock can cause skin breakdown as a result of friction within the socket. Some amputees also wear a nylon sheath beneath the residual limb sock to wick perspiration from the skin toward the sock and reduce friction on the skin.

For clients with AK amputations, the prosthetic knee system allows flexion and extension to accommodate sitting and a more natural gait while walking. The knee system connects the socket to the shank of the prosthesis (Fig. 26-14).

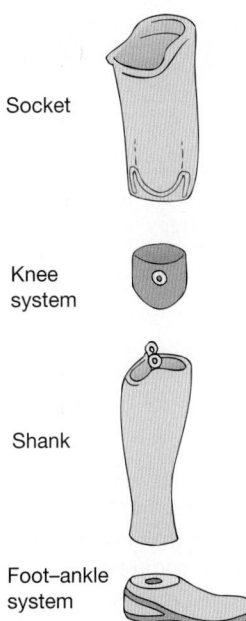

FIGURE 26-14 Components of a permanent prosthetic limb; a prosthesis for a BK amputation does not contain a knee system or a thigh socket.

The shank usually is shaped like a natural lower leg. It transfers the body weight to the walking surface. The shank is painted to resemble the client's skin color.

There are two basic types of ankle/foot systems: those that have one or more moving artificial joints (articulated systems) and those that do not. Although articulated systems allow more motion, the nonarticulated type has a cushion in the heel that permits compression during walking. The client wears a sock and shoe on the prosthetic foot. The client can vary their shoes, but all should be of similar height to ensure alignment of the prosthesis and a near-normal gait pattern.

Client Care

Nurses are responsible for managing the care of the residual limb and ensuring maintenance of the prosthesis (Skill 26-3).

Ambulation with a Lower Limb Prosthesis

Ambulation with a lower limb prosthesis requires strength and endurance. The more natural joints that are preserved, the more natural the gait appears and the more easily it is performed. To ensure as normal a gait as possible, clients learn to stand erect and look ahead when walking. They keep the feet slightly separated and take each step without hiking the hip unnaturally to swing the artificial limb forward. If using a cane, the client holds it in the hand opposite the prosthetic limb. When going up or down stairs, curbs, or hills, the client moves the unaffected leg first, followed by the one with the prosthesis.

People with amputations who wish to participate in strenuous activities such as skiing in the snow or running can use a sturdier modified prosthesis (Fig. 26-15).

NURSING IMPLICATIONS

Many nursing diagnoses are possible for clients who need to use an ambulatory aid. Applicable nursing diagnoses may include:

- Risk for activity intolerance
- Venous thromboembolism risk
- Perioperative positioning injury
- Deconditioning
- Fall risk

Nursing Care Plan 26-1 demonstrates how the nurse would devise a care plan for a client with the nursing diagnosis of activity intolerance, which is defined as the inability of an individual to perform or complete necessary activities due to insufficient physical or psychological energy. This may be due to recent surgery.

⟩⟩ Stop, Think, and Respond 26-2

Give some reasons why amputees may abandon rehabilitation and the use of a prosthesis; discuss how clients can overcome these impediments.

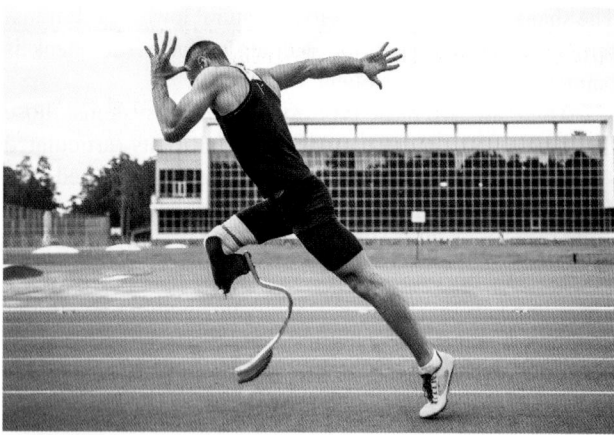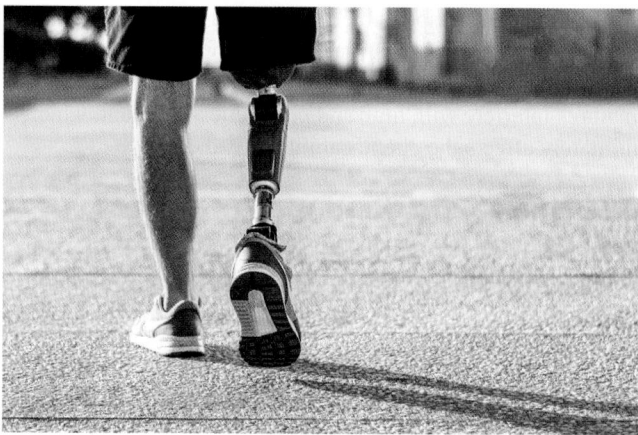

FIGURE 26-15 Different types of leg prostheses that allow the client to do more activities. (Left to right: 22Images Studio/Shutterstock; Real Sports Photos/Shutterstock.)

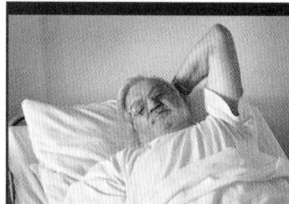

Clinical Scenario A 73-year-old male client has had a hip replacement to relieve pain and disability from osteoarthritis. He is anxious about upcoming physical therapy and resumption of his independent lifestyle.

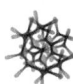

NURSING CARE PLAN 26-1 — Activity Intolerance

Assessment

- Assess motor strength and range of motion in both lower extremities.
- Observe the client's ability to turn themself, rise from a lying or sitting position, and move from one location to another.
- Watch the client walk, noting whether the client has a stable or unstable gait.
- Ask whether the client uses any type of ambulatory assistive device like crutches, cane, or walker.
- Inspect the client's lower extremities to determine whether the client wears a lower limb prosthesis or a mechanical brace.

- Review the client's health history for disorders that affect or impair mobility such as a previous stroke, joint disease like arthritis, or neurologic deficits that affect balance and coordination such as Parkinson disease.
- Gather information about the client's current use of prescription and nonprescription medications and research possible actions or side effects that can cause sedation, dizziness, and physical instability.

Nursing Diagnosis. Activity intolerance related to restricted positioning, limited weight-bearing, pain, and fear of ambulating as manifested by hip replacement surgery 3 days earlier, joint position of operative hip limited to extension, slight flexion, and continuous abduction, partial weight-bearing on operative leg with three-point gait following physical therapy instruction, and statement, "My hip hurts and I feel scared about walking."

Expected Outcome. The client will ambulate 6 ft with the assistance of a walker following physical therapy by the end of postoperative day 3.

Interventions	Rationales
Instruct and supervise the client to dorsiflex, plantar flex, and perform quad-setting exercises of both lower extremities every hour while awake.	Active exercise and range of motion promote joint flexibility and muscle tone.
Maintain abduction wedge between legs to keep knees apart at all times while in bed.	Maintaining abduction prevents the hip prosthesis from becoming displaced until healing is complete.
Keep flat with slight elevation (30–45 degrees) of head.	Preventing hip flexion helps maintain the placement of the hip prosthesis until healing is complete.
Encourage the use of a patient-controlled analgesia (PCA) pump at frequent intervals to control pain.	Relieving pain facilitates the client's comfort and cooperation in performing rehabilitative exercise and mobility.

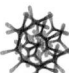

NURSING CARE PLAN 26-1 — Activity Intolerance (*continued*)

Transfer from the bed to a standing position at the bedside following these directions:
- Slide affected left leg to edge of bed; remove abduction wedge.
- Have client use trapeze or elbows and hands to slide buttocks and legs perpendicular to bed. Remind client to avoid leaning forward and praise efforts at moving.
- Lower unaffected right foot to floor and help with lowering affected left foot, keeping knees apart.
- Dangle at bedside for approximately 5 minutes.
- Apply walking safety belt around waist.
- Brace feet and pull forward on belt.
- Stand at bedside, putting only partial weight on left leg.
- Reverse actions for returning the client to bed.

Preventing hip flexion helps maintain the placement of the hip prosthesis until healing is complete.

Evaluation of Expected Outcome

- Client maintains postoperative positions as ordered by physician.
- Abduction wedge is in place while client is in bed.
- Client performs active isotonic and isometric quad-setting exercises.
- Use of PCA pump reduces pain to a level that facilitates exercise.
- Client can transfer from bed and stand at bedside following the procedure outlined in the written plan of care.
- Client alternates full weight-bearing on right leg with partial weight-bearing on left leg in preparation for ambulation in the physical therapy department.

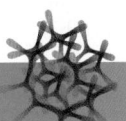

KEY POINTS

- Activities that prepare clients for ambulation
  - Exercise
  - Dangling
  - Using a tilt table
- Ambulatory assistive device
  - Walking/gait belt
  - Parallel bars
- Ambulatory aids: Consider the client's condition when determining which type of ambulatory aid would be best for the client. A client with poor balance needs an aid that would provide a strong base of support.
  - Canes
    - Half-circle
    - T-handle
    - Quad cane
- Walkers: The most stable form of ambulatory aid
- Crutches:
  - Four-point gait
  - Three-point gate
  - Two-point gait
  - Swing-through gait
- Prosthetic limbs
  - Temporary prosthesis: IPOP, facilitates early ambulation and promotes an intact body image
  - Permanent prosthesis: Custom-made to conform to the residual limb, mainly arms or legs; different options available depending on the needs of the client

CRITICAL THINKING EXERCISES

1. Compare the differences in using crutches and a walker as ambulatory aids.
2. Discuss stereotypes of people who use ambulatory aids.
3. What are some advantages of implementing an exercise regimen to promote early ambulation?
4. What rationales could the nurse offer a client for providing an immediate postoperative prosthesis on an amputated limb?

NEXT-GENERATION NCLEX-STYLE REVIEW QUESTIONS

1. What is the best evidence for a nurse that a client using a walker is performing a three-point partial weight-bearing gait correctly?
   a. The client advances the walker and the operative leg while putting most of the weight on the handgrips of the walker.
   b. The client advances the walker and the operative leg while putting most of the weight on the back legs of the walker.

c. The client advances the walker and the operative leg while putting most of the weight on the toes of the operative leg.

d. The client advances the walker and the operative leg while putting most of the weight on the heel of the inoperative leg.

Test-Taking Strategy: Analyze the choices and select the option that best describes a three-point partial weight-bearing gait.

2. When the nurse observes a client with arthritis using a cane, which findings indicate that the client needs more instruction about its use? Select all that apply.

   a. The client's cane tip is covered with a rubber cap.

   b. The client wears athletic shoes with nonskid soles.

   c. The client positions the cane on the painful side.

   d. The client's head is held up while looking straight ahead.

   e. The client moves the cane and stronger extremity together.

   Test-Taking Strategy: Analyze all the choices and select the options that are incorrect techniques when using a cane.

3. After a client undergoes a total hip replacement, which position of the operative hip is essential for the nurse to maintain?

   a. Adduction

   b. Abduction

   c. Flexion

   d. Rotation

   Test-Taking Strategy: Note the key word, "essential." Use the process of elimination to select the joint position that maintains the hip prosthesis within the acetabulum of the pelvis.

4. Which nursing activity is best for strengthening the muscles of a client before ambulating with crutches immediately after surgery?

   a. Standing at the side of the bed

   b. Balancing between parallel bars

   c. Lifting with the overbed trapeze

   d. Transferring from bed to a chair

Test-Taking Strategy: Note the key words, "best" and "immediately." Use the process of elimination to select the option that is better than any of the others to promote the ability to use crutches.

5. Which nursing observation is most indicative that the crutches a client is using need further adjustment?

   a. The client stands straight without bending forward.

   b. The elbows are slightly flexed when standing in place.

   c. The top bars of the crutches fit snugly into the axillae.

   d. The wrists are hyperextended when grasping the handgrips.

   Test-Taking Strategy: Note the key word and modifier, "most indicative." Use the process of elimination to select the option that provides the best evidence that crutches require readjustment.

NEXT-GENERATION NCLEX-STYLE CLINICAL SCENARIO QUESTIONS

Clinical Scenario:

A 73-year-old male client has had a hip replacement to relieve pain and disability from osteoarthritis. He is anxious about upcoming physical therapy and resumption of his independent lifestyle.

1. From the list below select some of the factors that may be contributing to the anxiety.

   a. Pain

   b. Muscle weakness

   c. Physical therapy exercises

   d. Inability to perform exercises

   e. Transportation to physical therapy

   f. Thinking that he may not be able to resume his independence

SKILL 26-1 Measuring for Crutches, Canes, and Walkers

Suggested Action	Reason for Action
ASSESSMENT	
Check the medical orders.	Nursing activities align with the medical treatment.
Determine the type of ambulatory aid the client will use.	Indicates the type of measurements needed
Check agency policy about personnel responsible for measuring and dispensing ambulatory aids.	Complies with agency procedures; clients in health care agencies sometimes are referred to personnel in the physical therapy department
Determine the strength of the client's arm and leg muscles.	Indicates the client's potential for weight-bearing; weakness suggests a need to measure the client in bed or for further collaboration with the physician concerning muscle strengthening
PLANNING	
Obtain a long tape measure.	Facilitates measuring clients with a range of heights
Wash your hands or use an alcohol-based hand rub (see Chapter 10).	Reduces the transmission of microorganisms
Assist the client with putting on socks and walking shoes if the client can stand for the measurement.	Aids in more accurate measurement that accommodates added height of the heel
IMPLEMENTATION	
Axillary Crutches	
Assist the client who can support their body weight to a standing position at the bedside with supportive shoes.	Positions the client in a posture for the actual use of crutches
Measure from the anterior skinfold of the axilla to approximately 4–8 in (10–20 cm) diagonally from the foot (Fig. A).	Approximates the length required for appropriate use

Anterior axillary fold

4–8 in (10–20 cm)

A

Measuring for crutches in a standing position.

Place a weak client in a supine position.	Simulates the client's height in a standing position

(continued)

SKILL 26-1 Measuring for Crutches, Canes, and Walkers (*continued*)

Suggested Action	Reason for Action
Measure the distance from the anterior skinfold of the axilla to heel and add 2 in (5 cm) or subtract 16 in (40 cm) from the client's height (Fig. B).	Accommodates for the added height of the heel

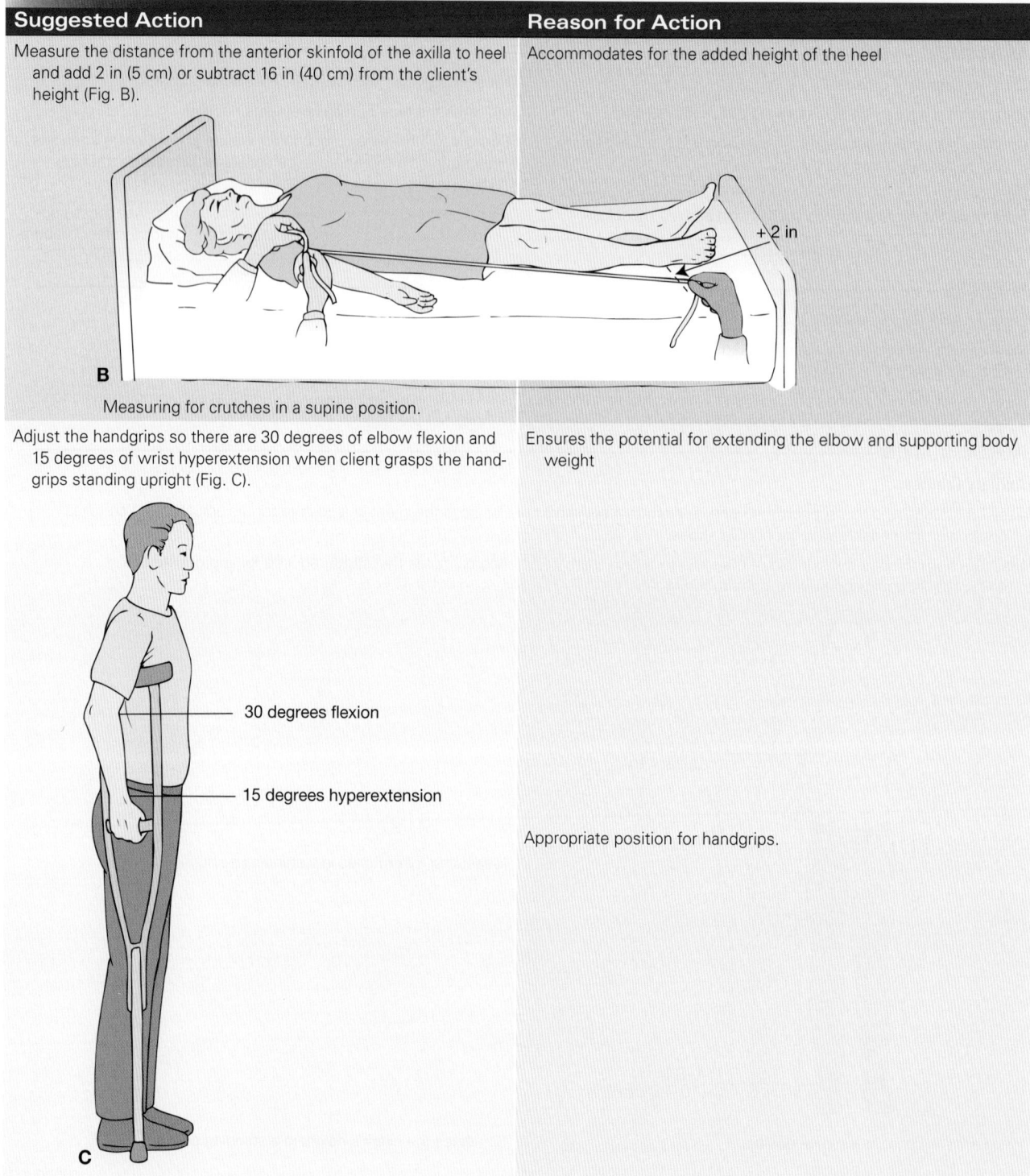

+ 2 in

B

Measuring for crutches in a supine position.

Suggested Action	Reason for Action
Adjust the handgrips so there are 30 degrees of elbow flexion and 15 degrees of wrist hyperextension when client grasps the handgrips standing upright (Fig. C).	Ensures the potential for extending the elbow and supporting body weight

— 30 degrees flexion

— 15 degrees hyperextension

Appropriate position for handgrips.

C

SKILL 26-1 Measuring for Crutches, Canes, and Walkers (*continued*)

Suggested Action	Reason for Action
Lengthen or shorten axillary crutches by removing wing nuts and replacing metal screws in the appropriate hole in the stem of the crutch. Adjust handgrips in the same way (Fig. D).	Customizes the length of the crutches according to the client's height

D

Adjusting length of an axillary crutch. (Photo by B. Proud.)

Forearm Crutches

Suggested Action	Reason for Action
Stand the client in shoes with the elbows flexed so the crease of the wrist is at the hip.	Simulates the appropriate posture when using forearm crutches
Measure the forearm from 3 in below the elbow, then add the distance between the wrist and floor (Fig. E).	Adjusts total length to accommodate for elbow and wrist flexion

E

Measuring forearm crutches. Total length C = sum of A (3 in below elbow to wrist) + B (wrist to floor).

Suggested Action	Reason for Action
Adjust the length of the forearm crutches by telescoping them up or down.	Customizes the final fit

Canes

Suggested Action	Reason for Action
Have the client stand erect in shoes that they wear most often for ambulating.	Incorporates the height of the client's shoes
Instruct the client to avoid leaning forward or elevating the shoulders.	Ensures an accurate measurement
Measure from the wrist to the floor.	Determines the appropriate length of the cane
Adjust the length of cane to provide 30 degrees of elbow flexion with the hand on the grip.	Customizes the final height of the cane

(*continued*)

SKILL 26-1 Measuring for Crutches, Canes, and Walkers (*continued*)

Suggested Action	Reason for Action
Walkers	
Have the client stand while wearing supportive shoes.	Accommodates for the added height of shoes
Measure from the mid-buttocks to the floor.	Facilitates the approximate height of the walker
Adjust the legs of the walker to provide approximately 30 degrees of elbow flexion.	Customizes the final fit of the walker

EVALUATION

- The client stands upright with the shoulders relaxed.
- With axillary crutches, there is space for two fingers between the axilla and axillary bar to prevent **crutch palsy** (a weakened forearm, wrist, and hand muscles from nerve impairment secondary to pressure on the brachial plexus of nerves in the axilla) from incorrectly fitted crutches or poor posture.
- There are 30 degrees of elbow flexion and slight hyperextension of the wrist when standing in place.

DOCUMENT

- Type of ambulatory aid
- Measurements for ambulatory aid
- Method for measuring client

SAMPLE DOCUMENTATION

Date and Time Measured for axillary crutches. Approximate length of crutches is 53 in (132.5 cm) based on length from axillary fold to heel (51 in) while in a supine position and the addition of 2 in. _____ J. Doe, LPN

SKILL 26-2 Assisting with Crutch-Walking

Suggested Action	Reason for Action
ASSESSMENT	
Review the medical orders for the type of activity and crutch-walking gait.	Reflects the implementation of the medical treatment
Read any previous nursing documentation regarding the client's efforts at crutch-walking.	Provides evaluative data and indicates the need to simulate or modify nursing interventions
Wash hands or use an alcohol-based hand rub (see Chapter 10).	Reduces the transmission of microorganisms
Observe the condition of the client's axillae and palms.	Provides objective data concerning the weight-bearing effects on the upper body
Ask the client whether there is any muscle or joint pain or tingling or numbness in the fingers.	Provides subjective data concerning the effects of crutch-walking and possible nerve irritation
Inspect the conditions of the axillary pads and rubber crutch tips.	Demonstrates concern for safety
PLANNING	
Consult with the client about the preferred time for ambulation.	Shows respect for individual decision-making
Assist the client with putting on clothes or a robe and supportive shoes or slippers with nonskid soles.	Demonstrates concern for modesty and safety
Apply a walking belt if the client is weak or inexperienced in using crutches.	Demonstrates concern for safety
Clear a pathway where the client will ambulate.	Demonstrates concern for safety
Review the technique for performing the prescribed crutch-walking gait.	Reinforces prior learning

SKILL 26-2 Assisting with Crutch-Walking (*continued*)

Suggested Action	Reason for Action
IMPLEMENTATION	
Help the client into a standing position.	Prepares the client for ambulation
Offer the crutches and observe that they are placed 4–8 in (10–20 cm) to the side of the feet (Fig. A).	Forms a triangle for good balance

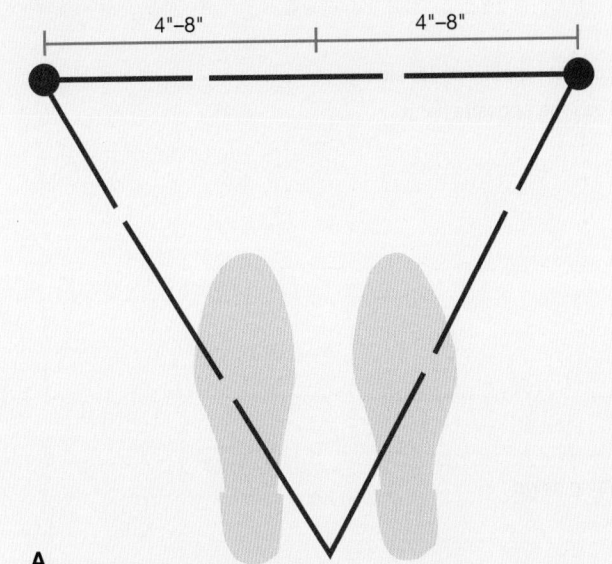

A tripod of support.

A

| Remind the client to stand straight with the shoulders relaxed. | Reduces muscle strain |
| Position yourself to the side and slightly behind the client on the weaker side (Fig. B). | Facilitates assistance without causing interference |

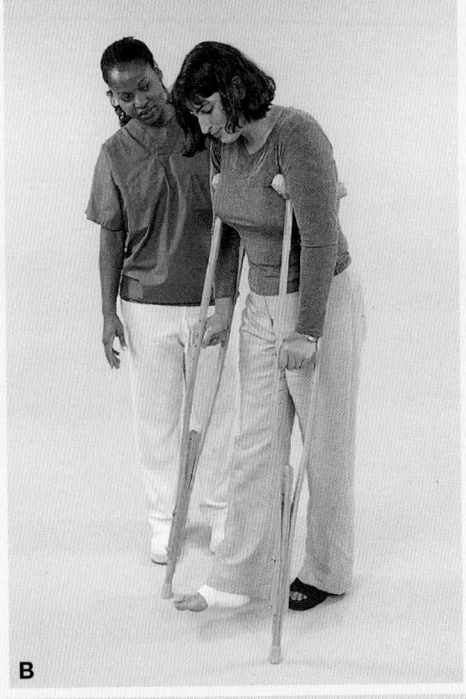

Positioning for assistance. (Photo by B. Proud.)

B

| Take hold of the walking belt. | Helps steady or support the client |

(*continued*)

SKILL 26-2 Assisting with Crutch-Walking (*continued*)

Suggested Action	Reason for Action
Instruct the client to advance the crutches, lean forward, put some weight on the handgrips, and move one or both feet depending on the prescribed gait.	Promotes walking
Remind the client to slow down if there is evidence of fatigue or intolerance to the activity.	Demonstrates concern for the client's well-being
For Sitting	
Recommend backing up to the seat of the chair.	Promotes a position for sitting
Have the client place both crutches in the hand on the same side as the weaker leg (Fig. C).	Frees the opposite hand

C

Sitting down

While using the handgrips on the crutches for support, have the client grasp one armrest with the free hand.	Reduces the potential for falling
When balanced, tell the client to lower themselves into the seat of the chair.	Facilitates sitting
To get up, help the client to the edge of the chair.	Facilitates using the stronger muscles of the thighs
Instruct the client to hold the crutches upright on the weaker side, balancing the crutches with one hand.	Positions crutches for support
Tell the client to position the weaker leg forward of the body and the stronger leg toward the base of the chair.	Helps distribute weight over the stronger leg
Tell the client to push on the handgrips and armrest, lean forward, and press down with the stronger leg.	Raises the client from the chair
To Climb Stairs	
Have the client use a handrail on the stronger side of the body, if possible.	Balances needed support
Have the client transfer both crutches to the hand opposite the handrail.	Frees one hand for grasping the handrail for support

SKILL 26-2 Assisting with Crutch-Walking (*continued*)

Suggested Action	Reason for Action
Tell the client to push down on the handrail and step up with the good leg (Fig. D).	Uses the stronger muscles for bearing weight
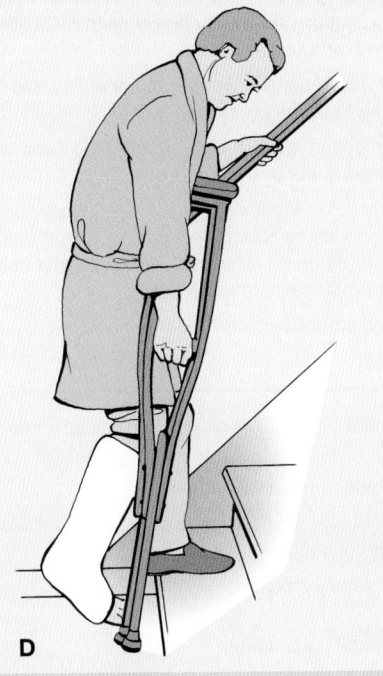 **D**	Climbing stairs
Follow by raising the weaker leg.	Brings both legs to the same stair
Remind the client that when going down the stairs, the weaker leg is advanced first with the support of the crutches or handrail; then the stronger leg is moved.	Enables a safe descent

EVALUATION

- Crutches fit appropriately.
- Client performs crutch-walking gait correctly.
- No fatigue or other symptoms develop.
- Client remains free of injury.

DOCUMENT

- Distance ambulated
- Gait used
- Response of the client

SAMPLE DOCUMENTATION

Date and Time Ambulated length of hospital corridor (approximately 100 ft) using crutches and a three-point non–weight-bearing gait. No breathlessness noted. States upper arms "ache" and attributes discomfort to "muscle strain" from previous day's ambulation efforts. Refuses medication for muscle discomfort. _____ J. Doe, LPN

SKILL 26-3 Applying a Leg Prosthesis

Suggested Action	Reason for Action
ASSESSMENT	
Wash hands or use an alcohol-based hand rub (see Chapter 10).	Reduces the transmission of microorganisms
Inspect the residual limb for evidence of bleeding, wound drainage, skin abrasions, blisters, and edema.	Detects complications that delay healing and rehabilitation or that interfere with ambulation
Weigh the client at regular intervals.	Helps detect fluctuations in weight that alter the size of the residual limb and the fit of the prosthesis
Observe the ease or difficulty of inserting the residual limb within the socket.	Indicates changes in residual limb size and the need to add or decrease the numbers or thickness of residual limb socks
Examine the joint connections in the prosthetic limb.	Determines whether lubrication or prosthetic maintenance is necessary; concerns about the mechanical features of the prosthesis or its fit are referred to a **prosthetist** (a person who constructs prostheses) immediately
Inspect the shoe on the prosthetic limb for signs of wear or moisture.	Establishes whether heels or the entire shoe needs to be replaced or dried
PLANNING	
Cleanse the skin on the residual limb each evening, not in the morning.	Allows sufficient time for the skin to be moisture-free
Rinse the soap from the residual limb and dry it well.	Avoids skin impairment and irritation
Encourage the client to lie supine or prone periodically during the day.	Promotes venous circulation, reduces residual limb edema, and avoids joint contractures
Instruct the client to avoid crossing the legs or keeping the natural knee flexed for a prolonged period.	Prevents circulatory problems
Wash the socket each evening with water and mild soap.	Removes soil and perspiration
Dry the socket well before application.	Prevents skin breakdown
Use a small brush to clean the valve on a prosthesis with a suction socket.	Removes dust and facilitates the formation of a vacuum
Keep a supply of clean residual limb socks to facilitate a daily change and a nylon sheath if one is used.	Promotes cleanliness and comfort
Store clean wool residual limb socks for several days before use.	Allows the restoration of wool fiber resiliency
Wash a nylon sheath in soapy lukewarm water, rinse well, and stretch it lengthwise before air-drying; never remove water by twisting the sheath.	Maintains shape and integrity
Advise the client with a new prosthesis to wear it for short periods initially and then increase the wearing time each day.	Prevents overexertion and impaired skin integrity
IMPLEMENTATION	
Cover the prosthetic foot with the stocking and shoe of choice.	Coordinates apparel and helps conceal the appearance of the prosthetic limb
Apply the nylon sheath if used and the appropriate number or ply of residual limb socks.	Promotes comfort and the fit of the residual limb within the prosthesis
Place a nylon stocking over the residual limb sock, allowing a long portion of the toe to extend from the base of the residual limb (Fig. A).	Helps slide the residual limb within the socket

A nylon stocking covers the residual limb sock.

A

SKILL 26-3 Applying a Leg Prosthesis (*continued*)

Suggested Action	Reason for Action
Stand and position the prosthetic limb next to the residual limb.	Facilitates application
Pull the toe of the nylon stocking through the valve at the base of the socket (Fig. B).	Locates the residual limb well within the lower area of the socket
	The nylon is pulled through the valve hole on the socket of the prosthesis.
Pump the residual limb up and down as the nylon stocking is completely removed.	Expels air and creates a vacuum that keeps the prosthesis attached to the residual limb
Replace the plug within the valve opening.	Ensures the retention of vacuum suction
Fasten all slings if other than a suction socket type of prosthesis is used.	Secures the prosthesis to the residual limb

B

EVALUATION

- Residual limb size is unchanged.
- Skin is intact.
- Circulation is adequate based on similar skin color in the residual limb and the remaining limb.
- Joints above the amputation have full range of motion.
- Prosthesis is mechanically sound.
- Client ambulates without discomfort or injury.

DOCUMENT

- Care and condition of the residual limb
- Care of residual limb socks
- Care and condition of the prosthesis
- Level of client performance in residual limb care and application of the prosthesis
- Client's performance in ambulation

SAMPLE DOCUMENTATION

Date and Time   Residual limb washed and dried by client. No evidence of skin breakdown. Soiled residual limb socks exchanged with spouse for supply of clean socks. Inside of prosthetic socket cleaned and dried. Client observed while independently putting on prosthesis. Procedure completed accurately and appropriately. Ambulated for approximately 15 minutes without loss of balance or other difficulties. _____ J. Doe, LPN

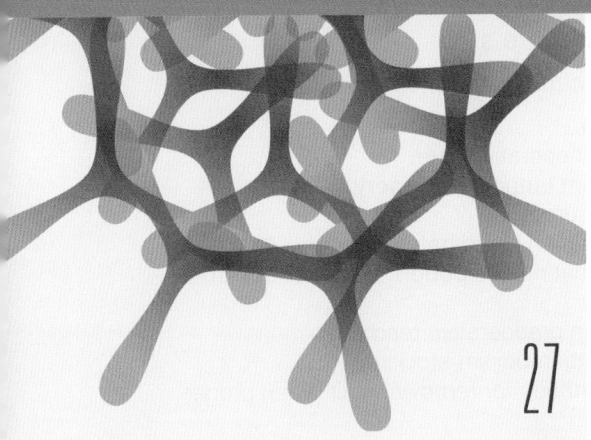

UNIT 7 | The Surgical Client

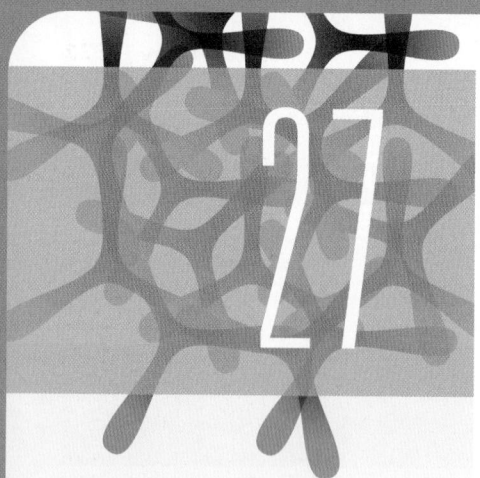

Perioperative Care

Words To Know

anesthesiologist
anesthetist
antiembolism stockings
atelectasis
autologous transfusion
conscious sedation
depilatory agent
directed donors
discharge instructions
emancipated minor
emboli
forced coughing
informed consent
inpatient surgery
intraoperative period
microabrasions
outpatient surgery
perioperative care
plume
pneumatic compression device
pneumonia
postanesthesia care unit
postoperative care
postoperative period
preoperative checklist
preoperative period
receiving room
reversal drugs
substituted judgment
surgical waiting area
thrombus
Universal Protocol

Learning Objectives

On completion of this chapter, the reader should be able to:

1. Define perioperative care.
2. Identify the phases of perioperative care.
3. Differentiate inpatient from outpatient surgery.
4. List advantages of laser surgery.
5. Discuss methods for donating blood before surgery.
6. Identify major activities that nurses perform for all clients immediately before surgery.
7. Name topics to address in preoperative teaching.
8. Explain the purpose of antiembolism stockings.
9. Name recommended methods for removing hair when preparing the skin for surgery.
10. List items that are verified on the preoperative checklist.
11. Discuss the purpose and information required during a presurgical time-out according to The Joint Commission's Universal Protocol.
12. Name the areas of the surgical department used during the intraoperative period.
13. Describe the focus of nursing care during the immediate postoperative period.
14. Give examples of common postoperative complications.
15. Discuss the purpose of a pneumatic compression device.
16. Describe information included in discharge instructions for postsurgical clients.
17. Discuss ways in which the surgical care of older adults differs from that of other age groups.

INTRODUCTION

Perioperative care (care that clients receive before, during, and after surgery) is unique. The current trend is to facilitate as short a perioperative period as possible. This trend is driven by efforts to control health care costs by facilitating the client's return to the comfort and support of their home environment. This chapter discusses the general responsibilities nurses assume when caring for clients during the preoperative, intraoperative, and postoperative periods of perioperative care.

 Gerontologic Considerations

■ Chronic health conditions may be present in older adults and may increase the complexity of the preoperative, intraoperative, and postoperative periods.

■ The older person should be educated about taking or omitting usual medications before surgical procedures and about resuming usual or new medications after surgery.

- Before any period of fluid restriction in older adults, it is important to assess vital signs, weight, and sternal skin turgor to establish a baseline for comparison.
- Older adults are also likely to be self-conscious when dentures are removed before surgery. Collaboration with operating room personnel regarding the removal of dentures, eyeglasses, and hearing aids is helpful to ensure their use as much or as long as possible.
- Older adults who rely on eyeglasses or hearing aids may experience sensory deprivation if these aids are removed before surgery or other procedures. Removal may interfere with communication or contribute to confusion and altered mental status.
- Ensure that dentures, eyeglasses, and hearing aids are labeled with the person's name.
- The cardiac status of older adults is monitored carefully after surgery because they may not be able to tolerate or eliminate intravenous (IV) fluids given at standard rates due to compromised cardiac or renal status.
- Wound healing in older adults may occur more slowly because of age-related skin changes and impaired circulation and oxygenation. Poor hydration and nutrition further interfere with wound healing. A registered dietitian can recommend nutritional interventions such as protein, zinc, and vitamin C to improve wound healing.
- If an indwelling catheter is inserted before surgery, it is best to remove it as soon as possible after surgery to prevent urinary tract infections. Careful assessment of urination pattern and volume is indicated to ensure adequate voiding amounts and timing, especially if a bedpan will be required during a period of ambulatory restrictions.
- Muscle atrophy occurs in older adults who have been on bed rest even for only 1 or 2 days. Range of motion and muscle tone can be maintained through routine active or passive range of motion exercises.
- Consider requesting a referral for physical therapy for older adults who have been on bed rest.
- If older adults develop postoperative infections, the manifestations are likely to be subtle or delayed. Older adults are likely to have a lower "normal" temperature. Therefore, it is imperative to document the client's usual baseline temperature so that deviations can be assessed. A change in mental status may be an early indicator of infection.
- A thorough assessment of an older client's support system must be done well before discharge. It should include the ability of the support system to provide assistance once the client is discharged. Support people should be included in discharge teaching, with plenty of time to provide any return demonstration of learning regarding the needs of the older adult. In addition, the home environment should be assessed before discharge for safety issues (e.g., use of scatter rugs, lighting, rails, grab bars).
- If the older person cannot manage their postoperative care independently or with the assistance of supportive family or friends, options relative to extended or skilled nursing care should be explored and discussed. Skilled nursing or rehabilitation therapists may be available from home care agencies and covered by health insurance for home settings.

PREOPERATIVE PERIOD

The **preoperative period** starts when clients learn that surgery is necessary and ends when clients are transported to the operating room. This period can be short or long; one major factor affecting its length is the urgency with which the surgery must be performed (Table 27-1).

Inpatient Surgery

Surgery is performed for various reasons (Table 27-2). **Inpatient surgery** is the term used for procedures performed on a client who is admitted to the hospital, expected to remain at least overnight, and in need of nursing care for more than 1 day after surgery. All, except the sickest of, clients are usually admitted the morning of the scheduled surgery.

Many people who have inpatient surgery undergo prior laboratory and diagnostic tests. Some have met with an **anesthesiologist** (a physician who administers chemical agents that temporarily eliminate sensation and pain; Table 27-3) or an **anesthetist** (a certified nurse specialist who administers anesthesia under the direction of a physician). Most clients will have received preoperative instructions from either the surgeon's office nurse or a hospital nurse.

Outpatient Surgery

Outpatient surgery, also called *ambulatory surgery* and *same-day surgery*, is the term used for operative procedures performed on clients who return home the same day. It is generally reserved for clients in an optimal state of health whose recovery is expected to be uneventful. Advantages and disadvantages of outpatient surgery are listed in Table 27-4.

Outpatient surgical units are located in either a hospital or a separate building that the hospital owns. Others are freestanding, privately owned facilities such as a surgeon's office that is not affiliated with a hospital. The client remains in the location of the surgery for a brief time and is able to return home by midafternoon or early evening when (1) the client is awake and alert, (2) vital signs are stable, (3) pain and nausea are controlled, (4) oral fluids are retained, (5) the client voids a sufficient quantity of urine, and (6) the client has received home care instructions. If a complication develops, the client is transferred and admitted to a hospital unit.

 Pharmacologic Considerations

Outpatients are frequently instructed to take preoperative or routine medications at home before procedures; this is especially important for those who take heart, hypertension, or diabetes medications. It is critical for the physician to know when and what dose was taken for appropriate monitoring during procedures.

Outpatient procedures have increased dramatically as a result of advances in techniques such as those using endoscopes, an instrument for performing internal procedures in lieu of those requiring an incision (see Chapter 14), and lasers; methods of anesthesia; prospective reimbursement;

TABLE 27-1 Types of Surgery According to Urgency

TYPE	DESCRIPTION	EXAMPLE
Optional	Surgery is performed at the client's request.	Surgery for cosmetic purposes
Elective	Surgery is planned at the client's convenience. Failure to have the surgery does not result in catastrophe.	Surgery for the removal of a superficial cyst
Required	Surgery is necessary and should be done relatively promptly.	Surgery for the removal of a cataract
Urgent	Surgery is required promptly, within 1 or 2 days if at all possible.	Surgery for the removal of a malignant tumor
Emergency	Surgery is required immediately for survival.	Surgery to relieve an intestinal perforation

managed care; and changes in Medicare and Medicaid provisions (Hinkle & Cheever, 2013).

Laser Surgery

Although now commonly used as a word in and of itself, "laser" is an acronym for **l**ight **a**mplification by the **s**timulated **e**mission of **r**adiation. Lasers convert a solid, gas, or liquid into light. When focused, the energy from the light is converted to heat, causing the vaporization of tissue and coagulation of blood vessels. Examples include the carbon dioxide laser, the argon laser, the ruby laser, and the yttrium–aluminum–garnet (YAG) laser.

Laser surgery is used as an alternative to many previously conventional surgical techniques, such as reattaching the retina, removing skin tattoos, and revascularizing ischemic heart muscle (instead of coronary artery bypass graft surgery). Laser surgery offers the following advantages:

- Cost-effectiveness
- Reduced need for general anesthesia
- Smaller incisions
- Minimal blood loss
- Reduced swelling
- Less pain
- Decreased incidence of wound infections
- Reduced scarring
- Less time recuperating

Laser technology requires unique safety precautions, such as eye, fire, heat, and vapor protection. Depending on the type of laser used, everyone—including the client—wears goggles. In some cases, prescription glasses with side shields are sufficient, but contact lenses are not allowed. Because lasers produce heat, fire, and electrical discharge, safety is paramount. Volatile substances such as alcohol and acetone are not used around lasers because of their flammability. Surgical instruments are coated black to avoid absorbing scattered light that causes them to retain heat. Sometimes even the client's teeth are covered with plastic or a rubber mouth guard to shield metal dental fillings. For the same reason, no jewelry is allowed.

When a laser is used, it releases a **plume** (a substance composed of vaporized tissue, carbon dioxide, and water) that may contain intact cells. Plumes, sometimes referred to as *surgical smoke*, are accompanied by an offensive odor and (for some) burning and itching eyes. The latter effects are not hazardous and usually can be reduced with the use of local exhaust ventilators and smoke evacuators. The greater concern involves the consequences of inhaling plumes. Airborne cells in the inhaled plume may contain viruses, such as human papillomavirus (HPV) and possibly human immunodeficiency virus (HIV). Although no cases of HIV transmission through lasers have been documented, protective masks that can filter particulate matter between 2 and 5 microns in size should be worn (UTMB, 2018) (see Chapter 22).

Informed Consent

Regardless of whether surgery is performed conventionally, endoscopically, or with a laser, clients are commonly fearful and anxious. They often have many questions and preconceived ideas about what surgery involves. Health care providers may answer some of these questions. Nevertheless, the physician is responsible for providing information that meets the criteria for **informed consent** (permission a client

TABLE 27-2 Reasons for Surgery

TYPE OF SURGERY	PURPOSE	EXAMPLES
Diagnostic	Removal and study of tissue to make a diagnosis	Breast biopsy Biopsy of skin lesion
Exploratory	More extensive means to diagnose a problem; usually involves exploration of a body cavity or use of scopes inserted through small incisions	Exploration of abdomen for unexplained pain Exploratory laparoscopy
Curative	Removal or replacement of defective tissue to restore function	Cholecystectomy Total hip replacement
Palliative	Relief of symptoms or enhancement of function without cure	Resection of a tumor to relieve pressure and pain
Cosmetic	Correction of defects, improvement of appearance, or change to a physical feature	Rhinoplasty Cleft lip repair Mammoplasty

TABLE 27-3 Types of Anesthesia

TYPE	DESCRIPTION
General anesthesia	Eliminates all sensation and consciousness or memory of the event
Inhalants	Includes gas or volatile liquids
Injectables	Administered intravenously
Regional anesthesia	Blocks sensation in an area but consciousness is unaffected
Spinal (includes epidural)	Eliminates sensation in lower extremities, lower abdomen, and pelvis
Local	Blocks sensation in a circumscribed area of skin and subcutaneous tissue
Topical	Inhibits sensation where directly applied in epithelial tissues such as skin and mucous membranes

gives after an explanation of the risks, benefits, and alternatives; see Chapter 14). A signed form, witnessed by a nurse, is evidence that consent has been obtained (Fig. 27-1).

If an adult client is confused, unconscious, or mentally incompetent, the client's spouse, nearest blood relative, or someone with a durable power of attorney for the client's health care must sign the consent form. If an adult client is under the influence of a mind-altering drug such as a narcotic or is alcohol intoxicated, obtaining consent must be delayed until the drug has been metabolized. In a life-threatening emergency, a court may waive the need to obtain a written or verbal consent from a client who requires immediate surgery on the basis of **substituted judgment**; that is, the court believes that if the client had the capacity to consent, they would have done so. Refer to Chapter 14 for the elements that constitute informed consent.

If the client is younger than 18 years, a parent or legal guardian must sign the consent form. In an emergency, health care personnel make every effort to obtain consent by telephone, telegram, or fax. Adolescents younger than 18

TABLE 27-4 Advantages and Disadvantages of Outpatient Surgery

ADVANTAGES	DISADVANTAGES
Lowers the surgical costs because of the reduced use of hospital services	Reduces the time for establishing a nurse–client relationship
Reduces the time spent away from home, school, or place of employment	Requires intensive preoperative teaching in a short amount of time
Interferes less with the client's usual daily routine	Reduces the opportunity for reinforcement of teaching and for answering questions
Provides the potential for more rest and sleep before and after surgery	Allows for fewer delays in assessing and preparing a client once they arrive for surgery
Allows more opportunity for family contact and support	Requires that care of the client after discharge be carried out by unskilled people

years, living independently, and supporting themselves are regarded as **emancipated minors** and may sign their own consent forms.

Each nurse must be familiar with agency policies and state laws regarding surgical consent forms. Clients must sign the consent form before receiving any preoperative sedatives. When the client or designated person has signed the permit, an adult witness also signs it to indicate that the client or designee signed voluntarily. This witness is usually a member of the health care team or an employee in the admissions department. The nurse is responsible for ensuring that all necessary parties have signed the consent form and that it is in the client's chart before the client goes to the operating room.

Preoperative Blood Donation

When the need for a blood transfusion during the perioperative period is anticipated, the low risk for acquiring HIV from a blood transfusion is sometimes discussed before the surgical procedure. Although publicly donated blood is tested for several pathogens including HIV and hepatitis B, the potential, though slight, of acquiring a blood-borne disease still exists. Therefore, some clients undergoing surgery donate their own blood preoperatively if it does not jeopardize their own health. Predonated blood is held on reserve in the event that the client needs a blood transfusion during or after surgery. Receiving one's own blood is called an **autologous transfusion** (self-donated blood). Autologous transfusions are also prepared by salvaging blood lost during or immediately after surgery. The salvaged blood is suctioned, cleaned, and filtered from drainage collection devices.

Clients who do not meet the time or health requirements for self-donation may select **directed donors** (blood donors chosen from among the client's relatives and friends). The client's siblings should not donate blood for the client. Doing so would rule them out as future organ or tissue donors for the client because antigens in the transfused blood would sensitize the recipient, increasing the risk for organ or tissue rejection. In addition, a male sexual partner of a woman in her reproductive years should not be a directed donor to avoid possible antibody reactions against a fetus in any future pregnancy.

Most authorities believe that receiving blood from directed donors is no safer than receiving blood from public donors. Although predonation of blood is available in the United States, the criteria for autologous and directed donors (Table 27-5) may vary among regions and hospitals. Because directed donors must meet the same requirements as public donors, if the intended recipient does not use the blood, it is released into the public pool and can be given to someone else.

Immediate Preoperative Care

Although some presurgical activities take place weeks in advance, others cannot be performed until just before surgery. During the immediate preoperative period—the few hours before the procedure—several major tasks must be completed: conducting a nursing assessment, providing preoperative teaching, performing methods of physical preparation, administering medications, assisting with psychosocial preparation, and completing the surgical checklist.

INFORMED CONSENT TO SURGERY

1. Title of Form.

This form is called an "Informed Consent Form." It is your doctor's obligation to provide you with the information you need in order to decide whether to consent to the surgery or special procedure that your doctors have recommended. The purpose of this form is to verify that you have received this information and have given your consent to the surgery or special procedure recommended to you. You should read this form carefully and ask questions of your doctors so that you understand the operation or procedure before you decide to give your consent. If you have questions, you are encouraged and expected to ask them before you sign this form.

2. Recommendation

Your doctors have recommended the following operation or procedure: _____
_____
_____

and the following type of anesthesia: _____.

Upon your authorization and consent, this operation or procedure, together with any different or further procedures which, in the opinion of the doctor(s) performing the procedure, may be indicated due to any emergency, will be performed on you. The operations or procedures will be performed by the doctor named below (or, in the event the doctor is unable to perform or complete the procedure, a qualified substitute doctor), together with associates and assistants, including anesthesiologists, pathologists, and radiologists from the medical staff of (name of hospital) _____
to whom the doctor(s) performing the procedure may assign designated responsibilities.

3. Standard Risks

All operations and procedures carry the risk of unsuccessful results, complications, injury or even death, from both known and unforeseen causes, and no warranty or guarantee is made as to result or cure. you have the right to be informed of:

- The nature of the operation or procedure, including other care, treatment or medications
- Potential benefits, risks or side effects of the operation or procedure, including potential problems that might occur with the anesthesia to be used and during recuperation
- The likelihood of achieving treatment goals
- Reasonable alternatives and the relevant risks, benefits and side effects related to such alternatives, including the possible results of not receiving care or treatment
- Any independent medical research or significant economic interests your doctor may have related to the performance of the proposed operation or procedure.

Except in cases of emergency, operations or procedures are not performed until you have had the opportunity to receive this information and have given your consent. You have the right to give or refuse consent to any proposed operation or procedure at any time prior to its performance.

4. Anesthesia

Your doctor will discuss with you the risks and benefits of the recommended operation or procedure, including the following (the patient's doctor is responsible for the content of the information provided below):

If your doctor determines that there is a reasonable possibility that you may need a blood transfusion as a result of the surgery or procedure to which you are consenting, your doctor will inform you of this and will provide you with information concerning the benefits and risks of the various options for blood transfusion, including predonation by yourself or others. You also have the right to have adequate time before your procedure to arrange for predonation, but you can waive this right if you do not wish to wait.

Transfusion of blood or blood products involves certain risks, including the transmission of disease such as hepatitis or human immunodeficiency virus (HIV), and you have a right to consent or refuse consent to any transfusion. You should discuss any questions that you may have about transfusions with your doctor.

Your signature on this form indicates that:
- You have read and understand the information provided in this form; • Your doctor has adequately explained to you the operation or procedure and the anesthesia set forth above, along with the risks, benefits, and the other information described above in this form; • You have had a chance to ask your doctors questions; • You have received all of the information you desire concerning the operation or procedure and the anesthesia; and • You authorize and consent to the performance of the operation or procedure and the anesthesia.

Date: _____   Time: _____   ☐ AM ☐ PM

Signature: _____ (Patient / Legal Representative)

If signed by someone other than the patient, indicate their name: _____

Relationship: _____

Physician Certification

I, the undersigned physician, hereby certify that I have discussed the procedure described in this consent form with this patient (or the patient's legal representative), including:

- The risks and benefits of the procedure
- Any adverse reactions that may reasonably be expected to occur
- Any alternative efficacious methods of treatment which may be medically viable
- The potential problems that may occur during recuperation
- Any research or economic interest I may have regarding this treatment.

I further certify that the patient was encouraged to ask questions and that all questions were answered

Date: _____   Time: _____   ☐ AM ☐ PM

FIGURE 27-1 A surgical consent form.

TABLE 27-5 American Red Cross Criteria for Autologous and Directed Blood Donation

AUTOLOGOUS DONATION	DIRECTED DONATION
To bank one's own blood, the donor must: Have a physician's recommendation Have a hematocrit within a safe range Be free of infection at the time of donation Meet the blood collection center's minimum weight requirement Donate 40 days before the anticipated date of use but not within 72 hours of the procedure Donate no more frequently than every 3–5 days; once per week is preferred Avoid acetaminophen (Tylenol), aspirin, and alcohol for 48 hours before a donation Assume responsibility for costs above the usual processing fees even if blood is not used Be advised that their blood will be discarded if unused	**To be a directed donor, the person must:** Be at least 17 years of age Meet all the criteria of a public donor Have the same blood type as the potential recipient or one that is compatible Not have received a blood transfusion within the last 6 months Donate 3–20 days before the anticipated use Be free of blood-borne pathogens and high-risk behaviors

Nursing Assessment

Nurses and physicians share the responsibility for assessing preoperative clients. The assessment varies depending on the urgency of the surgery and if the client is admitted the same day of surgery or earlier. Although assessment of the surgical client is always necessary, the particular circumstances dictate the extent of the process. There may not be time to perform a detailed assessment.

When surgery is not an emergency, the nurse performs a thorough history and physical examination. They assess the client's understanding of the surgical procedure, postoperative expectations, and ability to participate in recovery. The nurse also considers cultural needs, specifically as they relate to beliefs about surgery, personal privacy, and presence of family members during the preoperative and postoperative phases. Clients from different cultures may experience differences in postoperative pain sensitivity and analgesic requirements. The nurse may question the client regarding strong culturally influenced feelings about disposal of body parts and blood transfusions.

Upon admission, the nurse reviews preoperative instructions, such as diet and fluid restrictions, bowel and skin preparations, and the withholding or self-administration of medications, to ensure that the client has followed them. If the client has not carried out a specific portion of the instructions, the nurse immediately notifies the surgeon.

 Pharmacologic Considerations

When asked, some adults do not realize the anticoagulant (bleeding) effect of the medications and supplements routinely taken. They may not readily tell you about these preparations because they do not know what might constitute a postoperative risk for bleeding. Ask about the following items in addition to standard anticoagulant therapy (such as warfarin):

■ Low-dose aspirin self-therapy (anticoagulant)
■ Cold and cough product use (contains salicylates)
■ Nonsteroidal antiinflammatory drugs (NSAIDs) such as ibuprofen (Advil) and naproxen (Aleve) (increase gastrointestinal [GI] bleeding risk)
■ Health supplements used for memory improvement (e.g., ginkgo and ginseng) (anticoagulant)

The nurse identifies the client's potential risks for complications during or after the surgery. Certain surgical risk factors increase the likelihood of perioperative complications:

- Extremes of age; very young and very old
- Dehydration
- Malnutrition
- Obesity
- Smoking
- Diabetes
- Cardiopulmonary disease
- Drug and alcohol misuse
- Bleeding tendencies
- Low hemoglobin and red cells
- Pregnancy

Some problems, such as an unexplained elevation in temperature, abnormal laboratory data, current infectious disease, or significant deviations in vital signs, are causes for postponing or canceling the surgery (Table 27-6).

Preoperative Teaching

Preoperative teaching varies with the type of surgery and the length of hospitalization. Preoperatively, clients are alert and free from pain or currently in less pain, which facilitates their participation. Knowledge of what to expect on the part of clients and family can enhance recovery from surgery.

The following are examples of information to include in preoperative teaching:

- Preoperative medications—when they are given and their effects
- Postoperative pain control
- Explanation and description of the postanesthesia recovery room or postsurgical protocol
- Discussion of the frequency of assessing vital signs and the use of monitoring equipment

The nurse also explains and demonstrates how to perform deep breathing, coughing, and leg exercises.

Deep Breathing

Deep breathing, a form of controlled ventilation that opens and fills small air passages in the lungs (see Chapter 21), is especially advantageous for clients who receive general anesthesia or who breathe shallowly after surgery because

TABLE 27-6 Surgical Risk Factors and Potential Complications

VARIABLE	POTENTIAL COMPLICATION
Age	
Very young—Immaturity of organ systems and regulatory mechanisms	Respiratory obstruction, fluid overload, dehydration, hypothermia, and infection
Older adult—Multiple organ degeneration and slowed regulatory mechanisms	Decreased metabolism and excretion of anesthetics and pain medications, fluid overload, renal failure, formation of blood clots, delayed wound healing, infection, confusion, and respiratory complications
Nutritional Status	
Malnourished—Low weight and nutrient deficiencies	Fluid and electrolyte imbalances, cardiac dysrhythmias, delayed wound healing, and wound infections
Obese—Stressed cardiovascular system, decreased circulation, and decreased pulmonary function	Atelectasis, pneumonia, blood clots, delayed wound healing, wound infection, delayed metabolism, and excretion of anesthetics and pain medication
Substance Use	
Alcohol, tobacco, sedatives—Altered respiratory function, nutritional status, or liver function	Atelectasis, pneumonia, altered effectiveness of anesthetics and pain medications, drug interactions, and drug withdrawal
Medical Problems	
Immune—Allergies and immunosuppression secondary to corticosteroid therapy, transplants, chemotherapy, or diseases such as acquired immune deficiency disease	Adverse reactions to medications, blood transfusions, or latex; infection
Respiratory—Acute and chronic respiratory problems and history of tobacco use	Atelectasis, bronchopneumonia, and respiratory failure
Cardiovascular—Hypertension, coronary artery disease, and peripheral vascular disease	Hypotension, hypertension, fluid overload, congestive heart failure, shock, dysrhythmias, myocardial infarction, stroke, and blood clots
Hepatic—Liver dysfunction	Delayed drug metabolism leading to drug toxicity, disrupted clotting mechanisms leading to excessive bleeding or hemorrhage, confusion, and increased risk of infection
Renal—Kidney disease, chronic renal insufficiency, and renal failure	Fluid and electrolyte imbalances, congestive heart failure, dysrhythmias, delayed excretion of drugs leading to drug toxicity
Endocrine—Diabetes	Hypoglycemia, hyperglycemia, hypokalemia, infection, and delayed wound healing

of pain. Deep breathing reduces the postoperative risk for respiratory complications such as **atelectasis** (airless, collapsed lung areas) and **pneumonia** (lung infection), both of which can lead to hypoxemia.

The nurse practices deep breathing with clients before they undergo surgery (Fig. 27-2). Deep breathing involves inhaling deeply using the abdominal muscles, holding the breath for several seconds, and exhaling slowly. Pursing the lips may extend the period of exhalation. Incentive spirometers (see Chapter 21) are also used to promote deep breathing.

Coughing

Thickened respiratory secretions often accompany impaired ventilation. Coughing is a natural method for clearing secretions from the airways. Deep breathing alone is sometimes sufficient to produce a natural cough. **Forced coughing** (coughing that is purposely produced) may not be necessary for all postoperative clients. Forced coughing is most appropriate for clients who have diminished or moist lung sounds or who raise thick sputum. Nevertheless, all clients need to be prepared for the possibility of having to perform this technique and should receive instructions about it (see Client and Family Teaching 27-1).

Coughing is more painful for clients with abdominal or chest incisions. Administering pain medication approximately 30 minutes before coughing or splinting the incision during coughing can reduce discomfort. Methods of splinting include pressing on the incision with both hands, pressing on a pillow placed over the incision, or wrapping a bath blanket around the client (Fig. 27-3).

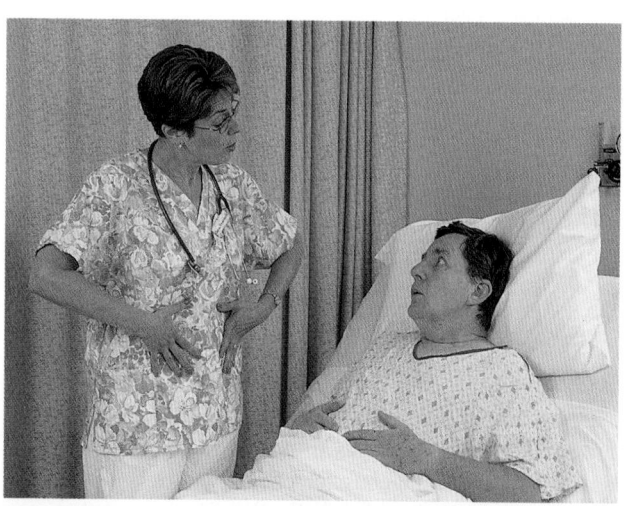

FIGURE 27-2 Teaching deep breathing. (Photo by B. Proud.)

Client and Family Teaching 27-1
Performing Forced Coughing

The nurse teaches the client and the family as follows:

- Sit upright.
- Take a slow, deep breath through the nose.
- Make the lower abdomen rise as much as possible.
- Lean slightly forward.
- Exhale slowly through the mouth.
- Pull the abdomen inward.
- Repeat, but this time cough three times in a row while exhaling.

Leg Exercises

Leg exercises help promote circulation and reduce the risk for forming a **thrombus** (a stationary blood clot) in the veins. Blood clots form when venous circulation is sluggish and when the fluid component of blood is reduced. Surgical clients are predisposed to both. Surgical clients have reduced circulatory volume because of the preoperative restriction of food and fluids and blood loss during surgery. In addition, blood tends to pool in the lower extremities because of the stationary position during surgery and the reluctance or inability to move afterward. With the use of leg exercises, efforts to reduce circulatory complications begin as soon as the client recovers from anesthesia (Client and Family Teaching 27-2).

Antiembolism stockings are knee-high or thigh-high elastic stockings. They are sometimes called *thromboembolic disorder* (TED) hose. These stockings help prevent thrombi and **emboli** (mobile blood clots) by compressing superficial veins and capillaries, redirecting more blood to larger and deeper veins, where it flows more effectively toward the heart. Intermittent pneumatic compression devices (discussed later in this chapter) are used for the same purpose but are applied postoperatively.

›› *Stop, Think, and Respond 27-1*

Discuss reasons why surgical clients are not as active and mobile as nonsurgical clients.

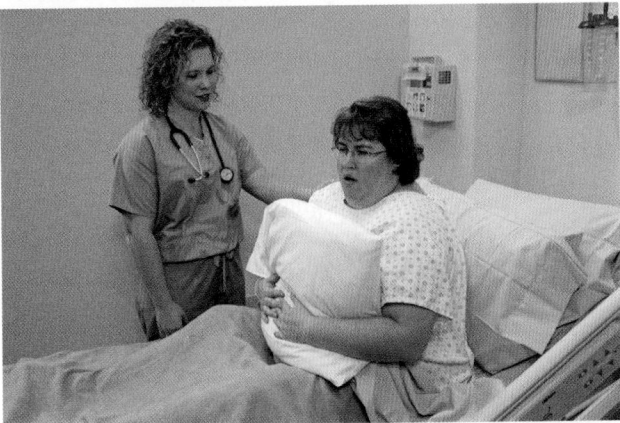

FIGURE 27-3 Teaching the client to splint the incision and to cough. (Photo by Ken Kasper.)

 Client and Family Teaching 27-2
Performing Leg Exercises

The nurse teaches the client and the family as follows:

- Sit with the head slightly raised.
- Bend one knee. Raise and hold the leg above the mattress for a few seconds (Fig. A).

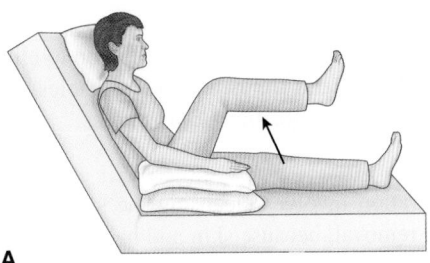

A

- Straighten the raised leg (Fig. B).

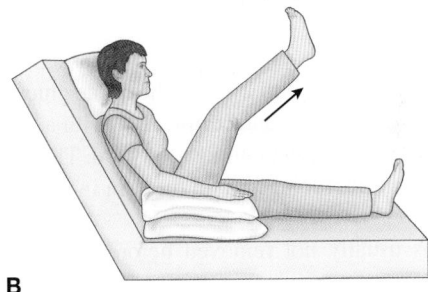

B

- Lower the leg back to the bed gradually (Fig. C).

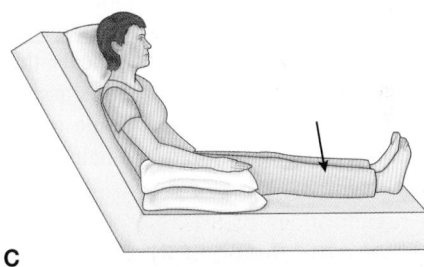

C

- Do the same with the other leg.
- Rest both legs on the bed.
- Point the toes toward the mattress and then toward the head (Fig. D).

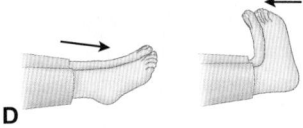

D

- Move both feet in clockwise and then counterclockwise circles (Fig. E).

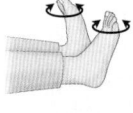

E

- Repeat the exercises five times at least every 2 hours while awake.

Figures from Taylor, C. R., Lynn, P., & Bartlett, J., (2018). *Fundamentals of nursing* (9th ed.). Lippincott Williams & Wilkins.

Antiembolism stockings must fit the client properly and be applied correctly (Skill 27-1). Stockings that become dirty are laundered, during which a second pair is used. If washed by hand, the stockings are laid flat to dry to prevent the loss of their elasticity.

Physical Preparation

Depending on the time of admission to the hospital or surgical facility, the nurse may perform some physical preparation that includes skin preparation, attention to elimination, restriction of food and fluids, care of valuables, putting on surgical attire, and disposition of prostheses.

Skin Preparation

Skin preparation involves cleansing the skin and, in some cases, hair removal, because skin and hair are reservoirs for microorganisms (Skill 27-2). The goal is to decrease transient and resident bacteria without compromising skin integrity. Reducing bacteria helps prevent postoperative wound infections.

For planned surgery, the client may be asked to bathe or shower twice at home with 2% chlorhexidine gluconate for a minimum of 2 minutes contact time; dry with a fresh, clean dry towel; and don clean clothing afterward. The soap leaves a persistent antimicrobial film on the skin in preparation for surgery.

Hair is usually not removed before surgery unless it is likely to interfere with the incision. Shaving causes **microabrasions** (tiny cuts that provide an entrance for microorganisms). For this reason, institutions generally use electric or battery-operated clippers rather than razors for hair removal. **Depilatory agents**, chemicals that remove hair, are another alternative, but their use is associated with skin irritation and allergic reactions. Some authorities believe that simply washing the skin and hair is sufficient to prevent infections.

≫ *Stop, Think, and Respond 27-2*

Correlate the potential for transmitting an infection using a razor for presurgical skin preparation with the chain of infection discussed in Chapter 10.

Elimination

The nurse may need to insert an indwelling urinary catheter (see Chapter 30) preoperatively for some surgeries, particularly of the lower abdomen. A distended bladder increases the risk of bladder trauma and difficulty in performing the procedure. The catheter keeps the bladder empty during surgery. If a catheter is not inserted, the nurse instructs the client to urinate immediately before receiving preoperative medication.

Enemas or a laxative may be ordered to clean the lower bowel (see Chapter 31) if the client is having abdominal or pelvic surgery. A clean bowel allows for improved visualization of the surgical site and prevents trauma to the intestines or accidental contamination of the abdominal cavity with feces. A cleansing enema or laxative is prescribed the evening before surgery and may be repeated the morning of surgery.

If bowel surgery is scheduled, IV antibiotics may be prescribed to destroy intestinal microorganisms.

Food and Fluids

The physician gives specific instructions about how long to restrict food and fluids preoperatively. Fasting from food and water from midnight onward before surgery is common, but the basis for the practice is now questionable. Fasting is used to reduce the potential for aspirating (inhaling) stomach contents while a client is anesthetized. However, aspiration is uncommon today with standard practices used by those administering general anesthesia. Consequently, the 2023 American Society of Anesthesiology's guidelines recommend that healthy preoperative clients can consume clear liquids 2 hours before elective surgery, have a light breakfast 6 hours before a surgical procedure, and eat a heavier meal 6 to 8 hours beforehand. Despite these newer recommendations, old practices persist. The nurse, therefore, encourages clients to maintain good nutrition and hydration before the restricted time to promote nutrients, such as protein and ascorbic acid (vitamin C), which are needed for healing.

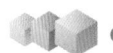 Concept Mastery Alert

Preoperative Intake

Despite current scientific evidence and recommendations that a healthy client can have clear liquids up to 2 hours prior to surgery, the old recommendation of nothing by mouth (NPO, *nil per os*) after midnight often persists in practice.

Valuables

The nurse instructs the client preoperatively to leave valuables at home. If the client forgets or does not follow this instruction, they must entrust valuables to a family member. Otherwise, health care agency personnel itemize them, place them in an envelope, and lock them in a designated area. The client signs a receipt, and the nurse notes the items' whereabouts in the client's medical record.

If the client is reluctant to remove a wedding band, the nurse may slip a ribbon of gauze under the ring and then loop the gauze around the finger and wrist or apply adhesive tape around a plain wedding band. The client also removes eyeglasses and contact lenses, which the nurse places in a safe location or gives to a family member.

Surgical Attire

Usually, clients wear a hospital gown and surgical cap to the operating room. The physician may order thigh-high or knee-high antiembolism stockings or order the client's legs wrapped in elastic roller bandages (see Chapter 28) before surgery to prevent venous stasis.

Hair ornaments are removed to avoid injury with equipment used to administer oxygen and inhalant anesthetics. Makeup and nail polish are omitted to facilitate assessing oxygenation. If a client has acrylic nails, one is usually removed to attach a pulse oximeter, which measures oxygen saturation (see Chapter 21).

Dentures and Prostheses

Depending on agency policy and the preference of the anesthesiologist or surgeon, the client removes full or partial dentures. Doing so prevents the dentures from causing airway obstruction during the administration of a general anesthetic. Some anesthesiologists prefer that well-fitting dentures remain in place to preserve facial contours, but that information must be communicated and well documented. When dentures are removed, they are placed in a denture container and stored at the client's bedside or with the client's belongings. Other prostheses, such as artificial limbs, are also removed unless otherwise ordered.

Preoperative Medications

The anesthesiologist or surgeon orders preoperative parenteral medications.

 Pharmacologic Considerations

Common preoperative medications include one or more of the following:

- *Antianxiety drugs*, such as lorazepam (Ativan), reduce preoperative anxiety, cause slight sedation, slow motor activity, and promote the induction of anesthesia.
- *Histamine-2 receptor antagonists*, such as cimetidine (Tagamet), decrease gastric acidity and volume.
- *Anticholinergics*, such as glycopyrrolate (Robinul), decrease respiratory secretions, dry mucous membranes, and prevent vagal nerve stimulation during endotracheal intubation.
- *Neuromuscular blocking agents*, such as succinylcholine (Anectine), promote skeletal muscle relaxation during the procedure and allow for rapid intubation.
- *Opioids*, such as fentanyl, sedate and decrease the amount of anesthesia.
- *Sedatives*, such as midazolam (Versed), promote sleep or amnesia and decrease anxiety.
- *Antibiotics*, such as kanamycin, destroy enteric microorganisms.

Before administering preoperative medications, the nurse uses at least two methods to verify the identity of the client. An example would be checking the client's identification bracelet and asking the client to state their name and date of birth (see Chapters 19, 32, and 34). The nurse asks about drug allergies, obtains vital signs, asks the client to void, and ensures that the surgical consent form has been signed.

Psychosocial Preparation

Preparing the client emotionally and spiritually is as important as doing so physically. Psychosocial preparation should begin as soon as the client is aware that surgery is necessary. If extreme, anxiety and fear can affect a client's condition during and after surgery. Anxious clients have a poor response to surgery and are prone to complications (Stamenkovic et al., 2018). Many clients are fearful because they know little or nothing about what will happen before, during, and after surgery. Careful listening and explaining by the nurse about what will happen and what to expect can help allay some of these fears and anxieties. The nurse also must assess methods the client uses for coping. Religious faith is a source of strength for many clients; therefore, nurses question the client as part of the spiritual assessment, then facilitate contact with a client's clergyperson or the hospital chaplain if requested.

Preoperative Checklist

A **preoperative checklist** (Fig. 27-4) is a form that identifies the status of essential presurgical activities and is completed before surgery. The nurse verifies the following:

- The history and physical examination have been documented.
- The name of the procedure on the surgical consent form matches that scheduled in the operating room.
- The surgical consent form has been signed and witnessed.
- All laboratory and diagnostic test results, such as a fasting blood sugar or electrocardiogram (ECG), have been returned and reported if abnormal.
- Allergies have been identified.
- The client is wearing an identification bracelet and allergy bracelet, if any exist.
- The client has had NPO since midnight or the number of hours prescribed.
- Skin preparation, if required, has been completed.
- Vital signs have been assessed and recorded.
- Nail polish, glasses, contact lenses, and hairpins have been removed.
- Jewelry has been removed, or the wedding ring has been secured.
- Dentures have been removed or left in place if requested by the person administering inhalant anesthesia.
- The client is wearing only a hospital gown and hair cover.
- The client has urinated.
- Location of IV site, type of solution, and rate of infusion are identified.
- The prescribed preoperative medication has been given.

The nurse is responsible for completing and signing the checklist. Operating room personnel review it when they arrive to transport the client. Surgery may be delayed if the checklist is incomplete.

Efforts have increased to ensure that the right client has the proper procedure at the correct site (if that applies). See Box 27-1 for the **Universal Protocol** developed by The Joint Commission (2024) to prevent errors in these categories.

INTRAOPERATIVE PERIOD

The **intraoperative period** (the time during which the client undergoes surgery) takes place in the operating suite. It involves transportation to a receiving room and then to the operating room where anesthesia is administered and the procedure is performed. The family is directed to a surgical waiting area during this time.

Receiving Room

The **receiving room** (Fig. 27-5) is a place in the surgery department where clients are observed until the operating room and surgical team are ready. In some hospitals, preoperative

COMPREHENSIVE SURGICAL CHECKLIST

PREPROCEDURE CHECK-IN	SIGN-IN	TIME-OUT	SIGN-OUT
In Preoperative Ready Area	Before Induction of Anesthesia	Before Skin Incision	Before the Patient Leaves the Operating Room
Patient or patient representative actively confirms with registered nurse (RN):	RN and anesthesia professional confirm:	Initiated by designated team member: All other activities to be suspended (except in case of life-threatening emergency)	RN confirms:
Identity ☐ Yes Procedure and procedure site ☐ Yes Consent(s) ☐ Yes Site marked ☐ Yes ☐ N/A by the person performing the procedure **RN confirms presence of:** History and physical ☐ Yes Preanesthesia assessment ☐ Yes Nursing assessment ☐ Yes Diagnostic and radiologic test results ☐ Yes ☐ N/A Blood products ☐ Yes ☐ N/A Any special equipment, devices, implants ☐ Yes ☐ N/A Include in Preprocedure check-in as per institutional custom: Beta-blocker medication given ☐ Yes ☐ N/A Venous thromboembolism prophylaxis ordered ☐ Yes ☐ N/A Normothermia measures ☐ Yes ☐ N/A	Confirmation of the following: identity procedure, procedure site, and consent(s) ☐ Yes Site marked ☐ Yes ☐ N/A by person performing the procedure Patient allergies ☐ Yes ☐ N/A Pulse oximeter on patient ☐ Yes Difficult airway or aspiration risk ☐ No ☐ Yes (preparation confirmed) Risk of blood loss (> 500 mL) ☐ Yes ☐ N/A # of units available_____ Anesthesia safety check completed ☐ Yes **Briefing:** All members of the team have discussed care plan and addressed concerns ☐ Yes	Introduction of team members ☐ Yes **All:** Confirmation of the following: identity procedure, incision site, consent(s) ☐ Yes Site is marked and visible ☐ Yes ☐ N/A Fire Risk Assessment and Discussion ☐ Yes (prevention methods implemented) ☐ N/A Relevant images properly labeled and displayed ☐ Yes ☐ N/A Any equipment concerns ☐ Yes ☐ N/A **Anticipated Critical Events** **Surgeon:** States the following: ☐ Critical or nonroutine steps ☐ Case duration ☐ Anticipated blood loss **Anesthesia professional:** Antibiotic prophylaxis within 1 hour before incision ☐ Yes ☐ N/A Additional concerns ☐ Yes ☐ N/A Scrub person and RN circulator: Sterilization indicators confirmed ☐ Yes Additional concerns ☐ Yes ☐ N/A **RN:** Documented completion of time-out ☐ Yes	Name of operative procedure: _____ Completion of sponge, sharp, and instrument counts ☐ Yes ☐ N/A Specimens identified and labeled ☐ Yes ☐ N/A Equipment problems to be addressed ☐ Yes ☐ N/A Discussion of Wound Classification ☐ Yes **To all team members:** What are the key concerns for recovery and management of this patient?_____ _____ _____ _____ _____ **Debriefing with all team members:** Opportunity for discussion of – team performance – key events – any permanent changes in the preference card

FIGURE 27-4 Combining guidance from the World Health Organization Surgical Safety Checklist and The Joint Commission Universal Protocol, the Association of PeriOperative Registered Nurses created a comprehensive surgical checklist (Reprinted with permission from AORN.org. Copyright © 2024, AORN, Inc. All rights reserved.).

BOX 27-1 Universal Protocol for Preventing Wrong Site, Wrong Procedure, Wrong Person Surgery

Conduct a Preprocedural Verification Process
- Address missing information or discrepancies before starting the procedure.
- Verify the correct procedure, for the correct patient, at the correct site.
- When possible, involve the patient in the verification process.
- Identify the items that must be available for the procedure.
- Use a standardized list to verify the availability of items for the procedure. (It is not necessary to document that the list was used for each patient.) At a minimum, these items include:
  - relevant documentation (e.g., history and physical, signed consent form, preanesthesia assessment)
  - labeled diagnostic and radiology test results that are properly displayed (e.g., radiology images and scans, pathology reports, biopsy reports)
- any required blood products, implants, devices, special equipment
- Match the items that are to be available in the procedure area to the patient.

Mark the Procedure Site
- At a minimum, mark the site when there is more than one possible location for the procedure and when performing the procedure in a different location could harm the patient.
- For spinal procedures: Mark the general spinal region on the skin. Special intraoperative imaging techniques may be used to locate and mark the exact vertebral level.
- Mark the site before the procedure is performed.
- If possible, involve the patient in the site marking process.

BOX 27-1   **Universal Protocol for Preventing Wrong Site, Wrong Procedure, Wrong Person Surgery (continued)**

- The site is marked by a licensed independent practitioner who is ultimately accountable for the procedure and will be present when the procedure is performed.
- In limited circumstances, site marking may be delegated to some medical residents, physician assistants (PA), or advanced practice registered nurses (APRN).
- Ultimately, the licensed independent practitioner is accountable for the procedure—even when delegating site marking.
- The mark is unambiguous and is used consistently throughout the organization.
- The mark is made at or near the procedure site.
- The mark is sufficiently permanent to be visible after skin preparation and draping.
- Adhesive markers are not the sole means of marking the site.
- For patients who refuse site marking or when it is technically or anatomically impossible or impractical to mark the site (see examples below): Use your organization's written, alternative process to ensure that the correct site is operated on. Examples of situations that involve alternative processes:
  - mucosal surfaces or perineum
  - minimal access procedures treating a lateralized internal organ, whether percutaneous or through a natural orifice
  - teeth
  - premature infants, for whom the mark may cause a permanent tattoo

Perform a Time-Out
- The procedure is not started until all questions or concerns are resolved.
- Conduct a time-out immediately before starting the invasive procedure or making the incision.
- A designated member of the team starts the time-out.
- The time-out is standardized.
- The time-out involves the immediate members of the procedure team: the individual performing the procedure, anesthesia providers, circulating nurse, operating room technician, and other active participants who will be participating in the procedure from the beginning.
- All relevant members of the procedure team actively communicate during the time-out.
- During the time-out, the team members agree, at a minimum, on the following:
  - correct patient's identity
  - correct site
  - procedure to be done
- When the same patient has two or more procedures: If the person performing the procedure changes, another time-out needs to be performed before starting each procedure.
- Document the completion of the time-out. The organization determines the amount and type of documentation.

medication is administered when clients reach the receiving room rather than before leaving the nursing unit. This practice coordinates the client's sedation more closely with the actual time of surgery.

Skin preparation may be delayed until this time as well. There is a direct relationship between the time the skin preparation is performed and the rate of microbial proliferation (Smith et al., 2013).

Operating Room

Eventually, clients are taken to the operating room, where their care and safety are in the hands of a team of experts including physicians and nurses. Anesthesia is administered in the operating room. Various types of anesthesia cause partial or complete loss of sensation with or without a loss of consciousness. They include general, regional, and local anesthesia.

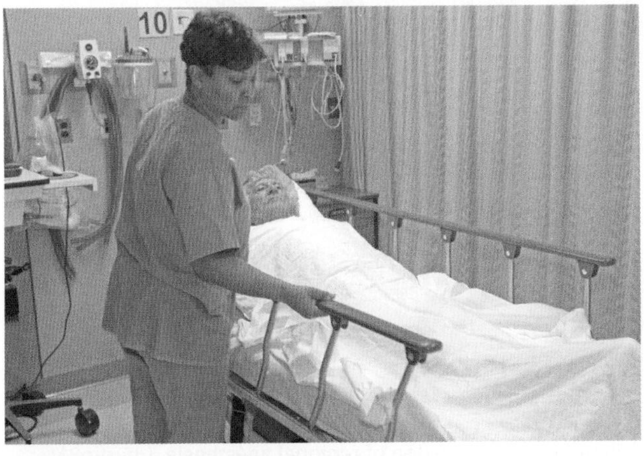

General Anesthesia

General anesthesia acts on the central nervous system to produce a loss of sensation, reflexes, and consciousness. General anesthetics are commonly administered via inhaled gases (Fig. 27-6) or a drug like propofol (Diprivan) IV.

Throughout the duration of and recovery from anesthesia, the client is monitored closely for effective breathing and oxygenation; effective circulatory status, including blood pressure (BP) and pulse within normal ranges; effective temperature regulation; and adequate fluid balance. During weaning from the anesthetic at the end of the surgery, the client's consciousness will be elevated sufficiently for them to follow commands and breathe independently. The recovery

FIGURE 27-5 A client awaiting surgery in a receiving room. (From Carter, P. J. [2019]. *Lippincott textbook for nursing assistants* [5th ed.]. Lippincott Williams & Wilkins.)

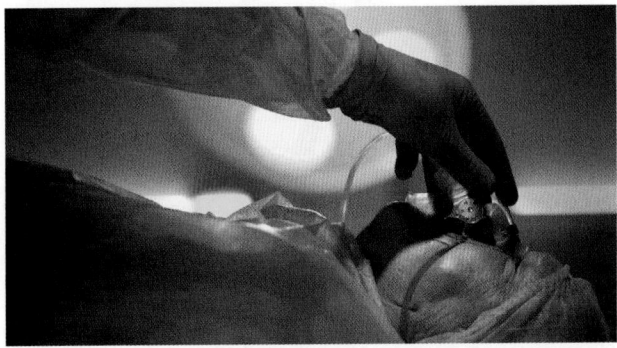

FIGURE 27-6 Client receiving inhaled general anesthesia. (TommyStockProject/Shutterstock.)

period can be brief or long. Many effects of general anesthesia take some time for the client to eliminate completely. Usually, clients do not remember much about the initial recovery period.

Regional Anesthesia

Regional anesthesia interferes with the conduction of sensory and motor nerve impulses to a specific area of the body. The client experiences loss of sensation and decreased mobility to the specific anesthetized area. They do not lose consciousness. Depending on the surgery, the client may receive a sedative to promote relaxation and comfort during the procedure. Types of regional anesthesia include local and spinal anesthesia and epidural and peripheral nerve blocks (Fig. 27-7).

The major advantage of regional anesthesia is the decreased risk for respiratory, cardiac, and GI complications. Team members must monitor the client for signs of allergic reactions, changes in vital signs, and toxic reactions. In addition, they must protect the anesthetized area if sensation is absent, because the client is at risk for injury.

Conscious Sedation

Conscious sedation refers to a state in which clients are sedated and in a state of relaxation and emotional comfort but are not unconscious. They are free of pain, fear, and anxiety and can tolerate unpleasant diagnostic and short therapeutic surgical procedures, such as endoscopies or bone marrow aspiration, while maintaining independent cardiorespiratory function. They can respond verbally and physically.

The IV route is used to administer medications that create conscious sedation. If other routes are used, the client must have venous access for the treatment of possible adverse effects, such as hypoxemia and central nervous system depression. The responsibility for ensuring client safety and comfort during sedation rests with the nurse directly involved in the client's care. Although numerous types of equipment for monitoring clients are available, no equipment replaces a nurse's careful observations. Clients are discharged shortly after the procedure in which conscious sedation is used.

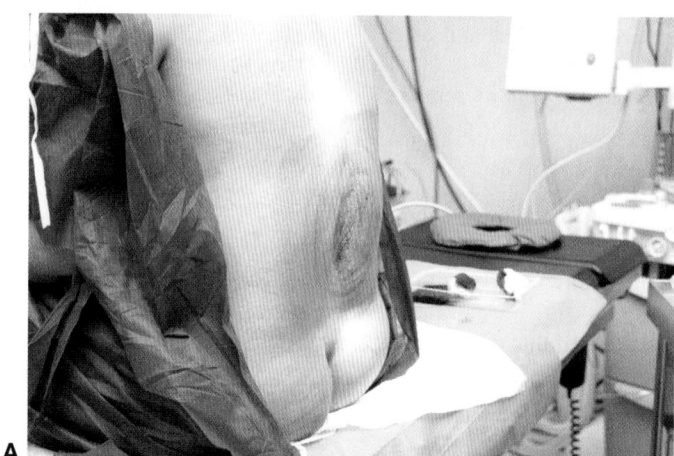

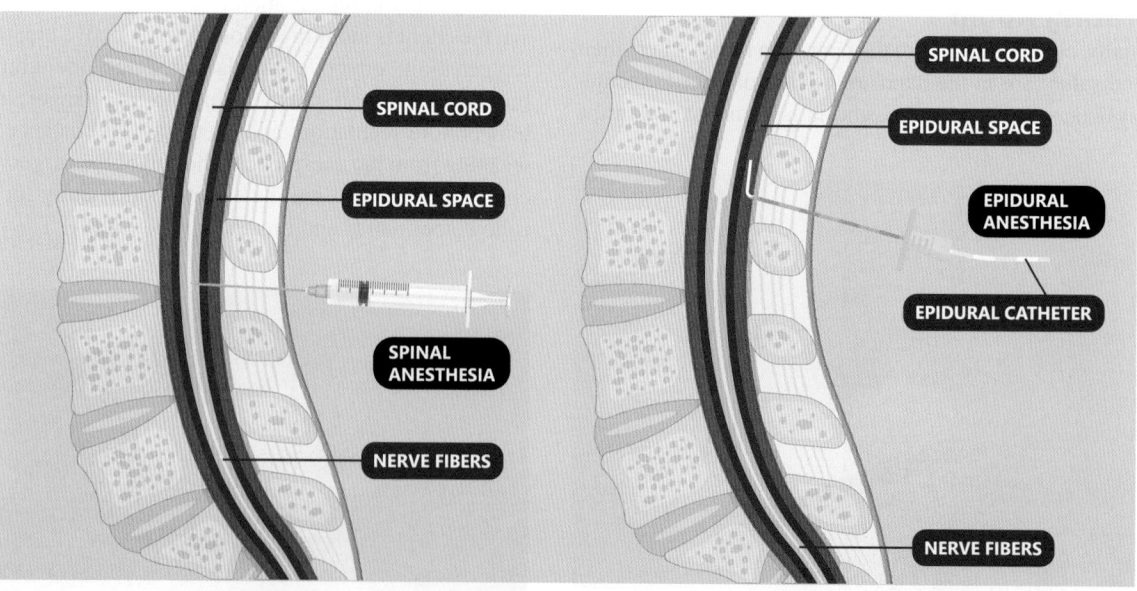

FIGURE 27-7 Administration of regional anesthesia. **A.** Preparing the client for administration of regional anesthesia. (martin81/ Shutterstock.) **B.** Types and injection locations for regional anesthesia. (Pepermpron/Shutterstock.)

Pharmacologic Considerations

Reversal drugs, medications that counteract the effects of those used for conscious sedation, must be readily available in case the client becomes overly sedated. Two examples of reversal drugs are naloxone (Narcan), which is the antagonist for opiates like morphine, and flumazenil (Romazicon), which reverses antianxiety drugs like midazolam (Versed).

Surgical Waiting Area

The **surgical waiting area** is the room where family and friends await information about the client. It is staffed by volunteers who provide comfort, support, and news about how the client's surgery is progressing. Many agencies provide food and beverages, public telephones, television, and magazines in this area. Often, the surgeon comes to the waiting area immediately after the procedure to contact the family. The family and surgeon generally go to a private room where the surgeon discusses the client's status and the procedure to ensure confidentiality.

POSTOPERATIVE PERIOD

The **postoperative period** begins after the operative procedure is completed and the client is transported to an area to recover from the anesthesia and ends when the client is discharged. The **postanesthesia care unit** (PACU), also known as the *postanesthesia reacting* (PAR) room or the *recovery room*, is the area in the surgical department where clients are intensively monitored (Fig. 27-8). Nurses in the PACU ensure the safe recovery of surgical clients from anesthesia.

Immediate Postoperative Care

The focus of **postoperative care** (nursing care after surgery) is different during the immediate postoperative period than it is later, when clients are more stable. The immediate

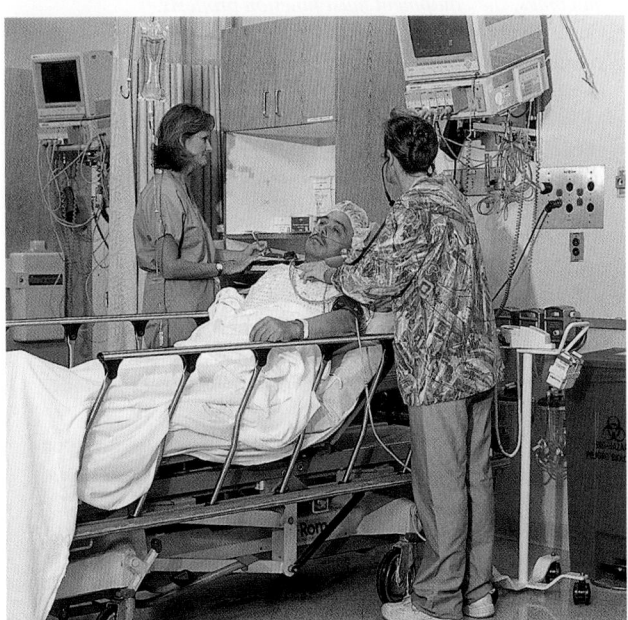

FIGURE 27-8 A postanesthesia care unit. (Photo by B. Proud.)

postoperative period refers to the first 24 hours after surgery. During this time, nurses monitor the client for complications as they recover from anesthesia and are sufficiently stable to be transferred to a nursing unit for continued assessment.

Initial Postoperative Assessments

The circulating surgical nurse or anesthesiologist reports pertinent information regarding the surgery and the client's condition to the nurse in the PACU. Once the care of the client is transitioned to the recovery room nurse, the PACU nurse's major responsibilities are to ensure a patent airway; maintain adequate circulation; prevent or assist with the management of shock; maintain proper positions and function of drains, tubes, and IV infusions; and detect evidence of any complications. The nurse systematically checks:

- Level of consciousness
- Vital signs
- Effectiveness of respirations
- Presence or need for supplemental oxygen
- Condition of the wound and dressing
- Location of drains and drainage characteristics
- Location, type, and rate of IV fluid
- Level of pain and need for analgesia
- Presence of a urinary catheter and urine volume

Continuing Postoperative Care

Once the client is stable, the client is readied for transport to the general surgical unit where the client's room is prepared and assessments will continue to prevent, detect, or minimize complications.

Preparing the Room

The next stage of care begins with getting the client's bed and the environment ready. The nurses fold the top bed linen toward the foot or side of the bed. They place the bed in a high position to facilitate transferring the client from the stretcher. Often, they keep additional blankets ready for use because some clients feel cold after being quiet and inactive.

In addition, nurses assemble bedside supplies and equipment that facilitate caring for the client. Potentially useful items include oxygen equipment (see Chapter 21), a pole or electronic infusion device for continuing the administration of IV fluids (see Chapter 16), an emesis basin if the client becomes nauseous, paper tissues, and a device for collecting and measuring urine (see Chapter 30). Suction canisters may be necessary for clients who have gastric tubes (see Chapter 29).

Monitoring for Complications

Postoperative clients are at risk for many complications (Table 27-7), some of which are more likely to develop soon after surgery. Frequently focused assessments of the client and equipment facilitate a safe postoperative recovery (Nursing Guidelines 27-1).

Providing Food and Oral Fluids

After surgery, the client needs to resume eating. Food and oral fluids are withheld until surgical clients are awake, free of nausea and vomiting, and bowel sounds are active.

TABLE 27-7 Postoperative Complications

COMPLICATION	DESCRIPTION	TREATMENT
Airway occlusion	Obstruction of throat	Tilt the head and lift the chin.
		Insert an artificial airway.
Hemorrhage	Severe, rapid blood loss	Control bleeding.
		Administer intravenous fluid.
		Replace blood.
Shock	Inadequate blood flow	Place the client in a modified Trendelenburg position.
		Replace fluids.
		Administer oxygen.
		Give emergency drugs.
Pulmonary embolus	Obstruction of circulation through the lung as a result of a wedged blood clot that began as a thrombus	Give oxygen.
		Administer anticoagulant drugs.
Hypoxemia	Inadequate oxygenation of blood	Give oxygen.
Adynamic ileus	Lack of bowel motility	Treat the cause.
		Give nothing by mouth.
		Insert a nasogastric tube and connect to suction.
		Administer intravenous fluid.
Urinary retention	Inability to void	Insert a catheter.
Wound infection	Proliferation of pathogens at or beneath the incision	Cleanse with antimicrobial agents.
		Open and drain incision.
		Administer antibiotics.
Dehiscence	Separation of incision	Reinforce wound edges.
		Apply a binder.
Evisceration	Protrusion of abdominal organs through separated wound	Cover with wet dressing.
		Reapproximate wound.

NURSING GUIDELINES 27-1

Providing Postoperative Care

- Obtain a summary report from a postanesthesia care unit (PACU) nurse. *This report provides current assessment data concerning the client's progress.*
- Check the postoperative medical orders on the chart. *The medical orders provide instructions for individualized care.*
- Assist PACU personnel to transfer the client to bed. *The client should be observed continuously at this time.*
- Observe the client's respiratory pattern and auscultate the lungs. *Maintaining breathing is a priority for care.*
- Check oxygen saturation using a pulse oximeter if the client seems hypoxic (see Chapter 21). *An oximeter indicates the quality of internal respiration.*
- Administer oxygen if the oxygen saturation is less than 90% or if prescribed by the physician. *Oxygen administration increases oxygen available for binding with hemoglobin and for becoming dissolved in the plasma.*
- Note the client's level of consciousness and response to stimulation. *Findings indicate the client's neurologic status.*
- Orient the client and instruct them to take several deep breaths as taught preoperatively. *Deep breathing improves ventilation and gas exchange.*
- Check vital signs. *Findings provide data for assessing the client's current general condition.*
- Repeat vital sign assessments at least every 15 minutes until they are stable; then follow agency policy and retake them every hour to every 4 hours depending on the client's condition or medical orders. *Repeat assessment of vital signs provides comparative data.*

- Check the incisional area and the dressing for drainage. *Findings provide data concerning the status of the wound and blood loss.*
- Inspect all tubes, insertion sites, and connections. *For optimal outcomes, the equipment must function properly.*
- Check the type of intravenous fluid, rate of administration, and volume that remains. *Findings provide data regarding fluid therapy.*
- Monitor urination; report failure to void within 8 hours of surgery. *Failure to void indicates urinary retention.*
- Auscultate bowel sounds. *Findings provide data concerning bowel motility.*
- Assess the client's level of pain, its location, and characteristics. *Pain indicates the need for analgesia.*
- Administer analgesic drugs according to prescribed medical orders if doing so is safe. *Analgesic drugs relieve pain.*
- Remind the client to perform leg exercises or apply antiembolism stockings. *Leg exercises and antiembolism stockings promote circulation.*
- Use a side-lying position if the client is lethargic or unresponsive. *This position prevents airway obstruction by the tongue and aspiration of emesis if vomiting occurs.*
- Raise the side rails unless providing direct care. *Keeping the side rails up ensures safety.*
- Fasten the signal device within the client's reach. *The signal device is a way for the client to communicate and obtain assistance.*

Postoperative clients usually progress from a clear liquid diet to more solid food unless complications develop. Nurses monitor fluid intake and output to ensure clients are adequately hydrated.

 Nutrition Notes

The postsurgical diet order may be "progress from clear liquids to a regular diet as tolerated." A quick progression to self-selected regular food by the second postsurgical meal is safe for most clients, even those who have had major GI surgery, and may even hasten recovery.

Promoting Venous Circulation

Surgical clients ambulate with assistance as soon as possible to reduce the potential for pulmonary and vascular complications. After some surgical procedures, however, antiembolism stockings, leg exercises, ambulation, and elevation of the lower extremities may not be enough to reduce swelling of the lower extremities and the potential for thrombus formation.

For clients who have the potential for impaired circulation in one or both extremities, a **pneumatic compression device**, a machine that promotes the circulation of venous blood and relocation of excess fluid into the lymphatic vessels, may be medically prescribed. Various companies make pneumatic compression devices, but they all consist of an extremity sleeve with tubes that connect to an electric air pump (Fig. 27-9). The device compresses the sleeved extremity either intermittently or sequentially from distal to proximal areas. Most devices cycle on for a few seconds and then cycle off for a longer period. Depending on the manufacturer, pumps may cycle one to four times/minute. The nurse is responsible for applying this device (Skill 27-3).

Other measures to prevent thrombi include drinking plenty of fluids, avoiding long periods of sitting, keeping the legs uncrossed (especially at the knees), ambulating, and changing position frequently.

≫ Stop, Think, and Respond 27-3
Compare the use of a TED hose with a pneumatic compression device; list advantages and disadvantages for each.

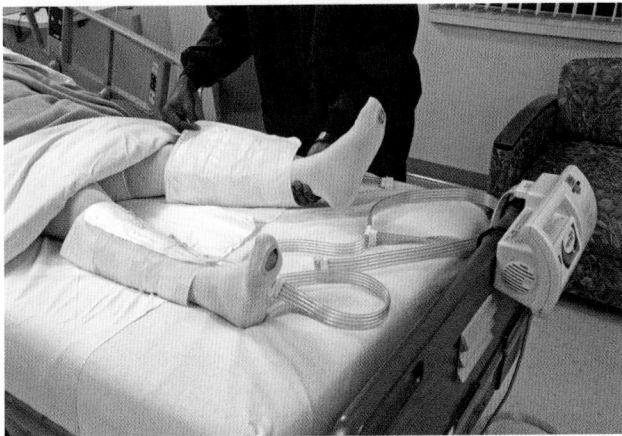

FIGURE 27-9 A pneumatic compression device.

Preventing Thrombus Formation

Postoperatively, clients are at risk for developing deep vein thromboses as a consequence of preoperative fluid restrictions, a decrease in blood volume due to fluid loss during the surgical procedure, and decreased activity following the surgery. The nurse encourages leg exercises that were taught prior to surgery and early ambulation and administers prophylactic antithrombotic medications as prescribed by the physician.

 Pharmacologic Considerations

Following major surgical procedures, a client typically receives an injectable anticoagulant, such as dalteparin (Fragmin) or fondaparinux (Arixtra), to prevent thrombus formation. This medication supports standard nursing postoperative care and is not a substitute for ambulation or other activities to promote venous circulation.

Performing Wound Management

Nurses assess the condition of the wound and the characteristics of drainage at least once in each shift. Dressings are reinforced or changed if they become loose or saturated. Eventually, sutures or staples are removed (see Chapter 28). Most hospitalized clients are discharged within 3 to 5 days of surgery or sooner to continue their recuperation at home.

Providing Discharge Instructions

The nurse provides **discharge instructions** (directions for managing self-care and medical follow-up) before the client leaves. Common areas to address when discharging clients who have undergone surgery include:

- How to care for the incision site
- Signs of complications to report
- What drugs to use to relieve pain
- How to self-administer prescribed drugs
- When normal activity can be resumed
- If and how much weight can be lifted
- Which foods to consume or avoid
- When and where to return for follow-up appointments

The nurse gives information both verbally and in written form.

NURSING IMPLICATIONS

Surgical clients offer unique nursing care problems. Applicable nursing diagnoses include:

- Fear
- Acute pain
- Ineffective airway clearance
- Altered body image perception
- Knowledge deficiency
- Infection risk
- Altered skin integrity risk
- Hypovolemia
- Altered breathing pattern
- impaired gas exchange

Nursing Care Plan 27-1 shows how the nurse can use the nursing process to identify and resolve a diagnosis of "altered body image perception," defined as a state of disturbance when the person's changed body image does not enable the person to experience their usual sense of self, or it inhibits their ability to engage in social interaction (Tadman et al., 2019). This diagnosis is especially pertinent to clients who have had their appearance altered as a result of surgery.

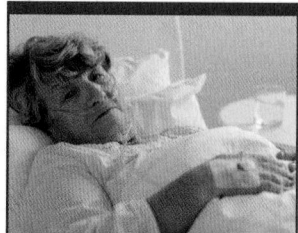

Clinical Scenario A 73-year-old female was diagnosed with a colorectal malignancy following a routine colonoscopy. She has become depressed during the postoperative recovery.

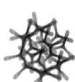

NURSING CARE PLAN 27-1 — Altered Body Image Perception

Assessment

- Observe the client's reaction to their body changes.
- Note if the client refuses to touch or look at the body part that has been altered.
- Scrutinize the client's involvement, or lack of it, in learning techniques for self-care or rehabilitation.
- Observe if the client seeks others to manage care for which they are capable.
- Watch the quality and quantity of the client's social interactions or avoidance of others.
- Listen for self-deprecating remarks or hostility toward others.

Nursing Diagnosis. Altered body image perception related to fear of rejection based on altered elimination secondary to a colectomy with ileostomy as evidenced by asking that room freshener be sprayed frequently, applying perfume heavily, positioning herself more than 5 ft from visitors, and stating, "I hate myself for agreeing to this operation. This thing fills up, it bulges, and it smells. No one will ever want to come near me again."

Expected Outcome. The client will demonstrate acceptance and less self-consciousness about changed body image by interacting with a visitor within 3 ft by 10/9.

Interventions	Rationales
Spend at least 15 minutes with the client midmorning, midafternoon, and early evening without performing direct care.	Social interaction not associated with performing a task communicates interest and acceptance of the client as a worthwhile person.
During interaction, sit within 3 ft of the client.	Sitting closely provides evidence that closeness is not a problem.
Acknowledge verbally that the ostomy and resulting change in elimination are difficult to accept.	Verbalizing what the client is implying nonverbally and actively demonstrating shows empathy.
Offer to contact another person with an ostomy through the United Ostomy Association.	Interacting with another person who is coping well with a similar change can help the client share feelings and acquire a different perspective from an objective role model.
Offer a referral to an enterostomal nurse therapist.	An enterostomal nurse therapist has knowledge and skills for managing problems experienced by clients with ostomies, such as odor control and other wound and skin impairments.
During ostomy teaching sessions and care of the stoma, avoid facial expressions that may communicate disgust or repulsion.	Nonverbal behavior is more accurate than verbal expressions during communication.
Use terminology such as "your stoma" and avoid any depersonalized or slang names for the changed body part.	Using inappropriate terms trivializes the significance of the issue with which the client is coping.

Evaluation of Expected Outcomes

- Client moved away to provide more distance during close interaction.
- Client looked at stoma while skin care and changing of appliance were demonstrated.
- Client read booklet provided by the United Ostomy Association.
- Client agreed to meet with the enterostomal therapist.

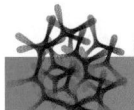

KEY POINTS

- Perioperative care: Care clients receive before, during, and after surgery
- Three phases of perioperative care
  - Preoperative: Begins when it becomes clear surgery is necessary and ends when clients are transported to the operating room
  - Intraoperative: The time during which the client undergoes surgery
  - Postoperative: After the operative procedure is completed
- Surgeries
  - Inpatient: Procedures performed on a client who is admitted to the hospital
  - Outpatient: Procedures performed on clients who return home the same day
- Preoperative blood donation
  - Some clients undergoing surgery donate their own blood preoperatively if it does not jeopardize their own health. Predonated blood is held on reserve in the event that the client needs a blood transfusion during or after surgery.
  - Autologous transfusion: Receiving one's own blood (self-donated blood). Autologous transfusions are also prepared by salvaging blood lost during or immediately after surgery. The salvaged blood is suctioned, cleaned, and filtered from drainage collection devices.
- Preoperative risk factors
  - Age
  - Nutritional status
  - Substance use
  - Medical problems
- Preoperative teaching
  - Preoperative medications
  - Postsurgical pain control
  - Vital signs and monitoring

- Deep breathing
- Coughing
- Leg exercises and antiembolism stockings to prevent blood clots
- Preoperative physical preparation
  - Skin preparation
  - Elimination
  - Food and fluids
  - Valuables
  - Surgical attire
  - Dentures and prosthesis
- Preoperative verification process
  - Marking the operative site
  - Time-out: Final verification of the correct client, procedure, and site
- Intraoperative period and areas
  - Receiving room
  - Operating room
  - Anesthesia
    - General
    - Regional
    - Conscious sedation
  - Surgical waiting room
- Postoperative period
  - Immediate postoperative period
  - Initial postoperative assessment
  - Monitoring for complications
  - Providing food and oral fluids
  - Promoting venous circulation
  - Preventing thrombus formation
  - Performing wound management
  - Providing discharge instructions

CRITICAL THINKING EXERCISES

1. The following data are reviewed by a nurse preparing a client for surgery: The client is 60 years old; weighs 205 lb; has a history of chronic pulmonary disease; quit smoking 10 years ago; vital signs are BP 140/88 mm Hg, temperature 101.8°F, pulse rate 92, and respiratory rate 28 breaths/minute. Which finding is most important to report to the surgeon?
2. A client reports having taken only one shower with chlorhexidine gluconate rather than two the night before surgery. What actions could the nurse take?
3. A nurse assesses a postoperative client and obtains the following data: BP 102/64 mm Hg, pulse rate 90, respirations 32 and shallow, responds when shaken, and experiences nausea. What finding is most serious at this time, and what nursing actions are appropriate?
4. A preoperative client who is Native American wants you to attach a dream catcher, a circular object with a woven web, to the IV pole. Based on principles of transcultural nursing, what is an appropriate way to respond to the client's request?

NEXT-GENERATION NCLEX-STYLE REVIEW QUESTIONS

1. Assuming a client is admitted the evening before surgery, when is it best for the nurse to perform preoperative skin antisepsis and hair removal, if the latter is necessary, on a client who is scheduled for a procedure at 1300?
   a. The night before surgery
   b. After the morning shower
   c. Before transport to the receiving area
   d. When in the operating room
   Test-Taking Strategy: Note the key word, "best." Select the option that is better than any of the others for reducing the risk of a surgical infection.
2. What information is essential to verify during a presurgical time-out? Select all that apply.
   a. The client's room number
   b. The client's identity
   c. The name of the surgeon
   d. The name of the procedure
   e. The type of anesthesia
   f. The site of the procedure

Test-Taking Strategy: Analyze the choices and select the options that comply with The Joint Commission's Universal Protocol that promotes the performance of safe surgery.

3. From whom is it most appropriate for the nurse to obtain consent to perform surgery on an adolescent?
   a. The client
   b. The client's physician
   c. The client's minister
   d. The client's parent
   Test-Taking Strategy: Note the key word and modifier, "most appropriate." Select the option that is better legally than any of the others.

4. What is the most important nursing action after administering a preoperative medication containing a narcotic?
   a. Raise the side rails on the bed.
   b. Help the client with using the toilet.
   c. Give the client a surgical gown.
   d. Apply an identification band.
   Test-Taking Strategy: Note the key word and modifier, "most important." Select the option that is better than any of the others when preparing a client for surgery.

5. When the nurse assesses a client during the immediate postoperative period, which assessment is most indicative of impending shock?
   a. Bounding pulse
   b. Slow respirations
   c. Low BP
   d. High body temperature
   Test-Taking Strategy: Note the key word and modifier, "most indicative." Eliminate choices until the option suggesting that the client is developing a postoperative complication of shock remains.

NEXT-GENERATION NCLEX-STYLE CLINICAL SCENARIO QUESTIONS

Clinical Scenario:

A 73-year-old female was diagnosed with a colorectal malignancy following a routine colonoscopy. She has become depressed during the postoperative recovery.

1. Select all of the nursing diagnoses that may be pertinent for this client.
   a. Fear
   b. Infection risk
   c. Altered body image perception
   d. Caregiver fatigue
   e. Bowel incontinence
   f. Denial
   g. Coping impairment

2. For each recommendation, use an "x" to indicate whether the interventions were effective or ineffective.

RECOMMENDATION	EFFECTIVE	INEFFECTIVE
Encourage the patient to acknowledge and discuss body changes and accompanying emotions.		
Keep personal items close to the patient.		
Allow the patient to express feelings, and actively listen.		
Provide support to the patient and family (as appropriate).		
Educate the patient and family (as appropriate) about expected changes in body function or appearance.		
Provide the patient with alternative ways of communicating.		

SKILL 27-1 Applying Antiembolism Stockings

Suggested Action	Reason for Action
ASSESSMENT	
Review the medical orders and the nursing plan for care.	Directs client care
Wash your hands or use an alcohol-based hand rub (see Chapter 10).	Reduces the transmission of microorganisms
Measure the client's leg from the flat of the heel to the bend of the knee or to midthigh (Fig. A). 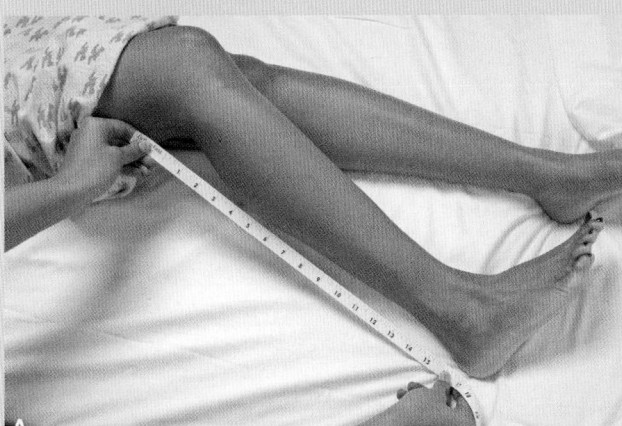	Determines the length needed for knee-high or thigh-high stockings Measuring the leg length from bottom of heel to back of knee. (From Springhouse. [2009]. *Lippincott's visual encyclopedia of clinical skills*. Lippincott Williams & Wilkins.)
Measure the calf or thigh circumference (Fig. B). 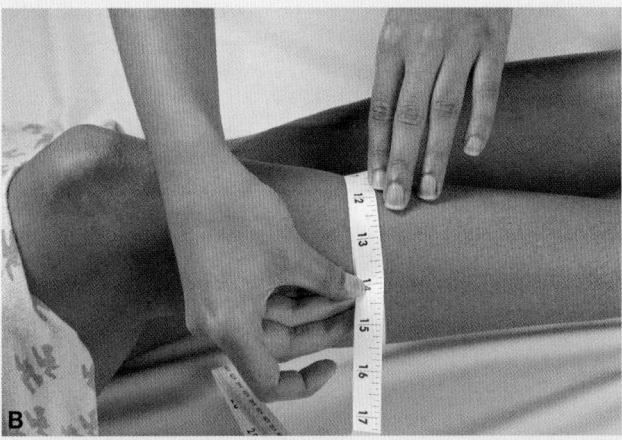	Determines the size needed Measuring the circumference at its widest point. (From Springhouse. [2009]. *Lippincott's visual encyclopedia of clinical skills*. Lippincott Williams & Wilkins.)
Assess the client's understanding of the purpose and use of elastic stockings.	Determines the type and amount of health teaching needed
Check the fit of stockings that the client is currently wearing.	Identifies the potential complications from tight, loose, or wrinkled stockings
PLANNING	
Obtain the correct size of stockings before surgery or as soon as possible after they are ordered.	Facilitates early preventive treatment
Plan to remove the stockings for 20 minutes once in each shift or at least twice a day and then reapply them.	Allows for assessment and hygiene
Elevate the legs for at least 15 minutes before applying the stockings if the client has been sitting or standing for some time.	Promotes venous circulation and avoids trapping venous blood in the lower extremities

(continued)

SKILL 27-1 Applying Antiembolism Stockings (*continued*)

Suggested Action	Reason for Action
IMPLEMENTATION	
Wash and dry the feet.	Removes dirt, skin oil, and some microorganisms
Apply cornstarch or talcum powder if desired (Fig. C).	Reduces friction when applying the stockings
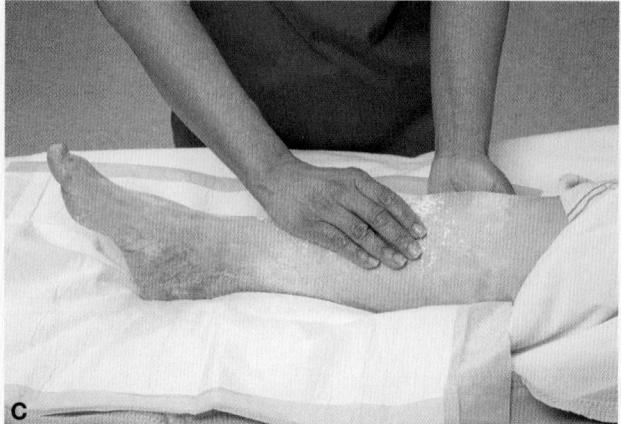 **C**	Powdering the skin. (From Craven, R. F., Hirnle, C. J., & Jensen, S. [2020]. *Fundamentals of nursing* [9th ed.]. Lippincott Williams & Wilkins.)
Avoid massaging the legs. Turn the stockings inside out (Fig. D).	Prevents dislodging a thrombus if one is present
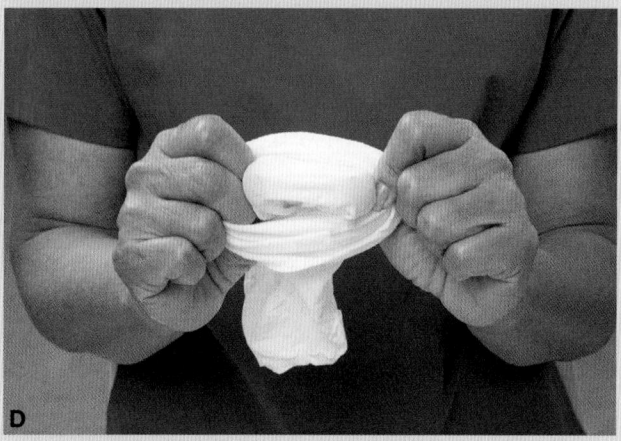 **D**	Turning the stockings inside out and tucking the heel inside.
Insert the toes and pull the stockings upward a few inches until it covers the foot (Fig. E).	Facilitates threading the stockings over the foot and leg
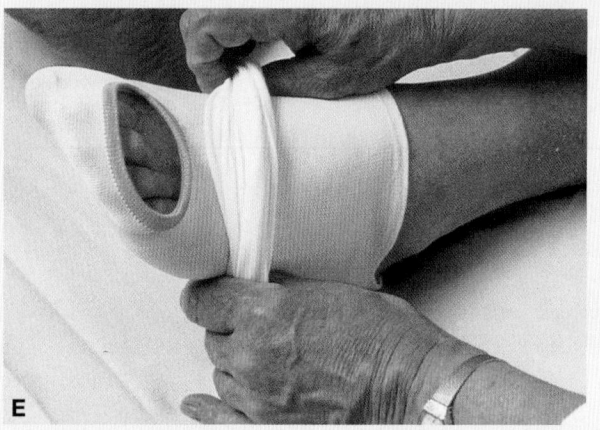 **E**	Easing the foot section over the toe and heel. (Photo by B. Proud.)
Gather the remaining length of the stockings and pull it upward a few inches at a time (Fig. F).	Reduces bunching and bulkiness, eases application, and avoids forming wrinkles

SKILL 27-1 Applying Antiembolism Stockings (*continued*)

Suggested Action	Reason for Action
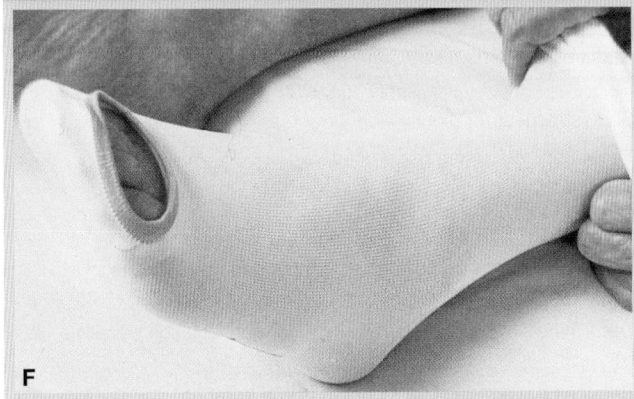**F**	Pulling the stockings upward over the rest of the leg. (Photo by B. Proud.)

EVALUATION

- Skin remains intact and circulation is adequate.
- Stockings are removed and reapplied at least twice daily.

DOCUMENT

- Assessment findings
- Removal and reapplication of elastic stockings

SAMPLE DOCUMENTATION

Date and Time   Toes are warm. Blood returns to nail beds within 3 seconds of compression. Skin over legs is smooth and intact. TED hose reapplied after bathing. _____ J. Doe, LPN

SKILL 27-2 Performing Presurgical Skin Preparation

Suggested Action	Reason for Action
ASSESSMENT	
Determine that the client has followed instructions regarding showering and avoiding shaving the surgical site before coming to the facility.	Washing and rinsing with an antiseptic removes microorganisms from the skin; shaving the surgical area hours or the day before surgery significantly increases the risk for a surgical site infection.
Consult the preoperative medical orders to determine whether it is necessary to remove hair in the area of the potential surgical incision.	Studies indicate that surgical site infections are reduced by omitting hair removal or only removing hair without a razor at or around the incision site if it will interfere with the procedure.
Wash your hands or use an alcohol-based hand rub (see Chapter 10).	Reduces the transmission of microorganisms
Assess the condition of the skin, looking especially for skin lesions.	Indicates areas that may bleed if irritated or provide a reservoir of microorganisms
Explore how much the client understands about the purpose and extent of skin preparation.	Helps identify the extent and level of health teaching needed
PLANNING	
Arrange to perform the skin preparation shortly before the client is transported for surgery.	Reduces the time during which microorganisms will recolonize the skin
Explain the procedure.	Reduces anxiety and promotes cooperation
Provide an opportunity for the client to don a hospital gown.	Protects personal clothing and provides access for care
Obtain electric or battery-operated clippers or depilatory agent, if ordered, a towel, a bath blanket, and gloves.	Provides essential supplies
Braid scalp hair or use a nonflammable gel to keep hair out of the way prior to surgical procedures in which an incision will be made in the scalp.	Leaving scalp hair in place has not been shown to increase the incidence of surgical site infections and promotes a client's self-esteem postoperatively.

(*continued*)

SKILL 27-2 Performing Presurgical Skin Preparation (*continued*)

Suggested Action	Reason for Action
IMPLEMENTATION	
Wash your hands or use an alcohol-based hand rub (see Chapter 10) and put on clean gloves.	Reduces the transmission of microorganisms
Provide privacy.	Shows respect for dignity
Position the client so the area to be prepared is accessible.	Facilitates performing the procedure
Drape the client with a bath blanket.	Maintains dignity as well as warmth
Protect the bed with towels or a disposable pad.	Contains the dispersal of loose hair
Use a single-use hair clipper or clipper with a reusable head that can be disinfected to remove hair from the designated area.	Prevents transmission of microorganisms to other clients
Follow the manufacturer's directions regarding skin testing in a small area if a depilatory is used.	Determines whether hypersensitivity or skin irritation develops
Keep a depilatory away from the client's eyes and genitalia.	Reduces the potential for skin and tissue irritation
Deposit or dispose of items used for skin antisepsis and hair removal in appropriate containers.	Confines sources of infectious disease transmission and restores comfort and orderliness
Remove the reusable head from a nondisposable hair clipper and follow the agency's policy for disinfection.	Reduces the transmission of microorganisms
Remove gloves and wash hands.	Reduces the transmission of microorganisms
Return reusable clippers to their designated location and recharge the battery.	Ensures that reusable hair clippers are in working condition for future use

EVALUATION

- Skin has been prepared according to policy and medical orders.
- Skin remains essentially intact.

DOCUMENT

- Assessment findings
- Technique for preoperative skin antisepsis (i.e., bathing, showers, hair removed with clippers, depilatory, or not removed)
- Area prepared

SAMPLE DOCUMENTATION

Date and Time   Client reports taking two showers with chlorhexidine gluconate the evening before surgery. No hair removed from the potential site of the incision. Skin is intact. No evidence of lesions or body piercings. _____ J. Doe, LPN

SKILL 27-3 Applying a Pneumatic Compression Device

Suggested Action	Reason for Action
ASSESSMENT	
Review the medical orders and the nursing plan for care.	Directs client care
Determine whether the device will be applied to one or both extremities.	Gives direction for gathering assessment data and applying the device
Wash your hands or use an alcohol-based hand rub (see Chapter 10).	Reduces the potential for the transmission of microorganisms
Assess the circulation of the toes and integrity of the skin.	Provides a baseline of data for future comparison
Measure the calf circumference and assess for pitting edema in extremities.	Provides a baseline of data for future comparison
Palpate the pedal pulses.	Validates arterial blood flow to the foot if present and strong
Assess the client's understanding of the purpose and use of a pneumatic compression device.	Determines the type and amount of health teaching needed

SKILL 27-3 Applying a Pneumatic Compression Device (*continued*)

Suggested Action	Reason for Action
PLANNING	
Obtain the extremity sleeves, electric air pump, and accompanying air tubes.	Facilitates expeditious implementation of the medical order
Assist the client with any elimination needs.	Avoids having to disconnect the equipment shortly after the device is applied
Arrange supplies the client may need within their reach, including the signal device.	Promotes independence yet ensures that the client can call for assistance
Help the client into a position of comfort such as a supine or low Fowler position.	Fosters rest and relaxation
IMPLEMENTATION	
Wrap the extremity sleeve snugly around the extremity (Fig. A).	Positions the sleeve where compression is desired
A Applying the extremity sleeve. (Photo by B. Proud.)	Applying the extremity sleeve. (Photo by B. Proud.)
Secure the sleeve once it encircles the leg; most are secured with Velcro.	Ensures that the sleeve will remain in the applied position
Secure the air pump to the bottom of the bed or a stable surface.	Protects the device from damage and prevents injury to staff or visitors
Attach the air tubes to the ports that extend from the sleeve and to the adapter within the air pump (Fig. B).	Provides a channel through which air is delivered to the extremity sleeve
B	Attaching air tubes so that the arrows align. (Photo by B. Proud.)
Check that the air tubes are unkinked and not compressed under the client or the wheels of the bed.	Ensures the unobstructed delivery of air
Plug the air pump into an electrical outlet.	Delivers power to the air pump motor

(continued)

SKILL 27-3 Applying a Pneumatic Compression Device (*continued*)

Suggested Action	Reason for Action
Set the pressure on the air pump to the amount prescribed (most medical orders range from 35 to 55 mm Hg with a common average of 40 mm Hg).	Provides intermittent compression at an appropriate pressure to promote venous circulation
Turn the power switch on and observe that the function lights illuminate during compression and turn off between compressions.	Indicates that the machine is operational
Assess the client's circulatory status and comfort every 2–4 hours throughout the therapeutic treatment, which is continuous for some clients.	Focuses assessment on signs that indicate adverse effects
Remove the extremity sleeve before ambulation or other out-of-bed activities.	Allows freedom of movement from the tether of the air tubes and pump
Discontinue the compressions if serious impairment of circulation and sensation, tingling, numbness, or leg pain occurs.	Helps to avoid serious complications
Remove the extremity sleeve and assess calf size and circulation to distal areas of the extremity at least once per day.	Provides comparative data with which to evaluate the therapeutic response
Apply elastic stockings and reinforce the need to perform leg exercises every hour when the machine is not in use.	Promotes venous circulation
Place equipment in a safe area where it is available for the next use.	Demonstrates regard for safety and efficient time management

EVALUATION

- Calf size is reduced or does not increase in diameter.
- Skin in lower extremity is intact, warm, and the appropriate color.
- Capillary refill is less than 2–3 seconds.
- Pedal pulses are present and strong.

DOCUMENT

- Assessment findings before and after application
- Extremity to which device was applied
- Setting and duration of application
- To whom abnormal assessment findings have been reported and the outcome of the communication

SAMPLE DOCUMENTATION

Date and Time   Right calf measures 18 in (45 cm). Left calf is 20 in (50 cm). Toes are warm. Blood returns to nail beds within 3 seconds of compression. Skin over legs is pink, warm, and intact. Homans sign is negative bilaterally. Pneumatic compression device applied to calves of both legs and set at a pressure of 40 mm Hg. _____ J. Doe, LPN

Date and Time   Pneumatic compression device removed after 2 hours of use to facilitate bathing and reapplied at 40 mm Hg. _____ J. Doe, LPN

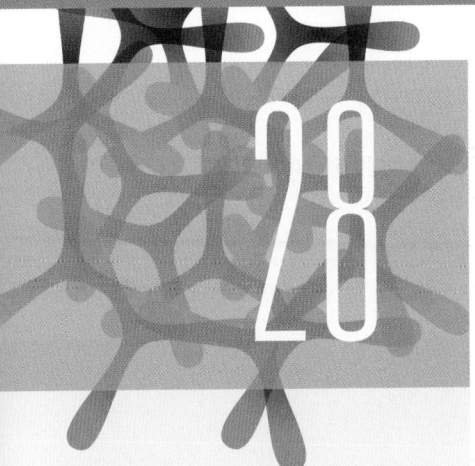

Wound Care

28

Words To Know

Learning Objectives

On completion of this chapter, the reader should be able to:

1. Define wound.
2. Name phases of wound repair.
3. Identify signs and symptoms classically associated with the inflammatory response.
4. Discuss the purpose of phagocytosis, including the types of cells involved.
5. Name ways in which the integrity of a wound is restored.
6. Explain first-, second-, and third-intention healing.
7. Name types of wound complications.
8. State purposes for using a dressing.
9. Explain the rationale for keeping wounds moist.
10. Describe types of drains, including the purpose of each.
11. Name the major methods for securing surgical wounds together until they heal.
12. Explain reasons for using a bandage or binder.
13. Discuss the purpose for using one type of binder.
14. Give examples of methods used to remove nonliving tissue from a wound.
15. List commonly irrigated structures.
16. State uses for applying heat and for applying cold.
17. Identify methods for applying heat and cold.
18. List risk factors for developing pressure ulcers.
19. Discuss techniques for preventing pressure ulcers.

INTRODUCTION

Body tissues have a remarkable ability to recover when injured. This chapter discusses several types of tissue injury, including those caused by surgical incisions and prolonged pressure. It also addresses nursing interventions to support the healing process and actions to prevent tissue injury.

 Gerontologic Considerations

■ Wound healing is delayed in older adults. Regeneration of healthy skin takes twice as long for an 80-year-old client as it does for a 30-year-old client.

■ Age-related changes that affect wound healing include diminished collagen and blood supply and decreased quality of elastin, necessary components for wound repair. Long-term exposure to ultraviolet rays from the sun compounds these age-related changes.

■ Factors such as depression, poor appetite, cognitive impairments, and physical or economic barriers that interfere with adequate nutrition

Words To Know (*continued*)
sutures
therapeutic baths
third-intention healing
trauma
undermining
vacuum-assisted wound closure
wound

in older adults may impair wound healing. These factors may be addressed by enlisting the assistance of registered dietitians, who can suggest appropriate nutritional interventions, and by making referrals to community resources, such as home-delivered meals or homemaker/home health aide services.

■ Diminished immune response from reduced T-lymphocyte cells predisposes older adults to wound infections.

■ Signs of inflammation may be subtle in older adults (see Chapter 27).

■ Diabetes or other conditions that may interfere with circulation increase the older adult's susceptibility to delayed wound healing and wound infections.

■ The risk for thermal skin injury is increased in older adults with impaired tactile sensation or sensory nerve damage because of circulatory or neurologic disorders. Older adults who have problems with the ability to sense temperatures need to take special precautions such as using a thermometer to ensure that applications involving heat are less than 100°F (38°C) to avoid burns or injury.

■ Age-related changes (i.e., a thinning dermal layer of skin, decreased subcutaneous tissue) result in increased susceptibility to pressure ulcers and shear-type injuries in older adults. Because of the decreased blood supply to the skin, an older adult may need position changes every 60 to 90 minutes, rather than every 120 minutes. Take special care when moving older adults to avoid friction on the skin.

■ Absorbent undergarments may contribute to skin breakdown because they may not allow for air circulation. Urine or feces next to the skin will cause damage and possible skin breakdown. Therefore, any incontinent older adult must be checked every 60 to 90 minutes to prevent skin damage. If urinary incontinence interferes significantly with wound healing, an indwelling catheter (see Chapter 30) may be necessary. It should be removed as soon as feasible, however, and efforts must be made to restore continence.

■ Older adults with diminished mobility require aggressive skin care to prevent pressure ulcers. The elbows, heels, coccyx, shoulder blades, and hips are especially vulnerable, as are the creases above the ears if oxygen tubing is in use. Special precautions include heel and elbow protectors, pressure relief pads, and mattresses, and a strict routine of changing the client's position at least every 2 hours or more frequently if the person's skin becomes reddened or darkened in a shorter period. Assessment of at-risk pressure point areas should be done before the 2-hour period.

WOUNDS

A **wound** (damaged skin or soft tissue) results from **trauma** (a general term referring to injury). Examples of tissue trauma include cuts, blows, poor circulation, strong chemicals, and excessive heat or cold. Such trauma produces two basic types of wounds: open and closed (Table 28-1).

An **open wound** is one in which the surface of the skin or mucous membrane is no longer intact. It may be caused accidentally or intentionally, as when a surgeon incises the tissue. In a **closed wound**, there is no opening in the skin or mucous membrane. Closed wounds occur more often from blunt trauma or pressure.

WOUND REPAIR

Regardless of the type of wound, the body immediately attempts to repair the injury and heal the wound. The process of wound repair proceeds in three sequential phases: inflammation, proliferation, and remodeling.

Inflammation

Inflammation, the physiologic process immediately after tissue injury, lasts approximately 2 to 5 days. Its purposes

TABLE 28-1 Types of Wounds

WOUND TYPES	DESCRIPTION
Open Wounds	
Incision	A clean separation of skin and tissue with smooth, even edges
Laceration	A separation of skin and tissue in which the edges are torn and irregular
Abrasion	A wound in which the surface layers of skin are scraped away
Avulsion	Stripping away of large areas of skin and underlying tissue, leaving cartilage and bone exposed
Ulceration	A shallow crater in which the skin or the mucous membrane is missing
Puncture	An opening of skin, underlying tissue, or mucous membrane caused by a narrow, sharp, pointed object
Closed Wounds	
Contusion	Injury to soft tissue underlying the skin from the force of contact with a hard object, sometimes called a *bruise*

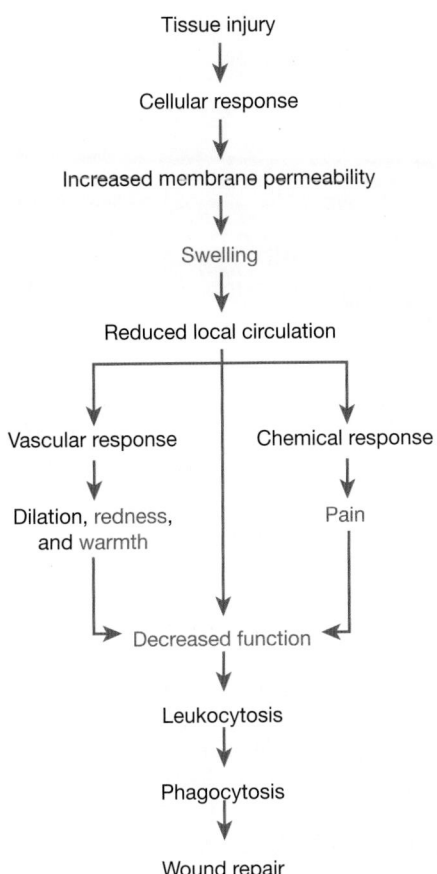

Tissue injury

↓

Cellular response

↓

Increased membrane permeability

↓

Swelling

↓

Reduced local circulation

Vascular response   Chemical response

↓   ↓

Dilation, redness,   Pain
and warmth

↓

Decreased function

↓

Leukocytosis

↓

Phagocytosis

↓

Wound repair

FIGURE 28-1 The inflammatory response. The words in *red* are the five classic signs and symptoms of inflammation.

are to (1) limit the local damage, (2) remove injured cells and debris, and (3) prepare the wound for healing. Inflammation progresses through multiple stages (Fig. 28-1).

During the first stage, local changes occur. Immediately following an injury, blood vessels constrict to control blood loss and confine the damage. Shortly thereafter, the blood vessels dilate to deliver platelets that form a loose clot. The membranes of the damaged cells become more permeable,

causing the release of plasma and chemical substances that transmit a sensation of discomfort. The local response produces the characteristic signs and symptoms of inflammation: *swelling, redness, warmth, pain,* and *decreased function.*

A second wave of defense follows the local changes when **polymorphonuclear leukocytes** (**neutrophils**) and **macrophages** (**monocytes**), types of white blood cells, migrate to the site of injury, and the body produces more and more white blood cells to take their place. **Leukocytosis** (an increased production of white blood cells) is confirmed and monitored by counting the number and type of white blood cells in a sample of the client's blood. The laboratory test is called a white blood cell count and differential count. Increased production of white blood cells, particularly neutrophils and monocytes, suggests an inflammatory and, in some cases, infectious process.

Neutrophils and monocytes are primarily responsible for **phagocytosis**, a process by which these cells emigrate from blood vessels to consume pathogens, coagulated blood, and cellular debris. Consumed substances are enclosed within **lysosomes**, enzymatic sacs inside the phagocytes that digest the engulfed matter. Once digestion occurs, the degraded products are released into extracellular fluid (Fig. 28-2). Collectively, neutrophils and monocytes clean the injured area and prepare the site for wound healing.

Proliferation

Proliferation (a period during which new cells fill and seal a wound) occurs from 2 days to 3 weeks after the inflammatory phase. It is characterized by the appearance of **granulation tissue** (a combination of new blood vessels, fibroblasts, and epithelial cells) that forms in the bed of an open wound. Granulation tissue has a somewhat irregular surface and looks bright pink to red because of the extensive projections of capillaries in the area (Fig. 28-3).

Granulation tissue grows from the wound margin toward the center. It is fragile and easily disrupted by physical or chemical means. As more and more fibroblasts produce **collagen** (a tough and inelastic protein substance), the adhesive strength of the wound increases. Toward the end of the

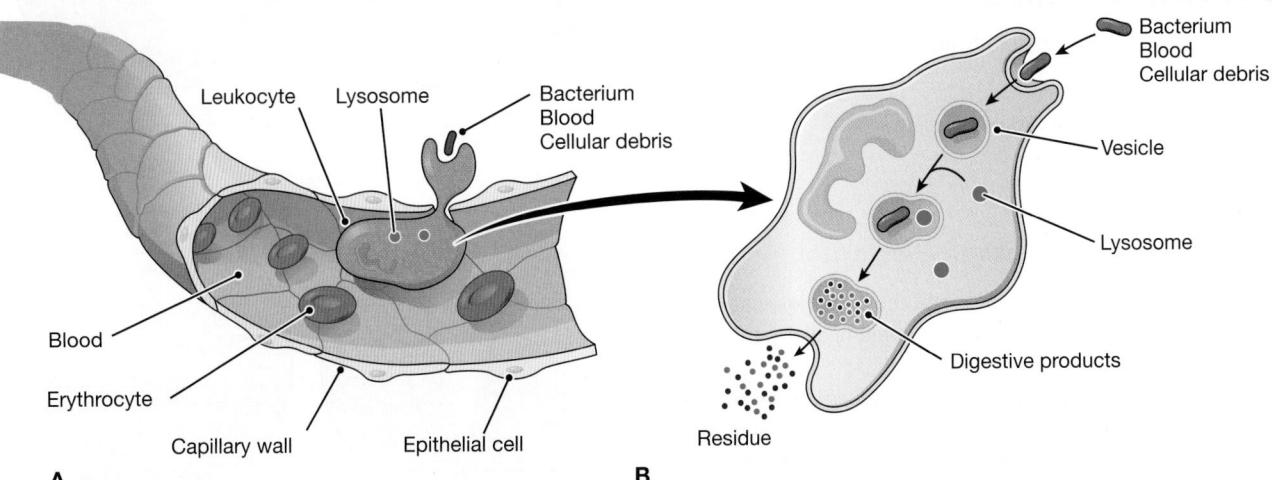

FIGURE 28-2 An example of the process of phagocytosis. **A.** A phagocytic leukocyte exits through a capillary wall. **B.** The debris is enclosed within a vesicle and digested by a lysosome. (From Cohen, B. J., & Hull, K., [2015]. *Memmler's structure and function of the human body* [11th ed.]. Lippincott Williams & Wilkins.)

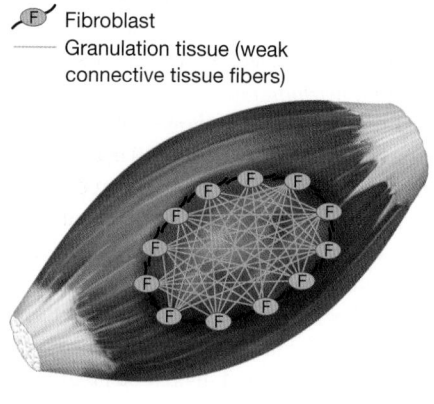

Fibroblast
Granulation tissue (weak connective tissue fibers)

A. Granulation

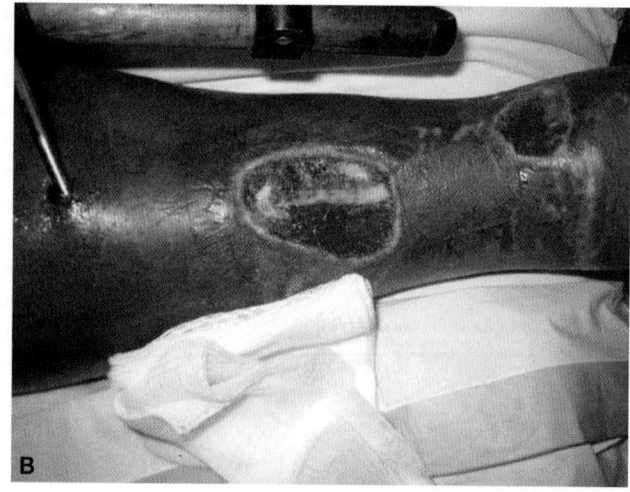

B

FIGURE 28-3 Wound repair. **A.** To promote tissue healing, phagocytes decrease and fibroblasts increase. The fibroblasts migrate to the perimeter forming a web of granulation fibers. **B.** A wound with healthy granulation tissue. (**A**, from Archer, P., & Nelson, L. A. [2012]. *Applied anatomy & physiology for manual therapists.* Lippincott Williams & Wilkins [PE]; **B**, from Sussman, C., & Bates-Jensen, B. [2012]. *Wound care* [4th ed.]. Lippincott Williams & Wilkins.)

proliferative phase, the new blood vessels degenerate, causing the previously pink color to regress. Epithelial cells fill the wound from its base with new tissue and vasculature and can typically fill any size wound (Alhajj & Goyal, 2022).

Generally, the integrity of skin and damaged tissue is restored by (1) **resolution** (a process by which damaged cells recover and reestablish their normal functions), (2) **regeneration** (cell duplication), or (3) **scar formation** (replacement of damaged cells with fibrous scar tissue). Fibrous scar tissue acts as a nonfunctioning patch. The extent of scar tissue that forms depends on the magnitude of tissue damage and the manner of wound healing (discussed later in this chapter).

Remodeling

Remodeling (a period during which the wound undergoes changes and maturation) follows the proliferative phase and may last 6 months to 2 years (Mercandetti & Molnar, 2021). During this time, the wound contracts and the scar shrinks.

WOUND HEALING

Several factors affect wound healing:

- Type of wound injury
- Expanse or depth of wound
- Quality of circulation
- Amount of wound debris
- Presence of infection
- Status of the client's health

The speed of wound repair and the extent of scar tissue that forms depend on whether the wound heals by first, second, or third intention (Fig. 28-4).

First-intention healing, also called *healing by primary intention*, is a reparative process in which the wound edges are directly next to each other. Because the space between the wound is so narrow, only a small amount of scar tissue forms. Most surgical wounds that are closely approximated heal by first intention (Fig. 28-5).

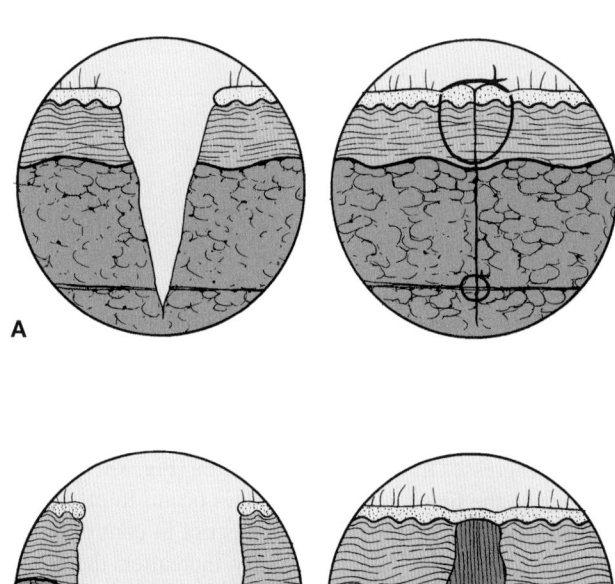

A

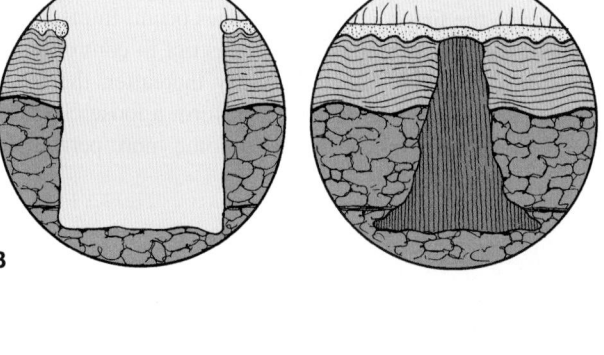

B

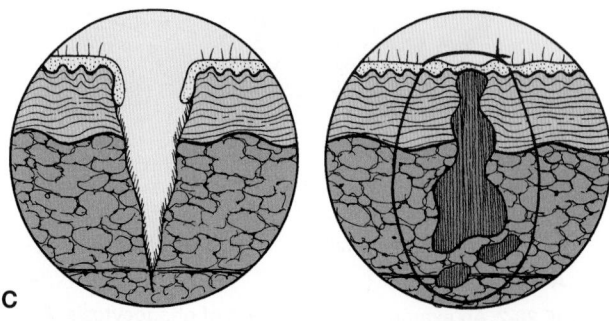

C

FIGURE 28-4 A. First-intention healing. **B.** Second-intention healing. **C.** Third-intention healing.

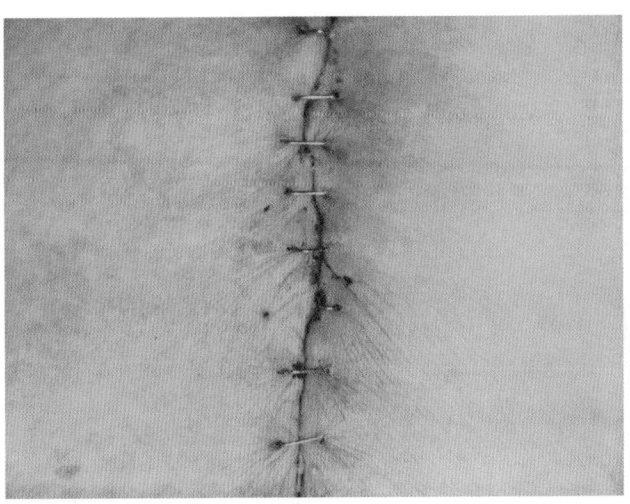

FIGURE 28-5 Example of a first-intention wound healing.

Nutrition Notes

■ Adequate protein, calories, and micronutrients are necessary for wound healing.

■ The extent to which healing increases nutrient needs is dependent upon the severity of the wound and the client's nutritional status. For instance, extensive burns may increase protein needs two to three times above normal, whereas minor surgery may have no impact on nutrient needs.

■ Although nutrient deficiencies are linked with poor wound healing, there is no magic bullet that will accelerate healing in an adequately nourished client.

In **second-intention healing**, the wound edges are widely separated, leading to a more time-consuming and complex reparative process. Because the margins of the wound are not in direct contact, the granulation tissue needs additional time to extend across the expanse of the wound. Generally, a conspicuous scar results. Healing by second intention is prolonged when the wound contains body fluid or other wound debris. Wound care must be performed cautiously to avoid disrupting the granulation tissue and retarding the healing process.

With **third-intention healing**, the wound edges are intentionally left widely separated and are later brought together with some type of closure material. This reparative process results in a broad, deep scar. Generally, wounds that heal by third intention are deep and are likely to contain extensive drainage and tissue debris. To speed up healing, they may contain drainage devices or be packed with absorbent gauze.

WOUND HEALING COMPLICATIONS

The key to wound healing is adequate blood flow to the injured tissue. Factors that may interfere include compromised circulation, infection, and purulent, bloody, or serous fluid accumulation that prevent skin and tissue approximation. In addition, excessive tension or pulling on wound edges contributes to wound disruption and delays healing. One or several of these factors may be secondary to poor nutrition, impaired inflammatory or immune responses related to drugs such as corticosteroids, and obesity (see discussion of surgical risks in Chapter 27).

The nurse assesses the wound to determine whether it is intact or shows evidence of unusual swelling, redness, warmth, drainage, and increasing discomfort. When assessing the wound, it is important to look for **undermining**, erosion of tissue from underneath intact skin at the wound edge; **slough**, which is dead tissue on the wound surface that is moist, stringy, yellow, tan, gray, or green; and **necrotic tissue**, which is dry, brown, or black devitalized tissue (Fig. 28-6). The latter two must be removed to facilitate wound healing (see the later discussion on debridement).

Two potentially serious surgical wound complications include **dehiscence** (the separation of wound edges) and **evisceration** (wound separation with the protrusion of organs) (Fig. 28-7). These complications are most likely within 7 to 10 days after surgery. They may be caused by

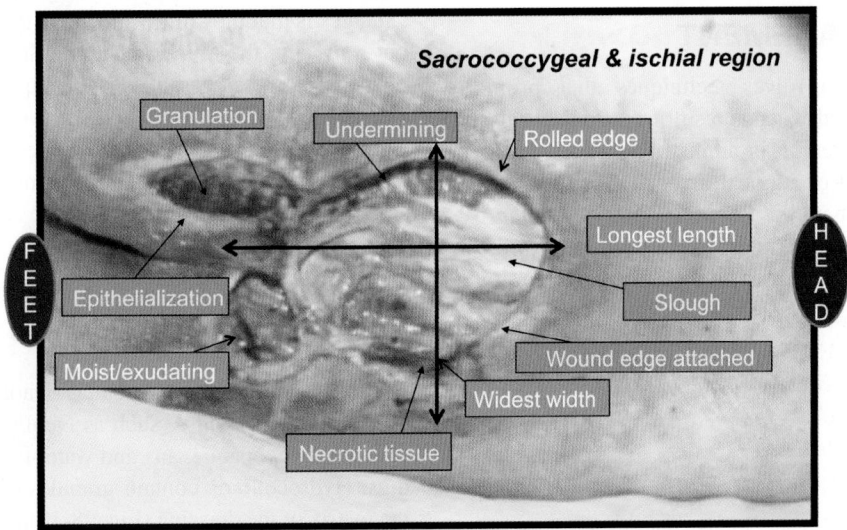

FIGURE 28-6 Components in wound assessment.

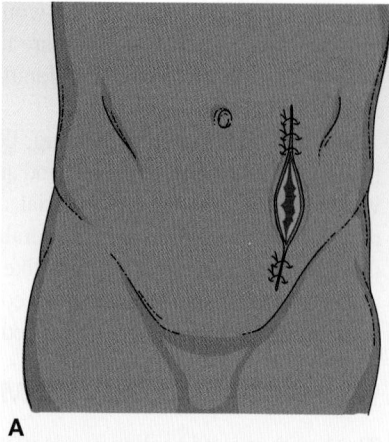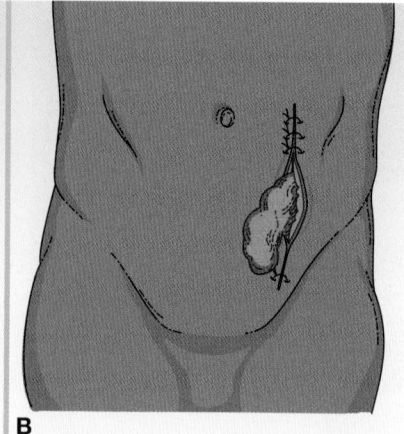

FIGURE 28-7 A. Wound dehiscence. **B.** Wound evisceration.

insufficient dietary intake of protein and sources of vitamin C; premature removal of sutures or staples; unusual strain on the incision from severe coughing, sneezing, vomiting, dry heaves, or hiccupping; weak tissue or muscular support secondary to obesity; distention of the abdomen from accumulated intestinal gas; or compromised tissue integrity from previous surgical procedures in the same area.

The client may describe that something has "given way." Pinkish drainage may appear suddenly on the dressing. If wound disruption is suspected, the nurse positions the client to put the least amount of strain on the open area. If evisceration occurs, the nurse places sterile dressings moistened with normal saline over the protruding organs and tissues. For any wound disruption, the nurse notifies the physician immediately. The nurse must be alert for signs and symptoms of impaired blood flow, such as swelling, localized pallor or mottled appearance, and coolness of the tissue in the area around the wound.

›› *Stop, Think, and Respond 28-1*

Discuss the signs and symptoms a person would exhibit if a wound were infected.

WOUND MANAGEMENT

Wound management involves techniques that promote wound healing. Surgical wounds result from incising tissue with a laser (see Chapter 27) or an instrument called a *scalpel.* The primary goal of surgical or open wound management is to reapproximate the tissue to restore its integrity. This involves changing dressings, caring for drains, removing sutures or staples when directed by the surgeon, applying bandages and binders, and performing wound irrigations.

Dressings

A **dressing** (the cover over a wound) serves one or more purposes:

- Keeping the wound clean
- Absorbing drainage
- Controlling bleeding
- Protecting the wound from further injury

- Holding medication in place
- Maintaining a moist environment

Types and sizes of dressings differ depending on their purpose. The most common wound coverings are gauze, transparent, hydrocolloid, hydrogel, and alginate dressings.

Gauze Dressings

Gauze dressings are made of woven cloth fibers. Their highly absorbent nature makes them ideal for covering fresh wounds that are likely to bleed or wounds that exude drainage. Unfortunately, gauze dressings obscure the wound and interfere with wound assessment. Unless an ointment is used on the wound or the gauze is lubricated with an ointment such as petroleum, granulation tissue may adhere to the gauze fibers and disrupt the wound when removed.

Gauze dressings are usually secured with tape. If gauze dressings need frequent changing, **Montgomery straps** (strips of tape with eyelets) may be used (Fig. 28-8). Another method may be necessary if the client is allergic to tape (see the discussion on "Bandages and Binders" section).

Transparent Dressings

Transparent dressings, such as OpSite and Tegaderm, are clear, acrylic film wound coverings. One of their chief advantages is that they allow the nurse to assess a wound without removing the dressing. In addition, they are less bulky than gauze dressings and do not require tape because they consist of a single sheet of adhesive material (Fig. 28-9). They are commonly used to cover peripheral and central intravenous insertion sites. Transparent dressings are nonabsorbent; therefore, if wound drainage accumulates, they tend to loosen. Once a dressing is no longer intact, many of its original purposes are defeated.

Hydrocolloid, Hydrogel, Alginate, and Collagen Dressings

Hydrocolloid dressings, such as DuoDerm and Tegasorb, and hydrogel dressings, such as DuoDerm and IntraSite, are self-adhesive, opaque, air- and water-occlusive wound coverings. Hydrocolloids contain granules of gelatin or pectin in the matrix of the dressing (Fig. 28-10). The granules in hydrocolloids become gelatinous when in contact with exudate in a wound, keeping the wound moist. Hydrogels, which contain

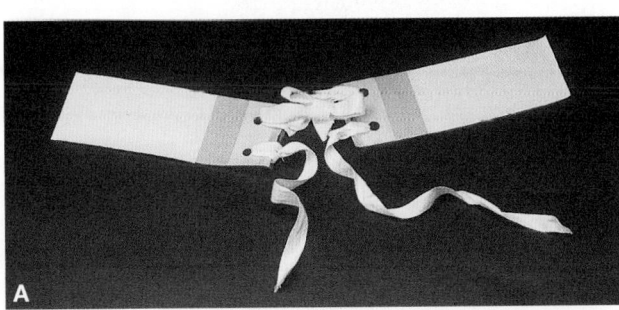

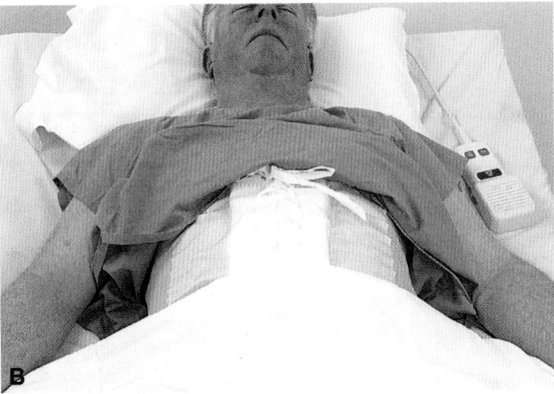

FIGURE 28-8 **A.** The adhesive outer edges of Montgomery straps are applied to either side of a wound. **B.** The inner edges of Montgomery straps are tied to hold a dressing over a wound. They prevent skin breakdown and wound disruption from repeated tape removal when checking or changing a dressing.

water and a network of fibers and alginates such as Algisite and Tegagel, which contain a seaweed component, have a similar function. Collagen dressings can be used for chronic wounds, pressure ulcers, transplant and surgical wounds, second-degree or higher burns, and wounds across large areas.

Moist wounds heal more quickly because new cells grow more rapidly in a wet environment. If the hydrocolloid dressing remains intact, it can be left in place for up to 1 week. Its occlusive nature also repels other body substances, such as urine or stool. For proper use, these dressings must be sized generously, allowing at least a 1-in margin of healthy skin around the wound.

Dressing Changes

Health care providers change dressings when a wound requires assessment or care and when the dressing becomes loose or saturated with drainage. In some cases, the physician may choose to assume total responsibility for changing the dressing—at least for the initial dressing change. Nurses, however, commonly *reinforce* dressings (apply additional absorbent layers) when dressings become moist. Reinforcing a dressing prevents wicking (absorbing or drawing) microorganisms toward the wound (see Chapter 10).

Because most surgical wounds are covered with gauze dressings, this example is used when describing the technique

for changing a dressing in Skill 28-1. When using dressings made of materials other than gauze, nurses can modify the technique by following the manufacturer's directions.

Drains

Drains are tubes that provide a means for removing blood and drainage from a wound. They promote wound healing by removing fluid and cellular debris. Although some drains are placed directly within a wound, the current trend is to insert them so that they exit from a separate location beside the wound. This approach keeps the wound margins approximated and avoids a direct entry site for pathogens. The physician may choose to use an open or closed drain.

Open Drains

Open drains are flat, flexible tubes that provide a pathway for drainage toward the dressing. Draining occurs passively by gravity and **capillary action** (the movement of a liquid at the point of contact with a solid, which in this case is the drain). Sometimes, a safety pin or long clip is attached to the drain as it extends from the wound. This prevents the drain from slipping within the tissue. As the drainage decreases, the physician may instruct the nurse to shorten the drain, enabling healing to take place from inside toward the outside of the wound. To shorten a drain, the nurse pulls it from the wound for the specified length. They then reposition the safety pin or clip near the wound to prevent the drain from sliding back internally within the wound (Fig. 28-11).

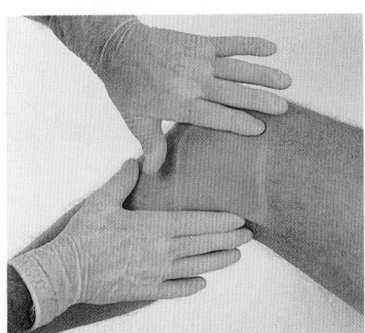

FIGURE 28-10 A hydrocolloid dressing absorbs drainage into its matrix.

FIGURE 28-9 A transparent dressing. (Photo by B. Proud.)

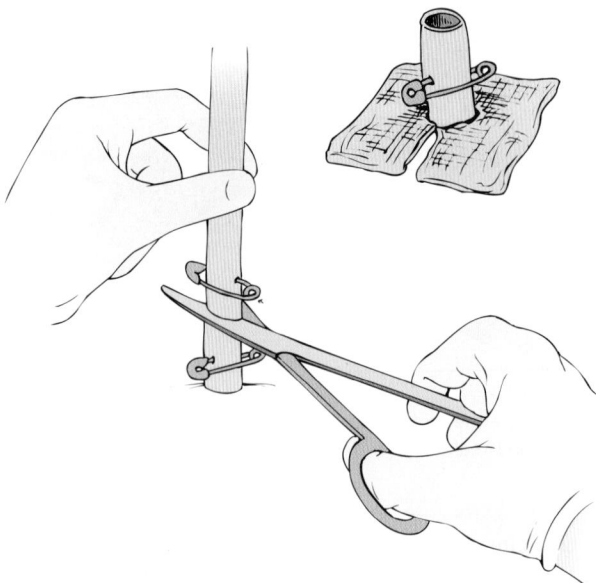

FIGURE 28-11 An open drain is pulled from the wound, and the excess portion is cut. A drain sponge is placed around the drain, and the wound is covered with a gauze dressing.

Closed Drains

Closed drains are tubes that terminate in a receptacle. Some examples of closed drainage systems are the Hemovac and the Jackson–Pratt drain (Fig. 28-12). Closed drains are more efficient than open drains because they pull fluid by creating a vacuum or negative pressure. This is done by opening the vent on the receptacle, compressing the drainage collection chamber, then capping the vent (Fig. 28-13).

When caring for a wound with a drain, the nurse cleans the insertion site in a circular manner from the center outward. After cleansing, they place a precut drain sponge or gauze, which is open to its center, around the base of the drain. An open drain may require additional layers of gauze because the drainage does not collect in a receptacle.

Vacuum-Assisted Closure

Wound healing is complicated when the edges are so widely separated that they cannot be approximated with sutures or staples. Consequently, reepithelialization across the surface

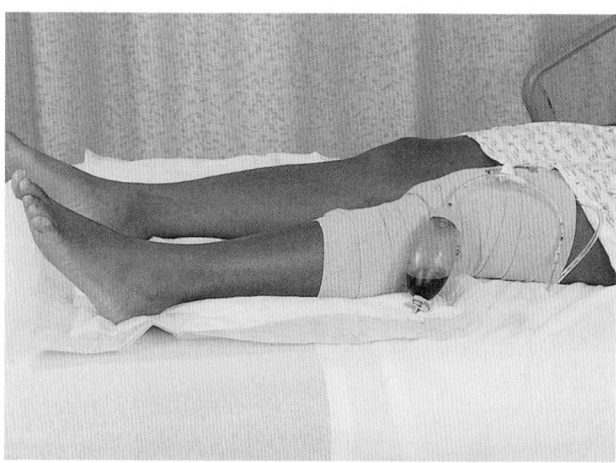

FIGURE 28-12 A Jackson–Pratt (closed) drain. (Photo by B. Proud.)

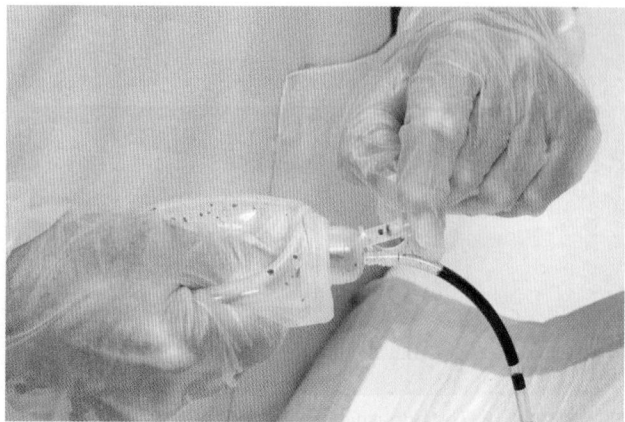

FIGURE 28-13 Compressing the bulb on a Jackson–Pratt drain and capping the vent reestablish negative pressure that allows the collection of wound drainage.

of the wound is delayed due to inadequate formation of new capillaries, the presence of cellular debris including an accumulation of tissue fluid, or an infectious process, any of which leads to a chronic wound.

Negative pressure wound therapy (NPWT), also called **vacuum-assisted wound closure** (VAC), refers to wound dressing systems that continuously or intermittently apply pressure to the system, which provides a positive pressure to the surface of a wound. NPWT has become a popular treatment modality for the management of many acute and chronic wounds (Gestring et al., 2023). With NPWT/VAC (Fig. 28-14), it is possible to promote more rapid wound healing. The process involves a foam filler within the wound that is covered with a sealed occlusive dressing connected to a suction tube and pump. When suction is applied either intermittently or continuously, fluid and debris in the entire wound bed are pulled through the foam filler into a collection canister. As a result, the wound gradually shrinks, cellular growth is promoted, blood flow increases, and healing improves. On average, the wound dressing is changed two or three times per week. Wound healing may take 6 months or longer.

Sutures, Staples, and Adhesives

Sutures, knotted ties that hold an incision together, are generally constructed from silk or synthetic materials, such as nylon. **Staples** (wide metal clips) perform a similar function. Staples do not encircle a wound like sutures; instead, they form a bridge that holds the two wound margins together. Staples are advantageous because they do not compress the tissue if the wound swells. Tissue adhesives (liquid stiches or surgical glues) are used to close minor and major wounds. Adhesives can result in lower rates of infection, less scarring, no needlesticks, and no stitches to remove when compared to sutures and staples.

Sutures and staples are left in place until the wound has healed sufficiently to prevent reopening. Depending on the location of the incision, this may be a few days to as long as 2 weeks. The physician may direct the nurse to remove sutures and staples (Fig. 28-15), sometimes every other one on one day and the other half on another day. Adhesive Steri-Strip skin closures, also known as *butterflies* because of their winged appearance, can hold a weak incision together

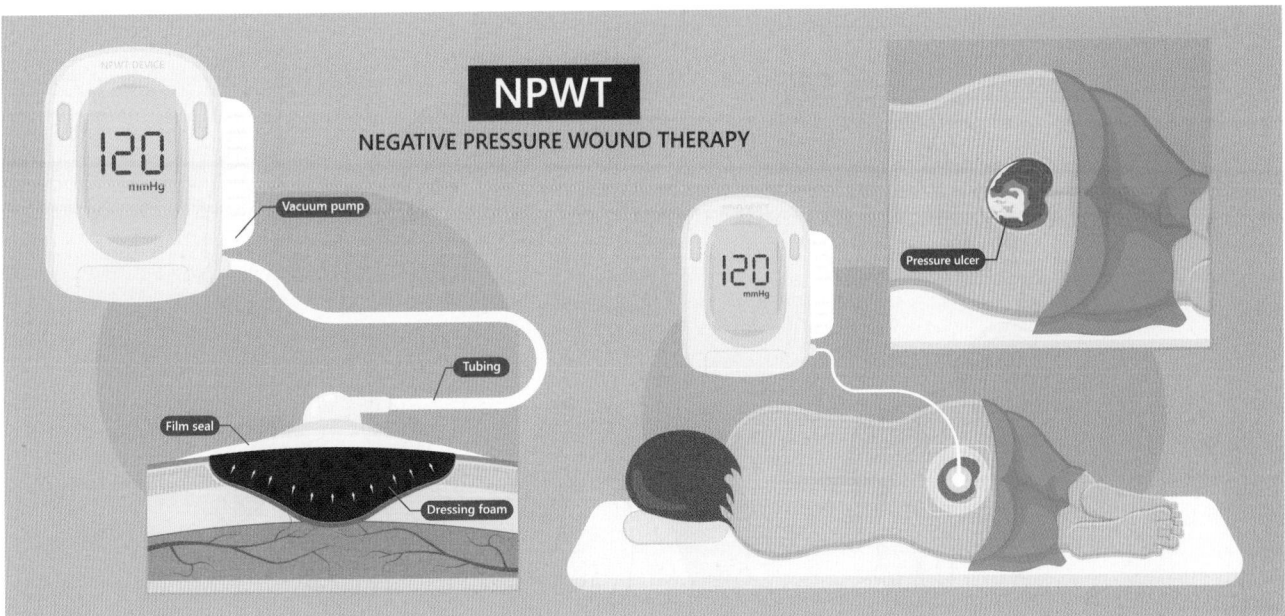

FIGURE 28-14 Negative pressure wound therapy with vacuum-assisted closure drain tube. (Pepermpron/Shutterstock.)

temporarily. Sometimes, Steri-Strips are used instead of sutures or staples to close superficial lacerations.

Bandages and Binders

A **bandage** is a strip or roll of cloth wrapped around a body part. One example is an Ace bandage. A **binder** is a type of cloth cover generally applied to a particular body part, such as the abdomen or breast. Bandages and binders are made from gauze, muslin, elastic rolls, and stockinette (see Chapter 25).

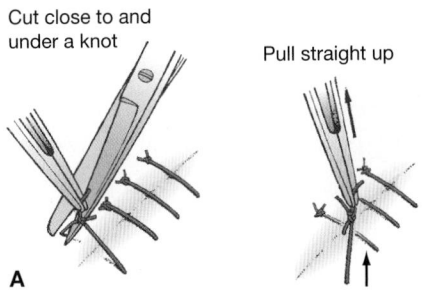

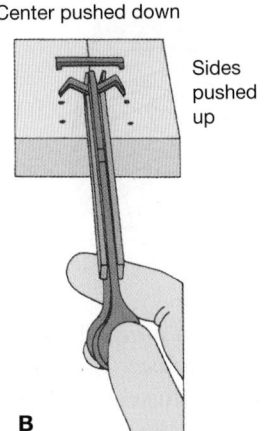

FIGURE 28-15 A. A technique for suture removal. **B.** A technique for staple removal.

Bandages and binders serve multiple purposes:

- Holding dressings in place, especially when tape cannot be used or if the dressing is extremely large
- Supporting the area around a wound or injury to reduce pain
- Limiting movement in the wound area to promote healing

 Concept Mastery Alert

Bandages and Dressings

Bandages do not help to keep a wound clean. Dressings do. Bandages hold dressings in place, support the area, and limit movement.

Roller Bandage Application

Most bandages are prepared in rolls of varying widths. The nurse holds the end in one hand while passing the roll around the part being bandaged. Nurses follow several principles when applying a roller bandage:

- Elevate and support the limb.
- Wrap from a distal to proximal direction.
- Avoid gaps between each turn of the bandage.
- Exert equal but not excessive tension with each turn.
- Keep the bandage free of wrinkles.
- Secure the end of the roller bandage with metal clips.
- Check the color and sensation of exposed fingers or toes often.

Remove the bandage for hygiene and replace at least twice a day.

Six basic techniques are used to wrap a roller bandage (Fig. 28-16): circular turn, spiral turn, spiral-reverse turn, figure-of-eight turn, spica turn, and recurrent turn.

A *circular turn* is used to anchor and secure a bandage where it starts and ends. It simply involves holding the free end of the rolled material in one hand and wrapping it around the area, bringing it back to the starting point.

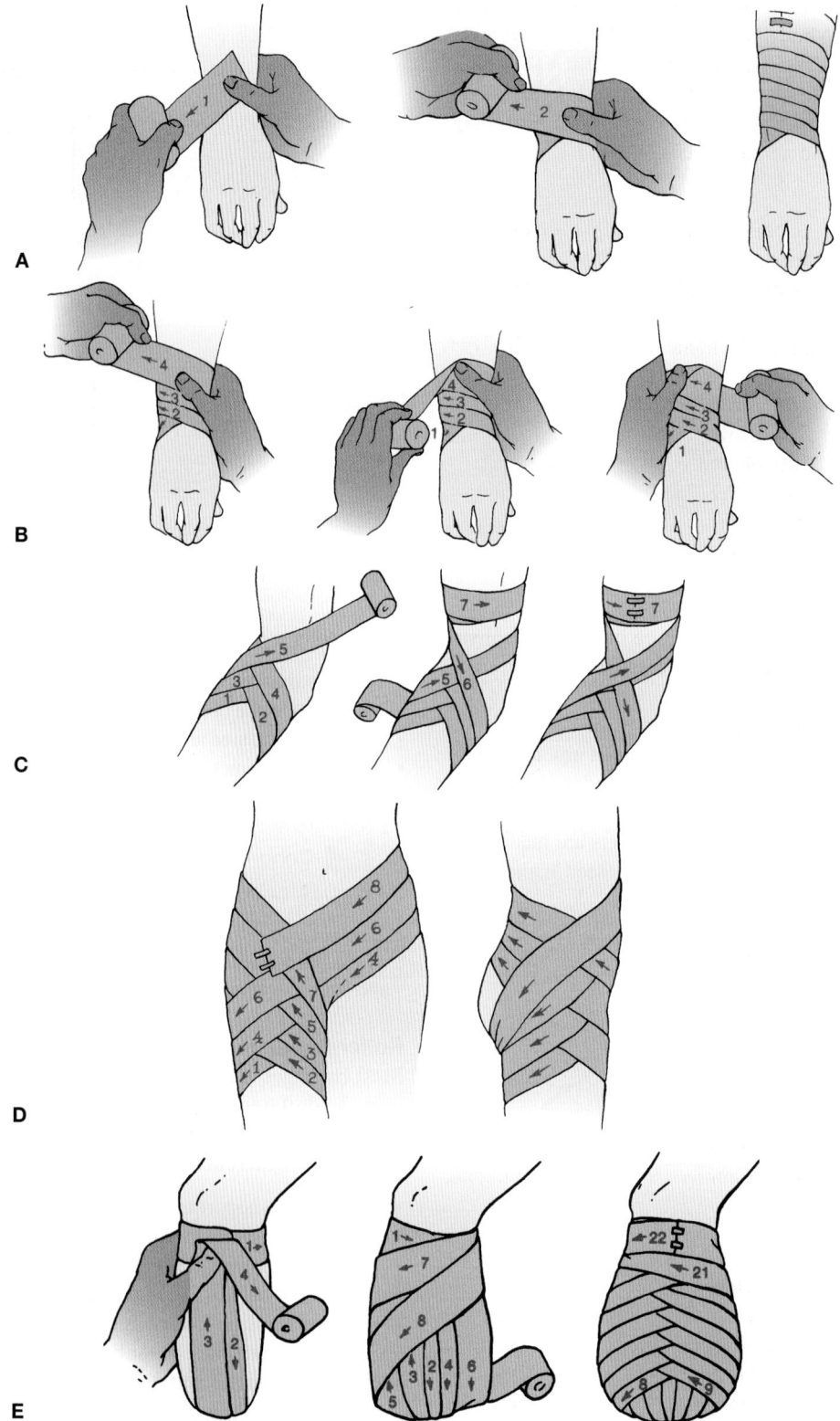

FIGURE 28-16 **A.** A circular and spiral turn. **B.** A spiral-reverse turn. **C.** A figure-of-eight turn. **D.** A spica turn. **E.** A recurrent turn.

A *spiral turn* partly overlaps a previous turn. The amount of overlapping varies from one half to three fourths of the width of the bandage. Spiral turns are used when wrapping cylindrical parts of the body, such as the arms and legs.

A *spiral-reverse turn* is a modification of a spiral turn. The roll is reversed or turned downward halfway through the turn.

A *figure-of-eight turn* is best when bandaging a joint such as the elbow or knee. This pattern is made by making oblique turns that alternately ascend and descend, simulating the number eight.

A *spica turn* is a variation of the figure-of-eight pattern. It differs in that the wrap includes a portion of the trunk or chest (see section "Spica Cast" in Chapter 25).

A *recurrent turn* is made by passing the roll back and forth over the tip of a body part. Once several recurrent turns are made, the bandage is anchored by completing the application with another basic turn, such as the figure-of-eight turn. A recurrent turn is especially beneficial when wrapping a residual limb after an amputation or the head.

Binder Application

Binders are not used as commonly as bandages; more convenient commercial devices have largely replaced binders. For example, brassieres are frequently used instead of breast binders. Sometimes after rectal or vaginal surgery, nurses apply a T-binder, which, as the name implies, looks like the letter T. T-binders are used to secure a dressing to the anus or perineum or within the groin. To apply a T-binder, the nurse fastens the crossbar of the T around the waist. Then, they pass the single or double tails between the client's legs and pin the tails to the belt (Fig. 28-17). Adhesive sanitary napkins worn inside underwear briefs are an alternative to a T-binder for stabilizing absorbent materials.

Debridement

Most wounds heal rapidly with conventional care. Nevertheless, some wounds require **debridement** (the removal of dead tissue) to promote healing. Four methods of debridement are sharp, enzymatic, autolytic, and mechanical.

Sharp Debridement

Sharp debridement is the removal of necrotic tissue from the healthy areas of a wound with sterile scissors, forceps, or other instruments (Fig. 28-18). This method is preferred if the wound is infected because it helps the wound heal more quickly. The procedure is done at the bedside or in the operating room if the wound is extensive. Sharp debridement is painful, and the wound may bleed afterward.

Enzymatic Debridement

Enzymatic debridement involves the use of topically applied chemical substances that break down and liquefy wound debris. A dressing is used to keep the enzyme in contact with the wound and to help absorb the drainage. This form of debridement is appropriate for uninfected wounds or for clients who cannot tolerate sharp debridement.

Autolytic Debridement

Autolytic debridement, or self-dissolution, is a painless, natural physiologic process that allows the body's enzymes to soften, liquefy, and release devitalized tissue. It is used when a wound is small and free of infection. The main disadvantage of autolysis is the prolonged time it takes to achieve the desired results. To accelerate autolysis, an occlusive or semiocclusive hydrocolloid, hydrogel, or calcium alginate dressing keeps the wound moist. Because removal of tissue debris is slow, the nurse monitors the client closely for signs of wound infection.

Mechanical Debridement

Mechanical debridement involves the physical removal of debris from nonhealing wounds. One technique is **maggot therapy**, which was approved by the U.S. Food and Drug

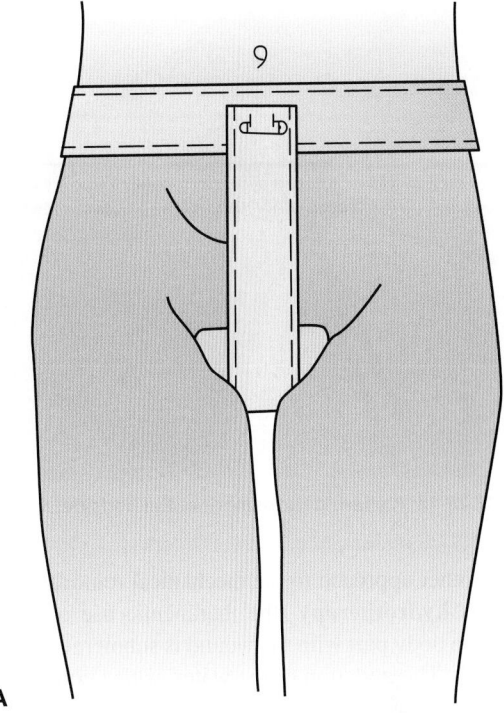

A

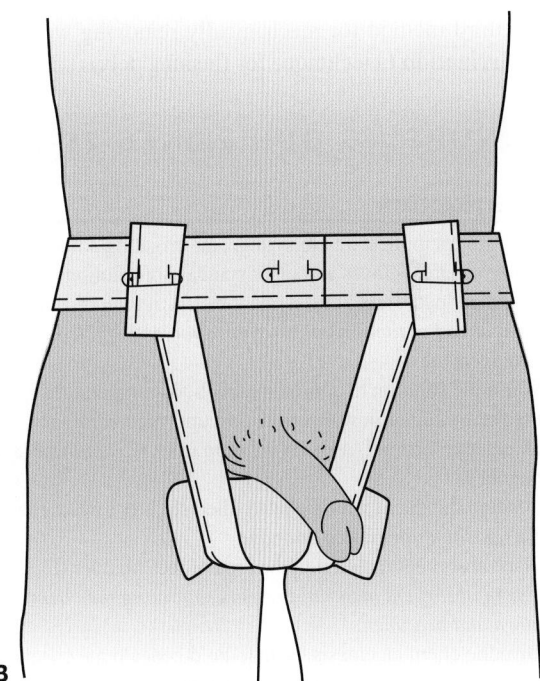

B

FIGURE 28-17 A. A single T-binder. **B.** A double T-binder. (From [2022]. *Lippincott's nursing procedures and skills* [9th ed.]. Lippincott Williams & Wilkins.)

Administration in 2004. Medical maggots are the larvae of a species of blow flies. Once the maggots are sterilized by a supplying laboratory, they are deposited into the wound. The maggots secrete an enzyme that dissolves dead tissue leaving healthy tissue alone. The maggots are confined beneath a dressing that provides air to the maggots and drainage of the liquefied tissue. When the debridement is completed, the maggots are transferred into a double-bagged biohazard bag.

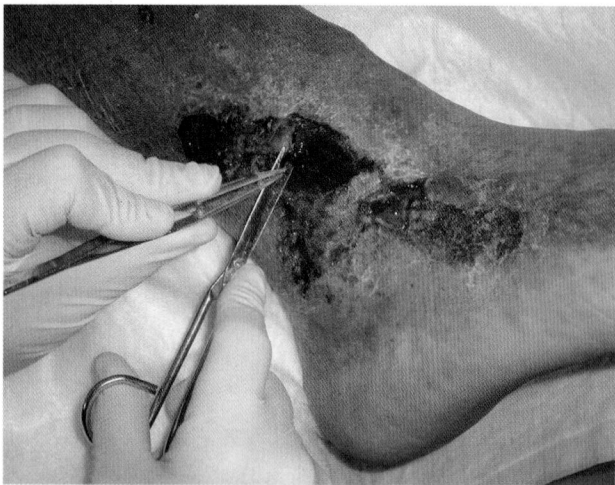

FIGURE 28-18 A sharp debridement at the bedside.

Another approach to the mechanical removal of wound debris is **hydrotherapy** (the therapeutic use of water), in which the body part with the wound is submerged in a whirlpool tank. The agitation of the water, which contains an antiseptic, softens the dead tissue. Loose debris that remains attached is removed afterward by sharp debridement.

A third method for mechanically removing wound debris is **irrigation** (a technique for flushing debris). Irrigation

is used when caring for a wound and also when cleaning an area of the body, such as the eyes, ears, and vagina.

Wet-to-dry dressings were used in the past as a form of debridement in which moist gauze was packed within the wound and allowed to dry. When the dry dressing was removed, dead tissue that was embedded within the dry gauze was also removed. This type of debridement is now considered substandard practice because it disrupts the formation of new blood vessels and increases costs and time as well as the risk of infection from multiple dressing changes.

≫ *Stop, Think, and Respond 28-2*
State an advantage and disadvantage of each method used for wound debridement.

Wound Irrigation
Wound irrigation (Skill 28-2) is generally carried out just before applying a new dressing. This technique is best used when granulation tissue has formed. Surface debris should be removed gently without disturbing the healthy proliferating cells.

Eye Irrigation
Eye irrigation flushes a toxic chemical from one or both eyes or displaces dried mucus or other drainage that accumulates from inflamed or infected eye structures (Nursing Guidelines 28-1).

 NURSING GUIDELINES 28-1

Eye Irrigation

- Assemble supplies: a bulb syringe, an irrigating solution, gauze squares, gloves and other standard precaution apparel, absorbent pads, and at least one towel. *Assembling equipment ahead of time ensures organization and efficient time management.*
- Warm the solution to approximately body temperature by placing the container in warm water, except when administering emergency first aid. *A warm solution is more comfortable for the client.*
- Position the client with the head tilted slightly toward the side. *This position facilitates drainage.*
- Place absorbent material in the area of the shoulder (Fig. A). *Use of absorbent material prevents saturating the client's gown and bed linen.*
- Give the client an emesis basin to hold beneath the cheek (Fig. B). *The basin can be used to collect the irrigating solution.*
- Wash hands or use an alcohol-based hand rub and put on gloves. *Hand hygiene and glove use reduce the transmission of microorganisms.*
- Open and prepare supplies. *This enables the nurse to perform the irrigation efficiently.*
- Wipe a moistened gauze square from the nasal corner of the eye toward the temple; use additional gauze squares one at a time as needed. *This removes gross debris.*
- Separate the eyelids widely with the fingers of one hand. *This action widens the exposed surface area.*
- Direct the solution onto the conjunctiva, holding the syringe or irrigating device about 1 in (2.5 cm) above the eye (Fig. C). *Holding the syringe away from the eye prevents injury to the cornea.*

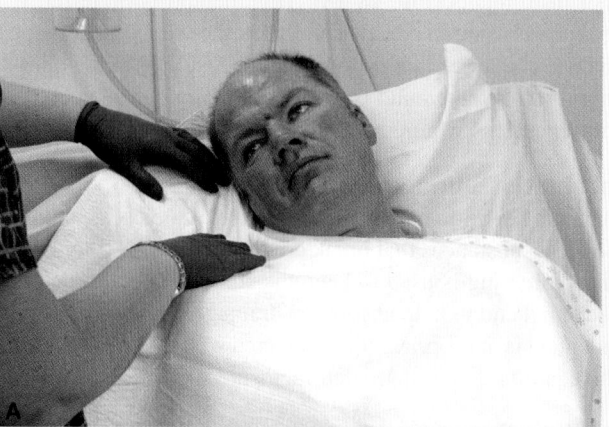

Protecting the client's gown and bed linen. (From [2022]. *Lippincott's nursing procedures and skills* [9th ed.]. Lippincott Williams & Wilkins.)

- Instruct the client to blink periodically. *Blinking distributes solution under the eyelid and around the eye.*
- Continue irrigating until the debris is removed. *This accomplishes the desired result.*
- Dry the client's face and replace a wet gown or linen. *These actions promote client comfort.*
- Dispose of soiled materials and gloves; wash hands. *These measures reduce the transmission of microorganisms.*
- Record assessment data, the specifics of the procedure, and the outcome. *Documentation records performance of the nursing intervention and the client's response.*

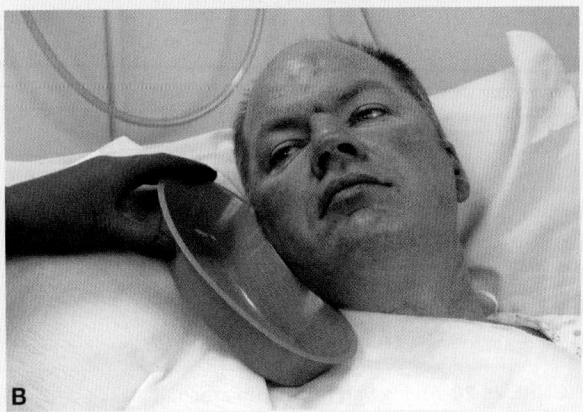

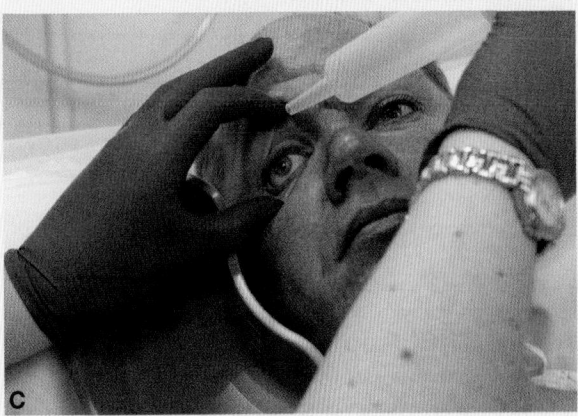

An emesis basin collects irrigant. (From [2022]. *Lippincott's nursing procedures and skills* [9th ed.]. Lippincott Williams & Wilkins.)

Instilling the irrigation onto the conjunctiva. (From [2022]. *Lippincott's nursing procedures and skills* [9th ed.]. Lippincott Williams & Wilkins.)

Ear Irrigation

Ear irrigation removes debris from the ear. Ear irrigation is contraindicated if the tympanic membrane (eardrum) is perforated. Performing a gross inspection of the ear is important if a foreign body is suspected because a bean, pea, or other dehydrated substance can swell if the ear is irrigated, causing it to become even more tightly fixed. Solid objects may require removal with an instrument.

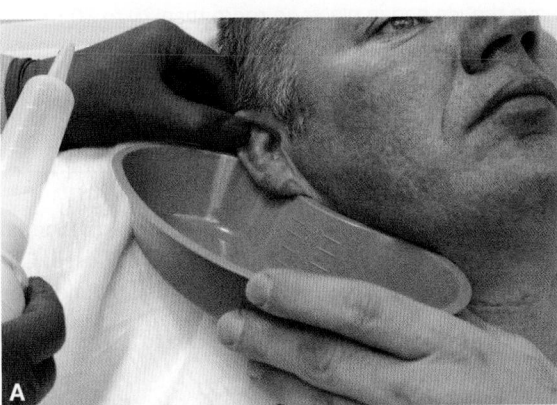

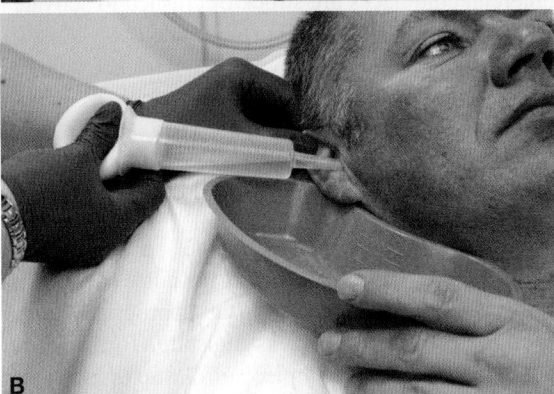

FIGURE 28-19 Ear irrigation. **A.** Position the emesis basin close the face under the ear and use the basin to collect the instilled solution after irrigation. **B.** Instill the solution with a syringe into the roof of the auditory canal.

If ear irrigation is not contraindicated, it is performed much like an eye irrigation, except that the nurse directs the solution toward the roof of the auditory canal (Fig. 28-19). In addition, the nurse takes care to avoid occluding the ear canal with the tip of the syringe because the pressure of the trapped solution could rupture the eardrum. After the irrigation, the nurse places a cotton ball loosely within the ear to absorb drainage, but not to obstruct its flow.

Vaginal Irrigation

Vaginal irrigation, also known as a **douche** (a procedure for cleansing the vaginal canal), is sometimes necessary to treat an infection (Client and Family Teaching 28-1).

Client and Family Teaching 28-1
Douching

The nurse teaches the client or the family as follows:

- Do not douche routinely because douching removes microbes called *Döderlein bacilli* that help prevent vaginal infections.
- Do not douche 24 to 48 hours before a Pap test (see Chapter 14). Douching may wash away diagnostic cells.
- Consult a physician about symptoms such as itching, burning, or drainage rather than attempting self-diagnosis.
- Find out from the physician if sexual partners also need to be treated with medications to avoid reinfection.
- Buy douching equipment from a drugstore; prefilled disposable containers are available.
- Warm the solution to a comfortable temperature (no more than 110°F [43.3°C]).
- Clamp the tubing (on reusable equipment) and fill the reservoir bag.
- Undress and lie down in the bathtub.
- Suspend the douche bag (if used) about 18 to 24 in (45 to 60 cm) above the hips.

- Insert the lubricated tip of the nozzle or the prefilled container downward and backward within the vagina about the distance of a tampon.
- Unclamp the tubing and rotate the nozzle as the fluid is instilled.
- Contract the perineal muscles as though trying to stop urinating and then relax the muscles. Repeat the exercise four or five times while douching.
- Sit up to facilitate drainage or shower afterward.
- Use a sanitary napkin or perineal pad to absorb residual drainage.

Heat and Cold Applications

Heat and cold have various therapeutic uses (Box 28-1), and each can be used in several ways. Examples include an ice bag, collar, chemical pack, compress, and aquathermia pad. Heat is also applied with soaks, moist packs, and therapeutic baths.

The terms *hot* and *cold* are subject to wide interpretation. Table 28-2 correlates common terms with temperature ranges. Because exposing the skin to extremes of temperature can result in injuries, the nurse assesses the temperature of the application and frequently monitors the condition of the skin. Direct contact between the skin and the heating or cooling device is avoided. Hot and cold applications are used cautiously in children younger than 2 years, older adults, clients with diabetes, and clients who are comatose or neurologically impaired.

Ice Bag and Ice Collar

Ice bags and ice collars are containers for holding crushed ice or small ice cubes (Fig. 28-20). Ice collars are usually applied after tonsil removal. Ice bags are applied to any small injury in the process of swelling. Although ice bags are commercially available, they can also be improvised. A rubber

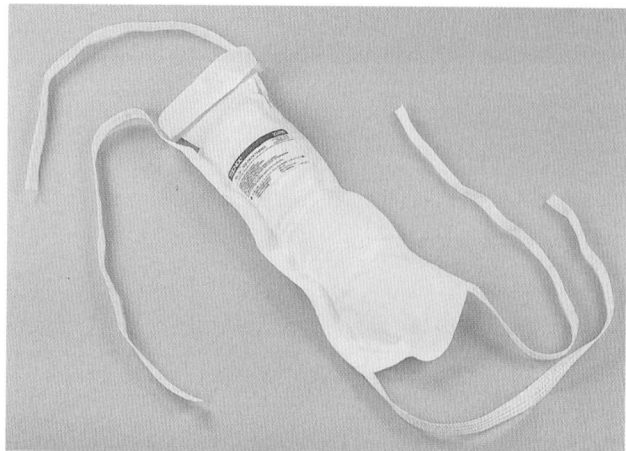

FIGURE 28-20 An ice bag filled with crushed ice.

 ### Client and Family Teaching 28-2 Using an Ice Bag

The nurse teaches the client or the family as follows:

- Test the ice bag for leaks.
- Fill it one half to two thirds full of crushed ice or small cubes so that it can be molded easily to the injured area.
- Eliminate as much air from the bag as possible.
- Pour water over the ice to provide slight melting. This tends to smooth the sharp edges from frozen ice crystals.
- Cover the ice bag with a layer of cloth before placing it on the body.
- Leave the ice bag in place no more than 20 to 30 minutes. Allow the skin and tissue to recover for at least 30 minutes before reapplying.
- If the skin becomes mottled or numb, remove the ice bag; it is too cold.

or plastic glove, a plastic bag with a zipper closure, or a bag of small frozen vegetables, such as peas, can be used. Client instruction minimizes the risk for injury (Client and Family Teaching 28-2).

Chemical Packs

Commercial cold packs are struck or crushed to activate the chemicals inside, causing them to become cool. Most first-aid kits generally include this type of cold pack. Commercial cold packs can be used only once. Gel packs, designed for cold or hot application, are reusable. They are stored in the freezer until needed or heated in a microwave.

Compresses

Compresses (moist, warm, or cool cloths) are applied to the skin. Before applying the compress, the nurse soaks it in tap water or a medicated solution at the appropriate temperature and then wrings out excess moisture. To maintain the moisture and temperature, a piece of plastic or plastic wrap is used to cover the compress, and the area is secured in a towel. As the compress material cools or warms outside the range of the intended temperature, the nurse removes it and reapplies it if necessary.

BOX 28-1	Common Uses for Heat and Cold Applications

Uses for Heat	Uses for Cold
Provides warmth	Reduces fevers
Promotes circulation	Prevents swelling
Speeds healing	Controls bleeding
Relieves muscle spasm	Relieves pain
Reduces pain	Numbs sensation

TABLE 28-2 Temperature Ranges for Applications of Heat and Cold

LEVEL OF HEAT OR COLD	TEMPERATURE RANGE
Very hot	40.5°–46.1°C (105°–115°F)
Hot	36.6°–40.5°C (98°–105°F)
Warm and neutral	33.8°–36.6°C (93°–98°F)
Tepid	26.6°–33.8°C (80°–93°F)
Cool	18.3°–26.6°C (65°–80°F)
Cold	10°–18.3°C (50°–65°F)
Very cold	<10°C (<50°F)

If the skin is not intact, as in the case of a draining wound, nurses wear gloves when applying a compress. They use aseptic surgical technique when applying compresses to an open wound.

Aquathermia Pad

An **aquathermia pad** (an electrical heating or cooling device) is sometimes called a *K-pad*. It resembles a mat but contains hollow channels through which heated or cooled distilled water circulates (Fig. 28-21). An aquathermia pad is used either alone or as a cover over a compress. A thermostat is used to keep the temperature of the water at a specified setting. As with other forms of hot and cold therapeutic devices, the nurse assesses the skin frequently and removes the device periodically.

Before placing the client on the aquathermia pad or wrapping it around a body part, the nurse covers the pad to help prevent thermal skin damage. A roller bandage may help hold the pad in place. The nurse positions the electrical unit slightly higher than the client to promote gravity circulation of the fluid.

Larger styles are used to warm clients who are hypothermic or to cool those with heat stroke. Because these clients have dangerously altered body temperatures, the nurse must monitor vital signs continuously.

Soaks and Moist Packs

A **soak** is a technique in which a body part is submerged in fluid to provide warmth or to apply a medicated solution. A **pack** (a commercial device for applying moist heat) can also be used. Moist heat is more comforting and therapeutic than dry heat.

A soak usually lasts 15 to 20 minutes. The nurse keeps the temperature of the fluid as constant as possible, which requires frequent emptying and refilling of the basin. The newly added water should not be too hot; overly hot water causes discomfort or tissue damage.

Packs differ from soaks in two major ways: the duration of the application is usually longer, and the initial application of heat is generally more intense. Packs are usually applied at temperatures as warm as the client can tolerate. Because of the potential for causing burns, a pack is never used on a client who is unresponsive or paralyzed and cannot perceive temperatures. The nurse must make frequent assessments and remove the pack if there is any likelihood of a thermal injury.

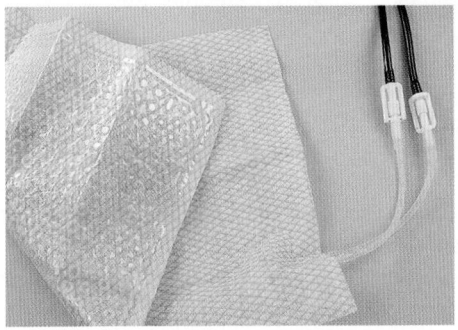

FIGURE 28-21 An aquathermia pad (K-pad). (Photo by B. Proud.)

Therapeutic Baths

Therapeutic baths (those performed for other than hygiene purposes) help reduce a high fever or apply medicated substances to the skin to treat skin disorders or discomfort. Examples are baths to which sodium bicarbonate (baking soda), cornstarch, or oatmeal paste is added.

The most common type of therapeutic bath is a **sitz bath** (a soak of the perianal area). Sitz baths reduce swelling and inflammation and promote healing of wounds after a *hemorrhoidectomy* (the surgical removal of engorged veins inside and outside the anal sphincter) or an *episiotomy* (an incision that facilitates vaginal birth). Some health care agencies have special tubs for administering sitz baths, but most provide clients with disposable equipment (Skill 28-3).

>>> *Stop, Think, and Respond 28-3*
What assessment findings suggest that a sitz bath is providing a therapeutic effect?

PRESSURE ULCERS

A **pressure ulcer**, also referred to as a *decubitus ulcer*, is a wound caused by prolonged capillary compression that is sufficient to impair circulation to the skin and underlying tissue. Pressure ulcers most often appear over bony prominences of the sacrum, hips, and heels. They can also develop in other locations such as the elbows, shoulder blades, the back of the head, and places where pressure is unrelieved because of infrequent movement (Fig. 28-22). The tissue in these areas is particularly vulnerable because body fat, which acts as a pressure-absorbing cushion, is minimal. Consequently, the tissue is compressed between the bony mass and a rigid surface such as a chair seat or a bed mattress. If the compression reduces the pressure in local capillaries to less than 32 mm Hg for 1 to 2 hours without intermittent relief, the cells die from a lack of oxygen and nutrients. The primary goal in managing pressure ulcers is prevention. Once a pressure ulcer forms, however, the nurse implements measures to reduce its size and restore skin and tissue integrity.

Stages of Pressure Ulcers

Pressure ulcers are grouped into four stages according to the extent of tissue injury (Fig. 28-23). Care and healing depend on the stage of injury. Without aggressive nursing care, early-stage pressure ulcers can easily progress to much more serious ones.

Stage I is characterized by intact but reddened or darkened skin. The hallmark of cellular damage is skin that remains red or darker and fails to resume its normal color when pressure is relieved.

A stage II pressure ulcer is red and accompanied by blistering or a **skin tear** (a shallow break in the skin) without slough. Impairment of the skin may lead to colonization and infection of the wound.

A stage III pressure ulcer has a shallow skin crater that extends to the subcutaneous tissue. It may be accompanied by **serous drainage** (leaking plasma), undermining, slough, or **purulent drainage** (white or greenish fluid) caused by a

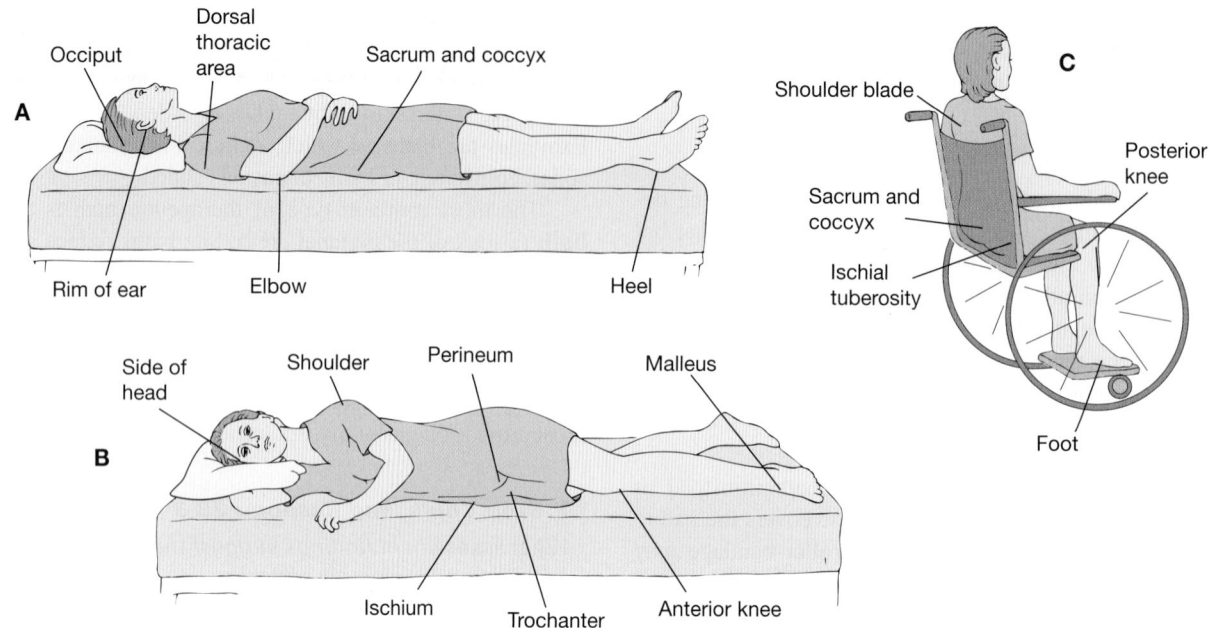

FIGURE 28-22 Locations where pressure ulcers commonly form. **A.** The supine position. **B.** A side-lying position. **C.** The sitting position.

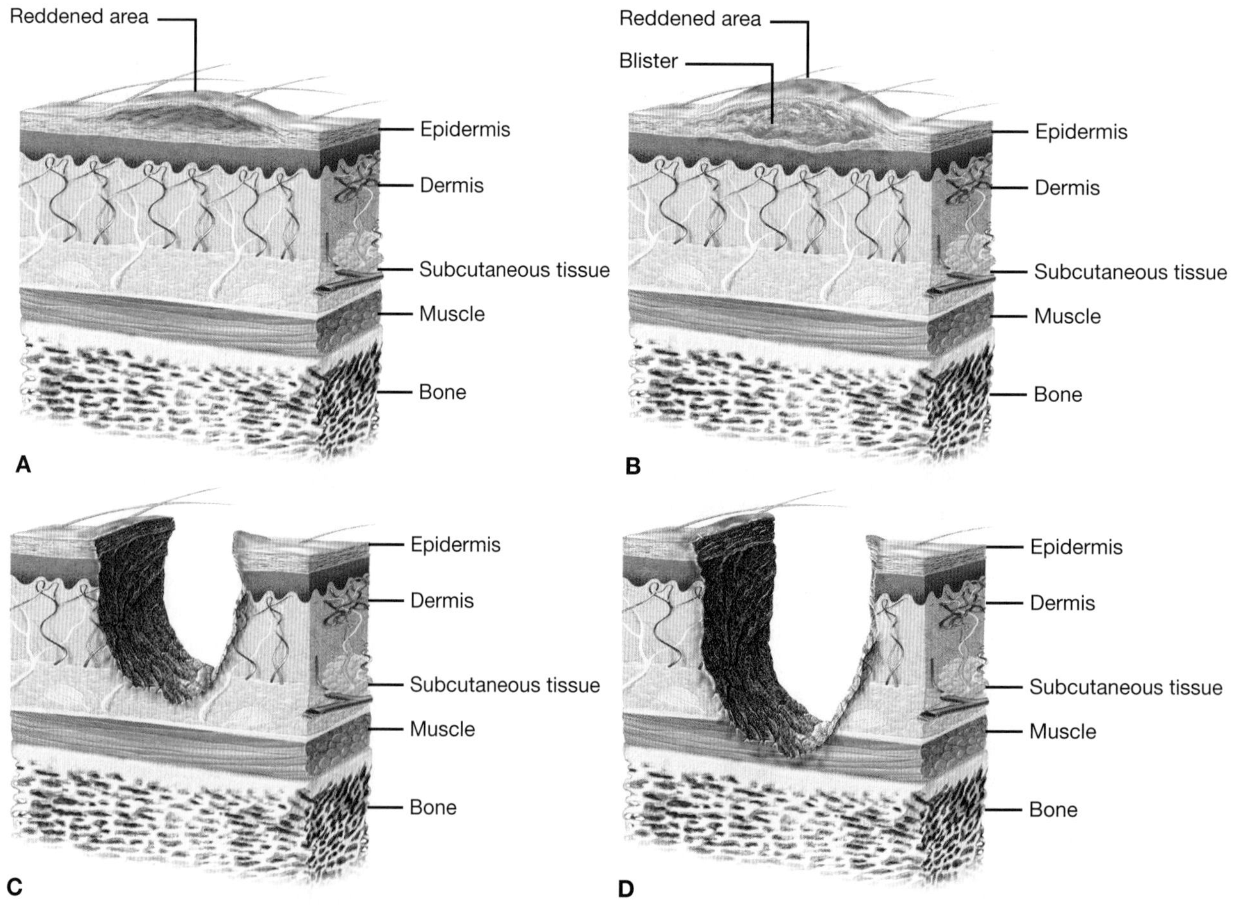

FIGURE 28-23 Pressure sore stages. **A.** Stage I. **B.** Stage II. **C.** Stage III. **D.** Stage IV.

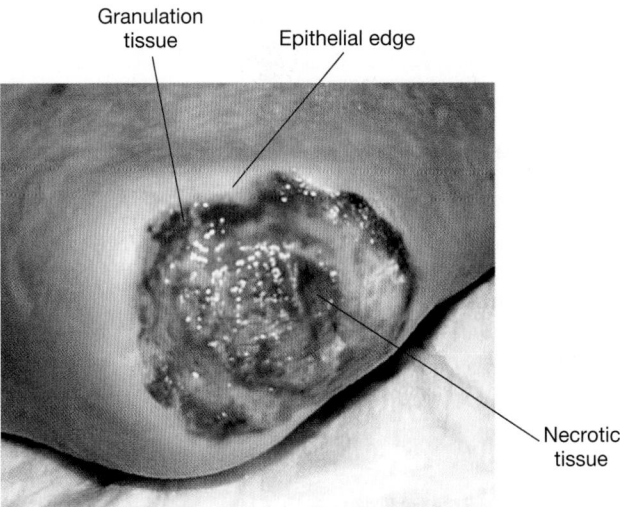

FIGURE 28-24 Example of stage IV pressure sore.

Labels on figure: Granulation tissue · Epithelial edge · Necrotic tissue

<table>
</table>

BOX 28-2	**Risk Factors for Developing Pressure Ulcers**

Inactivity
Immobility
Malnutrition
Emaciation
Diaphoresis
Incontinence
Vascular disease
Localized edema
Dehydration
Sedation
Age greater than 70 years (more likely to have fragile skin)
Obesity
Smoking
Not having enough nutrients in the diet
Having chronic conditions that can restrict blood circulation or limit mobility

wound infection. The area is relatively painless despite the severity of the ulcer.

Stage IV pressure ulcers are life-threatening. The tissue is deeply ulcerated, exposing muscle and bone (Fig. 28-24). Slough and necrotic tissue may be evident. The dead or infected tissue may produce a foul odor. If an infection is present, it easily spreads throughout the body, causing **sepsis** (a potentially fatal systemic infection).

Sometimes, it is not possible to measure the depth of a sore or the amount of tissue damage that has occurred, making the wound "unstageable." This makes it difficult to fully evaluate and stage an ulcer. It may be due to the presence of a hard plaque called an *eschar* inside the sore (Healthline, 2021).

Prevention and Treatment of Pressure Ulcers

The first step in prevention is to identify clients with risk factors for pressure ulcers (Box 28-2). The second step is to implement measures that reduce conditions under which pressure ulcers are likely to form (Nursing Guidelines 28-2).

NURSING GUIDELINES 28-2

Preventing Pressure Ulcers

• Change the bedridden client's position frequently. Remind a client who is sitting in a chair to stand and move hourly or at least to shift their weight every 15 minutes while sitting. *Changing positions relieves pressure and restores circulation.*

• Lift rather than drag the client during repositioning. *Dragging causes friction, which abrades the skin and damages underlying blood vessels.*

• Avoid using plastic-covered pillows when positioning clients. *Plastic prevents evaporation of perspiration because it is nonporous. It also raises skin temperature, further contributing to the growth of microorganisms.*

• Use positioning devices such as pillows to keep two parts of the body from direct contact with each other. *Such devices absorb perspiration, reduce localized heat, and avoid the compression of tissue between two body parts.*

• Use the lateral oblique position (see Chapter 23) rather than the conventional lateral position for side lying. *The lateral oblique position more effectively reduces the potential for pressure on vulnerable bony prominences.*

• Massage bony prominences only if the skin blanches with pressure relief. *Massage improves circulation to normal tissue but causes further damage to areas where pressure ulcers—even those that are stage I—are already established.*

• Keep the skin clean and dry especially when clients cannot control their bladder or bowel function. *Cleansing removes substances that chemically injure the skin.*

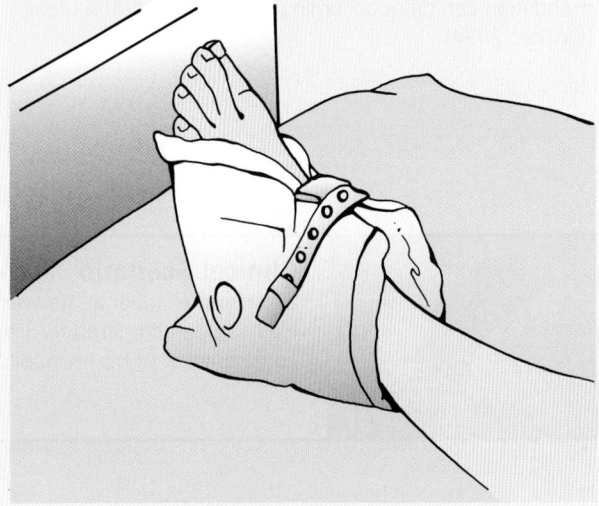

Heel and ankle protection.

(continued)

NURSING GUIDELINES 28-2 (*continued*)

- Use a moisturizing skin cleanser rather than soap if possible. *A nonsoap cleanser maintains skin hydration and avoids altering the skin's natural acidity, which protects it from bacterial colonization.*
- Rinse and dry the skin well. *Cleansing then drying removes chemical residues and surface moisture.*
- Use pressure-relieving devices such as special beds or mattresses (see Chapter 23). *These special devices maintain capillary blood flow by reducing pressure.*
- Pad body areas such as the heels, ankles, and elbows, which are vulnerable to friction and pressure (see figure). *Padding*

prevents friction and adds a cushioning layer over the bony prominence.
- Use seat cushions such as a commercial gel-filled pad when clients sit for extended periods. *These cushions distribute pressure over a wider area, relieving direct pressure on the coccyx.*
- Keep the head of the bed elevated no more than 30 degrees. *Sliding down in bed can produce a **shearing force** (the effect that moves layers of tissue in opposite directions).*
- Provide a balanced diet and adequate fluid intake. *Adequate nutrition maintains and restores cells and keeps tissues hydrated.*

Nutrition Notes

■ The precise amount of nutrients is not known, but nutritional intake to promote wound healing includes increased needs for energy, protein, zinc, and vitamins A, C, and E. High-protein oral nutritional supplements have been shown to successfully reduce the occurrence of pressure ulcers in patients at risk by 25%.

■ Vitamin C: fundamental for collagen formation and proper immune response; also helps with iron absorption

■ Zinc and copper: needed for healing by the growth of epithelium and granulation tissue formation

■ Vitamin E: essential for optimal immune function and assists with healthy tissue formation

■ Vitamin A: increases the inflammatory response and helps with collagen formation

■ Iron: required to assist with various mechanisms in the skin. Iron deficiencies can affect cell production and differentiation, protein synthesis, and regulation of macrophage function during the inflammatory phase (Manley & Mitchell, 2022).

■ The recommended protein intake for pressure ulcer healing is 1.25 to 1.5 g/kg of body weight per day. The recommendation can differ according to the stage of the ulcer (Kirman, 2024).

■ Malnutrition is detrimental to pressure ulcer healing. Unplanned weight loss is a risk factor for malnutrition and pressure ulcer development.

Kirman, C. N., et al. (2022). Pressure injuries (pressure ulcers) and wound care guidelines. *eMedicine.* https://emedicine.medscape.com/article/190115-guidelines; Manley, S., & Mitchell, A. (2022). The impact of nutrition on pressure ulcer healing. *British Journal of Nursing, 31*(12), S26–S30. https://www.britishjournalofnursing.com/content/nutrition/the-impact-of-nutrition-on-pressure-ulcer-healing

NURSING IMPLICATIONS

Clients with surgical wounds, pressure ulcers, or other types of tissue injury are likely to have one or more of the following nursing diagnoses:

- Acute pain
- Altered skin integrity risk
- Altered skin integrity
- Altered tissue perfusion
- Pressure injury risk
- Infection risk

Nursing Care Plan 28-1 shows how nurses use the nursing process to care for a client with altered skin integrity, defined as an increase in the chance of infection, impaired mobility, and decreased function and may result in the loss of limb or, sometimes, life. Skin is affected by both intrinsic and extrinsic factors, including altered nutritional status, vascular disease issues, and diabetes.

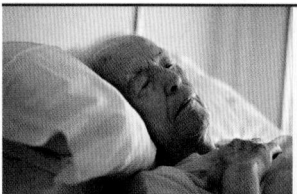

Clinical Scenario A 72-year-old male experienced paralysis below his neck following a fall from a ladder as he was cleaning leaves from the gutters on his home 2 years ago. He has been admitted for treatment of multiple pressure sores that have developed as a consequence of his immobility.

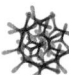

NURSING CARE PLAN 28-1 | Altered Skin Integrity

Assessment
- Inspect the skin, especially over bony prominences.
- Look for skin redness that does not blanch with relief of pressure, evidence of skin tears, or ulceration.
- Observe the client's ability to move and reposition themselves independently.
- Assess the status of the client's hydration and nutrition.
- Determine whether the client is incontinent or feverish or has other contributing factors to skin and tissue breakdown such as conditions accompanied by edema, those that require the application of devices such as a cast or traction, or treatments that increase the potential for impairment of the integument such as radiation cancer therapy.

Nursing Diagnosis. Altered skin integrity related to unrelieved pressure secondary to immobility from a spinal cord injury at the C7 (seventh cervical vertebrae) level 2 years ago as manifested by stage III pressure ulcer over the coccyx and a stage I ulcer over the bilateral heels and elbows

Expected Outcome. The skin integrity in the area of the coccygeal pressure ulcer will be restored as evidenced by the development of granulation tissue around the circumference of the wound by 8/30 and closure by 10/1. The elbows and heels will blanch with pressure relief by 8/18.

Interventions	Rationales
Reposition the client every 2 hours until an air-fluidized bed can be obtained.	Frequent repositioning maintains capillary pressure above 32 mm Hg to facilitate the oxygenation of tissue.
Use a 30-degree lateral oblique (tilted side-lying) position; alternate right and left sides or prone position if tolerated.	Relief of pressure prevents additional injury to tissues.
Avoid the supine and Fowler positions as much as possible.	These positions increase the potential for shear forces and pressure over bony prominences on posterior body areas such as the coccyx, shoulders, and heels.
Keep the heels elevated or resting on natural (not synthetic) sheepskin.	Elevation or natural sheepskin padding reduces pressure on tissue and promotes capillary blood flow.
After bathing, spray heels and elbows with Bard Barrier Film.	Skin products, such as Bard Barrier Film, form a clear, breathable film that is impervious to liquids and potential irritants and protects against skin abrasion and friction.

Care for the open coccygeal wound as follows:

Cleanse the wound with chlorhexidine antiseptic solution at the time of each dressing change.	An antiseptic reduces the transient and resident microorganisms that can increase the extent and severity of the pressure ulcer and delay healing.
Rinse with normal saline.	
Pack the wound with foam filler within the package that contains a negative pressure wound closure system.	The vacuum created by a negative pressure wound closure system shrinks the wound and promotes cellular growth to heal the impaired tissue.
After sealing the foam with an occlusive dressing, attach the suction tubing set at 125 mm Hg.	
Change the negative pressure wound closure dressing every 3 days.	

Once healing is evident:

Clean, dry, and cover wound with a hydrogel dressing and leave in place for 3 days.	A hydrogel dressing creates a moist environment that continues to accelerate the healing process.
If drainage collects, remove and reapply a new dressing.	Accumulation of fluid beneath the dressing increases the potential for loosening the wound cover. Changing the dressing restores the occlusive cover over the wound.
Measure the open pressure sore every 3 days (8/18, 8/21, etc.) during the day shift.	Regular assessment of the wound helps determine the need to continue or revise the plan for wound care.

Evaluation of Expected Outcome

- Pressure ulcer in area of coccyx measures 2 × 3 × 1/2 in on 8/18 with 1/16 in of granulation tissue around the circumference of the wound.
- Heels and elbows no longer appear red.

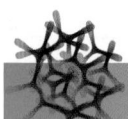

- Wound: Damaged skin or soft tissue resulting from an injury
  - Open wound: The surface of the skin or mucous membrane is no longer intact.
  - Closed wound: No opening in the skin or mucous membrane
- Three phases of wound repair: Inflammation, proliferation, and remodeling
- Factors that affect wound healing
  - Type of wound injury
  - Expanse or depth of wound
  - Quality of circulation
  - Amount of wound debris
  - Presence of infection
  - Status of the client's health
- Wound healing complications
  - Compromised circulation
  - Infection
  - Purulent, bloody, or serous fluid accumulation
  - Excessive tension or pulling on wound edges
    - Dehiscence: The separation of wound edges
    - Evisceration: Wound separation with the protrusion of organs
- Wound management
  - Keeping the wound clean
  - Absorbing drainage
  - Controlling bleeding
  - Protecting the wound from further injury
  - Holding medication in place
  - Maintaining a moist environment
  - Wound care

- Dressings
- Drains
- Sutures, staples, and adhesives
- Bandages and binders
- Debridement: The removal of dead tissue to promote healing
  - Sharp
  - Enzymatic
  - Autolytic
  - Mechanical
- Heat and cold applications
  - Cold: Ice bags or ice collars
  - Hot: Soaks, moist packs, therapeutic baths
  - Both: Chemical packs, aquathermia pads, compresses
- Pressure ulcer: Also referred to as a *decubitus ulcer*, a wound caused by prolonged capillary compression that is sufficient to impair circulation to the skin and underlying tissue
  - Stage I is characterized by intact but reddened or darkened skin.
  - A stage II pressure ulcer is red and accompanied by blistering or a skin tear without slough.
  - A stage III pressure ulcer has a shallow skin crater that extends to the subcutaneous tissue.
  - A stage IV pressure ulcer is life-threatening. The tissue is deeply ulcerated, exposing muscle and bone, and necrotic tissue may be evident.
- Prevention and treatment of pressure ulcers
  - The first step in prevention is to identify clients with risk factors for pressure.
  - The second step is to implement measures that reduce conditions under which pressure ulcers are likely to form.

CRITICAL THINKING EXERCISES

1. What nursing assessment findings would suggest that a wound is healing?
2. A nurse notes that the gauze dressing that covers a wound comes loose repeatedly. What measures could the nurse take?
3. Describe the wound care appropriate for a client with a stage I pressure ulcer, one with an abdominal incision, and one with a peripheral intravenous infusion site.
4. A 75-year-old client is admitted from a nursing home to have surgery to repair a fractured hip. Discuss factors that may threaten this client's wound healing.

NEXT-GENERATION NCLEX-STYLE REVIEW QUESTIONS

1. Which is the best body position the nurse can utilize to promote wound drainage from an abdominal incision with an open drain?

a. Lithotomy
b. Fowler
c. Recumbent
d. Trendelenburg

Test-Taking Strategy: Note the key term, "best." Eliminate options to select one that would promote gravity drainage.

2. When the nurse changes a client's dressing, which nursing action is correct?
   a. The nurse removes the soiled dressing with sterile gloves.
   b. The nurse frees the tape by pulling it away from the incision.
   c. The nurse encloses the soiled dressing within a latex glove.
   d. The nurse cleans the wound in circles toward the incision.

Test-Taking Strategy: Use the process of elimination to select the action that supports a principle for managing care of a wound.

3. When a nurse empties the drainage in a Jackson–Pratt reservoir, which nursing action is essential for reestablishing the negative pressure within this drainage device?
   a. The nurse compresses the bulb reservoir and closes the vent.
   b. The nurse opens the vent, allowing the bulb to fill with air.
   c. The nurse fills the bulb reservoir with sterile normal saline.
   d. The nurse secures the bulb reservoir to the skin near the wound.

   Test-Taking Strategy: Note the key word, "essential." Analyze the choices and select the option that must be performed in order to create negative pressure.

4. When the physician considers debriding a wound using an autolytic process, which interventions can the nurse expect to implement? Select all that apply.
   a. Removing necrotic tissue with scissors
   b. Applying a chemical enzyme to the wound
   c. Applying a dressing with a seaweed component
   d. Depositing live fly larvae within the wound
   e. Using a dressing that contains gelatin granules
   f. Flushing the wound with an irrigating solution

   Test-Taking Strategy: Analyze the choices and select options that promote self-dissolution of devitalized tissue.

5. Place the physiologic processes that occur during an inflammatory response in the order in which they occur.
   a. Leukocytosis occurs.
   b. There is increased cellular permeability.
   c. The area becomes red and warm.
   d. Local circulation is reduced.

Test-Taking Strategy: Analyze the options and place them in a sequence that begins shortly after tissue is injured through steps leading to wound repair.

NEXT-GENERATION NCLEX-STYLE CLINICAL SCENARIO QUESTIONS

Clinical Scenario:

A 72-year-old male experienced paralysis below his neck following a fall from a ladder as he was cleaning leaves from the gutters on his home 2 years ago. He has been admitted for treatment of multiple pressure sores that have developed as a consequence of his immobility.

1. Select all of the indicators that may suggest a cause for concern regarding an altered tissue perfusion.
   a. Paralysis below his neck
   b. Using an air mattress
   c. Immobility
   d. Multiple pressure sores
   e. Turning the client every 2 hours

2. Choose the most likely options for the information missing from the statement below by selecting from the list of options provided.

   The client's _____1_____ is contributing to the physical examination findings of _____2_____.

OPTION 1	OPTION 2
employment	multiple pressure sores
paralysis	poor nutritional status
body type	high cholesterol

SKILL 28-1 Changing a Gauze Dressing

Suggested Action	Reason for Action
ASSESSMENT	
Inspect the current dressing for drainage, integrity, and type of dressing supplies used.	Provides assessments indicating a need to change the dressing and supplies that may be needed
Check the medical orders for a directive to change the dressing.	Shows collaboration with the prescribed medical treatment
Determine whether the client has allergies to tape or antimicrobial wound agents.	Helps determine the dressing supplies to use
Assess the client's level of pain and its characteristics.	Determines whether analgesia will be beneficial before changing the dressing
PLANNING	
Explain the need and technique for changing the dressing.	Relieves anxiety and promotes cooperation
Consult the client on a preferred time for the dressing change if there is no immediate need for it.	Empowers the client to participate in decision-making
Give pain medication if needed 15–30 minutes before the dressing change.	Allows time for medication absorption and effectiveness
Gather the necessary supplies, which are likely to include a paper bag for the soiled dressing, clean and sterile gloves, individually packaged gauze dressings, tape, and, in some cases, an antimicrobial agent such as povidone–iodine swabs for wound cleansing.	Facilitates organization and efficient time management
IMPLEMENTATION	
Wash your hands or use an alcohol-based hand rub (see Chapter 10).	Reduces the transmission of microorganisms
Pull the privacy curtain.	Shows respect for the client's dignity
Position the client to allow access to the dressing.	Facilitates comfort and dexterity
Drape the client to expose the area of the wound.	Ensures modesty but facilitates care
Loosen the tape securing the dressing; pull the tape toward the wound (Fig. A).	Facilitates removal without separating the healing wound

Loosen the tape. (Photo by B. Proud.)

Put on at least one glove, and lift the dressing from the wound (Fig. B).	Provides a barrier against contact with blood and body substances

Remove the dressing.

SKILL 28-1 Changing a Gauze Dressing (*continued*)

Suggested Action	Reason for Action
Moisten the gauze with sterile normal saline if it adheres to the wound.	Prevents disrupting granulation tissue
Discard the soiled dressing in a paper bag or other receptacle along with the glove(s) (Fig. C).	Confines the sources of pathogens
	Dispose of the dressing.
Wash your hands again or repeat using the alcohol-based hand rub.	Removes transient microorganisms
Tear several long strips of tape and fold the ends over, forming tabs (Fig. D).	Facilitates handling tape later when wearing gloves and eases tape removal during the next dressing change
	Prepare the tape.
Open sterile supplies using the inside wrapper of one of the gauze dressings as a sterile field if needed.	Ensures an aseptic technique
Put on sterile gloves.	Ensures sterility
Inspect the wound.	Provides data for description and comparison
Cleanse the wound with the antimicrobial agent.	Removes drainage and microorganisms
Use a technique that prevents transferring microorganisms back to a cleaned area (Fig. E).	Supports principles of medical asepsis

C

D

E

Wound cleansing techniques.

| Use a single swab or a small gauze square for each stroke. | Prevents transferring microorganisms to clean areas |
| Allow the antimicrobial agent to dry. | Ensures that the tape will stay secured when applied |

(continued)

SKILL 28-1 Changing a Gauze Dressing (*continued*)

Suggested Action	Reason for Action
Cover the wound with the gauze dressing (Fig. F). **F**	Protects the wound Apply the dressing.
Secure the dressing with tape in the opposite direction of the incision or across a joint. Place a strip of tape at each end of the dressing and in the middle if needed (Fig. G). Correct—Gentle pressure in both directions away from injury Correct—tape covers ends of dressing Over joints, place tape at right angles to direction of motion **G**	Prevents loosening with activity; holds the dressing in place without exposing the wound or incision Secure with tape. (From Hinkle, J. L., Cheever, K. H., & Overbaugh, K. [2021]. *Brunner and Suddarth's textbook of medical-surgical nursing* [15th ed.]. Lippincott Williams & Wilkins.)
Remove and discard gloves.	Confines the sources of microorganisms
Rewash hands or repeat using the alcohol-based hand rub.	Removes transient microorganisms

EVALUATION

- Dressing covers the entire wound.
- Dressing is secure, dry, and intact.

DOCUMENT

- Type of dressing
- Antimicrobial agent used for cleansing
- Assessment data

SAMPLE DOCUMENTATION

Date and Time Gauze dressing changed over abdominal wound. Wound cleansed with povidone iodine. Incision is well approximated with sutures. No drainage, swelling, or tenderness observed. _____ J. Doe, LPN

SKILL 28-2 Irrigating a Wound

Suggested Action	Reason for Action
ASSESSMENT	
Check the medical orders for a directive to irrigate the wound.	Shows collaboration with the prescribed medical treatment
Determine how much the client understands about the procedure.	Indicates the level of health teaching needed
PLANNING	
Plan to irrigate the wound at the same time that the dressing requires changing.	Makes efficient use of time
Gather the equipment required, which is likely to include a container of solution, a basin, a bulb or Asepto syringe, gloves, and absorbent material including a towel to dry the skin.	Facilitates organization
Bring supplies for changing the dressing.	Makes efficient use of time
Consider additional items for standard precautions such as goggles or face shield and cover apron or gown.	Follows infection control guidelines when there is a potential for being splashed with blood or body substances
IMPLEMENTATION	
Wash your hands or use an alcohol-based hand rub (see Chapter 10).	Reduces the transmission of microorganisms
Pull the privacy curtain.	Shows respect for the client's dignity
Drape the client to expose the area of the wound.	Ensures modesty but facilitates care
Follow directions in Skill 28-1 for removing the dressing.	Provides access to the wound
Wash your hands or repeat the use of alcohol-based hand rub.	Reduces the transmission of microorganisms
Position the client to facilitate filling the wound cavity with solution.	Ensures contact between the solution and the inner area of the wound
Pad the bed with absorbent material, and place an emesis basin adjacent to and below the wound.	Reduces the potential for saturating the bed linens
Open and prepare supplies following the principles of surgical asepsis.	Confines and controls the transmission of microorganisms
Put on gloves and other standard precautions apparel.	Reduces the potential for contact with blood and body substances
Fill the syringe with solution, and instill it into the wound without touching the wound directly (Fig. A).	Dilutes and loosens debris

A

Instill the irrigant.

Hold the emesis basin close to the client's body to catch the solution as it drains from the wound (Fig. B).	Collects and contains the irrigating solution

B

Position the client to drain the irrigant.

Repeat the process until the draining solution seems clear.	Indicates the evacuation of debris
Tilt the client toward the basin.	Drains the remaining solution from the wound

(continued)

SKILL 28-2 Irrigating a Wound (*continued*)

Suggested Action	Reason for Action
Dry the skin.	Facilitates applying a dressing
Dispose of the drained solution, soiled equipment, and linens.	Reduces the potential for transmitting microorganisms
Remove gloves, wash hands, and prepare to change the dressing.	Provides for the absorption of residual solution and coverage of the wound

EVALUATION

- Irrigation solution shows evidence of debris removal.
- Wound shows evidence of healing.

DOCUMENT

- Assessment data
- Type and amount of solution
- Outcome of procedure

SAMPLE DOCUMENTATION

Date and Time   Dressing removed. Moderate purulent drainage on soiled dressing. Wound is separated 3 in. Approximately 300 mL of sterile NSS instilled within wound. Drained solution is cloudy with particles of debris. _____ J. Doe, LPN

SKILL 28-3 Providing a Sitz Bath

Suggested Action	Reason for Action
ASSESSMENT	
Check the medical orders for a directive to administer a sitz bath.	Shows collaboration with the prescribed medical treatment
Determine how much the client understands about the procedure.	Indicates the level of health teaching needed
Assess the condition of the rectal or perineal wound and the client's level of pain.	Provides baseline data for future comparisons; indicates if pain medication is needed
PLANNING	
Explain the procedure.	Relieves anxiety and promotes cooperation
Ask if the client prefers the sitz bath before or after routine hygiene.	Involves the client in the decision-making process
Obtain disposable equipment unless specially installed tubs are available.	Facilitates organization and efficient time management
Assemble other supplies such as a bath blanket and towels.	Prepares for maintaining warmth and provides a means for drying the skin
Inspect and clean the bathroom area or the tub room.	Supports principles of medical asepsis
Place the basin inside the rim of the raised toilet seat (Fig. A).	Allows for submerging the rectum and the perineum

A

Position the sitz bath basin.

SKILL 28-3 Providing a Sitz Bath (*continued*)

Suggested Action	Reason for Action
IMPLEMENTATION	
Wash your hands or use an alcohol-based hand rub (see Chapter 10).	Reduces the transmission of microorganisms
Help the client put on a robe and slippers.	Maintains warmth, safety, and comfort
Help the client ambulate to the location where the sitz bath will be administered.	Demonstrates concern for safety
Shut the door to the bathroom or tub room.	Provides privacy
Fill the container with warm water, no hotter than 110°F (43.3°C) (Fig. B).	Provides comfort without the danger of burning the skin
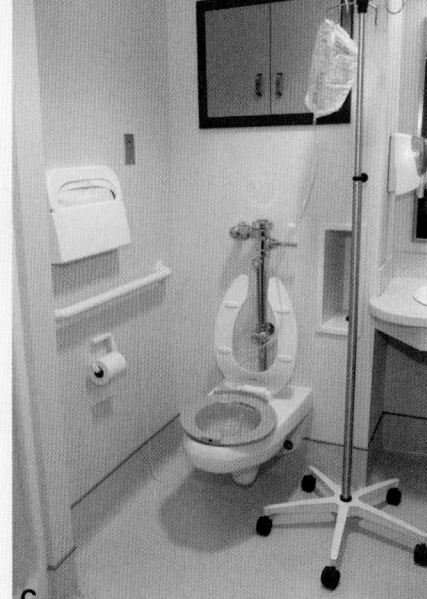 B	Fill the solution container.
Hang the bag above the toilet seat (Fig. C).	Facilitates gravity flow
C	Hang the bag and insert the tubing into the basin.
Help the client sit on the basin.	Facilitates filling the basin
Cover the client's shoulders with a bath blanket if the client feels chilled.	Promotes comfort
Instruct the client on how to signal for assistance.	Ensures safety
Leave the client alone, but recheck frequently to add more warm water to the reservoir bag.	Provides a sustained application of warm water
Help the client pat the skin dry after soaking for 20–30 minutes.	Restores comfort

SKILL 28-3 Providing a Sitz Bath (*continued*)

Suggested Action	Reason for Action
Assist the client back to bed.	Ensures safety in case the client feels dizzy from hypotension caused by peripheral vasodilation
Put on gloves and clean the equipment and bath area.	Supports principles of medical asepsis and infection control
Replace the sitz bath equipment in the client's bedside cabinet or leave it in the client's private bathroom.	Reduces costs by reusing disposable equipment

EVALUATION

- A sitz bath is administered according to the agency's policy or standards of care.
- Safety is maintained.
- The client reports that symptoms are relieved.

DOCUMENT

- Procedure
- Response of the client
- Assessment data

SAMPLE DOCUMENTATION

Date and Time Sitz bath provided over 30 minutes. Client states, "I always feel so good after this treatment." Perineum is slightly swollen. Margins of episiotomy are approximated. Continues to have moderate bloody vaginal drainage. _____ J. Doe, LPN

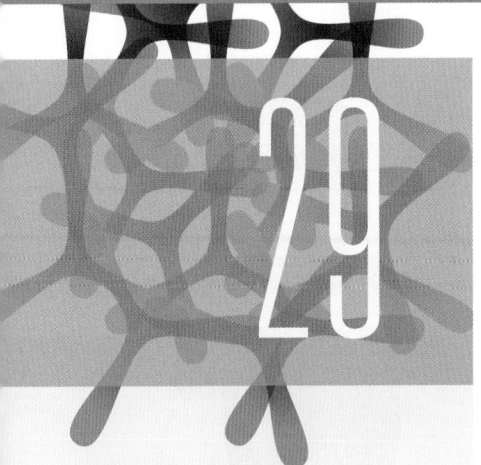

Gastrointestinal Intubation

Words To Know

bolus feeding
continuous feeding
cyclic feeding
decompression
dumping syndrome
enteral nutrition
gastric reflux
gastric residual
gastrostomy tube (G-tube)
gavage
intermittent feeding
intestinal decompression
intubation
jejunostomy tube (J-tube)
lavage
lumen
nasogastric intubation
nasogastric tube
nasointestinal intubation
nasointestinal tubes
nose-to-earlobe-to-the-xiphoid
(NEX) measurement
orogastric intubation
orogastric tube
ostomy
percutaneous endoscopic
gastrostomy (PEG) tube
percutaneous endoscopic
jejunostomy (PEJ) tube
pseudoconfirmatory gurgling
stylet
sump tubes
tamponade
transabdominal tubes

Learning Objectives

On completion of this chapter, the reader should be able to:

1. Define intubation and list reasons for gastrointestinal intubation.
2. Identify general types of gastrointestinal tubes.
3. Name assessments that are necessary before inserting a tube nasally.
4. Explain the purpose of and how to obtain a *n*ose-to-*e*arlobe-to-the-*x*iphoid (NEX) measurement.
5. Describe methods for determining distal placement in the stomach.
6. Discuss ways that nasointestinal feeding tubes or their insertion differs from their gastric counterparts.
7. Name schedules for administering tube feedings.
8. Explain the purpose of assessing gastric residual.
9. Name nursing activities involved in managing the care of clients who are being tube-fed.
10. Name nursing responsibilities for assisting with the insertion of a tungsten-weighted intestinal decompression tube.

INTRODUCTION

Clients, especially those undergoing abdominal or gastrointestinal (GI) surgery, may require some type of tube placed within the stomach or intestine. The use of a gastric or intestinal tube reduces or eliminates problems associated with surgery or conditions affecting the GI tract, such as impaired peristalsis, vomiting, or gas accumulation. Tubes can also be used to nourish clients who cannot eat. This chapter discusses the multiple uses for gastric and intestinal tubes and the nursing guidelines and skills for managing related client care.

 Gerontologic Considerations

■ An age-related reduction in the number of laryngeal nerve endings contributes to diminished efficiency of the gag reflex. Other conditions that can depress the gag reflex include neurologic disorders such as dementia, strokes, and Parkinson disease.

■ Long-term use of tube feedings in older adults with dementia or other chronic declining conditions involves many ethical considerations. Refusal to eat, which may be intentional or unintentional, is associated with a variety of conditions, including depression, suicidal behaviors, or advanced cognitive impairment.

■ Adults with decision-making capacity or the medical power of attorney for clients who lack capacity, along with the health care team, are the most appropriate people for weighing the risks and benefits of nutrition and hydration during end-of-life care. The client's choice must be respected (American Nurses Association, 2017).

■ Nurses need up-to-date knowledge about ethical and legal issues related to the use of tube feedings (see Chapter 3).

■ Tube-feeding formulas are prescribed based on the older client's condition (i.e., malabsorption syndromes, glucose intolerance). For example, lactose-free tube-feeding formulas may be beneficial to older clients who experience malabsorption syndromes.

■ Clients with or who are at risk for pressure sores benefit from formulas fortified with additional zinc, protein, and other nutrients.

■ In home and long-term care settings, registered dietitians may be helpful in the ongoing assessment of tube feedings.

■ Older adults tend to best tolerate small, continuous feedings.

■ Older adults are at increased risk for fluid and electrolyte disturbances and as a result may develop hyperglycemia (elevated blood glucose levels) when tube feedings are administered.

■ If an older client is receiving tube feedings with full-strength formula concentrations, it is important to check capillary blood glucose levels at intervals until the client's results are within a normal range.

■ Monitor older adults for agitation or confusion, which may cause them to pull out feeding tubes inadvertently. Also, a change in behavior or mental status may be an early indicator of a fluid or electrolyte imbalance.

■ When teaching older adults or older caregivers how to manage a G-tube or administer tube feedings at home, allow more time for processing information and include several practice sessions.

■ A referral for skilled nursing care, which may be covered by Medicare/Medicaid or private health insurance plans, may be appropriate for ongoing teaching and assessments for clients who require tube feedings after being discharged.

■ For older adults living on a fixed income, dietitians can suggest ways to prepare less costly, home-blended formulas that meet the client's nutritional needs.

INTUBATION

Intubation generally means the placement of a tube into a body structure; in this chapter, it refers specifically to insertion of a tube into the stomach or intestine by way of the mouth or nose. **Orogastric intubation** (the insertion of a tube through the mouth into the stomach), **nasogastric intubation** (the insertion of a tube through the nose into the stomach), and **nasointestinal intubation** (the insertion of a tube through the nose to the intestine) are performed to remove gas or fluids or to administer liquid nourishment.

A tube may also be inserted within an **ostomy** (a surgically created opening). A prefix identifies the anatomic site of the ostomy; for instance, a *gastrostomy* is an artificial opening into the stomach (Fig. 29-1).

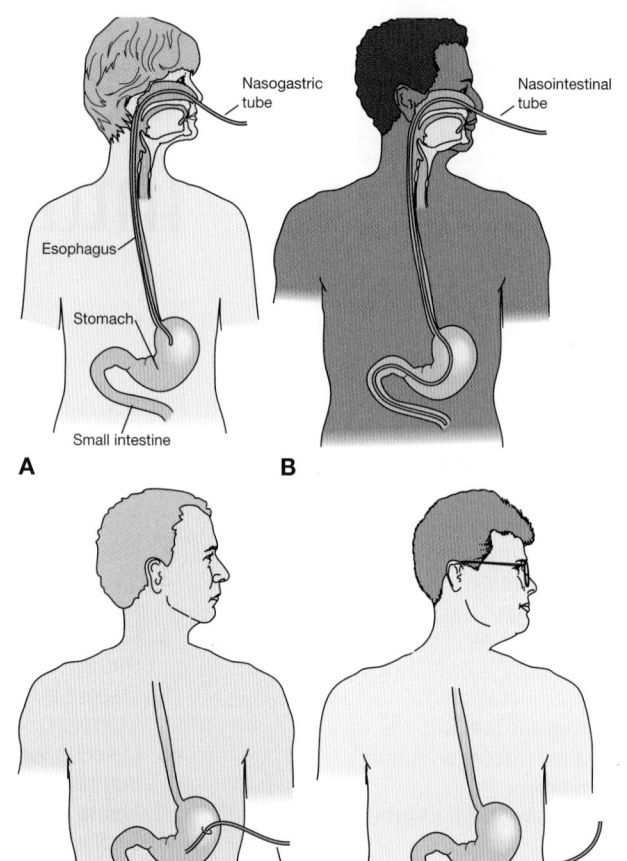

FIGURE 29-1 Examples of various methods of gastric and intestinal intubation. **A.** Nasogastric tube that terminates in the stomach. **B.** Nasogastric tube that terminates in the small intestine. **C.** Gastrostomy tube inserted surgically directly into the stomach. **D.** Jejunostomy tube inserted surgically into the jejunum of small intestine. (From Carter, P. [2019]. *Lippincott textbook for nursing assistants* [5th ed.]. Lippincott Williams & Wilkins.)

Gastric or intestinal tubes are used for a variety of reasons, including:

• Performing a **gavage** (providing nourishment)
• Administering oral medications that the client cannot swallow
• Obtaining a sample of secretions for diagnostic testing
• Performing a **lavage** (removing substances from the stomach, typically poisons)
• Promoting **decompression** (removing gas and liquid contents from the stomach or bowel)

Controlling gastric bleeding, a process called compression or **tamponade** (pressure)

TYPES OF TUBES

Although all gastric and intestinal tubes have proximal and distal ends, their sizes, constructions, and compositions vary according to their uses (Table 29-1). The outside diameter of most tubes is measured using the French scale, indicated

TABLE 29-1 Types of Gastrointestinal Tubes

TUBE	PURPOSE	CHARACTERISTICS
Orogastric		
Ewald	Lavage	Large diameter: 36–40 F Single lumen Multiple distal openings for drainage
Nasogastric		
Levin	Lavage Gavage Decompression Diagnostics	Usual adult size 14–18 F Single lumen 42–50 in (107–127 cm) long Multiple drain openings
Salem sump	Decompression	Same diameter as Levin Double lumen Pigtail vent 48 in (122 cm) long Marked at increments to indicate depth of insertion Radiopaque
Sengstaken–Blakemore	Compression Drainage	Usual diameter: 20 F 36 in (90 cm) long Triple lumen; two lead to balloons in the esophagus and stomach and the third is for removing gastric drainage; a fourth lumen may be used to remove pharyngeal secretions
Nasointestinal		
Keofeed	Gavage	Small diameter: 8 F 36 in (90 cm) long Polyurethane or silicone Weighted tip Extremely flexible and may require the use of a stylet during insertion Radiopaque Bonded lubricant that becomes activated with moisture
Maxter	Intestinal decompression	Usual size: 18 F 100 in (250 cm) long Double lumen Tungsten-weighted tip Graduated marks every 10 in (25 cm)
Transabdominal		
Gastrostomy	Gavage; may be used for decompression while the client is fed through a jejunostomy tube	Sizes 12–24 F for adults Rubber or silicone May have additional side ports for balloon inflation to maintain placement May be capped or plugged between feedings Radiopaque
Jejunostomy	Gavage	Sizes 5–14 F for adults Silicone or polyurethane Radiopaque

by a number followed by the letter F. Each number on the French scale equals approximately 0.33 mm. The larger the number, the larger the diameter of the tube.

Tubes can be identified according to the location of the insertion (mouth, nose, or abdomen) or the location of their distal end (stomach or intestine).

Orogastric Tubes

An **orogastric tube** (a tube inserted through the mouth into the stomach), such as an Ewald tube, is used in an emergency to remove toxic substances that have been ingested. The diameter of the tube is large enough to remove pill fragments and stomach debris. Because of its size, the tube is introduced through the mouth rather than the nose.

Nasogastric Tubes

A **nasogastric tube** (a tube placed through the nose and advanced to the stomach) is smaller in diameter than an orogastric tube but larger and shorter than a nasointestinal tube. Some nasogastric tubes have more than one **lumen** (channel) within the tube.

A Levin tube is a commonly used, single-lumen gastric tube with multiple uses, one of which is decompression. Gastric **sump tubes** (double-lumen tubes) are used almost exclusively to remove fluid and gas from the stomach (Fig. 29-2). The second lumen serves as a vent. The use of sump tubes decreases the possibility that the stomach wall will adhere to and obstruct the distal drainage openings when suction is applied.

Because nasogastric tubes remain in place for several days or more, many clients report nose and throat discomfort. If the tube's diameter is too large or pressure from the tube is prolonged, nasopharyngeal tissue irritation or breakdown may occur. Furthermore, gastric tubes tend to dilate the esophageal sphincter, also known as the cardiac valve, a circular muscle between the esophagus and stomach. The stretched opening may contribute to **gastric reflux** (the reverse flow of gastric contents), especially when the tube is used to administer liquid formula. If gastric reflux occurs, the liquid could enter the airway and interfere with respiratory function.

Nasointestinal Tubes

Nasointestinal tubes (tubes inserted through the nose for distal placement below the stomach) are longer than their gastric counterparts. The added length permits them to be

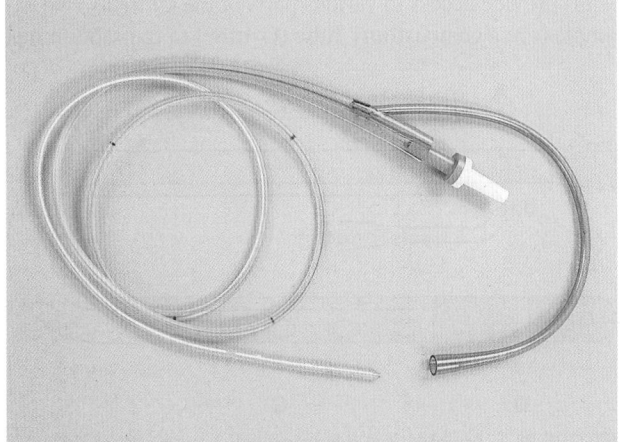

FIGURE 29-2 Vented nasogastric (Salem sump) tube with a one-way valve. (Photo by B. Proud.)

placed in the small bowel. They are used to provide nourishment (feeding tubes) or to remove gas and liquid contents from the small intestine (decompression tubes).

Feeding Tubes

Nasointestinal tubes used for nutrition, such as a Dobhoff tube, are usually small in diameter and made of a flexible substance such as polyurethane or silicone. Their narrow width and soft composition allow them to remain in the same nostril for 4 weeks or longer. In addition, they reduce the potential for gastric reflux because they deliver liquid nutrition beyond the stomach.

Narrow tubes are not problem-free. They tend to curl during insertion because they are so flexible. Therefore, some are supplied with a **stylet** (metal guidewire) that helps straighten and support them during insertion. Almost all have a weighted tip that helps them descend past the stomach. Checking the placement of the distal end is more difficult; these tubes also become obstructed more easily. Despite the problems associated with maintenance, small-diameter tubes are preferred for their comfort. They are ideal for providing a continuous infusion of nourishment.

Intestinal Decompression Tubes

Although surgery is often the most common intervention when a client has a partial or complete bowel obstruction, **intestinal decompression** (the removal of gas and intestinal contents) may also be used. A tube used for intestinal decompression has a double lumen and a weighted tip (Fig. 29-3). One lumen is used to suction the intestinal contents; the other acts as a vent to reduce suction-induced trauma to intestinal tissue. The weighted tip and peristalsis, if present, propel the tube beyond the stomach and into the intestine. The progress of the radiopaque tip through the GI tract is monitored by X-ray.

Intestinal tubes, like the Maxter tube (see Table 29-1) and the Anderson tube, are weighted with tungsten. Other weighted intestinal tubes are weighted at distal tip with water or saline.

Transabdominal Tubes

Transabdominal tubes (tubes placed through the abdominal wall) provide access to various parts of the GI tract. Two examples are a **gastrostomy tube (G-tube)** (a transabdominal

tube located within the stomach) and a **jejunostomy tube (J-tube)** (a transabdominal tube that leads to the jejunum of the small intestine).

A G-tube is placed surgically or with the use of an endoscope. A surgically inserted G-tube resembles a long rubber catheter sutured to the abdomen. A **percutaneous endoscopic gastrostomy (PEG) tube** (a transabdominal tube inserted under endoscopic guidance) is anchored with internal and external crossbars called bumpers (Fig. 29-4). A **percutaneous endoscopic jejunostomy (PEJ) tube** (a tube that is passed through a PEG tube into the jejunum) is small in diameter so that it can be inserted through the larger PEG tube.

Transabdominal tubes are used instead of nasogastric or nasointestinal tubes when clients require an alternative to oral feeding for more than 1 month.

NASOGASTRIC TUBE MANAGEMENT

Usually, nurses insert nasogastric tubes. Additional nursing responsibilities include keeping the tube patent (or unobstructed), implementing the prescribed use, and removing the tube when it has accomplished its therapeutic purpose.

Nasogastric Tube Insertion

Inserting a nasogastric tube involves preparing the client, conducting preintubation assessments, and placing the tube.

Client Preparation

Most clients are anxious about having to swallow a tube. Explaining that the diameter of the tube is smaller than most pieces of food may foster a positive outcome. Describing the procedure and giving instructions on how the client can assist while the tube is being passed may further reduce anxiety. One of the most important ways to support clients is to provide them with some means of control. The nurse can establish a signal, such as the client raising a hand, to indicate the need for a pause during the tube's passage.

Preintubation Assessment

Before insertion, the nurse conducts a focused assessment that includes the client's:

- Level of consciousness
- Weight
- Bowel sounds
- Abdominal distention
- Integrity of nasal and oral mucosa
- Ability to swallow, cough, and gag
- Any nausea and vomiting

Assessment findings serve as a baseline for future comparisons and may suggest a need to modify the procedure or the equipment used. One main goal of the assessment is to determine which nostril is best to use when inserting the tube and the length to which the tube will be inserted.

Nasal Inspection

After the client clears nasal debris by blowing into a paper tissue, the nurse inspects each nostril for size, shape, and

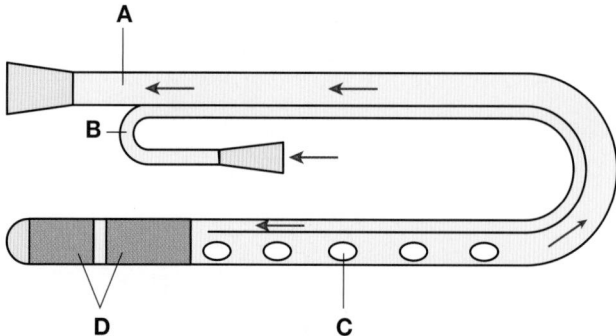

FIGURE 29-3 An intestinal decompression tube, including the suction lumen (**A**), the vent lumen (**B**), openings for suction (**C**), and the radiopaque tungsten tip (**D**).

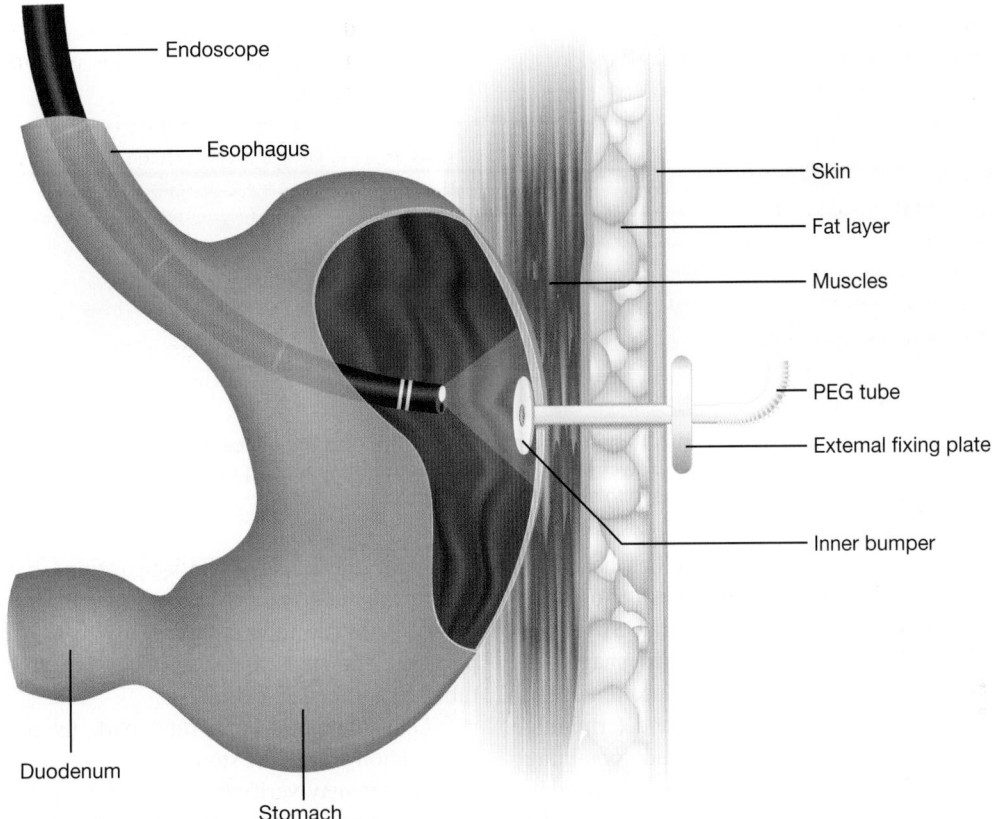

FIGURE 29-4 A percutaneous endoscopic gastrostomy tube. (Sezer33/Shutterstock.)

patency. The client should exhale while each nostril in turn is occluded. The presence of nasal polyps (small growths of tissue), a deviated septum (nasal cartilage deflected from the midline of the nose), or a narrow nasal passage excludes a nostril for tube insertion.

Nasogastric Tube Measurement

Some tubes are already marked to indicate the approximate length at which the distal tip will be located within the stomach. These markings, however, may not correlate exactly with the client's anatomy. Therefore, before inserting a tube, the nurse obtains the client's *nose-to-earlobe-to-the-xiphoid (NEX) measurement* (Fig. 29-5) and marks the tube appropriately.

The first mark on the tube is made at the measured distance from the nose to the earlobe. It indicates the distance to the nasal pharynx—a location that places the tip at the back of the throat but above where the gag reflex is stimulated. A second mark is made at the point where the tube reaches the xiphoid process, indicating the depth required to reach the stomach.

Nasogastric Tube Placement

When inserting a nasogastric tube, the nurse's primary concerns are to cause as little discomfort as possible, preserve the integrity of the nasal tissue, and locate the tube within the stomach, not in the respiratory passages.

Although several bedside physical assessment methods such as auscultating the abdomen while instilling air and

testing the pH of aspirated liquid have been used by nurses and may still be widely practiced to determine the distal location of a nasogastric tube, they do not always provide credible evidence. Current data indicate that testing the pH of aspirated fluid can be unreliable because the pH can be falsely altered by the aspiration of swallowed alkaline saliva,

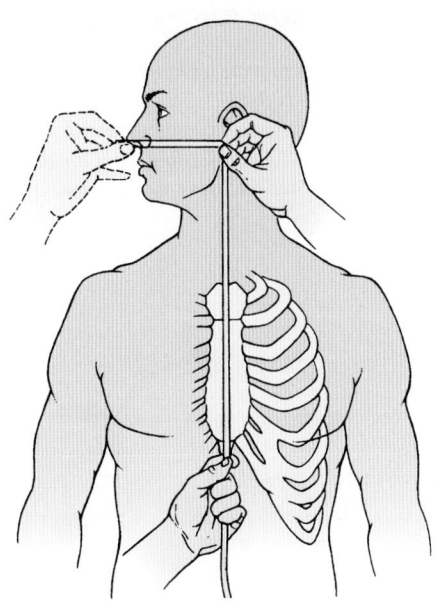

FIGURE 29-5 Obtaining the nose-to-earlobe-to-the-xiphoid (NEX) measurement.

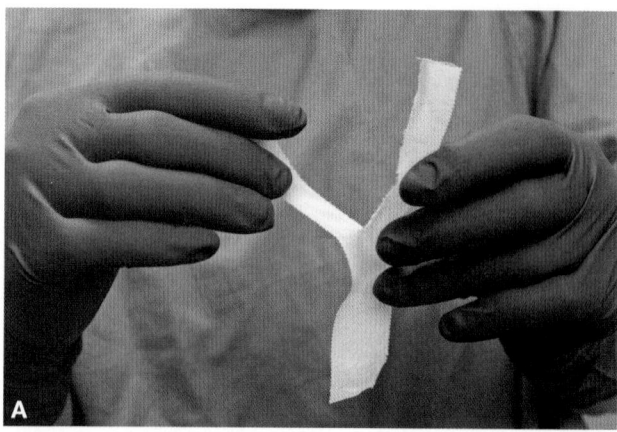
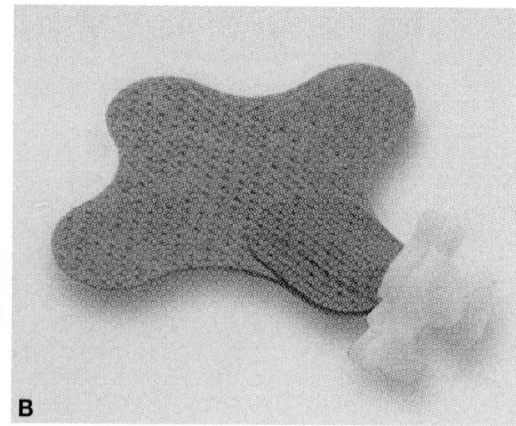

FIGURE 29-6 A. One end of a piece of tape is split, forming two narrower strips, and the opposite end is left intact. The wider intact end of the tape is applied to the nose, and the narrower strips are wound around the tube in opposite directions to secure the nasogastric tube. **B.** A commercial adhesive product used to secure a tube's placement.

refluxed acidic gastric secretions, and medications that make gastric secretions less acidic. In addition, auscultation over the abdomen while air is instilled is known to cause **pseudo-confirmatory gurgling** when air enters the esophagus or small intestine, thus misinterpreting a gastric location of the tube's tip. The only evidence-based methods for determining the distal location of a nasogastric tube include obtaining an abdominal X-ray after its initial insertion and monitoring the external tube length (the "X" marked component of the NEX measurement to the proximal end of the tube) after radiographic confirmation (Miller et al., 2015). The placement of weighted-tip feeding tubes may also be confirmed using bedside ultrasonography.

Once the nurse has confirmed stomach placement, they secure the tube to avoid upward or downward migration (Fig. 29-6). The tube is then ready to use for its intended purpose. The steps to follow when inserting a nasogastric tube are outlined in Skill 29-1.

Once the tube is at its final mark, the nurse must verify the location within the stomach.

Nurses may verify the tube's distal placement throughout its use by aspirating fluid from the tube after the initial X-ray using a large-volume (30- to 50-mL) syringe. The large-volume syringe creates less negative pressure during aspiration and therefore provides enough fluid to test the pH (Nursing Guidelines 29-1).

 NURSING GUIDELINES 29-1

Inserting a Nasointestinal Feeding Tube

- Wash hands or use an alcohol-based hand rub (see Chapter 10). *Hand hygiene reduces the transmission of microorganisms.*
- Put on gloves. *Gloves provide a physical barrier between the nurse's hands and body fluids.*
- Obtain a flexible small-gauge feeding tube with a stylet (Fig. A). *Flexible small-gauge feeding tubes are designed to remain in place longer and have less potential for nasal trauma.*

- Follow the manufacturer's suggestions for activating the lubricant bonded to the tube. Two common techniques are to instill water through the tube and to immerse the tip in water or dip the end of the tubing in the water-soluble gel (included in most kits) (Fig. B). *Water-soluble gel aids the insertion of the tube.*

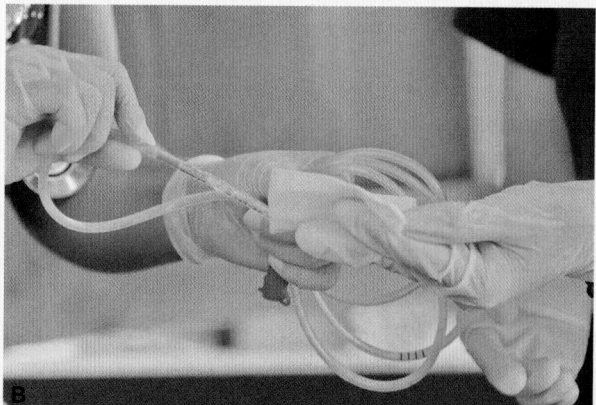

Preparing the nasogastric tube with water-soluble gel. (Anukool Manoton/Shutterstock.)

- Secure the stylet within the tube. *This measure stiffens the tube and facilitates insertion.*

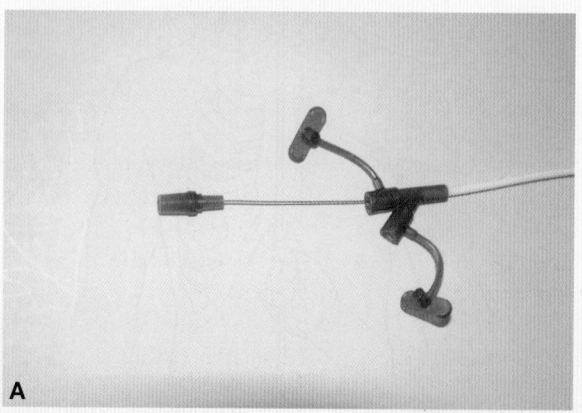

A small-gauge flexible feeding tube with stylet.

NURSING GUIDELINES 29-1

- Insert the tube into the nose (Fig. C) until it reaches the second mark. *Doing so places the tube in the presumed area of the stomach.*

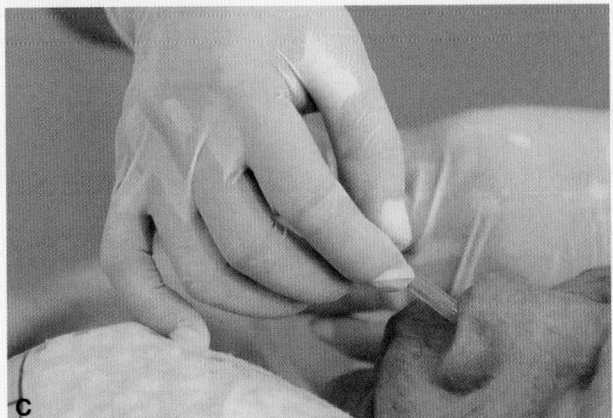

Inserting the feeding tube. (Anukool Manoton/Shutterstock.)

- Assess for signs of respiratory distress. *Coughing and difficulty breathing suggest the distal end of the tube is in the respiratory tract.*
- Aspirate fluid using a 30- to 50-mL syringe (Fig. D) and test the fluid pH (Fig. E).

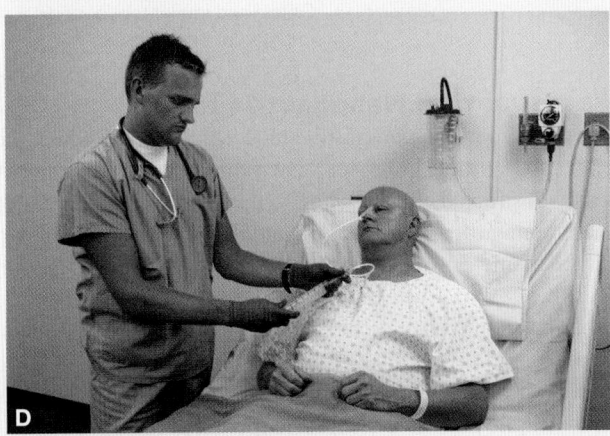

Aspirating fluid from the tube.

- Drop a sample of aspirated fluid onto an indicator strip (Fig. F). *This step initiates a chemical reaction on contact and saturation.*

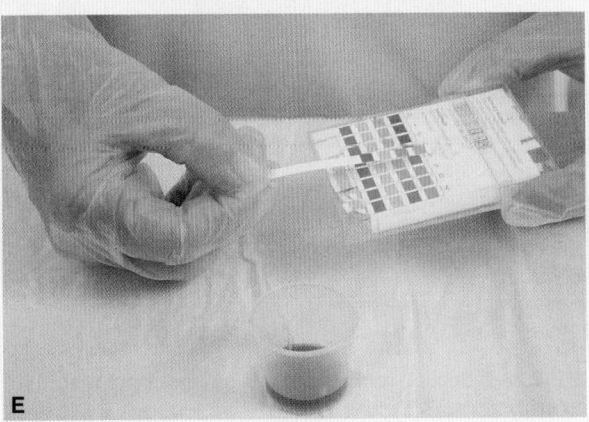

Checking the pH of aspirated fluid.

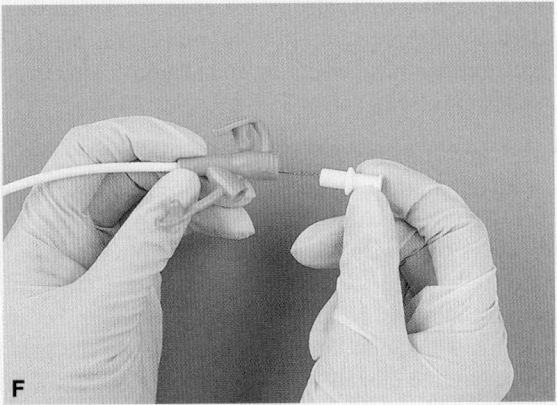

Removing the stylet.

- Compare the color on the test strip with the color guide on the container of reagent strips. *The color of the test strip changes according to the hydrogen ion concentration of the liquid. Stomach fluid usually has a pH of 5 or less even in those receiving gastric acid inhibitors; secretions from the small intestine have a pH of 6 or greater.*
- Loop the tubing if there is no respiratory distress and tape it temporarily to the cheek if the desired distal location is beyond the pyloric valve. *Looping provides slack so the tube can descend into the small intestine.*
- Ambulate or position the client on their right side for at least 1 hour or the time specified in the agency's policy. *This duration allows the tube to move by gravity through the pyloric valve.*

>>> ***Stop, Think, and Respond 29-1***

Discuss the consequences of inserting a nasogastric tube into the respiratory passages.

Use and Maintenance of Nasogastric Tubes

Nasogastric tubes are connected to suction for gastric decompression or are used for tube feeding.

Gastric Decompression

Suction is either continuous or intermittent. Continuous suctioning with an unvented tube can cause the tube to adhere to the stomach mucosa, resulting in localized irritation and interfering with drainage. Using a vented tube or intermittent suction prevents or minimizes these effects.

The tube is connected to a wall outlet or portable suction machine (Fig. 29-7). The suction setting is prescribed

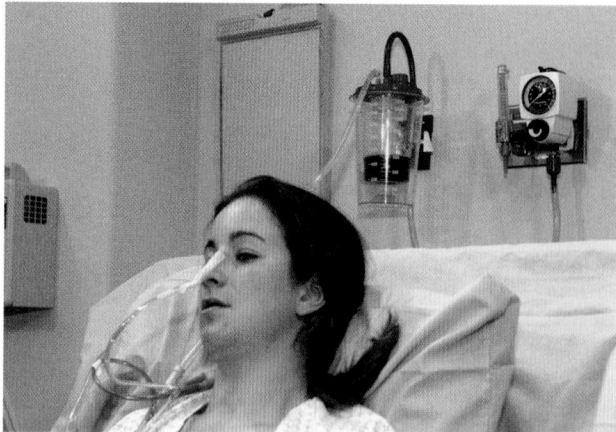

FIGURE 29-7 Suction removes liquids and gas from the stomach.

TABLE 29-2	Troubleshooting a Poorly Draining Nasogastric Tube	
POSSIBLE CAUSES	**SOLUTIONS**
The drainage holes are adhering to the gastric mucosal wall.	Turn the suction off momentarily. Change the client's position.
The tube is displaced above the esophageal sphincter.	If the measured mark is not at the tip of the nose, remove the tape, advance the tube, check placement, and resecure.
The portable suction machine is disconnected or turned off.	Replace the plug into the electrical outlet or turn on power.
The drainage container is filled beyond capacity.	Empty and record the amount of drainage in the suction container.
The vent is acting as a siphon.	Instill a bolus of air into the vent to restore patency.
The vent is capped or plugged.	Remove the cap and restore the port to atmospheric pressure.
The tubing is kinked or disconnected.	Straighten tubing or reconnect to the suction machine.
The suction is inadequate.	Check that the pressure is 40–60 mm Hg.
The cover on the suction container is loose.	Resecure the lid to the container.
A solid particle or thick mucus obstructs the lumen.	Increase suction pressure momentarily. Obtain and implement a medical order for an irrigation.

by the physician or indicated in the agency's standards for care. Usually low pressure (40 to 60 mm Hg) is used. The tube is clamped or plugged during ambulation or after instilling medications (see Chapter 32).

Promoting Patency

Even with intermittent suctioning, the tube may become obstructed. Giving ice chips or occasional sips of water to a client who is otherwise NPO (receives nothing by mouth) promotes tube patency. The fluid helps dilute the gastric secretions. Both must be given sparingly, however, because water is hypotonic and draws electrolytes into the gastric fluid. Because the diluted fluid is ultimately removed, giving the client liberal amounts of water can deplete serum electrolytes (see Chapter 16).

Restoring Patency

The nurse assesses tube patency frequently by monitoring the volume and characteristics of drainage and observing for signs and symptoms suggesting an obstruction (nausea, vomiting, and abdominal distention). Inspection of the equipment helps identify possible causes for the assessment findings (Table 29-2). Once the cause is identified, a variety of simple nursing interventions can resolve it. Sometimes the nasogastric tube must be irrigated to maintain or restore patency (Skill 29-2). The nurse must obtain a medical order before attempting an irrigation.

> **Stop, Think, and Respond 29-2**
>
> Explain the reason for using an isotonic saline solution, rather than a hypotonic or hypertonic solution, to irrigate a nasogastric tube.

Enteral Nutrition

Enteral nutrition (nourishment provided through the stomach or small intestine rather than by the oral route) is delivered by instilling formula through a tube. Although a nasogastric tube can be used, it is more likely that liquid formula will be administered through a nasointestinal or transabdominal tube. Both are discussed later in this chapter.

Removal of a Nasogastric Tube

Nurses remove a nasogastric tube (Skill 29-3) when the client's condition improves, when the tube becomes hopelessly obstructed, or according to the agency's standards for maintaining the integrity of the nasal mucosa. Unobstructed larger diameter tubes are usually removed and changed at least every 2 to 4 weeks for adults. Small-diameter, flexible tubes are removed and changed every 4 weeks to 3 months, depending on the agency's policy. Tubes used for pediatric clients are changed more frequently because the tissue is more fragile and there is a greater potential for infection.

Before permanent removal, some physicians prescribe a trial period during which the tube is clamped and the client is allowed to consume oral fluids. Remaining asymptomatic (i.e., no nausea, vomiting, or gastric distention) is a good indication that the client no longer requires intubation. If symptoms develop, the tube is already in place and can be easily reconnected to suction. This practice avoids subjecting the client to the discomfort associated with tube replacement.

> **Stop, Think, and Respond 29-3**
>
> If the client who has just had a nasogastric tube removed wants something to eat, what nursing actions are appropriate?

NASOINTESTINAL TUBE MANAGEMENT

Nurses also insert nasointestinal tubes that are used for enteral feeding.

Insertion of a Nasointestinal Tube

The techniques for client preparation, positioning, and advancement of nasointestinal tubes are similar to those for nasogastric tubes. Some modifications are necessary, however, because nasointestinal tubes are constructed differently (see Nursing Guidelines 29-1 and 29-2).

To estimate the length of tube required for an intestinal placement, the nurse determines the NEX measurement and adds 9 in (23 cm). They also mark the additional measurement on the tubing.

New technologies that promise to promote safety and efficacy in nasoenteric tube placement are becoming available. A computer system that uses electromagnetic technology to direct and locate a feeding tube has also been developed. It consists of an electronically modified feeding tube and a receiver that is placed externally over the midabdomen. A computer then converts the signal into a graphic display. This helps identify misplacement immediately, and subsequent use eliminates the need for repeated radiographic verification of its location.

NURSING GUIDELINES 29-2

Managing a Gastrostomy

- Wash hands or use an alcohol-based hand rub (see Chapter 10). *Hand hygiene reduces the transmission of microorganisms.*
- Put on gloves. *They provide a physical barrier between the nurse's hands and body fluids.*
- Assess and replace the gauze dressing over a new gastrostomy if it becomes moist; slight bleeding or a clear serous drainage from the wound is normal for a few weeks after the procedure. *These measures reduce the conditions that support the growth of microorganisms and maceration of the skin.*
- Remove and discontinue the dressing after the first 24 hours unless the physician orders otherwise. *This facilitates assessment.*
- Inspect the skin around the tube daily. *Regular monitoring provides assessment data about the status of wound repair* (Fig. A).
- Make sure that the sutures holding a surgically placed tube are intact. *Checking prevents tube migration.*
- Report any redness or tissue maceration. *These findings indicate early skin impairment.*
- Apply a skin barrier ointment such as zinc oxide, karaya gum wafer, hydrocolloid dressing, or ostomy pouch if the skin appears irritated (see section "Ostomy Care" in Chapter 31). *Such barriers protect the skin and promote healing.*
- Press down on the skin at the base of the tube. If the client has a PEG tube, compress the arms of the external bumper together and lift them about 1 in (2.5 cm) (Fig. B). *These steps aid in assessing for drainage, which normally disappears by the end of the first week.*
- Clean the skin with half-strength hydrogen peroxide or 0.9% saline. After 1 week, using soap and water is sufficient. Dry the skin well using air or a blow dryer on a cool or low-heat setting. *Appropriate cleaning removes secretions and reduces microorganisms.*

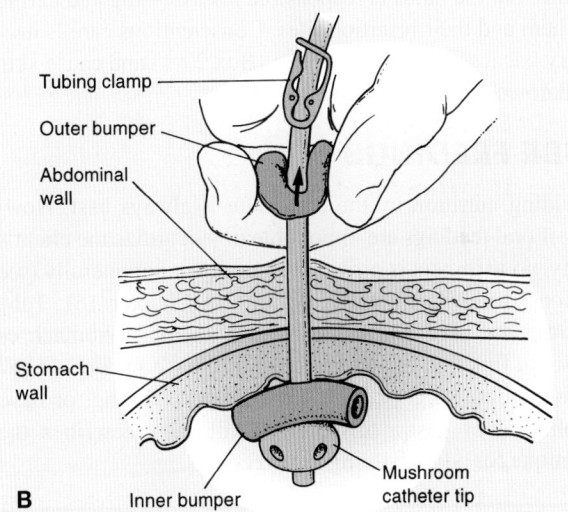

Inspecting the skin.

- Rotate the direction of the external bumper 90 degrees or other external retaining device at least once a day. *Doing so relieves pressure and maintains skin integrity.*
- Slide the external bumper down so it is flush with the skin. *Sliding restabilizes the tube.*
- Avoid placing any type of dressing material under the arms of the external bumper. *This helps avoid creating pressure on the internal bumper and damaging the tissue.*
- Replace the water in the balloon beneath the bumper weekly using a Luer-tip (not Luer-Lok) syringe. *This keeps the balloon fully inflated and prevents tube migration.*
- Tape the G-tube to the abdomen or secure it with an abdominal binder or commercial tube stabilizer. *Appropriately securing the tube maintains its position.*
- Make sure the tube is not kinked and the skin is not stretched. *These assessments ensure tube patency and skin integrity.*
- Insert a Foley catheter (see Chapter 30) if the client is not sensitive to latex, 2 to 5 in (5 to 10 cm) within the opening, and inflate the balloon if the tube comes out. *Doing so maintains temporary access to the stomach and, if done within 3 hours of accidental extubation, prevents the site from closing.*
- Use the G-tube in a manner similar to how a nasogastric tube is used for administering feedings. *The tube facilitates nourishment.*

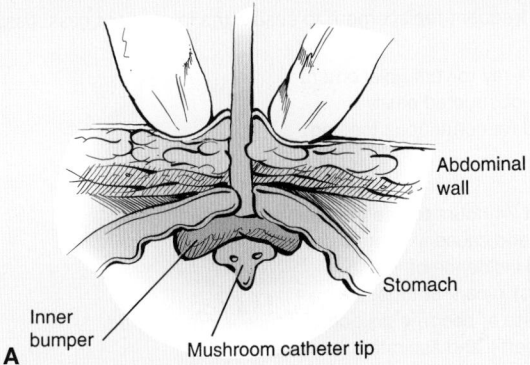

Inspecting for drainage.

- Disconnection between the feeding delivery tube and G-tube
- Clamped G-tube while tube feeding is infusing
- Mismatch between the size of the G-tube and stoma
- Increased abdominal pressure from formula accumulation, retching, sneezing, and coughing
- Underinflation of the balloon beneath the skin
- Less than optimal stoma or stomal location

TRANSABDOMINAL TUBE MANAGEMENT

The physician inserts transabdominal tubes, such as G- and J-tubes, but the nurse is responsible for assessing and caring for them and their insertion sites. Conscientious care is necessary because G-tubes may leak (Box 29-1) and cause skin breakdown.

TUBE FEEDINGS

Providing nutrition by the oral route is always best. However, if oral feedings are impossible or jeopardize the client's safety, nourishment is provided enterally or parenterally (see section "Total Parenteral Nutrition" in Chapter 16). Tube feedings are used when clients have an intact stomach or intestinal function but are unconscious, have undergone extensive mouth surgery, have difficulty swallowing, or have esophageal or gastric disorders. Skill 29-4 describes the technique for administering tube feedings.

Benefits and Risks of Tube Feedings

Tube feedings are delivered through a nasogastric, nasointestinal, or transabdominal tube. Each has its advantages and disadvantages (Table 29-3).

Instilling nutritional formulas into the stomach uses the body's natural reservoir for food. It also reduces the potential for enteritis (inflammation of the intestine) because the chemicals in the stomach tend to destroy microorganisms. Gastric feedings increase the potential for gastric reflux, however, because of their volume and temporary retention within the stomach.

Although the placement of tubes within the intestine reduces the risk for gastric reflux, it does not eliminate that risk. Additional problems are associated with intestinal tube feedings. For example, an intestinally placed tube may lead to **dumping syndrome** (a cluster of symptoms from the rapid deposition of calorie-dense nourishment into the small intestine). The symptoms, which include weakness, dizziness, sweating, and nausea, are caused by fluid shifts from the circulating blood to the intestine and a low blood glucose level related to a surge of insulin. Diarrhea may also result when administering hypertonic formula solutions.

Formula Considerations

In addition to the type of tube and the access site, the type of formula is also individualized based on the client's nutritional needs (Table 29-4). Factors include the client's weight, nutritional status, concurrent medical conditions, and the projected length of therapy. The feeding schedule also affects the choice of formula: calories may need to be concentrated if the client is being fed several times a day rather than continuously. Most formulas provide 0.5 to 2.0 kcal/mL with 750 to 800 mL of water per liter (nutrient component).

Nutrition Notes

- Specialty formulas are available with altered nutritional profiles for specific disease states, such as for clients with diabetes, renal failure, hepatic failure, respiratory insufficiency, and wound healing. Pediatric formulas are also available.

- Products like Boost, Carnation Breakfast Essentials, and Ensure are primarily intended as oral supplements, not for tube feedings.

TABLE 29-3 Comparison of Feeding Tubes

TUBE	ADVANTAGES	DISADVANTAGES
Nasogastric	Low incidence of obstruction Accommodates crushed medications Facilitates bolus or intermittent feedings Easy to check distal placement and gastric residual	Can damage nasal and pharyngeal mucosa from pressure or friction Dilates esophageal sphincter, potentiating gastric reflux Potential for aspiration Requires frequent replacement to ensure the integrity of nasal tissue
Nasointestinal	Easy to insert Comfortable Only slight dilation of esophageal sphincter Reduced danger for aspiration Can remain in place for 4 weeks or longer	Requires X-ray to verify placement Becomes obstructed easily Best used for continuous feeding
Gastrostomy	No nasal tube Easily concealed Accommodates long-term use Infrequent tube replacement Client can be taught self-care	Must wait 24 hours to use after initial placement May leak and cause skin breakdown Increased incidence of infection Requires skin care at tube site Can migrate or become dislodged if tube is not secured Gastric overfill and aspiration possible
Jejunostomy	Same as gastrostomy Reduced potential for reflux and aspiration	Same as gastrostomy

TABLE 29-4 Tube-Feeding Formulas

TYPE	EXAMPLES	DESCRIPTION
Standard, isotonic	Osmolite Isocal Nutren 1.0	Routine formulas for clients with normal digestion and absorption; do not alter water distribution. Provide approximately 1.0 cal/mL
High calorie	Comply Nutren 1.5 Nutren 2.0 Deliver 2.0	Provide up to double the amount of calories of standard formulas for clients who require a fluid restriction or have high-calorie needs
High protein	Promote Isocal HN Ultracal HN plus	Provide up to double the amount of protein of standard formulas
Fiber-containing	Jevity Compleat Ultracal	Provide fiber to normalize bowel function in clients with diarrhea or constipation
Partially hydrolyzed	Criticare HN Optimental Vivonex T.E.N.	Provide nutrients in simple form that require little or no digestion for clients with impaired digestion or absorption

Tube-Feeding Schedules

Tube feedings may be administered on bolus, intermittent, cyclic, or continuous schedules.

Bolus Feedings

A **bolus feeding** (the instillation of liquid nourishment in less than 30 minutes four to six times a day) usually involves 250 to 400 mL of formula per administration. This schedule is the least desirable because it distends the stomach rapidly, causing gastric discomfort and an increased risk for reflux. Bolus feedings may be used because to some extent, they mimic the natural filling and emptying of the stomach. Some clients experience discomfort from the rapid delivery of this quantity of fluid. Clients who are unconscious or who have delayed gastric emptying are at greater risk for regurgitation, vomiting, and aspiration with this method of administration.

Intermittent Feedings

An **intermittent feeding** (the gradual instillation of liquid nourishment four to six times a day) is administered over 30 to 60 minutes, the time most people spend eating a meal. The usual volume is 250 to 400 mL per administration. Intermittent feedings are generally given by gravity drip from a suspended container or with a feeding pump. Gradual filling of the stomach at a slower rate reduces the bloated feeling that can accompany bolus feedings. The container and feeding tube that holds the formula require thorough flushing after each feeding to reduce the growth of microorganisms. Tube-feeding administration sets are replaced every 24 hours regardless of the feeding schedule.

Cyclic Feedings

A **cyclic feeding** (the continuous instillation of liquid nourishment for 8 to 12 hours) is followed by a 16- to 12-hour

pause. This routine often is used to wean clients from tube feedings while continuing to maintain adequate nutrition. The tube feeding is given during the late evening and hours of sleep. During the day, clients eat some food orally. As oral intake increases, the volume and duration of the tube feeding gradually decreases.

Continuous Feedings

A **continuous feeding** (the instillation of liquid nutrition without interruption) is administered at a rate of approximately 1.5 mL/minute. A feeding pump is used to regulate the instillation. Because only a small amount of fluid is instilled at any one time, the formula does not need to be held in the reservoir of the stomach; it can be delivered directly into the small intestine. Instilling small amounts of fluid beyond the stomach reduces the risk of vomiting and aspiration. Continuous feeding creates some inconvenience, though, because the pump must go wherever the client goes.

Client Assessment

The following daily assessments are standard for almost every client who receives tube feedings: weight, fluid intake and output, bowel sounds, lung sounds, temperature, condition of the nasal and oral mucous membranes, breathing pattern, gastric complaints, status of abdominal distention, vomiting, bowel elimination patterns, and skin condition at the site of a transabdominal tube. Once tube feedings have been initiated, it is also necessary to routinely assess the client's **gastric residual** (the volume of liquid within the stomach). The nurse measures the gastric residual to determine whether the rate or volume of feeding exceeds the client's physiologic capacity. Overfilling the stomach can cause gastric reflux, regurgitation, vomiting, aspiration, and pneumonia. As a rule of thumb, the gastric residual should be no more than 100 mL or no more than 20% of the previous hour's tube-feeding volume. If the gastric residual is more than 200 mL, delay the feeding. If the gastric residual is high, the feeding is stopped and the gastric residual is rechecked every 30 minutes until it is within a safe volume for resuming the feeding (Nursing Guidelines 29-3).

⟫ *Stop, Think, and Respond 29-4*

If a client's nutritional needs are met entirely with tube feedings, what effects might that have on the person physically, emotionally, and socially?

Nursing Management

Caring for clients with feeding tubes generally involves maintaining tube patency, clearing any obstructions, providing adequate hydration, dealing with common formula-related problems, and preparing clients for home care.

Maintaining Tube Patency

Feeding tubes, especially those smaller than 12 F, are prone to obstruction. Common causes are using formulas with large-molecule nutrients, refeeding partially digested gastric residual, administering formula at a rate less than 50 mL/hour,

NURSING GUIDELINES 29-3

Checking the Gastric Residual

- Wash hands or use an alcohol-based hand rub (see Chapter 10). *Hand hygiene reduces the transmission of microorganisms.*
- Don gloves. *Gloves provide a physical barrier between the nurse's hands and body fluids.*
- Stop the infusion of the tube-feeding formula. *This measure facilitates assessment.*
- Aspirate fluid from the feeding tube using a 50-mL syringe. *Doing so allows for the collection of a large volume of fluid.*
- Continue aspirating until no more fluid is obtained. *This ensures an accurate assessment.*
- Measure the aspirated fluid and record the amount. *Documentation provides objective data for evaluation.*
- Reinstill the aspirated fluid. *This measure returns partially digested nutrients and electrolytes to the client.*
- Postpone tube feeding and report residual amounts that exceed agency guidelines or those established by the physician. *Doing so reduces the risk of aspiration.*
- Check gastric residual again in 30 minutes. *This duration allows time for part of the stomach contents to empty into the small intestine.*
- Provide or resume tube feeding if the gastric residual is within an acceptable range. *Doing so prevents overfeeding.*
- Flush a feeding tube with 30 mL of water with a large-volume syringe before and after an intermittent feeding or administration of medication, any interruption of feeding, and every 4 hours during a continuous feeding. *Clients require additional water for hydration and to prevent obstructions within the feeding tube.*
- Document the volume of flushes separately from the volume of formula. *Intake and output records facilitate monitoring clients for fluid volume excess or deficit.*

NURSING GUIDELINES 29-4

Clearing an Obstructed Feeding Tube

- Select a syringe with a 30- to 60-mL capacity. *This capacity reduces negative pressure during aspiration, which could lead to the collapse of the tube walls.*
- Wash hands or use an alcohol-based hand rub (see Chapter 10). *Hand hygiene reduces the transmission of microorganisms.*
- Don gloves. *They provide a physical barrier between the nurse's hands and potential contact with body fluids.*
- Aspirate as much as possible from the feeding tube. *Aspiration clears the path above the obstructing debris.*
- Instill 5 to 15 mL of the selected solution. *Instillation allows for direct contact between the irrigating solution and debris.*
- Clamp the tube and wait 15 minutes. *This duration gives the substance in the solution time to physically affect the obstructing debris.*
- Aspirate and flush the tube with water. *Repeat if necessary. Use of negative pressure or positive pressure restores patency.*
- Consult the physician if unable to clear the obstruction with instilled water. *Chemical and mechanical measures are alternative options for removing an obstruction in a tube.*

obstructions. One is a product called Bionix Feeding Tube Declogger, which is a stem with a "screw-and-thread design" that, when inserted, bends and conforms to the shape of the tube freeing the obstruction (Bionex, 2022). And similarly, the TubeClear system provides a stem with a wire encased within a sheath. A power source creates a jackhammer-like motion at the wire tip inside the obstructed tube (unclogging, 2019). When an obstruction cannot be cleared, the tube is removed and another is inserted rather than compromising nutrition by the delay.

Providing Adequate Hydration

Although tube feedings are approximately 80% water, clients usually require additional hydration. Adults require 30 mL of water per kilogram of body weight, or 1 mL/kcal, on a daily basis (Dudek, 2021).

To determine whether a client's hydration needs are being met, the nurse identifies the amount of water on the label of commercial formula. The nurse can then add this amount to the total volume of flush solution and compare it with the recommended amount. If there is a significant deficit, the nurse revises the plan of care to increase either the volume or, preferably, the frequency of flushing the tube. If the fluid volume is excessive, the nurse monitors the client's urine output and lung sounds to determine whether the client can excrete comparable amounts (see Chapter 16).

Handling Miscellaneous Problems

Clients who require enteral feeding experience several common or potential problems. Many are associated with tube-feeding formulas or the mechanical effects of the tubes themselves (Table 29-5). Nurses must report problems promptly and make necessary adjustments to the plan of care.

and instilling crushed or hydrophilic (water-absorbing) medications into the tube. To maintain patency, it is best to flush feeding tubes with 30 to 60 mL of water immediately before and after administering a feeding or medications, after any interruption in a feeding, every 4 hours if the client is being continuously fed, and after refeeding the gastric residual. Exceptions for varying the volume of flush solution would be for clients on fluid restrictions such as those with renal or heart failure.

Clearing an Obstruction

If an obstruction occurs, the nurse consults the physician. Occasionally, it is possible to clear the tube with a solution of warm water in a 30- to 60-mL syringe using a back-and-forth motion, withdrawing the instilled fluid, and repeating the process if necessary (Nursing Guidelines 29-4). Another option, if unclogging with water is unsuccessful, is instilling fluid-activated pancreatic enzyme combined with 1/8 tsp of sodium bicarbonate followed by letting it dwell for 30 minutes before attempting to flush the tube again (unclogging, 2019). The latter method requires a written medical order. There are other possible mechanical means for clearing

TABLE 29-5 Common Tube-Feeding Problems

PROBLEM	COMMON CAUSES	SOLUTIONS
Diarrhea	Highly concentrated formula Rapid administration Bacterial contamination Lactose intolerance Inadequate protein content Medication side effects	Dilute initial tube feeding to one-quarter to one-half strength. Start at 25 mL/hour and increase rate by 25 mL q12h. Hang no more than 4 hours' worth of formula. Wash hands. Change formula bag and tubing q24h. Refrigerate unused formula. Consult with the physician on using a milk-free formula. Raise serum albumin levels with total parenteral nutrition solutions containing supplemental protein or administer albumin intravenously. Consult with the physician about adjusting drug therapy or administering an antidiarrheal.
Nausea and vomiting	Rapid feeding Overfeeding Air in stomach Medication side effects	Instill bolus and intermittent feedings by gravity. Delay feeding until gastric residual is <100 mL or <20% of hourly volume. Maintain sitting position for at least 30 minutes after feeding. Consult with the physician about ordering medication that facilitates gastric emptying. Administer continuous feedings. Instill feedings within the small intestine. Keep tubing filled with formula or water. Consult with the physician about adjusting drug therapy or administering drugs to control symptoms.
Aspiration	Incorrect tube placement Vomiting	Check placement before instilling liquids. Keep head elevated at least 30 degrees during feedings and for 30 minutes afterward. Keep cuffed tracheostomy and endotracheal tubes inflated. Refer to measures for controlling vomiting.
Constipation	Lack of fiber Dehydration	Change formula. Increase supplemental water. Consult with the physician on giving a laxative, enema, or suppository.
Elevated blood glucose level	Calorie-concentrated formula	Instill diluted formula and gradually increase concentration. Administer insulin according to medical orders.
Weight loss	Inadequate calories	Increase calories in formula. Increase rate or frequency of feedings.
Elevated electrolytes	Dehydration	Increase supplemental water.
Dry oral and nasal mucous membranes	Mouth breathing Dried nasal mucus	Provide frequent oral and nasal hygiene.
Middle ear inflammation	Narrowing or obstruction of eustachian tube from presence of tube in pharynx	Turn from side to side q2h. Insert a small-diameter feeding tube. Use a small-diameter feeding tube.
Sore throat	Pressure and irritation from tube	Use liquid medications.
Plugged feeding tube	Instilling crushed or powdered medications through the tube Formula coagulation from drug–food interactions Kinked tube Large molecules in formula	Dilute crushed drugs. Flush the tubing liberally after drug administration. Flush tubing with water before and after drug administration. Follow agency policy for alternative flush solutions. Maintain neck in neutral position or change position frequently. Dilute formula. Flush tubing at least q4h. Use a larger diameter feeding tube.
Dumping syndrome	Rapid and large instillation of highly concentrated formula into the intestine	Administer small, continuous volume. Adjust glucose content of formula.

 Pharmacologic Considerations

Although liquid medications are preferred for enteral administration, they can cause GI distress. Sorbitol, an inactive ingredient, is used as a sweetener for oral liquid medications. In large amounts, such as multiple medications administered via enteral tube, sorbitol acts as an osmotic laxative. Tablets crushed and mixed with water may reduce diarrhea if it occurs.

Preparing for Home Care

Because of shortened lengths of stay in hospitals, some clients who continue to need tube feedings are discharged for self-care or with a caregiver when home. Before demonstrating the procedure to those who will administer tube feedings, the nurse provides a written instruction sheet that includes:

- Places to obtain equipment and formula
- The amount and schedule for each feeding and flush using household measurements

- Guidelines for delaying a feeding
- Special instructions for skin, nose, or stomal care, including frequency and types of products to use
- Problems to report such as weight loss, reduced urination, weakness, diarrhea, nausea and vomiting, and breathing difficulties
- Names and phone numbers of people to call if questions arise
- Date, time, and place for continued medical follow-up

Depending on the client's or caretaker's self-confidence and competence in self-administering tube feedings, health care providers often make a referral to a home health agency for postdischarge nursing support.

INTESTINAL DECOMPRESSION

Most nasogastric, nasointestinal, and transabdominal tubes are used for enteral feeding or gastric decompression. Sometimes, however, clients require intestinal decompression, which is performed with a tungsten-weighted tube (see Table 29-1). Intestinal decompression sometimes makes it possible to avoid surgery.

Nasointestinal Decompression Tube Insertion

A nasointestinal decompression tube is inserted in the same manner as a nasogastric tube. The nurse then promotes and monitors its passage into the intestine. In the presence of peristalsis, the weight of the tungsten propels the tip of the tube beyond the stomach. Openings through the distal end provide channels through which the intestinal contents are suctioned. An intestinal decompression tube generally remains in place until the intestinal lumen is patent or until surgical treatment is instituted (Nursing Guidelines 29-5).

Removal of an Intestinal Decompression Tube

Once the intestinal decompression tube has served its purpose, the nurse begins the process of removing it. An intestinal decompression tube is removed slowly because removal is in a reverse direction through the curves of the intestine and the valves of the lower and upper ends of the stomach.

First, the tube is disconnected from the suction source. Next, the tape that secures the tube to the face is removed and the tube is withdrawn 6 to 10 in (15 to 25 cm) at 10-minute intervals. When the last 18 in (45 cm) remains, the tube is pulled gently from the nose. Afterward, nasal and oral hygiene measures are provided. The tube cannot be removed nasally if the distal end descends below the ileocecal valve between the small and large intestine. Instead, the proximal end is cut and the tube is gradually removed manually or by peristalsis when it descends through the anus.

NURSING IMPLICATIONS

Depending on data collected during client care, the nurse may identify one or more of the following nursing diagnoses:

- Malnutrition risk
- Feeding ADL deficit
- Aspiration risk
- Diarrhea
- Constipation

Nursing Care Plan 29-1 is a model for managing the care of a client with a large gastric residual with a nursing diagnosis of aspiration risk, defined as, "breathing in a foreign object such as foods or liquids into the trachea and lungs [that] happens when protective reflexes are reduced or jeopardized" (Nurseslabs, 2022).

NURSING GUIDELINES 29-5

Inserting an Intestinal Decompression Tube

- Assemble all the necessary equipment as for any nasally inserted tube. *Doing so ensures organization and efficient time management.*
- Follow the techniques in Skill 29-1 for inserting a nasogastric tube. *The same principles are involved during the initial insertion.*
- Ambulate the client, if possible. *Ambulation helps the tube move through the pyloric valve into the small intestine.*
- When the radiograph indicates that the intestinal tube has advanced beyond the stomach, position the client on the right side for 2 hours, then on the back in a Fowler position for 2 hours, then on the left side for 2 hours. *Gravity and positioning promote movement through intestinal curves.*
- Follow agency policy or physician's instructions for manually advancing the tube several inches each hour. *This advancement supplements the natural peristaltic advancement.*
- Observe the graduated marks on the tube. *The marks provide a means for monitoring the tube's progression and approximate anatomic location.*
- Request an X-ray confirmation when the tube has reached the prescribed distance. *An X-ray provides objective evidence of the terminal location of the distal tip.*

- Secure the tube to the nose once its distal location has been confirmed. *This stabilizes the tube and prevents further migration.* (See figure.)
- Coil the excess tubing and attach it to the client's pajamas or gown. *Coiling and attachment prevent accidental extubation.*
- Connect the proximal end to a wall or a portable suction source. *Produces negative pressure to pull substances from the intestine.*

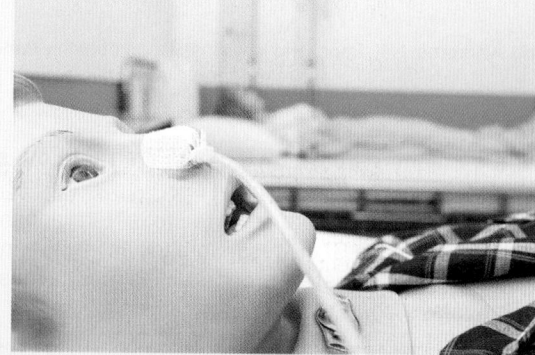

Secure the tube to the client's nose.
(Bangkoker/Shutterstock.)

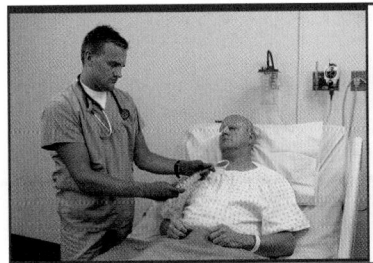

Clinical Scenario A 56-year-old male with metastatic cancer has been admitted while undergoing chemotherapy. He has been receiving bolus tube feedings due to side effects of his cancer treatment. Currently he has become nauseous and reports abdominal discomfort and the feeling that vomiting is imminent. Before administering the next bolus feeding, the nurse checks the client's gastric residual volume because overfeeding could lead to aspiration. The nurse obtains a gastric residual volume of 550 mL.

NURSING CARE PLAN 29-1 | Aspiration Risk

Assessment

- Measure the gastric residual before each bolus feeding and whenever the client develops gastric symptoms.
- Auscultate bowel sounds.
- Palpate the abdomen and measure abdominal girth for evidence of distention.

- Ask an alert client about feeling full, nauseous, or vomiting.
- Check if any medical orders restrict the positioning of a client in a Fowler position.

Nursing Diagnosis. Aspiration risk related to slow gastric emptying as manifested by the measurement of the gastric residual of 550 mL from a 16 F nasogastric tube and the development of feeling nauseous, bloated, and potential for vomiting 2 hours before a scheduled bolus feeding of 400 mL.

Expected Outcome. The client's risk for aspiration will be reduced as evidenced by a gastric residual of less than 500 mL within 30 minutes of a scheduled feeding.

Interventions	Rationales
Maintain head elevation at no less than 30 degrees at all times.	Elevating the upper body promotes the deposition of the tube-feeding formula within the stomach and movement toward the small intestine.
Monitor bowel sounds; report if absent or fewer than five per minute.	Active bowel sounds suggest that peristalsis is sufficient to facilitate gastric emptying and intestinal absorption and the elimination of liquid nourishment.
Measure the length of the tube as it exits the naris.	Checking the proximal length of a feeding tube provides evidence that the end of the tube has not migrated from its insertion location.
Measure gastric residual before all tube feedings.	This standard of care helps determine the client's response to liquid nourishment via a gastric tube.
Refeed gastric residual and follow with a 15- to 30-mL tap water flush for a total of no more than 500 mL.	Gastric residual contains partially digested nutrients that should not be discarded; flushing the tube following refeeding helps prevent obstruction within the tube and provides additional water intake.
Postpone tube feeding for 30 minutes if the gastric residual measures 500 mL.	Distention of the stomach with additional formula predisposes the client to regurgitation and the potential for aspiration.
Report the gastric residual volume to the physician if it remains above the maximum volume after delaying feeding for 30 minutes.	Sharing the assessment findings with the physician facilitates collaboration in modifying the plan of care by changing the type, volume, or frequency of the tube feeding or administering a medication that promotes gastric emptying.
Keep the client in a high Fowler position.	A Fowler position promotes forward movement of gastric contents toward the small intestine.
Maintain a suction machine at the bedside.	Having equipment for performing oral–pharyngeal suctioning ensures a rapid response for clearing the upper gastrointestinal tract and airway following episodes in which the client vomits.

Evaluation of Expected Outcome

- Gastric residual measures less than 500 mL.
- Bowel sounds are present and active in all quadrants.
- Head is elevated 30 degrees.
- Tube feeding has resumed on schedule.

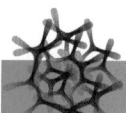

KEY POINTS

- Gastrointestinal intubation: The placement of a tube into the stomach or intestine by way of the mouth or nose
- Reasons for gastrointestinal intubation
  - Reducing or eliminating problems associated with surgery or conditions affecting the GI tract, such as impaired peristalsis, vomiting, or gas accumulation
  - Nourishing clients who cannot eat
  - Administering oral medications that the client cannot swallow
  - Obtaining a sample of secretions for diagnostic testing
  - Performing a lavage (removing substances from the stomach, typically poisons)
  - Promoting decompression (removing gas and liquid contents from the stomach or bowel)
  - Controlling gastric bleeding, a process called compression or tamponade (pressure)
- Types of tubes
  - Orogastric tube: A tube inserted through the mouth into the stomach
  - Nasogastric tube: A tube placed through the nose and advanced to the stomach
  - Nasointestinal tubes: Tubes inserted through the nose for distal placement below the stomach
    - Tubes used for nutrition
    - Intestinal decompression: The removal of gas and intestinal contents
  - Transabdominal tubes: Tubes placed through the abdominal wall
- Client preparation and preintubation assessment
  - Level of consciousness
  - Weight
  - Bowel sounds
  - Abdominal distention
  - Integrity of nasal and oral mucosa
  - Ability to swallow, cough, and gag
  - Any nausea and vomiting
- The only evidence-based methods for determining the distal location of a nasogastric tube include obtaining an abdominal X-ray after its initial insertion and monitoring the external tube length.
- Gastric decompression: Suction is either continuous or intermittent.
- Removal of nasogastric tube: Before permanent removal, some physicians prescribe a trial period during which the tube is clamped and the client is allowed to consume oral fluids.
- Four schedules for administering tube feedings
  - Bolus: The instillation of liquid nourishment in less than 30 minutes four to six times a day
  - Intermittent: The gradual instillation of liquid nourishment four to six times a day administered over 30 to 60 minutes, the time most people spend eating a meal
  - Cyclic: The continuous instillation of liquid nourishment for 8 to 12 hours
  - Continuous: The instillation of liquid nutrition without interruption
- Client assessment for tube feedings
  - Checking the gastric residual
  - Flushing a feeding tube with 30 mL of water with a large-volume syringe before and after an intermittent feeding or administration of medication
- Common tube-feeding problems
  - Diarrhea
  - Nausea and vomiting
  - Aspiration
  - Constipation
  - Elevated blood glucose levels
  - Weight loss
  - Elevated electrolytes
  - Dumping syndrome
  - Plugged feeding tube
- Nasointestinal decompression tube: The weight of the tungsten propels the tip of the tube beyond the stomach. Openings through the distal end provide channels through which the intestinal contents are suctioned. An intestinal decompression tube generally remains in place until the intestinal lumen is patent or until surgical treatment is instituted.

CRITICAL THINKING EXERCISES

1. What nutritional suggestions could a nurse make for a client who has a chronic disease that impairs the ability to swallow food?
2. When a client experiences persistent gagging during attempts to insert a nasogastric tube, what actions can the nurse take?
3. Describe the similarities and differences between inserting a tube for gastric decompression and one for intestinal decompression.
4. What questions would be important to ask if a client receiving tube feedings at home calls to report the onset of diarrhea?

NEXT-GENERATION NCLEX-STYLE REVIEW QUESTIONS

1. Place an X on the image where the nurse determines the distal measurement on a nasogastric tube prior to its insertion.

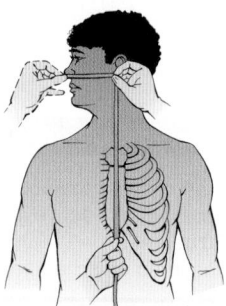

Test-Taking Strategy: Recall the components of the sternum and their locations.

2. When a practical nurse assists with the insertion of a single-lumen nasogastric tube, what instruction is correct when the tube is in the client's oropharynx?
   a. Breathe deeply as the tube is advanced.
   b. Hold your head in a sniffing position.
   c. Press your chin to your upper chest.
   d. Avoid coughing until the tube is down.
   Test-Taking Strategy: Use the process of elimination to select the option that is better than any of the others for facilitating the insertion of a nasogastric tube.

3. What is the most definitive technique for determining whether the distal end of a tube for gastric decompression is in the stomach?
   a. Obtaining an abdominal X-ray
   b. Checking the pH of aspirated fluid
   c. Instilling 100 mL of tap water into the tube
   d. Feeling for air at the tube's proximal end
   Test-Taking Strategy: Note the key term and modifier, "most definitive." Select the option that provides the most valid evidence that the nasogastric tube is in the stomach.

4. Immediately after insertion of a transabdominal G-tube, which finding should the nurse consider normal when assessing the gastrostomy site?
   a. Milky-appearing drainage
   b. Serosanguineous drainage
   c. Green-tinged drainage
   d. Bright bloody drainage
   Test-Taking Strategy: Note the key words, "immediately" and "normal." Analyze the choices and select the option that the nurse should consider an appropriate appearance to drainage around a newly inserted G-tube.

5. When a client with a nasogastric tube for gastric decompression indicates they are very thirsty, which nursing intervention is most appropriate to add to the plan of care?
   a. Offer fluids at least every 2 hours.
   b. Provide crushed ice in sparse amounts.
   c. Increase oral liquids on the dietary tray.
   d. Refill the water carafe twice each shift.
   Test-Taking Strategy: Note the key word and modifier, "most appropriate." Use the process of elimination to select the option that is better than any of the others.

NEXT-GENERATION NCLEX-STYLE CLINICAL SCENARIO QUESTIONS

Clinical Scenario:
A 56-year-old male with metastatic cancer has been admitted while undergoing chemotherapy. He has been receiving bolus tube feedings due to side effects of his cancer treatment. Currently he has become nauseous and reports abdominal discomfort and the feeling that vomiting is imminent. Before administering the next bolus feeding, the nurse checks the client's gastric residual volume because overfeeding could lead to aspiration. The nurse obtains a gastric residual volume of 550 mL.

1. Select all of the indicators that may suggest a cause for concern regarding a risk for aspiration.
   a. Chemotherapy
   b. Pressure sores
   c. Nauseousness
   d. Bolus tube feedings
   e. Gastric residual >250 mL
   f. Gastric residual <80 mL
   g. Viscosity of tube feedings

2. Place an "x" under "effective" identifying actions that would help prevent aspiration. Place an "x" under "ineffective" identifying actions that may contribute to aspiration.

ACTIONS	EFFECTIVE	INEFFECTIVE
Maintain head elevation >30 degrees during feedings		
Measure gastric residual before feedings		
Flush the tube feeding with 100 mL of tap water		
Keep client in high Fowler's position during feedings		
Client lies flat during tube feedings		
Residual amount not measured before tube feeding		

SKILL 29-1 Inserting a Nasogastric Tube

Suggested Action	Reason for Action
ASSESSMENT	
Check that a medical order has been written.	Ensures that care is within the legal scope of practice
Determine the reason for the nasogastric tube.	Facilitates the evaluation of outcomes
Identify the client.	Ensures that the procedure will be performed on the correct client
Assess how much the client understands about the procedure.	Indicates the need for and the level of health teaching
Inspect the nose after the client blows into a paper tissue (Fig. A).	Provides data that will determine which naris to use

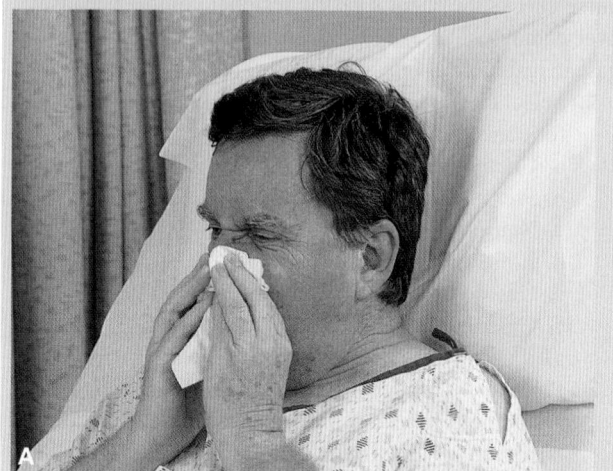

Clearing the nose. (Photo by B. Proud.)

Suggested Action	Reason for Action
Unwrap and uncoil the tube.	Straightens the tube and releases bends from product packaging
Obtain the NEX measurements (Fig. B).	Determines length for insertion

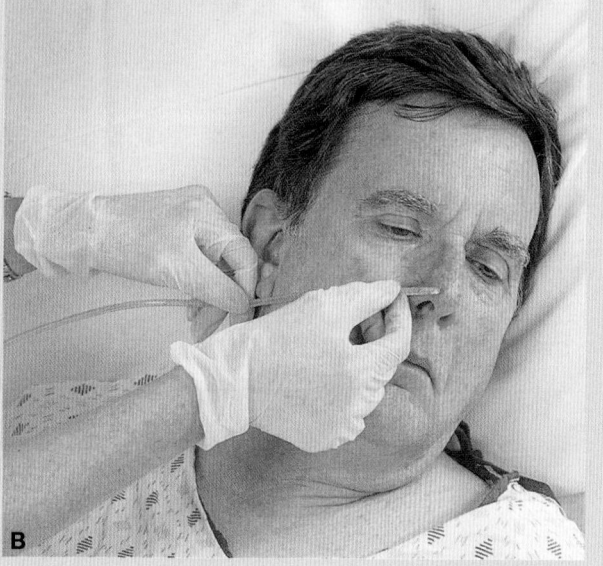

Obtaining the NEX measurement. (Photo by B. Proud.)

SKILL 29-1 Inserting a Nasogastric Tube (*continued*)

Suggested Action	Reason for Action
Mark the tube at the NE (nose-to-ear) and EX (ear-to-xiphoid) measurements (Fig. C).	Provides a guide during insertion

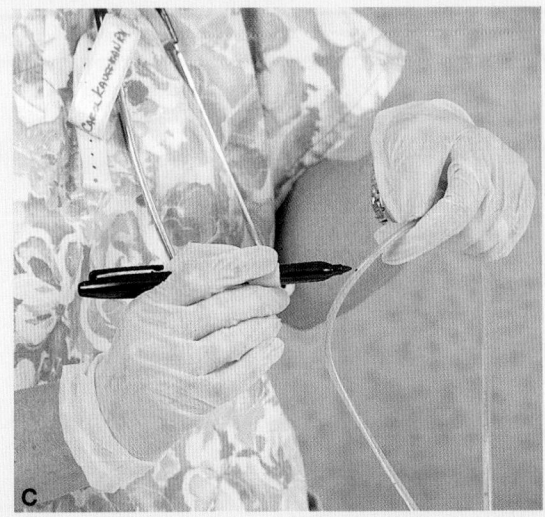

Marking the tube. (Photo by B. Proud.)

PLANNING

If a plastic tube feels rigid, place it in or flush it with warm water.	Promotes flexibility
Assemble the following equipment in addition to the tube: water, straw, towel, lubricant, tissues, tape, emesis basin, flashlight, stethoscope, clean gloves, and 50-mL syringe.	Contributes to organization and efficient time management
Place a suction machine at the bedside if the client is unresponsive or has difficulty swallowing.	Provides a method for clearing the client's airway of vomitus
Remove dentures.	Avoids choking should they become loose or displaced
Establish a hand signal for pausing.	Relieves anxiety by providing the client with some locus for control

IMPLEMENTATION

Wash your hands or use an alcohol-based hand rub (see Chapter 10).	Reduces the transmission of microorganisms
Pull the privacy curtain.	Demonstrates respect for the client's dignity
Assist the client to sit in semi-Fowler or high Fowler position and hyperextend the neck as if in a sniffing position.	Ensures the visualization of the nasal passageway to facilitate inserting the tube
Protect the client, bed clothing, and linen with a towel.	Avoids linen changes
Put on gloves.	Reduces the transmission of microorganisms
Lubricate the tube with water-soluble gel over 6–8 in (15–20 cm) at the distal tip.	Reduces friction and tissue trauma
Insert the tube into the nostril while pointing the tip backward and downward (Fig. D).	Follows the normal contour of the nasal passage

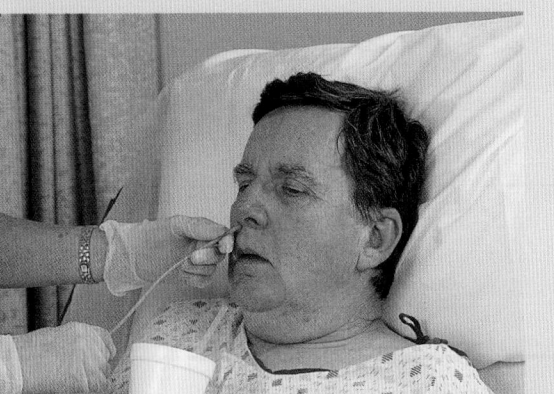

Preparing to insert the tube. (Photo by B. Proud.)

Do not force the tube. Relubricate or rotate it if there is resistance.	Prevents trauma

(*continued*)

SKILL 29-1 Inserting a Nasogastric Tube (*continued*)

Suggested Action	Reason for Action
Stop when the first mark on the tube is at the tip of the nose.	Places the tip above the area where the gag reflex may be stimulated
Use a flashlight to inspect the back of the throat.	Confirms that the tube has been maneuvered around the nasal curve
Instruct the client to lower their chin to the chest and swallow sips of water.	Narrows the trachea and opens the esophagus; helps advance the tube
Advance the tube 3–5 in (7.5–12.5 cm) each time the client swallows.	Coordinates insertion; reduces the potential for gagging or vomiting
Pause if the client gives the preestablished signal.	Demonstrates respect and cooperation
Discontinue the procedure and raise the tube to the first mark if there are signs of distress such as gasping, coughing, a bluish skin color, or the inability to speak or hum.	Indicates that the tube is possibly in the airway
Assess placement according to agency policy when the second mark is reached.	Provides data on distal placement
Withdraw the tube to the first mark and reattempt insertion if the assessment findings are inconclusive or consult with the physician about obtaining an X-ray.	Ensures safety
Proceed to secure the tube if the data indicate the tube is in the stomach (Fig. E).	Prevents tube migration

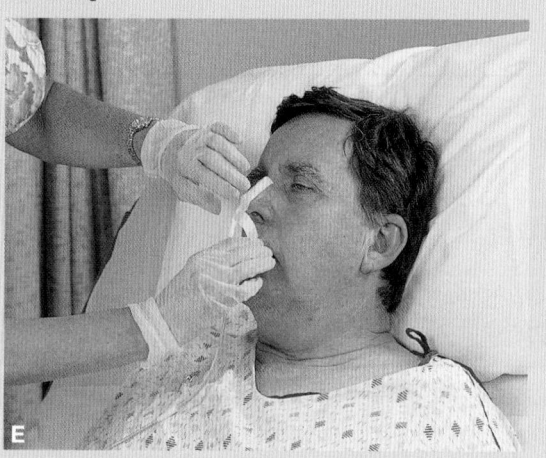

Securing the tube. (Photo by B. Proud.)

Suggested Action	Reason for Action
Connect the tube to suction or clamp it while awaiting further orders.	Promotes gastric decompression or potential use
Remove gloves and wash your hands or use an alcohol-based hand rub.	Reduces the transmission of microorganisms
Position the client with a minimum head elevation of 30 degrees.	Prevents gastric reflux
Remove equipment from the bedside.	Restores orderliness and supports the principles of medical asepsis
Measure and record the volume of drainage at least every 8 hours.	Provides data for evaluating fluid balance

EVALUATION ──────────────────────────────

- Distal placement within the stomach is confirmed.
- Client exhibits no evidence of respiratory distress.
- Client can speak or hum.
- Lung sounds are present and clear bilaterally.
- No bleeding or pain is noted in the area of nasal mucosa.

DOCUMENT ──────────────────────────────

- Type of tube
- Outcomes of the procedure
- Method for determining placement and outcome of assessment
- Description of drainage
- Type and amount of suction if the tube is used for decompression

SAMPLE DOCUMENTATION

Date and Time A 16 F nasogastric tube inserted without difficulty. No respiratory distress. Can talk and hum following insertion. Placement verified by radiograph evaluation. Salem sump tube secured to nose and connected to low, intermittent wall suction. Positioned with the head of bed elevated 30 degrees. _____ J. Doe, LPN

SKILL 29-2 Irrigating a Nasogastric Tube

Suggested Action	Reason for Action
ASSESSMENT	
Monitor the client's symptoms, the volume and rate of drainage, and evidence of abdominal distention.	Provides data for future comparisons
Check that a medical order has been written if that is the agency's policy.	Complies with the legal scope of the nursing practice
Identify the client.	Ensures that the procedure will be performed on the correct client
Assess how much the client understands about the procedure.	Provides an opportunity for client teaching
PLANNING	
Assemble the following equipment: Asepto or irrigating syringe, irrigating fluid (isotonic saline solution), container, clean towel or pad, clean gloves, and cover or plug for end of tube.	Contributes to organization and efficient time management
Turn off the suction.	Facilitates implementation
IMPLEMENTATION	
Pull the privacy curtain.	Demonstrates respect for the client's dignity
Wash your hands or use an alcohol-based hand rub (see Chapter 10).	Reduces the transmission of microorganisms
Place a clean pad or towel beneath where the tube will be separated.	Avoids changing bed linens and protects the client from soiling
Put on clean gloves.	Complies with standard precautions
Disconnect the nasogastric tube from the suction tubing and apply cover or insert plug into suction tubing.	Keeps the connection area clean
Confirm that the external tube length has not changed.	Ensures safety
Fill irrigating syringe with 30–60 mL of normal saline solution.	Provides an adequate quantity of isotonic solution to clear tubing
Insert the tip of the syringe within the proximal end of the tube and allow the solution to flow in by gravity or apply gentle pressure (Fig. A).	Dilutes and mobilizes debris

Instilling the irrigation solution. (Photo by B. Proud.)

A

Aspirate after the fluid has been instilled.	Removes substances that may impair future drainage
Reconnect the tube to the source of suction.	Resumes therapeutic management
Observe the characteristics of the aspirated solution; measure and discard.	Provides data for evaluating the effectiveness of the procedure

(continued)

SKILL 29-2 Irrigating a Nasogastric Tube (*continued*)

Suggested Action	Reason for Action
Monitor for the flow of drainage through the suction tubing (Fig. B).	Provides evidence that patency is being maintained
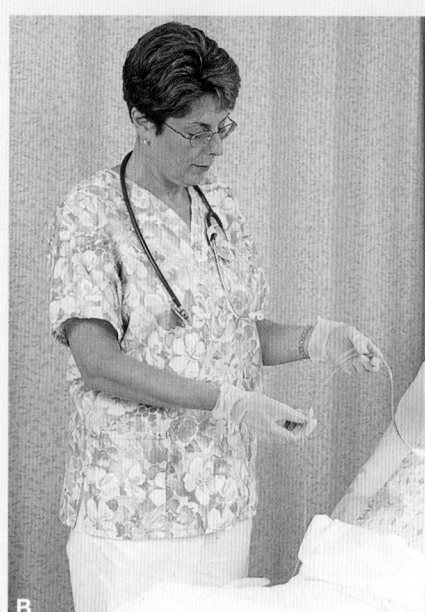	Monitoring drainage. (Photo by B. Proud.)
Remove gloves and perform hand hygiene.	Reduces the transmission of microorganisms
Record the volume of instilled and drained fluid on the bedside intake and output sheet.	Provides accurate data for determining fluid balance

EVALUATION

- Drainage is restored.
- Nausea and vomiting are relieved.
- Abdominal distention is reduced.

DOCUMENT

- Volume and type of fluid instilled
- Appearance and volume of returned drainage
- Response of client

SAMPLE DOCUMENTATION

Date and Time Nasogastric tube irrigated with 60 mL of normal saline. Solution instilled with slight pressure. 100 mL of solution returned with several large mucus particles. Reconnected to low, intermittent suction. Gastric tube draining well at the present time. Abdomen is soft. No vomiting. _____ J. Doe, LPN

SKILL 29-3 Removing a Nasogastric Tube

Suggested Action	Reason for Action
ASSESSMENT	
Assess bowel sounds, the condition of the mouth and nasal mucosa, the level of consciousness, and gag reflex.	Provides data for future comparisons and may affect how the procedure is performed
Check that a medical order has been written.	Complies with the legal scope of nursing practice
Identify the client.	Ensures that the procedure will be performed on the correct client
Assess how much the client understands the procedure.	Provides an opportunity for client teaching
PLANNING	
Assemble the following equipment: towel, emesis basin, cotton-tipped applicator sticks, oral hygiene equipment, and clean gloves.	Contributes to organization and efficient time management
IMPLEMENTATION	
Pull the privacy curtain.	Demonstrates respect for dignity
Wash your hands or use an alcohol-based hand rub (see Chapter 10).	Reduces the transmission of microorganisms
Place the client in a sitting position if alert or in a lateral position if not.	Prevents aspiration of stomach contents
Cover the chest with a clean towel and place the emesis basin and tissues within easy reach.	Prepares for possible vomiting and protects the client from soiling
Remove the tape securing the tube to the client's nose.	Facilitates pulling the tube from the stomach
Put on clean gloves.	Complies with standard precautions
Turn off the suction and separate the tube.	Prepares for removal
Instill a bolus of air into the lumen that drains gastric secretions.	Prevents residual fluid from leaking as the tube is withdrawn
Clamp, plug, or pinch the tube (Fig. A).	Prevents fluid from leaking as the tube is withdrawn

A

Occluding the tube. (Photo by B. Proud.)

Instruct the client to take a deep breath and hold it just before removing the nasogastric tube.	Reduces the risk for aspirating gastric fluid
Remove the tube from the client's nose gently and slowly.	Lessens the potential for trauma
Enclose the tube within the towel or glove and discard the tube in a covered container (Fig. B).	Provides a transmission barrier against microorganisms

B

Enclosing the tube. (Photo by B. Proud.)

(continued)

SKILL 29-3 Removing a Nasogastric Tube (*continued*)

Suggested Action	Reason for Action
Empty, measure, and record the drainage in the suction container.	Provides data for evaluating the client's fluid status
Remove gloves and perform hand hygiene.	Reduces the transmission of microorganisms
Offer an opportunity for oral hygiene.	Removes disagreeable tastes from the client's mouth
Encourage the client to clear the nose of mucus and debris with paper tissues or cotton-tipped applicators.	Promotes the integrity of nasal tissue
Discard disposable equipment; rinse and return portable suction equipment.	Preserves cleanliness and orderliness in the client's unit; demonstrates accountability for equipment

EVALUATION

- The tube is removed.
- The client resumes eating and drinking fluids.
- The client experiences no nausea or vomiting.
- The airway remains clear.
- The nasal mucosa is moist and intact.

DOCUMENT

- Type of tube removed
- Response of client
- Appearance and volume of drainage
- Appearance of nose and nasopharynx

SAMPLE DOCUMENTATION

Date and Time   Nasogastric tube removed. Brief period of retching during removal. Total of 75 mL clear green drainage emptied from suction container. Oral care provided. L naris swabbed with applicator lubricated with petroleum jelly. Mucosa is red but intact. _____ J. Doe, LPN

SKILL 29-4 Administering Tube Feedings

Suggested Action	Reason for Action
Bolus Feeding	
ASSESSMENT	
Check the medical order for the type of nourishment, volume, and schedule to follow.	Complies with the legal scope of nursing practice
Check the date and identifying information on the container of tube-feeding formula.	Ensures accurate administration and avoids using outdated formula
Wash your hands or use an alcohol-based hand rub (see Chapter 10).	Reduces the transmission of microorganisms
Identify the client.	Ensures that the procedure will be performed on the correct client
Distinguish the tubing for gastric or intestinal feeding from the tubing to instill intravenous solutions.	Prevents administering nutritional formula into the vascular system
Assess bowel sounds.	Provides data indicating the safety for instilling liquids through the tube
Validate that the external length of the feeding tube has not migrated internally upward or downward.	Supports that the feeding tube remains in the desired anatomic location

SKILL 29-4 Administering Tube Feedings (*continued*)

Suggested Action	Reason for Action
Measure gastric residual if a 12 F or larger tube is in place (Fig. A).	Determines if the stomach has the capacity to manage the next instillation of formula; aspiration of fluid may be impossible with small-lumen tubes

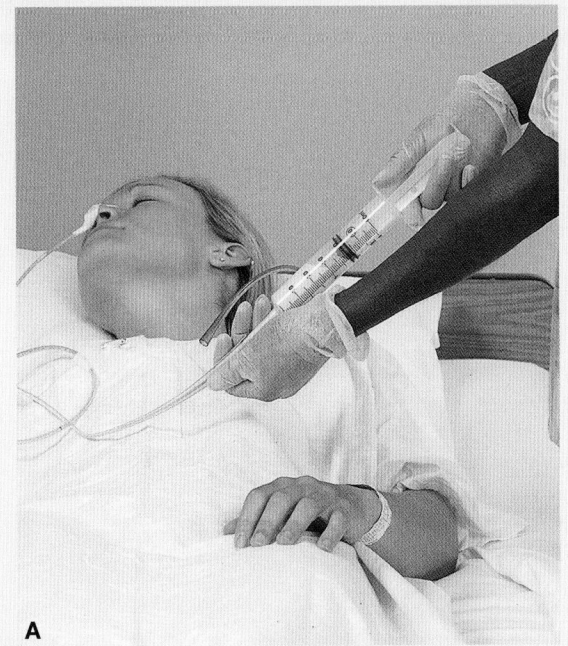

Measuring gastric residual. (Photo by B. Proud.)

A

Suggested Action	Reason for Action
Flush the feeding tube with 30 mL of water.	Prevents an obstruction of the tube
Measure capillary blood glucose or glucose in the urine.	Provides data indicating response to caloric intake
Assess how much the client understands the procedure.	Provides an opportunity for client teaching

PLANNING

Replace any unused formula and feeding bag every 24 hours.	Reduces the potential for bacterial growth
Wait and recheck gastric residual in 30 minutes if it exceeds 500 mL.	Avoids overfilling the stomach
Assemble the following equipment: Asepto syringe, formula, tap water.	Contributes to organization and efficient time management
Warm refrigerated nourishment to room temperature in a basin of warm water.	Prevents chilling and abdominal cramping

IMPLEMENTATION

Perform hand hygiene.	Reduces the transmission of microorganisms
Place the client in a 30- to 90-degree sitting position.	Prevents regurgitation and aspiration
Reinstill gastric residual by gravity flow if volume is less than 500 mL.	Returns predigested nutrients without excessive pressure
Pinch the tube just before all the residual has instilled (Fig. B).	Prevents air from entering the tube

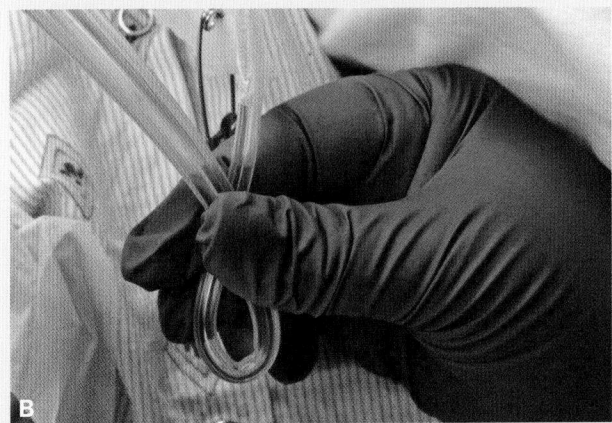

Pinch the tubing before it becomes empty.

B

(*continued*)

SKILL 29-4 Administering Tube Feedings (*continued*)

Suggested Action	Reason for Action
Add fresh formula to the syringe and adjust the height to allow a slow but gradual instillation (Fig. C).	Provides nourishment
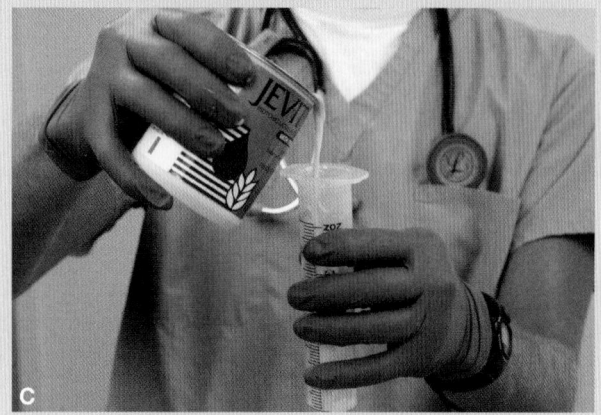	Administering a bolus feeding.
Continue filling the syringe for a bolus feeding before it becomes empty.	Prevents air from entering the tube
If a gastrostomy tube is being used, tilt the barrel of the syringe during the feeding (Fig. D).	Permits air displacement from the stomach
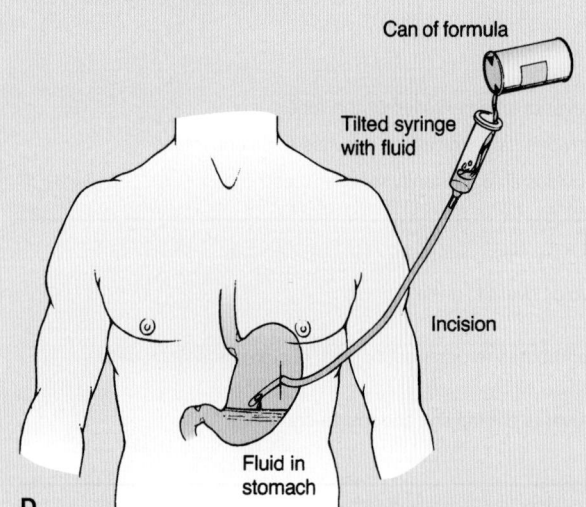	Bolus feeding through a gastrostomy tube (G-tube).
Flush the tubing with at least 30–60 mL of water after each feeding or follow the agency's policy for suggested amounts (Fig. E).	Ensures all nourishment has entered the stomach; prevents fermentation and coagulation of formula in the tube; provides water for fluid balance
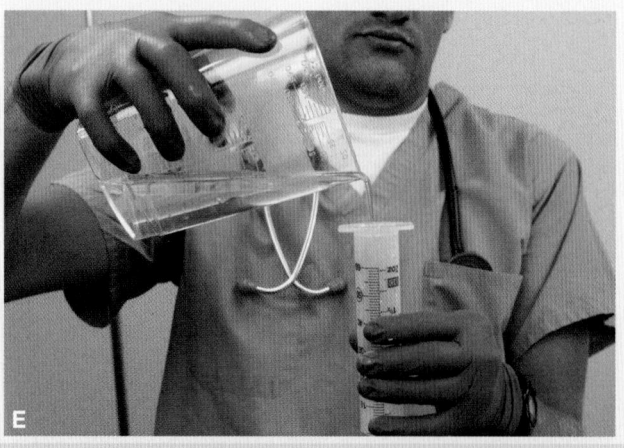	Instilling water to flush the tubing.
Plug or clamp the tube as the water leaves the syringe.	Prevents air from entering the tubing; maintains patency

Figure D labels: Can of formula; Tilted syringe with fluid; Incision; Fluid in stomach

SKILL 29-4 Administering Tube Feedings (*continued*)

Suggested Action	Reason for Action
Keep the head of the bed elevated for at least 30–60 minutes after a feeding.	Prevents gastric reflux
Wash and dry the feeding equipment. Return items to the bedside.	Supports principles of medical asepsis
Record the volume of formula and water administered on the bedside intake and output record.	Provides accurate data for assessing fluid balance and caloric value of nourishment
Provide oral hygiene at least twice daily.	Removes microorganisms and promotes comfort and hygiene of the client

Intermittent Feeding

ASSESSMENT

Follow the previous sequence for assessment.	Principles remain the same

PLANNING

In addition to those activities listed for bolus feeding, replace unused formula, feeding containers, and tubing every 24 hours.	Reduces the potential for bacterial growth

IMPLEMENTATION

Fill the feeding container with room-temperature formula (Fig. F).	Prevents administration of cold formula, which can cause cramping; room-temperature formula will be instilled before supporting bacterial growth

F

Filling a formula infusion bag. (From LifeART copyright 2016. Lippincott Williams & Wilkins. All rights reserved.)

Gradually open the clamp on the tubing.	Purges air from the tube
Connect the tubing to the nasogastric or nasoenteral tube.	Provides access to formula
Open the clamp and regulate the drip rate according to the physician's order or the agency's policy.	Supports safe administration of liquid nourishment
Check at 10-minute intervals (Fig. G).	Ensures early identification of infusion problems

G

Checking the rate of flow.

(continued)

SKILL 29-4 Administering Tube Feedings (*continued*)

Suggested Action	Reason for Action
Flush the tubing with water after the formula has infused (Fig. H).	Clears the tubing of formula, prevents obstruction, and provides water for fluid balance

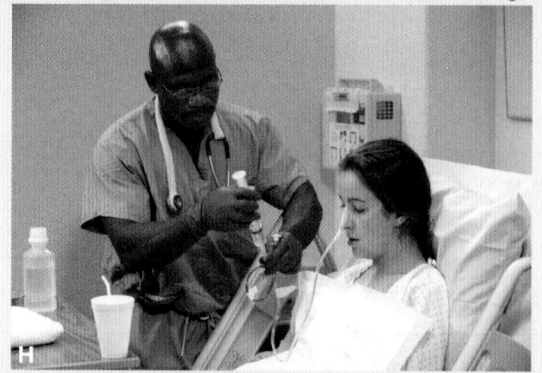

Flushing the tubing following feeding.

Suggested Action	Reason for Action
Pinch the feeding tube just as the last volume of water is administered.	Prevents air from entering the tube
Clamp or plug the feeding tube.	Prevents leaking
Record the volume of formula and water instilled.	Provides accurate data for assessing fluid balance and caloric value of nourishment
Follow recommendations for postprocedural care as described with a bolus feeding.	Principles for care remain the same

Continuous Feeding

ASSESSMENT ――――――――――――――――――――――――――――

In addition to previously described assessments, check the gastric residual every 4–6 hours or according to agency policy.	Principles remain the same; ensures a routine pattern for assessment to accommodate the schedule of continuous feedings and prevents inadvertent overfeeding

PLANNING ―――――――――――――――――――――――――――――――

In addition to previously described planning activities, obtain equipment for regulating continuous infusion (e.g., tube-feeding pump).	Aids in an accurate administration and sounds an alarm if the infusion is interrupted
Replace unused formula, feeding containers, and tubing every 24 hours.	Reduces the potential for bacterial growth
Label the date and attach a time tape on the feeding container.	Facilitates periodic assessment

IMPLEMENTATION ――――――――――――――――――――――――――――

Flush the new feeding container with water.	Reduces surface tension within the tube and enhances the passage of large protein molecules
A feeding container filled with refrigerated formula may hang for no more than 4 hours. Commercially prepared, sterilized containers of formula or a formula that is kept iced while infusing may hang for longer periods.	Prevents growth of bacteria; body heat will warm cold formula when infused at a slow rate
Purge the tubing of air.	Prevents distention of the stomach or intestine
Thread the tubing within the feeding pump according to the manufacturer's directions (Fig. I).	Ensures the correct mechanical operation of equipment and accurate administration to the client

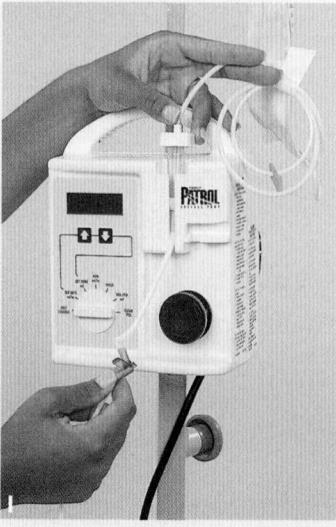

Preparing the pump. (Photo by B. Proud.)

SKILL 29-4 Administering Tube Feedings (*continued*)

Suggested Action	Reason for Action
Connect the tubing from the feeding pump to the client's feeding tube (Fig. J). 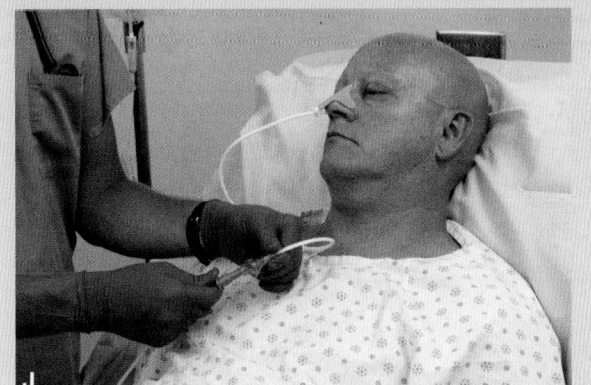	Provides access to formula
	Connecting the feeding tube to the pump.
Set the prescribed rate on the feeding pump (Fig. K). 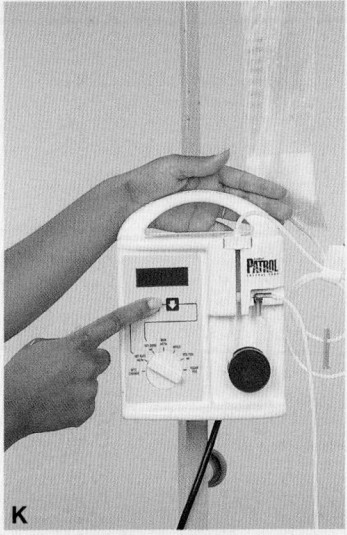	Complies with the medical order
	Programming the pump. (Photo by B. Proud.)
Open the clamp on the feeding tube and start the pump (Fig. L). 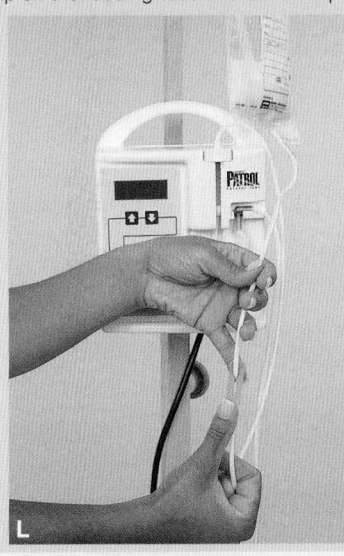	Initiates infusion
	Releasing the clamp. (Photo by B. Proud.)
Keep the client's head elevated at all times.	Prevents reflux and aspiration
Flush the tubing with 30–60 mL of water or more every 4 hours after checking and refeeding gastric residual and after administering medications.	Promotes patency and contributes to the client's fluid balance

(*continued*)

SKILL 29-4 Administering Tube Feedings (*continued*)

Suggested Action	Reason for Action
Record the instilled volume of formula and water.	Provides accurate data for assessing fluid balance and caloric value of nourishment
Follow recommendations for postprocedural care as described with a bolus feeding.	Principles for care remain the same.

EVALUATION

- The client receives a prescribed volume of formula according to an established feeding schedule.
- The client's weight remains stable or the client reaches the target weight.
- The lungs remain clear.
- Bowel elimination is within normal parameters for client.
- The client has a daily fluid intake between 2,000 and 3,000 mL unless intake is otherwise restricted.

DOCUMENT

- Volume of gastric residual and actions taken, if excessive
- Type and volume of formula
- Rate of infusion, if continuous
- Volume of water used for flushes
- Response of client; if symptomatic, describe actions taken and results

SAMPLE DOCUMENTATION

Date and Time Exit length of tube corresponds with insertion measurement. Gastric residual of 50 mL obtained by aspiration. Residual reinstilled and tube flushed with 30 mL of tap water. A 480 mL of Enrich with Fiber placed in tube-feeding bag. Formula infusing at 120 mL/hour. No diarrhea or gastric complaints at this time. _____ J. Doe, LPN

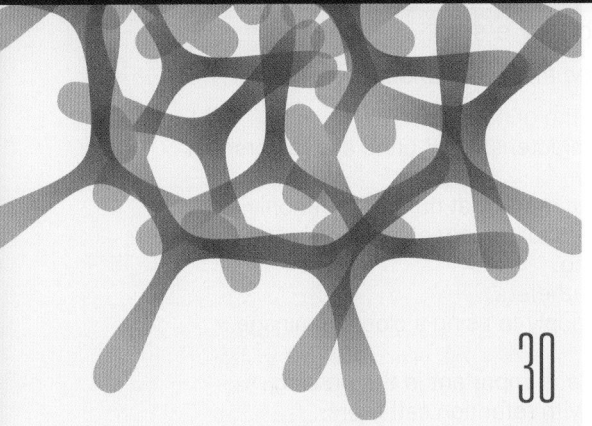

UNIT 8 | Promoting Elimination

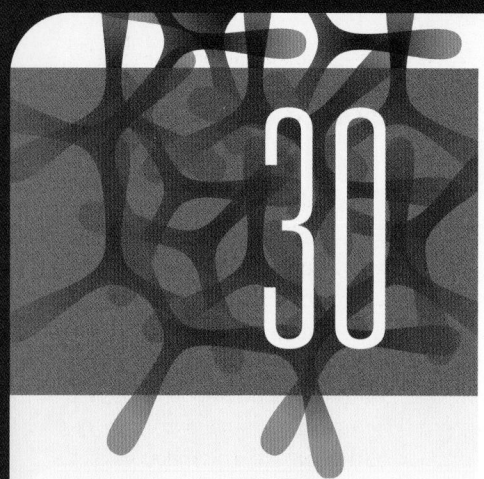

Urinary Elimination

Words To Know

24-hour specimen
anuria
bedpan
catheter-associated urinary tract infections (CAUTIs)
catheter care
catheter irrigation
catheterization
clean-catch specimen
closed drainage system
commode
continence training
continuous irrigation
Credé maneuver
cutaneous triggering
dysuria
external catheter
fenestrated drape
frequency
incontinence
nocturia
oliguria
pelvic floor muscle exercises
peristomal skin
polyuria
residual urine
retention catheter
stasis
straight catheter
urgency
urinal
urinary diversion
urinary elimination
urinary retention
urine
urostomy
voided specimen
voiding reflex

Learning Objectives

On completion of this chapter, the reader should be able to:

1. Identify the functions of the urinary system.
2. Describe the physical characteristics of urine and factors that affect urination.
3. Name types of urine specimens that nurses commonly collect.
4. Identify alternative devices for urinary elimination.
5. Define continence training.
6. Name types of urinary catheters.
7. Describe principles that apply to using a closed drainage system.
8. Explain why catheter care is important in the nursing management of clients with retention catheters.
9. Discuss the purpose of irrigating a catheter and methods for performing this skill.
10. Define urinary diversion.
11. Discuss factors that contribute to impaired skin integrity in clients with a urostomy.

INTRODUCTION

This chapter reviews the process of urinary elimination and describes the nursing skills for assessing and maintaining urinary elimination.

 Gerontologic Considerations

■ Older adults are more likely to have chronic residual urine (excessive urine in the bladder after urinating), which increases the risk for urinary tract infections (UTIs).

■ Maintenance of good perineal hygiene is one intervention for preventing UTIs. Females should always clean from the urinary area back toward the rectal area to prevent organisms from the stool entering the bladder. In addition, thorough handwashing by the client and caregiver is necessary.

■ Older adults may benefit from learning double voiding in which the person voids, then waits a few more minutes to allow any residual urine to be voided (Elist, 2022).

■ Older adults are likely to experience urinary urgency and frequency because of normal physiologic changes such as diminished bladder capacity and degenerative changes in the cerebral cortex. Subsequently, when they perceive the urge to void, they need to access a bathroom as soon as possible.

■ Age-related changes, such as a diminished bladder capacity and a relaxation of the pelvic floor muscle tone, increase the risk for incontinence.

- Fluid restriction may be used in an attempt to control urination, but it may instead contribute to incontinence by causing concentrated urine and eliminating the normal perception of a full bladder.

- Loss of control over urination often threatens an older adult's independence and self-esteem. It may also cause an older adult to restrict activities, possibly contributing to depression. Teaching older adults to structure activities with planned toileting breaks every 60 to 90 minutes results in less urine in the bladder and thus diminishes urge incontinence.

- Older adults who experience difficulty controlling urine need an evaluation to identify and treat contributing factors, such as constipation, UTI, and side effects from medications.

- Older adults need encouragement to discuss urinary incontinence with a knowledgeable, nonjudgmental health care provider. If they understand that urinary incontinence is a condition that frequently responds to medication or behavioral retraining, they are more likely to seek professional help.

- Many resources are available to assist older adults in evaluating and treating incontinence. For example, some health care facilities offer special incontinence clinics and physical therapy departments to teach pelvic muscle exercises. The National Association for Continence (http://www.nafc.org) is an excellent source of information for products, resources, and continence programs. Nurses can encourage older adults to take advantage of these kinds of resources rather than accepting incontinence as an inevitable condition that compromises quality of life.

- When efforts to restore continence are unsuccessful, nurses can encourage older adults to verbalize their feelings and identify interventions helpful in maintaining dignity, ultimately enabling older adults to participate in meaningful activities.

- An individualized toileting schedule should be maintained, for example, at intervals of every 90 to 120 minutes for clients who have difficulty maintaining continence.

- Absorbent products may interfere with the person's independence in toileting and may lead to skin breakdown. Incontinence products are never used primarily for staff convenience in institutional settings. In addition, an older person should never be reprimanded for an episode of incontinence.

- Enlargement of the prostate, a common problem among older males, can obstruct urinary outflow and make catheterization difficult or impossible. Insertion of a urinary catheter should never be forced. Sometimes, a malecot catheter is inserted into the bladder through the abdominal wall (suprapubic catheterization) when it cannot be inserted into a narrowed urethra.

- Indwelling catheters should be avoided if at all possible because older people have increased susceptibility to UTIs. Bladder training or other interventions are much more desirable.

- If indwelling catheters are necessary, meticulous daily care is required. The tubing should never be placed higher than the bladder to prevent any backflow of urine into the bladder.

OVERVIEW OF URINARY ELIMINATION

The urinary system (Fig. 30-1) consists of the kidneys, ureters, bladder, and urethra. These major components, along with some accessory structures, such as the ring-shaped muscles called the *internal and external sphincters*, work together to produce **urine** (fluid within the bladder), collect it, and excrete it from the body.

Urinary elimination (the process of releasing excess fluid and metabolic wastes), or urination, occurs when urine is excreted. Under normal conditions, the average person eliminates approximately 1,500 to 3,000 mL of urine each day. The consequences of impaired urinary elimination can be life-threatening.

Urination takes place several times each day. The need to urinate becomes apparent when the bladder distends with approximately 150 to 300 mL of urine. The distention with urine causes increased fluid pressure, stimulating stretch receptors in the bladder wall and creating a desire to empty it of urine.

CHARACTERISTICS OF URINE

The physical characteristics of urine include its volume, color, clarity, and odor. Variations in what is considered normal are wide (Table 30-1).

FACTORS AFFECTING URINARY ELIMINATION

Patterns of urinary elimination depend on physiologic, emotional, and social factors. Examples include (1) the degree of neuromuscular development and the integrity of the spinal cord; (2) the volume of fluid intake and the amount of fluid losses, including those from other sources; (3) the amount and type of food consumed; and (4) the person's circadian rhythm, habits, opportunities for urination, and anxiety.

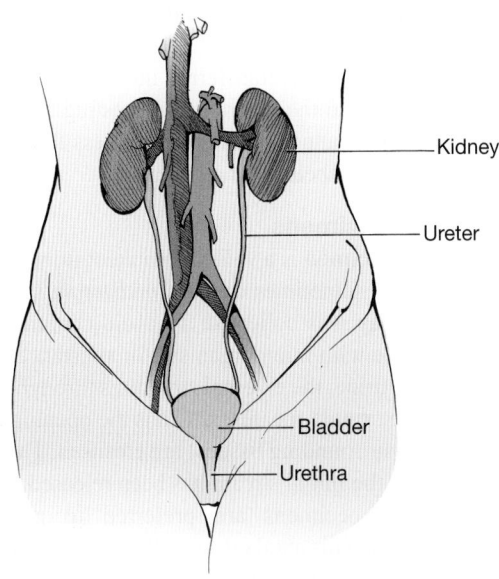

FIGURE 30-1 The major structures of the urinary system.

TABLE 30-1 Characteristics of Urine

CHARACTERISTIC	NORMAL	ABNORMAL	COMMON CAUSES OF VARIATIONS
Volume	500–3,000 mL/day 1,200 mL/day average	<400 mL/day	Low fluid intake Excess fluid loss Kidney dysfunction
		>3,000 mL/day	High fluid intake Diuretic medication Endocrine diseases
Color	Light yellow	Dark amber	Dehydration
		Brown	Liver/gallbladder disease
		Reddish brown	Blood
		Orange, green, blue	Water-soluble dyes
Clarity	Transparent	Cloudy	Infection Stasis
Odor	Faintly aromatic	Foul	Infection
		Strong	Dehydration
		Pungent	Certain foods

General measures to promote urination include providing privacy, assuming a natural position for urination (sitting for females, standing for males), maintaining adequate fluid intake, and using stimuli such as running water from a tap to initiate voiding.

Urine Specimen Collection

Health care providers collect urine specimens, or samples of urine, to identify microscopic or chemical constituents. Common urine specimens that nurses collect include voided specimens, clean-catch specimens, catheter specimens, and 24-hour specimens.

Voided Specimens

A **voided specimen** is a sample of fresh urine collected in a clean container. The first voided specimen of the day is preferred because it is most likely to contain substantial urinary components that have accumulated during the night. Nevertheless, a specimen can be voided and collected at any time it is needed.

The sample of urine is transferred into a specimen container and delivered to the laboratory for testing and analysis. If the specimen cannot be examined in less than 1 hour after collection, it is labeled and refrigerated.

Clean-Catch Specimens

A **clean-catch specimen** is a voided sample of urine considered sterile and is sometimes called a *midstream* specimen because of the way it is collected. To avoid contaminating the voided sample with microorganisms or substances other than those in the urine, the external structures through which urine passes (the urinary meatus, which is the opening to the urethra, and the surrounding tissues) are cleansed. The urine is collected after the initial stream has been released.

Clean-catch specimens are preferred to randomly voided specimens. This method of collection is also preferable when a urine specimen is needed during a client's menstrual period. As soon as the specimen is collected, it is labeled and taken to the laboratory. A clean-catch urine specimen is refrigerated if the analysis will be delayed more than 1 hour.

Collecting a specimen midstream after the use of soap, tap water, and nonsterile gauze for perineal cleansing provides reliable results and, in some cases, is more reliable than when an antiseptic solution is used. Nurses should follow their agency's policy for collecting midstream voided specimens. When a clean-catch specimen is needed, nurses can instruct clients who are capable of performing the procedure on the collection technique (Client and Family Teaching 30-1).

Client and Family Teaching 30-1
Collecting a Clean-Catch Specimen

The nurse teaches the female client as follows:
- Wash your hands.
- Remove the lid from the specimen container.
- Rest the lid upside down on its outer surface, taking care not to touch the inside areas.
- Sit on the toilet and spread your legs.
- Separate your labia with your fingers.
- Cleanse each side of the urinary meatus with a separate swab, wiping from front to back toward the vagina.
- Use the final clean, moistened swab to wipe directly down the center of the separated tissue.
- Begin to urinate.
- After releasing a small amount of urine into the toilet, catch a sample of urine in the specimen container.
- Take care not to touch the mouth of the specimen container to your skin.
- Place the specimen container nearby on a flat surface.
- Release your fingers and continue voiding normally.
- Wash your hands.
- Cover the specimen container with the lid.

The male client should follow the same steps as earlier but should perform the following cleansing routine:

- Retract your foreskin if you are uncircumcised or cleanse in a circular direction around the tip of the penis toward its base using a premoistened swab.
- Repeat with another swab.
- Continue retracting the foreskin while initiating the first release of urine and until you have collected the midstream specimen.

Catheter Specimens

A urine specimen can be collected under sterile conditions using a catheter, but this is usually done when clients are catheterized for other reasons, such as to control incontinence in an unconscious client. For clients who are already catheterized, the nurse clamps the drainage tube for 30 minutes and then aspirates a sample through the lumen of a latex catheter or from a self-sealing port that has been cleansed with an alcohol pad (Fig. 30-2).

24-Hour Specimens

The nurse collects, labels, and delivers a **24-hour specimen** (a collection of all urine produced in a full 24-hour period) to the laboratory for analysis. Because the contents in urine decompose over time, the nurse places the collected urine in a container with a chemical preservative or puts the container in a basin of ice or in a specimen-dedicated refrigerator.

To establish the 24-hour collection period accurately, the nurse instructs the client to urinate just before starting the test and then discards that urine. All urine voided thereafter becomes part of the collected specimen. Exactly 24 hours later, the nurse asks the client to void one last time to complete the test collection. The final urination and all collected voidings from the preceding 24 hours represent the total specimen, which the nurse labels and takes to the laboratory.

Abnormal Characteristics of Urine

Laboratory analysis is a valuable diagnostic tool for identifying abnormal characteristics of urine. Specific terms describe particular abnormal characteristics of urine and

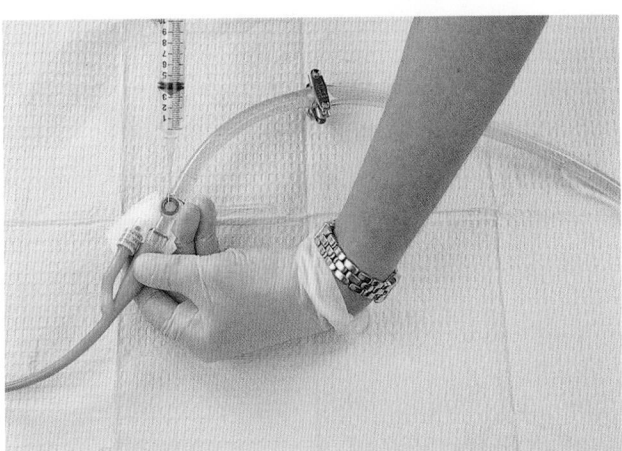

FIGURE 30-2 The location for collecting a urine specimen from a catheter. (Photo by B. Proud.)

urination. Many terms use the suffix *-uria*, which refers to urine or urination. For example,

- Hematuria: urine containing blood
- Pyuria: urine containing pus
- Proteinuria: urine containing plasma proteins
- Albuminuria: urine containing albumin, a plasma protein
- Glycosuria: urine containing glucose
- Ketonuria: urine containing ketones

ABNORMAL PATTERNS OF URINARY ELIMINATION

Assessment findings may indicate abnormal patterns of urinary elimination. Some common problems include anuria, oliguria, polyuria, nocturia, dysuria, and incontinence.

Anuria

Anuria means the absence of urine or a volume of 100 mL or less in 24 hours. It indicates that the kidneys are not forming sufficient urine. In this case, the term "urinary suppression" is used. In urinary suppression, the bladder is empty; therefore, the client feels no urge to urinate. This distinguishes anuria from **urinary retention**, in which the client produces urine but does not release it from the bladder. A sign of urinary retention is a progressively distending bladder.

Oliguria

Oliguria, urine output less than 400 mL in 24 hours, indicates the inadequate elimination of urine. Sometimes, oliguria is a sign that the bladder is being only partially emptied during voidings. **Residual urine**, or more than 50 mL of urine that remains in the bladder after voiding, can support the growth of microorganisms, leading to infection. In addition, when there is urinary **stasis** (a lack of movement), dissolved substances such as calcium can precipitate, leading to urinary calculi (stones).

Polyuria

Polyuria means greater than normal urinary elimination and may accompany minor dietary variations. For example, consuming higher than normal amounts of fluids, especially those with mild diuretic effects (e.g., coffee and tea), or taking certain medications can increase urination. Ordinarily, urine output is nearly equal to fluid intake. When the cause of polyuria is not apparent, excessive urination may be the result of a disorder. Common disorders associated with polyuria include *diabetes mellitus*, an endocrine disorder caused by insufficient insulin or insulin resistance, and *diabetes insipidus*, an endocrine disease caused by insufficient antidiuretic hormone.

Nocturia

Nocturia (nighttime urination) is unusual because the rate of urine production is normally reduced at night. Consequently, nocturia suggests an underlying medical problem. In aging males, an enlarging prostate gland, which encircles the urethra, interferes with complete bladder emptying. As a result, there is a need to urinate more frequently, including during the usual hours of sleep.

Pharmacologic Considerations

Nurses who are pregnant or may become pregnant should not handle crushed or broken dutasteride (Avodart) tablets or capsules, which can be used to treat an enlarged prostate. Absorption of the drug poses a substantial risk for abnormal growth to a male fetus.

Dysuria

Dysuria is difficult or uncomfortable voiding and a common symptom of trauma to the urethra or a bladder infection. **Frequency** (the need to urinate often) and **urgency** (a strong feeling that urine must be eliminated quickly) often accompany dysuria.

 Nutrition Notes

- Chemicals in cranberries keep bacteria from sticking to the cells in the urinary tract. However, they do not seem to be able to remove bacteria that are already stuck to these cells. This might explain why cranberry helps prevent UTIs but does not help treat them (WebMD, 2023).
- Problems with assessing cranberry efficacy include the difficulty in standardizing dosing because cranberry is available in various forms, such as juice, capsules, tablets, and extract.

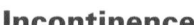

Incontinence

Incontinence is the inability to control either urinary or bowel elimination and is abnormal after a person has achieved earlier continence. The term *urinary incontinence* should not be used indiscriminately; anyone may be incontinent if their need for assistance goes unnoticed. Once the bladder becomes extremely distended, spontaneous urination may be more of a personnel problem than a client problem; the client may not be incontinent if staff members are attentive to their need to urinate.

 Pharmacologic Considerations

- Drug therapy can increase the risk for urinary incontinence, especially in older adults when cognitive/mobility issues hamper the ability to void in a timely manner. Drugs that increase urinary incontinence include:

- High blood pressure drugs—vasodilate and put more fluid into the vascular system

- Antidepressants—impair bladder contraction and worsen overflow incontinence symptoms

- Diuretics (water pills)—pull excess water and salt into the bladder

- Sleeping pills—clients do not respond and waken to void with a full bladder at night

- Client care includes more frequent voiding, especially within 2 hours of diuretic administration.

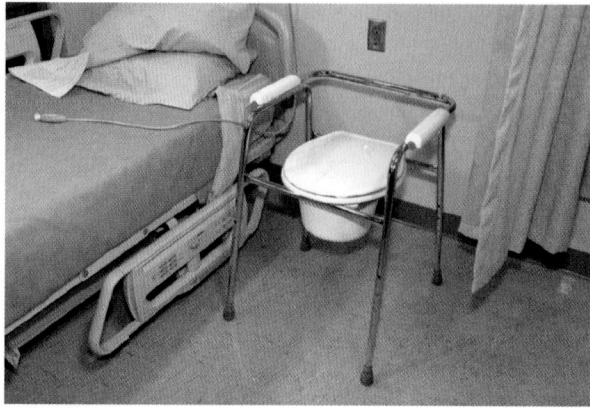

FIGURE 30-3 A bedside commode.

ASSISTING CLIENTS WITH URINARY ELIMINATION

Stable clients who can ambulate are assisted to the bathroom to use the toilet. Clients who are weak or cannot walk to the bathroom may need a commode. Clients confined to the bed use a urinal or bedpan.

Commode

A **commode** (a chair with an opening in the seat under which a receptacle is placed) is located beside or near the bed (Fig. 30-3). It is used for eliminating urine or stool. Immediately afterward, the waste container is removed, emptied, cleaned, and replaced.

Urinal

A **urinal** is a cylindrical container for collecting urine. It is more easily used by males. When given to the client, the urinal should be empty; otherwise, the bed linen may become wet and soiled. If the client needs help placing the urinal,

- Pull the privacy curtain.
- Put on gloves.
- Ask the client to spread their legs.
- Hold the urinal by its handle.
- Direct the urinal at an angle between the client's legs so that the bottom rests on the bed (Fig. 30-4).
- Lift the penis and place it well within the urinal.

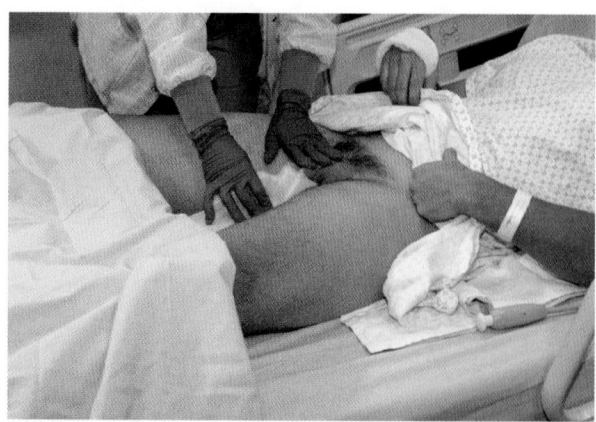

FIGURE 30-4 Placement of a urinal.

After use, the nurse promptly empties the urinal. They measure and record the volume of urine if the client's intake and output are being monitored (see Chapter 16). The nurse washes their hands and always offers the client an opportunity to wash their hands after voiding.

Using a Bedpan

A **bedpan** (a seat-like container for elimination) is used to collect urine or stool. Most bedpans are made of plastic and are several inches deep. A *fracture pan*, a modified version of a conventional bedpan, is flat on the sitting end rather than rounded (Fig. 30-5). Clients with musculoskeletal disorders who cannot elevate their hips and sit on a bedpan in the usual manner use a fracture pan. When a client confined to bed feels the need to eliminate, the nurse places a bedpan under the buttocks (Skill 30-1).

>> *Stop, Think, and Respond 30-1*

Describe measures that may reduce a client's concerns when they require a bedpan.

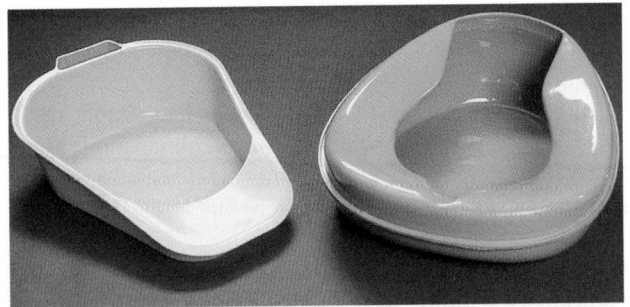

FIGURE 30-5 Two types of bedpans: a fracture pan (left) and a conventional bedpan (right). (Photo by B. Proud.)

MANAGING INCONTINENCE

Urinary incontinence, depending on its type, may be permanent or temporary. The six types of urinary incontinence are stress, urge, reflex, functional, total, and overflow (Table 30-2).

The management of incontinence is complex because there are so many variations. Treatment is further

TABLE 30-2 Types of Incontinence

TYPE	DESCRIPTION	EXAMPLE	COMMON CAUSES	NURSING APPROACH
Stress	The loss of small amounts of urine when intra-abdominal pressure rises	Dribbling is associated with sneezing, coughing, lifting, laughing, or rising from a bed or chair.	Loss of perineal and sphincter muscle tone secondary to childbirth, menopausal atrophy, prolapsed uterus, or obesity	Pelvic floor muscle strengthening Weight reduction
Urge	Need to void perceived frequently with short-lived ability to sustain control of the flow	Voiding commences when there is a delay in accessing a toilet.	Bladder irritation secondary to infection; loss of bladder tone from recent continuous drainage with an indwelling catheter	Restriction of fluid intake of at least 2,000 mL/day Omit bladder irritants, such as caffeine or alcohol. Administration of diuretics in the morning
Reflex	Spontaneous loss of urine when the bladder is stretched with urine but without prior perception of a need to void	The person automatically releases urine and cannot control it.	Damage to motor and sensory tracts in the lower spinal cord secondary to trauma, a tumor, or other neurologic conditions	Cutaneous triggering Straight intermittent catheterization
Functional	Control over urination lost because of inaccessibility of a toilet or a compromised ability to use one	Voiding occurs while attempting to overcome barriers such as doorways, transferring from a wheelchair, manipulating clothing, acquiring assistance, or making needs known.	Impaired mobility, impaired cognition, physical restraints, inability to communicate	Clothing modification Access to a toilet, commode, or urinal Assistance to a toilet according to a preplanned schedule
Total	Loss of urine without any identifiable pattern or warning	The person passes urine without any ability or effort to control.	Altered consciousness secondary to a head injury, loss of sphincter tone secondary to prostatectomy, anatomic leak through a urethral/vaginal fistula	Absorbent undergarments External catheter Indwelling catheter
Overflow	Urine leakage because the bladder is not completely emptied; bladder distended with retained urine	The person voids small amounts frequently, or urine leaks around a catheter.	Overstretched bladder or weakened muscle tone secondary to obstruction of the urethra by debris within a catheter, an enlarged prostate, distended bowel, or postoperative bladder spasms	Hydration Adequate bowel elimination Patency of catheter Credé maneuver

complicated when clients have more than one type of incontinence; for example, stress incontinence often accompanies urge incontinence.

Some forms of incontinence respond to simple measures, such as modifying clothing to make elimination easier. Other forms improve only with a more regimented approach like continence training.

Continence Training

Continence training to restore the control of urination involves teaching the client to refrain from urinating until an appropriate time and place. This process is sometimes referred to as *bladder retraining*, but this term is inaccurate because the various techniques used involve mechanisms other than those unique to the bladder.

Continence training primarily benefits clients with the cognitive ability and desire to participate in a rehabilitation program. This includes clients with lower body paralysis who wish to facilitate urination without the use of urinary

BOX 30-1	Technique for Performing Pelvic Floor Muscle Exercises (Kegel Exercises)

- Tighten the internal muscles used to prevent urination or interrupt urination once it has begun.
- Keep the muscles contracted for at least 10 seconds.
- Relax the muscles for the same period.
- Repeat the pattern of contraction and relaxation 10 to 25 times.
- Perform the exercise regimen three or four times a day for 2 weeks to 1 month.

drainage devices, such as catheters. Clients who are not candidates for continence training require alternative methods, such as absorbent undergarments.

Continence training is often a slow process that requires the combined effort and dedication of the nursing team, client, and family (Nursing Guidelines 30-1; Box 30-1).

NURSING GUIDELINES 30-1

Providing Continence Training

- Compile a log of the client's urinary elimination patterns. *The data can help reveal the client's type of incontinence.*
- Set realistic, specific, short-term goals with the client. *Short-term goals prevent self-defeating consequences and promote client control.*
- Discourage strict limitation of liquid intake. *Intake maintains fluid balance and ensures adequate urine volume.*
- Plan a trial schedule for voiding that correlates with the times when the client is usually incontinent or experiences bladder distention. *This schedule reduces the potential for accidental voiding or sustained urinary retention.*
- In the absence of any identifiable pattern, plan to assist the client with voiding every 2 hours during the day and every 4 hours at night. *This duration provides time for urine to form.*
- Communicate the plan to nursing personnel, the client, and the family. *Collaboration promotes continuity of care and dedication to reaching goals.*
- Assist the client to a toilet or commode; position the client on a bedpan or place a urinal just before the scheduled time for trial voiding. *These measures prepare the client for releasing urine.*
- Simulate the sound of urination such as by running water from the faucet. *Doing so simulates relaxation of the sphincter muscles, allowing the release of urine.*
- Suggest performing **Credé maneuver** (the act of bending forward and applying hand pressure over the bladder; see figure). *Credé maneuver increases abdominal pressure to overcome the resistance of the internal sphincter muscle.*
- Instruct paralyzed clients to identify any sensation that precedes voiding such as a chill, muscular spasm, restlessness, or spontaneous penile erection. *These cues can help the client anticipate urination.*
- Suggest that paralyzed clients with reflex incontinence use **cutaneous triggering** (lightly massaging or tapping the skin above the pubic area). *Cutaneous triggering initiates urination*

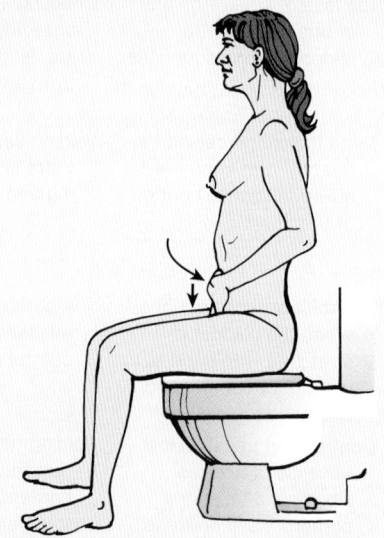

A Credé maneuver.

in clients who have retained a **voiding reflex** *(the spontaneous relaxation of the urinary sphincter in response to physical stimulation).*

- Teach clients with stress incontinence to perform **pelvic floor muscle exercises** (Kegel exercises), which are isometric exercises to improve the ability to retain urine within the bladder; see Box 30-1. *Pelvic floor muscle exercises strengthen and tone the pubococcygeal and levator ani muscles used voluntarily to hold back urine and intestinal gas or stool.*
- Assist clients with urge incontinence to walk slowly and concentrate on holding their urine when nearing the toilet. *These measures reverse previous mental conditioning in which the urge to urinate becomes stronger and more overpowering close to the toilet.*

Pharmacologic Considerations

■ Pharmacologic therapy may be an option for female clients with urinary incontinence:
■ Topical estrogen (creams or Estring vaginal ring) to treat stress incontinence
■ Antispasmodics (oxybutynin [Ditropan]) to treat urge incontinence
■ Tricyclic antidepressants (imipramine [Tofranil]) to treat mixed incontinence issues

CATHETERIZATION

Catheterization (the act of applying or inserting a hollow tube), in this case, refers to using a device inside the bladder or externally about the urinary meatus. A urinary catheter is used for various reasons:

• Keeping incontinent clients dry (catheterization is a last resort that is used only when all other continence measures have been exhausted)
• Relieving bladder distention when clients cannot void
• Assessing fluid balance accurately
• Keeping the bladder from becoming distended during procedures such as surgery
• Measuring the residual urine
• Obtaining sterile urine specimens
• Instilling medication within the bladder

Types of Catheters

There are a variety of urinary catheters, but the three most common types are external, straight, and retention. Most catheters are made of latex. For clients who are sensitive or allergic to latex, latex-free catheters such as those made of silicone are used.

External Catheters

An **external catheter**, also known as a *condom* catheter (a urine-collecting device applied to the skin), is not inserted within the bladder; instead, it surrounds the penis (Fig. 30-6). An external catheter is more effective for male clients.

Condom catheters are helpful for clients receiving care at home because they are easy to apply. A condom catheter has a flexible sheath that is unrolled over the penis. The narrow end is connected to tubing that serves as a channel for draining urine. The drainage tube may be attached to a leg bag (Fig. 30-7) or connected to a larger urine collection device.

Three potential problems accompany the use of condom catheters. First, the sheath may be applied too tightly, restricting blood flow to the skin and tissues of the penis. Second, moisture tends to accumulate beneath the sheath, leading to skin breakdown. Third, condom catheters frequently leak. Applying the catheter correctly and managing care appropriately can prevent these problems (Skill 30-2).

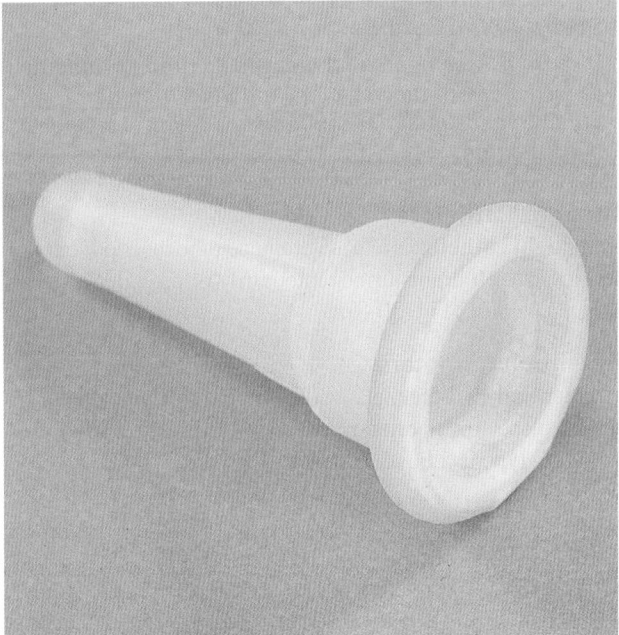

FIGURE 30-6 A condom catheter is an example of an external urine collection device. (Photo by B. Proud.)

Nurses may apply an external collection device called a *urinary bag* (U bag). A urinary bag serves as a disposable container for collecting a urine specimen from a male or female infant who has not developed the ability to achieve continence. The upper portion of the bag has a self-adherent pad that covers the pubic area. The bag encircles the penis or labia. A diaper is applied over the U bag to ensure that it does not become loose or removed by the infant. Once the specimen is obtained, the U bag is removed and discarded.

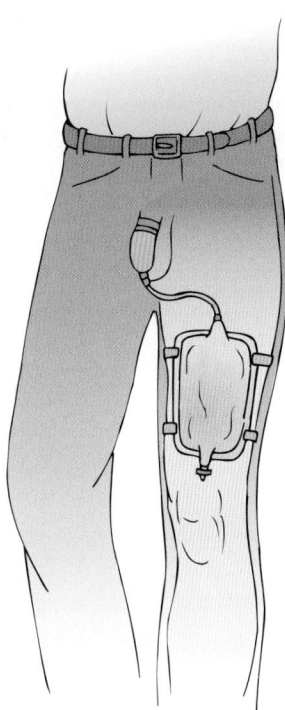

FIGURE 30-7 A leg bag collects urine from a catheter but is concealed under clothing.

>>> *Stop, Think, and Respond 30-2*
Discuss assessments that indicate common problems associated with the use of a condom catheter and nursing measures that can reduce or eliminate negative outcomes.

Straight Catheters
A **straight catheter** is a urine drainage tube inserted, but not left in place. It drains urine temporarily or provides a sterile urine specimen (Fig. 30-8).

Retention Catheters
A **retention catheter**, also called an *indwelling* catheter, is left in place for a period of time (see Fig. 30-8). The most common type is a Foley catheter.

Unlike straight catheters, retention catheters are secured with a balloon that is inflated once the distal tip is within the bladder. Both straight and retention catheters are available in various diameters, sized according to the French (F) scale (see Chapter 29). For adults, sizes 14, 16, and 18 F are commonly used.

Inserting a Catheter
The techniques for inserting straight and retention catheters are similar, though the steps for inflating the retention balloon do not apply to a straight catheter. When inserting a straight or a retention catheter in a health care setting, the nurse uses sterile technique. In the home setting, nurses and clients who self-catheterize use clean technique because most clients have adapted to the organisms in their own

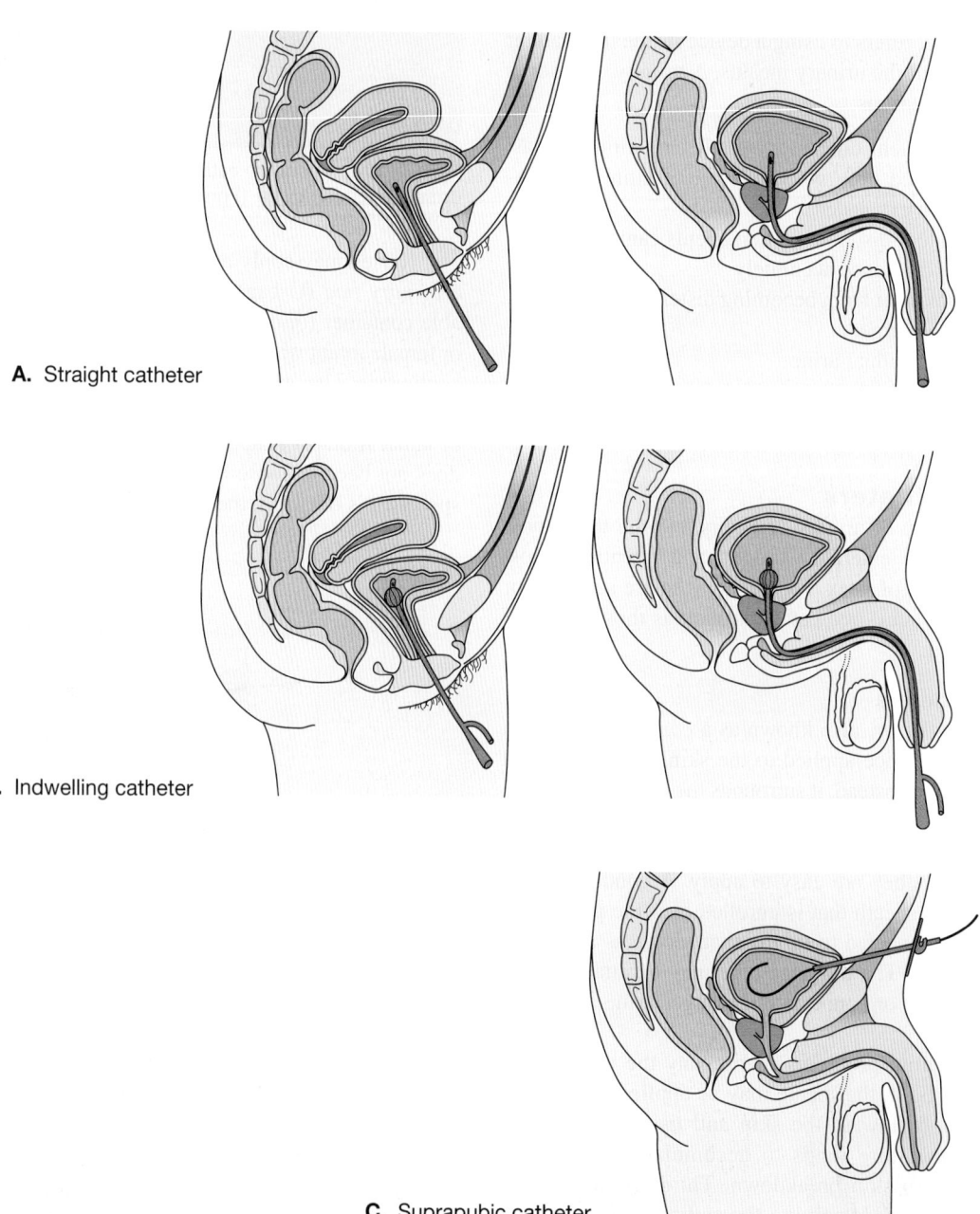

A. Straight catheter

B. Indwelling catheter

C. Suprapubic catheter

FIGURE 30-8 Types of urinary catheters. **A.** Straight catheter, a temporary catheter, is also used to collect a sterile specimen. **B.** Retention (Foley) catheter with balloon is a continuous dwelling catheter. **C.** Suprapubic catheter is inserted surgically directly into the bladder.

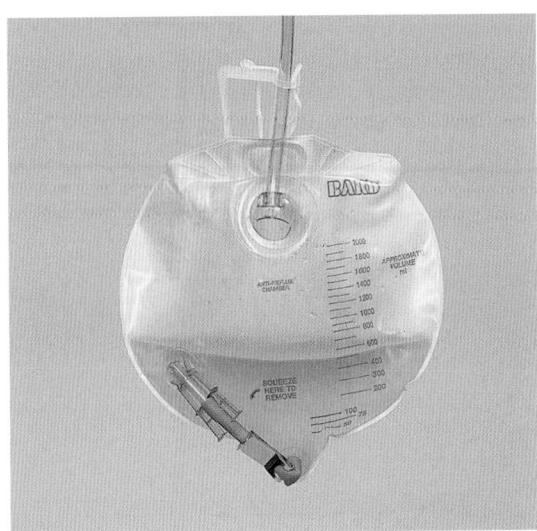

FIGURE 30-9 A closed urine drainage system.

environment. Because of anatomic differences, techniques for insertion differ in male and female clients and are described in Skills 30-3 and 30-4.

>>> **Stop, Think, and Respond 30-3**
Discuss factors that predispose a female with a Foley catheter to develop a UTI.

Connecting a Closed Drainage System

A **closed drainage system** (a device used to collect urine from a catheter) consists of a calibrated bag, which can be opened at the bottom; tubing of sufficient length to accommodate for turning and positioning clients; and a hanger from which to suspend the bag from the bed (Fig. 30-9). The nurse coils excess tubing on the bed but keeps the section from the bed to the collection bag vertical. Dependent loops in the tubing interfere with gravity flow. The nurse also takes care

to avoid compressing the tubing, which can obstruct drainage. Placing the tubing over the client's thigh is acceptable.

The nurse always positions the drainage system lower than the bladder to avoid a backflow of urine. When transporting the client in a wheelchair, the nurse suspends the drainage bag from the chair below the level of the bladder. When the client is ambulating, the nurse secures the drainage bag to the lower part of an intravenous (IV) pole or allows the client to carry the bag by hand (Fig. 30-10).

>>> **Stop, Think, and Respond 30-4**
Discuss possible explanations for why urine may not flow from a catheter.

To reduce the potential for the drainage system becoming a reservoir of pathogens, the entire drainage system is replaced whenever the catheter is changed and at least every 2 weeks in clients with a UTI.

Catheter-Associated Urinary Tract Infections

Those who are catheterized are at risk for acquiring UTIs. Approximately 80% of health care-associated UTIs are related to the use of indwelling urinary catheters (IUCs); catheter-associated UTIs have been associated with increased morbidity, mortality, length of stay, and hospital costs (Lachance & Grobelna, 2019). In an effort to prevent **catheter-associated urinary tract infections** (CAUTIs), the American Nurses Association (2020) has recommended specific goals to reduce their incidence:

1. Placement of fewer IUCs
2. More timely removal of IUCs per the Centers for Disease Control and Prevention (CDC) guidelines
3. Consistent, timely evidence-based nursing assessments and interventions for adequate bladder emptying

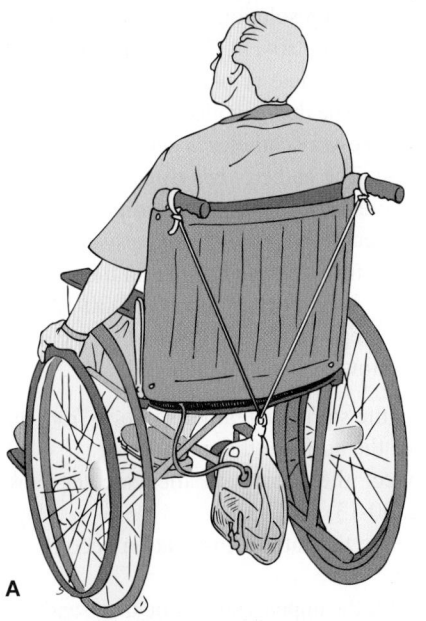
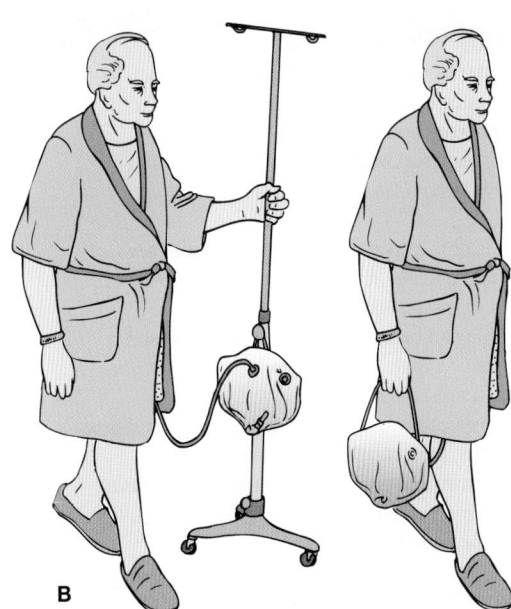

FIGURE 30-10 Techniques for suspending a drainage system below the bladder. **A.** A patient who uses a wheelchair. **B.** An ambulating patient with and without an intravenous pole.

Providing Catheter Care

A retention catheter keeps the meatus slightly dilated, providing pathogens with a direct pathway to the bladder where an infection could develop. Adhering to catheter care recommendations of hand hygiene and catheter maintenance can help decrease the incidences of CAUTI.

Catheter care (hygiene measures used to keep the meatus and adjacent area of the catheter clean) helps deter the growth and spread of colonizing pathogens. Nursing Guidelines 30-2 describes the technique for providing catheter care. Nurses must follow agency policy for using antiseptic and antimicrobial agents because the use of these substances is not a standard recommendation by the CDC.

Catheter Irrigation

Catheter irrigation (flushing the lumen of a catheter) is a technique for restoring or maintaining catheter patency. A catheter that drains well, however, does not need to be irrigated. A generous oral fluid intake is usually sufficient to produce dilute urine, which keeps small shreds of mucus or tissue debris from obstructing the catheter. Occasionally, however, the catheter may need to be irrigated, such as after a surgical procedure that results in bloody urine.

Depending on the type of indwelling catheter, nurses irrigate continuously through a three-way catheter or periodically using an open system or a closed system (Skill 30-5).

Using an Open System

An open system is one in which the retention catheter is separated from the drainage tubing to insert the tip of an irrigating syringe. Opening the system creates the potential for infection because it provides an opportunity for pathogens to enter the exposed connection. Consequently, it is the least desirable of the three methods.

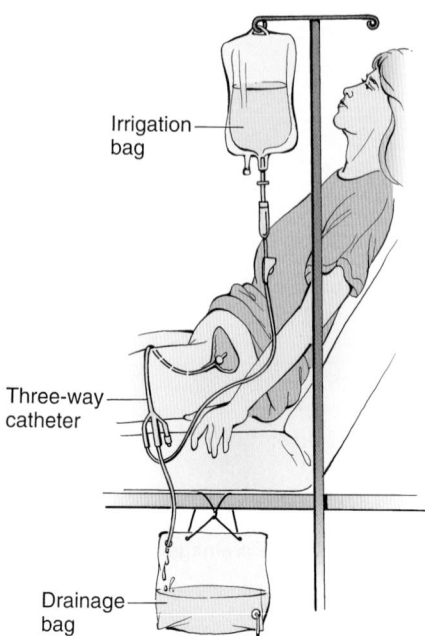

FIGURE 30-11 Bladder irrigation using a three-way catheter.

Using a Closed System

A closed system is irrigated without separating the catheter from the drainage tubing. To do so, the catheter or drainage tubing must have a self-sealing port. After cleansing the port with an alcohol swab, the nurse pierces the port with an 18- or 19-gauge, 1.5-in needle (see Chapter 34). They attach the needle to a 30- to 60-mL syringe containing a sterile irrigation solution. The nurse pinches or clamps the tubing beneath the port and instills the solution, then releases the tubing for drainage. The nurse records the volume of irrigant as fluid intake or subtracts it from the urine output to maintain an accurate intake and output record.

Continuous Irrigation

Continuous irrigation (the ongoing instillation of solution) instills irrigation solution into a catheter by gravity over a period of days (Fig. 30-11). Continuous irrigations keep a catheter patent after prostate or other urologic surgery in which blood clots and tissue debris collect within the bladder and catheter.

A three-way catheter is necessary to provide continuous irrigation. The catheter has three lumens or channels within the catheter, each leading to a separate port. One port connects the catheter to the drainage system; another provides a means for inflating the balloon in the catheter; and the third instills the irrigation solution (Fig. 30-12).

The steps involved in providing a continuous irrigation are as follows:

- Hang the sterile irrigating solution from an IV pole.
- Purge the air from the tubing.
- Connect the tubing to the catheter port for irrigation (Fig. 30-13).
- Regulate the rate of instillation according to the medical order.
- Monitor the appearance of the urine and volume of urinary drainage.

NURSING GUIDELINES 30-2

Providing Catheter Care

- Plan to cleanse the meatus and a nearby section of the catheter at least once a day. *Regular cleansing reduces colonizing microorganisms.*
- Gather clean gloves, soap, water, washcloth, towel, and a disposable pad. *Organization facilitates efficient time management.*
- Wash your hands or use an alcohol-based hand rub (see Chapter 10). *Hand hygiene reduces the potential for transmitting microorganisms.*
- Place a disposable pad beneath the hips of a female and beneath the penis of a male. *The pad protects the bed linen from becoming wet or soiled.*
- Put on clean gloves and wash the meatus, the catheter where it meets the meatus, the genitalia, and the perineum (in that order) with warm, soapy water. Rinse and dry. *Routine hygiene removes gross secretions and transient microorganisms while following the principles of asepsis.*
- Remove soiled materials and gloves, and repeat hand hygiene measures. *These steps remove colonizing microorganisms.*

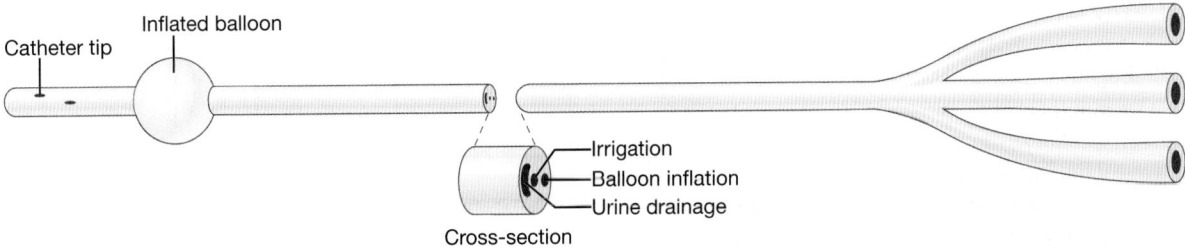

FIGURE 30-12 Components of a three-way catheter.

Irrigation
Balloon inflation
Urine drainage
Cross-section

>>> Stop, Think, and Respond 30-5

Discuss what actions might be appropriate if irrigating a catheter is unsuccessful in promoting catheter patency.

Indwelling Catheter Removal

A catheter is removed when it needs to be replaced or when its use is discontinued. The best time to remove a catheter is in the morning when there is more opportunity to address any urination difficulties without depriving a client of sleep (Nursing Guidelines 30-3).

URINARY DIVERSIONS

In a **urinary diversion**, one or both ureters are surgically implanted elsewhere. This procedure is done for various life-threatening conditions. The ureters may be brought to and through the skin of the abdomen (Fig. 30-14) or implanted within the bowel (called an *ileal conduit*). A **urostomy** (a urinary diversion that discharges urine from an opening in the abdomen) is the focus of this discussion.

Care for an ostomy, a surgically created opening, is discussed in more detail in Chapter 31 because those formed for bowel elimination are more common. Chapter 31 also provides a detailed description of an ostomy appliance, the device used for collecting stool or urine, and the manner in which it is applied and removed from the skin.

Caring for a urostomy and changing a urinary appliance are more challenging than the care of intestinal stomas. Urine drains continuously from a urostomy, increasing the

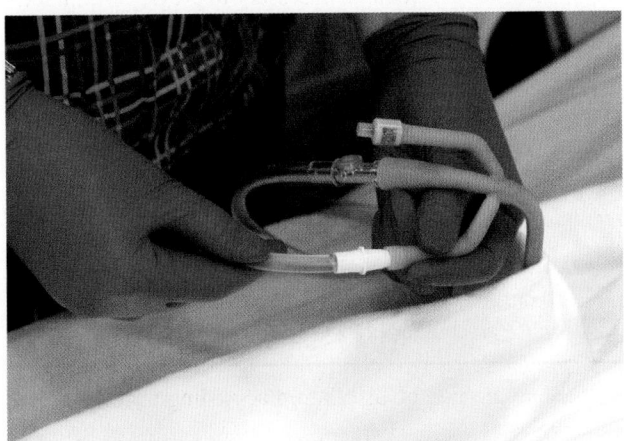

FIGURE 30-13 Attaching irrigation tubing to a port on a three-way catheter.

NURSING GUIDELINES 30-3

Removing a Foley Catheter

- Wash your hands or use an alcohol-based hand rub (see Chapter 10) and put on clean gloves. *These measures follow standard precautions.*
- Empty the balloon by aspirating the fluid with a syringe. *This step ensures that all the fluid has been withdrawn.*
- Gently pull the catheter near the point where it exits from the meatus. *Doing so facilitates withdrawal.*
- Inspect the catheter and discard if it appears to be intact. *This ensures safety.*
- Clean the urinary meatus. *This promotes comfort and hygiene.*
- Monitor the client's voiding, especially for the next 8–10 hours; measure the volume of each voiding. *Findings determine whether elimination is normal as well as the characteristics of the urine.*

risk for skin breakdown. In addition, because moisture and the weight of the collected urine tend to loosen the appliance from the skin, a urinary appliance may need to be emptied and changed more frequently. When changing the appliance, it may help to place a tampon within the stoma to absorb urine temporarily while the skin is cleansed and prepared for another appliance.

It is often difficult to maintain the integrity of the **peristomal skin** (the skin around the stoma) because of the frequent appliance changes and the ammonia in urine. Skin barrier products are used, and sometimes, an antibiotic or steroid ointment is applied.

NURSING IMPLICATIONS

Clients with urinary elimination problems may have one or more of the following nursing diagnoses:

- Toileting activity of daily living (ADL) deficit
- Urinary retention
- Infection risk
- Reflex urinary incontinence
- Functional urinary incontinence

Nursing Care Plan 30-1 is developed for a client with reflex urinary incontinence, defined as the contraction of the bladder muscle and leakage of urine (often in large amounts) without any warning or urge.

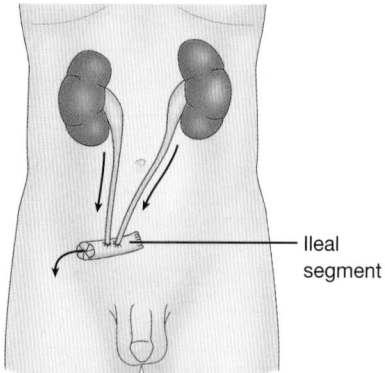

A: Conventional ileal conduit.
The surgeon transplants the ureters to an isolated section of the terminal ileum (ileal conduit), bringing one end to the abdominal wall. The ureter may also be transplanted into the transverse sigmoid colon (colon conduit) or proximal jejunum (jejunal conduit).

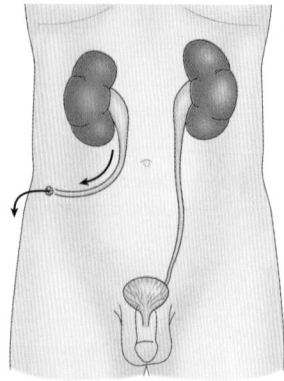

B: Cutaneous ureterostomy.
The surgeon brings the detached ureter through the abdominal wall and attaches it to an opening in the skin.

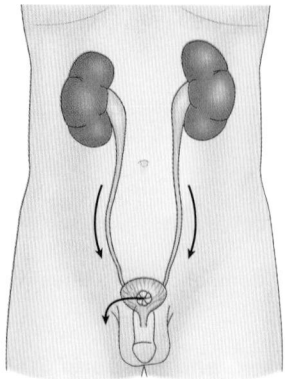

C: Vesicostomy.
The surgeon sutures the bladder to the abdominal wall and creates an opening (stoma) through the abdominal and bladder walls for urinary drainage.

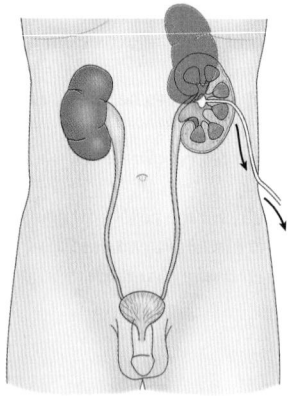

D: Nephrostomy.
The surgeon inserts a catheter into the renal pelvis via an incision into the flank or, by percutaneous catheter placement, into the kidney.

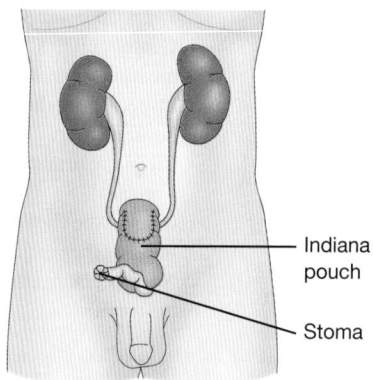

E: Indiana pouch.
The surgeon introduces the ureters into a segment of ileum and cecum. Urine is drained periodically by inserting a catheter into the stoma.

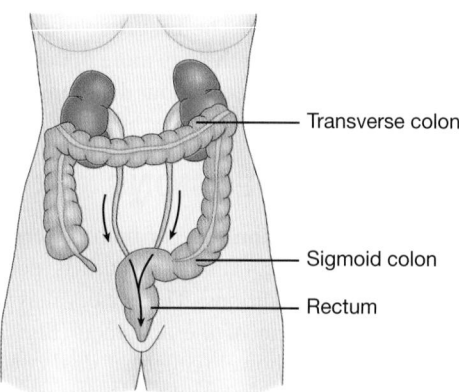

F: Ureterosigmoidostomy.
The surgeon introduces the ureters into the sigmoid colon, thereby allowing urine to flow through the colon and out of the rectum.

FIGURE 30-14 Examples of urinary diversions. **A.** An ileal conduit. **B.** A cutaneous ureterostomy. **C.** Vesicostomy. **D.** Nephrostomy. **E.** Indiana pouch. **F.** Ureterosigmoidostomy. (From Hinkle, J. L., & Cheever, K. H. [2021] *Brunner and Suddarth's textbook of medical-surgical nursing* [15th ed.]. Lippincott Williams & Wilkins.)

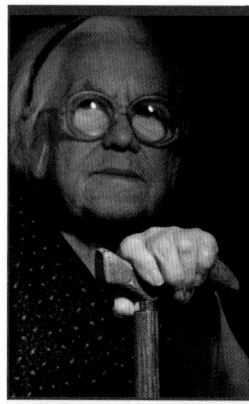

Clinical Scenario Nursing staff in a nursing home note that an 85-year-old female client frequently requires changes in her underclothing because she cannot ambulate to the toilet in time to void. The client is embarrassed because others notice a wet patch of urine on the floor and her wet outer garments.

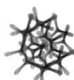

NURSING CARE PLAN 30-1 — Reflex Urinary Incontinence

Assessment

- Inquire about the number of voidings per day; voiding more than eight times in 24 hours or waking up two or more times at night to urinate, or urinating soon after the bladder has been emptied suggests a pattern of urgency or what has also been referred to as an overactive bladder.

- Identify the interim the client can wait to postpone urination following the sensation of a need to empty the bladder.
- Ask the client if the need to urinate is less easily controlled as the person gets nearer to the location of a toilet.
- Determine whether the client experiences accidental loss of urine when there is an almost unstoppable need to urinate.

Nursing Diagnosis. Reflex urinary incontinence related to uninhibited bladder muscle contractions as manifested by 14–18 voidings per day including awakening three times at night to urinate; daily episodes of urinary incontinence with impaired ability to delay the urge to void

Expected Outcome. The client will report a decrease in the number of daily voidings to fewer than eight per day; absence or limited occasions of nocturia; ability to delay urination by 15 minutes or more when urination seems imminent; and absence of urinary incontinence within 6–8 weeks of implementing therapeutic interventions, for example, by 9/15.

Interventions	Rationales
Keep a record of the frequency of voidings and the length of time between the warning sign for voiding and actual voiding for 3 days beginning 8/1 through 8/3.	Documenting the client's unique pattern of urination facilitates appropriate nursing interventions.
Alert all nursing team members to respond as soon as possible to the client's signal for assistance.	Responding promptly reduces episodes of incontinence and demonstrates a united effort to help the client achieve control of urination.
Instruct the client to restrain urination as long as possible after the warning sign is perceived.	Efforts to delay urination help reverse an established habit of overresponding to an urgent need to void.
Suggest that the client uses a technique such as breathing deeply, singing a song, or talking about family to delay voiding.	Focusing thoughts on something other than urination may provide sufficient distraction to extend the interval between the warning sign and actual voiding.
Encourage the client to eliminate the intake of beverages that contain caffeine or alcohol.	Caffeine promotes urination; alcohol inhibits the antidiuretic hormone, which prevents the reabsorption of water in the nephrons and leads to an increased formation of urine.
Ensure an oral fluid intake of at least 1,500–2,000 mL/day.	An adequate fluid intake reduces the potential for urinary infection or renal stone formation.
Assist the client to the toilet for the purpose of urination at a frequency that corresponds with the client's preconditioning pattern of urination (i.e., approximately q1½h), and extend the time by 15 minutes until there is an interval of 2 hours between voidings.	Increasing the length of time between voidings reduces chronic low-volume voiding, improves bladder muscle tone, and increases bladder capacity, which potentiates achieving continence.
Continue to extend the intervals between voiding until the client is voiding no more frequently than q4h in a 24-hour period.	Reconditioning the control of urination is facilitated by repetition and gradually extending the efforts to control voiding.
Praise the client every time a short-term goal of delaying or controlling urination is achieved.	Positive reinforcement helps motivate the client to continue efforts to control incontinence.
Share the client's progress with the physician.	Medical interventions such as prescribing a medication that blocks acetylcholine (anticholinergic agent) may help inhibit bladder muscle contractions and promote contraction of the urinary sphincter.

Evaluation of Expected Outcome

- The client is able to gradually delay urination.
- Nocturia is reduced to once per night.
- The client has fewer to no episodes of incontinence.

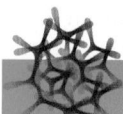

KEY POINTS

- Urination becomes apparent when the bladder distends with approximately 150 to 300 mL of urine, causing pressure on the bladder receptors for the urge to empty it.
- Physical characteristics of urine
  - Normal amount: 500 to 3,000 mL/day
  - Normal color: Light yellow
  - Normal clarity: Transparent
  - Normal odor: Faintly aromatic
- Factors affecting urinary elimination include physiologic, emotional, and social factors.
  - The degree of neuromuscular development and the integrity of the spinal cord
  - The volume of fluid intake and the amount of fluid losses, including those from other sources
  - The amount and type of food consumed
  - Circadian rhythm
  - Habits
  - Opportunities for urination
  - Anxiety
- Specimen types
  - Voided specimen: Fresh urine in a clean container
  - Clean-catch specimen: Voided sample of urine considered sterile; clean external structure and have the client start to void, obtaining specimen after the initial stream has begun
  - Catheter specimen: Using a urinary catheter to obtain a sample from the self-sealing port on the catheter
  - 24-hour urine specimen: Have the client void and discard the first urine, then start the collection and continue for 24 hours.
- Abnormal urinary elimination patterns
  - Anuria: The absence of urine or a volume of 100 mL or less in 24 hours

- Oliguria: Urine output less than 400 mL in 24 hours
- Polyuria: Greater than normal urinary elimination
- Nocturia: Nighttime urination
- Dysuria: Difficult or uncomfortable urination
- Urinary incontinence, depending on its type, may be permanent or temporary.
  - Stress
  - Urge
  - Reflex
  - Functional
  - Total
  - Overflow
- Urinary catheterization: The act of applying or inserting a hollow tube into the bladder via the external meatus
  - External catheter (condom catheter): Applied to the skin
  - Straight catheter: A temporary inserted catheter not left in place
  - Retention catheter (indwelling catheter): Left in place for a period of time
- CAUTIs prevention
  - Provide catheter care.
  - Secure the catheter appropriately.
  - Maintain the drainage bag below the level of the bladder.
  - Empty the drainage bag regularly.
  - Keep the tube from twisting or kinking.
  - Provide perineal care at least daily.
- Urinary diversion: One or both ureters are surgically implanted elsewhere; the ureters may be brought to and through the skin of the abdomen or implanted within the bowel (called an ileal conduit).
- A urostomy is a urinary diversion that discharges urine from an opening in the abdomen.

CRITICAL THINKING EXERCISES

1. During a nursing assessment, a female client reports periodic dribbling of urine. What additional information is important to obtain?
2. An older adult client confides that they would like to participate in activities outside their home, but they are worried that others will notice their problem with urinary incontinence. What response might help this client? What suggestions could you offer?
3. A resident in a nursing home who has had a retention catheter for the last 6 months says, "I'd do anything if I didn't have to have this catheter." What suggestions would be appropriate at this time?
4. The physician orders the removal of a urinary retention catheter. What actions should the nurse take?

NEXT-GENERATION NCLEX-STYLE REVIEW QUESTIONS

1. What is the most important nursing assessment before beginning continence retraining?
   a. Recording the time when the client is incontinent
   b. Checking the results of a routine urinalysis
   c. Palpating the extent of bladder distention
   d. Observing the characteristics of the client's urine
   Test-Taking Strategy: Note the key word and modifier, "most important assessment." Analyze the choices and select the option that is better than any of the others.

2. During continence retraining, what is the best nursing response when a client wants to restrict fluid intake to remain dry for longer periods?
   a. Encourage the practice because it shows evidence of client cooperation.
   b. Encourage the practice because it leads to accomplishing the goal.
   c. Discourage the practice because it contributes to constipation.
   d. Discourage the practice because it predisposes the client to fluid imbalance.
   Test-Taking Strategy: Note the key word and modifier, "best nursing response." Consider the pros and cons regarding restricting fluids to achieve continence, then select the option that is better than any of the others.

3. When applying an external condom catheter, which nursing action is correct?
   a. Lubricate the penis before applying the catheter.
   b. Measure the length and circumference of the penis.
   c. Leave space between the penis and the bottom of the catheter.
   d. Retract the foreskin and roll the catheter over the penis.
   Test-Taking Strategy: Note the key word, "correct." Review the choices and eliminate those that are incorrect.

4. When the nurse instructs a female client on the technique for collecting a clean-catch midstream urine specimen for routine urinalysis, which statement is correct?
   a. Cleanse the urethral area using several circular motions.
   b. Void into the plastic liner that is under the toilet seat.
   c. After voiding a small amount, collect a sample of urine.
   d. Mix the antimicrobial solution with the collected urine specimen.
   Test-Taking Strategy: Note the key word, "correct." Review the choices and eliminate those that are incorrect.

5. Identify the female urinary meatus by placing an X on the diagram.

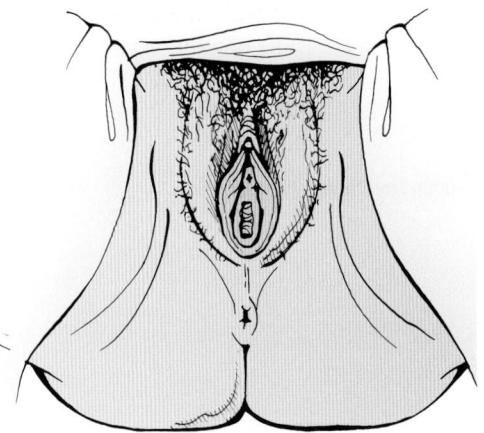

Test-Taking Strategy: Examine the diagram and identify anatomic structures. Mark the location where the nurse inserts a urinary catheter.

NEXT-GENERATION NCLEX-STYLE CLINICAL SCENARIO QUESTIONS

Clinical Scenario:
Nursing staff in a nursing home note that an 85-year-old female client frequently requires changes in her underclothing because she cannot ambulate to the toilet in time to void. The client is embarrassed because others notice a wet patch of urine on the floor and her wet outer garments.

1. Select all of the indicators that may suggest a cause for concern regarding the client's worry about incontinence.
   a. Frequently changing underclothing
   b. Not being able to ambulate to the bathroom
   c. Not drinking enough fluids throughout the day
   d. Drinking too many fluids prior to bedrest
   e. Smell of urine on the client's clothes
   f. Taking medicines that may cause incontinence

2. Place an "x" under "effective" identifying actions that would help the client with her incontinence. Place an "x" under "ineffective" identifying actions that may contribute to the client's incontinence.

ACTIONS	EFFECTIVE	INEFFECTIVE
Encourage the client to decrease the intake of beverages that contain caffeine or alcohol.		
Teach continence training to the client.		
Decrease the amount of fluids the clients drink.		
Assist the client to the toilet for the purpose of urination frequently.		
Change the client's diet.		
Keep a record of the frequency of voidings.		

SKILL 30-1 Placing and Removing a Bedpan

Suggested Action	Reason for Action
ASSESSMENT	
Ask the client if they feel the need to void.	Anticipates elimination needs
Palpate the lower abdomen for signs of bladder distention.	Indicates bladder fullness
Determine whether a fracture pan is necessary or if there are any restrictions in turning or lifting.	Prevents injury
PLANNING	
Gather needed supplies such as clean gloves, bedpan, toilet tissue, and a disposable pad.	Promotes organization and efficient time management
Warm the bedpan by running warm water over it, especially if it is made of metal.	Demonstrates concern for the client's comfort
IMPLEMENTATION	
Wash your hands or use an alcohol-based hand rub (see Chapter 10); put on clean gloves.	Reduces the transmission of microorganisms
Place the adjustable bed in high position.	Promotes the use of good body mechanics
Close the door and pull the privacy curtains.	Demonstrates concern for the client's right to privacy and dignity
Raise the top linen enough to determine the location of the client's hips and buttocks.	Prevents unnecessary exposure
Instruct the client to bend the knees and press down with the feet.	Helps elevate the hips
Place a disposable pad over the bottom sheets if necessary.	Protects bed linen from becoming wet and soiled
Slip the bedpan beneath the client's buttocks (Fig. A).	Ensures proper placement

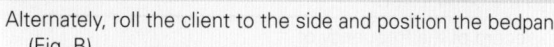

Placing a bedpan.

Suggested Action	Reason for Action
Alternately, roll the client to the side and position the bedpan (Fig. B).	Reduces work effort and the potential for a work-related injury; aids in placement if client cannot lift buttocks

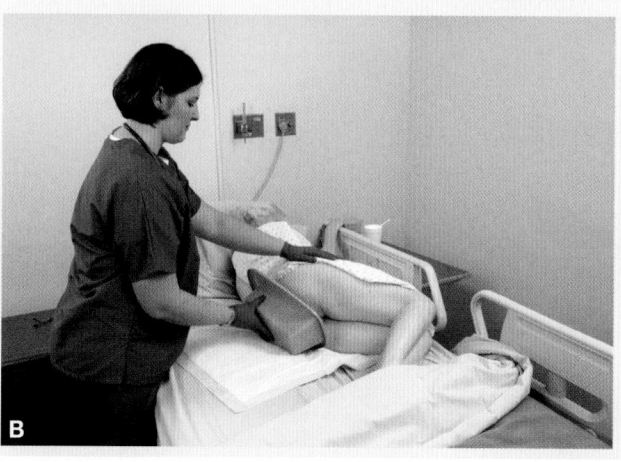

Placing a bedpan from a side-lying position.

SKILL 30-1 Placing and Removing a Bedpan (*continued*)

Suggested Action	Reason for Action
Raise the head of the bed (Fig. C).	Simulates the natural position for elimination
C	The position for elimination.
Ensure toilet tissue is within the client's reach.	Provides supplies for hygiene
Identify the location of the signal device and leave the client if doing so is safe.	Respects privacy yet provides a mechanism for communicating a need for assistance
Return and remove the bedpan.	Prevents discomfort
Assist with removing residue of urine from the skin if necessary.	Prevents offensive odors and skin irritation
Wrap the gloved hand with toilet tissue and wipe from the meatus of a female toward the anal area.	Supports principles of medical asepsis
Place soiled tissue in the bedpan unless it requires measuring.	Contains soiled tissue until the time of disposal
Help the client into a comfortable position.	Ensures the client's well-being
Provide supplies for hand hygiene.	Removes residue from elimination and colonizing microorganisms
Measure the volume of urine if the client's intake and output are being monitored.	Ensures accurate data collection
Save a sample of urine if it appears abnormal in any way.	Facilitates laboratory examination or further assessment
Empty the urine into a toilet and flush.	Facilitates disposal
Clean the bedpan and replace it in a place that is separate from clean supplies.	Supports the principles of asepsis
Remove gloves and repeat hand hygiene.	Removes colonizing microorganisms

EVALUATION

- Bedpan is positioned without injury.
- Urine is eliminated.
- Hygiene measures are performed.

DOCUMENT

- Volume of urine eliminated (for monitoring intake and output)
- Appearance and other characteristics of the urine

SAMPLE DOCUMENTATION

Date and Time Assisted to use the bedpan. Voided 300 mL of clear, amber urine without difficulty.
—————————————————— J. Doe, LPN

SKILL 30-2 Applying a Condom Catheter

Suggested Action	Reason for Action
ASSESSMENT	
Wash your hands or use an alcohol-based hand rub (see Chapter 10).	Reduces the potential for transmitting microorganisms
Assess the penis for swelling or skin breakdown.	Provides data for future comparison or a basis for using some other method for urine collection
Determine the client's understanding about the application and use of an external catheter.	Provides an opportunity for health teaching
Verify the client's willingness to use a condom catheter.	Respects the client's right to participate in making decisions
Check the medical record to determine whether the client has a latex allergy.	Maintains client safety and prevents possible allergic reaction
PLANNING	
Gather supplies such as soap, water, a towel, a condom catheter, drainage tubing, a collection device, and clean gloves. Some devices come packaged with an adhesive strip or Velcro for securing the catheter.	Promotes organization and efficient time management
Provide privacy.	Demonstrates respect for the client's dignity
Place the client in a supine position and cover them with a bath blanket.	Facilitates the application of the catheter and maintains privacy
IMPLEMENTATION	
Wash your hands or use an alcohol-based hand rub (see Chapter 10) and put on clean gloves.	Reduces the transmission of microorganisms and follows standard precautions
Wash and dry the penis well.	Promotes skin integrity
Wind the adhesive strip in an upward spiral around the penis (Fig. A).	Reduces the potential for restricting blood flow

Applying the adhesive strip in a spiral.

Ensure that the wider end of the condom catheter is rolled to the narrower tip (Fig. B).	Facilitates application to the penis

A rolled condom sheath.

SKILL 30-2 Applying a Condom Catheter (*continued*)

Suggested Action	Reason for Action
Hold ~1–2 in (2.5–5 cm) of the lower sheath below the tip of the penis and unroll the sheath upward (Fig. C).	Leaves space below the urethra to prevent the irritation of the meatus
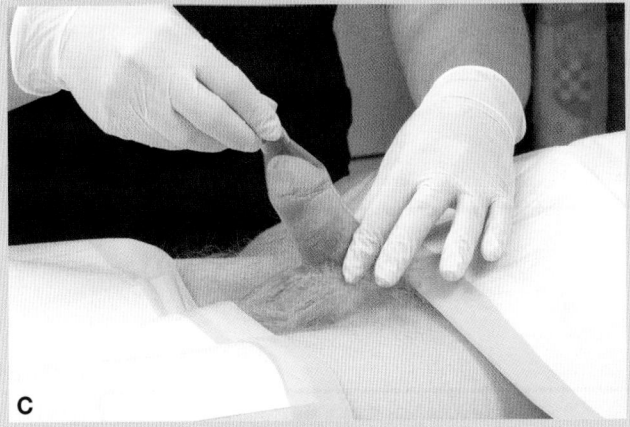

C | Unrolling the condom catheter sheath over the penis. |
| Secure the upper end of the unrolled sheath to the skin firmly with a second strip of adhesive or a Velcro strap, but not so tight as to interfere with circulation (Fig. D).

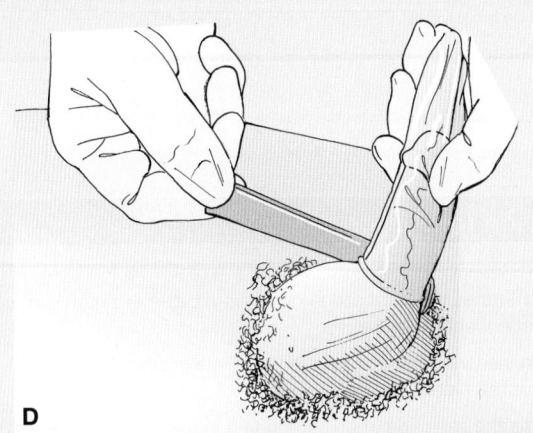

D | Ensures the catheter will remain in place

Securing a condom catheter. |
| Connect the drainage tip to a drainage collection device (Fig. E).

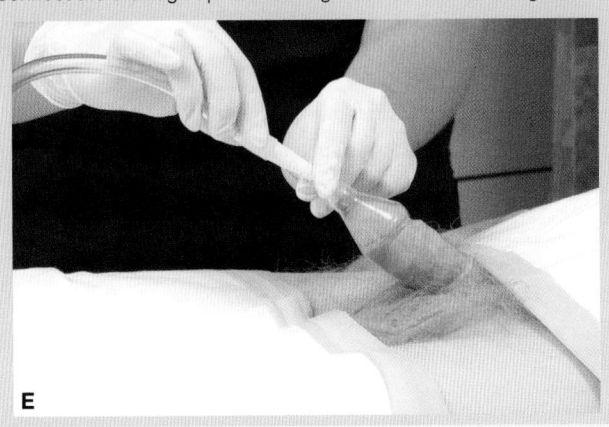

E | Allows for urine drainage and collection

Connecting the condom catheter to a drainage collection system. |
Keep the penis in a downward position.	Promotes urinary drainage
Assess the penis at least every 2 hours.	Ensures prompt attention to signs of impaired circulation
Check that the catheter has not become twisted.	Maintains catheter patency
Empty the leg bag, if one is used, as it becomes partially filled with urine.	Ensures that the catheter will not be pulled from the penis by the weight of the collected urine
Remove and change the catheter daily or more often if it becomes loose or tight.	Maintains skin integrity

(*continued*)

SKILL 30-2 Applying a Condom Catheter (*continued*)

Suggested Action	Reason for Action
Substitute a waterproof garment during periods of nonuse.	Provides a mechanism for absorbing urine
Wash the catheter and collection bag with mild soap and water and rinse with a 1:7 solution of vinegar and water.	Extends the use of the equipment and reduces offensive odors

EVALUATION

- Catheter remains attached to the penis.
- Penis exhibits no evidence of skin breakdown, swelling, or impaired circulation.
- Linen and clothing remain dry.

DOCUMENT

- Preapplication assessment data
- Hygiene measures performed
- Time of catheter application
- Content of teaching
- Postapplication assessment data

SAMPLE DOCUMENTATION

Date and Time Penis washed with soap and water. Penile skin is intact. No discoloration or lesions noted. Condom catheter applied and connected to a leg bag. Instructed to report any swelling or local discomfort. _____ J. Doe, LPN

SKILL 30-3 Inserting a Foley Catheter in a Female Client

Suggested Action	Reason for Action
ASSESSMENT	
Check the client's record to verify that a medical order has been written.	Demonstrates the legal scope of nursing; catheterization is not an independent measure
Inspect the medical record to determine whether the client has a latex allergy.	Determines whether it is safe to use a latex catheter or if a latex-free type is needed
Determine the type of catheter that has been prescribed.	Ensures the selection of an appropriate catheter
Review the client's record for documentation of genitourinary problems.	Provides data by which to modify the procedure or equipment
Assess the client's age, size, and mobility.	Influences the size of the catheter and the need for additional assistance
Assess the time of the last voiding.	Indicates how full the bladder may be
Determine how much the client understands about catheterization.	Provides an opportunity for health teaching
Familiarize yourself with the anatomic landmarks (Fig. A).	Facilitates insertion in the appropriate location

Clitoris
Urinary meatus
Labia minora
Labia majora
Vagina
Anus

Female anatomic landmarks.

A

SKILL 30-3 Inserting a Foley Catheter in a Female Client (*continued*)

Suggested Action	Reason for Action
PLANNING	
Gather supplies, which include a catheterization kit, a bath blanket, and additional light if necessary.	Promotes organization and efficient time management
IMPLEMENTATION	
Close the door and pull the privacy curtain.	Demonstrates concern for the client's dignity
Raise the bed to a high position.	Prevents back strain
Wash your hands or use an alcohol-based hand rub (see Chapter 10).	Reduces the potential for transmitting microorganisms
Cover the client with a bath blanket and pull the top linen to the bottom of the bed.	Avoids unnecessary exposure
Position an additional light at the bottom of the bed or ask an assistant to hold a flashlight.	Ensures good visualization
Use the corners of the bath blanket to cover each leg.	Provides warmth and maintains modesty
Place the client in a dorsal recumbent position with the feet about 2 ft apart (Fig. B).	Provides access to the female urinary system

A client draped and placed in a dorsal recumbent position.

Use a lateral or Sims position for clients who have difficulty maintaining a dorsal recumbent position.	Provides access to the female urinary system, but neither is the preferred position
If the client is soiled, put on gloves, wash the client, remove gloves, and perform hand hygiene measures again.	Supports the principles of asepsis
Remove the wrapper from the catheterization kit and position it nearby.	Provides a receptacle for collecting soiled supplies
Unwrap the sterile cover to maintain the sterility of the supplies inside (see Chapter 10) (Fig. C).	Prevents contamination and the potential for infection

Opening the sterile catheter tray.

Remove and put on the packaged sterile gloves (see Chapter 10).	Facilitates handling the remaining equipment without transferring microorganisms

(continued)

SKILL 30-3 Inserting a Foley Catheter in a Female Client (*continued*)

Suggested Action	Reason for Action
Remove the sterile towel from the kit and place it beneath the client's hips (Fig. D).	Provides a sterile field

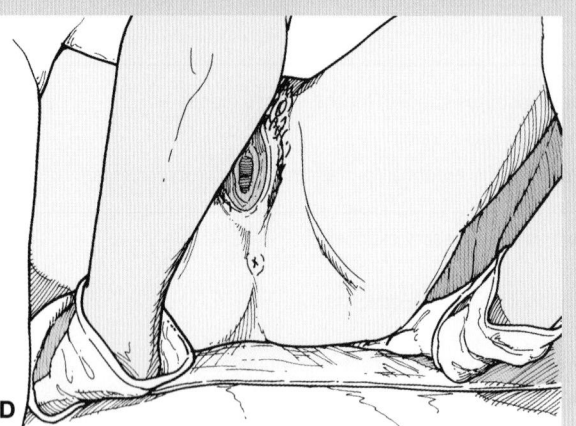

Placing a sterile towel.

Suggested Action	Reason for Action
Place a **fenestrated drape** (one with an open circle in its center) over the perineum (Fig. E).	Provides a sterile field

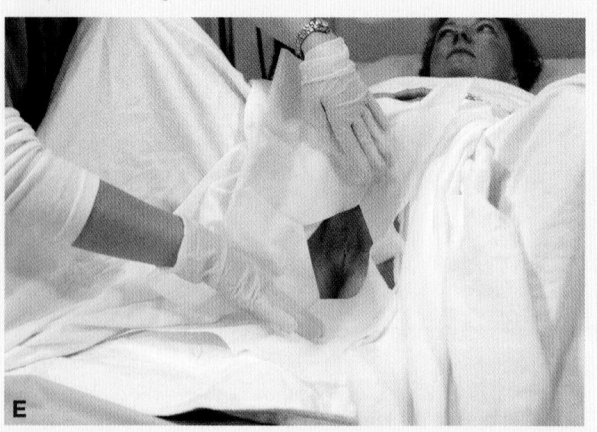

Placing a fenestrated drape over the perineum.

Suggested Action	Reason for Action
Open and pour the packet of antiseptic solution (Betadine) over the cotton balls. Spread lubricant on the tip of the catheter (Fig. F).	Prepares the sterile supplies before contaminating one of two hands later in the procedure

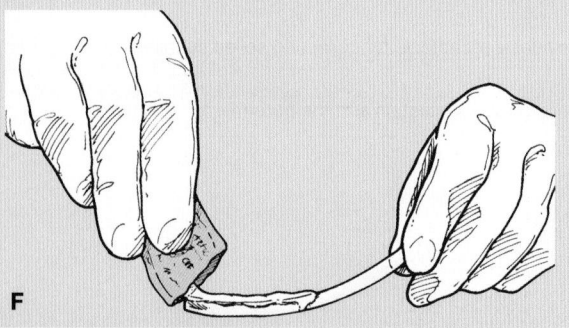

Lubricating the catheter.

Suggested Action	Reason for Action
Place the catheterization tray on top of the sterile towel between the client's legs.	Promotes access to supplies and reduces the potential for contamination
Pick up a moistened cotton ball with the sterile forceps and wipe one side of the labia majora from an anterior to posterior direction.	Cleanses outer skin before cleansing deeper areas of tissue
Discard the soiled cotton ball in the outer wrapper of the catheterization kit; repeat cleansing the other side of the labia majora.	Completes the bilateral outer cleansing

SKILL 30-3 Inserting a Foley Catheter in a Female Client (*continued*)

Suggested Action	Reason for Action
Separate the labia majora and minora with the thumb and fingers of the nondominant hand, exposing the urinary meatus (Fig. G).	Facilitates the visualization of anatomic landmarks and prevents contaminating the catheter during insertion
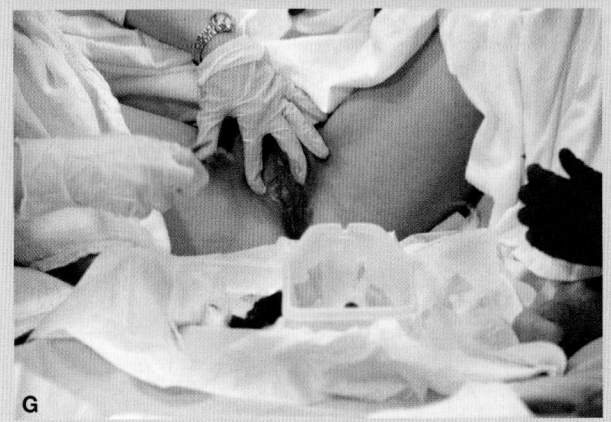 G	Separating the labia.
Consider the hand separating the labia to be contaminated.	Avoids transferring microorganisms to sterile equipment and supplies
Clean each side of the labia minora with a separate cotton ball while continuing to retract the tissue with the nondominant hand.	Removes colonizing microorganisms
Use the last cotton ball to wipe centrally, starting above the meatus down toward the vagina (Fig. H).	Completes the cleaning of external structures
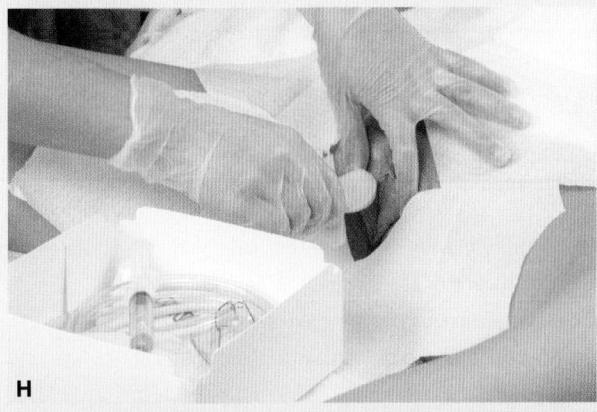 H	Wiping from above the meatus downward.
Discard the forceps with the last cotton ball into the wrapper for contaminated supplies.	Follows the principles of asepsis
Keep the clean tissue separated.	Prevents recontamination
Pick up the catheter, holding it ~3–4 in (7.5–10 cm) from its tip (Fig. I).	Facilitates control during insertion
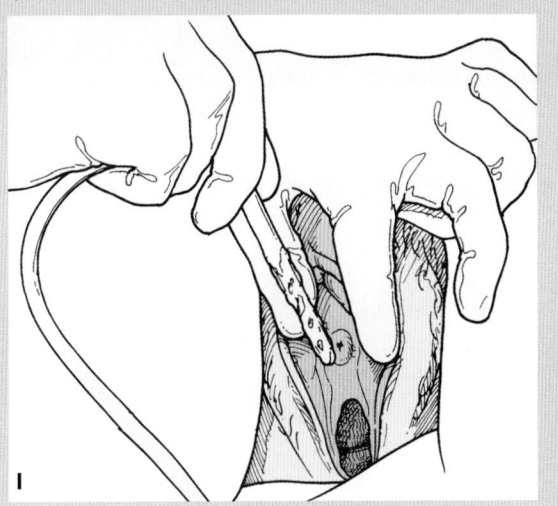 I	Preparing to insert the catheter.

(continued)

SKILL 30-3 Inserting a Foley Catheter in a Female Client (*continued*)

Suggested Action	Reason for Action
Insert the tip of the catheter into the meatus ~2–3 in (5–7.5 cm) or until urine begins to flow.	Locates the tip beyond the length of the female urethra, which is ~1.5–2.5 in (4–6.5 cm)
Recheck anatomic landmarks if there is no evidence of urine; remove an incorrectly placed catheter and repeat using another sterile catheter.	Indicates one of two possibilities: either the bladder is empty or the catheter has been placed within the vagina by mistake; ensures sterility of equipment
Advance the catheter another 0.5–1 in (1.3–2.5 cm) after urine begins to flow.	Ensures that the catheter is well within the bladder where the balloon can be safely inflated
Direct the end of the catheter so that it drains into the equipment tray or specimen container.	Avoids wetting the linens
Hold the catheter in place with the fingers and thumb that were separating the labia.	Stabilizes the catheter externally
Pick up the prefilled syringe with the sterile, dominant hand, insert it into the opening of the balloon, and instill the fluid (Fig. J).	Stabilizes the catheter internally

J

Inflating the balloon.

Suggested Action	Reason for Action
Withdraw the fluid from the balloon if the client describes feeling pain or discomfort, advance the catheter a little more, and try again.	Prevents internal injury
Tug gently on the catheter after the balloon has been filled.	Tests whether the catheter is well anchored within the bladder
Connect the catheter to a urine collection bag.	Provides a means of assessing the urine and its volume
Wipe the meatus and labia of any residual lubricant.	Demonstrates concern for the client's comfort
Secure the catheter to the leg with tape or other commercial device (Fig. K).	Prevents pulling on the balloon within the catheter

K

Securing the catheter to the thigh.

Suggested Action	Reason for Action
Hang the collection bag below the level of the bladder; coil excess tubing on the mattress.	Ensures gravity drainage
Discard the catheterization tray and wrapper with soiled supplies.	Follows the principles of asepsis
Remove your gloves and perform hand hygiene.	Removes colonizing microorganisms
Remove the drape, restore the top sheets, make the client comfortable, and lower the bed.	Restores comfort and safety

SKILL 30-3 Inserting a Foley Catheter in a Female Client (*continued*)

Suggested Action	Reason for Action

EVALUATION

- The catheter is inserted under aseptic conditions.
- The urine is draining from the catheter.
- The client exhibits no evidence of discomfort during or after the insertion.

DOCUMENT

- Preassessment data
- Size and type of catheter
- Amount and appearance of urine
- Client's response

SAMPLE DOCUMENTATION

Date and Time   Unable to void in past 8 hours. Bladder feels distended. Dr. Peter notified. 16-F Foley catheter inserted per order and connected to gravity drainage. 550 mL of urine drained from bladder at this time. Urine appears light amber. No discomfort reported. _____ J. Doe, LPN

SKILL 30-4 Inserting a Foley Catheter in a Male Client

Suggested Action	Reason for Action
ASSESSMENT	
Check the client's record to verify that a medical order has been written.	Demonstrates the legal scope of nursing; catheterization is not an independent measure
Inspect the medical record to determine if the client has a latex allergy.	Determines whether it is safe to use a latex catheter or if a latex-free type is needed
Determine the type of catheter that has been prescribed.	Ensures the selection of the appropriate catheter
Review the client's record for documentation of genitourinary problems.	Provides data by which to modify the procedure or equipment
Assess the client's age, size, and mobility.	Influences the size of the catheter and need for additional assistance
Assess the time of the last voiding.	Indicates the potential fullness of the bladder
Determine how much the client understands about catheterization.	Provides an opportunity for health teaching
Familiarize yourself with the anatomic landmarks (Fig. A, diagrams a and b).	Facilitates insertion

a: Coronal ridge, Glans penis, Scrotum. *b*: Foreskin (prepuce), Urethral meatus. A

(*continued*)

SKILL 30-4 Inserting a Foley Catheter in a Male Client (*continued*)

Suggested Action	Reason for Action
PLANNING	
Gather supplies, which include a catheterization kit, a bath blanket, and additional light.	Promotes organization and efficient time management
IMPLEMENTATION	
Close the door and pull the privacy curtain.	Demonstrates concern for the client's dignity
Raise the bed to a high position.	Prevents back strain
Perform handwashing or use an alcohol-based hand rub (see Chapter 10).	Reduces the potential for transmitting microorganisms
Place the client in a supine position.	Provides access to the male urinary system
Cover the client's upper body with a bath blanket and lower the top linen to expose just the penis.	Provides minimal exposure
Position an additional light at the bottom of the bed or ask an assistant to hold a flashlight.	Ensures good visualization
If the client is soiled, put on gloves, wash the client, remove gloves, and repeat hand hygiene measures.	Supports the principles of asepsis
Remove the wrapper from the catheterization kit and position it nearby.	Provides a receptacle for collecting soiled supplies
Unwrap the sterile inner cover so as to maintain the sterility of the supplies inside (see Chapter 10).	Prevents contamination and the potential for infection
Remove and put on the packaged sterile gloves (see Chapter 10).	Facilitates handling the remaining equipment without transferring microorganisms
Place the fenestrated drape over the client's penis without touching the upper surface of the drape (Fig. B).	Provides a sterile field

Bath blanket
Drape
Sheet

Placing a fenestrated drape.

B

Open and pour the packet of antiseptic solution (Betadine) over the cotton balls.	Prepares sterile supplies before contaminating one of two hands later in the procedure
Place the catheterization tray between the client's thighs.	Promotes ease of access to supplies and reduces the potential for contamination
Lift the penis at its base with the nondominant hand; retract the foreskin if the client is uncircumcised.	Promotes visualization and support during catheter insertion
Consider the gloved hand holding the penis to be contaminated.	Avoids transferring microorganisms to sterile equipment and supplies

SKILL 30-4 Inserting a Foley Catheter in a Male Client (*continued*)

Suggested Action	Reason for Action
Pick up a moistened cotton ball with the sterile forceps and wipe the penis in a circular manner from the meatus toward the base; repeat using a different cotton ball each time (Fig. C).	Moves microorganisms away from the meatus

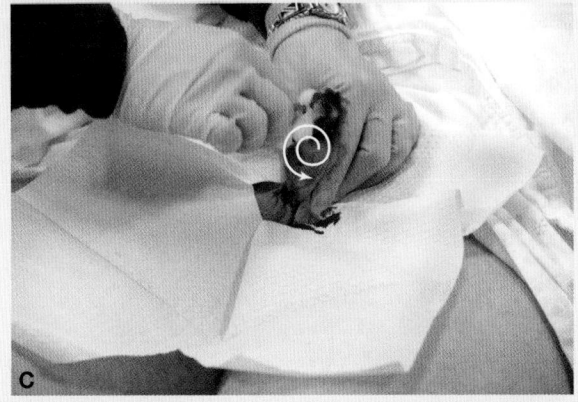

C

Cleaning the penis.

Discard the forceps with the last cotton ball into the wrapper for contaminated supplies.	Follows the principles of asepsis
Apply gentle traction to the penis by pulling it straight up with the nondominant gloved hand.	Straightens the urethra
Instill the contents of a prefilled syringe containing 5–10 mL of water-soluble lubricant or water-soluble 2% lidocaine gel directly through the meatus into the urethra (Fig. D).	Avoids trauma to the urethra caused by insufficient lubrication; this technique replaces the traditional practice of lubricating the outer surface of the catheter, which resulted in its accumulation at the meatus only (Gerard & Sueppel, 1997; Society of Urologic Nurses and Associates, 2021)

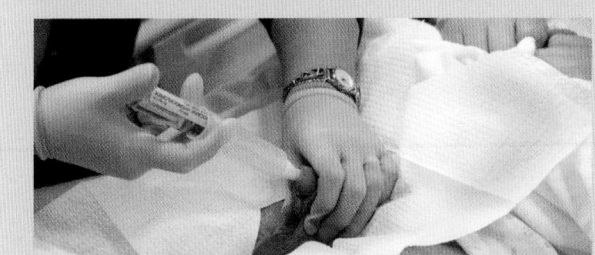

D

Instilling lubricant.

Insert but never force the catheter; rather, rotate the catheter, apply more traction to the penis, encourage the client to breathe deeply, or angle the penis toward the toes (Fig. E).	Adjusts for passing the catheter beyond the prostate gland

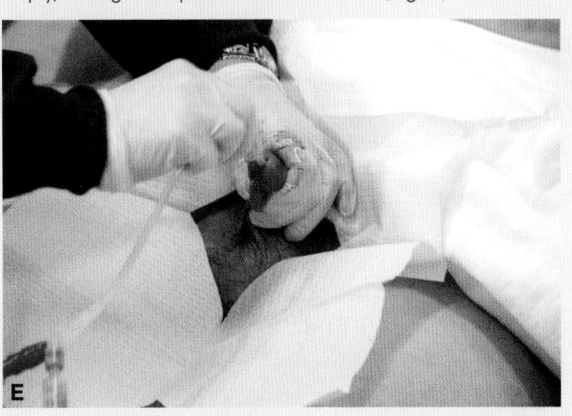

E

Catheter insertion.

Continue insertion until only the inflation and drainage ports are exposed and urine flows.	Locates the tip beyond the length of the male urethra

(*continued*)

SKILL 30-4 Inserting a Foley Catheter in a Male Client (*continued*)

Suggested Action	Reason for Action
Pick up the prefilled syringe with the sterile, dominant hand, insert it into the opening of the balloon, and instill the fluid (Fig. F).	Stabilizes the catheter internally
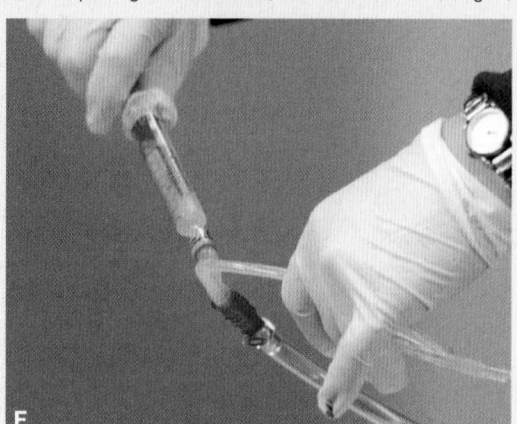	Inflating the balloon.
Withdraw the fluid from the balloon if the client describes feeling pain or discomfort, advance the catheter a little more, and try again.	Prevents internal injury
Tug gently on the catheter after the balloon has been filled.	Tests whether the catheter is well anchored within the bladder
Connect the catheter to a urine collection bag.	Provides a means of assessing the urine and its volume
Wipe the meatus and penis of any residual lubricant.	Demonstrates concern for the client's comfort
Secure the catheter to the leg or abdomen with tape or other commercial device (Fig. G).	Prevents pulling on the balloon within the catheter
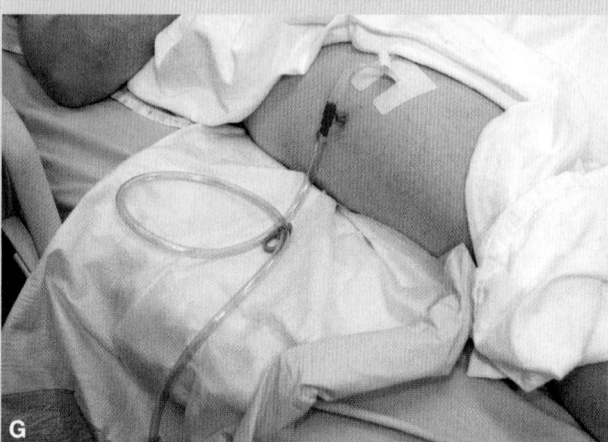	Securing a catheter.
Hang the collection bag below the level of the bladder; coil excess tubing on the mattress.	Ensures gravity drainage
Discard the catheterization tray and wrapper with soiled supplies.	Follows the principles of asepsis
Remove your gloves and repeat hand hygiene measures.	Removes colonizing microorganisms
Remove the drape, restore the top sheets, make the client comfortable, and lower the bed.	Restores comfort and safety

---

SKILL 30-4 Inserting a Foley Catheter in a Male Client (*continued*)

Suggested Action	Reason for Action

EVALUATION

- The catheter is inserted under aseptic conditions.
- The urine is draining from the catheter.
- The client demonstrates no evidence of discomfort during or after insertion.

DOCUMENT

- Preassessment data
- Size and type of catheter
- Amount and appearance of urine
- Client's response

SAMPLE DOCUMENTATION

Date and Time 16 F Foley catheter inserted before surgery according to preoperative orders. 350 mL of urine obtained before connecting the catheter to gravity drainage. Urine appears light yellow and clear. _____ J. Doe, LPN

SKILL 30-5 Irrigating a Foley Catheter

Suggested Action	Reason for Action
ASSESSMENT	
Check the client's record to verify that a medical order has been written.	Demonstrates the legal scope of nursing; a catheter irrigation is not an independent measure
Verify the type of irrigating solution prescribed, or follow the standard for practice, which usually advises using sterile normal saline solution.	Complies with the medical directives or standards of care
Assess the urine characteristics.	Provides a baseline for assessing the outcome of the procedure
Determine how much the client understands about a catheter irrigation.	Provides an opportunity for health teaching
Locate the port on the drainage tube through which fluid can be instilled (Fig. A).	Ensures a safe procedure and maintains the integrity of the catheter
A	Identifying the self-sealing irrigation port.
PLANNING	
Gather necessary equipment and supplies: an irrigation kit, a flask of sterile irrigating solution, a 30- to 60-mL syringe, and alcohol swabs.	Promotes organization and efficient time management

(continued)

SKILL 30-5 Irrigating a Foley Catheter (*continued*)

Suggested Action	Reason for Action
IMPLEMENTATION	
Wash hands or use an alcohol-based hand rub (see Chapter 10).	Follows the principles of asepsis and standards of practice
Raise the height of the bed.	Reduces back strain
Pull the privacy curtain.	Demonstrates concern for the client's dignity
Add 100–200 mL of solution to the irrigating basin.	Avoids contaminating and wasting all the solution in the flask
Put on gloves kept at the bedside or within the irrigation kit.	Complies with standard precautions
Fill the syringe with 30–60 mL of solution (Fig. B).	Provides a means for penetrating the self-sealing port

B

Filling the syringe with solution.

Clean the port on the catheter with an alcohol swab (Fig. C).	Removes gross debris and colonizing microorganisms

C

Cleaning the irrigation port.

Clamp or kink the tubing below the port through which the irrigating solution will be instilled (Fig. D).	Ensures that the solution will move forward into the catheter and not into the drainage system

D

Clamping the drainage tubing.

SKILL 30-5 Irrigating a Foley Catheter (*continued*)

Suggested Action	Reason for Action
While holding the catheter with one hand, insert the syringe into the port (Fig. E).	Maintains sterility
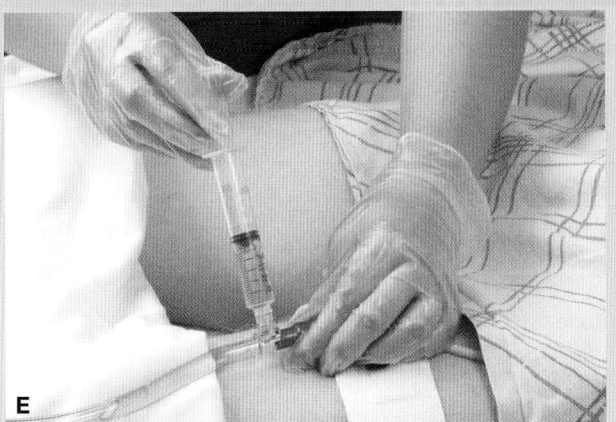	Instilling the irrigation solution.
Gently instill the solution.	Clears the catheter of debris and dilutes particles within the catheter
Remove the syringe.	Prevents leaking
Release the clamp from the drainage tubing and observe the flow of urine through the tubing (Fig. F).	Facilitates gravity drainage
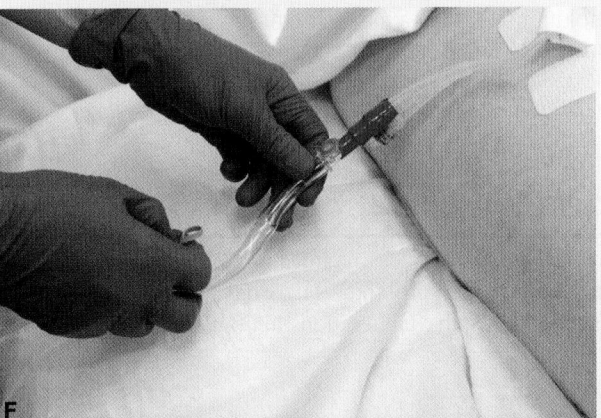	Draining the irrigation solution.
Repeat the instillation and drainage if the urine appears to contain appreciable debris.	Promotes patency
Record the volume of instilled solution as fluid intake.	Maintains accurate assessment data
Discard or protect the sterility of the irrigating equipment, which may be reused for the next 24 hours as long as it is not contaminated.	Complies with the principles of infection control

EVALUATION

- The prescribed amount and type of solution are instilled.
- The principles of asepsis have been maintained.
- The urine continues to drain well through the catheter.
- The client reports no discomfort.

DOCUMENT

- Preassessment data
- Volume and type of solution
- Volume and appearance of drainage

SAMPLE DOCUMENTATION

Date and Time Urine appears amber with some evidence of white particles. 60 mL of sterile normal saline solution instilled into catheter. 120 mL drainage returned. Urine appears to have less sediment. Catheter remains patent.
————————————————————— J. Doe, LPN

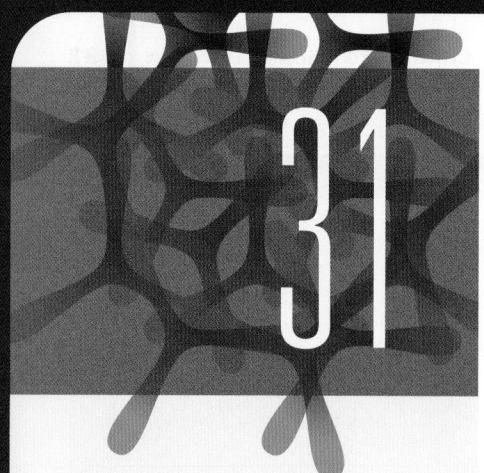

Bowel Elimination

Words To Know
anal sphincters
appliance
colonography
colonoscopy
colostomy
constipation
continent ostomy
defecation
diarrhea
enema
enterostomal therapist
excoriation
fecal immunochemical test (FIT)
fecal impaction
fecal incontinence
fecal occult blood test (FOBT)
feces
flatulence
flatus
gastrocolic reflex
globin
heme
ileostomy
melena
ostomy
peristalsis
retention enema
sigmoidoscopy
stoma
suppository
Valsalva maneuver

Learning Objectives

On completion of this chapter, the reader should be able to:

1. Describe the process of defecation.
2. Name components of a bowel elimination assessment.
3. List common alterations in bowel elimination.
4. Name types of constipation.
5. Identify measures within the scope of nursing practice for treating constipation.
6. Identify interventions that promote bowel elimination when it does not occur naturally.
7. Name categories of enema administration.
8. List common solutions used in a cleansing enema.
9. Explain the purpose of an oil retention enema.
10. Describe nursing activities involved in ostomy care.

INTRODUCTION

This chapter briefly reviews the process of intestinal elimination and discusses nursing measures to help promote it. It also describes nursing skills that may assist clients who have alterations in bowel elimination.

Gerontologic Considerations

■ Age-related changes, such as a loss of elasticity in the intestinal walls and slower motility throughout the gastrointestinal (GI) tract, predispose older adults to constipation. Such changes alone, however, do not cause constipation. Other factors, such as adverse medication effects, diminished physical activity, and diets that are low in fiber, fresh fruits, and vegetables, contribute to the development of constipation.

■ If older adults use laxatives or enemas, it is important to teach about healthier alternatives, such as increasing dietary fiber, for example, by incorporating more fresh fruits and vegetables in the daily diet. A natural laxative, such as "power pudding," consists of 1 cup wheat bran, 1 cup applesauce, and 1 cup prune juice. Ingredients can be mixed thoroughly and refrigerated. The older person can begin with 1 tbsp per day and increase the amount by small increments daily until ease of bowel movement is achieved and no disagreeable symptoms occur.

■ Older adults may have benign lesions such as hemorrhoids or polyps in the lower bowel, which may interfere with the passage of stool. If the digital removal of an impaction is required, gentle manipulation within the rectum should be used to prevent bleeding and tissue trauma.

■ Diarrhea can easily lead to dehydration and electrolyte imbalances (especially hypokalemia) in older adults, who tend to have less body fluid reserve than younger people.

■ Musculoskeletal disorders, such as arthritis of the hands or neurologic disorders, may interfere with an older person's ability to care for an ostomy appliance or perform colostomy irrigations.

■ An occupational or enterostomal therapist can offer suggestions for promoting self-care. In addition, a wound, ostomy, and continence nurse may be available for consultation and patient teaching.

DEFECATION

Defecation (bowel elimination) is the act of expelling **feces** (stool) from the body. To do so, all structures of the GI tract, especially the components of the large intestine (also referred to as the *bowel* or *colon*), must function in a coordinated manner (Fig. 31-1). In the large intestine, 10% or approximately a pint to a quart of water is removed from the remnants of digestion, causing the bowel's contents to become a consolidated mass of residue before being eliminated.

Peristalsis is the rhythmic contractions of intestinal smooth muscle that facilitate defecation. Peristalsis moves fiber, water, and nutritional wastes along the ascending, transverse, descending, and sigmoid colon toward the rectum. Peristalsis becomes even more active during eating; this increased peristaltic activity is called the **gastrocolic reflex**.

The gastrocolic reflex usually precedes defecation. Its accelerated wave-like movements, sometimes perceived as slight abdominal cramping, propel stool forward, packing it within the rectum. As the rectum distends, the person feels the urge to defecate. Stool is eventually released when the **anal sphincters** (ring-shaped bands of muscles) relax. Performing the **Valsalva maneuver** (closing the glottis and contracting the pelvic and abdominal muscles to increase abdominal pressure) facilitates this process. Several dietary, physical, social, and emotional factors can influence the bowel's mechanical function (Table 31-1).

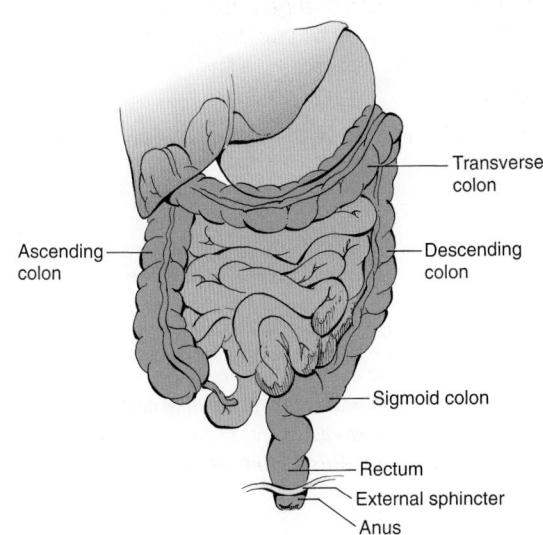

FIGURE 31-1 The large intestine.

TABLE 31-1 Common Factors Affecting Bowel Elimination	
FACTOR	**EFFECT**
Types of food consumed	Influence color, odor, volume, and consistency of stool as well as fecal velocity
Fluid intake	Influences moisture content of stool
Drugs	Slow or speed motility
Emotions	Alter bowel motility
Neuromuscular function	Affects the ability to control rectal muscles
Abdominal muscle tone	Affects the ability to increase intra-abdominal pressure (Valsalva maneuver)
Opportunity for defecation	Inhibits or facilitates elimination

ASSESSMENT OF BOWEL ELIMINATION

A comprehensive assessment of bowel elimination involves collecting data about the client's elimination patterns (bowel habits) and the actual characteristics of the feces.

Elimination Patterns

Because various elimination patterns can be normal, it is essential to determine the client's usual patterns, including the frequency of elimination, the effort required to expel stool, and what elimination aids, if any, they use. Health education regarding bowel elimination includes the following points: (1) adults should identify their own patterns of bowel regularity, which can range from three times a day to three times a week; (2) include daily exercise; (3) eat high-fiber foods on a regular basis; (4) drink 8 to 10 glasses of liquid a day (unless contraindicated); and (5) respond to the urge to defecate as soon as possible.

 Nutrition Notes

■ Fiber is found only in plant foods, most abundantly in wheat bran, whole grains (e.g., brown rice, whole wheat bread, oatmeal), dried peas and beans (e.g., kidney beans, garbanzo beans, lentils), and the skins and seeds of fresh fruits and vegetables (e.g., pears and apples).

■ Eating a variety of high-fiber foods is recommended. Americans consume approximately half the recommended amount of fiber daily. Tolerance to a high-fiber diet may improve by increasing fiber intake gradually.

■ Adequate fluid is needed for maximum benefit.

Stool Characteristics

Health care providers can obtain objective data about stool characteristics by inspecting the stool or asking the client to describe its appearance. Information that is particularly diagnostic includes stool color, odor, consistency, shape, and unusual components (Table 31-2). Any change in bowel elimination that does not respond to simple dietary or lifestyle changes requires further investigation.

TABLE 31-2 Characteristics of Stool

CHARACTERISTIC	NORMAL	ABNORMAL
Color	Brown	Black
		Clay colored (tan)
		Yellow
		Green
Odor	Aromatic	Foul
Consistency	Soft, formed	Soft, bulky
		Hard, dry
		Watery
		Paste like
Shape	Round, full	Unformed
		Flat
		Pencil shaped
		Stone like
Components	Undigested fiber	Worms
		Blood
		Pus
		Mucus

Whenever stool appears abnormal, a sample is saved in a covered container for the physician's inspection. In some instances, nurses may independently perform screening tests on stool samples, such as those that determine the presence of blood (Nursing Guidelines 31-1). Nurses

then report the results, which can be falsely positive, to the physician, who may order more specific laboratory or diagnostic tests.

Testing for Colorectal Disorders

The incidence of colorectal cancer increases with age; it is the third most common cancer diagnosed in the United States and the second most common cause of death from cancer among men and women combined (American Cancer Society, 2023). An early sign of colorectal cancer is a change in bowel elimination patterns and stool characteristics. Blood in stool (**melena**) is an abnormal characteristic that may be invisible to the naked eye. The death rate from colorectal cancer has decreased among both men and women for the past several decades. There are a number of possible reasons for this, including detection of polyps during screening, leading to early removal and improved colorectal cancer treatment (American Cancer Society, 2023).

Fecal Occult Blood Test

A **fecal occult blood test (FOBT)**, a self-collected screening test from three separate stools, may be obtained by clients to detect **heme**, an iron compound in blood present within stool as it passes through the small and large intestines. An FOBT requires some drug and dietary restrictions prior to collecting samples of stool (Client and Family Teaching 31-1).

 NURSING GUIDELINES 31-1

Testing Stool for Occult Blood

- Collect stool within a toilet liner or bedpan. *Use of such devices prevents mixing stool with water or urine.*
- Put on gloves and use an applicator stick to collect the specimen. *These measures reduce the transmission of microorganisms.*
- Take a sample from the center area of the stool. *A sample from here provides more diagnostic value because it is not superficially tainted with blood from local tissue.*
- Apply a thin smear of stool onto the test area supplied with the screening kit (Fig. A). *Correct use of the kit ensures thorough contact with the chemical reagent.*

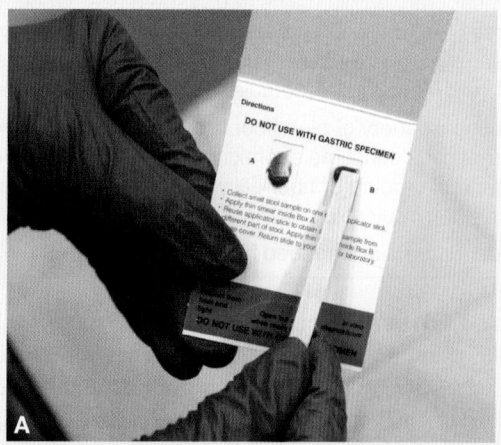

Stool is applied to the paper within the test kit. (From Wolters Kluwer Health. [2013]. *Lippincott's visual encyclopedia of clinical skills.* Wolters Kluwer Health.)

- Cover the entire test space. *Doing so ensures more accurate findings.*
- Place two drops of the chemical reagent onto the test space (Fig. B). *This step promotes a chemical reaction.*

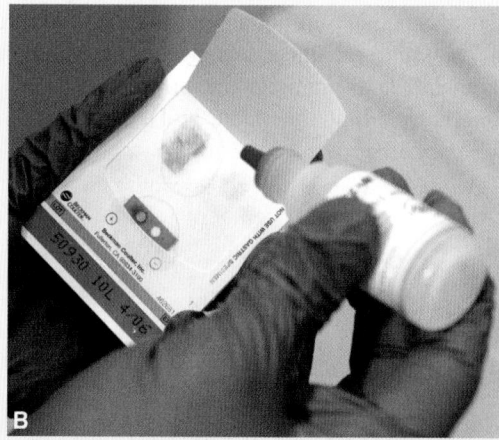

A drop of chemical reagent is applied to the collected stool specimen. (From Wolters Kluwer Health. [2013]. *Lippincott's visual encyclopedia of clinical skills.* Wolters Kluwer Health.)

- Wait for 60 seconds. *This duration is the time needed for chemical interaction with the stool.*
- Observe for a blue color. *This finding indicates blood is present.*

Client and Family Teaching 31-1
Preparation for Collecting a Fecal Occult Blood Test

The nurse teaches the client to do the following:

• Stop taking nonsteroidal antiinflammatory drugs (NSAIDs), such as more than one adult aspirin, ibuprofen, or naproxen, for 7 days before self-collecting stool. Acetaminophen (Tylenol) can be taken as needed.

• Avoid taking more than 250 mg of vitamin C or consuming citrus fruits or juices for 3 days before beginning the test.

• Eat a high-fiber diet containing whole grains; cook vegetables and fruits well.

• Refrain from eating red meat for 3 days before testing; poultry and fish are allowed.

• Do not eat raw turnips, radishes, broccoli, beets, carrots, cauliflower, cucumbers, or mushrooms for 2 to 3 days before the test.

Fecal Immunochemical Test

A **fecal immunochemical test (FIT)** uses antibodies to detect blood in the stool. It is done once a year in the same way as an FOBT (MedlinePlus, 2023). The FIT is more specific than an FOBT because it uses antibodies to detect **globin**, a protein removed from heme, which is present exclusively in the lower intestine. Advantages of the FIT test are that there are no dietary or medication restrictions, only one or two specimens need to be collected, and it has a high rate of specificity for colorectal cancer (MedlinePlus, 2023). Collection of the specimen and application to a test card are similar to FOBT.

Stool DNA Test

The FIT-DNA test, also referred to as the *stool DNA test*, combines FIT with a test that detects altered DNA in the stool. For this test, an entire bowel movement is collected and checked for cancer cells (CDC, 2023). Collection does not require any preparation, diet, or medication changes. Clinical studies have shown a 92% detection of colon cancers as well as precancerous conditions.

Endoscopic Examinations

Older asymptomatic adults are advised to have regular **colonoscopy** examinations, a visual inspection of the interior colon using a flexible lighted endoscope, which is considered the most accurate test for detecting colorectal cancer. Colonoscopy examinations should begin at 50 years of age and every 10 years thereafter. Those with colorectal cancer risk factors, such as a family history of colorectal cancer or polyps, should undergo colonoscopies earlier and more frequently (CDC, 2024). An alternative to a colonoscopy is to schedule a flexible **sigmoidoscopy**, visual endoscopic inspection limited to the sigmoid portion of the large intestine, every 5 to 10 years (Fig. 31-2). Other alternatives recommended by the American Cancer Society include a barium enema every 5 years or a **colonography**, a computed tomography scan without a colonoscope, sometimes referred to as a *virtual colonoscopy*, every 5 years.

COMMON ALTERATIONS IN BOWEL ELIMINATION

Clients often have temporary or chronic problems with bowel elimination and intestinal function, such as constipation, fecal impaction, flatulence, diarrhea, and fecal incontinence. By analyzing assessment findings, nurses may help physicians diagnose a medical problem or use the conclusions to identify alterations within the independent scope of nursing management. If these conditions are a component of a serious disorder, nurses and physicians collaborate to address them.

Constipation

Constipation is an elimination problem characterized by dry, hard stool that is difficult to pass. Various accompanying signs and symptoms include:

• Reports of abdominal fullness or bloating
• Abdominal distention
• Reports of rectal fullness or pressure
• Pain with defecation
• Decreased frequency of bowel movements
• Inability to pass stool
• Changes in stool characteristics, such as oozing, liquid stool, or hard, small stool

Constipation is classified into one of three distinct types (primary, secondary, and iatrogenic) according to the underlying cause.

The infrequent elimination of stool does not necessarily indicate that a person is constipated. Some people may be constipated, even though they have a daily bowel movement, while others who defecate irregularly may have normal bowel function.

The incidence of constipation tends to be high among those whose dietary habits lack adequate fiber (such as not eating sufficient raw fruits and vegetables, whole grains, seeds, and nuts). Dietary fiber, which includes undigested cellulose, is important because it attracts water within the bowel, resulting in bulkier stool that is more quickly and easily eliminated.

Some researchers speculate that a shortened transit time—the time between when a person eats food and eliminates stool—protects against serious medical disorders. They argue that the longer the stool is retained, the more contact with and absorption of toxic substances takes place that may contribute to the development of colorectal cancer (The Life Today, 2023).

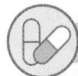

P h a r m a c o l o g i c   C o n s i d e r a t i o n s

When clients experience constipation, diarrhea, loss of appetite, or other GI distress, always ask about medications taken. GI distress is one of the most frequent side effects with many drugs.

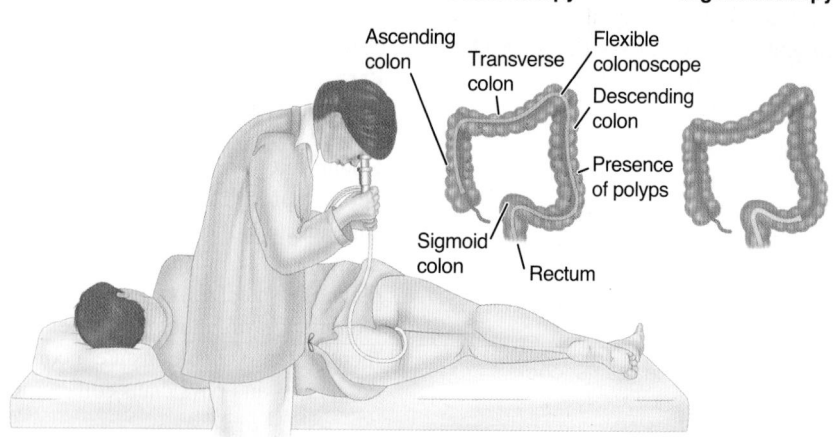

FIGURE 31-2 Flexible endoscopes are used during a colonoscopy to visualize the length of the large intestine or to visualize the lower bowel and sigmoid section during a sigmoidoscopy. (From Hinkle, J. L., & Cheever, K. H. [2021]. *Brunner & Suddarth's textbook of medical-surgical nursing* [15th ed.]. Lippincott Williams & Wilkins.)

Primary Constipation

Primary or simple constipation is well within the treatment domain of nurses. It results from lifestyle factors, such as inactivity, inadequate intake of fiber, insufficient fluid intake, or ignoring the urge to defecate.

Secondary Constipation

Secondary constipation is a consequence of a pathologic disorder, such as a partial bowel obstruction. It usually resolves when the primary cause is treated.

 Pharmacologic Considerations

Caution adults to avoid self-administration of mineral oil to relieve constipation as it interferes with absorption of fat-soluble vitamins (A, D, E, and K).

Iatrogenic Constipation

Iatrogenic constipation occurs as a consequence of other medical treatments. For example, prolonged use of narcotic analgesia tends to cause constipation. These and other drugs slow peristalsis, delaying transit time. The longer the stool remains in the colon, the drier it becomes, making it more difficult to pass.

 Concept Mastery Alert

Laxative Misuse

Many individuals believe that a daily bowel movement is the norm and turn to laxative use to promote a daily bowel movement. If a client reports chronic constipation, investigate the client's use of laxatives. Laxatives, like many medications, can lead to dependence with long-term use.

 Pharmacologic Considerations

■ Laxative misuse is possible among older adults experiencing changes in bowel routine. Some adults may become bowel conscious and overuse laxatives or have sustained laxative abuse. Bowel assessment can discover these issues for appropriate intervention.

■ Older adults can develop healthier bowel elimination habits through use of bulk-forming products containing psyllium or polycarbophil, which are more effective and less irritating than other types of laxatives. Examples of these agents include Metamucil and FiberCon.

Fecal Impaction

Fecal impaction occurs when a large, hardened mass of stool interferes with defecation, making it impossible for the client to pass feces voluntarily. Fecal impaction results from unrelieved constipation, retained barium from an intestinal X-ray, dehydration, and weakness of abdominal muscles.

Clients with fecal impaction usually report a frequent desire to defecate but an inability to do so. Rectal pain may result from unsuccessful efforts to evacuate the lower bowel. Some clients with an impaction pass liquid stool, which may be misinterpreted as diarrhea. Forceful muscular contractions of peristalsis in higher bowel areas, where the stool is still fluid, cause the liquid stool. These contractions send the liquid around the margins of the impacted stool, but this passage of liquid stool does not relieve the initial condition.

To determine whether fecal impaction is present, it may be necessary to insert a lubricated, gloved finger into the rectum. If the rectum is filled with a mass of stool, the nurse implements measures for its removal. Sometimes, nurses administer enemas, first oil retention, and then cleansing. These therapeutic measures are discussed later in this chapter. Another intervention is to remove the stool digitally (Nursing Guidelines 31-2).

Flatulence

Flatulence or **flatus** (an excessive accumulation of intestinal gas) results from swallowing air while eating or from sluggish peristalsis. Another cause is the gas that forms as a byproduct of bacterial fermentation in the bowel. Vegetables such as cabbage, cucumbers, and onions are commonly known for producing gas. Beans are other gas formers. Eating beans creates intestinal gas because humans lack an enzyme to completely digest its particular form of complex carbohydrate.

Regardless of its cause, flatus may be expelled rectally, thus reducing intestinal accumulation and distention.

Sometimes, however, this is not sufficient to eliminate the cramping pain or other symptoms. When clients are extremely uncomfortable and ambulating does not eliminate flatus, the nurse may insert a rectal tube to help the gas escape (Skill 31-1).

Diarrhea

Diarrhea is the urgent passage of watery stool and is commonly accompanied by abdominal cramping. Simple diarrhea usually begins suddenly and lasts for a short period. Other associated signs and symptoms include nausea and vomiting and blood or mucus in the stools.

>>> *Stop, Think, and Respond 31-1*

Discuss measures to include in a teaching plan that would help clients reduce or eliminate intestinal gas.

 NURSING GUIDELINES 31-2

Removing a Fecal Impaction

- Wash your hands or use an alcohol-based hand rub (see Chapter 10). *Hand hygiene reduces the transmission of microorganisms.*
- Put on clean examination gloves. *Doing so complies with standard precautions by providing a barrier between the hands and a substance that contains body fluid.*
- Provide privacy. *Privacy demonstrates respect for the client's dignity.*
- Place the client in a Sims position (Fig. A; see Chapter 14). *This position facilitates access to the rectum.*

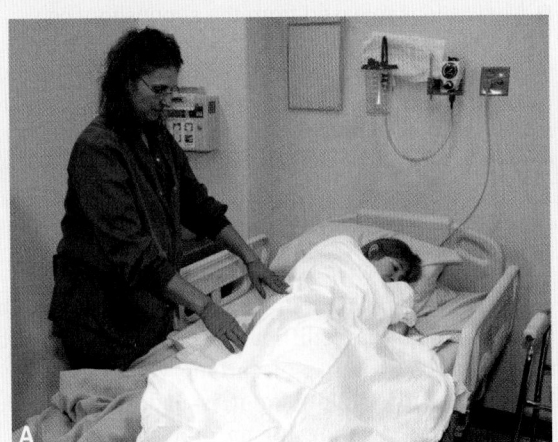

The client is in a Sims position. (From Rosdahl, C. B., [2021]. *Textbook of basic nursing* [12th ed.]. Lippincott Williams & Wilkins.)

- Cover the client with a drape and place a disposable pad under the client's hips. *Use of these materials prevents soiling.*
- Place a bedpan conveniently on the bed. *The bedpan acts as a container for removed stool.*
- Lubricate the forefinger of your dominant gloved hand. *Lubrication eases insertion within the rectum.*

- Insert your lubricated finger within the rectum to the level of the hardened mass. *Insertion to this level facilitates digital manipulation of the stool.*
- Move your finger about slowly and carefully to break up the mass of stool. *Movement facilitates removal or voluntary passage.*
- Withdraw segments of the stool (Fig. B) and deposit them in the bedpan. *Removal reduces the internal mass of stool.*

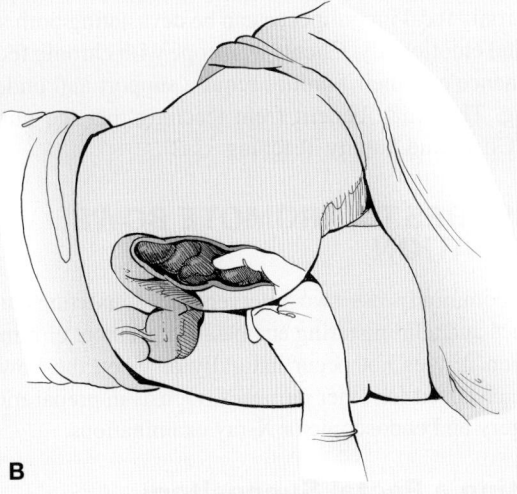

B

Stool is removed digitally.

- Provide periods of rest but continue until the mass has been removed or sufficiently reduced. *Doing so restores patency to the lower bowel.*
- Clean the client's rectal area; dispose of the stool and soiled gloves and repeat hand hygiene measures. *These measures support the principles of medical asepsis.*

Nutrition Notes

Probiotics are beneficial bacteria present in some commercial products like yogurt that contain live cultures. These bacteria survive digestion and colonize within the bowel, making bowel contents more acidic. The lowered intestinal pH creates a hostile environment for unhealthy bacteria. Eating products containing probiotics is believed to regulate and improve elimination, thus reducing symptoms of diarrhea, constipation, intestinal gas, and bloating.

Usually, diarrhea is a means of eliminating an irritating substance such as tainted food or intestinal pathogens. Diarrhea may also result from emotional stress, dietary indiscretions, laxative misuse, or bowel disorders.

Resting the bowel temporarily may relieve simple diarrhea. This means the person drinks clear liquids but avoids solid foods for 12 to 24 hours. Resumed eating begins with bland foods and those low in residue, such as bananas, applesauce, and cottage cheese. If diarrhea is not relieved within 24 hours, it is best to consult a physician.

Fecal Incontinence

Fecal incontinence is the inability to control the elimination of stool. It does not necessarily imply that stool is loose or watery, though that may be the case. In some instances, bowel function is normal, but incontinence results from neurologic changes that impair muscle activity, sensation, or thought processes. Even a fecal impaction may be an underlying cause of incontinence. Incontinence may also occur when a person cannot reach a toilet in time to eliminate, such as after taking a harsh laxative.

Chronic fecal incontinence can be devastating both socially and emotionally. Clients who cope with chronic fecal incontinence and their families require support and understanding. They may benefit from teaching that the nurse offers (Client and Family Teaching 31-2).

MEASURES TO PROMOTE BOWEL ELIMINATION

Nurses commonly use two interventions—inserting suppositories and administering enemas—to promote elimination when it does not occur naturally or when the bowel must be cleansed for other purposes, such as in preparation for surgery and endoscopic or X-ray examinations.

Inserting a Rectal Suppository

A **suppository** (an oval—or cone-shaped mass that melts at body temperature) is inserted into a body cavity, such as the rectum. The most common reason for inserting a suppository is to deliver a drug that will promote the expulsion of feces. Other medications, such as drugs to control vomiting and reduce fever, are also available in suppository form.

Client and Family Teaching 31-2 Managing Fecal Incontinence

The nurse teaches the client and the family as follows:

- Eat regularly and nutritiously.
- Monitor the pattern of incontinence to determine whether it occurs at a similar time each day.
- Sit on the toilet or bedside commode before the time elimination tends to occur.
- Consult the physician about inserting a suppository or administering an enema every 2 to 3 days to establish a pattern for bowel elimination.
- Use moisture-proof undergarments and absorbent pads to protect clothing and bed linens.
- Teach caregivers to do the following:

  - Do not imply verbally or nonverbally that the client is to blame for the incontinence or that cleaning them is disgusting.
  - Avoid anything that connotes diapering to preserve the client's dignity and self-esteem.

Pharmacologic Considerations

■ Suppositories are used for both systemic and local effects:

　■ Antipyretics are frequently used rectally when fever reduction cannot be managed orally.

　■ Constipation can be relieved locally in the rectum when used to soften or stimulate defecation.

　■ Medications released from the suppository can have local or systemic effects. Depending on the drug, local effects may include softening and lubricating dry stool, irritating the wall of the rectum and anal canal to stimulate smooth muscle contraction, and liberating carbon dioxide, thus increasing rectal distention and the urge to defecate.

Drugs administered in suppository form are chosen when clients have difficulty retaining or absorbing oral medications because of chronic vomiting or an impaired ability to swallow, or it is undesirable to delay defecation while waiting for an oral medication to act. Administering a suppository is a form of medication administration (Skill 31-2). For additional principles, refer to Chapters 32 and 33.

>> *Stop, Think, and Respond 31-2*

Discuss appropriate actions if a mass of stool is felt when inserting a suppository.

TABLE 31-3 Types of Cleansing Enema Solutions

SOLUTION	AMOUNT (mL)	MECHANISM OF ACTION
Tap water	500–1,000	A tap water enema can relieve constipation symptoms by distending the rectum and moistening the stool.
Normal saline	500–1,000	Normal saline solution. It is a combination of salt and water. The salt of the mixture sends the body's water into the bowels to make the feces soft, and distends rectum.
Soap and water (Castile soap)	500–1,000	It is a mild soap made of many oils, such as olive oil. This mild soap is added to saline solution, which is then inserted through an enema. This solution stimulates the bowel to create movements. It distends the rectum, moistens stool, and may irritate local tissue.
Hypertonic saline	120	Irritates local tissue and draws water into the bowel and helps to increase the intestinal motility and passage of stool into the colon
Mineral, olive, or cottonseed oil	120–180	The oil lubricates the inside of the intestine and any stool that is present, making the stool easier to pass or remove. Oil retention enemas are useful for helping to remove fecal impactions.
Glycerin	250	It activates the lining of the colon to cause bowel movements.
Coffee	950	It is a mixture of brewed coffee and water, used to eliminate bile from the colon.
Phosphate solution	118	A phosphate solution enema draws water into the bowel to soften the hardened feces. Too much phosphate in your body may cause health risks. A phosphate enema is also not recommended for people with kidney problems.

Administering an Enema

An **enema** introduces a solution into the rectum (Skill 31-3). Nurses give enemas to:

- Cleanse the lower bowel (most common reason).
- Soften feces.
- Expel flatus.
- Soothe irritated mucous membranes.
- Outline the colon during diagnostic X-rays.
- Treat worm and parasite infestations.

Cleansing Enemas

Cleansing enemas use different types of solutions to remove feces from the rectum (Table 31-3). Defecation usually occurs within 5 to 15 minutes after administration.

Large-volume cleansing enemas may create discomfort because they distend the lower bowel. Nurses must administer them cautiously to clients with intestinal disorders such as colitis (inflammation of the colon) because large-volume enemas may rupture the bowel or cause other secondary complications. In many health agencies and in the home, commercially prepared disposable administration sets have become the method of choice for cleansing the bowel. Their smaller volumes make them less fatiguing and distressing than large-volume enemas, and they can be easily self-administered (Fig. 31-3).

Tap Water and Normal Saline Enemas

Tap water and normal saline solutions are preferred for their nonirritating effects, especially for clients with rectal diseases or those being prepared for rectal examinations. Tap water and normal saline appear to have about the same degree of effectiveness for cleansing the bowel.

Because tap water is hypotonic, the fluid can be absorbed through the bowel. Consequently, if several enemas are administered in succession, fluid and electrolyte imbalances may occur (see Chapter 16). Therefore, to ensure client safety, if stool continues to be expelled after the administration of three enemas, the nurse consults the physician before administering more.

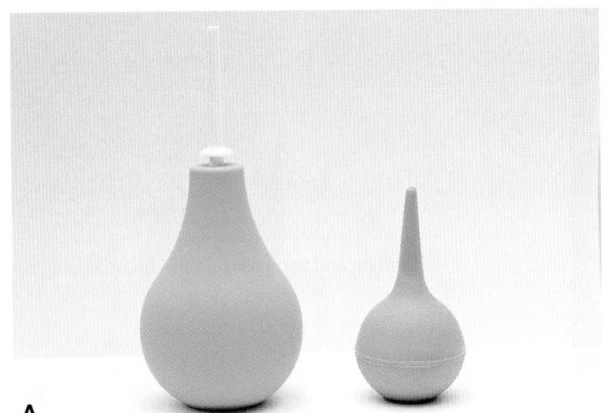

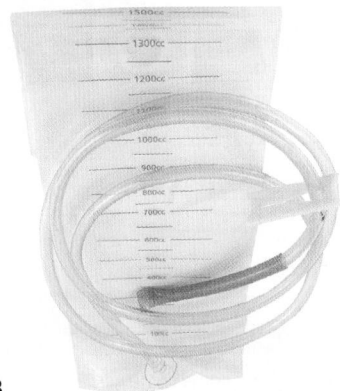

FIGURE 31-3 A. Pear shaped enemas (Andrei Sitnikov/Shutterstock). **B.** Enema bag with flush tubing (MARGRIT HIRSCH/Shutterstock).

Soap Solution Enemas

A soap solution enema is a mixture of water and soap. Many disposable enema kits contain an envelope of soap, which is mixed with up to 1 qt (1,000 mL) of water. If these soap packets are not available, a comparable mixture is 1 mL of mild liquid soap per 200 mL of solution, or a ratio of 1:200. Therefore, 5 mL of soap is added to prepare a volume of 1,000 mL.

Soap causes chemical irritation of the mucous membranes. Adding too much soap or using strong soap can potentiate the irritating effect.

Hypertonic Saline Enemas

A hypertonic saline (sodium phosphate) enema draws fluid from body tissues into the bowel. This increases the fluid volume in the intestine beyond what was originally instilled. The concentrated solution also acts as a local irritant on the mucous membranes.

Hypertonic enema solutions are available in commercially prepared disposable containers holding approximately 4 oz (120 mL) of solution. The container, which has a lubricated tip, substitutes for enema equipment and tubing (Nursing Guidelines 31-3).

Retention Enemas

A **retention enema** uses a solution held within the large intestine for a specified period, usually at least 30 minutes. Some retention enemas are not expelled at all. One type of retention enema is called an *oil retention enema* because the fluid instilled is mineral, cottonseed, or olive oil. Oils lubricate and soften the stool, so it can be expelled more easily.

The oil may come in a prefilled container similar to those that contain hypertonic saline. If disposable equipment is not available, the nurse lubricates and inserts a 14- to 22-F tube in the rectum. A small funnel or large syringe is attached to the tube, and the nurse instills approximately 100 to 200 mL of warmed oil slowly to avoid stimulating an urge to defecate. Premature defecation defeats the purpose of retaining the oil.

>> **Stop, Think, and Respond 31-3**
List measures for preventing constipation.

OSTOMY CARE

A client with an **ostomy** (a surgically created opening to the bowel or other structure; see Chapter 30) requires additional care for promoting bowel elimination. Two examples of intestinal ostomies are an **ileostomy** (a surgically created opening to the ileum) and a **colostomy** (a surgically created opening to a portion of the colon; Fig. 31-4). Materials enter and exit through a **stoma** (the entrance to the opening).

NURSING GUIDELINES 31-3

Administering a Hypertonic Enema Solution

- Warm the container of solution if it is cold by placing it in a basin or sink of warm water. *Warmth promotes comfort.*
- Assist the client into a Sims position or use a knee–chest position (see Chapter 14). *These positions promote gravity distribution of the solution.*
- Wash hands or use an alcohol-based hand rub (see Chapter 10) and put on gloves. *Hand hygiene reduces transmission of microorganisms; gloves provide a barrier from contact with a substance that contains body fluid.*
- Remove the cover from the lubricated tip (Fig. A). *This step facilitates administration.*
- Cover the tip with additional lubricant. *Lubricant eases insertion.*
- Invert the container and compress the fluid toward the enema tip (Fig. B). *Inversion causes air in the container to rise toward the upper end.*

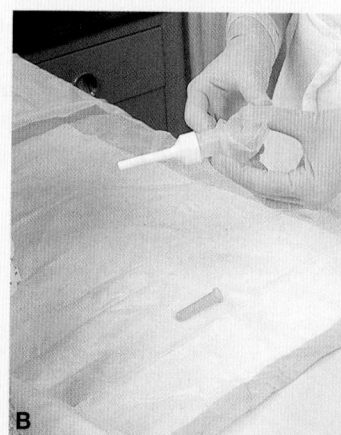

Inverting and compressing the enema container.

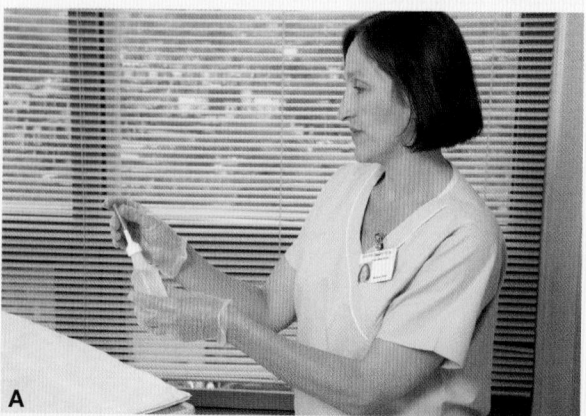

Removing the cap from the enema container. (From Lynn, P. [2022]. *Taylor's clinical nursing skills* [6th ed.]. Lippincott Williams & Wilkins.)

NURSING GUIDELINES 31-3 (*continued*)

- Insert the full length of the tip within the rectum (Fig. C). *This positioning places the tip at a level that promotes effectiveness.*

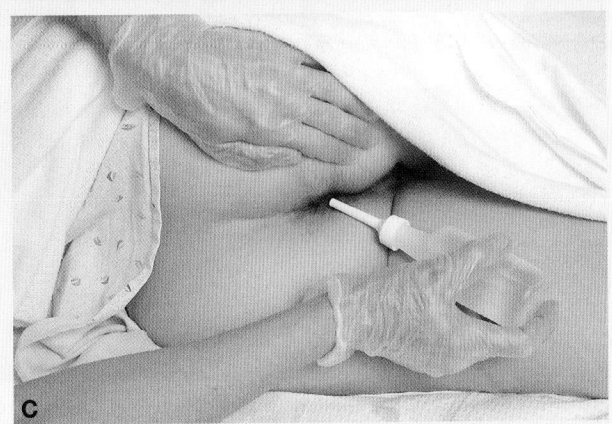

C

Inserting the enema tip within the rectum.

- Apply gentle, steady pressure on the solution container for 1 to 2 minutes or until the solution has been completely administered. *This method instills a steady stream of solution.*
- Compress the container as the solution instills (Fig. D). *Compression provides positive pressure rather than gravity to instill fluid.*

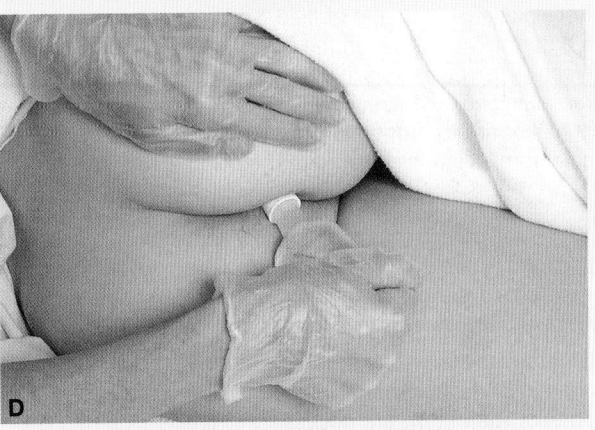

D

Compressing the container to instill the solution.

- Encourage the client to retain the solution for 5 to 15 minutes. *This duration promotes effectiveness.*
- Clean the client and position for comfort. *These measures demonstrate concern for the client's well-being.*
- Discard the container, remove gloves, and perform hand hygiene measures. *Doing so follows the principles of medical asepsis.*

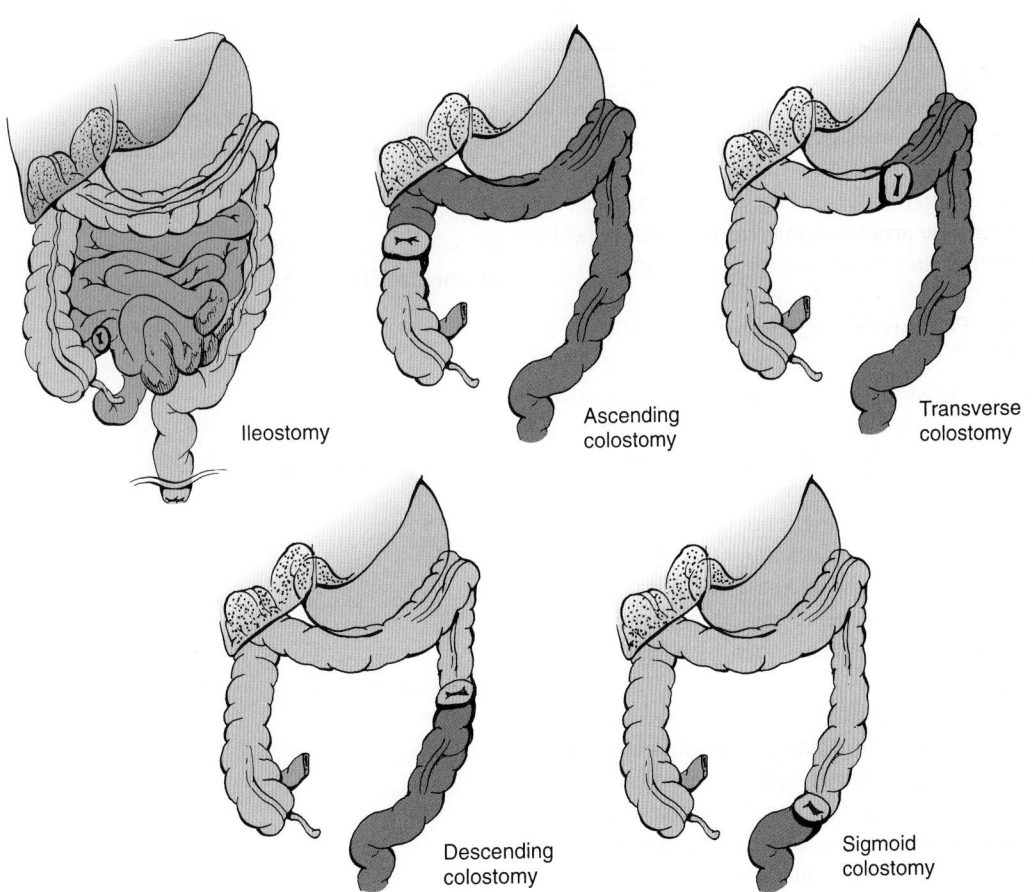

Ileostomy

Ascending colostomy

Transverse colostomy

Descending colostomy

Sigmoid colostomy

FIGURE 31-4 The locations of intestinal ostomies.

Nutrition Notes

- Because large amounts of fluid, sodium, and potassium are normally absorbed in the colon, the risk of fluid and electrolyte imbalances increases as the length of the remaining colon decreases. Clients with ileostomies are at higher risk of nutritional problems than are clients with colostomies in which some of the colon is retained.

- Clients with ileostomies are encouraged to consume 8 to 10 glasses of fluid daily to maintain a normal urine output and to minimize the risk of renal calculi. Assure clients that excess fluid is excreted through the kidneys, not the stoma. A liberal salt intake may be needed to replenish losses.

- Ileostomies are placed before the terminal ileum where vitamin B_{12} is absorbed. Nasal sprays or parenteral injections of vitamin B_{12} are necessary to prevent vitamin B_{12} deficiency anemia.

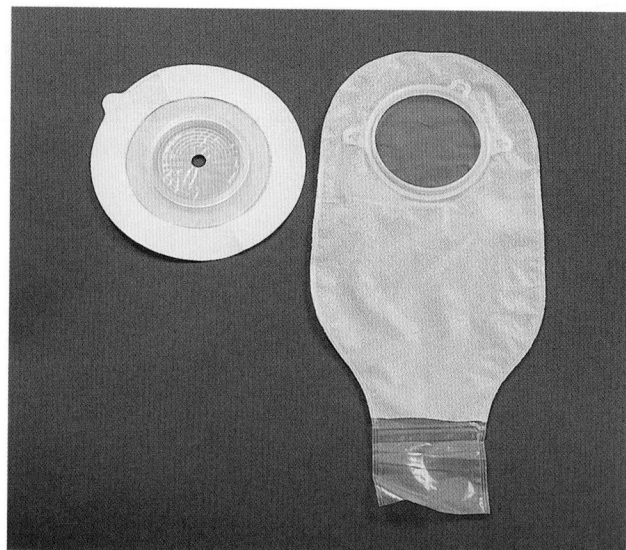

FIGURE 31-5 An ostomy appliance: a faceplate and pouch. (Photo by B. Proud.)

Most people who have ostomies wear an **appliance** (a bag or collection device over the stoma) to collect stool. Depending on the type and location of the ostomy, client care may involve providing peristomal care, applying an appliance, draining a continent ileostomy, and, for clients with colostomies, administering irrigations through the stoma.

Providing Peristomal Care

Preventing skin breakdown is a major challenge in ostomy care. Enzymes in the stool can quickly cause **excoriation** (chemical injury of the skin). Washing the stoma and the surrounding skin with mild soap and water, and patting it dry can preserve skin integrity. Another way to protect the skin is to apply barrier substances such as *karaya*, a plant substance that becomes gelatinous when moistened, and commercial skin preparations around the stoma. An **enterostomal therapist**, a nurse certified in caring for ostomies and related skin problems, may be consulted regarding skin and stomal care.

Securing an Ostomy Appliance

Various appliances are available, but all consist of a pouch for collecting stool and a faceplate, or disk, that attaches to the abdomen. The stoma protrudes through an opening in the center of the appliance (Fig. 31-5). The pouch fastens into position when pressed over the circular support on the faceplate. Some clients prefer a type that also fastens to an elastic belt worn around the waist. The belt helps support the weight of the fecal material and prevents the faceplate from being pulled away from the abdomen. The client empties the pouch by releasing the clamp at the bottom.

The faceplate usually remains in place for 3 to 5 days unless it becomes loose or causes skin discomfort. Pouches are emptied and rinsed or detached and replaced periodically. The client empties the pouch when it is one third to one half full; otherwise, it may become too heavy and pull the faceplate from the skin. Although design of the equipment varies, almost all types of appliances are changed similarly (Skill 31-4).

Draining a Continent Ileostomy

A **continent ostomy** (a surgically created opening that controls the drainage of liquid stool or urine by siphoning it from an internal reservoir) is also referred to as a *Kock pouch*, after the surgeon who developed the technique (Fig. 31-6). This type of ostomy requires no appliance; however, the client must drain the accumulating liquid stool or urine approximately every 4 to 6 hours. The client can use a gravity drainage system at night (Client and Family Teaching 31-3).

Irrigating a Colostomy

Clients with colostomies whose stool is more solid sometimes require the instillation of fluid to promote elimination. Colostomy irrigation involves instilling the solution through the stoma into the colon, a process similar to administering an enema (Skill 31-5).

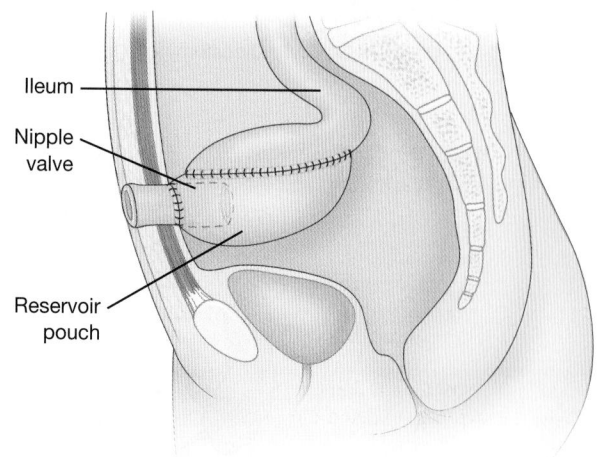

Ileum

Nipple valve

Reservoir pouch

FIGURE 31-6 A continent ileostomy.

Client and Family Teaching 31-3
Draining a Continent Ileostomy

The nurse teaches the client and the family as follows:

- Assume a sitting position.
- Insert a lubricated 22- to 28-F catheter into the stoma.
- Expect resistance after inserting the tube approximately 2 in; this is the location of the valve that controls the retention of liquid stool or urine.
- Gently advance the catheter through the valve at the end of exhalation, while coughing, or while bearing down as if to pass stool.
- Lower the external end of the catheter at least 12 in below the stoma.
- Direct the end of the catheter into a container or toilet as stool or urine begins to flow.
- Allow at least 5 to 10 minutes for complete emptying.
- Remove the catheter and clean it with warm soapy water.
- Place the clean catheter in a sealable plastic bag until its next use.
- Cover the stoma with a gauze square or a large bandage.
- If the catheter becomes plugged with stool or mucus:
  - Bear down as if to have a bowel movement.
  - Rotate the catheter tip inside the stoma.
  - Milk the catheter.
  - If these are not successful, remove the catheter, rinse it, and try again.
  - Notify the physician if these efforts do not result in drainage.
- Never wait longer than 6 hours without obtaining drainage.

The purpose of the irrigation is to remove formed stool and, in some cases, to regulate the timing of bowel movements. With regulation, a client with a sigmoid colostomy may not need to wear an appliance. The colostomy irrigation helps train the bowel to eliminate formed stool following the irrigation. Once the client has eliminated the stool, they will expel no more until the next irrigation. This mimics the pattern of natural bowel elimination for most people. Because of the predictability of bowel elimination, some clients with sigmoid colostomies feel it is unnecessary to wear an appliance.

>>> *Stop, Think, and Respond 31-4*
Discuss the various ways an ostomy affects the lives of clients.

NURSING IMPLICATIONS

While assessing and caring for clients with altered bowel elimination, the nurse may identify one or more of the following nursing diagnoses:

- Constipation
- Constipation risk
- Perceived constipation
- Diarrhea
- Fecal impaction
- Bowel incontinence
- Toileting activity of daily living (ADL) deficit
- Situational low self-esteem

Nursing Care Plan 31-1 reflects the nursing process as it applies to a client with constipation. *Constipation* is defined as infrequent, irregular, or difficult evacuation of the bowels.

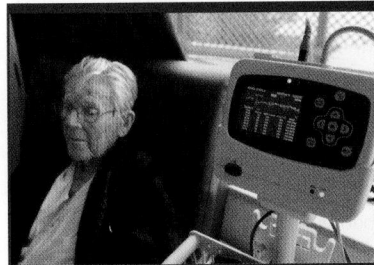

Clinical Scenario A 79-year-old widower has been hospitalized for 4 days. He lives alone and has come to the hospital because he has not been feeling well. During morning rounds, he reports to the nurse that he feels bloated and attributes his discomfort to being constipated.

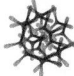

NURSING CARE PLAN 31-1 Constipation

Assessment
- Note the frequency, amount, and texture of the expelled stool.
- Ask the client about the effort required to eliminate stool.
- Inquire as to whether the client feels they empty the bowel during stool elimination and if there is any discomfort in the rectal area.
- Auscultate bowel sounds daily.
- Palpate the abdomen to determine whether there is any distention.
- Determine if any of the client's medications are constipating.

- Ask the client about measures they use to promote bowel elimination and their frequency.
- Ask the client to describe their daily intake of fluid and food, including types of beverages and foods commonly eaten.
- Explore lifestyle patterns that may interfere with bowel elimination such as a lack of privacy or lengthy travel that interferes with accessing a toilet when there is a need to eliminate stool.
- Note if any physical problems may compromise bowel elimination such as impaired physical mobility or dementia.

(continued)

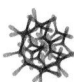

NURSING CARE PLAN 13-1 — Constipation (*continued*)

Nursing Diagnosis. Constipation related to inadequate dietary habits as manifested by a distended abdomen; hypoactive bowel sounds in all four quadrants; and client's statement: "I've got a problem. I haven't had a bowel movement in 4 days even though I've felt like I need to pass stool. I sit and strain but I only pass a small amount of hard stool. I used to have a problem now and then when I was a kid, but since I'm living alone, it's getting to be very frequent. Maybe it's because I don't eat regularly, and when I do, it's a lot of convenience food."

Expected Outcome. The client will have a bowel movement within 24 hours and will list three ways to improve the regularity of bowel elimination by 10/25.

Interventions	Rationales
Give an oil retention enema as ordered for prn administration.	This type of enema lubricates the bowel and softens the stool for easier expulsion.
Give prescribed laxative at bedtime 10/23 if no bowel movement has occurred.	Laxatives facilitate bowel elimination in various ways; some common mechanisms of action include increasing intestinal peristalsis, irritating the bowel, and attracting water into the large intestine.
Encourage drinking at least 8–10 glasses of fluid per day; offer prune juice or apple juice.	Oral fluid promotes hydration and avoids dry stool; prune juice has a laxative effect, and apple juice contains pectin, which also adds bulk to the stool.
Educate about high-fiber foods and that their intake should be gradually increased as tolerated until the desired effect is achieved.	Intestinal fiber adds bulk by pulling water into stool; a bulky, soft stool distends the rectum and promotes the urge to defecate.

Evaluation of Expected Outcomes

- The client eliminated moderate amount of brown formed stool approximately 6 hours following the administration of the oil retention enema.
- The client identified a minimum goal of consuming eight 8-oz glasses of fluid daily.
- The client can name sources of fiber, such as wheat bran, whole wheat bread, whole grain cereal, fresh fruits and vegetables, dried peas and beans, and nuts.
- The client stated that increasing active exercise for a total of 30 minutes each day either all at once or divided and performed several times during the day promotes bowel elimination.

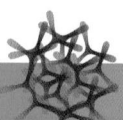

KEY POINTS

- Gastrocolic reflex: Accelerated wave-like movements, sometimes perceived as slight abdominal cramping that propel stool forward, packing it within the rectum; as the rectum distends, the person feels the urge to defecate.
- Valsalva maneuver: Closing the glottis and contracting the pelvic and abdominal muscles to increase abdominal pressure
- Factors affecting bowel elimination
  - Types of food
  - Fluid intake
  - Drugs
  - Emotions
  - Neuromuscular function
  - Abdominal muscle tone
  - Opportunity for defecation
- Stool characteristics
  - Color
  - Odor
  - Consistency
  - Shape
  - Components
- The incidence of colorectal cancer increases with age; it is the third most common cancer diagnosed in men and women in the United States and the second most common cause of deaths from cancer.

- Constipation: An elimination problem characterized by dry, hard stool that is difficult to pass:
  - Primary
  - Secondary
  - Iatrogenic
- Diarrhea: The urgent passage of watery stool that is commonly accompanied by abdominal cramping
- Fecal impaction occurs when a large, hardened mass of stool interferes with defecation, making it impossible for the client to pass feces voluntarily.
- Measures to promote bowel elimination
- Rectal suppository
- Enema
  - Tap water and normal saline
  - Soap solution
  - Hypertonic saline
  - Retention
- Ostomy: A surgically created opening to the bowel or other structure; it requires additional care for promoting bowel elimination.
  - Ileostomy: A surgically created opening to the ileum
  - Colostomy: A surgically created opening to a portion of the colon
  - Stoma: The entrance to the opening where materials enter and exit

CRITICAL THINKING EXERCISES

1. When inserting a rectal suppository, the nurse feels a hard mass of stool. What actions should be taken next?
2. What are some possible consequences of chronic constipation?
3. Formulate suggestions to promote bowel continence among older adults with impaired cognition, such as those with Alzheimer disease.
4. What nursing actions are appropriate when peristomal skin appears red and excoriated?

NEXT-GENERATION NCLEX-STYLE REVIEW QUESTIONS

1. When a client tells the nurse they cannot have a bowel movement without taking a daily laxative, what information is essential for the nurse to explain?
   a. The chronic use of laxatives impairs natural bowel tone.
   b. Stool softeners are likely to be less harsh.
   c. Daily enemas are more preferable than laxatives.
   d. Dilating the anal sphincter may aid bowel elimination.
   Test-Taking Strategy: Note the key word, "essential." Use the process of elimination to exclude explanations that are incorrect or of lesser importance.
2. Which assessment is the best indication that a client has a fecal impaction?
   a. The client passes liquid stool frequently.
   b. The client has extremely foul breath.
   c. The client requests medication for a headache.
   d. The client has not been eating well lately.
   Test-Taking Strategy: Note the key word and modifier, "best indication." Review the choices and select the option that provides the most objective evidence that correlates with a fecal impaction.
3. Before inserting a rectal tube, which nursing measure is most helpful for eliminating intestinal gas?
   a. Ambulate the client in the hall.
   b. Provide a carbonated beverage.
   c. Restrict the intake of solid food.
   d. Administer a narcotic analgesic.
   Test-Taking Strategy: Note the key word and modifier, "most helpful." Use the process of elimination to select the option that is better than any of the others for relieving intestinal gas.
4. When a nurse is assigned to care for a client with an ascending colostomy, place an X on the diagram where the colostomy would be located.

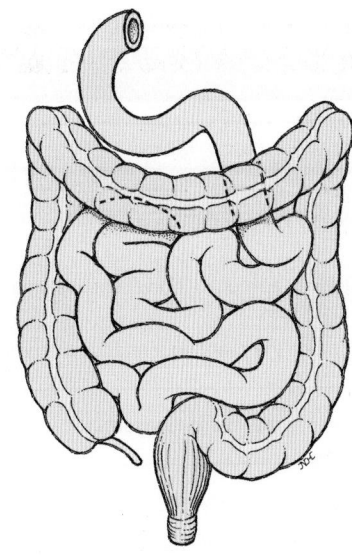

Test-Taking Strategy: Recall the names and locations of structures that make up the large intestine.

NEXT-GENERATION NCLEX-STYLE CLINICAL SCENARIO QUESTIONS

Clinical Scenario:
A 79-year-old widower has been hospitalized for 4 days. He lives alone and has come to the hospital because he has not been feeling well. During morning rounds, he reports to the nurse that he feels bloated and attributes his discomfort to being constipated.

1. Select all of the indicators that may suggest a cause for the client's constipation.
   a. Hospitalized for 4 days
   b. Feeling bloated
   c. Not eating healthy meals
   d. Not drinking enough fluids
   e. Client exercises every day.
   f. Client is nonambulatory.
2. The client has been given a kit for collecting stool specimens for occult blood. Which foods should the nurse inform the client to avoid for 3 days prior to collecting a specimen? Select all that apply.
   a. Beets
   b. Citrus fruits
   c. Beef
   d. Poultry
   e. Oatmeal
   f. Cheese
   Test-Taking Strategy: Review the list of food items and eliminate any options that are not contraindicated when a specimen for fecal occult blood is collected.

SKILL 31-1 Inserting a Rectal Tube

Suggested Action	Reason for Action
ASSESSMENT	
Check the medical orders.	Ensures collaboration between nursing activities and the medical treatment
Use two methods to identify the client.	Supports the principles of safety recommended by The Joint Commission
Inspect the abdomen, auscultate bowel sounds, and gently palpate for distention and fullness.	Provides baseline data for future comparisons
Determine how much the client understands the procedure.	Provides an opportunity for health teaching
PLANNING	
Obtain a 22- to 32-F catheter and lubricant.	Ensures proper size and easy insertion
IMPLEMENTATION	
Wash your hands or use an alcohol-based hand rub (see Chapter 10); put on gloves.	Reduces the transmission of microorganisms
Pull the privacy curtain.	Demonstrates respect for the client's dignity
Place the client in a Sims position.	Facilitates access to the rectum
Lubricate the tip of the tube generously (Fig. A).	Eases insertion

Lubricating the rectal tube.

Separate the buttocks well so that the anus is in plain view (Fig. B). — Helps visualize the insertion location

Separating the buttocks.

SKILL 31-1 Inserting a Rectal Tube (*continued*)

Suggested Action	Reason for Action
Insert the tube 4–6 in (10–15 cm) in an adult (Fig. C).	Places the distal tip above the sphincter muscles, stimulates peristalsis, and prevents displacement of the tube

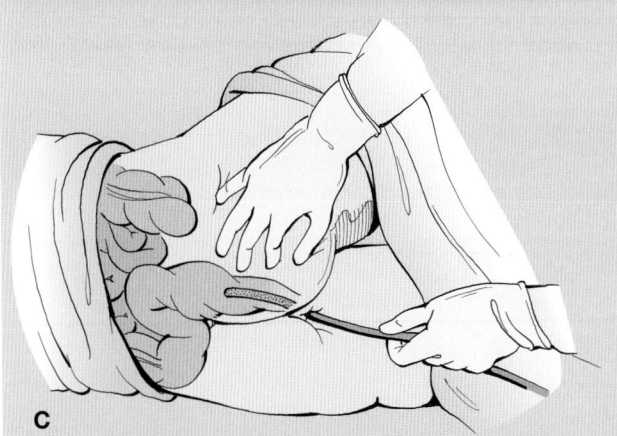

Inserting the rectal tube.

Suggested Action	Reason for Action
Enclose the free end of the tube within a clean, soft washcloth, disposable bed pad, or gauze square (Fig. D).	Provides a means for absorbing stool should it drain from the tube

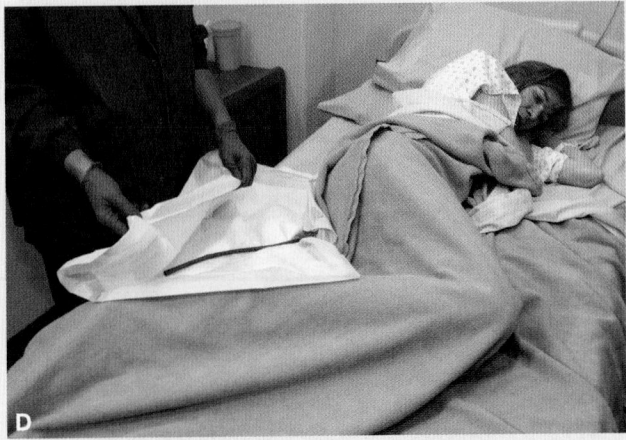

Enclosing the rectal tube.

Suggested Action	Reason for Action
Tape the tube to the buttocks or inner thigh.	Allows the client to ambulate or change positions without tube displacement
Leave the rectal tube in place no longer than 20 minutes.	Reduces the risk for impairing the sphincter
Reinsert the tube every 3–4 hours if discomfort returns.	Reinstitutes therapeutic management

EVALUATION ————————————————————————————————

- Intestinal gas is eliminated.
- The client states symptoms are relieved.
- The client reports no ill effects.

DOCUMENT ————————————————————————————————

- Assessment data
- Intervention
- Length of time tube was in place
- Client response

SAMPLE DOCUMENTATION

Date and Time Abdomen round, firm, and tympanic. Bowel sounds present in all four quadrants, but difficult to hear because of distention. States, "I can't hardly stand the pain anymore." Ambulated without relief. 26-F straight catheter inserted into rectum for 20 minutes. Flatus expelled during tube insertion. Abdomen softer. _____ J. Doe, LPN

SKILL 31-2 Inserting a Rectal Suppository

Suggested Action	Reason for Action
ASSESSMENT	
Check the medical orders.	Ensures collaboration between nursing activities and the medical treatment
Compare the medication administration record (MAR) with the written medical order.	Ensures accuracy
Read and compare the label on the suppository with the MAR at least three times—before, during, and after preparing the drug.	Prevents errors
Use two methods to identify the client.	Supports the principles of safety recommended by The Joint Commission
Determine how much the client understands the purpose and technique for administering a suppository.	Provides an opportunity for health teaching
PLANNING	
Prepare to administer the suppository according to the time prescribed by the physician.	Complies with medical orders
Obtain clean gloves and lubricant.	Facilitates insertion
IMPLEMENTATION	
Wash your hands or use an alcohol-based hand rub (see Chapter 10).	Reduces the transmission of microorganisms
Read the name on the client's identification band.	Prevents errors
Pull the privacy curtain.	Demonstrates respect for the client's modesty and dignity
Place the client in a Sims position.	Facilitates access to the rectum
Drape the client to expose only the buttocks.	Ensures modesty and dignity
Put on gloves.	Reduces the transmission of microorganisms and complies with standard precautions
Lubricate the suppository and index finger of the dominant hand (Fig. A).	Reduces friction and tissue trauma

The suppository and insertion finger are lubricated. (From Taylor, C., Lynn, P., & Bartlett, J. L. [2022]. *Fundamentals of nursing: The art and science of person-centered care* [10th ed.]. Lippincott Williams & Wilkins.)

Separate the buttocks so that the anus is in plain view.	Enhances visualization
Instruct the client to take several slow, deep breaths. Introduce the suppository, tapered end first, beyond the internal sphincter, about the distance of the finger (Fig. B).	Promotes muscle relaxation and places the suppository in the best location for achieving a local effect

Anal-rectal ridge
Anal sphincter
Suppository
Rectum

The suppository is inserted beyond the internal anal sphincter. (From Craven, R. F., Hirnle, C. J., & Jensen, S. [2020]. *Fundamentals of nursing* [9th ed.]. Lippincott Williams & Wilkins.)

Avoid placing the suppository within stool.	Reduces effectiveness

SKILL 31-2 Inserting a Rectal Suppository (*continued*)

Suggested Action	Reason for Action
Wipe excess lubricant from around the anus with a paper tissue.	Promotes comfort
Tell the client to try to retain the suppository for at least 15 minutes.	Enhances effectiveness
Suggest contracting the gluteal muscles if there is a premature urge to expel the suppository.	Tightens the anal sphincters
Ask the client to wait to flush the toilet until the stool has been inspected.	Provides an opportunity for evaluating the drug's effectiveness
Remove your gloves and wash your hands.	Reduces the transmission of microorganisms

EVALUATION

- The client retains the suppository for 15 minutes.
- Bowel elimination occurs.

DOCUMENT

- Drug, dose, route, and time (see Chapter 32)
- Outcome of drug administration

SAMPLE DOCUMENTATION

Date and Time Bisacodyl (Dulcolax) suppository inserted within rectum. Large brown formed stool expelled.
_____ J. Doe. LPN

SKILL 31-3 Administering a Cleansing Enema

Suggested Action	Reason for Action
ASSESSMENT	
Check the medical orders for the type of enema and prescribed solution.	Ensures collaboration between nursing activities and the medical treatment
Check the date of the client's last bowel movement.	Helps determine the need to check for an impaction or the basis for realistic expected outcomes
Use two methods to identify the client.	Supports the principles of safety recommended by The Joint Commission
Wash hands or use an alcohol-based hand rub (see Chapter 10).	Reduces the transmission of microorganisms
Auscultate bowel sounds.	Establishes the status of peristalsis
Determine how much the client understands the procedure.	Provides an opportunity for health teaching
PLANNING	
Plan the location where the client will expel the enema solution and stool.	Determines whether a bedpan is necessary
Obtain the appropriate equipment including an enema set, solution, an absorbent pad, lubricant, a bath blanket, and gloves.	Facilitates organization and efficient time management
Plan to perform the procedure according to the time specified by the physician or when it is most appropriate during client care.	Demonstrates collaboration and participation of the client in decision-making
Prepare the solution and equipment in the utility room (Fig. A).	Provides access to supplies

Preparing the enema solution. (From Lynn, P. [2022]. *Taylor's clinical nursing skills* [6th ed.]. Lippincott Williams & Wilkins.)

A

(*continued*)

SKILL 31-3 Administering a Cleansing Enema (*continued*)

Suggested Action	Reason for Action
Warm the solution to approximately 105°–110°F (40°–43°C).	Promotes comfort and safety
Clamp the tubing on the enema set (Fig. B).	Prevents the loss of fluid

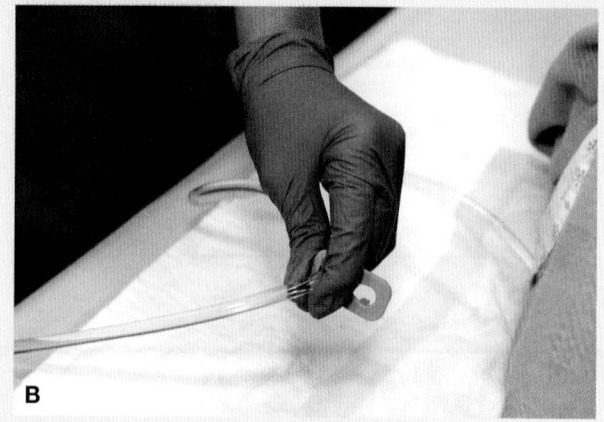

B

Clamping the administration tubing. (From Lynn, P. [2022]. *Taylor's clinical nursing skills* [6th ed.]. Lippincott Williams & Wilkins.)

Fill the container with the specified solution.	Provides the mechanism for cleansing the bowel

IMPLEMENTATION —————————————————————————

Pull the privacy curtain.	Demonstrates respect for the client's dignity
Place the client in a Sims position.	Facilitates access to the rectum
Drape the client, exposing the buttocks, and place a waterproof pad under the hips (Fig. C).	Preserves modesty and protects bed linen

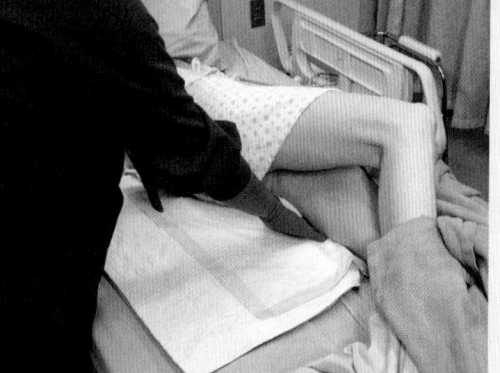

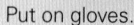
C

Draping for an enema.

Put on gloves.	Reduces the transmission of microorganisms and complies with standard precautions
Place (or hang) the solution container so that it is 12–20 in (30–50 cm) above the level of the client's anus (Fig. D).	Facilitates gravity flow

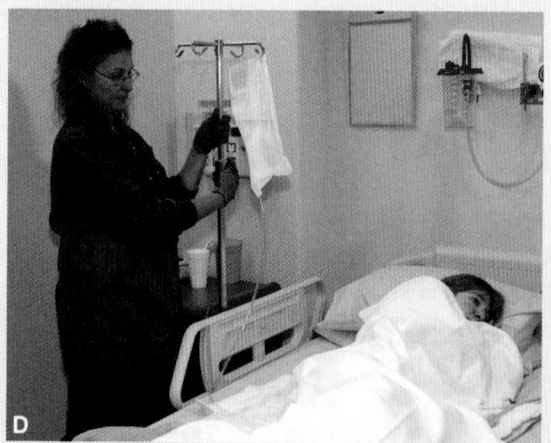

D

Hanging the enema administration bag.

SKILL 31-3 Administering a Cleansing Enema (*continued*)

Suggested Action	Reason for Action
Open the clamp and fill the tubing with solution. Reclamp (Fig. E).	Purges air from the tubing
 Purging air.	
Lubricate the tip of the tube generously (Fig. F).	Eases insertion
 Lubricating the tube.	
Separate the buttocks well so that the anus is in plain view.	Helps visualize insertion
Insert the tube 3–4 in (7–10 cm) in an adult.	Places the distal tip above the sphincters
Direct the tubing at an angle pointing toward the umbilicus (Fig. G).	Follows the contour of the rectum
 Inserting the enema tube. (From Lippincott Williams & Wilkins. [2022]. *Nursing procedures* [9th ed.]. Lippincott Williams & Wilkins.)	
Hold the tube in place with one hand (Fig. H).	Avoids displacement
 Holding the tube in place.	

(*continued*)

SKILL 31-3 Administering a Cleansing Enema (*continued*)

Suggested Action	Reason for Action
Release the clamp.	Promotes instillation
Instill the solution gradually over 5–10 minutes (Fig. I).	Fills the rectum

Instilling the enema solution.

Suggested Action	Reason for Action
Clamp the tube for a brief period while the client takes deep breaths and contracts the anal sphincters if cramping occurs.	Avoids further stimulation
Resume instillation when the cramping is relieved.	Facilitates effectiveness
Clamp and remove the tubing after sufficient solution has been instilled or the client states they cannot retain more.	Completes the procedure
Encourage the client to retain the solution for 5–15 minutes.	Promotes effectiveness
Hold the enema tubing in one hand and pull a glove over the inserting end of the tubing.	Prevents direct contact
Remove and discard the remaining glove and dispose of the enema equipment.	Follows the principles of medical asepsis
Assist the client to sit while eliminating the solution and stool.	Aids in defecation
Examine the expelled solution.	Provides data for evaluating the effectiveness of the procedure
Clean and dry the client; help them into a comfortable position.	Demonstrates concern for the client's well-being

EVALUATION

- A sufficient amount of solution is instilled.
- A comparable amount of solution is expelled.
- The client eliminates stool.

DOCUMENT

- Type of enema solution
- Volume instilled
- Outcome of procedure

SAMPLE DOCUMENTATION

Date and Time   1,000 mL tap water enema administered. Large amount of brown formed stool expelled.
_____ J. Doe, LPN

SKILL 31-4 Changing an Ostomy Appliance

Suggested Action	Reason for Action
ASSESSMENT	
Wash hands or use an alcohol-based hand rub (see Chapter 10).	Reduces the transmission of microorganisms and complies with standard precautions
Use two methods to identify the client.	Supports the principles of safety recommended by The Joint Commission
Inspect the faceplate, pouch, and peristomal skin.	Determines the necessity for changing the appliance and provides data about the condition of the stoma and the surrounding skin
Determine how much the client understands about stomal care and changing an ostomy appliance.	Provides an opportunity for health teaching; prepares the client for assuming self-care
PLANNING	
Obtain replacement equipment, supplies for removing the adhesive (e.g., the manufacturer's recommended solvent if appropriate), and products for skin care.	Facilitates organization and efficient time management
Plan to replace the appliance immediately if the client has localized symptoms.	Prevents complications
Schedule an appliance change for an asymptomatic client before a meal.	Coincides with a time when the gastrocolic reflex is less active
Plan to empty the pouch just before the appliance will be changed.	Prevents soiling
IMPLEMENTATION	
Pull the privacy curtain.	Demonstrates respect for the client's dignity
Place the client in a supine or dorsal recumbent position.	Facilitates access to the stoma
Wash your hands or use an alcohol-based hand rub; put on gloves.	Reduces the transmission of microorganisms; complies with standard precautions
Unfasten the pouch and discard it in a lined receptacle or waterproof container.	Facilitates access to the faceplate
Gently peel the faceplate from the skin (Fig. A).	Prevents skin trauma

A

Removing the faceplate. (Photo by B. Proud.)

Wash the peristomal area with water or mild soapy water using a soft washcloth or gauze square.	Cleans mucus and stool from the skin
Suggest that the client shower or bathe at this time.	Provides an opportunity for daily hygiene and will not affect the exposed stoma

(continued)

SKILL 31-4 Changing an Ostomy Appliance (*continued*)

Suggested Action	Reason for Action
After or instead of bathing, pat the peristomal skin dry.	Promotes the potential for adhesion when the faceplate is applied
Measure the stoma using a stomal guide (Fig. B).	Determines the size of the stomal opening in the faceplate

Measuring the stoma. (Photo by B. Proud.)

Suggested Action	Reason for Action
Trim the opening in the faceplate to the measured diameter plus approximately in larger (Fig. C).	Avoids pinching of or pressure on the stoma and causing circulatory impairment

Trimming the stomal opening. (Photo by B. Proud.)

Suggested Action	Reason for Action
Attach a new pouch to the ring of the faceplate (Fig. D).	Avoids pushing the pouch into place after the faceplate has been applied

Attaching the pouch. (Photo by B. Proud.)

Suggested Action	Reason for Action
Fold and clamp the bottom of the pouch (Fig. E).	Seals the pouch so leaking will not occur

Sealing the pouch. (Photo by B. Proud.)

SKILL 31-4 Changing an Ostomy Appliance (*continued*)

Suggested Action	Reason for Action
Peel the backing from the adhesive on the faceplate (Fig. F).	Prepares the appliance for application
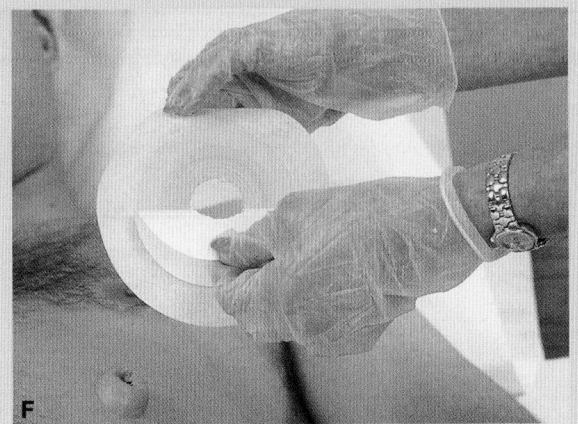 F	Removing the adhesive backing. (Photo by B. Proud.)
Have the client stand or lie flat.	Keeps the skin taut and avoids wrinkles
Position the opening over the stoma and press into place from the center outward (Fig. G).	Prevents air gaps and skin wrinkles
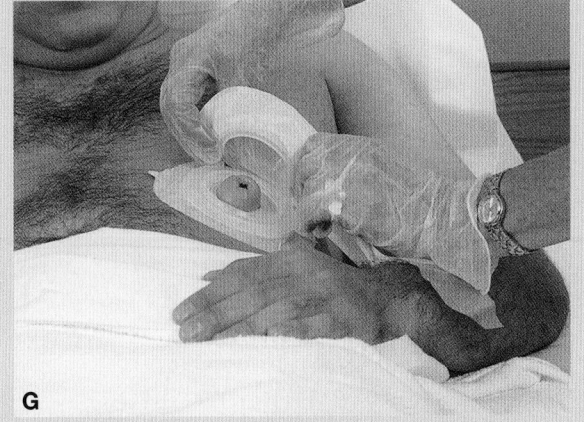 G	Attaching the appliance. (Photo by B. Proud.)
Perform hand hygiene after removing gloves.	Removes transient microorganisms

EVALUATION

- The stoma appears pink and moist.
- The skin is clean, dry, and intact with no evidence of redness, irritation, or excoriation.
- The new appliance adheres to the skin without wrinkles or gaps.

DOCUMENT

- Assessment data
- Peristomal care
- Application of new appliance

SAMPLE DOCUMENTATION

Date and Time Ostomy appliance removed. Peristomal skin cleansed with soapy water and patted dry. Stoma is pink and moist. Peristomal skin is intact and painless. New appliance applied over stoma. _____ J. Doe, LPN

SKILL 31-5 Irrigating a Colostomy

Suggested Action	Reason for Action
ASSESSMENT	
Check the medical orders to verify the written order and type of solution to use.	Ensures collaboration between nursing activities and the medical treatment
Use two methods to identify the client.	Supports the principles of safety recommended by The Joint Commission
Determine how much the client understands about colostomy irrigation.	Provides an opportunity for health teaching; prepares the client to assume self-care
PLANNING	
Obtain an irrigating bag and sleeve, lubricant, and a belt (Fig. A). A bedpan will be needed if the client is confined to the bed.	Promotes organization and efficient time management

A

Irrigation bag

Irrigation sleeve

Stoma cone

Irrigation equipment. (From Craven, R. F., Hirnle, C. J., & Jensen, S. [2020]. *Fundamentals of nursing* [9th ed.]. Lippincott Williams & Wilkins.)

Suggested Action	Reason for Action
Prepare the irrigating bag with solution in the same way as for an enema set (see Skill 31-3).	Provides the mechanism for cleansing the bowel
Unclamp the tubing and fill it with solution.	Purges air from the tubing
IMPLEMENTATION	
Assist the client into a sitting position in bed, in a chair in front or beside the toilet, or on the toilet itself.	Facilitates collecting drainage
Place absorbent pads or towels on the client's lap.	Prevents soiling of linen or clothing
Hang the container approximately 12 in (30 cm) above the stoma.	Facilitates gravity flow
Wash your hands or use an alcohol-based hand rub; don gloves.	Reduces the transmission of microorganisms; complies with standard precautions
Empty and remove the pouch from the faceplate if the client is wearing one.	Provides access to the stoma
Secure the sleeve over the stoma and fasten it around the client with an elastic belt (Fig. B).	Provides a pathway for drainage

Positioning the irrigation sleeve.

B

SKILL 31-5 Irrigating a Colostomy (*continued*)

Suggested Action	Reason for Action
Place the lower end of the sleeve into the toilet, commode, or bedpan (Fig. C).	Collects drainage

Placing the distal end of the sleeve.

C

Suggested Action	Reason for Action
Lubricate the cone at the end of the irrigating bag.	Facilitates insertion
Open the top of the irrigating sleeve.	Provides access to the stoma
Insert the cone into the stoma (Fig. D).	Dilates the stoma and provides a means for instilling fluid

Inserting the irrigation cone.

D

Suggested Action	Reason for Action
Hold the cone in place and release the clamp on the tubing.	Prevents expulsion of the cone and initiates the instillation
Clamp the tubing and wait if cramping occurs.	Interrupts the instillation while the bowel adjusts
Release the clamp and continue once the discomfort disappears.	Resumes instilling the fluid without discomfort to the client
Clamp the tubing and remove the cone when the irrigating solution has been instilled.	Discontinues the administration of solution
Close the top of the irrigating sleeve.	Keeps drainage in a downward direction
Give the client reading materials or hygiene supplies.	Provides diversion or uses time for other productive activities
Remove the belt and sleeve when the draining has stopped.	Eliminates unnecessary equipment
Clean the stoma and pat it dry.	Maintains tissue integrity

(continued)

SKILL 31-5 Irrigating a Colostomy (*continued*)

Suggested Action	Reason for Action
If the client is wearing an appliance, place a clean pouch over the stoma or cover the stoma temporarily with a gauze square.	Collects fecal drainage
Repeat hand hygiene measures after removing gloves.	Removes transient microorganisms

EVALUATION

- A sufficient amount of solution is instilled.
- A comparable amount of solution is expelled.
- Stool is eliminated.

DOCUMENT

- Type of irrigation solution
- Volume instilled
- Outcome of procedure

SAMPLE DOCUMENTATION

Date and Time Colostomy irrigated with 500 mL of tap water. Instilled without difficulty. Moderate amount of semiformed stool expelled with solution. Stoma cleansed with water and dried. Covered with a gauze square. _____ J. Doe, LPN

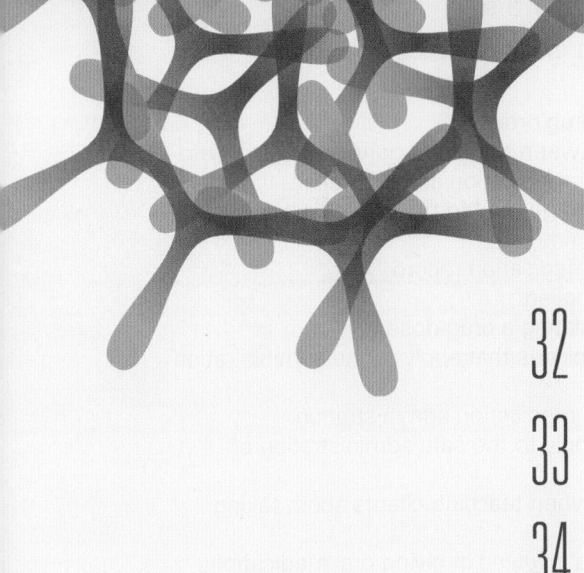

UNIT 9 | Medication Administration

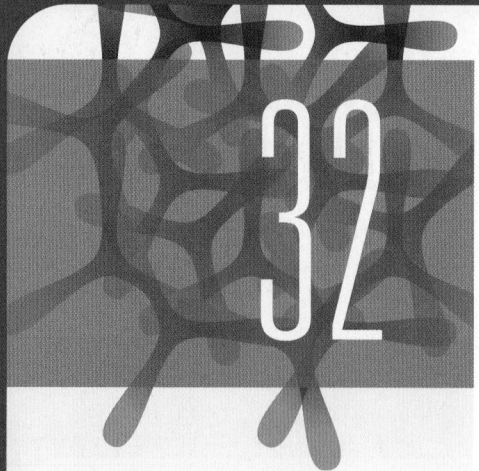

Oral Medications

Words To Know

automated medication-dispensing systems
barcode medication administration system
computerized provider order entry
continuous release
controlled substances
dose
drug diversion
enteric-coated tablets
extended release
generic name
individual supply
medication administration record
medication order
medications
opioids
oral route
over-the-counter medications
polypharmacy
route of administration
scored tablet
stock supply
sustained release
trade name
unit dose supply
xerostomia

Learning Objectives

On completion of this chapter, the reader should be able to:

1. Define medication.
2. Name components of a drug order.
3. Explain the difference between trade and generic drug names.
4. Name common routes for medication administration.
5. Describe the oral route and general forms of medication administered this way.
6. Explain the purpose of a medication record.
7. Name ways drugs are supplied.
8. Give the formula for calculating a drug dose.
9. Discuss nursing responsibilities that apply to the administration of opioids.
10. Name the five "rights" of medication administration.
11. Discuss guidelines that apply to the safe administration of medications.
12. Discuss points to stress when teaching clients about taking medications.
13. Explain the circumstances involved in giving oral medications by an enteral tube and commonly associated problems.
14. Describe appropriate actions in the event of a medication error.

INTRODUCTION

One of the nurse's most important responsibilities is the administration of **medications** (chemical substances that change body function). This chapter emphasizes the safe preparation and administration of medications, particularly those given by the oral route. This chapter uses the terms *medications* and *drugs* synonymously; information on specific drugs can be found in pharmacology texts or in drug reference manuals.

 Gerontologic Considerations

■ Older people who have had cerebrovascular accidents (or strokes) or who are experiencing middle-to-late stages of dementia may have dysphagia (impaired swallowing). Speech therapists are helpful in evaluating dysphagia and recommending safe and effective methods of administering oral medications.

■ Some older adults have diminished salivary gland secretions and develop **xerostomia** (dry mouth). Offering a sip of water before administering medications or mixing oral medications with some soft food (such as applesauce) may prevent medication from adhering to the tongue and thus facilitate administration.

■ If an older person has difficulty comprehending information about medication routines, include a responsible person in the discharge instructions to ensure client safety. A referral for skilled nursing visis is appropriate for homebound older adults who need additional instructions about medication routines after discharge.

■ Older people should be taught to carry a current list of all their medications, dosages, times of administration, and names of the prescribing provider. Should an older client be found wandering or unconscious, an evaluation for possible medication adverse effects can happen more quickly if such information is readily available.

■ Older people should use eyeglasses or hearing aids as needed to optimize their learning conditions. Other important considerations for the teaching–learning environment are adequate nonglare lighting and little, if any, background noise.

■ An evaluation of comprehension may be best done by having the older person repeat instructions after they are provided. Reinforce verbal instructions with written instructions at the older person's reading level. A copier may be used to enlarge instructions for clients with visual impairments. Written instructions are particularly important for clients with hearing impairments. They provide a reference for older adults with difficulty recalling or comprehending information. In addition, written instructions serve as a point of reference for caregivers who may assist with medication administration.

■ Older adults who have problems with manual dexterity or strength may request that pharmacists use easy-to-open caps on their prescription containers.

■ Clients with visual impairments may benefit from methods of identifying their medication containers other than reading labels. Suggestions include using rubber bands or textured materials on certain containers or using bright colors to mark the labels. Many simple-to-use medication management systems, sometimes called pill organizers, are available. Often, a family member is helpful in setting up weekly medication management systems. For example, a family member may set out the medications in specially designed containers weekly. This method enables others to monitor patterns and the adherence to the medication regimen and may be especially helpful when working with older people experiencing memory impairments.

■ Older adults with insurance coverage for prescriptions may find it easier and more economic to have prescriptions filled every 3 months. It may also be more economic to purchase prescriptions by mail or internet if the insurance provider approves this option.

■ Encourage older adults to ask their primary health care providers about prescribing generic forms of medication for cost savings.

MEDICATION ORDERS

A **medication order** lists the drug name and directions for its administration. Usually, physicians or dentists provide medication orders either written or signed electronically via a secured computer program. Other health care providers, such as a physician's assistant or an advanced practice nurse, can also provide medication orders if legally designated to do so by state statutes. Medication orders in the client's medical record are used here for the purposes of discussion.

Components of a Medication Order

All medication orders must have seven components:

1. The client's name
2. The date and time the order is written
3. The drug name
4. The dose to be administered
5. The route of administration
6. The frequency of administration
7. The signature of the person ordering the drug

If any one of these components is absent, the nurse must withhold administering the drug until they have obtained the missing information. Medication errors are serious. *Nurses never implement a questionable medication order until after consulting with the person who has written the order.*

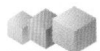 Concept Mastery Alert

Questionable Medication Orders

A nurse is legally responsible for ensuring that all components of a medication order are present and correct before administering any drug. If there is any question in the nurse's mind about the order as it is written, whether it be misleading or difficult to understand, the nurse must get clarification from the person who wrote the order. Remember, the client's safety is the primary concern.

Drug Name

Most drugs have a **trade name** (the name by which a pharmaceutical company identifies its drug). A trade name is sometimes called a brand or proprietary name. A drug's trade name is generally capitalized and followed by an R within a circle, as in ®.

Drugs also have a **generic name** (a chemical name not protected by a company's trademark), which is written in lowercase letters. For example, Demerol® is a trade name used by Winthrop Pharmaceuticals for the generically named drug meperidine hydrochloride. The NCLEX examination is using generic names and omitting trade names in the current test plan.

Look-Alike and Sound-Alike Drug Names

Physicians, nurses, and pharmacists must be aware that there are many look-alike and sound-alike drug names. The Institute for Safe Medication Practices (ISMP) requires hospitals to develop a list of look-alike/sound-alike medications they store, dispense, or administer in an effort to promote the safe administration of medications. The ISMP provides a list of confused drug names that is available as a resource (see examples in Box 32-1). Everyone involved in prescribing and administering medications should refer to a compiled list. The list should be updated at least yearly.

Avoiding abbreviations for drug names, such as "MS" for "morphine sulfate," and indicating the purpose for the drug with the medication order may also help avoid any misinterpretation. For example, a prescription for Lunesta written "for sleep" would not be confused with Neulasta, which

BOX 32-1	Examples of Confused Drug Names

Drug Name	Look-Alike and Sound-Alike Drug
Adderall	Inderal
Apidra	Spiriva
Celexa	Zyprexa
Bupropion	Buspirone
Cozaar	Zocor
Ephedrine	Epinephrine

TABLE 32-2 Routes of Drug Administration

ROUTE	METHOD OF ADMINISTRATION
Oral	Swallowing
	Instillation through an enteral tube
Sublingual	Under the tongue
Buccal	Between the gum and the inner cheek
Topical	Application to skin or mucous membrane
Inhalant	Aerosol
Parenteral	Injection: intravenous, intramuscular, subcutaneous

is prescribed to increase a client's white blood cell count. Some agencies have a policy that only the generic name can be prescribed or that the prescription include both the generic name and the trade name.

Drug Dose

The **dose** means the amount of drug to administer and is prescribed using the metric system. Some drugs are also prescribed in units, milliunits, international units, and milliequivalents (mEq), a unique measurement used primarily for chemical compounds such as potassium chloride.

The ISMP has identified additional error-prone abbreviations, symbols, and dose designations on their website. Other recommendations from the ISMP relate to high-alert medications in acute care settings, oral dosage forms that should not be crushed, and high-alert medications in long-term care settings. Additionally, refer to Table 32-1 for The Joint Commission's "Do Not Use" abbreviations in prescribed medications.

For home use, drug dosages are converted to household measurements that are more easily interpreted by nonprofessionals.

Route of Administration

The **route of administration** refers to how a drug is given, which may be by an oral, topical, inhalant, or parenteral route (Table 32-2). Topical and inhalant routes of administration are discussed in Chapter 33; parenteral administration is described in Chapters 34 and 35.

Oral Route

The **oral route** (the administration of drugs by swallowing or instillation through an enteral tube) facilitates drug absorption through the gastrointestinal tract. It is the most common route for medication administration because it is safer, more economic, and more comfortable than others. Medications administered by the oral route come in both solid and liquid forms.

Solid medications include tablets and capsules. A **scored tablet** (a solid drug manufactured with a groove in the center) is convenient when only part of a tablet is needed so it can be easily halved. **Enteric-coated tablets** (a solid drug covered with a substance that dissolves beyond the stomach) are manufactured for drugs that cause irritation of the stomach. Enteric-coated tablets are never cut, crushed, or chewed because when the integrity of the coating is impaired, the drug dissolves prematurely in gastric secretions. Some tablets and capsules are considered modified release and may be identified as **sustained release** (SR), sustained action (SA), **extended release** (ER, XR, or XL) or use similar abbreviations like **continuous release** (CR), which indicates that the drug is designed to dissolve slowly and be released over time. Modified-release drugs alter drug release and absorption, may improve patient adherence, improve effectiveness, maintain a steadier drug level in the body, and reduce adverse events (GoodRx Health, 2023). Sustained-, extended-, and continuous-release medications are never crushed; doing so affects the rate of drug absorption.

Liquid forms of oral drugs include syrups, elixirs, and suspensions. Nurses measure and administer liquid

TABLE 32-1 The Joint Commission's Official "Do Not Use" List of Abbreviations

DO NOT USE	POTENTIAL PROBLEM	USE INSTEAD
U (unit)	Mistaken for "0" (zero), the number "4" (four), or "cc"	Write "unit."
IU (international unit)	Mistaken for IV (intravenous) or the number 10 (ten)	Write "international unit."
Q.D., QD, q.d., qd (daily)	Mistaken for each other	Write "daily."
Q.O.D., QOD, q.o.d., qod (every other day)	Period after the Q mistaken for "I" and the "O" mistaken for "I"	Write "every other day."
Trailing zero (X.0 mg) in any medication order or medication-related documentation	Decimal point is missed	Write X mg.
Lack of leading zero (.X mg)	Decimal point is missed	Write 0.X mg.
MS	Can mean morphine sulfate or magnesium sulfate	Write "morphine sulfate"
MSO_4 and $MgSO_4$	Can be confused for one another	or "magnesium sulfate."

From The Joint Commission. (2022). *"Do Not Use" list of abbreviations.* http://www.jointcommission.org/topics/patient_safety.aspx

medications in calibrated cups, droppers, or syringes or with a dosing spoon (Fig. 32-1).

 Pharmacologic Considerations

Polypharmacy (the administration of four or more medications to the same person) increases the risk of drug interactions and adverse reactions. Almost 50% of people over 65 take five or more medications weekly. This can lead to drug interactions that are hard to identify due to the different drugs that could be the cause. Therefore, medication reconciliation should be done any time an unanticipated change in a client's status is observed.

Effects of Reduced Organ Function on Drugs

There are a number of pharmacokinetic changes that may result from the reduced function of different organs in the body, such as the kidneys and liver (Table 32-3).

Frequency of Administration

The frequency of drug administration refers to how often and how regularly the medication is to be given. Frequency of administration is written using standard abbreviations of Latin origin. Some common examples include:

- Stat—immediately
- b.i.d.—twice a day
- t.i.d.—three times a day
- q.i.d.—four times a day
- q.h.—hourly
- q4h—every 4 hours
- p.r.n.—as needed

Chapter 9 and Appendix list other common abbreviations.

When the medication order is implemented, drug administration is scheduled according to the prescribed frequency. The health agency sets a predetermined timetable for drug administrations; hours of administration may vary among agencies. For example, if a physician orders a q.i.d. (four times a day) administration of a medication, it may be scheduled for administration at 8 AM, noon, 4 PM, and 8 PM; at 10 AM, 2 PM, 6 PM, and 10 PM; or at 6 AM, noon, 6 PM, and midnight.

 Pharmacologic Considerations

To simplify a complex medication regimen, a number of drugs consistently prescribed together are made in combination form. An example is Namzaric, which combines memantine and donepezil, two drugs used to treat Alzheimer disease. This can reduce administration of three pills daily to one pill daily.

Verbal and Telephone Orders

Verbal orders are instructions for client care that are given during face-to-face conversations. Telephone orders are obtained from a physician during a telephone conversation. Both types of orders are more likely to result in misinterpretation than are written orders. However, there are circumstances when verbal and telephone orders are justified:

- When a physician or provider is involved in a procedure they cannot leave

TABLE 32-3 Effects of Reduced Organ Function on Drugs in the Body

CHANGES IN ORGAN SYSTEMS	CHANGES IN DRUG ABSORPTION, DISTRIBUTION, METABOLISM, AND EXCRETION
Reduced kidney/liver function	Increased circulatory drug concentration
Increased water and reduced fat in tissue (children/elders)	Hamper drug concentration in tissues
Decreased blood albumin levels	Reduced protein binding of medications
Decreased gastric secretions	Delayed drug absorption
Reduced urinary function	Higher bladder concentration of drugs

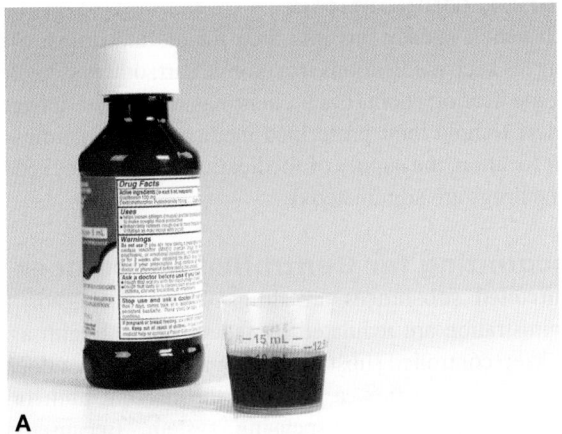

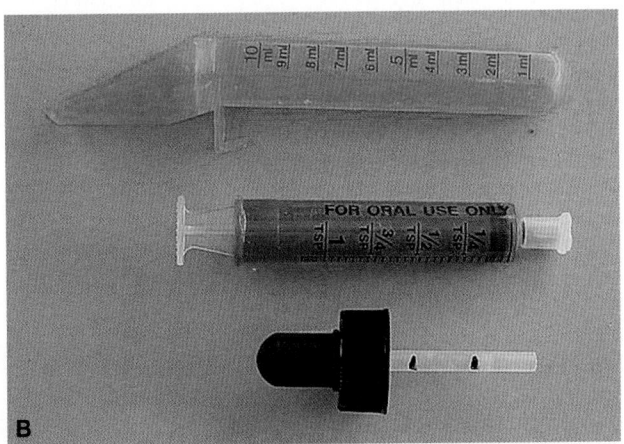

FIGURE 32-1 Equipment used to measure liquid medication. **A.** Calibrated medication cup. **B.** Dosing spoon, oral syringe, and medication dropper. (**A:** Cheryl Casey/Shutterstock. **B:** from Buchholz, S. [2019]. *Henke's med-math* [9th ed.]. Lippincott Williams & Wilkins.)

- When a physician or provider is managing the urgent care of another client
- When a **computerized provider order entry** (CPOE) is unavailable or the physician or provider is unable to access it
- When a delay in obtaining an order would cause harm to a client or result in a negative outcome

If a prescriber is physically present, it is appropriate to ask tactfully that the order be handwritten (Nursing Guidelines 32-1).

Documentation in the Medication Administration Record

Once the nurse has obtained the medication order, they transcribe it to the **medication administration record** (MAR; agency form used to document drug administration). Use of the MAR ensures timely and safe medication administration. Some agencies use a form on which nurses transcribe the

NURSING GUIDELINES 32-1

Obtaining Telephone Orders

- Always identify yourself, your agency, and the unit on which you are working. *This orients the provider as to who is requesting or receiving a medical order.*
- Identify the client, the situation, background circumstances, pertinent assessments, and recommendation (SBAR) concerning care. *SBAR is The Joint Commission's recommended practice for spoken communication among health care members.*
- Verify the identity of the prescriber with a call-back telephone number or a specific number on record at the agency. *Authenticating the prescriber's identity provides evidence that the order has reliably been obtained from the responsible provider or someone covering in their absence.*
- Have a second nurse listen simultaneously on an extension. *A second nurse serves as a witness to the communication.*
- Record the date and time with the drug order directly on the client's medical record as it is received. *A written recording avoids errors in memory.*
- Make sure the order includes the essential components. *Doing so complies with standards for care.*
- Clarify or spell drug names, especially those that sound similar, such as Celebrex and Celebrex, or Nicobid and Nitro-Bid. *Checking avoids medication errors.*
- Spell or repeat numbers to avoid misinterpretation, such as 15 (one, five) and 50 (five, zero). *This step avoids medication errors.*
- Read back the written information to the prescriber. *Repetition clarifies understanding and accuracy.*
- Use the abbreviation "T.O." at the end of the order. *This abbreviation indicates the order is a telephone order.*
- Write the prescriber's name and cosign with your name and title. *This step complies with legal standards and demonstrates accountability for the communication.*
- Remind the prescriber that the order must be signed as soon as possible according to the agency's policy. *This confirms responsibility for the order.*

drug order by hand; others use a computer-generated form (Fig. 32-2). Regardless of the type, all MARs provide a space for documenting when a drug is given, along with a place for the signature, title, and initials of each nurse who administers a medication or documenting the nurse who administers the medication automatically when barcodes are scanned electronically. The MAR being used is usually kept separate from the client's medical record, but it eventually becomes a permanent part of it.

METHODS OF SUPPLYING MEDICATIONS

After transcribing the medication order to the MAR, the nurse requests the drug from the pharmacy with a paper, computer, or a facsimile (fax) transmission request. Drugs are supplied, or dispensed, in three major ways. An **individual supply** is a container with enough of the prescribed drug for several days or weeks, which is common in long-term care facilities such as nursing homes (Fig. 32-3). A **unit dose supply** (a self-contained packet that holds one tablet or capsule) is most common in acute care hospitals that stock drugs for individual clients several times in 1 day (Fig. 32-4). In long-term care facilities, single doses of drugs may be packaged in a multidose blister pack. A **stock supply** (large number of stored drugs) remains on the nursing unit for use in an emergency so that a nurse can give a drug without delay.

Some facilities use **automated medication-dispensing systems** (Fig. 32-5). These systems usually contain frequently used medications for that unit, any as-needed (p.r.n.) medications, controlled drugs, and emergency medications. The nurse accesses the system by using a personal password and then selects the appropriate choice from a computerized menu. This type of system automatically keeps a record of dispensed medications and records the password, username, and title. To avoid **drug diversion**, a term used by the U.S. Drug Enforcement Administration (DEA) when referring to the theft or possession of drugs (usually controlled substances prescribed for someone else), the user's password should never be shared with anyone.

Storing Medications

Each health agency has one area for storing drugs. Some agencies keep medications in a mobile cart; others store them in a medication room. Each client has a separate drawer or cubicle to hold their prescribed medications. Regardless of their location, the supply of medications remains locked until the drugs are administered.

Accounting for Controlled Substances

Controlled substances are drugs whose possession and administration are regulated by federal laws. Health agencies keep controlled substances such as **opioids** in a double-locked drawer, a box, a room in the nursing unit, or an automated medication-dispensing system. Because controlled substances are usually delivered by stock supply, nurses are responsible for an accurate account of their use. They keep a record of each drug used from the stock supply.

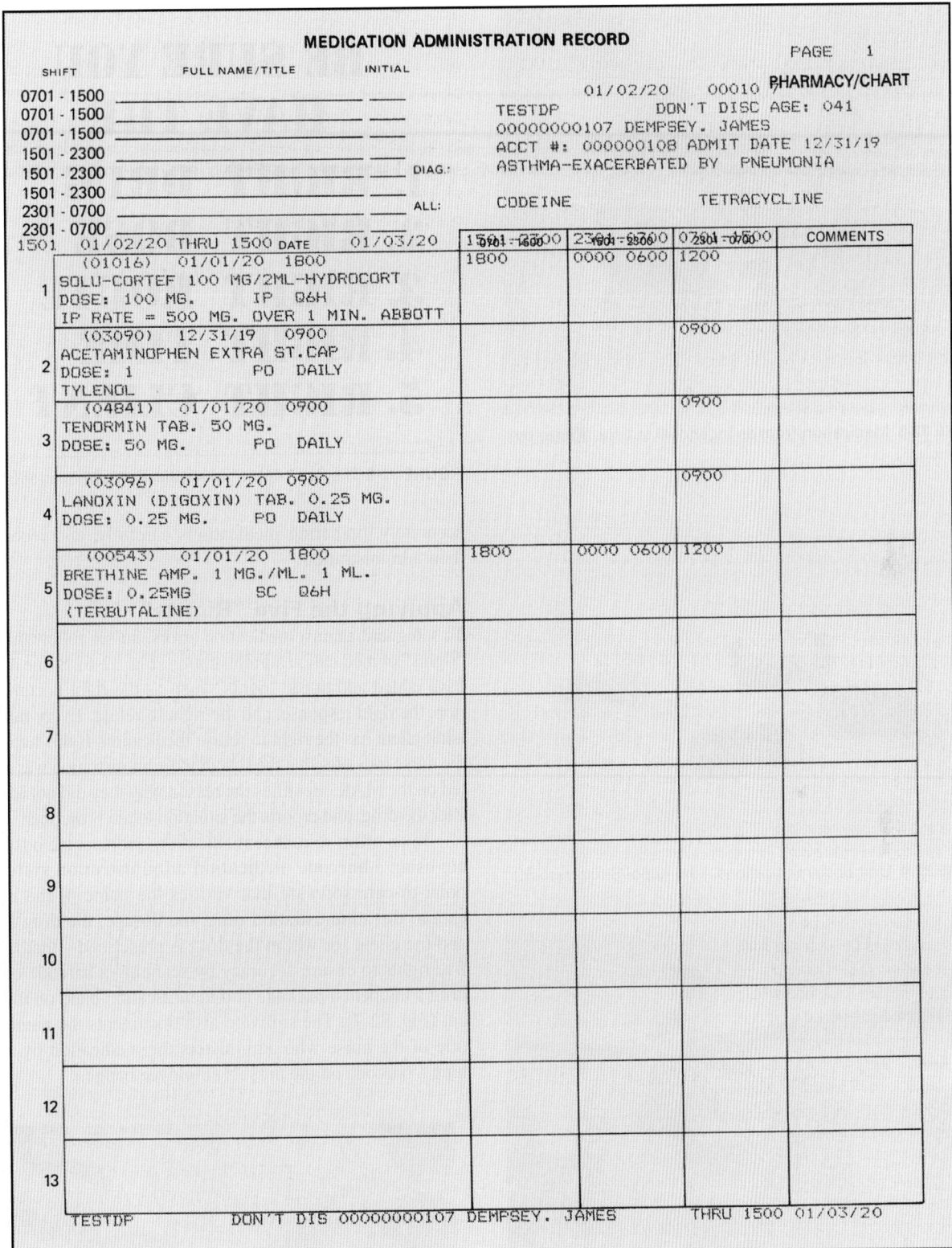

FIGURE 32-2 A computer-generated medication administration record.

Any controlled substance that is wasted in whole or in part must be cosigned by a witness.

Nurses count controlled substances regularly, usually at each change of shift. One nurse counts the number in the supply, while another checks the record of their administration or amounts that have been wasted. Both counts must agree with inconsistencies accounted for as soon as possible.

MEDICATION ADMINISTRATION

Safety is the main concern in medication administration. Taking various precautions before, during, and after each administration reduces the potential for medication errors. Some precautions include ensuring the five "rights" of medication administration, calculating drug dosages

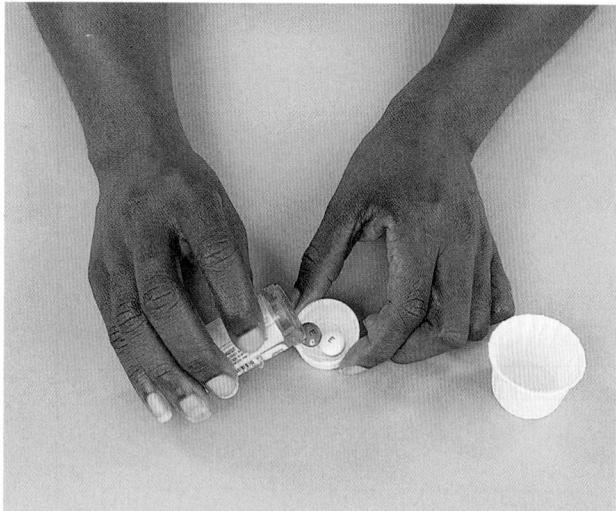

FIGURE 32-3 Medication from an individual supply. (Photo by B. Proud.)

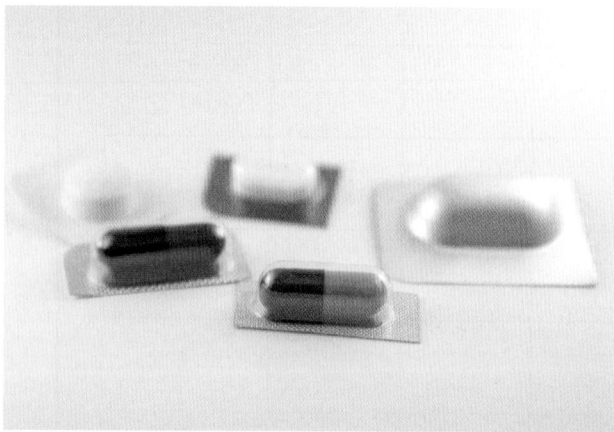

FIGURE 32-4 Unit dose medications. (khuntapol/Shutterstock.)

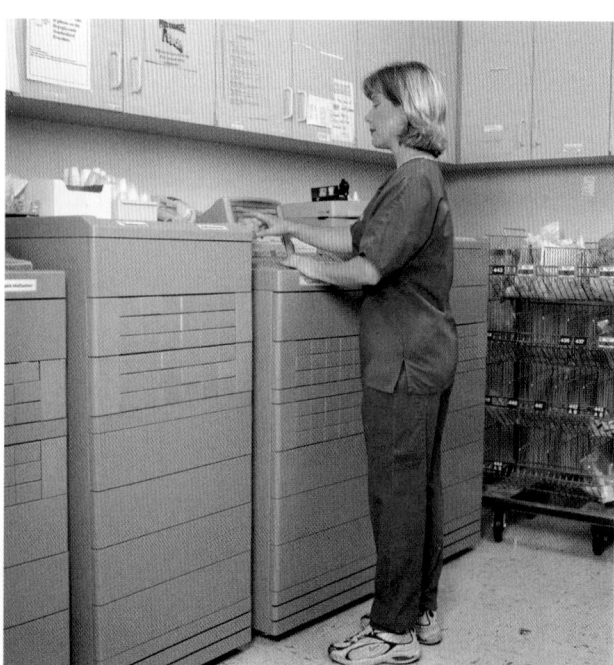

FIGURE 32-5 An automated medication-dispensing system.

BE SURE YOU HAVE THE
1. RIGHT DRUG
2. RIGHT DOSE
3. RIGHT ROUTE
4. RIGHT TIME
5. RIGHT CLIENT

FIGURE 32-6 The five "rights" of medication administration.

accurately, preparing medications carefully, and recording their administration.

Applying the Five "Rights"

To safeguard against medication errors, nurses follow the five "rights" of medication administration (Fig. 32-6). Some nurses have added additional "rights" such as the right documentation, the right response, and the right to refuse. Every rational adult client has the right to refuse medication. If this happens, the nurse indicates that the scheduled administration was omitted on the MAR, identifies the reason why they did not administer the drug, and reports the situation to the prescriber.

In an effort to reduce medication errors, some hospitals are using a **barcode medication administration system**, a point-of-care software that verifies the name of the medication, the administration time, the dosage, the drug form, and the client for whom the drug is prescribed—that is, the five rights to ensure accuracy by scanning a barcode on the drug's unopened package and identification band on the client (Fig. 32-7). The software also documents the name and title of the nurse who administers the medication by scanning a barcode on the nurse's employee badge.

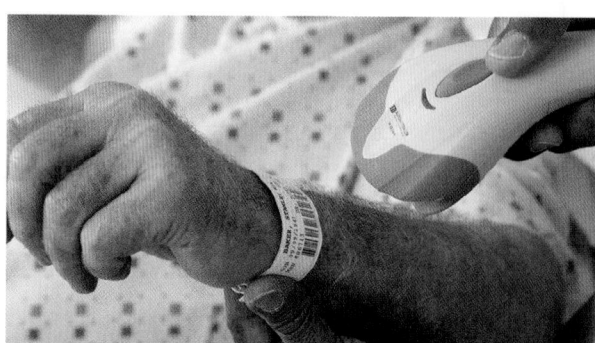

FIGURE 32-7 A client's identification bracelet is scanned prior to administering a medication. (From Craven, R. F., Hirnle, C., & Henshaw, C. M. [2020]. *Fundamentals of nursing* [9th ed.]. Lippincott Williams & Wilkins.)

BOX 32-2   Drug Calculation Formula

$$\frac{D}{H} \times Q = \frac{\text{Desired dose}}{\text{Dose on hand (supplied dose)}} \times \text{Quantity}$$

Example
Drug order: Tetracycline 500 mg (desired dose) by mouth q.i.d.
Dose supplied: 250 mg (dose on hand) per 5 mL (quantity)

$$\text{Calculation}: \frac{500\,\text{mg}}{250\,\text{mg}} \times 5\,\text{mL} = 10\,\text{mL}$$

Calculating Dosages

One of the major nursing responsibilities, and one of the five rights, is preparing the dose accurately. Preparing an accurate dose sometimes requires the nurse to convert doses between metric and household equivalents. Once the prescribed and supplied amounts are in the same measurements and system of measurement, the quantity for administration can be easily calculated using a standard formula (Box 32-2, Nursing Guidelines 32-2).

Administering Oral Medications

Nurses prepare and bring oral medications to the client in a paper or a plastic cup (Skill 32-1). The nurse administers only those medications that they have personally prepared, *never administering medications prepared by another nurse.* Once at the bedside, it is also important for the nurse to remain with the client while the client takes medications.

If a client is not on the unit at the time of medication administration, the nurse returns the medications to the medication cart or room. Leaving medications unattended may result in their loss or accidental ingestion by someone else.

 ## NURSING GUIDELINES 32-2

Preparing Medications Safely

- Prepare medications under well-lit conditions.
  Light improves the ability to read labels accurately.
- Work alone without interruptions and distractions.
  This promotes concentration.
- Check the label of the drug container three times: (1) when reaching for the medication, (2) just before placing the medication into an administration cup, and (3) when returning the medication to the client's drawer. *Checking ensures attention to important information.*
- Avoid using medications from containers with a missing or obliterated label. *This eliminates speculating on the drug name or dose.*
- Return medications with dubious or obscured labels to the pharmacy. *This step facilitates replacement or new labeling.*
- Never transfer medications from one container to another. *Such transfers could lead to mismatching contents.*
- Check the expiration dates on liquid medications. *Doing so ensures administration at desired potency.*
- Inspect the medication and reject any that appear to be decomposing. *This step promotes appropriate absorption.*

 ### Pharmacologic Considerations

Many drugs are absorbed better from the gastrointestinal tract when taken before or 1 to 2 hours after meals. Be sure and check for appropriate timing of oral drug administration for best absorption.

Many opportunities exist for teaching when administering medications. Teaching is especially important before discharge because the client often receives prescriptions for oral medications. Providing health teaching helps ensure clients administer their own medications safely, follow instructions, and adhere to the medication regimen. Even clients who purchase **over-the-counter medications** (nonprescription drugs) may benefit from instruction (Client and Family Teaching 32-1).

Administering Oral Medications by Enteral Tube

When a client cannot swallow oral medications, they can be instilled by enteral tube (Skill 32-2). Because the lumen of a tube is smaller than the esophagus, special techniques may be required to avoid obstruction (Nursing Guidelines 32-3).

 ### Client and Family Teaching 32-1
Taking Medications

The nurse teaches the client and the family as follows:
- Inform the prescriber of all other drugs that you are currently taking.
- Have prescriptions filled at the same pharmacy so that the pharmacist can spot any potential drug interactions.
- Consider asking for a new prescription to be partially filled. This provides an opportunity to evaluate the drug's effect and side effects before purchasing the full amount.
- Read and follow the label directions carefully.
- Take the prescription medication for the full time that it has been prescribed.
- Check with the prescriber before combining nonprescription and prescription drugs.
- Dispose of old prescription drugs and outdated over-the-counter medications; they tend to disintegrate or change in potency.
- Consult with the prescriber if a drug does not relieve symptoms or causes additional discomfort.
- Ask the prescriber or pharmacist whether it is appropriate to take specific medications with food or on an empty stomach.
- Drink a liberal amount of water or other fluids each day to assist with the appropriate absorption and elimination of drugs.
- Do not take drugs prescribed for someone else, even if your symptoms are similar.
- Wear a MedicAlert tag if you are taking prescription drugs on a regular and long-term basis.
- Use a pill organizer if you have trouble remembering whether you took a medication.

NURSING GUIDELINES 32-3

Preparing Medications for Enteral Tube Administration

- Use the liquid form of the drug whenever possible. *This promotes tube patency.*
- Add 15 to 60 mL of water to thick liquid medications. *Water dilutes the medication and facilitates instillation.*
- Pulverize tablets with a pill crusher (see figure) except those that are enteric-coated. *Pulverizing creates small granules that may instill more readily.*
- Open the shell of a capsule to release the powdered drug. *This step facilitates mixing into a liquid form.*
- Avoid crushing sustained-release pellets. *Keeping them whole ensures their sequential rate of absorption.*
- Mix each drug separately with at least 15 to 30 mL of water. *Water provides a medium and dilute volume for administration.*
- Use warm water when mixing powdered drugs. *It promotes dissolving the solid form.*
- Pierce the end of a sealed gelatin capsule and squeeze out the liquid medication or aspirate it with a needle and syringe. *These measures facilitate access to the medication.*
- As an alternative, soak a soft gelatin capsule in 15 to 30 mL of warm water for approximately 1 hour. *Soaking dissolves the gelatin seal.*
- Avoid administering bulk-forming laxatives through an enteral tube. *Such laxatives could obstruct the tube.*
- Interrupt a tube feeding for 15 to 30 minutes before and after administration of a drug that should be given on an empty stomach. *Doing so facilitates the drug's therapeutic action or its absorption.*
- Clamp a nasogastric tube that is being used to suction gastric secretions for 30 minutes after administering medication. *Keeping the tubing temporarily clamped allows time for the medication to move beyond the stomach and be absorbed.*

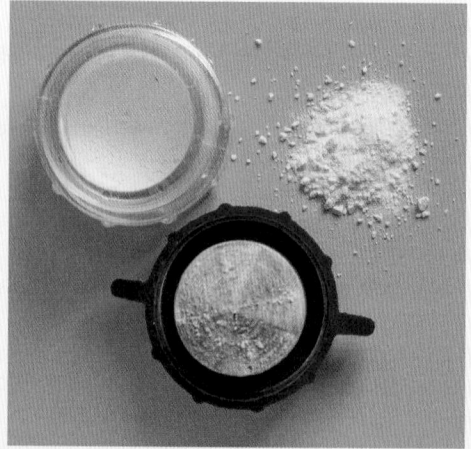

Crushing solid oral medications, with a pill crusher/grinder. (Zagorulko Inka/Shutterstock.)

Nurses use slightly different techniques for administering medications through an enteral tube used for nourishment than they do for tubes used for decompression (suctioning) (see Chapter 29). After administering the medications through an enteral tube used for decompression, the nurse clamps or plugs the tube for at least 30 minutes to prevent removal of the drug before it leaves the stomach. Nurses can administer medications while a client is receiving tube feedings, but they instill the medications separately—that is, they do not add the medications to the formula. This is done for two reasons. First, some drugs may physically interact with the components in the formula, causing it to curdle or otherwise change its consistency. Also, a slow infusion would alter the rate of absorption of the drug.

 Stop, Think, and Respond 32-1

What actions are appropriate if a client cannot swallow medications prescribed by the oral route?

Documentation

If the nurse is not using a barcode medication system that documents drug administration immediately and automatically, the nurse should document medication administration manually on the MAR, the client's chart, or both as soon as possible (Fig. 32-8). Timely documentation prevents medication errors; if the nurse does not record the dose, another nurse may assume that the client has not received the medication and may give a second dose.

If a nurse withholds a medication, they document its omission according to agency policy. A common method of such documentation is to circle the time of administration and initial the entry. The nurse may document the reason for the omission in a comments section on the MAR or elsewhere in the client's medical record.

Pharmacologic Considerations

■ Medication in liquid form is preferred for enteral tube administration when possible because it is less likely to cause tube occlusion.

■ Two important safety points to remember: (1) draw up drug solutions only in oral syringes to avoid the accidental parenteral administration of an oral preparation; (2) never crush extended—or timed-release medications for enteral tube administration; it could cause an overdose of the drug.

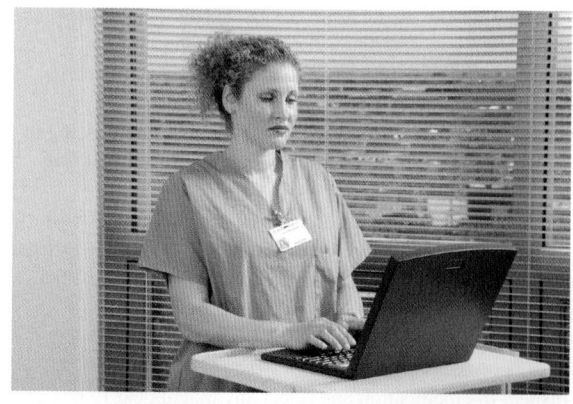

FIGURE 32-8 Documentation of the medication administration is an important nursing requirement. (Photo by B. Proud.)

Medication Errors

Medication errors happen too often. When errors occur, whether as a result of a prescriber's order, drug supplied by the pharmacy, or nursing drug administration, nurses have an ethical and legal responsibility to report the error to maintain the client's safety.

As soon as an error is recognized, the nurse checks the client's condition and reports the mistake to the prescriber and the supervising nurse immediately. Health care agencies have a form for reporting medication errors, called an incident sheet or accident sheet (see Chapter 3). The incident sheet is not a part of the client's permanent record, nor does the nurse make any reference in the chart to the fact that they have completed an incident sheet. The completed incident report is generally reviewed by the agency's risk management committee (see Chapter 3).

The purpose of the incident sheet is to understand the circumstances surrounding the error and prevent them in the future; *it is not intended to accuse or blame the involved health care provider. The desired outcome is to ensure the safety of clients and identify ways to prevent a similar reoccurrence.* However, if the same person makes repeated errors, the agency may recommend a period of retraining or supervision.

NURSING IMPLICATIONS

Whenever nursing care involves the administration of medications, one or more of the following nursing diagnoses may be applicable:

- Knowledge deficiency
- Aspiration risk
- Nonadherence
- Polypharmacy
- Altered health maintenance

Nursing Care Plan 32-1 shows how nurses can follow the steps in the nursing process to manage the care of a client with the nursing diagnosis of altered health maintenance, defined as a change in an individual's ability to perform the functions necessary to maintain health or wellness.

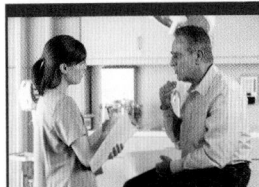

Clinical Scenario A nurse reviews a 58-year-old client's postoperative recovery following heart surgery. When the client is asked to review his current medications, the fails to identify taking medications for controlling hypertension and elevated lipids.

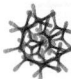

NURSING CARE PLAN 32-1 | Altered Health Maintenance

Assessment
- Check whether the client is returning for scheduled appointments with the prescribing physician or health care provider.
- Assess the current status of the client's health problem to determine whether the response to the prescribed plan of care is that which is expected.
- Ask to examine the client's containers of medications.
- Review the labels attached to prescription medications.
- Have the client identify the number of pills or capsules per dose, the frequency of self-administration, and time of the last dose.

- Determine by the dates on the containers and the number of medications in the container(s) whether the client is using or partially using medication.
- Encourage the client to relate problems encountered with self-administration of medications such as intolerance of side effects, an inability to pay for refills, a belief that the medication is ineffective, difficulty remembering the dosing schedule, and trouble opening the containers.

Nursing Diagnosis. Altered health maintenance related to an inaccurate belief regarding the use and benefit of prescribed medication therapy as manifested by pulse rate of 94 bpm at rest, blood pressure of 178/94 in R arm while sitting, dyspnea following coronary bypass surgery, beta-blocker, diuretic, cholesterol lowering, and elevated cholesterol test results. The client states, "I didn't get my prescriptions filled last week. I wasn't having any chest pain and I figured the surgery fixed my heart."

Expected Outcome. The client will (1) explain the purpose of prescribed medications and possible consequences if they are not taken and (2) resume taking prescribed medications within 24 hours (3/7).

Interventions	Rationales
Provide the client with the following information: The purpose for the prescribed beta-blocker and diuretic medications is to reduce the work of the heart. The diuretic helps lower blood pressure, so the heart does not have to pump as much circulating blood and can eject the blood from the heart more easily. Easing the work of the heart reduces the potential for recurring chest pain, a subsequent myocardial infarction (heart attack), or congestive heart failure. Cholesterol-lowering medication reduces the deposition of fatty plaque in arteries.	Health teaching helps clarify the rationale for medication therapy and promotes adherence.

(continued)

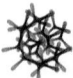

NURSING CARE PLAN 32-1 — Altered Health Maintenance (*continued*)

Interventions	Rationales
Have the client rephrase explanations for drug therapy in their own words.	Rephrasing provides evidence that the client has understood the nurse's explanation.
Note the client's level of understanding.	Doing so indicates whether or not the nurse needs to clarify misinformation.
Acknowledge when the client's explanation is accurate or reexplain information that continues to be misunderstood.	These measures reinforce learning.
Go over the schedule of medication administration with the client.	Reviewing the schedule helps the client plan a routine for self-administration.
Suggest that the client discuss any deviations in medication schedule or dosage with the physician.	This offers an alternative if the client feels a need to alter or discontinue self-administration.

Evaluation of Expected Outcome

- The client correctly paraphrased information regarding drug therapy.
- The client states, "I know people take nitroglycerin for heart problems, but I didn't know how important these other drugs are. I'd rather take some pills than to have to go back to the hospital again."
- The client plans to have prescriptions filled before returning home following the office visit.
- The client indicates that he will take one beta-blocker each morning if his heart rate is at least 60 bpm and one diuretic tablet every other day, which correlates with the dosing regimen.
- The client states that he will take his lipid-lowering medication every evening and return for a repeat laboratory test in 6 months.
- The client is scheduled for another office checkup in 1 month. He states, "I'll be sure to call if I think there's a reason I can't take my medications."

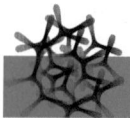

KEY POINTS

- A medication order lists the drug name and directions for its administration.
- Components of a medication order
  - The client's name
  - The date and time the order is written
  - The drug name
  - The dose to be administered
  - The route of administration
  - The frequency of administration
  - The signature of the person ordering the drug
- Drug names
  - Trade name: The name by which a pharmaceutical company identifies its drug
  - Generic name: A chemical name not protected by a company's trademark
- Four routes of administration
  - Oral
  - Topical
  - Inhalant
  - Parenteral route
- MAR: Written or computerized form used to document drug administration
- Methods of supplying medications
  - Individual supply: A container with enough of the prescribed drug for several days or weeks; common in long-term care facilities such as nursing homes

- Unit dose supply: A self-contained packet that holds one tablet or capsule and is most common in acute care hospitals that stock drugs for individual clients several times in 1 day
- Stock supply: Large number of stored drugs that remain on the nursing unit for use in an emergency so that a nurse can give a drug without delay
- Five "rights" of medication administration
  - Right drug
  - Right dose
  - Right route
  - Right time
  - Right client
- Medication administrations via enteral tube
  - Use liquid form of the medication if available.
  - Pulverize medication to make it easier to pass through the tube.
  - Add 15 to 60 mL of water as needed to thicken medication.
  - After administering medication through the tube, clamp the tube for 30 minutes to a tube used for suctioning.
- Medication errors
  - If an error occurs, first check the client.
  - Report mistake to the provider and nursing supervisor.
  - Complete an incident/accident report form.
  - No mention of the incident/accident report is included in the client chart.

CRITICAL THINKING EXERCISES

1. The nurse is administering medications to a client. The client says, "I've never taken that little yellow pill before." What actions are appropriate next?
2. A client who lives alone says, "You have to be a genius to keep all these pills straight." How could you help this client organize the medication regimen?
3. What action(s) are appropriate if a barcode medication administration system sounds an alert to a problem during the process of administering medication to a client?
4. What response would be appropriate if an experienced nurse asked you to document being a witness to a wasted controlled substance medication you did not observe?

NEXT-GENERATION NCLEX-STYLE REVIEW QUESTIONS

1. If a physician orders 250 mg of a drug, and it is supplied in 500-mg scored tablets, which nursing action is best?
   a. Ask the pharmacist to provide 250-mg tablets instead.
   b. Consult the physician about the prescribed dose.
   c. Give the client half of the 500-mg tablet.
   d. Check whether the drug is manufactured in a smaller dose.
   Test-Taking Strategy: Note the key word, "best." Use the process of elimination and select the option that is better than any of the others.
2. Which action is best when a nurse brings medication to a room for a client named Anna Jones, but the client in that room is not wearing an identification bracelet?
   a. The nurse asks the client, "Are you Anna Jones?"
   b. The nurse asks the client, "What is your name?"
   c. The nurse asks a nursing assistant to identify the client.
   d. The nurse asks the client, "What medications do you take?"

Test-Taking Strategy: Note the key word, "best." Use the process of elimination to select the option that is better than any of the others.

3. When a nurse observes that a client has difficulty swallowing a capsule of medication, which action is most appropriate?
   a. Soak the capsule in water until soft.
   b. Tell the client to chew the capsule.
   c. Empty the capsule in the client's mouth.
   d. Offer the client water before giving the capsule.
   Test-Taking Strategy: Note the key word and modifier, "most appropriate." Analyze the options and select the action that is better than any of the others.
4. A nurse is teaching a mother about administering liquid medication to a toddler. The medication is supplied with a dosing spoon shown here. Mark an "X" on the image indicating the equivalent of 1 tsp.

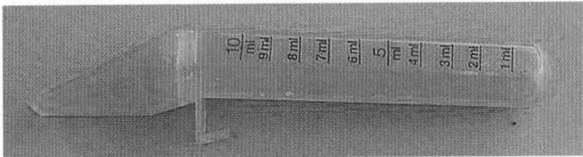

   Test-Taking Strategy: Review the metric milliliter (mL) equivalent for 1 tsp.
5. A nurse must administer a series of medications through a nasogastric tube that is being used for decompression. Place the nursing actions in the sequence they should be performed. Use all of the options.
   a. Clamp the tube for 30 minutes.
   b. Flush the tube with at least 5 mL of water.
   c. Add diluted medication to the tube.
   d. Check the distal location of the tube.
   e. Reconnect the tube to suction.
   Test-Taking Strategy: Recall the steps that should be followed when administering medications into a nasogastric tube; then place the options in their appropriate order.

SKILL 32-1 Administering Oral Medications

Suggested Action	Reason for Action
ASSESSMENT	
Compare the medication administration record (MAR) with the written medical order.	Prevents medication errors
Review the client's drug, allergy, and medical history.	Avoids potential complications
Consult a current drug reference concerning the drug's action, side effects, contraindications, and administration information.	Ensures appropriate administration based on a thorough knowledge base
PLANNING	
Plan to administer medications within 30–60 minutes of their scheduled time.	Demonstrates a timely administration and compliance with the medical order
Allow sufficient time to prepare the medications in a location with minimal distractions.	Promotes safe preparation of drugs
Make sure that there is a sufficient supply of paper and plastic medication cups.	Facilitates organization and efficient time management
Chill oily medications.	Reduces their unpleasant odor and improves palatability
IMPLEMENTATION	
Wash your hands or perform an alcohol-based hand rub (see Chapter 10).	Removes colonizing microorganisms
Read and compare the label on the drug with the MAR at least three times—before, during, and after preparing the drug (Fig. A).	Ensures that the *right drug* is given at the *right time* by the *right route*

Comparing the drug label and the MAR. (Photo by B. Proud.)

Calculate doses.	Complies with the medical order and ensures that the *right dose* is given
Place medications or unit dose packets within a paper or plastic cup without touching the medication itself.	Supports principles of asepsis
Keep drugs that require special assessments or special administration techniques in a separate cup.	Helps identify drugs that require special nursing actions
Pour liquids with the drug label toward the palm of the hand.	Prevents liquid from running onto the label
Hold the cup for liquid medications at eye level when pouring (Fig. B).	Facilitates accurate measurement

Ensuring accuracy by measuring liquids in a medicine cup at eye level.

SKILL 32-1 Administering Oral Medications (*continued*)

Suggested Action	Reason for Action
Prepare a supply of soft-textured food such as applesauce or pudding, according to the client's individual needs.	Facilitates the administration for clients with impaired swallowing
Help the client into a sitting position.	Facilitates swallowing and prevents aspiration
Identify the client using at least two methods, for example, checking the wristband and asking the client's name and birthdate (Fig. C).	Ensures that medications are given to the *right client; complies with the National Patient Safety Goals*

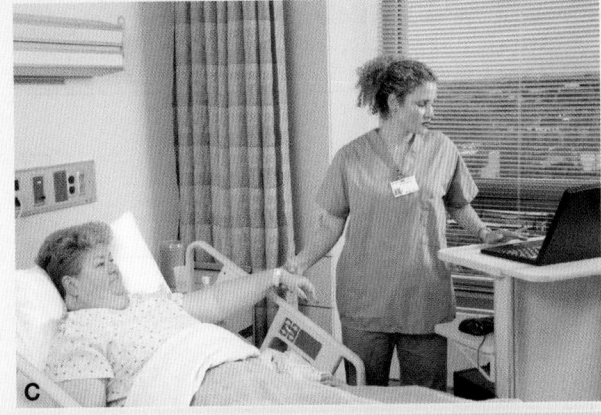

C

Checking the identification band. (Photo by B. Proud.)

Offer a cup of water with solid forms of oral medications (Fig. D).	Water moistens mucous membranes and prevents medication from sticking.

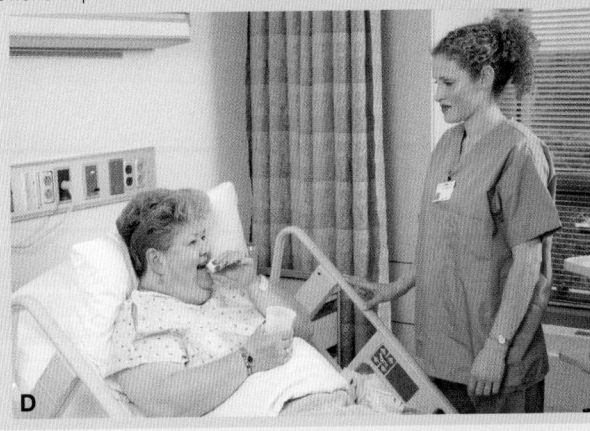

D

Offering the patient medication and water. (Photo by B. Proud.)

Advise the client to take medications one at a time or in amounts easily swallowed.	Prevents choking
Encourage the client to keep their head in a neutral position or one of slight flexion, rather than hyperextending the neck (Fig. E).	Protects the airway

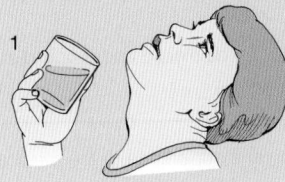
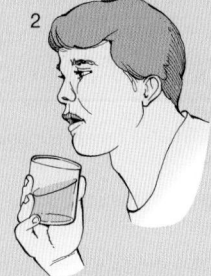
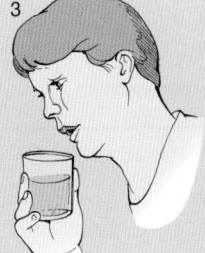

1, inappropriate neck position; 2 and 3, appropriate neck positions.

E

(*continued*)

SKILL 32-1 Administering Oral Medications (*continued*)

Suggested Action	Reason for Action
Remain with the client until they have swallowed the medications.	Ensures the appropriate administration
Restore the client to a position of comfort and safety.	Shows concern for the client's well-being
Record the volume of fluid consumed on the intake and output record.	Demonstrates responsibility for accurate fluid assessment
Record the administration of the medication.	Prevents medication errors
Assess the client in 30 minutes for desired and undesired drug effects.	Aids in evaluating the client's response and the effect of drug therapy

EVALUATION

- The five "rights" are upheld.
- The client experiences no choking or aspiration.
- The client exhibits a therapeutic response to the medication.
- The client demonstrates minimal or absent side effects.

DOCUMENT

- Preassessment data, if indicated
- Date, time, drug, dose, route, signature, title, and initials (usually on the MAR)
- Evidence of client's response, if it can be determined

SAMPLE DOCUMENTATION

Date and Time Temp. 103.8°F. Tylenol tabs given by mouth for relief of fever. Fever reduced to 103°F 30 minutes later.
_____ J. Doe, LPN

SKILL 32-2 Administering Medications through an Enteral Tube

Suggested Action	Reason for Action
ASSESSMENT	
Check the medication administration record (MAR) and compare the information with the written medical order.	Prevents medication errors
Review the client's drug, allergy, and medical history.	Avoids potential complications
Consult a current drug reference concerning the drug's action, side effects, contraindications, and administration information.	Ensures the appropriate administration based on a thorough knowledge base
Verify the location of the tube by comparing the length of the external tube with its measurement at the time of insertion.	Ensures airway protection and proper tube placement in the event that the tube has migrated
Inspect the client's mouth and throat.	Determines whether the tube has been displaced and is coiled at the back of the throat
PLANNING	
Plan to administer medications within 30–60 minutes of the scheduled time.	Demonstrates timely administration and adherence to the medical order
Separate and clamp or plug a feeding tube for 15–30 minutes if the drug will interact with food.	Ensures that the stomach will be relatively empty
Allow sufficient time to prepare the medications in a location with minimal distractions.	Promotes the safe preparation of drugs
Make sure there is a sufficient supply of plastic medication cups.	Facilitates organization and efficient time management
IMPLEMENTATION	
Wash your hands or perform an alcohol-based hand rub (see Chapter 10).	Removes colonizing microorganisms

SKILL 32-2 Administering Medications through an Enteral Tube (*continued*)

Suggested Action	Reason for Action
Read and compare the label on the drug with the MAR at least three times—before, during, and after preparing the drug.	Ensures the *right drug* is given at the *right time* by the *right route*
Prepare each drug separately.	Prevents potential physical changes when some drugs are combined
Take the cups containing diluted medications to the bedside, along with water for flushing, a 30- to 50-mL syringe, a towel or disposable pad, and clean gloves.	Facilitates instillation
Identify the client using at least two methods, for example, checking the wristband and asking the client's name and birthdate.	Ensures medications are given to the *right client; complies with the National Patient Safety Goals*
Help the client into a Fowler position.	Prevents gastric reflux
Put on clean gloves.	Prevents contact with body fluids
Insert the syringe into the tube, and instill 15–30 mL of water by gravity (Fig. A).	Flushes and reduces the surface tension of the tube

A

Instilling the medication. (From Lippincott Williams & Wilkins. [2008]. *Lippincott's nursing procedures and skills.* Author.)

Suggested Action	Reason for Action
Add the diluted medication to the syringe as it becomes nearly empty (Fig. B).	Prevents instilling air

B

Pouring medication into the tube. (From Lippincott Williams & Wilkins. [2022]. *Lippincott's nursing procedures and skills.* Author.)

Suggested Action	Reason for Action
Apply gentle pressure with the plunger or bulb of a syringe if the medication fails to instill easily.	Provides positive pressure
Flush with at least 5 mL of water between each instillation of medication and as much as 30 mL after instilling all the medications.	Prevents drug interactions and obstruction of the tube; fully instills all the prescribed drug
Pinch the tube as the syringe empties.	Prevents distending the stomach with air; maintains patency of the tube

(continued)

SKILL 32-2 Administering Medications through an Enteral Tube (*continued*)

Suggested Action	Reason for Action
Clamp or plug the tube for 30 minutes before reconnecting a tube to the suction (Fig. C).	Prevents removing the medication after it has been instilled
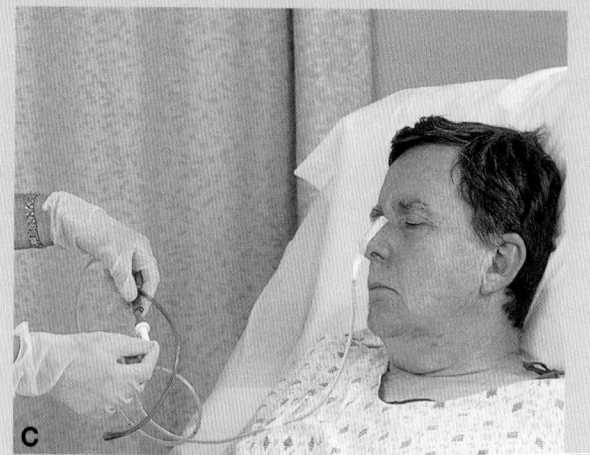	Plugging a gastric tube. (Photo by B. Proud.)
Connect a tube used for nourishment immediately if the medication and formula will not interact.	Facilitates the primary purpose of the enteral tube
Keep the head of the bed elevated with the client on the right side for at least 30 minutes (Fig. D).	Reduces the potential for esophageal reflux and aspiration
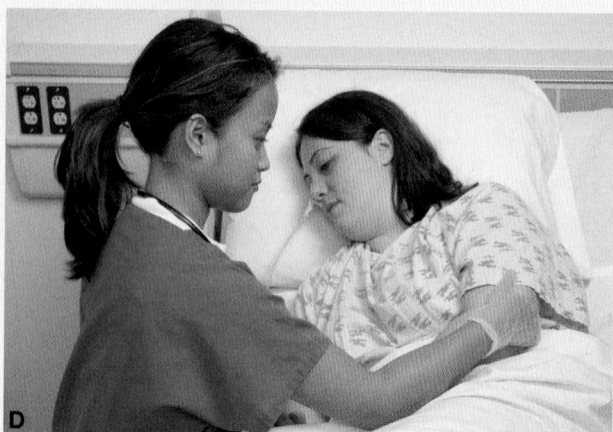	Positioning the client on the right side. (From Lippincott Williams & Wilkins. [2022]. *Lippincott's nursing procedures and skills*. Author.)

EVALUATION

- The tube placement is verified.
- The five rights are upheld.
- The medications instill freely and are flushed afterward.
- The client experiences no abdominal distention, nausea, vomiting, or other undesirable effects.
- The tube remains patent.

DOCUMENT

- Preadministration assessment data
- Medication administration on the MAR
- Volume of fluid instilled with the medication as well as for flushing the tube on the bedside intake and output record
- Response of the client

SAMPLE DOCUMENTATION

Date and Time   Placement of nasogastric tube verified by auscultation. No evidence of tube migration. Medications administered (see MAR) per nasogastric tube. Flushed with 30 mL after instilling medications. Tube clamped at this time. No evidence of nausea or distention. _____ J. Doe, LPN

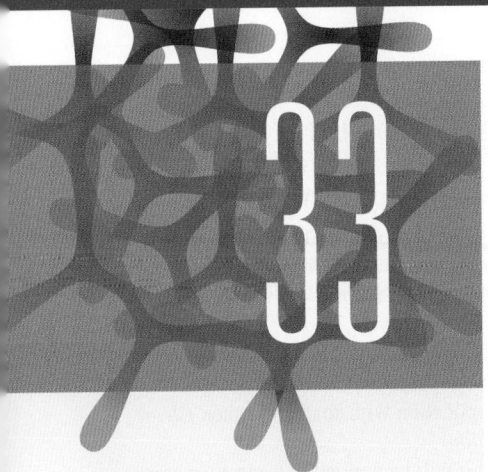

33

Topical and Inhalant Medications

Words To Know

aerosol
buccal application
dry powder inhaler
inhalant route
inhalers
metered-dose inhaler
nebulizer
ophthalmic application
otic application
paste
percutaneous application
rebound effect
skin patches
spacer
sublingual application
topical route
tragus
transdermal application

Learning Objectives

On completion of this chapter, the reader should be able to:

1. Explain how topical medications are administered and commonly applied.
2. Identify forms of drugs applied by the transdermal route and principles to follow when applying a skin patch.
3. Describe where eye medications are applied.
4. Explain how the administration of ear medications differs for adults and children.
5. Explain the rebound effect that accompanies the administration of nasal decongestants.
6. Describe the difference between sublingual and buccal administration.
7. Name a common reason for vaginal applications.
8. Give the form of medication used most often for rectal administration.
9. Explain why inhalation is a good route for medication administration.
10. Name types of inhalers and alternatives for administering inhaled medications.

INTRODUCTION

Drugs are administered by routes other than oral (see Chapter 32). This chapter describes the techniques used to administer drugs by the topical and inhalant routes.

 Gerontologic Considerations

■ The onset of drug action may be faster when administering topical medications to older adults because of their diminished subcutaneous fat, which leads to a more rapid absorption of topical medications.

■ Some older adults use two or more types of eye medications once or several times daily. If the caps of the eye medications are not color coded, suggest ways to color-code the containers or distinguish them in some other way such as using a rubber band on the container of one to help differentiate the medications.

■ Some older clients have difficulty reaching areas of the body to which topical drugs are applied. For example, arthritis may interfere with applying medication within the vagina or rectum or to skin lesions on the lower extremities.

■ Monitoring the heart rate and blood pressure of older adults who use inhaled bronchodilators is important because these medications commonly cause tachycardia and hypertension. Either or both of these effects increase the risks for complications, especially in older adults with an underlying cardiovascular disease.

737

TOPICAL ROUTE

Drugs given by the **topical route** (the administration of medications to the skin or mucous membranes) can be applied externally or internally (Table 33-1). Topically applied drugs have a local or systemic effect. Many are administered to achieve a direct effect on the tissue to which they are applied.

Percutaneous Applications

Percutaneous applications are drugs rubbed into or placed in contact with the skin. They include ointments, patches, and pastes.

Ointment Applications

An ointment is a topical preparation rubbed into the skin for administration of a medication (also called *oils, lotions, and creams*). Alert clients may self-administer an ointment after receiving proper instruction. In that situation, the nurse teaches proper application techniques and checks that the client has applied the medication appropriately and as often as prescribed. For clients who cannot perform their own topical ointments, the nurse does so (Nursing Guidelines 33-1).

Transdermal Applications

A **transdermal application** refers to drugs that are applied to and absorbed through the skin. Examples include skin patches and pastes.

Skin Patches

Skin patches are drugs bonded to an adhesive and applied to the skin for systemic distribution (Fig. 33-1). When applied,

NURSING GUIDELINES 33-1

Applying a Percutaneous Application

- Wash your hands or use an alcohol-based hand rub (see Chapter 10). *Hand hygiene removes colonizing microorganisms.*
- Check the identity of the client. *Doing so prevents administering the medication to the wrong person.*
- Put on clean gloves if your skin or that of the client is not intact. *Gloves provide a barrier to pathogens.*
- Cleanse the area of application with soap and water. *Clean skin promotes absorption.*
- Warm the substance if it will be applied to a sensitive area of the skin by holding it temporarily in your hands or placing the sealed container in warm water. *Warmth promotes comfort.*
- Shake the contents of liquids. *Shaking mixes the contents uniformly.*
- Apply the percutaneous substance to the skin with the fingertips, a cotton ball, or a gauze square. *Correct application distributes the substance over a wide area.*
- Rub the substance into the skin. *Rubbing promotes absorption.*
- Apply local heat to the area if desired (see Chapter 28). *Heat dilates peripheral blood vessels and speeds absorption.*

the patch stays in place for a number of hours and the drug migrates through the skin, absorbed at a rate that maintains a consistent drug level in the bloodstream.

Transdermal patches are typically applied to the chest, buttocks, stomach, and upper arms. The patch is marked

TABLE 33-1 Topical Medications

ROUTES	LOCATION	VEHICLE	EXAMPLES
Cutaneous	Skin	Ointment	Hydrocortisone (Cortaid)
	Skin	Cream	Benzocaine (Lanacane)
	Scalp	Liquid	Permethrin (Nix)
	Skin	Lotion	Lubriderm[a]
	Skin	Patch	Estrogen (Estraderm)
	Skin	Paste	Nitroglycerin (Nitrol)
	Oral mucous membrane	Gel	Benzocaine (Anbesol)
Ophthalmic	In the eye	Drops	Timolol (Timoptic)
		Ointment	Polymyxin, neomycin, bacitracin (Neosporin)
Otic	In the ear	Drops	Hydrocortisone, neomycin, polymyxin (Cortisporin Otic)
		Irrigation	Carbamide peroxide (Debrox)
Nasal	In the nose	Spray	Oxymetazoline (Afrin)
		Drops	Oxymetazoline (Neo-Synephrine)
Sublingual	Under the tongue	Tablet	Nitroglycerin (Nitrostat)
		Spray	Nitroglycerin (Nitrolingual)
Buccal	Between the cheek and gum	Tablet	Nitroglycerin (Nitrogard)
		Lozenge	Cepacol[a]
Vaginal	In the vagina	Douche	Povidone iodine (Massengill-medicated douche)
		Cream	Clotrimazole (Gyne-Lotrimin)
		Suppository	Fluconazole (Monistat)
Rectal	To or within the rectum	Irrigation	Sodium phosphate (Fleet Enema)
		Suppository	Bisacodyl (Dulcolax)
		Ointment	Hydrocortisone (Anusol)

[a]A nonprescription item that is a combination of ingredients.

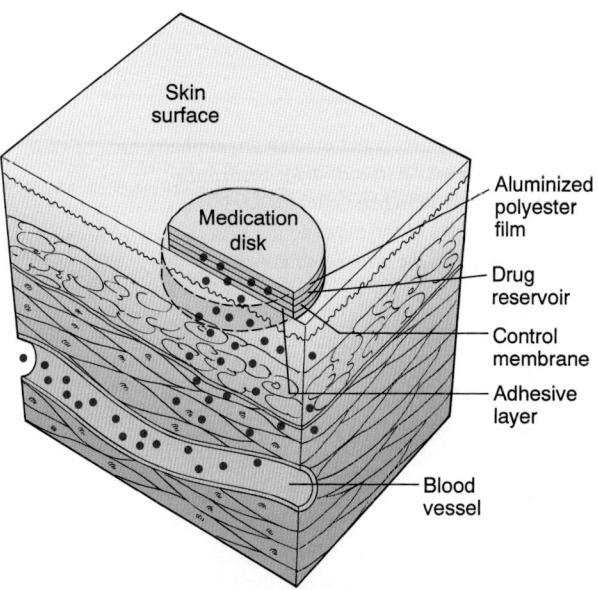

FIGURE 33-1 The pathway of absorption from a transdermal skin patch.

Labels on figure: Skin surface; Medication disk; Aluminized polyester film; Drug reservoir; Control membrane; Adhesive layer; Blood vessel

with date and time of administration, and the location is documented in the medication administration record. Each time a new patch is applied, it is placed in a slightly different location. Clipping hairy skin areas before an application may help adhesion. After initial application of a patch, it may take 30 minutes to 8 hours for the drug to reach a therapeutic level.

Because scopolamine, a drug used to prevent motion sickness, is a small, round patch, it is typically applied behind the ear. To maintain consistent blood levels of pain medication, fentanyl patches that are 100 times the strength of morphine are used around the clock. A nitroglycerin patch that is used to prevent and relieve chest pain is used for 12 to 14 hours and then removed for the same amount of time. When removed, patches should be closed with the adhesive edges together, preventing accidental exposure to others. Teach clients to dispose of patches away from children and pets.

 Pharmacologic Considerations

When clients are cognitively impaired, use the upper back for transdermal placement. This prevents the client from picking at and removing the patch.

Drug Pastes

A **paste** contains a drug within a thick base and is applied to but not rubbed into the skin. Nitroglycerin can be applied as a paste. Although sometimes the product is referred to as an *ointment*, this is a misnomer because the skin is not massaged once the drug is applied (Nursing Guidelines 33-2).

Nitroglycerin paste has a shorter duration of action than that supplied in a transdermal patch. Consequently, it must be applied more frequently to provide a sustained effect.

 Pharmacologic Considerations

■ Clients prescribed nitroglycerin in any form should not use a drug or herbal preparation for erectile dysfunction because the combination may contribute to severe hypotension due to the combined vasodilation effect.

■ Always use gloves when applying patches and pastes, and wash hands with soap and water after glove removal. This prevents accidental absorption of the drug by the provider.

Ophthalmic Applications

An **ophthalmic application** is a method of applying drugs onto the mucous membrane of one or both eyes (Skill 33-1). The mucous membrane of the eyes is called the *conjunctiva*. It lines the inner eyelids and the anterior surface of the *sclera*.

Ophthalmic medications are either supplied in liquid form and instilled as drops or applied as ointments along the lower lid margin. Blinking, rather than rubbing, distributes the drug over the surface of the eye. The eye is a delicate structure susceptible to infection and injury, just like any other tissue. Therefore, nurses take care to keep the applicator tip of the medication container sterile.

 Pharmacologic Considerations

Complex ophthalmic medication regimens can involve the instillation of multiple types of drops up to four times daily. When more than one eye medication is prescribed, it is best to wait 5 minutes between instillation of eye drops. For people having difficulty instilling eye medications independently, devices are available that can facilitate administration. Eye drop solutions should be disposed of every 28 days to prevent bacterial contamination of the eye.

>>> *Stop, Think, and Respond 33-1*

What actions should the nurse take if the tip of the ophthalmic medication becomes contaminated?

 Concept Mastery Alert

Distributing Eye Medications

When administering eye medications, it is important to ensure that the medication is distributed over the surface of the eye. The first instinct may be to rub the eye, but this would cause further trauma and irritation. Instead, have the client blink to distribute the eye medication.

Otic Applications

An **otic application** is a drug instilled in the outer ear. It is usually administered to moisten impacted cerumen or to instill medications to treat a local bacterial or fungal infection.

If drainage is present, put on gloves and clean the ear with a swab or face cloth. Warm the medication container

NURSING GUIDELINES 33-2

Applying Nitroglycerin Paste

- Wash your hands or perform an alcohol-based hand rub (see Chapter 10). *Hand hygiene removes colonizing microorganisms.*
- Use two methods for checking the client's identity. *Doing so prevents administering the medication to the wrong person.*
- Put on clean gloves. *Gloves act as a barrier preventing self-contact and absorption of the nitroglycerin.*
- Squeeze the prescribed amount of paste from the tube onto an application paper (Fig. A). *This complies with the medication order, which usually specifies the dose in inches.*

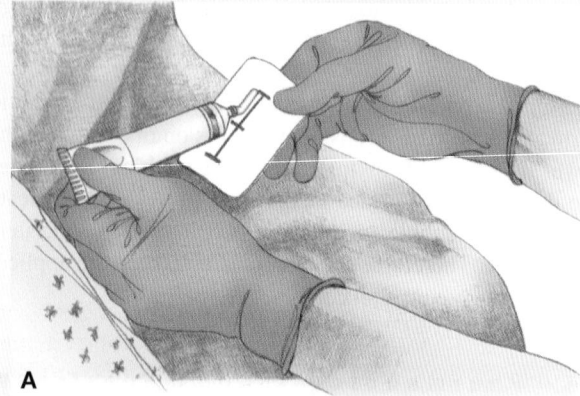

A

Applying paste to application paper. (From Springhouse. [2018]. *Lippincott's visual encyclopedia of clinical skills.* Wolters Kluwer Health.)

- Fold the paper or use a wooden applicator to spread the paste over approximately a 2.25 in × 3.5 in (5.6 cm × 8.8 cm) area of the paper. *These techniques facilitate distributing the drug over a wide area for quick absorption.*

- Place the application paper on a clean, nonhairy area of skin. *Such a placement facilitates drug absorption.*
- Cover the paper with plastic wrap, a transparent dressing, or tape all the edges of the paper to the skin (Fig. B). *This seals the drug between the paper and the skin.*

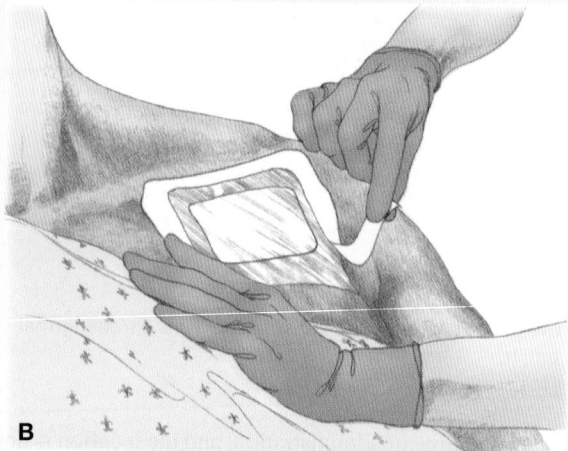

B

Covering the application paper with plastic wrap or a transparent semipermeable dressing. (From Springhouse. [2018]. *Lippincott's visual encyclopedia of clinical skills.* Wolters Kluwer Health.)

- Remove one application before applying another and remove any residue remaining on the skin. *Careful application prevents excessive drug levels.*
- Rotate the sites of medication placement. *Site rotation reduces the potential for skin irritation.*
- Remove the application if the client becomes flushed, hypotensive, or develops a severe headache.

to minimize the client's potential discomfort. Manipulate the ear to straighten the auditory canal. The technique varies depending on whether the client is a young child (the nurse pulls the ear down and back) or an adult (the nurse pulls the ear up and back; see Chapter 13).

Tilt the client's head away from the ear into which the medication will be instilled. Compress the container and instill the prescribed number of drops on the side of the ear canal rather than directly onto the tympanic membrane (Fig. 33-2). Press and release the **tragus**, the projection of skin-covered cartilage at the opening of the external ear, to facilitate moving the medication toward the eardrum. Place a small cotton ball loosely in the ear to absorb excess medication (Fig. 33-3). If a bilateral administration is prescribed, wait at least 5 minutes before instilling medication in the opposite ear. Briefly postponing the application within the second ear avoids displacing the initially instilled medication when repositioning the client.

Nasal Applications

Topical medications are dropped or sprayed within the nose (Skill 33-2). A proper instillation is important to avoid

displacing the medication into nearby structures, such as the back of the throat. Adults often self-administer their own nasal medications, but sometimes, nurses assist older adults and children.

Damage to the nasal passage from drug overuse can cause irritation of the nares and an inability to respond to the drug. This can happen when drugs are used more frequently

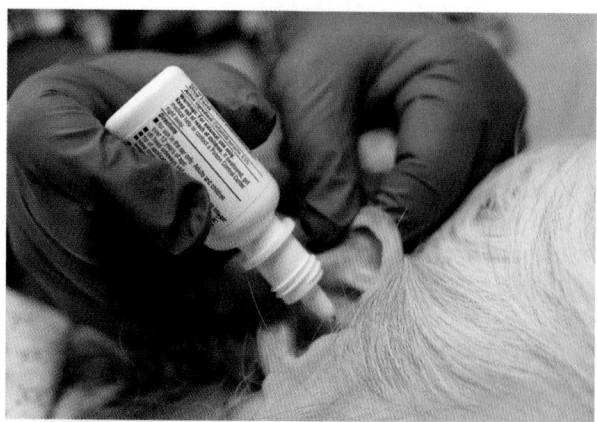

FIGURE 33-2 Instill eardrops with the affected ear uppermost.

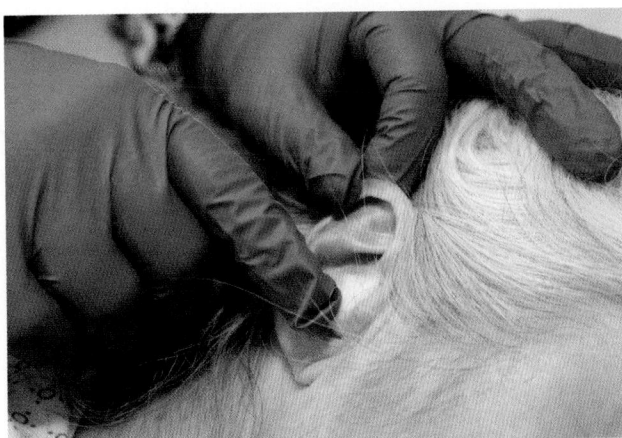

FIGURE 33-3 Insert a cotton ball loosely with the opening to the ear canal.

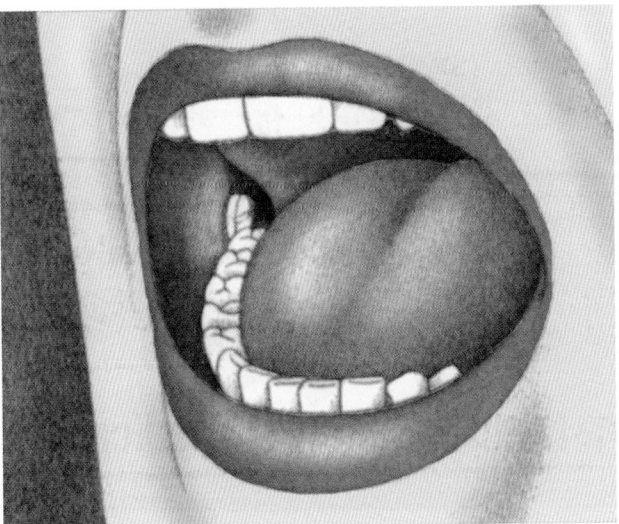

FIGURE 33-5 Site for buccal medication administration. (From Lippincott Williams & Wilkins. [2022]. *Lippincott's nursing procedures and skills*. Author.)

than prescribed and potentiated when people misinterpret the nasal congestion to be caused by cold or allergy rather than the drug itself and continue to use the drug to treat damaged nasal passages.

 Pharmacologic Considerations

Rebound nasal congestion also known as a **rebound effect** (rhinitis medicamentosa) results in nasal swelling when topical nasal decongestants are used more frequently than recommended.

Sublingual and Buccal Applications

A tablet given by **sublingual application** (a drug placed under the tongue) is left to dissolve slowly and becomes absorbed by the rich blood supply in the area (Fig. 33-4). Some drugs in spray form are also administered sublingually. A **buccal application** (a drug placed against the mucous

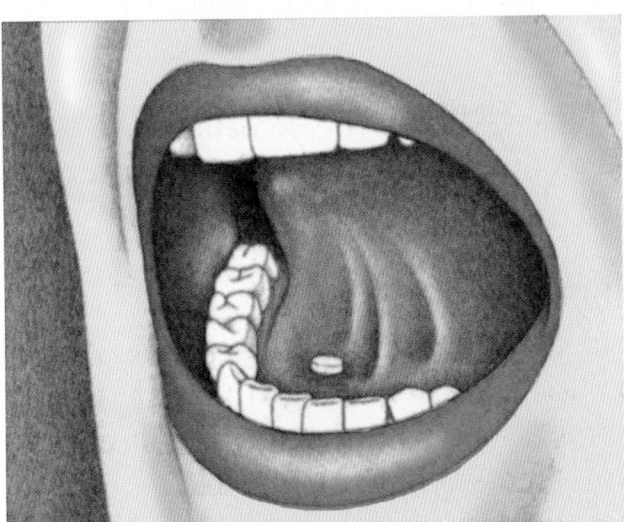

FIGURE 33-4 Site for sublingual medication administration. (From Lippincott Williams & Wilkins. [2022]. *Lippincott's nursing procedures and skills*. Author.)

membranes of the inner cheek) is another method of drug administration (Fig. 33-5).

During sublingual or buccal administration, the client is instructed not to chew or swallow the medication. Eating and smoking are also contraindicated during the brief time needed for a solid medication to dissolve.

Vaginal Applications

Topical applications are often used to treat local vaginal infections. Vaginal infections are common and usually the result of colonization by microorganisms such as yeasts that are abundant in stool. The microorganisms may get transferred during bowel elimination if the client wipes stool from the rectal area toward (not away from) the vagina. Yeast infections also occur when the pH balance of the vagina is disrupted, as can be caused by a number of different factors, including antibiotic use. Symptoms of a yeast infection include intense vaginal itching and a white, cheese-like vaginal discharge. Another common type of vaginitis is caused by a protozoan known as *Trichomonas vaginalis,* which is transmitted from an infected to an uninfected person during sex.

Several nonprescription antibiotic drugs such as metronidazole (Flagyl), miconazole (Monistat), and clotrimazole (Lotrimin) are useful in treating vaginal infections and are available in suppository, dissolvable vaginal tablet, gel, and cream form (Fig. 33-6). Early and appropriate self-treatment restores normal tissue integrity. Providing clients with instructions about how to administer vaginal medications for the most effective action may be helpful (Client and Family Teaching 33-1).

If the client cannot self-administer a vaginal medication, the nurse wears gloves to avoid contact with secretions (Fig. 33-7). After removing the gloves, handwashing or an alcohol-based hand rub is critical. The same advice holds true for rectal applications.

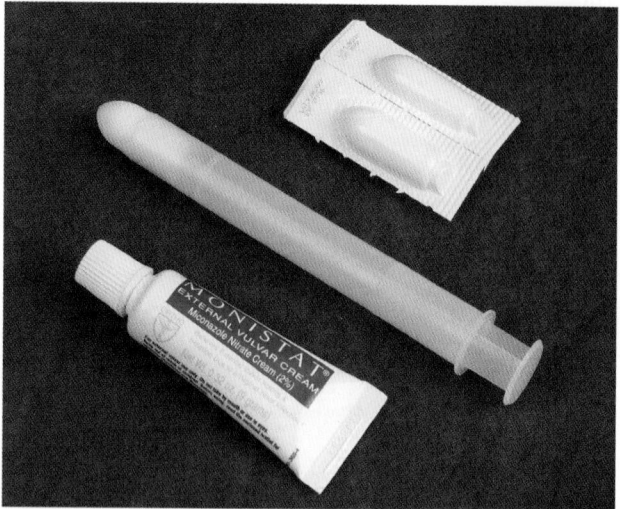

FIGURE 33-6 A vaginal applicator and forms of vaginal medications. (From Kronenberger, J., & Ledbetter, J. [2015]. *Lippincott Williams & Wilkins' comprehensive medical assisting* [5th ed.]. Lippincott Williams & Wilkins.)

Rectal Applications

Drugs administered rectally are usually in the form of suppositories (see Chapter 31); however, creams and ointments may also be prescribed. The technique for using a rectal applicator is similar to that of using a vaginal applicator.

Client and Family Teaching 33-1
Administering Medications Vaginally

The nurse teaches the client as follows:

- Obtain a form of medication based on personal preference; all come with a vaginal applicator.
- Plan to instill the medication before going to bed so that it can be retained for a prolonged period.
- Empty the bladder just before inserting the medication.
- Place the drug in the applicator (Fig. A).

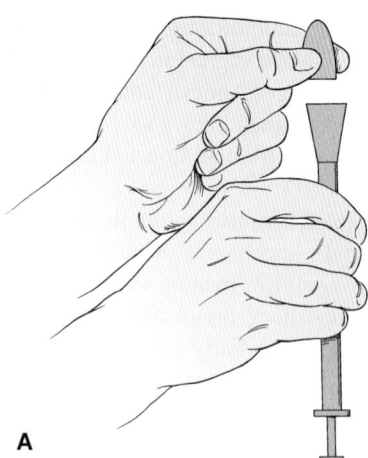

A

- Lubricate the applicator tip with a water-soluble lubricant.
- Lie down, bend your knees, and spread your legs.
- Separate the labia and insert the applicator into the vagina to the length recommended in the package directions, usually 2 to 4 in (5 to 10 cm) (Fig. B).

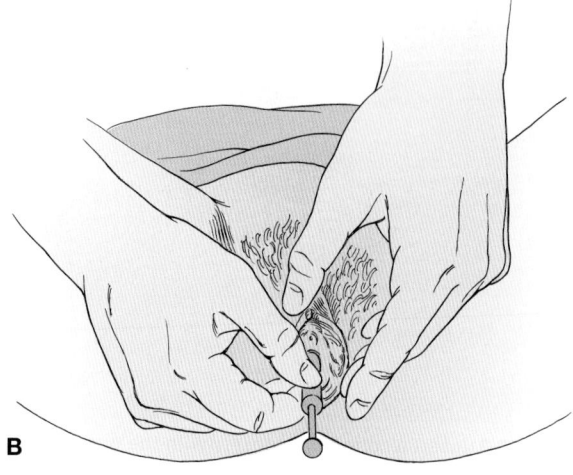

B

- Depress the plunger once it reaches the proper distance within the vagina to insert the medication.
- Remove the applicator and place it on a clean tissue.
- Apply a sanitary pad if you prefer.
- Remain recumbent for at least 10 to 30 minutes.
- Discard the applicator if it is disposable. Wash a reusable applicator with soap and water when you wash your hands.
- Consult a physician if symptoms persist.

INHALANT ROUTE

The **inhalant route** administers drugs to the lower airways. This method of medication administration is effective because the lungs provide an extensive area from which the circulatory system can quickly absorb the drug.

A simple method of administering inhaled medications is through an inhaler. **Inhalers** are handheld devices for delivering medication into the respiratory passages. They consist of a container of medication and a holder with a mouthpiece through which the drug is inhaled (Fig. 33-8).

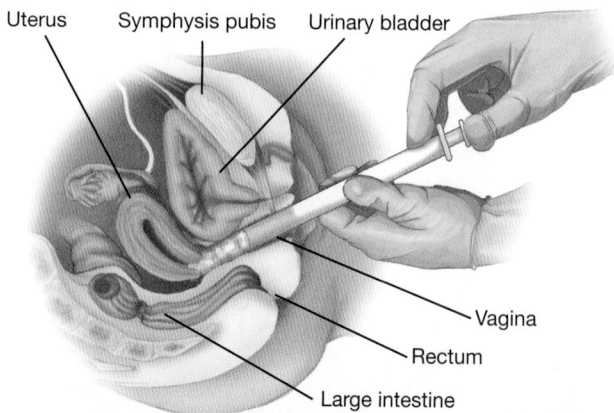

FIGURE 33-7 Insertion of vaginal medication by a nurse. (From Kronenberger, J., & Ledbetter, J. [2015]. *Lippincott Williams & Wilkins' comprehensive medical assisting* [5th ed.]. Lippincott Williams & Wilkins.)

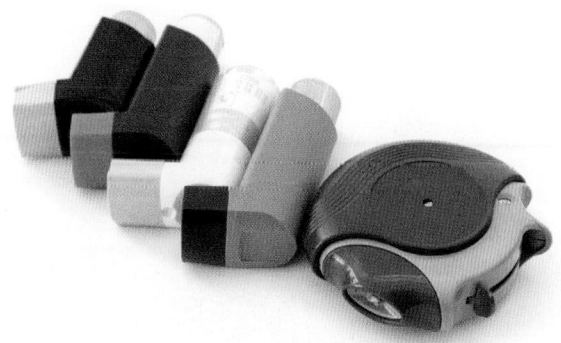

FIGURE 33-8 A variety of devices used for inhaled medications, both metered-dose and dry powder.

There are two types of inhalers: (1) a **dry powder inhaler** holds a reservoir of pulverized drug and a carrier substance and (2) a **metered-dose inhaler** delivers aerosolized medication, which is a liquid drug forced through a narrow channel via a chemical propellant.

 Pharmacologic Considerations

Traditionally, metered-dose inhalers have been propelled with chlorofluorocarbons, which contribute to environmental pollution. Current global regulations require them to be reformulated to contain substances that are safer for the environment.

Dry powder inhalers depend on the client's inspiratory effort to deliver the medication into the lungs. If the inspiratory effort is ineffective, the dose of the drug is reduced. A metered-dose inhaler contains medication under pressure within a canister. The canister is placed into a holder containing a mouthpiece; when the container is compressed, a measured volume (the metered dose) of aerosolized drug is released. Clients who use metered-dose inhalers do not always do so correctly. As a result, they may swallow, rather than inhale, much of the medication. As a result, their respiratory symptoms may not be relieved (Client and Family Teaching 33-2).

 Client and Family Teaching 33-2 Using an Inhaler

The nurse teaches the client and the family as follows:
- Insert the canister into the holder.
- Shake the canister to distribute the drug in the pressurized chamber.
- Remove the cap from the mouthpiece.
- Tilt your head back slightly and exhale slowly through pursed lips.
- Place the inhaler in your mouth and close your lips around the mouthpiece or place the inhaler 1 to 2 in away.
- Press down on the canister once to release the medication (Fig. A).

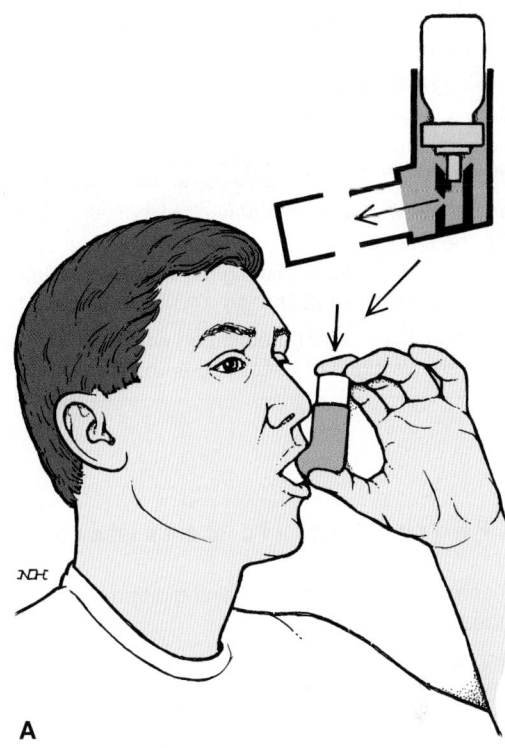

A

A metered-dose inhaler can be used by holding the mouthpiece 1 to 2 in away prior to depressing the canister and inhaling, or the mouthpiece can be placed in the mouth and sealed by the lips prior to administering the drug. (From Neil O. Hardy. Westport, CT.)

- As the medication is released, breathe in slowly through your mouth for approximately 3 to 5 seconds.
- Hold your breath for 10 seconds to let the medication reach your lungs (Fig. B).

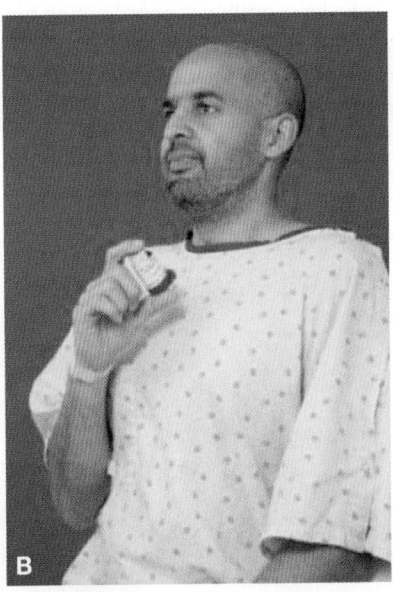

Client demonstrating his skill using a metered-dose inhaler. (From Craven, R. F., Hirnle, C. J., & Henshaw, C. M. [2020]. *Fundamentals of nursing* [9th ed.]. Lippincott Williams & Wilkins.)

- Exhale slowly through pursed lips.
- Wait 1 full minute before doing another inhalation if more than one is ordered.
- Clean the inhaler (holder and mouthpiece) daily by rinsing it in warm water and weekly with mild soap and water. Allow the inhaler to air-dry. Have another inhaler available to use while the first is drying.
- Check the amount of medication in the canister by floating it in a bowl of water; the higher the canister floats, the less medication it contains.
- Obtain a refill of inhalant medication when the current canister shows signs of becoming empty.

 Pharmacologic Considerations

■ Sometimes, two inhalers containing different drugs are prescribed.

■ During teaching sessions, it is important to educate how and when each drug is used, and the anticipated action. For example, one drug may act to expand the bronchioles and would improve the overall outcome to be administered before a medication that loosens secretions.

■ Providing simple written instructions with each medication is also helpful.

Some clients find that the inhaled drug leaves an unpleasant aftertaste. Gargling with salt water may diminish this. Drug residue may accumulate in the mouthpiece; therefore, the client should rinse the mouthpiece in warm water after use.

Clients who have problems coordinating breathing with the use of an inhaler may not receive the full dose of **aerosol.** A **spacer** (a chamber attached to an inhaler; Fig. 33-9) can be helpful in this situation. Spacers provide a reservoir for the aerosol medication. As the client takes additional

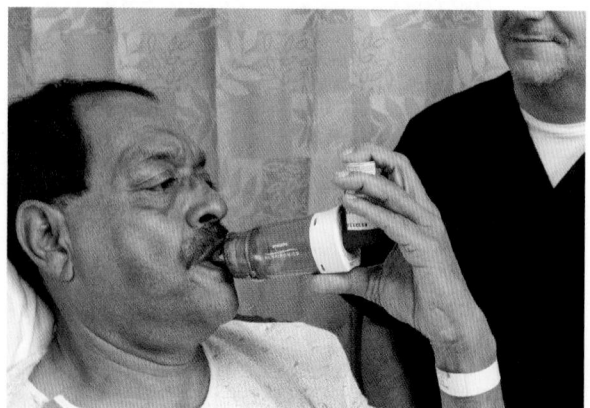

FIGURE 33-9 Using a metered-dose inhaler with a spacer.

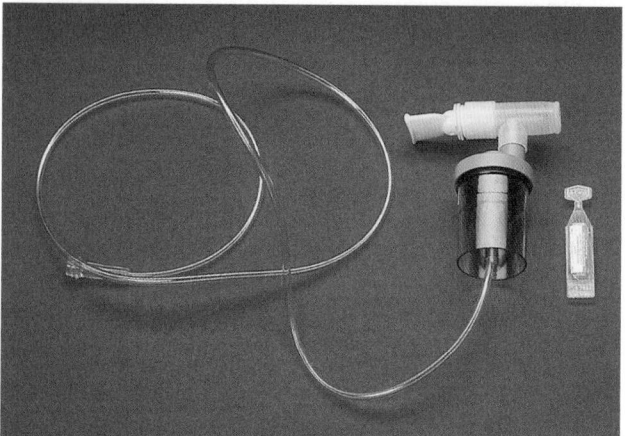

FIGURE 33-10 A nebulizer consists of a cup to which liquid medication is added, a mouthpiece, and tubing that connects to an electric or a battery-operated source for compressed air.

breaths, they continue to inhale the medication held in the reservoir. This tends to maximize drug absorption because it prevents drug loss. Some clients also find that prolonging inhalation of the drug reduces side effects such as tachycardia or tremulousness.

Some clients, such as infants, young children, and older adults who have difficulty coordinating inspiration with the use of a handheld inhaler, may use a nebulizer as an alternative to administering an inhalant. A **nebulizer,** sometimes called a "breathing machine," is a device that converts liquid medication to an aerosol using compressed air. The aerosol is inhaled through a mouthpiece or a face mask over 10 to 20 minutes until the mist is no longer visible (Fig. 33-10). The components of the nebulizer are cleaned after each use with soapy water and a small brush. After rinsing the cleaned parts, they are allowed to air-dry before storing them in a closed container.

NURSING IMPLICATIONS

When administering topical or inhalant drugs, nurses often assess and take steps to maintain the integrity of the skin and mucous membranes. Health teaching may be important to prevent improper self-administration. Applicable nursing diagnoses may include:

- Knowledge deficiency
- Impaired gas exchange
- Altered skin integrity
- Altered tissue integrity risk
- Altered breathing pattern

Nursing Care Plan 33-1 shows how nurses use the steps of the nursing process when managing the care of a client with the diagnosis of altered breathing pattern, defined as an abnormal respiratory rate and rhythm and changes in the amount of air exchanged during breathing.

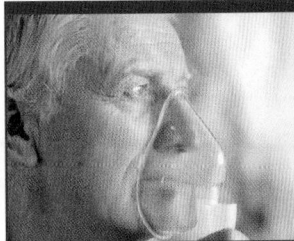

Clinical Scenario A 59-year-old male client who has chronic lung disease as a consequence of smoking for 40 years has recently acquired an upper respiratory infection. Despite administration of prescribed medications, his breathing has become labored. He now requires oxygen to relieve his shortness of breath. The nurse reviews the list of the client's self-administered medications and notes that he is reluctant to use his prescribed inhalant medications. The technique he describes using is not accurate.

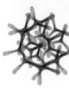

NURSING CARE PLAN 33-1   Altered Breathing Pattern

Assessment
- Count the client's respiratory rate for a full minute.
- Observe the client's pattern of respirations such as effort, nasal or mouth breathing, position used to enhance breathing, and use of accessory muscles.
- Establish if the client feels comfortable or anxious with regard to breathing.
- Measure the client's hemoglobin saturation with a pulse oximeter.
- Determine techniques the client uses to restore quiet, effortless breathing.

Nursing Diagnosis. Altered breathing pattern related to an improper technique using metered-dose inhaler to manage shortness of breath and mild hypoxemia associated with underlying lung disease as manifested by the client's statement, "I struggle to breathe and my chest gets tight even though I use the inhaler my doctor prescribed 2 days ago."

Expected Outcome. The client's breathing pattern will be effective as evidenced by quiet, effortless breathing at a respiratory rate between 16 and 28 breaths/minute with the correct use of the metered-dose inhaler.

Interventions	Rationales
Redemonstrate the correct use of a metered-dose inhaler.	Visual and verbal techniques enhance learning.
Observe the client's technique when using the metered-dose inhaler at least four times after demonstration.	Observation provides a means for evaluating the client's level of understanding.
Monitor the client's SpO_2 with a pulse oximeter before and after the use of the metered-dose inhaler.	Results will help evaluate the client's technique using a metered-dose inhaler and the drug's effectiveness.
Discuss the use of a spacer to assist with using the metered-dose inhaler.	A spacer facilitates a continuous inhalation of medication for clients who have difficulty inhaling while depressing the canister in the inhaler.

Evaluation of Expected Outcome

- The client is shown how to use a metered-dose inhaler.
- The client has been observed to perform the technique appropriately with each of the two puffs from the inhaler.
- Breathing changes from 32 breaths/minute with effort and an SpO_2 of 88% to 28 quiet breaths per minute and an SpO_2 of 90% within 15 minutes of using the inhaler.
- The client's physician has been contacted for a trial use of a spacer.

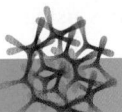

KEY POINTS

- Topical route: Administration of medications to the skin or mucous membranes that can be applied externally or internally
  - Cutaneous
  - Ophthalmic
  - Otic
  - Nasal
  - Sublingual
  - Buccal
  - Vaginal
  - Rectal
- Percutaneous applications are drugs rubbed into or placed in contact with the skin.
  - Ointment application: Rubbed into the skin
  - Transdermal application: Applied to the skin via patch or paste

- Ophthalmic application: Instilled into the mucous membranes of the eye
- Otic application: Instilled into the outer ear
- Nasal application: Dropped or sprayed into the nose
- Sublingual application: Under the tongue
- Buccal application: Against the mucous membranes of the inner cheek
- Vaginal application: Instilled into the vagina using an applicator
- Rectal application: Suppository, cream, or ointment instilled into the rectum, sometimes by using an applicator
- Inhalant route: Administration to the lower airways via inhaler or nebulizer
  - Dry powder inhaler
  - Metered-dose inhaler

CRITICAL THINKING EXERCISES

1. Before discharge from the hospital, a client who has had a heart attack says, "You nurses always put my nitroglycerin patches on my back. How can I do that when I have to do it myself?" How would you respond?
2. How might a nurse help a legally blind client identify two different containers of eye medication?
3. How can a nurse prevent eye drops from rolling down a client's cheek?
4. What questions would be important to ask if a client's symptoms persist after being treated for a vaginal infection with a regimen of self-administered medication?

NEXT-GENERATION NCLEX-STYLE REVIEW QUESTIONS

1. The nurse prepares to apply a transdermal patch of nitroglycerin to a client. Which locations on the client's body are appropriate sites? Select all that apply.
   a. The anterior thigh
   b. The upper chest
   c. The upper back
   d. The forearm
   e. The lower abdomen
   f. The upper arm
   Test-Taking Strategy: Use the process of elimination to select parts of the body that are used to apply nitroglycerin paste.
2. The nurse monitors the effect of a nitroglycerin paste application on the client. Which assessments indicate that the applicator paper and medication should be removed from the client's skin? Select all that apply.
   a. The client becomes restless.
   b. The client's blood pressure falls.
   c. The client says his skin is numb under the application.
   d. The client has developed a severe headache.
   e. The client appears flushed.
   f. The client's heart rate has slowed below normal.
   Test-Taking Strategy: Use the process of elimination to select signs and symptoms of vasodilation related to the application of nitroglycerin paste on the skin.
3. The nurse plans to teach a client how to self-administer vaginal medication. Which instruction is most accurate?
   a. Place the applicator just inside the vaginal opening.
   b. Insert the applicator while sitting on the toilet.
   c. Instill the medication just before retiring for sleep.
   d. Put on disposable gloves before applying the drug.
   Test-Taking Strategy: Note the key word and modifier, "most accurate." Analyze the choices and select the option that is better than any of the others.
4. The nurse administers eye drops to a client. Place an "X" on the diagram where slight pressure should be placed to avoid possible systemic absorption of ophthalmic medication.

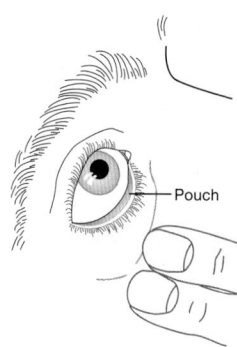

Test-Taking Strategy: Recall the external anatomic structure of the eye.

5. The nurse instills medication within a client's ear. After instilling the medication, what instruction is most appropriate for the nurse to give to the client?
   a. Remain in position for at least 5 minutes.
   b. Pack a cotton pledget tightly in the ear.
   c. Do not blow your nose for at least 1 hour.
   d. Avoid drinking very warm or cold beverages.
   Test-Taking Strategy: Note the key word and modifier, "most appropriate." Analyze the choices and select the option that is better than any of the others.

NEXT-GENERATION NCLEX-STYLE CLINICAL SCENARIO QUESTIONS

Clinical Scenario:
A 59-year-old male client who has chronic lung disease as a consequence of smoking for 40 years has recently acquired an upper respiratory infection. Despite administration of prescribed medications, his breathing has become labored. He now requires oxygen to relieve his shortness of breath. The nurse reviews the list of the client's self-administered medications and notes that he is reluctant to use his prescribed inhalant medications. The technique he describes using is not accurate.

1. From the following list, select the risk factors that may contribute to the client's upper respiratory infection.
   a. Chronic lung disease
   b. Oxygen therapy
   c. Use of prescribed inhalers
   d. Not using prescribed inhalers
   e. Smoking for 40 years
   f. Client's age
2. For each teaching guideline, use an "x" to indicate whether the action was effective (helped to meet expected outcome), ineffective (did not help with expected outcome), or unrelated (unrelated to expected outcome).

   Expected outcome: The client is shown how to use a metered-dose inhaler, and the client has been observed performing the technique appropriately.

TEACHING GUIDELINE	EFFECTIVE	INEFFECTIVE	UNRELATED
Shake the canister to distribute the drug in the pressurized chamber.			
Use the chin to neck position to inhale the medication accurately.			
Tilt your head back slightly and exhale slowly through pursed lips.			
As the medication is released, breathe in slowly through your mouth for approximately 3–5 seconds.			
Cough prior to medication administration.			
Hold your breath for 10 seconds to let the medication reach your lungs.			
Wait 10 full minutes before doing another inhalation if more than one is ordered.			
Exhale slowly through pursed lips.			

SKILL 33-1 Instilling Eye Medications

Suggested Action	Reason for Action
ASSESSMENT	
Compare the medication administration record (MAR) with the written medical order.	Prevents medication errors
Review the client's drug, allergy, and medical history.	Avoids potential complications
Consult a current drug reference concerning the drug's action, side effects, contraindications, and administration information.	Ensures appropriate administration based on a thorough knowledge base
PLANNING	
Plan to administer medications within 30–60 minutes of their scheduled time.	Demonstrates timely administration and compliance with the medical order
Allow sufficient time to prepare medications in a location with minimal distractions.	Promotes the safe preparation of drugs
Warm eye drops and ointments by holding the container between the hands if they have not been stored at room temperature.	Promotes comfort
Read and compare the label on the drug with the MAR at least three times—before, during, and after preparing the drug.	Ensures that the *right drug* is given at the *right time* by the *right route*
IMPLEMENTATION	
Wash your hands or use an alcohol-based hand rub (see Chapter 10).	Removes colonizing microorganisms
Identify the client using at least two methods, for example, checking the wristband and asking the client's name and birthdate.	Ensures that medications are given to the *right client;* complies with the National Patient Safety Goals
Position the client supine or sitting with the head tilted back and slightly to the side into which the medication will be instilled (Fig. A).	Prevents the drug from passing into the nasolacrimal duct or being blinked onto the cheek

Positioning for eye medication instillation. (From Springhouse. [2018]. *Lippincott's visual encyclopedia of clinical skills*. Wolters Kluwer Health.)

Suggested Action	Reason for Action
Put on clean gloves.	Acts as a barrier to pathogens in body fluids
Clean the lids and lashes if they contain debris. Use a face cloth, cotton ball, or tissue moistened with water (Fig. B).	Promotes comfort and maximizes the potential for absorption

Cleaning away debris. (From Springhouse. [2018]. *Lippincott's visual encyclopedia of clinical skills*. Wolters Kluwer Health.)

Suggested Action	Reason for Action
Wipe the eye from the corner by the nose, the inner canthus, toward the corner near the temple, and the outer canthus.	Moves debris away from the nasolacrimal duct

SKILL 33-1 Instilling Eye Medications (*continued*)

Suggested Action	Reason for Action
Instruct the client to look toward the ceiling.	Prevents looking directly at the applicator, which usually causes a blinking reflex as it comes close to the eye
Make a pouch in the lower lid by pulling the skin downward over the bony orbit (Fig. C).	Provides a natural reservoir for depositing liquid medication

Creating a pouch. (From Buchholz, S. [2019]. *Henke's med-math.* [9th ed.]. Wolters Kluwer Health.)

Suggested Action	Reason for Action
Move the container of medication from below the client's line of vision or from the side of the eye.	Prevents a blink reflex
Steady the container above the location for instillation without touching the eye surface.	Prevents injury and contamination of the tip of the dropper
Instill the prescribed number of drops into the appropriate eye within the conjunctival pouch (Fig. D).	Complies with the medical order by administering the *right dose*

Instilling eye drops. (From Ford, S. M. [2021]. *Introductory clinical pharmacology* [12th ed.]. Wolters Kluwer Health.)

Suggested Action	Reason for Action
Instruct the client to gently close the eyelid.	Prevents medication dripping onto the cheek
Apply gentle pressure to the inner canthus while the client closes their eyes (Fig. E).	Prevents systemic absorption through the tear duct

Applying pressure (From Springhouse. [2018]. *Lippincott's visual encyclopedia of clinical skills.* Wolters Kluwer Health.)

Suggested Action	Reason for Action
Wait at least 5 minutes before instilling a different type of medication into the eye.	Allows time for the medication to be distributed within the eye

(*continued*)

SKILL 33-1 Instilling Eye Medications (*continued*)

Suggested Action	Reason for Action
If using ointment, squeeze a ribbon onto the lower lid margin (Fig. F).	Applies the ointment to the conjunctiva

Administering eye ointment. (From Hatfield, N. T., & Kincheloe, C. A. [2021]. *Introductory maternity and pediatric nursing* [5th ed.]. Wolters Kluwer Health.)

Suggested Action	Reason for Action
Instruct the client to close the eyelids temporarily.	Distributes the drug
Wipe the eyes with a clean tissue.	Removes excess drug and promotes comfort

EVALUATION

- The five rights are upheld.
- The tip of the container remains uncontaminated.
- A sufficient amount of the drug is distributed within the eye.

DOCUMENT

- Assessment data
- Medication administration on the MAR

SAMPLE DOCUMENTATION

Date and Time Prescribed eye medication instilled into left eye before cataract surgery (see MAR). Conjunctiva appears pink and intact. Lens is opaque. Eyelashes have been clipped. _____ J. Doe, LPN

SKILL 33-2 Administering Nasal Medications

Suggested Action	Reason for Action
ASSESSMENT	
Compare the medication administration record (MAR) with the written medical order.	Prevents medication errors
Review the client's drug, allergy, and medical history.	Avoids potential complications
Consult a current drug reference concerning the drug's action, side effects, contraindications, and administration information.	Ensures appropriate administration based on a thorough knowledge of the drug
PLANNING	
Plan to administer medications within 30–60 minutes of their scheduled time.	Demonstrates timely administration and compliance with the medical order
Allow sufficient time to prepare the medications in a location with minimal distractions.	Promotes the safe preparation of drugs
Read and compare the label on the drug with the MAR at least three times—before, during, and after preparing the drug.	Ensures that the *right drug* is given at the *right time* by the *right route*
IMPLEMENTATION	
Wash your hands or use an alcohol-based hand rub (see Chapter 10).	Removes colonizing microorganisms

SKILL 33-2 Administering Nasal Medications (*continued*)

Suggested Action	Reason for Action
Identify the client using at least two methods, such as scanning or reading the wristband and asking the client's name and birthdate.	Ensures that medications are given to the *right client;* complies with the National Patient Safety Goals
Help the client into a sitting or lying position with their head tilted backward or to the side if the drug needs to reach one or the other sinuses.	Facilitates depositing the drug where its effect is desired
Place a rolled towel or pillow beneath the neck if the client cannot sit.	Provides support and aids in positioning
Remove the cap from the liquid medication exposing the outlet for the medication.	Provides a means for administering the drug
Aim the tip of the container or dropper toward the nasal passage and squeeze to administer the number of drops prescribed (Fig. A).	Deposits the drug within the nose rather than into the throat and ensures administering the *right dose*

Instilling nasal medication with a dropper.

Instruct the client to breathe through the mouth as the drops are instilled.	Prevents inhaling large droplets
If the drug is in a spray form, place the tip of the container just inside the nostril (Fig. B).	Confines the spray within the nasal passage

Instilling nasal medication with a spray applicator. (From Craven, R. F., Hirnle, C. J., & Henshaw, C. M. [2020]. *Fundamentals of nursing* [9th ed.]. Lippincott Williams & Wilkins.)

Occlude the opposite nostril.	Administers medication to one and then the other nasal passage
Instruct the client to inhale as the container is squeezed.	Distributes the aerosol
Repeat in the opposite nostril.	Deposits the drug bilaterally for maximum effect
Advise the client to remain in position for approximately 5 minutes.	Promotes local absorption
Recap the container and replace it where the medications are stored.	Supports the principles of asepsis and demonstrates responsibility for the client's property

(*continued*)

SKILL 33-2 Administering Nasal Medications (*continued*)

Suggested Action	Reason for Action

EVALUATION

- The five rights are upheld.
- A sufficient amount of the drug is distributed within the nose.
- The client reports decreased nasal congestion.

DOCUMENT

- Assessment data
- Medication administration on the MAR

SAMPLE DOCUMENTATION

Date and Time Indicates nasal passages are congested. Observed to be breathing through the mouth. Nasal medication administered (see MAR). States symptoms are relieved. _____ J. Doe, LPN

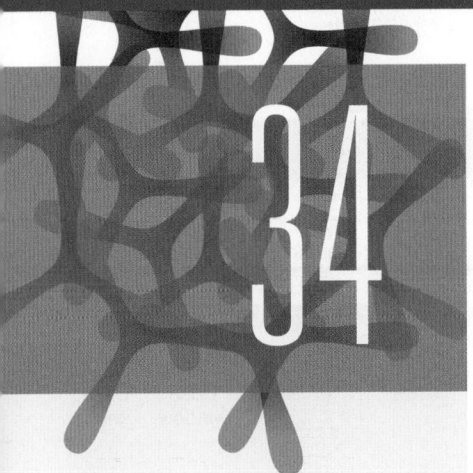

34

Parenteral Medications

Learning Objectives

On completion of this chapter, the reader should be able to:

1. Name the parts of a syringe.
2. List factors to consider when selecting a syringe and needle.
3. Explain the rationale for redesigning conventional syringes and needles.
4. Name ways pharmaceutical companies prepare parenteral drugs.
5. Discuss an appropriate action before combining two drugs in a single syringe.
6. List injection routes.
7. Identify common sites for intradermal, subcutaneous, and intramuscular (IM) injections.
8. Name types of syringe commonly used to administer an intradermal, subcutaneous, and IM injection.
9. Describe the angles of entry for intradermal, subcutaneous, and IM injections.
10. Discuss why most insulin combinations must be administered within 15 minutes of being mixed.
11. Describe techniques for preventing bruising when administering heparin subcutaneously.

INTRODUCTION

The **parenteral route** is a route of drug administration other than oral or through the gastrointestinal tract. "Parenteral" is commonly used when referring to medications given by injection. This chapter discusses techniques for administering injections. The preparation and administration of injections follow the principles of asepsis and infection control.

 Gerontologic Considerations

■ Older clients with diabetes often have visual problems interfering with their ability to fill their own syringes. They are candidates for using an insulin pen or a loading gauge that prevents filling a syringe with more than the prescribed dose. Sight centers are a good resource for obtaining assistive devices to facilitate self-administration of insulin.

■ Older adults learning to administer insulin may benefit from a referral for skilled nursing or diabetic health education following discharge. These services are generally covered by health insurance plans.

■ Selection and identification of injection site landmarks may be difficult when working with older adults experiencing dementia or musculoskeletal deformities such as contractures. Assistance from a second person to maintain the required position for an injection may be helpful.

An explanation of what will be done is always indicated before the intervention. The second person may be able to assist with providing comfort.

■ If an older person has decreased subcutaneous fat, pinching the muscular tissue together may be needed to avoid striking bone when administering an intramuscular (IM) injection.

■ The deltoid or ventrogluteal muscles may be the preferred IM sites for older adults experiencing impaired mobility.

 Pharmacologic Considerations

■ When the parenteral route is used for drug administration, the drug filtering performed by the liver does not occur. Therefore, more active drugs will be in circulation, and the intended and adverse drug effects can be more pronounced than when a drug is taken orally.

■ Clients, particularly children and older adults, should be monitored closely for drug effects.

PARENTERAL ADMINISTRATION EQUIPMENT

The major equipment used to administer parenteral drugs consists of a syringe and a needle. Numerous types of syringes and needles are available.

Syringes

Syringes contain a **barrel** (the part of the syringe that holds the medication), a **plunger** (the part of the syringe within the barrel that moves back and forth to withdraw and instill the medication), and a **tip** (the part of the syringe to which the needle is attached; Fig. 34-1). Syringes are calibrated in milliliters (mL) or cubic centimeters (cc) and units (U).

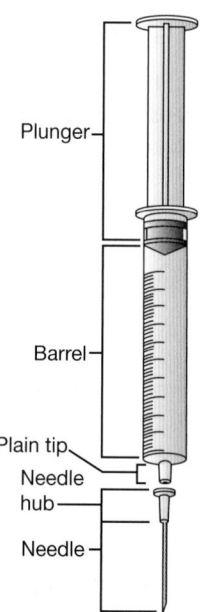

FIGURE 34-1 The parts of a syringe. (From Rosdahl, C. B. [2021]. *Textbook of basic nursing* [12th ed.]. Lippincott Williams & Wilkins.)

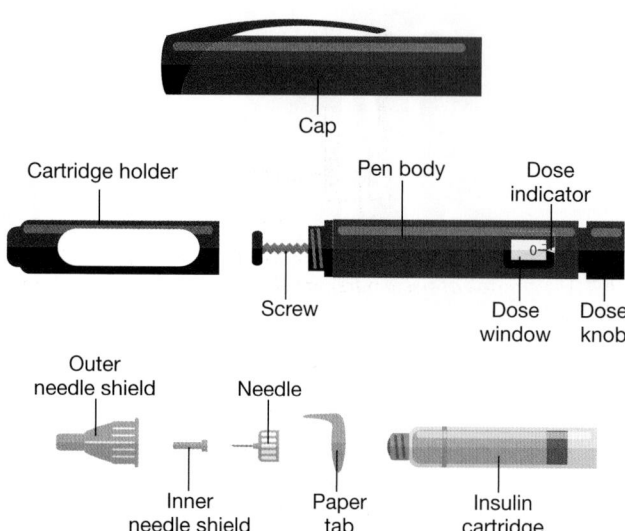

FIGURE 34-2 Parts of an insulin pen. (Alka5051/Shutterstock.)

When drugs are administered parenterally, syringes that hold 1 mL or its equivalent in units, and up to 3 to 5 mL are most commonly used.

Insulin Pens

Insulin pens have simplified how clients self-administer their medication. An **insulin pen** is a hard plastic cylinder that looks much like a fountain pen, hence its name. The cylinder contains a prefilled reservoir of insulin. The dose of insulin is dialed and displayed in a window at the end of the syringe. When selecting the prescribed dose, each unit of insulin is accompanied by a clicking sound in the pen, which is advantageous for patients with diabetes who have low vision. The pen automatically resets the dose window to zero following the injection. The insulin in prefilled pens is stable for up to 30 days.

A disposable needle is attached to the pen each time it is used. The insulin is released into the client's tissue by pressing an injection button at the end of the syringe (Fig. 34-2). Many clients prefer to use an insulin pen rather than a syringe and insulin vial, described later, based on a variety of advantages (Box 34-1).

BOX 34-1	Advantages and Disadvantages of Insulin Pens
Advantages	**Disadvantages**
• Easier to learn how to use than a syringe and vial	• More expensive than insulin vials
• Easily transported on one's person	• Cannot mix different types of insulin
• Insulin is self-contained within the pen.	• Not covered by some insurance plans
• Large variety of insulin types available	
• Dose is easily read with large numbers.	

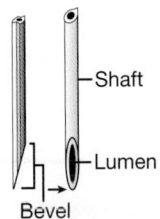

FIGURE 34-3 Parts of injection needle. (From Rosdahl, C. B. [2021]. *Textbook of basic nursing* [12th ed.]. Lippincott Williams & Wilkins.)

Needles

Needles are supplied in various lengths and gauges. The **shaft** (the length of the needle) depends on the depth to which the medication will be instilled. Needle lengths vary from approximately ½ to 2½ in. The tip of the shaft is beveled, or slanted, to pierce the skin more easily (Fig. 34-3). **Filter needles** contain a membrane that acts as a barrier blocking the entrance of glass shards when withdrawing medication from a glass ampule (Fig. 34-4). Ampules are discussed later in this chapter.

The needle **gauge** (diameter) refers to its width. For most injections, 18- to 27-gauge needles are used; the smaller the number, the larger the diameter. For example, an 18-gauge needle is wider than a 27-gauge needle. A wider diameter provides a larger lumen, or opening, through which drugs are administered into the tissue. Needles used on insulin pens are generally 31-gauge and have a very short length (3/16 to 5/16 in), which makes the injection less painful but just as effective as with the needles used for traditional subcutaneous injections. Several factors are considered when selecting a syringe and a needle:

- The type of medication
- The depth of tissue
- The volume of prescribed drug
- The viscosity of the drug
- The size of the client

Table 34-1 lists common sizes of syringes and needles used for various types of injections.

Modified Safety Injection Equipment

Conventional syringes and needles are being redesigned to avoid needlestick injuries, thus reducing the risk of acquiring a blood-borne viral disease such as hepatitis B virus (HBV), hepatitis C virus (HCV), and human immunodeficiency virus/acquired immunodeficiency syndrome (HIV/AIDS). Currently, there are three different safety injection devices: (1) those with plastic shields that cover the needle after its

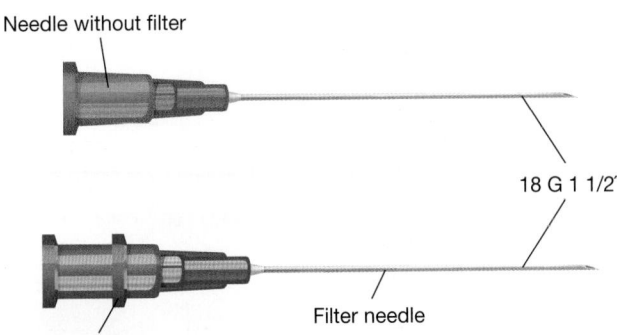

FIGURE 34-4 A needle without a filter and a filter needle.

use (Fig. 34-5), (2) those with needles that retract into the syringe, and (3) gas-pressured devices that inject medications without needles. Most health agencies are already using one or several types of modified equipment to enclose or cover the needle. Some syringes contain blunt substitutes for needles that can pierce laser-cut rubber ports.

Minimum federal needle safety regulations were established following the congressional passage of the Needlestick Safety and Prevention Act in 2000. Since then, 29 states have passed additional needle safety legislation that is more stringent, for example, requiring safety needles or needleless devices for administering medications and withdrawing bodily fluids (OSHA, 2023).

If modified safety injection devices are not available or not used, there are two techniques to prevent needlestick injuries with standard equipment:

- *Before administering an injection*, the protective cap covering a needle is replaced by using the **scoop method** (the technique of threading the needle within the cap without touching the cap itself; Fig. 34-6).
- *After administering an injection*, the needle is left uncapped and deposited in the nearest **biohazard container** (Fig. 34-7), which is usually mounted on the wall within the client's room.

Should an accidental injury occur, health care providers should follow the following recommendations:

- Report the injury to a supervisor immediately.
- Document the injury in writing.
- Identify the client if possible.
- Obtain HIV and HBV client status results if it is legal to do so.
- Obtain counseling on the potential for infection.
- Receive the most appropriate postexposure drug treatment prophylaxis.

TABLE 34-1 Common Sizes of Syringes and Needles

TYPE OF INJECTION	SIZES OF SYRINGES	SIZES OF NEEDLES
Intradermal (tuberculin)	1 mL calibrated in 0.01 mL	25-, 26-, or 27-gauge, 1/2–5/8 in
Subcutaneous	1, 2, 2.5, or 3 mL calibrated in 0.1 mL	23-, 25-, or 26-gauge, 1/2–5/8 in
Insulin, given subcutaneously	1 mL calibrated in units	25- or 27-gauge, 1/2–5/8 in
Intramuscular	3 or 5 mL calibrated in 0.2 mL	20-, 21-, 22-, or 23-gauge, 1½ or 2 in

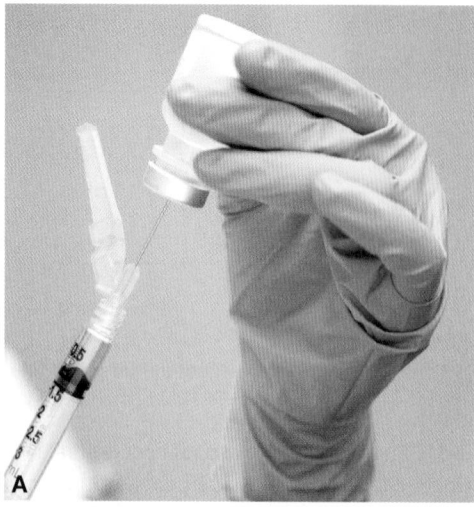

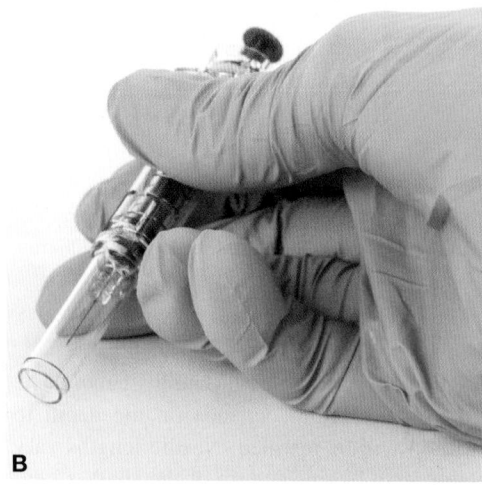

FIGURE 34-5 Safety injection devices. **A.** A syringe with an articulated levered shield that glides over the needle after it is used. (Marlon Lopez MMG1 Design/Shutterstock.) **B.** A syringe with a circular sleeve that covers the needle. (Warren Price Photography/Shutterstock.)

- Be tested for the presence of antibodies at appropriate intervals.
- Monitor for potential symptoms and obtain a medical follow-up.

DRUG PREPARATION

Drug preparation involves withdrawing medication from an ampule or vial or assembling a prefilled syringe cartridge (Fig. 34-8).

Ampules

An **ampule** (a sealed glass drug container) must be broken to withdraw the medication (Nursing Guidelines 34-1).

Vials

A **vial** (a glass or plastic container of parenteral medication with a self-sealing rubber stopper) must be pierced with a needle or a needleless adapter to remove medication. The amount of drug in a vial may be enough for one or multiple doses. Any unused drug is dated before it is stored for future use (Nursing Guidelines 34-2).

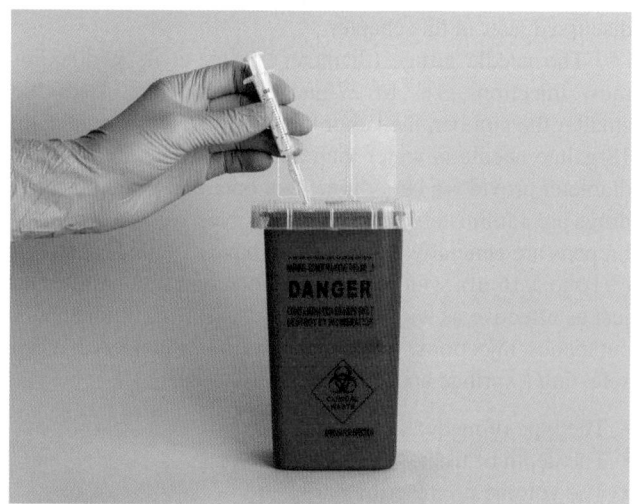

FIGURE 34-7 Syringes and all sharps are deposited in a puncture-proof container. (New Africa/Shutterstock.)

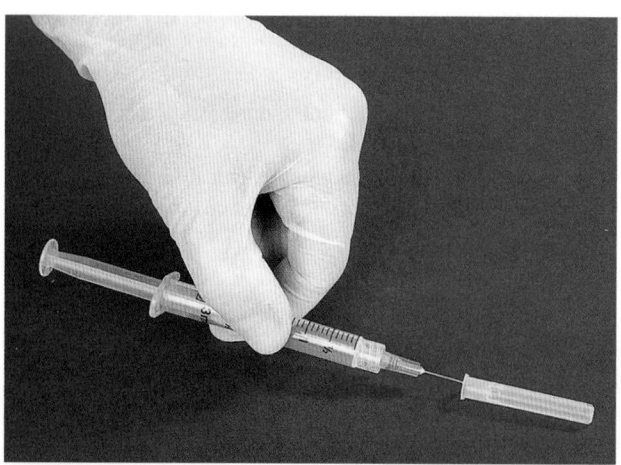

FIGURE 34-6 The scoop method for covering a needle. (Photo by B. Proud.)

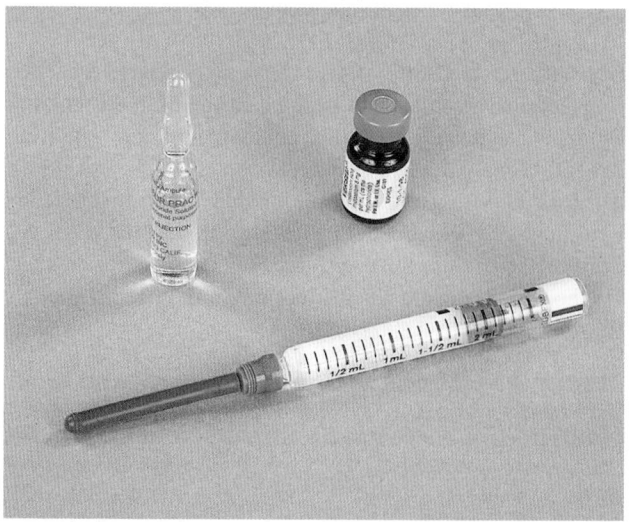

FIGURE 34-8 An ampule, a vial, and a prefilled cartridge. (Photo by B. Proud.)

NURSING GUIDELINES 34-1

Withdrawing Medication from an Ampule

- Select an appropriate syringe and filter needle. *Proper equipment ensures appropriate drug administration and prevents aspirating glass particles within the barrel of the syringe.*
- Tap the top of the ampule (Fig. A). *Tapping distributes all the medication to the lower portion of the ampule.*

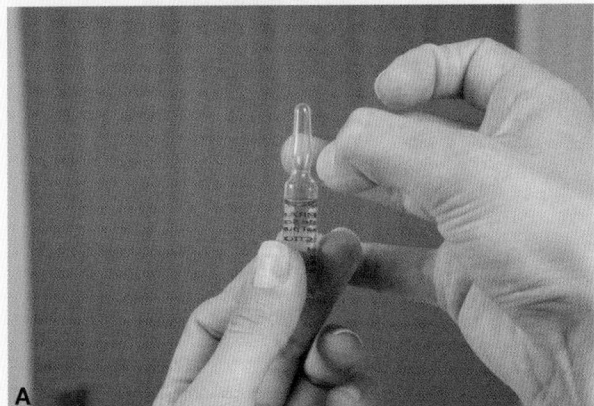

Tapping an unbroken ampule. (From Taylor, C. R., Lynn, P. B., & Bartlett, J. L. [2022]. *Fundamentals of nursing* [10th ed.]. Lippincott Williams & Wilkins.)

- Protect your thumb and fingers with a gauze square or alcohol swab (Fig. B). *These devices reduce the potential for injury.*

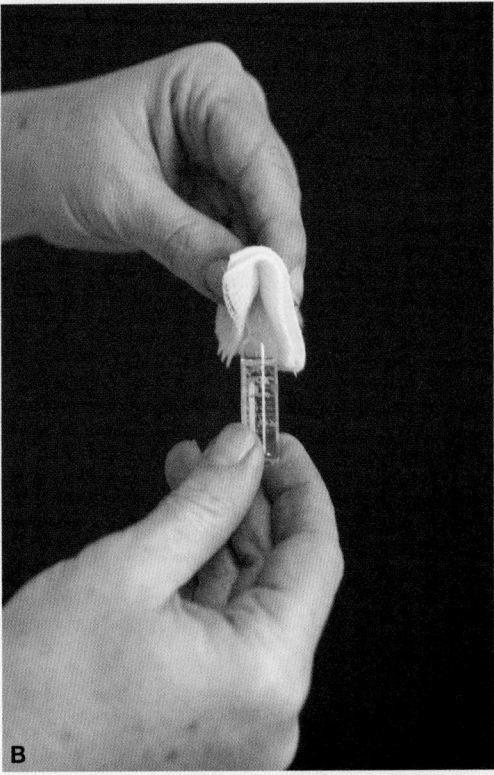

Protecting thumb and fingers. (From Ryan, T. A. [2023]. *Torres' patient care in imaging technology* [10th ed.]. Lippincott Williams & Wilkins.)

- Snap the neck of the ampule away from your body (Fig. C). *Doing so avoids accidental injury.*

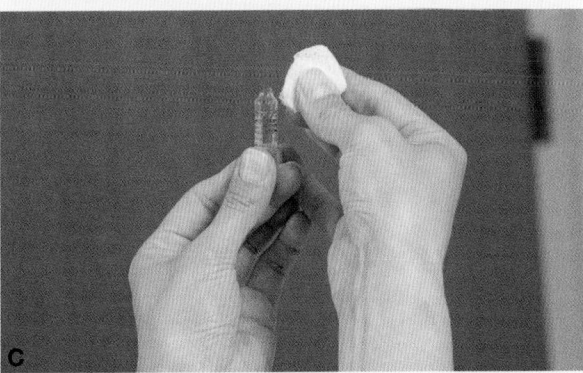

Breaking the ampule. (From Craven, R. F., Hirnle, C. J., & Henshaw, C. [2019]. *Fundamentals of nursing* [9th ed.]. Lippincott Williams & Wilkins.)

- Insert the filter needle attached to a syringe into the ampule. Avoid touching the outside of the ampule. *These methods ensure sterility of the needle.*
- Invert the ampule (Fig. D). *Inversion facilitates withdrawing the medication.*

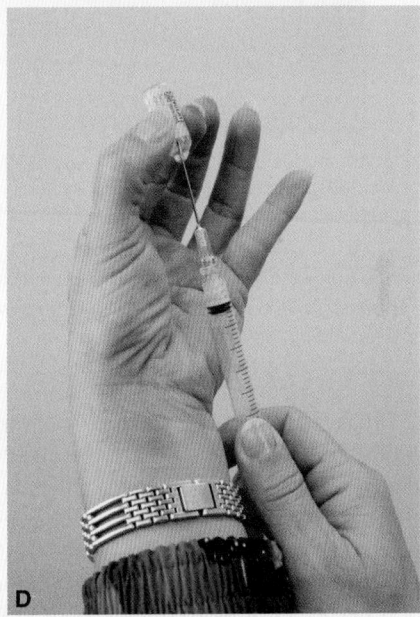

Withdrawing the drug from an ampule.

- Pull back on the plunger. *This step fills the syringe.*
- Remove the needle from the ampule when the volume has been withdrawn. *This prepares for drug administration.*
- Tap the barrel of the syringe near the hub. *Tapping moves air toward the needle.*
- Push carefully on the plunger. *Pushing expels air or excess medication.*
- Empty the unused portion of medication from the syringe. *Doing so prevents illegal drug use.*
- Discard the glass ampule in a puncture-resistant container. *Proper disposal prevents accidental injury.*
- Remove the filter needle and attach a sterile needle for administering the injection. *These techniques prevent injecting glass particles into the client.*

NURSING GUIDELINES 34-2

Withdrawing Medication from a Vial

- Select an appropriate syringe and needle. *The correct equipment ensures appropriate drug administration.*
- Remove the metal cover from the rubber stopper. *This step facilitates inserting the needle or needleless adaptor.*
- Clean a preopened vial with an alcohol swab. *Alcohol swabs remove colonizing microorganisms.*
- Fill the syringe with a volume of air equal to the volume that will be withdrawn from the vial. *This step provides a means for increasing pressure within the vial.*
- Pierce the rubber stopper with the needle or tip of a needleless syringe and instill the air (Fig. A). *Doing so facilitates the withdrawal of the drug.*

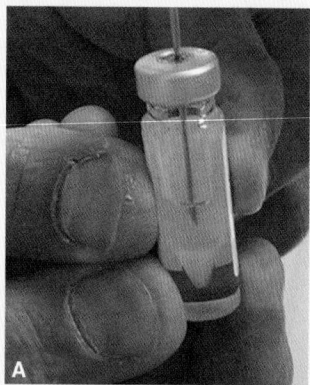

Piercing the rubber stopper on a vial. (From Wiesel, S. W. [2021]. *Operative techniques in orthopedic surgery, four-volume set* [3rd ed.]. Lippincott Williams & Wilkins.)

- Invert the vial, hold, and brace it while pulling on the plunger (Fig. B). *This step locates medication near the tip of the needle or needleless adaptor to facilitate its withdrawal.*

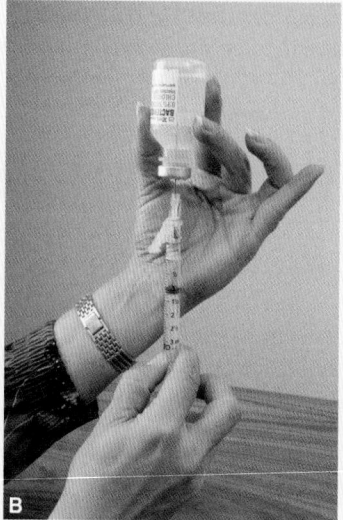

Withdrawing a drug from a vial.

- Remove the needle or adaptor when the desired volume has entered the barrel of the syringe. *Doing so leaves the remaining drug for additional administration.*
- If the medication is a controlled substance such as a narcotic, aspirate the entire contents from the vial. *Full aspiration prevents illegal drug use.*
- Discard any excess medication; if the drug is a narcotic, have someone witness this action. *These measures comply with federal laws to prevent illegal drug use.*
- Cover the needle or needleless adaptor and care for the used supplies as described in the guidelines for withdrawing from an ampule. *Nurses follow aseptic and safety principles.*
- Date and initial the vial if the remaining drug will be used in the near future. *Doing so supports the principles of asepsis.*

Usually, drugs in vials are in liquid form, but sometimes, they are supplied as powders that must be dissolved. **Reconstitution** (the process of adding liquid, known as *diluent*, to a powdered substance) is done before administering the drug parenterally. Common diluents for injectable drugs are sterile water or sterile normal saline. Reconstituting a drug just before it is needed ensures maximum potency. When reconstitution is necessary, the drug label lists:

- The type of diluent to use
- The amount of diluent to add
- The dosage per volume after reconstitution
- Directions for storing the drug

If the medication will be used for more than one administration, the preparer writes the date and time on the vial label and initials it. In some cases, when the directions provide several options in diluent volumes, the preparer also writes the amount on the vial.

Prefilled Cartridges

Pharmaceutical companies supply some drugs in a **prefilled cartridge** (a sealed glass cylinder of parenteral medication).

The cartridge comes with an attached needle. The cylinder is made so that it fits in a specially designed syringe.

Combining Medications in One Syringe

Sometimes, it is necessary or appropriate to combine more than one drug in a single syringe. Exact amounts must be withdrawn from each drug container because once the drugs are in the barrel of the syringe, there is no way to expel one without expelling some of the other (see section "Mixing Insulins"). Before mixing any drugs, however, the nurse consults a drug reference or compatibility chart because some drugs interact chemically when combined. The chemical reaction often causes the formation of a **precipitate** (liquid that contains solid particles).

INJECTION ROUTES

There are four injection routes for parenteral administration: **intradermal injections** (injections between the layers of the skin), **subcutaneous injections** (injections beneath the skin but above the muscle), **intramuscular injections** (injections in muscle tissue), and **intravenous injections** (injections

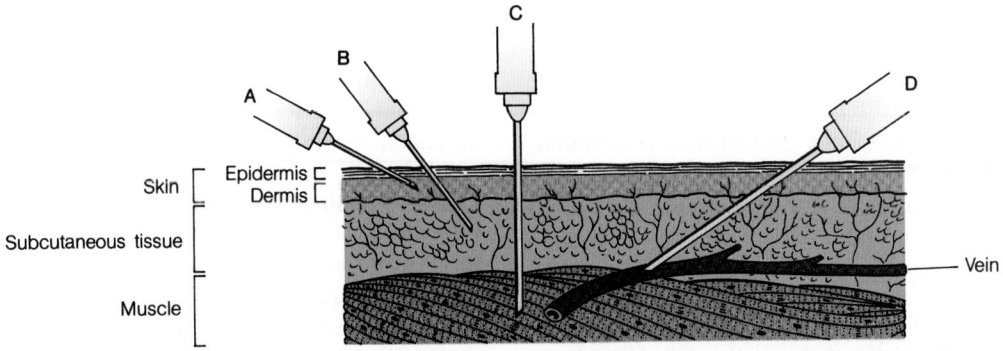

FIGURE 34-9 Injection routes: intradermal (**A**), subcutaneous (**B**), intramuscular and subcutaneous (**C**), and intravenous (**D**).

instilled into veins; Fig. 34-9). Each site requires a slightly different injection technique. Intravenous medication administration is discussed in Chapter 35.

Intradermal Injections

Intradermal injections are commonly used for diagnostic purposes. Examples include tuberculin tests and allergy testing. Small volumes, usually 0.01 to 0.05 mL, are injected because of the small tissue space.

Injection Sites

A common site for an intradermal injection is the inner aspect of the forearm. Other areas that may be used are the back, posterior upper arm, and upper chest (Fig. 34-10).

Injection Equipment

A **tuberculin syringe** holds 1 mL of fluid and is calibrated in 0.01-mL increments (Fig. 34-11). It is used to administer

intradermal injections. A 25- to 27-gauge needle measuring half an inch in length is commonly used when administering an intradermal injection.

>> ***Stop, Think, and Respond 34-1***

What actions are appropriate if the client shows signs of an allergic reaction to an agent given intradermally?

Injection Technique

When giving an intradermal injection, the nurse instills the medication shallowly at a 10- to 15-degree angle of entry (Skill 34-1).

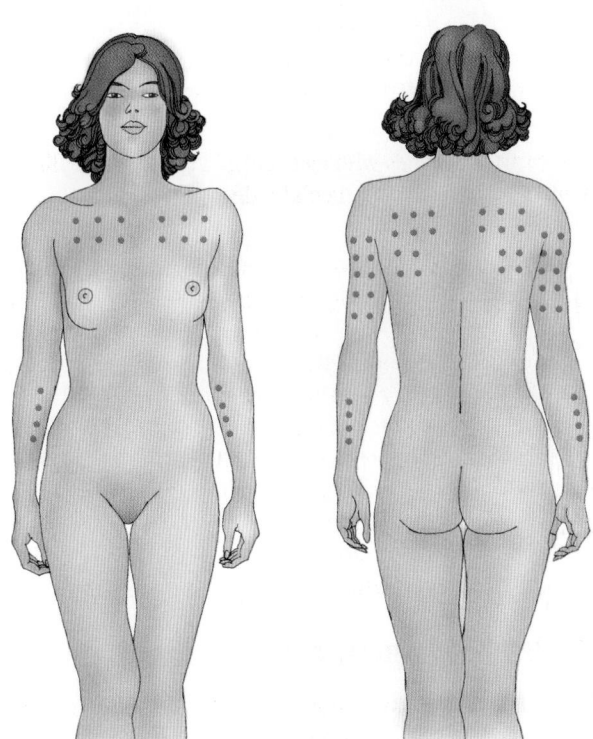

FIGURE 34-10 Intradermal injection sites. (From Lippincott Williams & Wilkins. [2018]. *Lippincott's nursing procedures.* Author.)

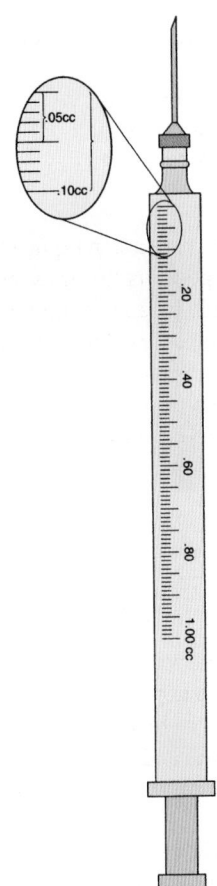

FIGURE 34-11 A tuberculin syringe.

Subcutaneous Injections

A subcutaneous injection is administered more deeply than an intradermal injection. Medication is instilled between the skin and the muscle and absorbed fairly rapidly; the medication usually begins acting within 15 to 30 minutes of administration. The volume of a subcutaneous injection is usually up to 1 mL. The subcutaneous route is commonly used to administer insulin and heparin.

Injection Sites

Subcutaneous injection sites are shown in Figure 34-12. The rate of drug absorption varies at the different sites in the body, from fastest to slowest. The site with the fastest absorption rate is the abdomen, then, in order to the slowest, the outer back area of the upper arm, where it is fleshier; the anterior upper areas of the thigh; and the upper ventral gluteal area of the buttocks.

Insulin Injection Sites

The preferred site for giving a subcutaneous injection of insulin is the abdomen. Rotating within one injection site, preferably the abdomen, is recommended rather than rotating to a different area with each injection. When the abdominal site

is used, insulin is absorbed at a more consistent rate from one injection to the next. Rotating sites avoids tissue injury. When rotating within one injection site, keep injections an inch from a previous site (Drugs.com, 2023). When using the abdomen, avoid a 2-in central area around the umbilicus.

Injection Equipment

Equipment used for a subcutaneous injection may depend on the type of medication prescribed. Insulin is prepared in an **insulin syringe** (see section "Administering Insulin"). Heparin is prepared in a tuberculin syringe, or it may be supplied in a prefilled cartridge. A 25-gauge needle is used most often because medications administered subcutaneously are usually not viscous. Needle lengths may vary from 1/2 to 5/8 in.

Injection Technique

To reach subcutaneous tissue in a person with average weight or a person with excess weight who has a 2-in tissue fold when it is bunched, the nurse inserts the needle at a 90-degree angle. For lower weight clients who have a 1-in fold of tissue, the nurse inserts the needle at a 45-degree angle (Fig. 34-13). Skill 34-2 describes the technique for administering a subcutaneous injection.

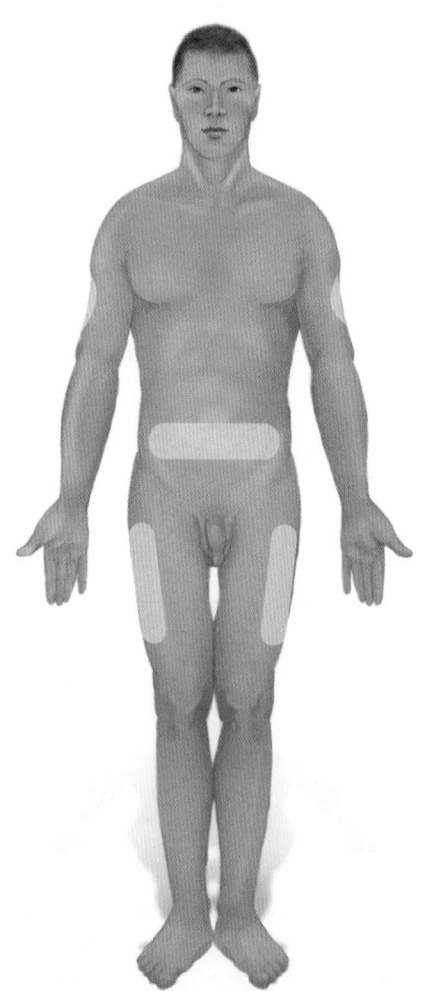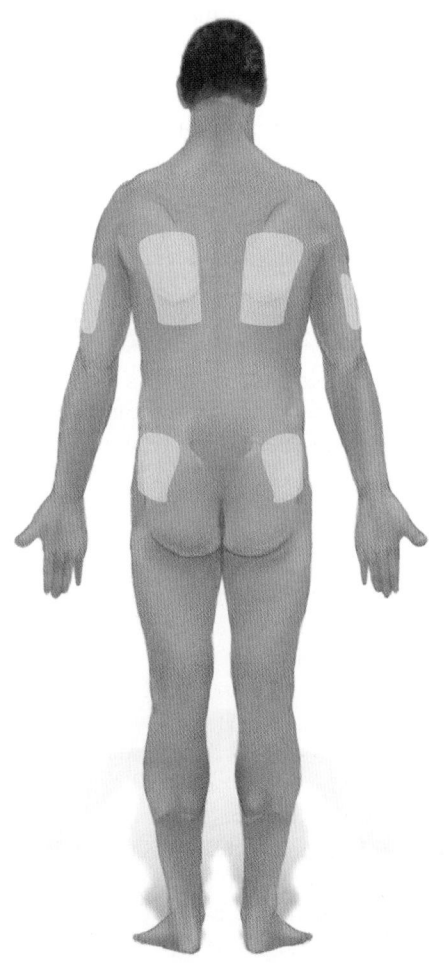

FIGURE 34-12 Subcutaneous injection sites.

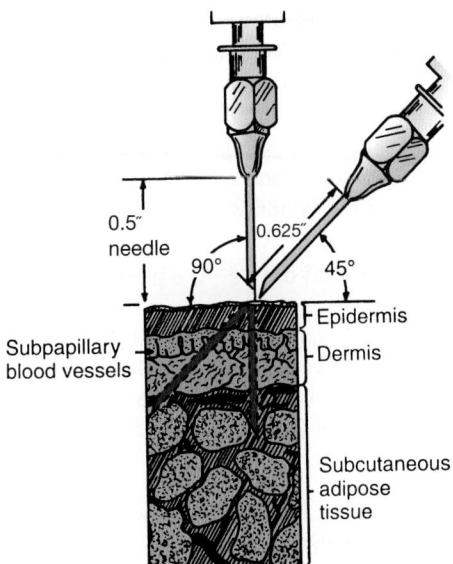

FIGURE 34-13 Angles and needle lengths for subcutaneous injections.

 Pharmacologic Considerations

■ Subcutaneous medications (other than insulin) should never be given using an insulin syringe. These syringes are calibrated for units of insulin only, which are not the same as other drugs such as heparin or vitamins, which also use the term "unit" for measurement.

■ Teach clients proper care of medication when self-administration is recommended. Biologics are typically refrigerated, whereas insulin is not when the vial is opened. Biologics may be fragile, and vigorous shaking is not recommended.

The tissue is usually bunched between the thumb and the fingers before administering the injection to avoid instilling insulin within the muscle. Bunching is unnecessary when injecting insulin with an insulin pen because the needle is only 5 mm long and unlikely to enter a muscle.

Administering Insulin

The most common route of administration of insulin is by subcutaneous or intravenous injection. Injectable insulin is supplied and prescribed in a dosage strength called *units* (U); a special syringe called an *insulin syringe* (a syringe calibrated in units) is used. Various insulin syringes hold volumes of 0.3, 0.5, and 1 mL. The standard dosage strength of insulin is 100 units/mL. Typically, low-dose insulin syringes are used to deliver insulin dosages of 30 to 50 units or less. A standard insulin syringe can administer up to 100 units of insulin (Fig. 34-14).

Clients who require insulin receive one or more daily injections. Over time, the injection sites tend to undergo changes that interfere with insulin absorption. To avoid **lipoatrophy** (the breakdown of subcutaneous fat at the site of repeated insulin injections) and **lipohypertrophy** (the thickening of subcutaneous fat at the site of repeated insulin injections), the sites are rotated each time an injection is administered.

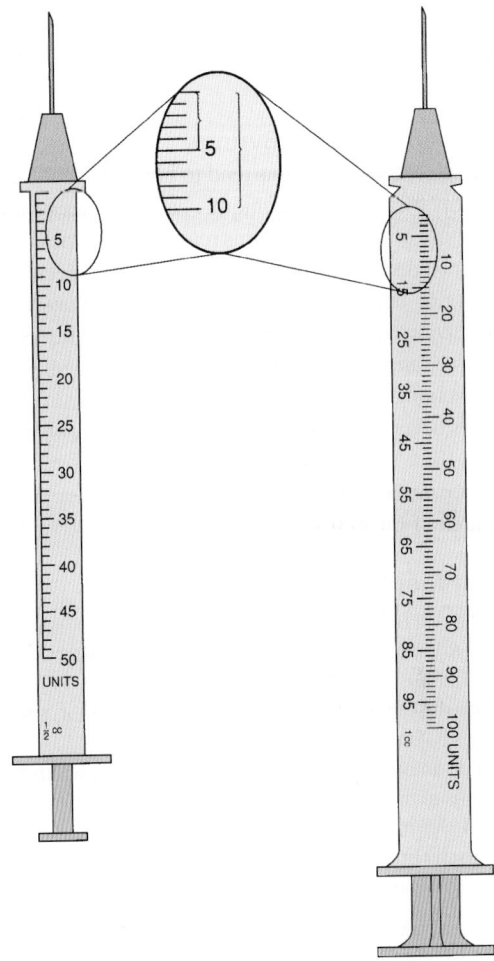

FIGURE 34-14 Low-dose and standard insulin syringes.

 Pharmacologic Considerations

■ Insulin pens are used for ease and convenience by an individual client. Although needles are removed immediately to prevent air backflow, that does not make them multipatient devices.

■ Transmission of blood-borne pathogens has been linked to multiple client use of the insulin pen. Pens should be clearly labeled for each client and separated from each other if used institutionally.

››› *Stop, Think, and Respond 34-2*

In addition to documenting the site of an insulin injection, discuss additional techniques a nurse can use for ensuring a rotation of sites with each subsequent injection.

Preparing Insulin from Vials

Types of insulin vary in their onset, peak effect, and duration of action. The nurse must read the vial labels carefully because they look similar. Some preparations of insulin contain an additive that delays its absorption. Insulin and the additive tend to separate on standing. Therefore, when preparing other than rapid- and short-acting insulin or the long-acting insulin glargine (Lantus), the nurse rotates the vial between the palms to redistribute the additive and insulin before filling the syringe.

Mixing Insulins in One Syringe

When mixed together, insulins tend to bind and become equilibrated. This means that the unique characteristics of each are offset by those of the other. For this reason, most types of insulin are combined just before administration. When injected within 15 minutes of being combined, they act as if they had been injected separately. Rapid- and short-acting insulin, which are additive free, are often combined with an intermediate-acting insulin (Nursing Guidelines 34-3). The long-acting insulin, glargine, is never mixed with any other type of insulin.

Pharmaceutical companies provide some combinations of insulin premixed in a single vial. Novolin 70/30 contains 70% of an intermediate-acting insulin and 30% of a short-acting insulin. Humulin 50/50 contains equal amounts of intermediate- and short-acting insulin. Commercially premixed insulins are stable and can be administered without concern for time after withdrawal from the respective vial.

Pharmacologic Considerations

Long-acting insulins, also called *basal* insulins—glargine (Lantus) or detemir (Levemir)—should never be mixed with any other insulins. Always check with the clinical pharmacist or a reference manual if you question the safety of combining drugs before mixing.

NURSING GUIDELINES 34-3

Mixing Insulins

- Roll the vial of insulin containing an additive between the palms. *Rolling between the palms mixes the insulin without damaging the protein molecules.*
- Cleanse the rubber stoppers of both vials of insulin. *Cleaning removes colonizing microorganisms.*
- Instill an amount of air equal to the volume that will be withdrawn from the vial containing the insulin with the additive labeled "N" in the photo. Do not insert the needle into the insulin itself (Fig. A). *This avoids coating the needle with insulin that contains the additive.*

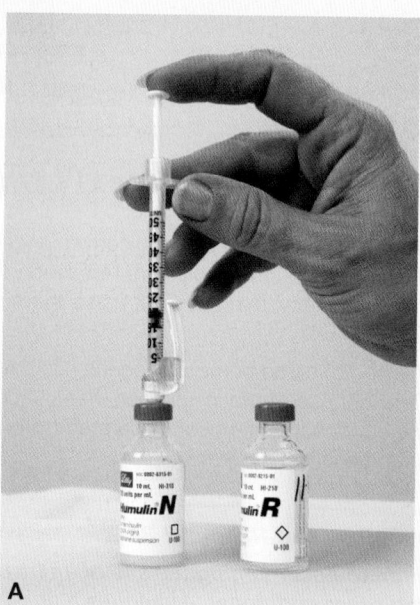

A

Instilling air into the vial containing insulin with additive. (From Evans-Smith, P. [2005]. *Taylor's clinical nursing skills* [pp. 128–129]. Lippincott Williams & Wilkins.)

- Withdraw the needle and use the same syringe to repeat the previous step in the vial containing the additive-free (clear) insulin labeled "R." *Ensures the needle is free of insulin containing an additive.*
- Ask another nurse to check the label on the insulin and the number of units in the syringe. *An additional check helps prevent a medication error.*

- Swab the rubber stopper of the other vial and pierce it with the needle of the partially filled syringe. *This step facilitates withdrawing the other type of insulin.*
- Invert the vial with additive-containing insulin and withdraw the second amount (Fig. B).

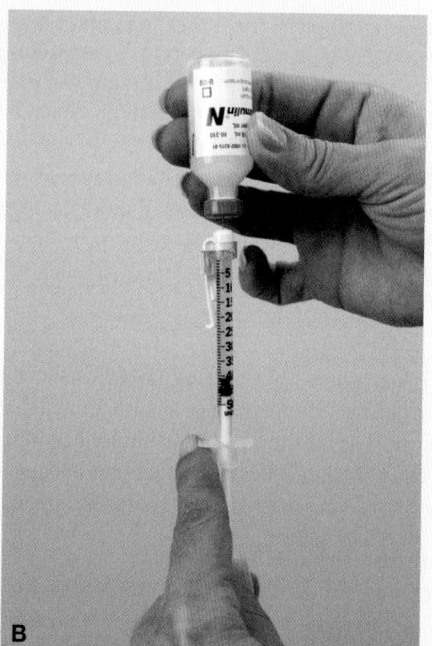

B

Adding insulin with an additive to syringe. (From Evans-Smith, P. [2005]. *Taylor's clinical nursing skills* [pp. 128–129]. Lippincott Williams & Wilkins.)

- Withdraw the specified number of units from the vial containing the insulin with the additive. *Doing so prepares the full prescribed dose.*
- Ask another nurse to check the label on the insulin and the number of units in the syringe. *This step prevents a medication error.*
- Administer within 15 minutes of mixing. *Prompt administration avoids equilibration.*

Insulin Pumps

Some diabetics use an insulin pump rather than a syringe and needle or insulin pen to self-administer insulin. An **insulin pump** is a small, programmable, computed device that contains 180 to 315 units of rapid-acting insulin that can be refilled from vials. Insulin is released from the device through a catheter attached to a needle in the skin (Fig. 34-15). The pump acts similar to a natural pancreas; it releases small amounts of insulin continuously and can release an additional amount manually after a meal or snack. It eliminates the need to self-administer individual injections. The infusion set and infusion site are changed every 2 to 3 days. The catheter can be temporarily disconnected from the pump when bathing, showering, or swimming. Some models have a glucose meter within the pump that can record blood glucose readings.

Administering Heparin

Heparin is an anticoagulant drug, meaning that it prolongs the time it takes for blood to clot. Heparin is frequently administered subcutaneously as well as intravenously. Its unique characteristics require special techniques when using the subcutaneous route for administration.

Heparin is supplied in multiple dose vials or prefilled cartridges. The dosages are very small volumes that may require a tuberculin syringe to ensure accuracy. The nurse removes the needle after withdrawal of the drug from a multidose vial and replaces it with another before administration.

Certain modifications are necessary for the prevention of bruising in the area of the injection. The nurse changes the needle after filling the syringe with the dose of heparin, that is, before injecting the client. The injection site is not cleaned with an alcohol wipe. The nurse does not aspirate with the plunger. The needle is left in place for 5 seconds. Bleeding or oozing following the injection can be controlled by pressing on the injection site with gauze, but it is never rubbed because this can increase the tendency for local bleeding. The nurse rotates the sites with each injection to avoid a previous area where there has been local bleeding.

The dose of unfractionated (standard) heparin may change on a daily or even hourly basis depending on the route of administration. The dose is determined after reporting laboratory test results of the client's partial thromboplastin time to the physician. Some clients are prescribed one of several low-molecular-weight heparins (LMWHs), such as enoxaparin (Lovenox). LMWH has the advantage of being prescribed in a consistent daily dose with no or fewer required anticoagulation blood tests, has less risk for side effects than standard heparin, and can be self-administered outside the hospital.

 Pharmacologic Considerations

Up to 30% of hospitalized clients will be ordered heparin therapy. Be aware that vials of heparin come in various dosages, for example, 20,000, 10,000, 5,000, and 1,000 units/mL. Carefully examine orders and vials supplied when administering the drug.

Intramuscular Injections

An IM injection is the administration of up to 3 mL of medication into one muscle or muscle group. Because deep muscles have few nerve endings, irritating medications are commonly given IM. Except for medications injected directly into the bloodstream, absorption from an IM injection occurs more rapidly than from the other parenteral routes. Injections should not be administered into the limbs that are paralyzed, inactive, or affected by poor circulation. If an older client has had a mastectomy or has a vascular site for hemodialysis, the arm on the affected side should be avoided, if possible.

Injection Sites

The four IM injection sites are named for the muscles into which the medications are injected: the ventrogluteal, the vastus lateralis, the rectus femoris, and the deltoid.

Ventrogluteal Site

The **ventrogluteal site** uses the gluteus medius and gluteus minimus muscles in the hip for injection. This site has several advantages; it has no large nerves or blood vessels, and it is usually less fatty and cleaner because fecal contamination is rare at this site. This is the favored injection site for adults, but it is also safe for use in children. Its main disadvantage is that there is only a small area for administering the injection.

To locate the ventrogluteal site:

- Place the palm of the hand on the greater trochanter and the index finger on the anterior–superior iliac spine (Fig. 34-16).

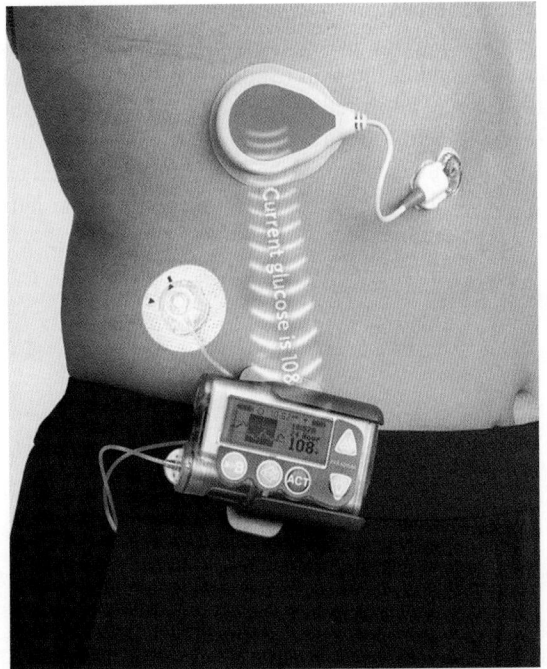

FIGURE 34-15 A continuous subcutaneous insulin infusion pump. (From Nath, J. [2019]. *Programmed learning approach to medical terminology* [3rd ed.]. Lippincott Williams & Wilkins.)

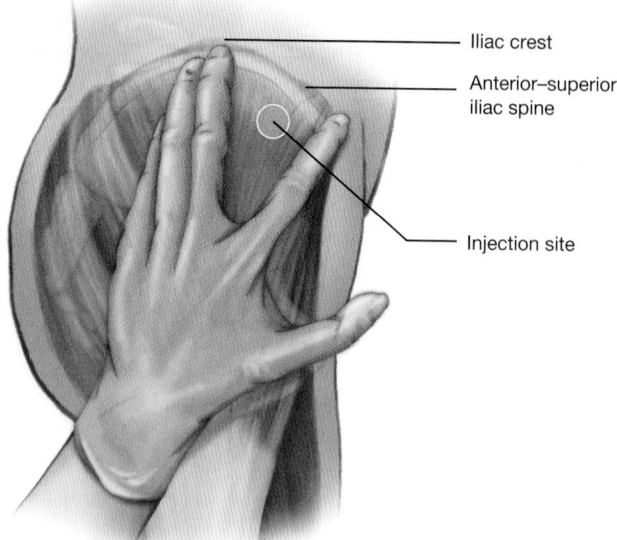

FIGURE 34-16 The ventrogluteal site.

- Move the middle finger away from the index finger as far as possible along the iliac crest.
- Inject into the center of the triangle formed by the index finger, the middle finger, and the iliac crest.

Vastus Lateralis Site

The **vastus lateralis site** uses the vastus lateralis muscle— one of the muscles in the quadriceps group of the outer thigh. Large nerves and blood vessels are usually absent in this area, which makes it safer. It is a particularly desirable site for administering injections to infants and small children and clients who are thin or debilitated with poorly developed gluteal muscles.

The nurse locates the vastus lateralis site by placing one hand above the knee and one hand just below the greater trochanter at the top of the thigh. The nurse then inserts the needle into the lateral area of the thigh (Fig. 34-17).

Rectus Femoris Site

The **rectus femoris site** is in the anterior aspect of the thigh. This site may be used for infants. The nurse places an injection in this site in the middle third of the thigh with the client sitting or supine (Fig. 34-18).

Deltoid Site

The **deltoid site** in the lateral aspect of the upper arm (Fig. 34-19) is the least used IM injection site because it is a smaller muscle than the others. It is used for children beginning at age 4 as well as for adults. Because of its small capacity, IM injections into this site are limited to 1 mL of solution.

There is a risk of damaging the radial nerve and artery if the deltoid site is not well identified. To use this site safely:

- Have the client lie down, sit, or stand with the shoulder well exposed.
- Palpate the lower edge of the acromion process.
- Draw an imaginary line at the axilla.
- Inject in the area between these two landmarks.

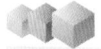 Concept Mastery Alert

Choosing an IM Injection Site

When administering an IM injection, adequate muscle mass and movement are needed to promote the distribution of the medication. Keep in mind that with an older adult client, muscle mass may be decreased. If this client also has impaired mobility, any site that will not receive sufficient movement should be avoided. Therefore, for an older adult client with impaired mobility, use the deltoid or ventrogluteal sites for IM injections.

Injection Equipment

Generally, 3- to 5-mL syringes are used to administer medications by the IM route. A 22-gauge needle that is 1½ to 2 in long is usually adequate for depositing medication in most sites.

Injection Technique

When administering IM injections, nurses use a 90-degree angle for piercing the skin (Skill 34-3). Nurses administer drugs that may be irritating to the upper levels of tissue by the **Z-track technique** (a technique for manipulating the tissue to seal a medication in the muscle). Sometimes called the *zigzag* technique, the maneuver resembles the letter Z (Nursing Guidelines 34-4).

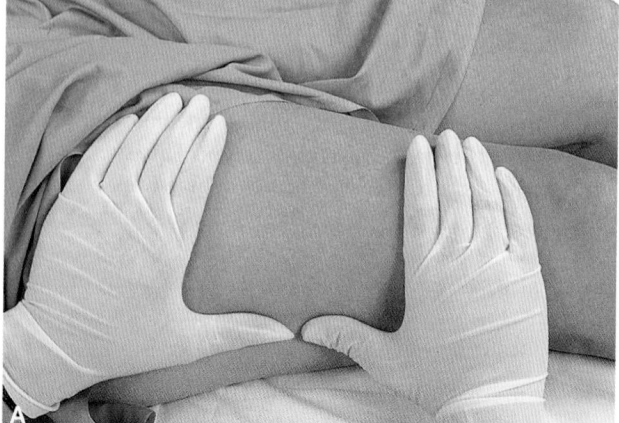
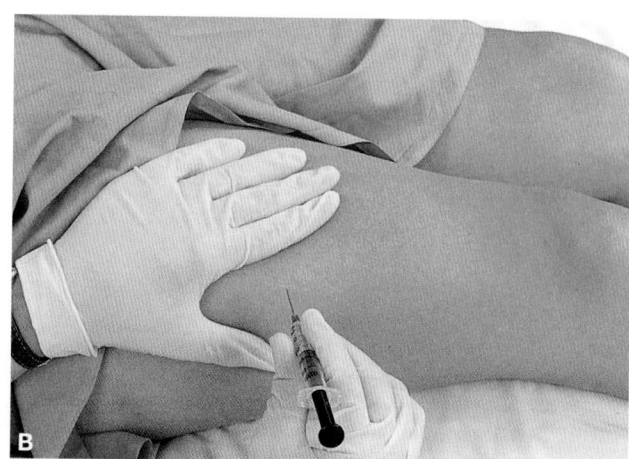

FIGURE 34-17 **A.** Locating the vastus lateralis muscle. **B.** Spreading the skin at the vastus lateralis site and darting the tissue.

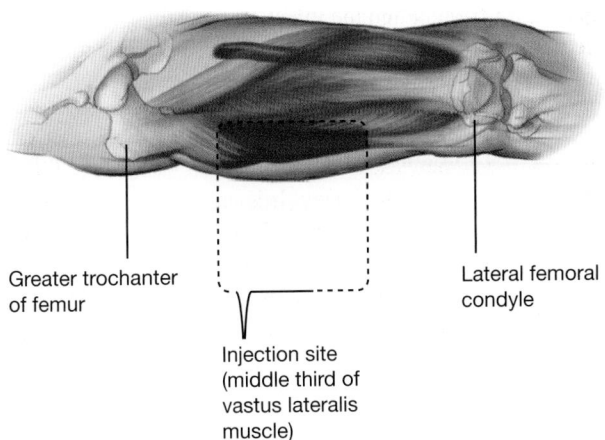

Greater trochanter of femur

Lateral femoral condyle

Injection site (middle third of vastus lateralis muscle)

FIGURE 34-18 The rectus femoris injection site is on the lateral aspect of the anterior thigh.

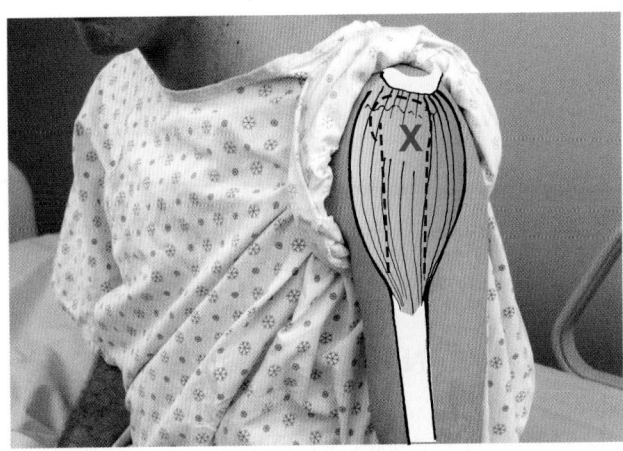

FIGURE 34-19 The deltoid injection site.

 NURSING GUIDELINES 34-4

Giving an Injection by the Z-Track Technique

- Fill the syringe with the prepared drug and then change the needle. *This measure prevents tissue contact with the irritating drug.*
- Attach a needle at least 1½ to 2 in long. *The correct needle length helps deposit the drug deep within the muscle.*
- Add a 0.2-mL bubble of air in the syringe. *Air flushes all the medication from the syringe during the injection.*
- Select a large muscular injection site such as the ventrogluteal site. *A large site provides a location with the capacity for depositing and absorbing the drug.*
- Wash your hands and don gloves. *These measures reduce the transmission of microorganisms.*
- Use the side of the hand to pull the tissue laterally about 1 in (2.5 cm) until the tissue is taut (Fig. A). *Taut tissue creates the mechanism for sealing the drug within the muscle.*
- Insert the needle at a 90-degree angle while continuing to hold the tissue laterally. *Correct placement directs the tip of the needle well within the muscle.*
- Steady the barrel of the syringe with the fingers and use the thumb to manipulate the plunger (Fig. B). *These measures avoid releasing the tissue held taut by the nondominant hand.*

- Aspirate for a blood return. *Doing so determines whether the needle is in a blood vessel.*
- Instill the medication by depressing the plunger with the thumb. *This measure deposits the medication into the muscle.*
- Wait 10 seconds with the needle still in place and the skin held taut. *This duration provides time to distribute the medication in a larger area.*
- Withdraw the needle and immediately release the taut skin. *Doing so creates a diagonal path that prevents leaking into the subcutaneous and dermal layers of tissue* (Fig. C).
- Apply pressure, but do not massage the site. *This ensures the medication remains sealed.*
- Discard the syringe without recapping the needle. *Proper disposal reduces the potential for a needlestick injury.*
- Remove gloves and wash your hands or use an alcohol-based hand rub. *These measures reduce the transmission of microorganisms.*
- Document the medication administration. *Proper recording maintains a current record of client care.*

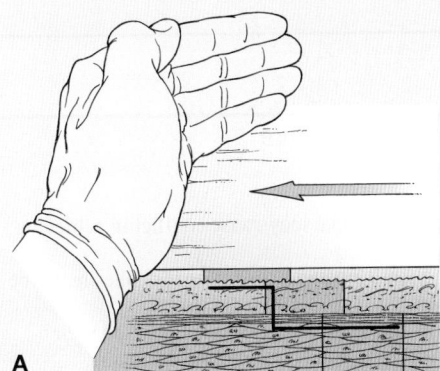

A Stretching the muscle laterally forming a "Z."

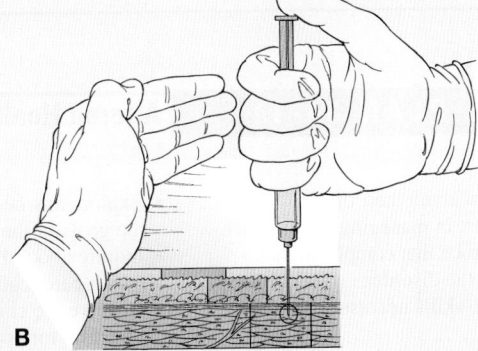

B Manipulating the plunger.

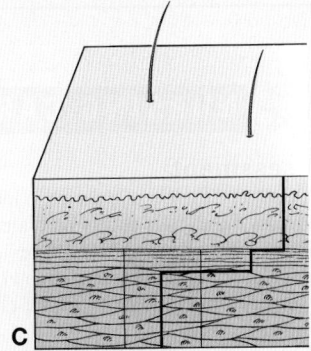

C The released tissue seals the pathway of injected medication.

Nurses can give any IM injection by the Z-track technique. Clients report slightly less pain during and the next day after a Z-track injection compared with the usual IM injection technique.

>>> **Stop, Think, and Respond 34-3**
What could occur if parenteral medication intended for the IM route is instilled into a blood vessel? How could this be prevented?

REDUCING INJECTION DISCOMFORT

All injections cause discomfort, and some cause more than others. The nurse can use the following alternative techniques to reduce discomfort associated with injections:

• Use the smallest gauge needle appropriately.
• Change the needle before administering a drug that is irritating to tissue.
• Select a site that is free of irritation.
• Rotate injection sites.
• Numb the skin with an ice pack before the injection.
• Insert and withdraw the needle without hesitation.
• Instill the medication slowly and steadily.
• Use the Z-track technique for IM injections.
• Apply pressure to the site during needle withdrawal.
• Massage the site afterward if appropriate.

The client can also assist in minimizing the pain associated with injections. Instructions commonly focus on positioning and relaxation techniques include:

• Perform deep breathing and other relaxation techniques before receiving an injection.

• Avoid watching when the injection is given.
• Ambulate or move the extremity where the injection was given as much as possible.

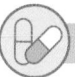 **Pharmacologic Considerations**

■ For clients who fear IM injections, products are available that produce local anesthesia when applied to the skin or mucous membranes. One example is eutectic mixture of local anesthetic (or EMLA), which reduces or eliminates the local discomfort of invasive procedures that pierce the skin, thereby eliminating the fear. To take effect, application of EMLA cream needs to be 1 to 2 hours before the injection.

■ EMLA is best suited for multiple administrations such as weekly IM interferon injections to treat multiple sclerosis.

NURSING IMPLICATIONS

Nurses who administer parenteral medications may identify applicable nursing diagnoses as follows:

• Acute pain
• Acute anxiety
• Fear
• Altered skin integrity risk
• Altered tissue integrity risk
• Nonadherence
• Knowledge deficiency

Nursing Care Plan 34-1 demonstrates the nursing process for a client with the nursing diagnosis risk for altered health maintenance, defined as reducing risk factors and assisting the client to achieve optimum levels of function and independence within the limits of defined health maintenance alterations.

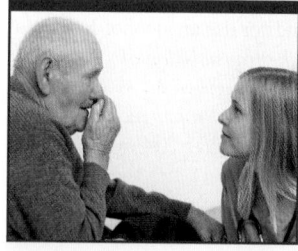 **Clinical Scenario** A 73-year-old male client has been referred to the diabetic clinic after being discharged 3 weeks ago. His record of glucometer readings has fluctuated above and below his target goals. His fasting blood sugar remains elevated despite the fact that he skips meals. He lives alone and relies on commercially prepared food. He reports experiencing palpitations, sweating, and difficulty processing information when his blood sugar is abnormally low. He feels he will never be able to manage his diabetes according to the prescribed regimen.

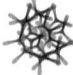 **NURSING CARE PLAN 34-1** | **Altered Health Maintenance**

Assessment

• Determine the client's desire to learn about their illness.
• Assess the client's ability and interest in managing the disorder.
• Review the client's history for evidence that complications developed from mismanagement of the disorder.
• Consider the complexity of self-care skills necessary after the client is discharged.
• Identify any problems that may pose a barrier in carrying out a regimen of self-care (e.g., dementia, physical weakness, pain, diminished self-confidence).

• Explore any health beliefs that may cause conflict in achieving the goals of therapy.
• Inquire about the client's financial resources for adhering to the health care regimen.
• Observe the client's network of significant others and their potential for providing physical and emotional support.
• Evaluate the client's level of understanding of ongoing health teaching throughout the period of nursing care.

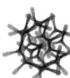

NURSING CARE PLAN 34-1 · Altered Health Maintenance (*continued*)

Nursing Diagnosis. Altered Health Maintenance related to dietary practices that interfere with regulating insulin therapy with daily food intake

Expected Outcome. The client will describe the need to eat food within 30 minutes of an insulin injection and ways to raise blood glucose levels if symptoms of hypoglycemia develop.

Interventions	Rationales
Review onset, peak, and duration of Humulin N insulin each morning when administering the client's dose of insulin.	The repetition of information enhances learning.
Emphasize that breakfast is required within 30 minutes of injecting the prescribed dose of insulin.	Demonstrating a regular pattern between administering insulin and eating food shortly afterward reinforces learning.
Reinforce that the client should eat meals three times a day at approximately the same time from day to day.	Eating consistently helps keep blood sugar stable throughout the day.
Assist the client with testing their own blood glucose level before and 2 hours after meals.	Testing capillary blood glucose provides objective evidence of the relationship between blood glucose levels before and after eating.
Review the signs and symptoms of low blood glucose levels; ask the client to recall as many signs and symptoms as possible.	Providing information and testing the client's ability to accurately recall the information measure the client's learning.
Give the client a list of foods or beverages that can raise blood glucose levels when signs or symptoms of low blood glucose levels occur.	Identifying techniques for resolving the problem of low blood glucose levels provides the client with options for managing self-care.

Evaluation of Expected Outcomes

- Client noted time of insulin administration at 0730 hours and eating breakfast between 0730 and 0800 hours.
- Client stated, "I will eat a meal within a half hour of giving myself my morning insulin."
- Client observed that blood glucose level was 98 mg/dL before eating breakfast and increased to 122 mg/dL 2 hours later.
- Client named grape juice, orange juice, regular soft drinks, and hard candies as foods or beverages to consume if he experiences symptoms of low blood glucose levels.

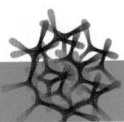

KEY POINTS

- Parenteral medications: Medications administered by injection
- Equipment
  - Syringe: Sizes 1 to 5 mL or units
  - Needle: Various lengths and gauges
  - Filtered needle: A membrane that acts as a barrier blocking the entrance of glass shards when withdrawing medication from a glass ampule
  - Insulin pen: Cylinder containing a prefilled reservoir of insulin; a disposable needle is attached to the pen each time it is used
  - Ampule: A sealed glass drug container that must be broken to withdraw the medication
  - Vial: A glass or plastic container of parenteral medication with a self-sealing rubber stopper that must be pierced with a needle or a needleless adapter to remove medication
  - Prefilled cartridge: A sealed glass cylinder of parenteral medication, the cartridge comes with an attached needle
- Combining medications in one syringe: At times, it is necessary or appropriate to combine more than one drug in a single syringe. Exact amounts must be withdrawn from each drug container because once the drugs are in the barrel of the syringe, there is no way to expel one without expelling some of the other.
- Injection routes
  - Intradermal injection: Between the layers of the skin (e.g., tuberculin syringe)
  - Subcutaneous injection: Beneath the skin but above the muscle
    - Insulin
    - A 25-gauge needle is used most often because medications administered subcutaneously are usually not viscous.
    - Needle lengths may vary from 1/2 to 5/8 in.
    - Insert at a 45- to 90-degree angle.
    - Insulin pump: A small, programmable, computed device that contains insulin and can be refilled from vials; insulin is released from the device through a catheter attached to a needle in the skin.
- Heparin: In order to prevent bruising in the area of the injection:
  - Change the needle after filling the syringe with the dose of heparin.
  - Do not clean the injection site with an alcohol wipe.
  - Do not aspirate with the plunger.

- Leave the needle in place for 5 seconds.
- Bleeding or oozing following the injection can be controlled by pressing on the injection site with gauze, but it is never rubbed because this can increase the tendency for local bleeding.
- Rotate the sites with each injection to avoid a previous area where there has been local bleeding.
- Insert at a 45- to 90-degree angle.
- IM injections: Injections in muscle tissue with 3- to 5-mL syringes, 22-gauge 1½- to 2-in needle, 90-degree angle or Z-track

- Ventrogluteal site: The gluteus medius and gluteus minimus muscles in the hip
- Vastus lateralis site: The vastus lateralis muscle, one of the muscles in the quadriceps group of the outer thigh
- Rectus femoris site: In the anterior aspect of the thigh, may be used for infants
- Deltoid site: The lateral aspect of the upper arm; IM injections into this site are limited to 1 mL of solution
- Intravenous injections: Injections instilled into veins

CRITICAL THINKING EXERCISES

1. How does administration of an IM injection differ for a 3-year-old client versus a 33-year-old client?
2. You are to administer an IM injection to a 76-year-old client. What factors are important to consider before choosing the equipment and injection site?
3. What information would be appropriate for the nurse to provide to a client who repeatedly administers insulin in nearly the exact same location with each injection?
4. What techniques might a nurse use to avoid injecting into a muscle when giving a thin client a subcutaneous injection?

NEXT-GENERATION NCLEX-STYLE REVIEW QUESTIONS

1. The nurse chooses to inject a prescribed IM medication into the ventrogluteal site. Which area is most descriptive of the site location?
   a. Upper hip
   b. Top arm
   c. Anterior thigh
   d. Posterior buttock
   Test-Taking Strategy: Analyze the descriptors and select the body site that correlates with the portion of the iliac crest above the head of the femur.
2. What techniques help reduce discomfort when giving an IM injection? Select all that apply.
   a. Withdraw the needle without hesitation.
   b. Use the smallest needle appropriately.
   c. Add a local anesthetic to the syringe.
   d. Tell the client to hold their breath.
   e. Rotate injection sites for repeated injections.
   f. Pierce the injection site quickly like a dart.
   Test-Taking Strategy: Use the process of elimination to select actions that are standard nursing procedures when administering injections.

3. The nurse plans to inject an irritating medication using the Z-track technique. Just before inserting the needle into the muscle, in which direction is the nurse correct in pulling the tissue at the injection site?
   a. Laterally
   b. Diagonally
   c. Downward
   d. Upward
   Test-Taking Strategy: Use the process of elimination to select the option that displaces the tissue before inserting the needle.
4. When administering an intradermal tuberculin skin test, which angle of needle insertion is correct?
   a. 180-degree angle
   b. 90-degree angle
   c. 45-degree angle
   d. 10-degree angle
   Test-Taking Strategy: Note the key word, "correct." Exclude angles that are used when administering subcutaneous and IM injections or are otherwise incorrect.
5. The nurse must mix a short- and intermediate-acting insulin in the same syringe. Place the actions in the correct sequence.
   a. The nurse instills air into the intermediate-acting insulin vial.
   b. The nurse rolls the vial of intermediate-acting insulin to mix it with its additive.
   c. The nurse instills air into the vial of short-acting insulin.
   d. The nurse inverts and withdraws the specified amount from the intermediate-acting insulin vial.
   e. The nurse inverts and withdraws the specified amount from the short-acting insulin vial.
   Test-Taking Strategy: Analyze the actions in each of the options and place them in order when mixing two insulins each of which acts at a different rate.

NEXT-GENERATION NCLEX-STYLE CLINICAL SCENARIO QUESTIONS

Clinical Scenario:

A 73-year-old male client has been referred to the diabetic clinic after being discharged 3 weeks ago. His record of glucometer readings has fluctuated above and below his target goals. His fasting blood sugar remains elevated despite the fact that he skips meals. He lives alone and relies on commercially prepared food. He reports experiencing palpitations, sweating, and difficulty processing information when his blood sugar is abnormally low. He feels he will never be able to manage his diabetes according to the prescribed regimen.

1. Select all of the indicators that may be a cause for concern regarding the client's knowledge of his diabetes diagnosis.
   a. Fluctuating glucometer readings
   b. Elevated blood sugar levels
   c. Palpitations and sweating
   d. Diet
   e. Confusion during times of low blood sugar

2. Place an "x" under "effective" identifying actions that would help the client with his diabetes. Place an "x" under "ineffective" identifying actions that may contribute to the client's fluctuating blood sugar levels.

ACTIONS	EFFECTIVE	INEFFECTIVE
Meeting with a nutritionist to help with the client's diet		
Telling the client about the side effects of high/low blood glucose levels		
Reviewing with a significant other and writing down the side effects of high/low blood glucose levels		
Refer the client and (if available, a significant other) to a diabetic educator		
Have the client keep a record of blood glucose levels and medications		

SKILL 34-1 Administering Intradermal Injections

Suggested Action	Reason for Action
ASSESSMENT	
Check the medical orders.	Collaborates the nursing activities with the medical treatment
Compare the medication administration record (MAR) with the written medical order.	Ensures accuracy
Read and compare the label on the drug with the MAR at least three times—before, during, and after preparing the drug.	Prevents errors
Check for any documented allergies to food or drugs.	Ensures safety
Determine how much the client understands about the purpose and technique for administering the injection.	Provides an opportunity for health teaching
PLANNING	
Prepare to administer the injection according to the schedule prescribed.	Complies with medical orders
Obtain clean gloves, a tuberculin syringe, the appropriate needle, and alcohol swabs.	Facilitates drug preparation and administration
Prepare the syringe with the medication.	Fills the syringe with the appropriate volume
IMPLEMENTATION	
Wash your hands or use an alcohol-based hand rub (see Chapter 10); put on gloves.	Reduces the transmission of microorganisms
Identify the client using at least two methods, for example, checking the wristband and asking the client's name and birthdate.	Ensures that medications are given to the *right client*; complies with the National Patient Safety Goals
Pull the privacy curtain.	Demonstrates respect for the client's dignity
Select an area on the inner aspect of the forearm, approximately a hand's breadth above the client's wrist.	Provides a convenient and easy location for accessing intradermal tissue
Cleanse the area with an alcohol swab using a circular motion outward from the site where the needle will pierce the skin (Fig. A).	Removes microorganisms following the principles of asepsis

Cleaning the forearm. (From Lippincott Williams & Wilkins. [2018]. *Lippincott's nursing procedures.*)

Allow the skin to dry.	Reduces tissue irritation
Hold the client's arm and stretch the skin taut.	Helps control the placement of the needle

SKILL 34-1 Administering Intradermal Injections (*continued*)

Suggested Action	Reason for Action
Hold the syringe almost parallel to the skin at a 10- to 15-degree angle with the bevel pointing upward. Then insert the needle 1/8 in (Fig. B).	Facilitates delivering the drug between the layers of the skin and advances the needle to the desired depth

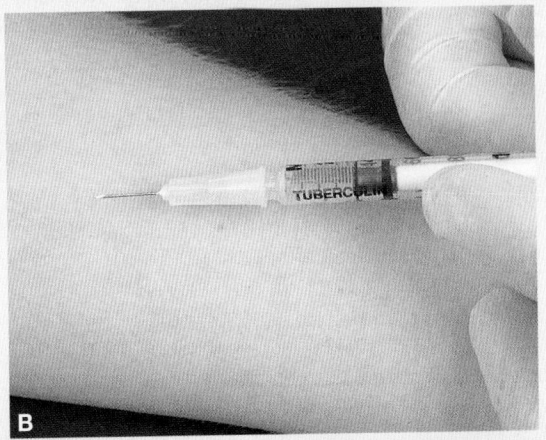

Entering the skin. (Photo by B. Proud.)

Push the plunger of the syringe and watch for a small **wheal** (elevated circle) to appear (Fig. C).	Verifies the correct injection of the drug

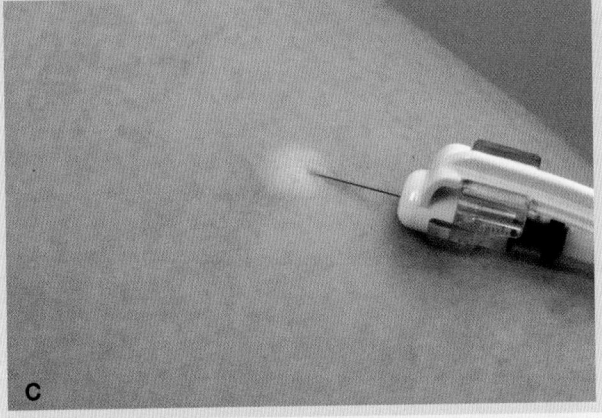

Producing a wheal. (From Lippincott Williams & Wilkins. [2018]. *Lippincott's nursing procedures*.)

Withdraw the needle at the same angle at which it was inserted.	Minimizes tissue trauma and discomfort
Do not massage the area after removing the needle.	Prevents interfering with test results if the purpose of the injection is to identify an allergen or response to a tuberculin test
Deposit the uncapped needle and syringe in a puncture-resistant container.	Prevents a needlestick injury
Remove gloves and perform hand hygiene.	Reduces the risk for the transmission of microorganisms
Observe the client's condition for at least the first 30 minutes after performing an allergy test.	Ensures emergency treatment can be quickly administered
Observe the area for signs of a local reaction at standard intervals such as 24 and 48 hours after a tuberculin test.	Determines the extent to which the client responds to the injected substance

EVALUATION

- The injection is administered.
- The client remains free of any untoward effects.

DOCUMENT

- The date, time, drug, dose, route, and specific site
- Client response

SAMPLE DOCUMENTATION

Date and Time Tuberculin skin test administered intradermally in L forearm with no immediate untoward effects. Instructed to return in 48 hours for inspection of site. _____ J. Doe, LPN

SKILL 34-2 Administering Subcutaneous Injections

Suggested Action	Reason for Action
ASSESSMENT	
Check the medical orders.	Collaborates the nursing activities with the medical treatment
Compare the medication administration record (MAR) with the written medical order.	Ensures accuracy
Read and compare the label on the drug with the MAR at least three times—before, during, and after preparing the drug.	Prevents errors
Check for any documented allergies to food or drugs.	Ensures safety
Determine where the last injection was given to ensure site rotation.	Prevents tissue injury
Determine how much the client understands about the purpose and technique for administering the injection.	Provides an opportunity for health teaching
Inspect the potential injection site for signs of bruising, swelling, redness, warmth, or tenderness.	Indicates injured tissue areas to avoid
PLANNING	
Prepare to administer the injection according to the schedule prescribed.	Complies with medical orders
Obtain clean gloves, the appropriate syringe and needle, and alcohol swabs.	Facilitates drug preparation and administration
Prepare the syringe with the medication.	Fills the syringe with the appropriate volume
Add 0.1–0.2 mL of air to the syringe.	Flushes all the medication from the syringe at the time of the injection
IMPLEMENTATION	
Wash your hands or use an alcohol-based hand rub (see Chapter 10); put on gloves.	Reduces the transmission of microorganisms
Identify the client using at least two methods, for example, checking the wristband and asking the client's name and birthdate.	Ensures that medications are given to the *right client*; complies with the National Patient Safety Goals
Pull the privacy curtain.	Demonstrates respect for the client's dignity
Select and prepare an appropriate site by cleansing it with an alcohol swab (Fig. A).	Removes colonizing microorganisms

Cleaning the injection site. (From Lynn, P. [2022]. *Taylor's clinical nursing skills* [6th ed.]. Lippincott Williams & Wilkins.)

Suggested Action	Reason for Action
Allow the skin to dry.	Reduces tissue irritation
Bunch the skin (Fig. B).	Facilitates placement in the subcutaneous level of tissue

Bunching the tissue. (From Lynn, P. [2022]. *Taylor's clinical nursing skills* [6th ed.]. Lippincott Williams & Wilkins.)

SKILL 34-2 Administering Subcutaneous Injections (*continued*)

Suggested Action	Reason for Action
Pierce the skin at a 45-degree (Fig. C) or 90-degree (Fig. D) angle of entry.	Facilitates placement in the subcutaneous level of tissue according to the length of the needle used and the client's body composition

Entering the tissue at a 45-degree angle. (Photo by B. Proud.)

Entering the tissue at a 90-degree angle. (Photo by B. Proud.)

Suggested Action	Reason for Action
Release the tissue once the needle is inserted; use the hand to support the syringe at its hub.	Steadies the syringe
Do not aspirate.	Subcutaneous tissue does not contain major blood vessels, which negates the need to aspirate
Inject the medication 5 seconds after the needle has been embedded within the tissue by pushing on the plunger.	Ensures complete delivery of the insulin
Withdraw the needle quickly while applying pressure against the medication site.	Controls bleeding
Massage the site unless contraindicated.	Promotes absorption and relieves discomfort
Deposit the uncapped needle and syringe in a puncture-resistant container.	Prevents injury
Remove gloves; perform hand hygiene.	Reduces the transmission of microorganisms
Assess the client's condition at least 30 minutes after giving the injection.	Aids in evaluating the drug's effectiveness

SKILL 34-2 Administering Subcutaneous Injections (*continued*)

Suggested Action	Reason for Action

EVALUATION

- The injection is administered.
- The client experiences no untoward effects.

DOCUMENT

- The date, time, drug, dose, route, and specific site
- Site assessment data
- Client's response

SAMPLE DOCUMENTATION[a]

Date and Time 10 units of regular insulin administered subcutaneously in 3 o'clock position in abdomen. Site appears free of redness, swelling, warmth, tenderness, and bruising. Alert and oriented 30 minutes after injection. _____ J. Doe, LPN

[a]The administration of drugs is usually documented on the MAR.

SKILL 34-3 Administering Intramuscular Injections

Suggested Action	Reason for Action
ASSESSMENT	
Check the medical orders.	Collaborates the nursing activities with the medical treatment
Compare the medication administration record (MAR) with the written medical order.	Ensures accuracy
Read and compare the label on the drug with the MAR at least three times—before, during, and after preparing the drug.	Prevents errors
Check for any documented drug allergies.	Ensures safety
Determine where the last injection was given.	Prevents tissue injury
Determine how much the client understands about the purpose and technique for administering the injection.	Provides an opportunity for health teaching
Inspect the potential injection site for signs of bruising, swelling, redness, warmth, tenderness, or **induration** (hardness).	Determines tissue integrity
PLANNING	
Prepare to administer the injection according to the schedule prescribed.	Complies with medical orders
Obtain clean gloves, the appropriate syringe and needle, and alcohol swabs.	Facilitates drug preparation and administration
Prepare the syringe with the medication.	Fills the syringe with the appropriate volume
Add 0.2 mL of air to the syringe.	Flushes all the medication from the syringe at the time of the injection
IMPLEMENTATION	
Wash your hands or perform an alcohol-based hand rub (see Chapter 10); put on gloves.	Reduces the transmission of microorganisms
Identify the client using at least two methods, for example, checking the wristband and asking the client's name and birthdate.	Ensures that medications are given to the *right client*; complies with the National Patient Safety Goals
Pull the privacy curtain.	Demonstrates respect for the client's dignity

SKILL 34-3 Administering Intramuscular Injections (*continued*)

Suggested Action	Reason for Action
Select an appropriate site such as the ventrogluteal site (Fig. A).	Supports the evidence that the ventrogluteal site is one of the best for all ages because it is free of major nerves and blood vessels and has a well-developed muscle mass

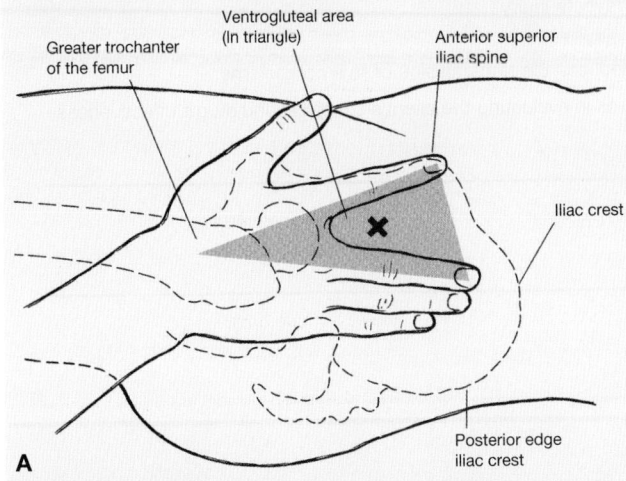

Identifying the ventrogluteal injection site. (Ryan, T. A. [2023]. *Torres' patient care in imaging technology* [10th ed.]. Lippincott Williams & Wilkins.)

A

Suggested Action	Reason for Action
Prepare the site by cleansing it with an alcohol swab.	Removes colonizing microorganisms
Allow the skin to dry.	Reduces tissue irritation
Spread the tissue taut.	Facilitates placement in the muscle
Hold the syringe like a dart and pierce the skin at a 90-degree angle (Fig. B).	Reduces discomfort

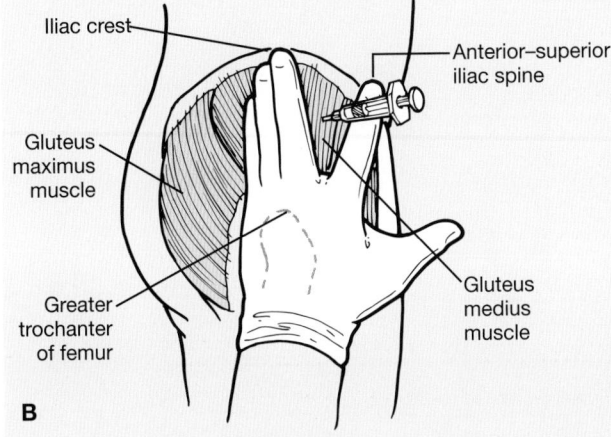

Inserting the needle. (From Lippincott Williams & Wilkins. [2016]. *LifeART*. All rights reserved.)

B

Suggested Action	Reason for Action
Depress the plunger on the syringe.	Deposits the drug into the muscle
Withdraw the needle quickly at the same angle it was inserted while applying pressure against the site (Fig. C).	Reduces discomfort and controls bleeding

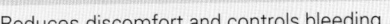

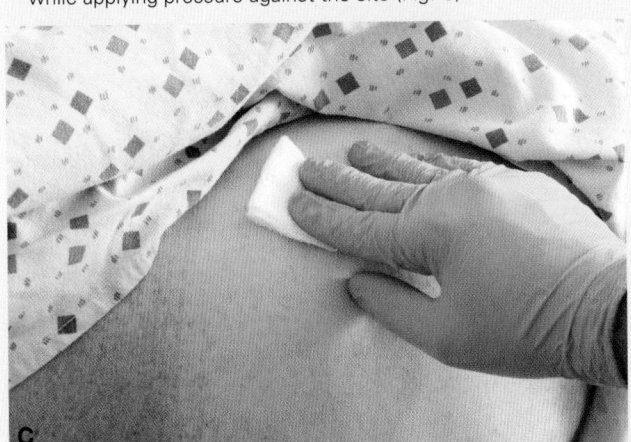

Applying pressure at injection site. (From Lynn, P. B. [2018]. *Taylor's clinical nursing skills* [5th ed.]. Wolters Kluwer.)

C

SKILL 34-3 Administering Intramuscular Injections (*continued*)

Suggested Action	Reason for Action
Massage the injection site with the alcohol swab.	Distributes the medication and reduces discomfort
Deposit the uncapped needle and syringe in a puncture-resistant container.	Prevents injury
Remove gloves; perform hand hygiene.	Reduces the transmission of microorganisms
Assess the client's condition at least 30 minutes after giving the injection.	Aids in evaluating the client's condition and drug's effectiveness

EVALUATION

- The injection is administered.
- The client experiences no untoward effects.

DOCUMENT

- The date, time, drug, dose, route, and specific site
- Site assessment data
- Client's response

SAMPLE DOCUMENTATION[a]

Date and Time Demerol 50 mg given IM into R ventrogluteal site for pain rated as 8 on a scale of 0–10. No signs of irritation at the injection site. Rates pain at a "5," 30 minutes after injection. _____ J. Doe, LPN

[a]The administration of drugs is usually documented on the MAR; as-needed drugs may be documented in both the nurse's notes and the MAR.

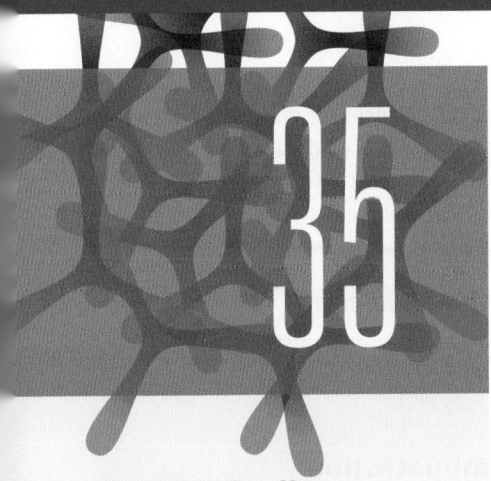

35

Intravenous Medications

Words To Know

antineoplastic drugs
bolus administration
central venous catheter
continuous infusion
implanted catheter
intermittent infusion
intravenous route
medication lock
noncoring needle
nontunneled percutaneous
catheter
port
secondary infusion
tunneled catheter
volume-control set

Learning Objectives

On completion of this chapter, the reader should be able to:

1. Name the types of veins into which intravenous (IV) medications are administered.
2. Describe appropriate situations for administering IV medications.
3. Describe one method for giving bolus administrations of IV medications.
4. Name ways by which IV medications are administered.
5. Describe methods for administering medicated solutions intermittently.
6. Explain the technique for administering a secondary piggyback infusion.
7. Discuss purposes for using a volume-control set.
8. Describe a central venous catheter (CVC).
9. Name types of CVCs.
10. Discuss techniques for protecting oneself when administering antineoplastic drugs.

INTRODUCTION

The **intravenous route** (drug administration through peripheral and central veins) provides an immediate effect. Consequently, this route of drug administration is the most dangerous. Drugs given in this manner cannot be retrieved once they have been delivered. Hence, only specially qualified nurses are permitted to administer intravenous (IV) medications. Those responsible for IV medication administration must use extreme caution in preparation and instillation.

Administering IV solutions (see Chapter 16) is also considered a form of IV medication administration. The focus of this chapter, however, is on the methods for administering IV drugs, not fluid replacement solutions, and the techniques for using various venous access devices.

 Gerontologic Considerations

■ Older adults are sometimes reluctant to ask questions of health care providers. Therefore, it is imperative that nurses explain the purpose and potential side effects for each drug administered, especially by the IV route.

■ Older adults tend to metabolize and excrete drugs at slower rates. This factor may predispose them to toxic effects from an accumulation of medications. This toxicity may occur more rapidly when the drug is administered IV. Adjustments may be needed in the amount or frequency of dosing. Older adults require frequent and comprehensive assessments during and after IV medication administration.

■ Older adults with dementia often experience more confusion and disorientation with an acute illness. Any change in mental status requires a comprehensive assessment of contributing conditions and the implementation of interventions to ensure the safe administration of IV medications and maintenance of the IV insertion site to prevent displacement of the venipuncture device.

■ Older adults comprise the largest age group of clients cared for in acute and long-term health care facilities. The administration of IV medications is quite common in older clients. Increased emphasis on early discharges may require teaching older adults, family caregivers, or both how to flush venous access equipment.

■ Older adults who are discharged with medical devices for medications or treatments are likely to qualify for skilled nursing for follow-up in home or other independent settings, such as assisted living facilities.

■ The veins of older adults tend to be fragile. Inserting a percutaneous central venous catheter (CVC) is often better than risking the trauma of repeated attempts at restarting or changing peripheral IV sites.

 Pharmacologic Considerations

■ Children and older adults are likely to experience greater effects of drugs, especially when given IV.

■ Drugs become inactive when they bind to protein in the bloodstream. Both children and older adults have fewer proteins in their blood, meaning more active drug circulates in the circulatory system. Immature (child) or diminished (older adult) liver and kidney function also results in less metabolized or excreted drug, again keeping drugs in the circulating blood. Together, this causes greater intended and adverse effects of the drug.

INTRAVENOUS MEDICATION ADMINISTRATION

Despite its risks, IV administration given either continuously or intermittently is the route chosen when:

• A quick response is needed during an emergency.
• Clients have disorders (e.g., serious burns) that affect the absorption or metabolism of drugs.
• Blood levels of drugs are needed to maintain a consistent therapeutic level, such as when treating infections caused by drug-resistant pathogens or providing pain relief.
• It is in the client's interest to avoid the discomfort of repeated intramuscular injections.
• A mechanism is needed to administer drug therapy over a prolonged period, as with cancer.

Continuous Administration

A **continuous infusion** (instillation of a parenteral drug over several hours), also called a *continuous drip*, involves adding medication to a large volume (500 to 1,000 mL) of IV solution (Skill 35-1). Drugs may be added to a new container of

IV solution or to an existing infusion if there is a sufficient volume to dilute the drug. After the medication is added, the solution is administered by gravity infusion or more commonly with an electronic infusion device such as a controller or pump (see Chapter 16).

>>> **Stop, Think, and Respond 35-1**
What are some advantages of administering an IV medication by a continuous infusion?

Intermittent Administration

Intermittent infusion is a short-term (from minutes up to 1 hour), parenteral administration of IV medication. Intermittent infusions are administered in three ways: bolus administrations, secondary administrations, and those in which a volume-control set is used.

Bolus Administration

The term *bolus* refers to a substance given all at one time. A **bolus administration** (an undiluted or a diluted medication given into a vein in 1 minute or more) is sometimes described as a drug given by IV push. Although the term "push" is used, the medication is administered at the rate specified in a drug reference or at a rate of 1 mL/minute if no information is available.

Bolus administrations are given in one of two ways: through a port in an existing IV line or through a medication lock (see Chapter 16).

 Pharmacologic Considerations

Specific drugs, such as diazepam or phenytoin, will crystallize (precipitate) in IV tubing solution. Therefore, they are given in the IV port closest to the client's body. Always check for solution compatibility before administering any IV medication.

Using an Intravenous Port

A **port** (sealed opening) extends from the IV tubing (Fig. 35-1). The seal is made of latex or another substance that can be pierced with a needle or needleless adapter (Nursing Guidelines 35-1).

Because the entire dose is administered quickly, a bolus administration has the greatest potential for causing life-threatening changes should a drug reaction occur. If the client's condition changes for any reason, the administration is ceased immediately, and emergency measures are taken to protect the client's safety.

Using a Medication Lock

A medication lock is also called a *saline or heparin lock* or an *intermittent infusion device*. The insertion and technique for maintaining the patency of a medication lock are described in Chapter 16.

Briefly, a **medication lock** is a plug that when inserted into the end of an IV catheter allows for instant access to the

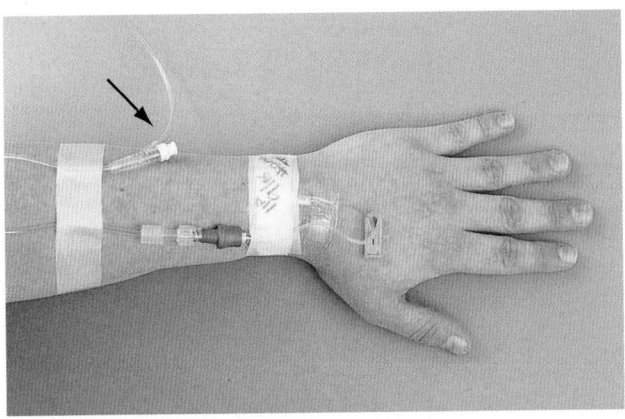

FIGURE 35-1 An intravenous port. (Photo by B. Proud.)

venous system (Fig. 35-2). One of its best features is that it eliminates the need for a continuous and sometimes unnecessary administration of IV fluid.

Instilling IV medication through a lock is similar to the routine for keeping it patent (see Skill 16-7). The technique varies depending on whether the agency's policy is to maintain patency with a 0.9% normal saline solution or heparin. The trend is to use saline.

Nurses use the mnemonic *SAS* or *SASH* as a guide to the steps involved in administering IV medication into a lock. "SAS" stands for flush with *s*aline, *a*dminister the drug, and flush again with *s*aline; "SASH" refers to flush with *s*aline, *a*dminister the drug, flush again with *s*aline, and instill

NURSING GUIDELINES 35-1

Administering Medications through an Intravenous Port

- Prepare the medication in a syringe. *This provides a means for accessing the port.*
- Check the client's identity using at least two methods, for example, checking the wristband and asking the client's name. *This ensures medications are given to the right client and complies with the National Patient Safety Goals.*
- Locate the port nearest to the IV insertion site. *This location provides the most rapid placement of medication in the circulatory system.*

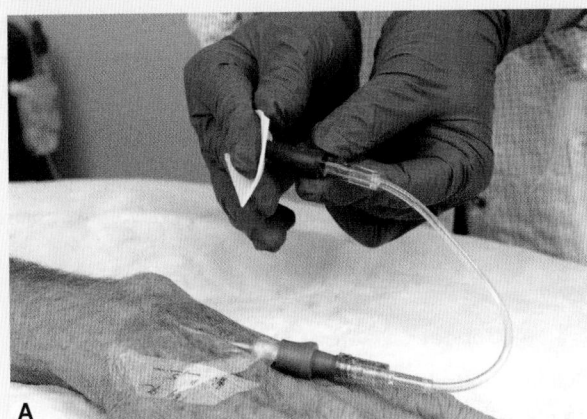

A

Swabbing the injection port on an infusing intravenous tubing.

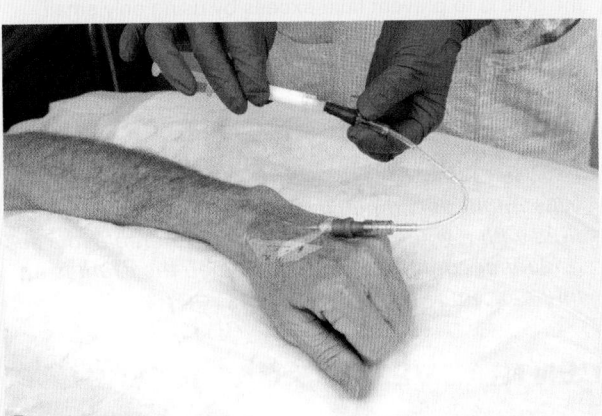

B

Inserting the syringe into the injection port.

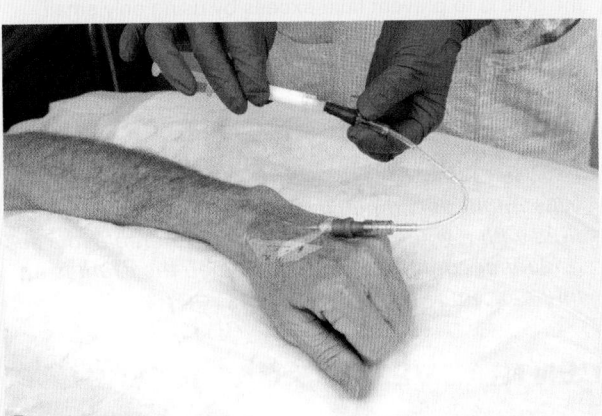

C

Clamping the tubing above the injection port.

- Swab the port with an alcohol sponge (Fig. A). *Alcohol swabbing removes colonizing microorganisms.*
- Pierce the port with the needle or a needleless adapter (Fig. B). *Piercing provides access to inside the tubing.*
- Pinch the tubing above the access port (Fig. C). *Pinching temporarily stops the flow of the IV fluid.*
- Pull back on the plunger of the syringe. *Pulling back creates negative pressure.*
- Observe for blood in the tubing near the IV catheter or insertion device. *Blood validates that the IV catheter is in the vein.*
- Gently instill a few tenths of a milliliter of medication. *This amount initiates the bolus administration.*
- Release the tubing. *Releasing allows some IV fluid to flow.*
- Continue the pattern of pinching the tubing, instilling a small amount of drug, and releasing the tubing until the medication has been administered over the specified period. *This method delivers the drug gradually and keeps the catheter or venous insertion device patent when medication is not being instilled. Pinching the tubing while instilling the drug ensures the administration of the drug to the client rather than backfilling the tubing.*

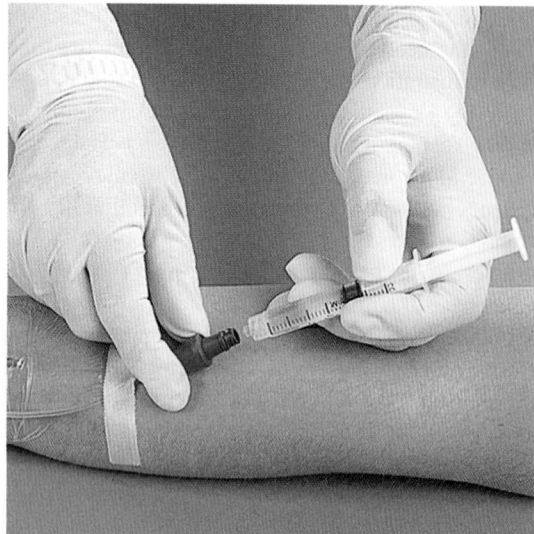

FIGURE 35-2 Accessing a medication lock. (From Craven, R. F., Hirnle, C. J., & Henshaw, C. M. [2019]. *Fundamentals of nursing* [9th ed.]. Lippincott Williams & Wilkins.)

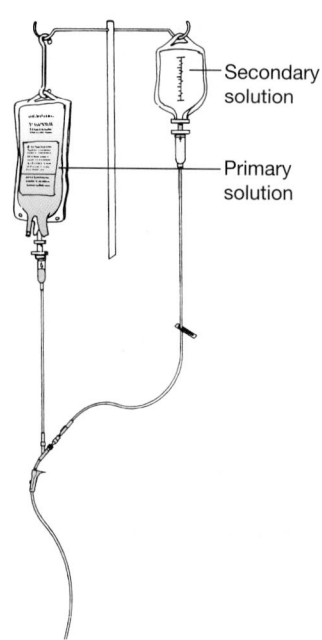

FIGURE 35-3 A secondary solution is hung higher than the primary solution, which is sometimes referred to as a piggyback arrangement. (From Nettina, S. M. [2018]. *Lippincott manual of nursing practice* [11th ed.]. Lippincott Williams & Wilkins. Adapted from Abbott Laboratories.)

*h*eparin. To maintain patency, nurses usually flush medication locks after each use with saline or heparin or every 8 to 12 hours if the lock has been unused. The flushing technique is the same, except only one syringe of flush solution is required.

Nurses change medication locks when changing the IV site or at least every 72 hours. If the nurse cannot verify patency by obtaining a blood return, and if there is resistance or leaking when administering the flush solution, they remove the IV catheter, change the site, and replace the lock.

Secondary Infusions

A **secondary infusion** is the administration of a parenteral drug that has been diluted in a small volume of IV solution, usually 50 to 100 mL, over 30 to 60 minutes. It is also called a *piggyback infusion* because it is administered in tandem with a primary IV solution (Fig. 35-3). Both are misnomers when the small volume of medicated solution is administered through a medication lock or the port of a CVC (discussed later). When administered this way, the medications are actually independent of a primary infusion. There are also instances when small volumes of medicated solution are given simultaneously with a primary infusion. This method involves using dual types of electronic infusion devices. Skill 35-2 describes how nurses administer secondary infusions by gravity in tandem with a currently infusing primary solution.

 Stop, Think, and Respond 35-2

Other than using a drug reference book, whom or what might you consult to determine the compatibility of two drugs that will infuse through the same IV tubing?

Volume-Control Set

A **volume-control set** is a chamber in IV tubing that holds a portion of the solution from a larger container. It is known by various names, such as volutrol, soluset, and buretrol. A volume-control set is used to administer IV medication in a small volume of solution at intermittent intervals and to avoid accidentally overloading the circulatory system. The volume-control set essentially substitutes for the separate secondary container of solution, therefore eliminating the need for additional fluid.

When caring for clients who are at risk for or manifest signs of fluid excess, it is appropriate to consult the physician and pharmacy department about using a volume-control set to administer intermittent IV medications.

Concept Mastery Alert

Volume Control

As the name implies, "volume control" equals small amounts intermittently. When using a volume-control set, the goal is to prevent fluid excess by using only small amounts of solution to give a medication at intermittent intervals.

》 **Stop, Think, and Respond 35-3**

Why might the administration of IV medications and fluid with a volume-control set be preferable to a secondary or continuous infusion when the client is an infant or small child?

CENTRAL VENOUS CATHETERS

A **central venous catheter** (CVC; a venous access device that provides access to larger veins leading to the superior vena cava) provides a means of administering parenteral medication in a large volume of blood. A CVC is used when:

- Clients require long-term IV fluid or medication administration.
- IV medications are irritating to peripheral veins.
- It is difficult to insert or maintain a peripherally inserted venous catheter.

CVCs have single or multiple lumens (Fig. 35-4). With multiple lumens, incompatible substances or more than one solution or drug can be given simultaneously. Each infuses through a separate channel and exits the catheter at a different location near the heart. Thus, the drugs or solutions never interact. When a lumen is used only intermittently, it is capped with a medication lock. The unused lumen is kept patent by scheduled flushes with normal saline or heparin.

There are three types of CVCs: percutaneous, tunneled, and implanted.

Pharmacologic Considerations

Heparin comes in vials for therapeutic use (1,000 units/1 mL up to 20,000 units/1 mL) and for IV line flushes (10 units/1 mL to 100 units/1 mL). Always verify the strength of the drug in the vial or prepared syringe before flushing an IV line.

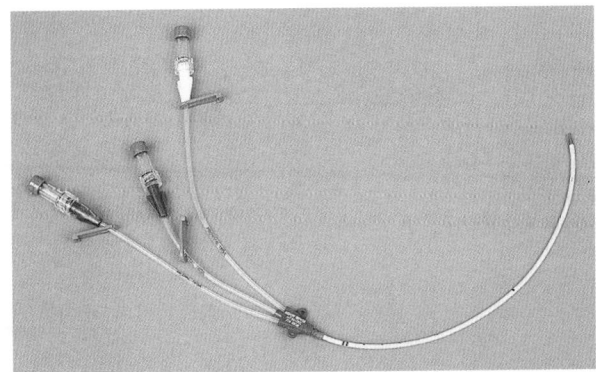

FIGURE 35-4 A triple-lumen central venous catheter showing the gauge size of each lumen and the outflow ports at the distal end of the catheter. (From Craven, R. F., Hirnle, C. J., & Henshaw, C. M. [2019]. *Fundamentals of nursing* [9th ed.]. Lippincott Williams & Wilkins.)

Nontunneled Percutaneous Catheters

A **nontunneled percutaneous catheter** is inserted through the skin in a peripheral vein (e.g., the basilic, cephalic, jugular, or subclavian vein) with the distal end terminating in the axillary vein, subclavian vein, or superior vena cava (see Chapter 16) (Fig. 35-5). Nontunneled percutaneous catheters are used when clients require short-term fluid therapy, parenteral nutrition, or medication therapy lasting a few days or weeks.

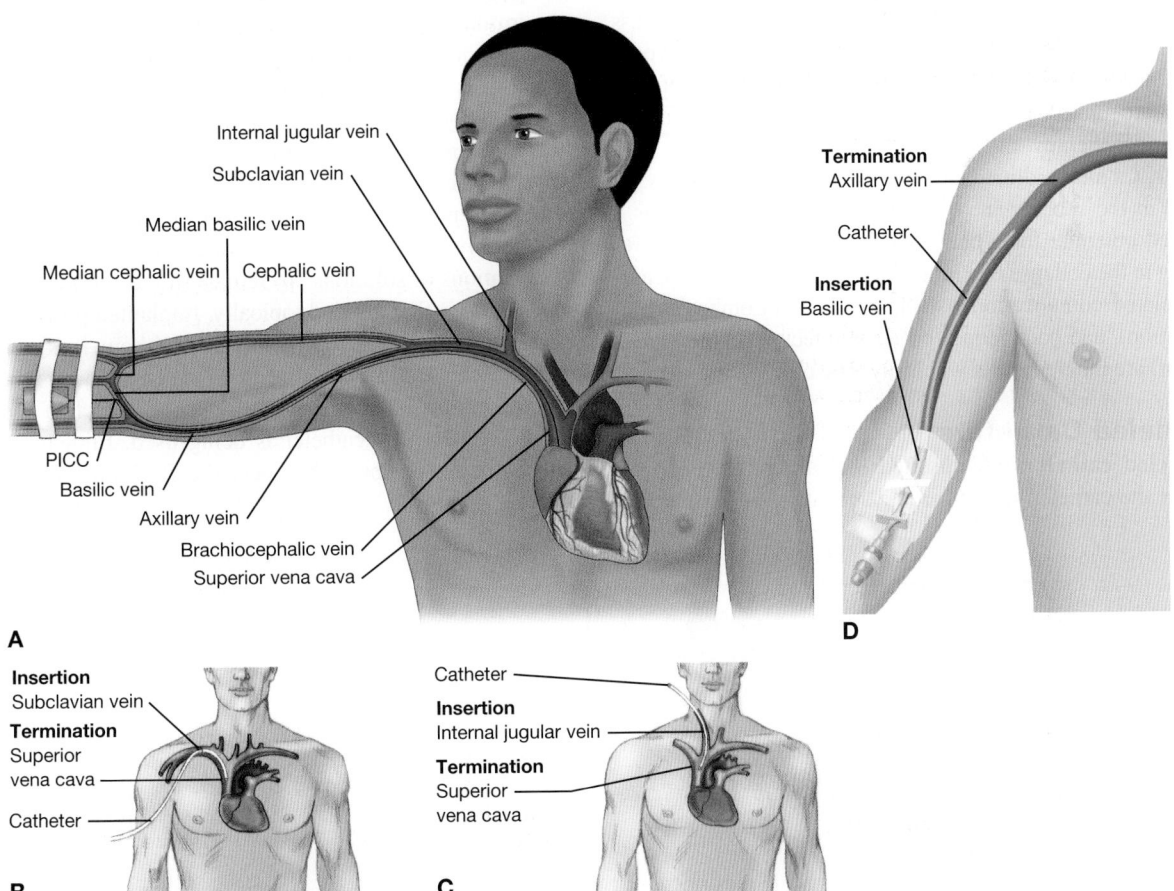

FIGURE 35-5 A. The location of a peripherally inserted central catheter. **B.** The location of a percutaneous catheter inserted in the subclavian vein. **C.** The location of a percutaneous catheter inserted in the jugular vein. **D.** The location of a midline catheter in the basilic vein. PICC, peripherally inserted central catheter. (**D**: From Donnelly-Moreno, L., & Moseley, B. [2023]. *Introductory medical-surgical nursing* [12th ed.]. Lippincott Williams & Wilkins.)

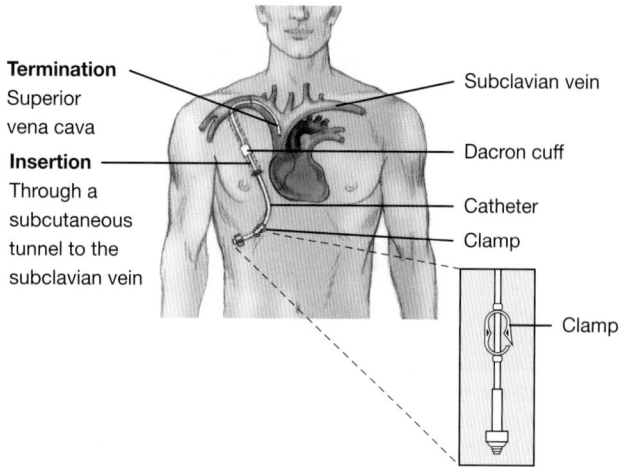

Termination
Superior
vena cava

Insertion
Through a
subcutaneous
tunnel to the
subclavian vein

Subclavian vein

Dacron cuff

Catheter

Clamp

Clamp

FIGURE 35-6 A tunneled catheter.

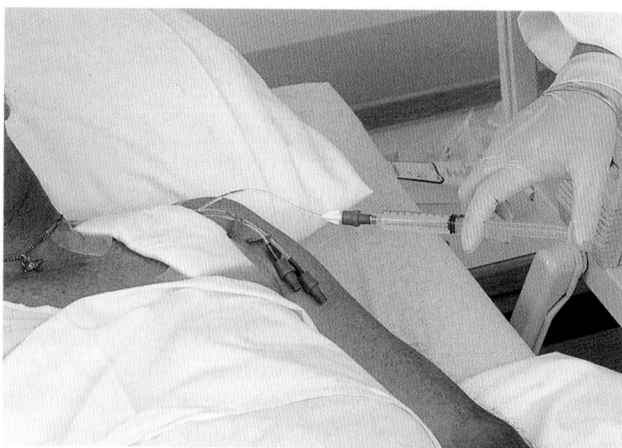

FIGURE 35-8 Flushing the lumen. (Photo by B. Proud.)

Registered nurses who are certified may insert a midline and peripherally inserted central catheter (PICC) after completing an infusion training program. Depending on the nurse practice act in the state of licensure, licensed practice nurses (LPNs) may administer medicated and unmedicated solutions through most peripheral venous access lines, including midline catheters. LPNs are generally not allowed to administer IV chemotherapy, blood, or blood products; to push IV medications; or to administer medications and flushes through tunneled or implanted central venous access devices. The scope of practice for LPN and licensed vocational nurses (LVNs) differs from state to state, so refer to your state's nurse practice act for rules and regulations regarding IV therapy.

PICCs and midline catheters are safer than catheters inserted in the subclavian or jugular veins because there is a reduced potential for a pneumothorax (punctured pleura resulting in the collapse of a lung) at the time of insertion. Catheter-related complications, such as venous thrombosis (clot formation), and bacteremia (bacterial infection in the bloodstream) are inherent risks when any type of CVC is used.

Tunneled Catheters

Tunneled catheters are inserted into a central vein with part of the catheter secured in the subcutaneous tissue. The

end of the catheter exits from the skin lateral to the xiphoid process (Fig. 35-6). Tunneled catheters are used when the client requires extended therapy. Tunneling helps stabilize the catheter and also reduces the potential for infection because an internal cuff acts as a barrier against migrating microorganisms. Some examples of tunneled catheters are the Hickman, Broviac, and Groshong catheters.

Implanted Catheters

An **implanted catheter** is sealed beneath the skin (Fig. 35-7) and provides the greatest protection against infection because it is totally confined internally without any exposed external portion.

Implanted catheters have a self-sealing port pierced through the skin with a special **noncoring needle** (a needle that does not remove a plug from the septum of the port, commonly called a *Huber needle*) when administering IV medications or solutions. To reduce skin discomfort, a local anesthetic is first applied topically. Implanted ports can sustain approximately 2,000 punctures without leaking; thus, the catheter can remain in place for several years, barring complications. A dressing is applied only when the port is pierced and the catheter is being used. Implanted catheters remain patent with a periodic flushing with heparin (Fig. 35-8).

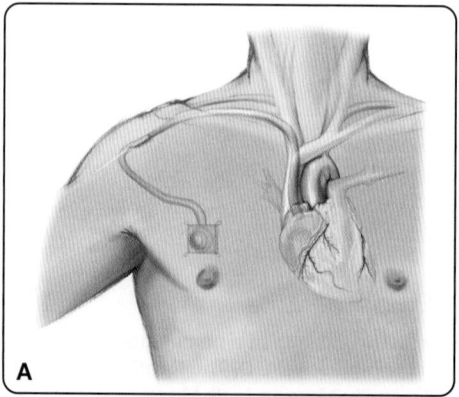

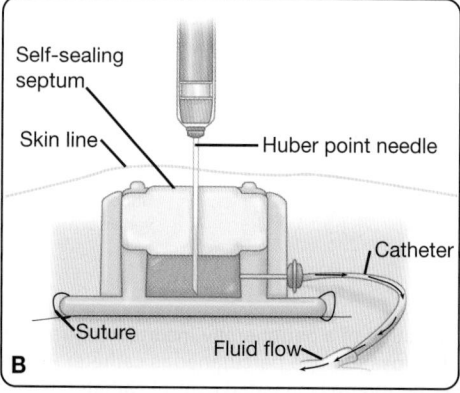

Self-sealing
septum

Skin line

Huber point needle

Catheter

Suture

Fluid flow

A

B

FIGURE 35-7 **A.** The placement of an implanted catheter with access via a port. **B.** Noncoring (Huber) needle used to access the port. (From Craven, R. F., Hirnle, C. J., & Henshaw, C. M. [2019]. *Fundamentals of nursing* [9th ed.]. Lippincott Williams & Wilkins.)

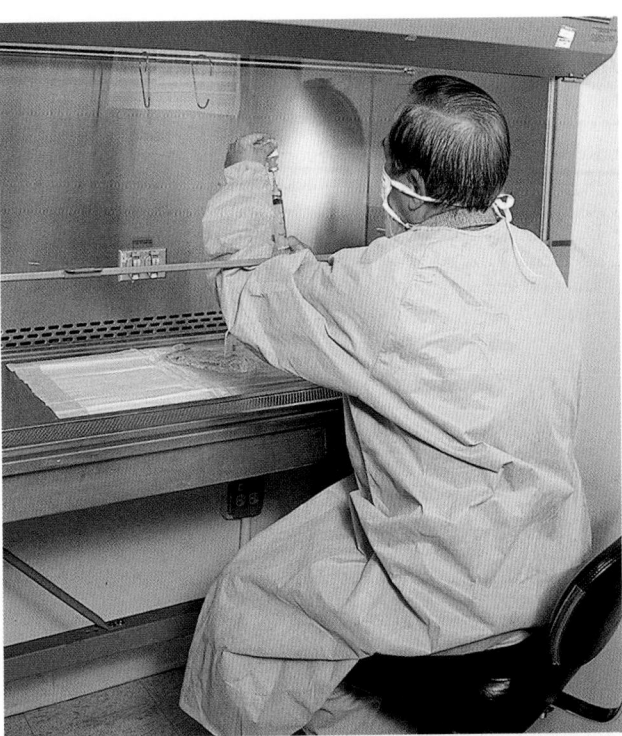

FIGURE 35-9 A pharmacy preparation of antineoplastic drugs using self-protective garments and equipment. (Photo by B. Proud.)

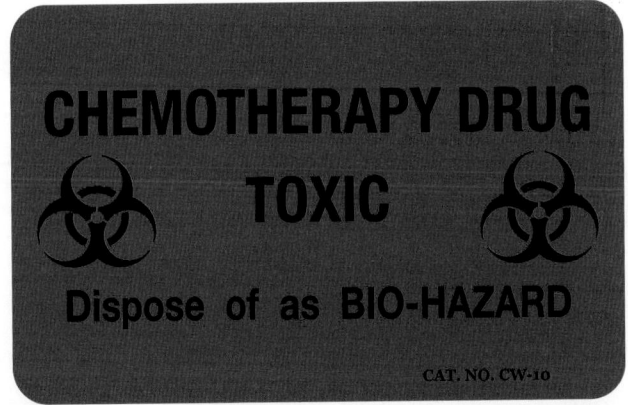

FIGURE 35-10 Example of a chemotherapy warning label that is attached to intravenous solutions containing an antineoplastic drug. (Photo by Ken Timby.)

In most cases, these drugs are reconstituted or diluted with sterile IV solutions in the pharmacy. The specifically trained pharmacist wears protective clothing when preparing the drugs under a vertical flow containment hood or biologic safety cabinet (Fig. 35-9). The pharmacist usually attaches a label to warn nurses to take special precautions during drug administration (Fig. 35-10).

NURSING IMPLICATIONS

Although the administration of all parenteral drugs involves specialized skills, the administration of IV medications in general and antineoplastic drugs in particular requires extreme caution and competency validation. Nurses may identify the following nursing diagnoses:

- Acute anxiety
- Infection risk
- Fear
- Fluid overload risk
- Injury risk
- Altered tissue integrity risk

Nursing Care Plan 35-1 demonstrates the nursing process as applied to a client with the nursing diagnosis altered tissue integrity risk, defined as impairment or a break in the skin's line of defense, causing impairment of tissue integrity. The most common causes include physical trauma. Other causes can be related to thermal factors or chemical injury (e.g., adverse reactions to drugs), infection, nutritional imbalances, fluid imbalances, and altered circulation.

Antineoplastic Drug Administration

Antineoplastic drugs (medications used to destroy or slow the growth of malignant cells) are also commonly referred to as *chemotherapy* or just *chemo*. CVCs are often used to administer antineoplastic drugs to clients with cancer.

Antineoplastic agents are toxic to both normal and abnormal cells. These drugs can even cause adverse effects on the pharmacists who mix them and on the nurses who administer them. Caregivers can absorb antineoplastic drugs through skin contact, inhalation of tiny fluid droplets or dust particles on which the droplets fall, or oral absorption of drug residue during hand-to-mouth contact. When transferred to the caregiver, these drugs can cause headaches, nausea, dizziness, and burning or itching of the skin. Long-term exposure can lead to changes in fast-growing body cells, including sperm, ova, or fetal tissue. It is important, therefore, that nurses certified to administer chemotherapy use safety measures like double gloving when administering these drugs and avoid exposure and contact with hazardous materials.

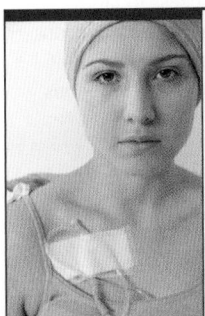

Clinical Scenario A 17-year-old female is being treated by an oncologist with combinations of antineoplastic drugs for a form of lymphatic cancer. The client presented with swollen lymph nodes in her neck and underarm. The client has a CVC inserted in her right subclavian vein. The drugs have caused hair loss and mouth sores. The client says she feels "sick, tired, and run-down."

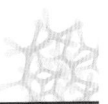

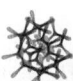

NURSING CARE PLAN 35-1 | Altered Tissue Integrity Risk

Assessment

- Review laboratory findings for evidence of decreased white blood cells (WBCs), review differential, reduced platelets, insufficient erythrocytes, and hemoglobin.
- Read the client's history for information indicating increased risk for infection.
- Analyze the client's weight in relation to height or calculate body mass index for evidence of inadequate nutrition.

- Refer to the client's medical record for current diagnoses such as cancer, alcohol misuse or other forms of substance misuse, and immune-related disorders.
- Determine whether the client is undergoing therapeutic management of disorders with drugs that suppress bone marrow function, cause immunosuppression, or interfere with fighting infection.

Nursing Diagnosis. Altered tissue integrity risk related to a debilitated state and a tendency for a decrease in tissue integrity due to chemotherapy for Hodgkin lymphoma as manifested by enlarged cervical and axillary lymph nodes, complete blood count (CBC) that reveals thrombocytopenia, and the client's statement: "I haven't been eating much. It's difficult to swallow. As a result, I'm losing weight and feeling very weak." The client has a central venous catheter (CVC) inserted in the right subclavian vein, for medication infusions.

Expected Outcome. The client will maintain effective protection from infection as evidenced by maintaining a sufficient WBC and differential count, platelet count within a normal range, and intact skin.

Interventions	Rationales
Monitor platelet count from a specimen drawn from CVC.	Platelets play a role in blood clotting; the normal range of platelets is 150,000–250,000/mm³.
Report platelet counts below normal and expect that chemotherapy will be withheld if the count is less than 100,000/mm³.	The nurse informs the physician of data that put the client at risk for complications; withholding a chemotherapeutic drug that suppresses bone marrow function protects the client by avoiding a further decline in platelets.
Assess skin for bruising and intactness and the central catheter site for any signs of infection.	Physical assessments provide data that indicate evidence of infection.
Consult the physician if they prescribe medications that can cause tissue extravasation.	Questioning an order for a medication that interferes with circulation and immunologic defenses helps ensure tissue integrity.

Evaluation of Expected Outcome

- Platelet count remains in low normal range or higher.
- WBC and differential are with normal limits.
- There is no evidence of infection at the CVC site.
- No bruises are noted on the skin, and skin is intact.

KEY POINTS

- The IV route: Drug administration through peripheral and central veins; provides an immediate effect, consequently, potentially the most dangerous
- Types of IV medication administration
  - Continuous infusion: Instillation of a parenteral drug over several hours, also called a continuous drip
  - Intermittent infusion: A short-term (from minutes up to 1 hour), parenteral administration of IV medication
  - Bolus administration: A substance given all at one time (e.g., IV push medications)
    - Port: A sealed opening, extends from the IV; the seal is made of latex or another substance that can be pierced with a needle or needleless adapter.
    - Medication lock: Also called a saline or heparin lock or an intermittent infusion device
  - Secondary infusion: The administration of a parenteral drug that has been diluted in a small volume of IV

solution, usually 50 to 100 mL over 30 to 60 minutes, also called a piggyback infusion
- Volume-control set: A chamber in IV tubing that holds a portion of the solution from a larger container, used to administer IV medication in a small volume of solution at intermittent intervals
- CVC: Venous access device that provides access to larger veins leading to the superior vena cava that provides a means of administering parenteral medication in a large volume of blood; some CVCs have multiple lumens for several venous access ports. CVCs are used for:
- Long-term IV fluids or medications
- IV medications that are irritating to peripheral veins
- Difficulty when inserting or maintaining a peripheral IV
- Types of CVCs
- Nontunneled percutaneous catheter: Inserted through the skin in a peripheral with the distal end terminating in the

axillary vein, subclavian vein, or superior vena cava; used when clients require short-term fluid therapy, parenteral nutrition, or medication therapy lasting a few days or weeks (e.g., PICC or midline)

- Tunneled catheters: Inserted into a central vein with part of the catheter secured in the subcutaneous tissue; used when the client requires extended therapy

- Implanted catheter: Sealed beneath the skin, provides the greatest protection against infection because it is totally confined internally without any exposed external portion
- Antineoplastic drugs: Medications used to destroy or slow the growth of malignant cells, are also commonly referred to as chemotherapy or just chemo. CVCs are often used to administer antineoplastic drugs to clients with cancer.

CRITICAL THINKING EXERCISES

1. Discuss the advantages and disadvantages of giving IV medications to older adults.
2. When preparing to administer an IV medication through an IV port or lock, you find no blood return on aspiration. Discuss the significance of this finding and appropriate actions.
3. If the volume of an IV medication is 4 mL by bolus administration but there is no published recommended period of time for its administration, how long should the nurse allow when instilling the drug?
4. Why do many oncology departments have a policy of excluding the employment of nurses who are currently pregnant?

NEXT-GENERATION NCLEX-STYLE REVIEW QUESTIONS

1. Which action is essential before a nurse administers an IV medication by bolus through a port of an infusing solution that also contains a medication?
   a. Dilute the bolus drug in a small volume of solution.
   b. Consult a drug-compatibility reference.
   c. Stop the infusing solution for approximately 3 minutes.
   d. Flush the port with 5 mL of sterile normal saline.
   Test-Taking Strategy: Note the key word, "essential," which indicates one option is a required action.
2. When the nurse instills a medication by bolus administration, which technique is correct for determining that the IV catheter is within the vein?
   a. The nurse increases the rate of infusion and looks for edema at the site.
   b. The nurse inspects the site looking for redness along the course of the vein.
   c. The nurse palpates the area of the infusion to note a difference in temperature.
   d. The nurse pulls back on the plunger of the syringe and looks for a blood return.
   Test-Taking Strategy: Eliminate options that are incorrect. Select the option that provides the most objective evidence.

3. Place the following nursing actions in the correct sequence when instilling a medication through an intermittent peripheral infusion device (medication lock).
   a. Withdraw the syringe with saline while instilling the final amount.
   b. Insert a syringe containing sterile normal saline into the lock.
   c. Instill saline followed by the medication into the lock.
   d. Aspirate by pulling back on the syringe plunger.
   e. Wipe the medication lock with an alcohol swab.
   Test-Taking Strategy: Read all the options, then select the options in the order that they are performed.
4. What is the best answer the nurse can provide when a client asks why the physician recommended inserting an implanted CVC for administering cancer medications?
   a. An implanted catheter has the lowest incidence of infection.
   b. An implanted catheter is best for short-term use.
   c. An implanted catheter will never need to be removed.
   d. An implanted catheter is easy to cover with a dressing.
   Test-Taking Strategy: Note the key word and modifier, "best answer." Use the process of elimination to select the option that is better than any of the others.
5. Which nursing action is best for avoiding self-contamination with IV antineoplastic drugs?
   a. Stay at least 5 ft away from a client receiving an infusion of an antineoplastic drug.
   b. Wear a high-efficiency air filter respirator while in the area where an antineoplastic drug is being given.
   c. Perform meticulous handwashing for about 5 minutes after handling a container of antineoplastic drugs.
   d. Put on two pairs of nonpowdered gloves when administering an antineoplastic drug.
   Test-Taking Strategy: Note the key word, "best." Analyze the choices and select the option that is better than any of the others.

NEXT-GENERATION NCLEX-STYLE CLINICAL SCENARIO QUESTIONS

Clinical Scenario:

A 17-year-old female is being treated by an oncologist with combinations of antineoplastic drugs for a form of lymphatic cancer. The client presented with swollen lymph nodes in her neck and underarm. The client has a CVC inserted in her right subclavian vein. The drugs have caused hair loss and mouth sores. The client says she feels "sick, tired, and run-down."

1. Select all of the indicators that may suggest a cause for concern regarding the use of antineoplastic drugs and her current symptoms.
   a. Swollen glands
   b. Edema in her extremities
   c. Hair loss
   d. Thickened nails
   e. Mouth sores
   f. Difficulty breathing
   g. Heat intolerance

2. From the following list, select measures that may assist the client in decreasing the symptoms of the antineoplastic drugs.
   a. Eat soft, nonspicy foods
   b. Increase fluid intake
   c. Discuss with provider about planning ahead for treatment symptoms
   d. Decrease exposure to infections
   e. Eat three full meals daily
   f. Discuss with provider the need for medication to help with treatment symptoms

SKILL 35-1 Administering Intravenous Medication by Continuous Infusion

Suggested Action	Reason for Action
ASSESSMENT	
Check the medical orders.	Collaborates nursing activities with medical treatment
Compare the medication administration record (MAR) with the written medical order.	Ensures accuracy
Read the label on the drug and compare it with the MAR (Fig. A).	Prevents errors

A

Comparing the drug label with the medication administration record. (Photo by B. Proud.)

Suggested Action	Reason for Action
Make sure the drug label indicates that it is for IV use.	Prevents injuring the client
Check for any documented drug allergies.	Ensures safety
Review the drug action and side effects.	Promotes safe client care
Consult a compatibility chart or drug reference.	Determines whether the solution and drug are known to interact when mixed
Determine how much the client understands about the purpose and technique for administering the medication.	Provides an opportunity for health teaching
Perform assessments that will provide a basis for evaluating the drug's effectiveness.	Provides a baseline for future comparisons
Inspect the current infusion site for swelling, redness, and tenderness.	Determines if a site change is needed
PLANNING	
Prepare the medication, taking care to read the medication label at least three times. Note: In most instances, IV solutions with medications already added are provided by the pharmacy.	Avoids medication errors
Have a second nurse double-check your drug calculations.	Ensures accuracy
IMPLEMENTATION	
Wash your hands or use an alcohol-based hand rub (see Chapter 10).	Reduces the transmission of microorganisms
Identify the client using at least two methods, for example, checking the wristband and asking the client's name and birthdate (Fig. B).	Ensures that medications are given to the *right client*; complies with the National Patient Safety Goals

B

Checking the client's identification band. (Photo by B. Proud.)

(continued)

SKILL 35-1 Administering Intravenous Medication by Continuous Infusion (*continued*)

Suggested Action	Reason for Action
Clamp or stop the current infusion of fluid.	Prevents administering a concentrated amount of medication while it is being added to the solution
Swab the appropriate port on the container of IV fluid (Fig. C).	Removes colonizing microorganisms

Swabbing the port on the container. (Photo by B. Proud.)

| Instill the medication through the port into the full container of fluid (Fig. D). | Promotes the dilution of concentrated additive |

Instilling the medication. (Photo by B. Proud.)

Lower the bag and gently rotate it back and forth.	Distributes the medication equally throughout the fluid
Suspend the solution and release the clamp.	Facilitates infusion
Regulate the rate of flow by using the roller clamp or programming the rate on the electronic infusion device (Fig. E).	Promotes a continuous infusion at the prescribed rate

Programming the rate. (Tyler Olson/Shutterstock.)

SKILL 35-1 Administering Intravenous Medication by Continuous Infusion (*continued*)

Suggested Action	Reason for Action
Record the medication administration in the MAR.	Documents the nursing care; avoids medication errors
Check the client and the progress of the infusion at least hourly.	Promotes early intervention for complications

EVALUATION
- Medication instills at a prescribed rate.
- Client remains free of any adverse effects.

DOCUMENT
- Client and site assessment data
- The date, time, drug, dose, and initials
- Solution to which the drug has been added
- Client's response

SAMPLE DOCUMENTATION[a]

Date and Time IV infusing in L forearm. No tenderness, swelling, or redness observed. KCl 20 mEq added to 1,000 mL of D5/W. IV infusing at 125 mL/hour. Heart rate is regular and ranges between 65 and 75 bpm. _____ J. Doe, LPN

[a]The administration of drugs is usually documented on the MAR.

SKILL 35-2 Administering an Intermittent Secondary Infusion

Suggested Action	Reason for Action
ASSESSMENT	
Check the medical orders.	Collaborates nursing activities with the medical treatment
Compare the medication administration record (MAR) with the written medical order.	Ensures accuracy
Read the label on the medicated solution and compare it with the MAR.	Prevents errors
Check for any documented drug allergies.	Ensures safety
Inspect the current infusion site for swelling, redness, and tenderness.	Determines whether a site change is needed
Review the drug action and side effects.	Promotes safe client care
Consult a compatibility chart or drug reference.	Determines whether the drug in the secondary solution may interact when mixed with the solution in the primary tubing
Determine how much the client understands about the purpose and technique for administering the medication.	Provides an opportunity for health teaching
Perform assessments that will provide a basis for evaluating the drug's effectiveness.	Provides a baseline for future comparisons
PLANNING	
Plan to administer the secondary infusion within 30–60 minutes of the scheduled time for drug administration established by the agency.	Complies with agency policy
Remove a refrigerated secondary solution at least 30 minutes before administration.	Warms the solution slightly to promote comfort during instillation
Check the drop factor on the package of secondary (short) intravenous (IV) tubing and calculate the rate of infusion (see Chapter 16).	Ensures that the secondary infusion will be instilled within the specified time
Have a second nurse double-check your calculations for the rate of infusion.	Ensures accuracy
Attach the tubing to the solution (see Skill 35-2), fill the drip chamber, and purge the air from the tubing.	Prepares the medicated solution for administration
Attach a needleless adapter.	Facilitates accessing the port

(continued)

SKILL 35-2 Administering an Intermittent Secondary Infusion (*continued*)

Suggested Action	Reason for Action
IMPLEMENTATION	
Wash your hands or use an alcohol-based hand rub (see Chapter 10).	Reduces the transmission of microorganisms
Identify the client using at least two methods, for example, checking the wristband and asking the client's name and birthdate.	Ensures that medications are given to the *right client*; complies with the National Patient Safety Goals
Hang the secondary solution on the IV pole or standard.	Prepares the solution for administration
Wipe the *uppermost port* on the primary tubing with an alcohol swab.	Removes colonized microorganisms
Insert modified adapter within the port.	Provides access to the venous system
Lock the connection.	Prevents separation from the port
Connect the secondary tubing to the primary tubing (Fig. A).	Initiates the infusion

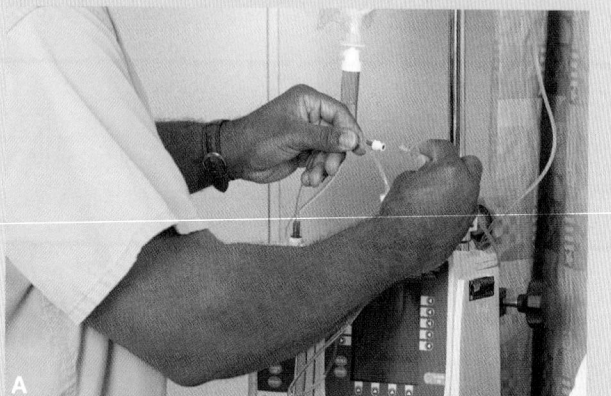

Attaching secondary tubing. (From Craven, R. F., Hirnle, C. J., & Henshaw, C. M. [2019]. *Fundamentals of nursing* [9th ed.]. Lippincott Williams & Wilkins.)

Program the rate of infusion (Fig. B).	Establishes the maintenance rate of flow to instill the solution in the time specified

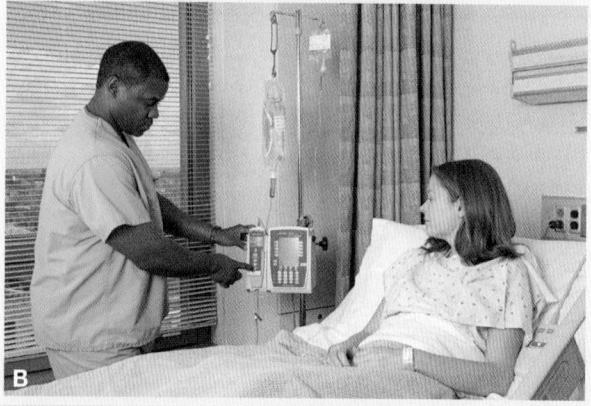

Programming the rate of infusion with an electronic device. (From Craven, R. F., Hirnle, C. J., & Henshaw, C. M. [2019]. *Fundamentals of nursing* [9th ed.]. Lippincott Williams & Wilkins.)

Clamp the tubing when the solution has instilled.	Prevents backfilling with the primary solution
Rehang the primary container of solution and readjust the rate of flow.	Continues the fluid replacement therapy at its appropriate rate
Leave the secondary tubing in place within the port if another secondary infusion of the same medication is scheduled again within the next 24 hours.	Controls health care costs without jeopardizing client safety; different tubing, however, is used if other drugs are administered as secondary infusions

EVALUATION

- The secondary infusion instills at the prescribed rate.
- The client remains free of any adverse effects.

DOCUMENT

- Client and site assessment data
- The date, time, drug, dose, and initials
- Client's response

SAMPLE DOCUMENTATION[a]

Date and Time IV infusing in L forearm. No tenderness, swelling, or redness observed. Vancomycin 1 g administered in 100 mL of normal saline solution as a secondary infusion over 60 minutes without signs of a reaction. _____ J. Doe, LPN

[a] The administration of drugs is usually documented on the MAR.

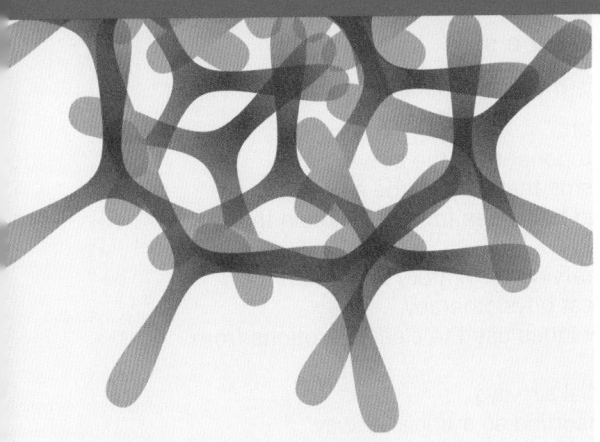

UNIT 10 | Intervening in Emergency Situations

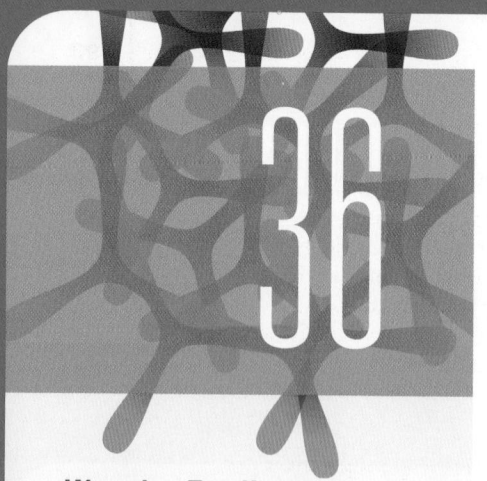

Airway Management

Words To Know

airway
airway management
chest physiotherapy
fenestrated tracheostomy tube
inhalation therapy
inner cannula
mucus
nasopharyngeal suctioning
nasotracheal suctioning
obturator
oral airway
oral suctioning
oropharyngeal suctioning
outer cannula
percussion
postural drainage
speaking valve
sputum
suctioning
tracheostomy
tracheostomy care
tracheostomy tube
ventilation
vibration

Learning Objectives

On completion of this chapter, the reader should be able to:

1. Define airway management.
2. Identify the structural components of the airway.
3. Discuss natural mechanisms that protect the airway.
4. Explain the methods used by nurses to help maintain the natural airway.
5. Name techniques for liquefying respiratory secretions.
6. Explain techniques of chest physiotherapy.
7. Describe suctioning techniques used to clear secretions from the airway.
8. Name examples of artificial airways.
9. Discuss indications for inserting an artificial airway.
10. Identify components of tracheostomy care.

INTRODUCTION

The primary function of the respiratory system is to permit **ventilation** (the movement of air in and out of the lungs) for an appropriate exchange of oxygen and carbon dioxide at the cellular level (see Chapter 21). A clear **airway** (collective system of tubes in the upper and lower respiratory tracts) is necessary for adequate ventilation. Many factors can jeopardize airway patency:

- An increased volume of **mucus** (a mixture of water, mucin, white blood cells, electrolytes, and cells that have been shed through the natural process of tissue replacement)
- Thick mucus
- Fatigue or weakness
- A decreased level of consciousness
- An ineffective cough
- An impaired airway

Consequently, nurses sometimes need to assist clients with measures that support or replace their own natural efforts. This chapter focuses on **airway management**, or those essential nursing skills that maintain natural or artificial airways for compromised clients.

 Gerontologic Considerations

■ Conditions affecting the respiratory system are among the most common life-threatening disorders that older adults experience. The severity of chronic pulmonary diseases increases with age.

■ Many older adults with pathologic pulmonary changes have a history of smoking cigarettes since youth, working in occupations where they inhaled pollutants that affected their lungs, or living for an extended time in industrial areas known for high levels of toxic emissions.

■ Inquiring about a current history of coughing, determining how long the cough has been present, and observing and describing any sputum are important when assessing older adults.

■ If not relieved quickly, a persistent, dry cough may consume the older adult's energy and result in fatigue.

■ Reduced air exchange and a reduced efficiency in ventilation are age-related changes affecting the older adult's respiratory system.

■ The muscular structures of the larynx tend to atrophy with age, which can affect the ability to clear the airway.

■ Usually, the bases of the older adult's lungs receive less ventilation, contributing to the retention of secretions, decreased air exchange, and compromised ventilation. Respiratory cilia become less efficient with age, predisposing older adults to a high incidence of pneumonia.

■ Diminished strength of accessory muscles for respiration, an increased rigidity of the chest wall, and a diminished cough reflex make it difficult for older adults to cough productively and effectively.

■ Older adults with difficulty swallowing (dysphagia), often associated with strokes or middle and late stages of dementia, are more vulnerable to aspiration pneumonia. An evaluation of the dysphagia is important for implementing appropriate interventions to prevent aspiration.

■ Deep breathing exercises may improve an older adult's ability to clear respiratory secretions.

■ Older adults are at increased risk for cardiac dysrhythmias during suctioning because many have preexisting hypoxemia from illnesses and age-related changes in ventilation.

THE AIRWAY

The upper airway consists of the nose and pharynx, which is subdivided into the nasopharynx, oropharynx, and laryngopharynx. The lower airway consists of the trachea, bronchi, bronchioles, and alveoli. Gases travel through these structures to and from the blood (Fig. 36-1).

Certain structures protect the airway from a wide variety of inhaled substances. These structures include the epiglottis, tracheal cartilage, mucous membrane, and cilia. The *epiglottis* is a protrusion of flexible cartilage above the larynx. It acts as a lid that closes during swallowing, helping to direct fluid and food toward the esophagus rather than the respiratory tract. The rings of *tracheal cartilage* ensure that the trachea, the portion of the airway beneath the larynx, remains open. The *mucous membrane*, a type of tissue from which mucus is secreted, lines the respiratory passages. The sticky mucus traps particulate matter. Hair-like projections called *cilia* beat debris that collects in the lower airway upward (Fig. 36-2).

Various mechanisms keep the airway open. For example, sneezing or blowing the nose can clear debris in nasal passages. Coughing, expectoration, or swallowing clears **sputum** (mucus raised to the level of the upper airways).

Concept Mastery Alert

Effective Coughing

It may appear that as individuals age, they produce more mucus, and as a result, their ability to cough effectively is diminished. However, this is not the case. Remember, effective coughing requires strong accessory muscles, an elastic chest wall, and adequate cough reflex. Older adults experience a change in these areas, often compromising their ability to cough effectively and productively.

NATURAL AIRWAY MANAGEMENT

The most common methods of maintaining the natural airway are keeping respiratory secretions liquefied, promoting their mobilization and expectoration with chest physiotherapy, and mechanically clearing mucus from the airway by suctioning.

Pharmacologic Considerations

■ Acute bronchospasm may cause airway constriction. Quick-relief medications include inhaled short-acting beta-2 agonists (SABAs) and oral steroids. Albuterol, a rescue inhalant drug for quickly relieving asthmatic symptoms, is an example of a SABA drug.

■ Long-acting bronchodilators, such as salmeterol, a drug in many inhalers used daily for preventing asthma attacks or exercise-induced bronchospasm, are not used in emergent situations.

Liquefying Secretions

The body continually produces mucus. The volume of water in mucus affects its *viscosity* or thickness. *Hydration*, the process of providing adequate oral fluid intake, tends to keep mucous membranes moist and the mucus thin. A thin consistency promotes expectoration (see Chapter 16). An essential nursing activity is ensuring that clients are well hydrated.

In addition, nurses may assist with **inhalation therapy** (respiratory treatments that provide a mixture of oxygen, humidification, and aerosolized medications directly to the lungs). The aerosol is delivered through a mask or a handheld mouthpiece (Fig. 36-3; also see Chapter 33). Aerosol therapy improves breathing, encourages spontaneous coughing, and helps clients raise sputum for diagnostic purposes (Nursing Guidelines 36-1).

Mobilizing Secretions

To help clients mobilize secretions from distal airways, health care providers often use **chest physiotherapy** (techniques including postural drainage, percussion, and vibration). Chest physiotherapy is usually indicated for clients with chronic respiratory diseases who have difficulty coughing or raising thick mucus.

Postural Drainage

Postural drainage is a positioning technique that promotes the drainage of secretions from various lobes or segments of

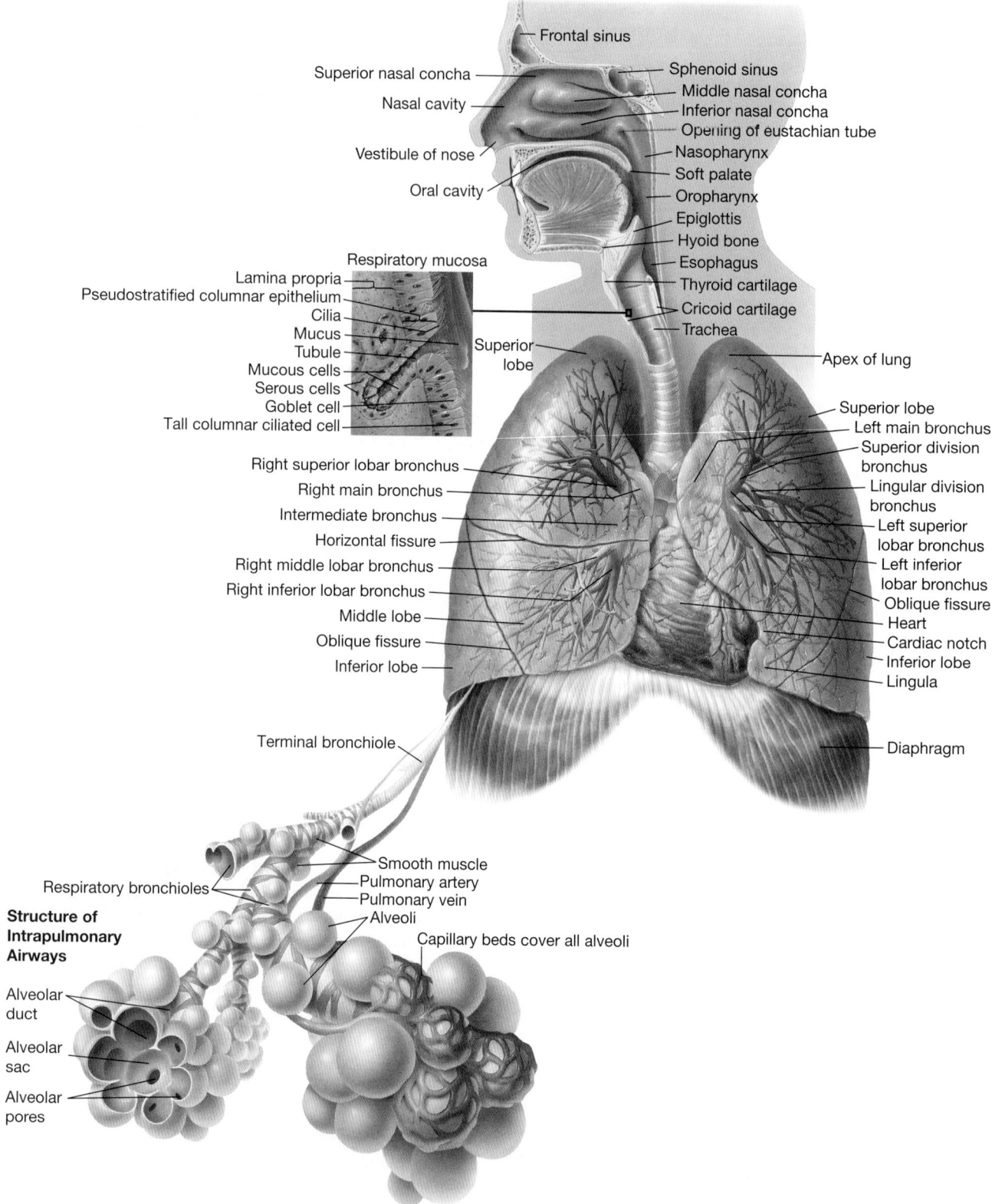

FIGURE 36-1 The airway and related structures. (From the Anatomical Chart Company. [2023]. *Respiratory system anatomical chart*. Lippincott Williams & Wilkins.)

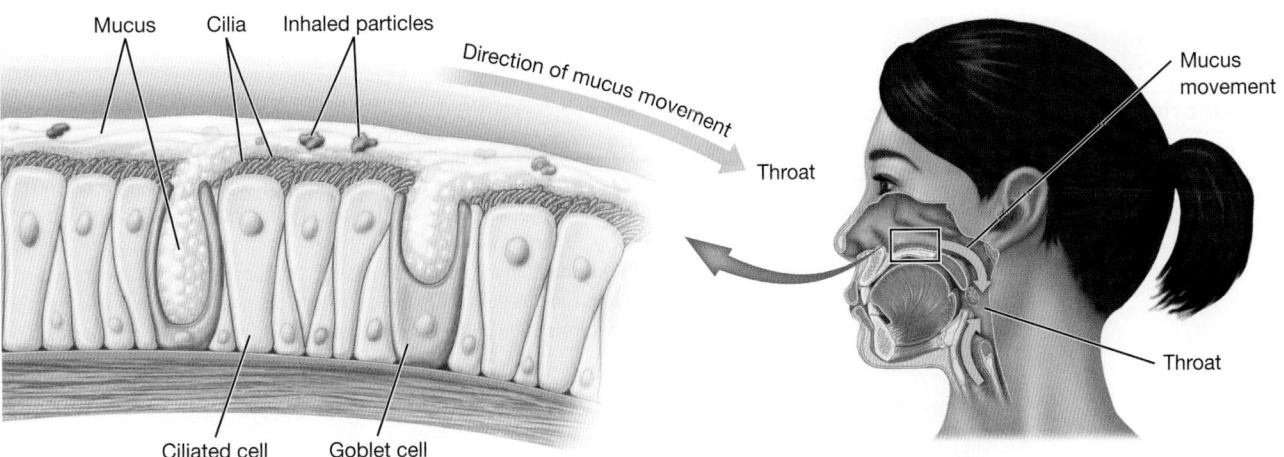

FIGURE 36-2 The cilia and mucus-producing cells. (From Archer, P., & Nelson, L. A. [2012]. *Applied anatomy & physiology for manual therapists.* Lippincott Williams & Wilkins.)

the lungs with the use of gravity (Fig. 36-4). In most hospitals, respiratory therapists are responsible for postural drainage. In long-term care facilities and home health care, however, nurses may teach clients and families to perform this technique (see Client and Family Teaching 36-1). Combining postural drainage with percussion and vibration enhances overall effectiveness.

Percussion

Percussion (the rhythmic striking of the chest wall) helps dislodge respiratory secretions that adhere to the bronchial walls. To perform percussion, the nurse cups the hands, keeping the fingers and thumb together, as if carrying water. They then apply the cupped hands to the client's chest as if trapping air between them and the

thoracic wall (Fig. 36-5). The nurse performs percussion for 3 to 5 minutes in each postural drainage position, taking care to avoid striking the breasts of female clients and any areas of chest injury or bone disease.

Vibration

Vibration uses the palms of the hands to shake underlying tissue and loosen retained secretions. The nurse positions the hands on the client's chest or back during inhalation and then vibrates them as the client exhales to increase the intensity of expiration (Fig. 36-6). Vibration is used with or as an alternative to percussion, especially for frail clients.

Suctioning Secretions

Suctioning relies on negative (vacuum) pressure to remove liquid secretions with a catheter. The amount of negative

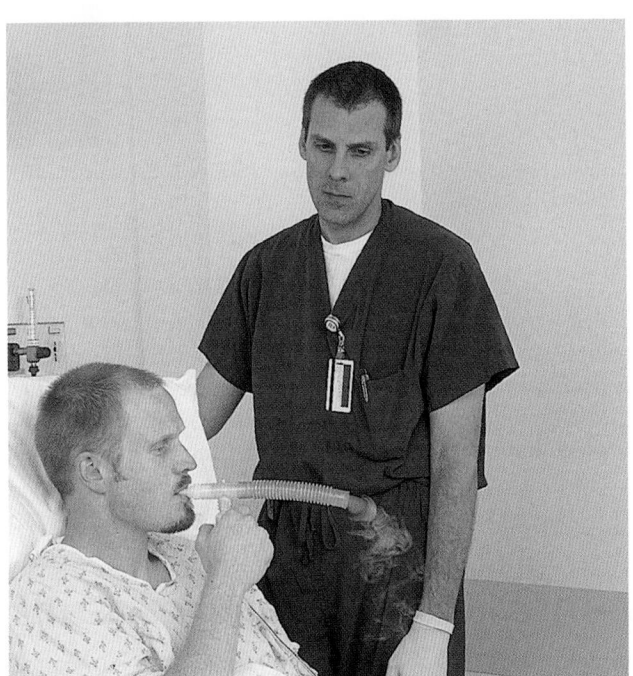

FIGURE 36-3 Aerosol therapy. (Photo by B. Proud.)

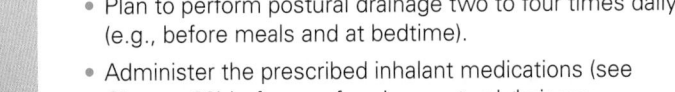

Client and Family Teaching 36-1
Considerations Performing Postural Drainage

The nurse teaches the client and family as follows:

- Plan to perform postural drainage two to four times daily (e.g., before meals and at bedtime).
- Administer the prescribed inhalant medications (see Chapter 33) before performing postural drainage.
- Have paper tissues and waterproof container nearby for collecting expectorated sputum.
- Position yourself to drain the appropriate lung areas.
- Cough and expectorate secretions that drain into the upper airway.
- Remain in each prescribed position for 15 to 30 minutes (no longer than 45 minutes).
- Resume a comfortable position after expectorating the usual volume of sputum or if you become tired, feel lightheaded, or have a rapid pulse rate, difficulty breathing, or chest pain.

NURSING GUIDELINES 36-1

Collecting a Sputum Specimen

- Plan to collect a sputum specimen just after the client awakens or after an aerosol treatment. *This timing allows for a collection when more mucus is available or is in a thinner state.*
- Obtain a sterile sputum specimen cup (Fig. A). *Sterility prevents contamination of the specimen.*

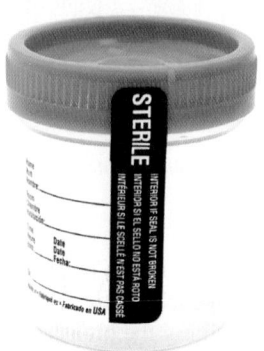

A

- A sterile sputum specimen cup. (ImagePixel/Shutterstock.)
- Help the client to a sitting position. *Sitting provides for an increased volume of inspired air and more forceful coughing to expel mucus.*
- Encourage the client to rinse the mouth with tap water. *Tap water removes some microorganisms and food residue.*
- Explain that the desired specimen should be from deep within the respiratory passages, not saliva from within the mouth. *The correct instruction helps prevent inconclusive or invalid test results.*
- Instruct the client to take several deep breaths, attempt a forceful cough, and expectorate into the specimen container. *These measures help mobilize secretions from the lower airway.*
- Collect at least a 1- to 3-mL (nearly a half teaspoon) specimen. *This quantity is sufficient for analysis.*
- Use a suction catheter with a mucus trap if the client cannot produce sufficient sputum for a specimen (Fig. B). *Negative pressure pulls mucus into the trap.*
- Put on gloves, cover or detach the mucus trap, and enclose the specimen container in a clear plastic bag (Fig. C). *These steps reduce the potential for the transmission of microorganisms.*
- Offer oral hygiene. *It promotes comfort and well-being.*

- Attach a label and laboratory request form to the specimen. *Doing so ensures the correct specimen identification and test procedure.*
- Take the specimen to the laboratory immediately. *Prompt delivery facilitates a timely and accurate analysis of the specimen.*
- Document in the client's medical record the appearance of the specimen and its delivery to the laboratory. *Such recording provides assessment data and information about the disposition of the specimen.*

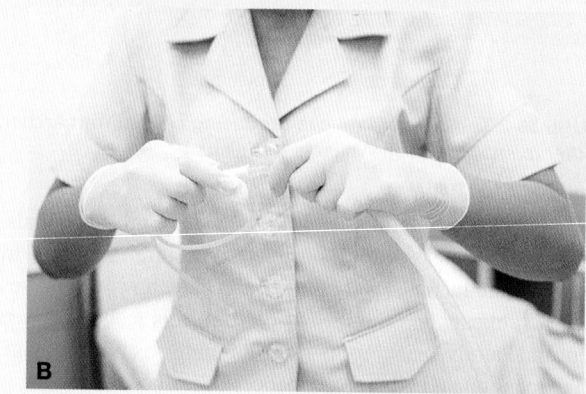

B

A suction catheter with a mucus trap. (Bangkoker/Shutterstock.)

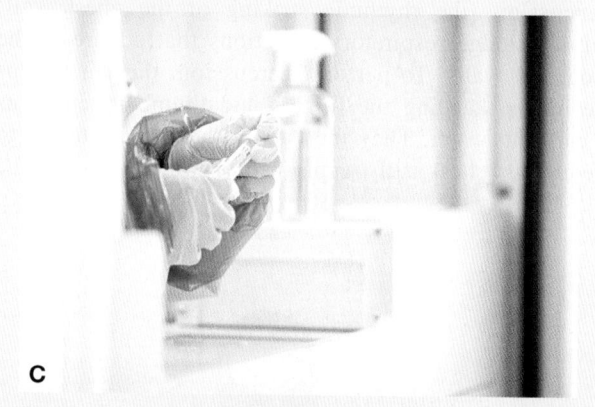

C

Sealing the specimen in the mucus trap. (SURAKIT SAWANGCHIT/ Shutterstock.)

pressure varies depending on the client and the type of suction equipment (Table 36-1). Nurses may suction the upper airway, lower airway, or both. In all cases, they suction the airway from the nose or mouth (Skill 36-1).

⟩⟩ *Stop, Think, and Respond 36-1*

In addition to an SpO_2 less than 90%, what signs or symptoms does a person with hypoxia manifest?

Nasopharyngeal suctioning (removing secretions from the throat through a nasally inserted catheter) is more common than **nasotracheal suctioning** (removing secretions from the upper portion of the lower airway through a nasally inserted catheter). A nasopharyngeal airway, sometimes

called a *trumpet* (Fig. 36-7), can be used to protect the nostril if frequent suctioning is necessary. An alternative method is **oropharyngeal suctioning** (removing secretions from the throat through an orally inserted catheter). Nurses perform **oral suctioning** (removing secretions from the mouth) with a suctioning device called a *Yankauer-tip or tonsil-tip catheter* (Fig. 36-8).

ARTIFICIAL AIRWAY MANAGEMENT

Clients at risk for airway obstruction or who require long-term mechanical ventilation are candidates for an artificial airway. Two common types are an oral airway and a tracheostomy tube.

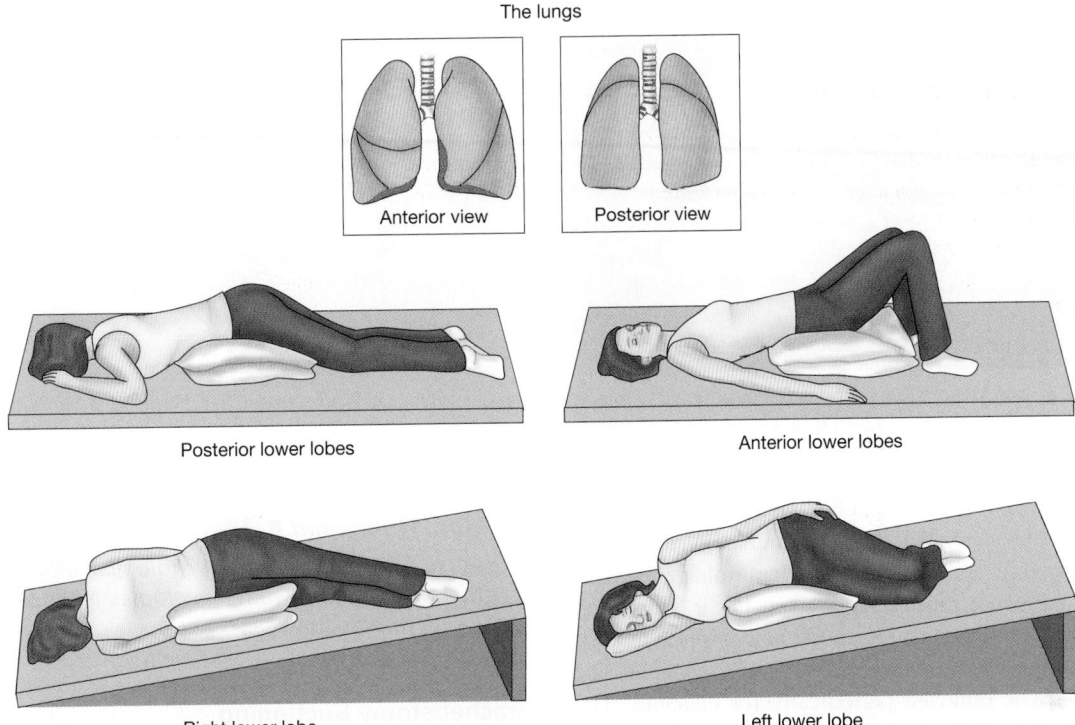

The lungs

Anterior view

Posterior view

Posterior lower lobes

Anterior lower lobes

Right lower lobe

Left lower lobe

FIGURE 36-4 Postural drainage. The four positions that use the force of gravity to assist the drainage of secretions from the smaller bronchial airways are shown.

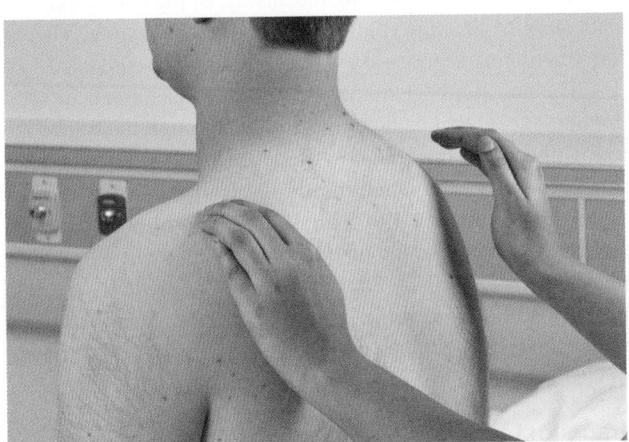

FIGURE 36-5 Performing percussion.

FIGURE 36-6 Performing vibration.

Oral Airway

An **oral airway** is a curved device that keeps a relaxed tongue positioned forward within the mouth, preventing the tongue from obstructing the upper airway (Fig. 36-9). It is most commonly used in clients who are unconscious and cannot protect their own airways, such as those recovering from general anesthesia or a seizure. Nurses insert oral airways, which are usually in place for only a brief time (Nursing Guidelines 36-2).

Tracheostomy

Clients who are less stable, who have an upper airway obstruction, or who require prolonged mechanical ventilation and oxygenation are more likely to be candidates for a **tracheostomy** (a surgically created opening into the trachea). A

tube is inserted through the opening to maintain the airway and provide a new route for ventilation.

Tracheostomy Tube

A **tracheostomy tube** (a curved, hollow plastic tube) is also called a *cannula*. Older metal tracheostomy tubes have largely been replaced by devices made of silicone or

TABLE 36-1 Variations in Suction Pressure

AGE	WALL SUCTION (MM HG)	PORTABLE SUCTION MACHINE (MM HG)
Adults	100–140	10–15
Children	95–100	5–10
Infants	50–95	2–5

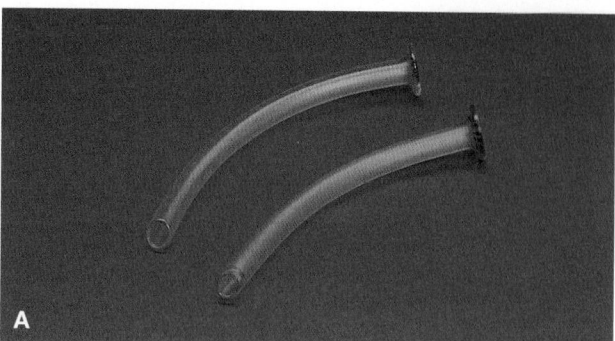
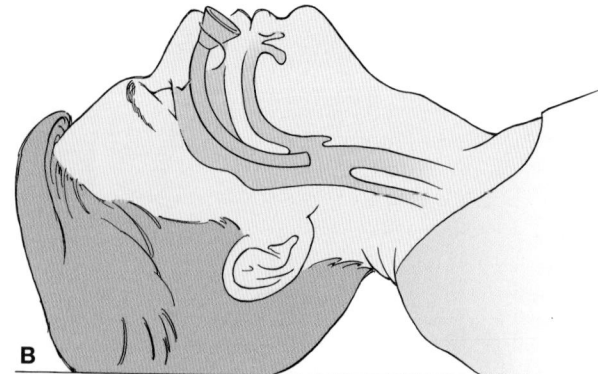

FIGURE 36-7 A. Nasopharyngeal trumpet. **B.** Placement of a nasopharyngeal trumpet. (**A:** From Craven, R. F., Hirnle, C. J., & Henshaw, C. M. [2019]. *Fundamentals of nursing* [9th ed.]. Lippincott Williams & Wilkins.)

polyvinyl chloride that softens at body temperature. Tracheostomy tubes have three parts: inner cannula, outer cannula, and obturator (Fig. 36-10). The **outer cannula** remains in place until the entire tube is replaced. It has a flange that accommodates cloth ties that keep the tube in place as well as a locking mechanism that retains the inner cannula. The **inner cannula** is removed periodically for cleaning. The **obturator** is a curved guide with a bullet-shaped tip. The obturator is used at the time of tube insertion to prevent the edge of the cannula from traumatizing tracheal tissue. Once the tube is in place, the obturator is removed, placed in a plastic bag, and retained at the bedside in the event of an accidental extubation. An alternative is to place a second tracheostomy set at the bedside. Tracheostomy tubes may also have a balloon cuff that, when inflated, seals the upper airway to prevent aspiration of oral fluids and to provide more efficient ventilation.

Because a tracheostomy tube is below the level of the larynx, clients cannot speak. One exception is if they have a **fenestrated tracheostomy tube** (one with holes in the outer cannula), which allows air to pass through the vocal cords allowing speech. A second option is to insert a **speaking valve**, a device that directs exhaled air through the upper airway. In the majority of cases, communication involves writing or reading the client's lips. Being unable to call for help is frightening for a speechless client; therefore, the nurse should check these clients frequently. Providing clients who are unable to vocalize with a bell can reduce their anxiety. When the bell is used, staff must respond as rapidly as possible.

>>> **Stop, Think, and Respond 36-2**
Discuss the physical and psychological effects a client with a tracheostomy may develop as a consequence of being unable to speak.

Tracheostomy Suctioning

Most clients with a tracheostomy require frequent suctioning because the tracheostomy tube irritates the tracheal tissue. Although clients can cough, the force of the cough may be ineffective in completely clearing the airway, or the cough may be inadequate to clear the volume of respiratory secretions. Therefore, suctioning is necessary when secretions are copious.

Tracheostomy suctioning is similar to nasotracheal suctioning, except that catheter insertion is through the tracheostomy tube rather than the nose (Fig. 36-11). When suctioning a tracheostomy, the nurse inserts the catheter a shorter distance (approximately 4 to 5 in [10 to 12.5 cm] or until resistance is felt) because the tube already lies in the trachea. The resistance is caused by contact between the catheter tip and the carina, the ridge at the lower end of the tracheal cartilage where the bronchi branch into each lung. The nurse then raises the catheter about 0.5 in (1.25 cm) and applies suction.

Tracheostomy Care

Tracheostomy care means cleaning the skin around the stoma, changing the dressing, and cleaning the inner cannula

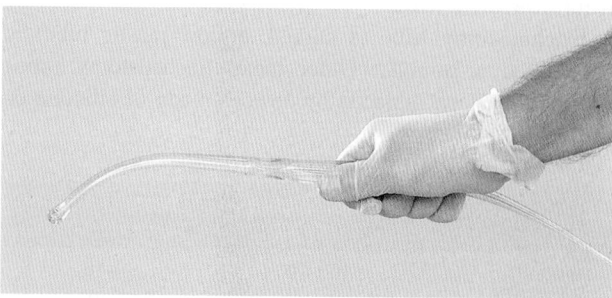

FIGURE 36-8 A Yankauer-tip suction device for oral suctioning. (Photo by B. Proud.)

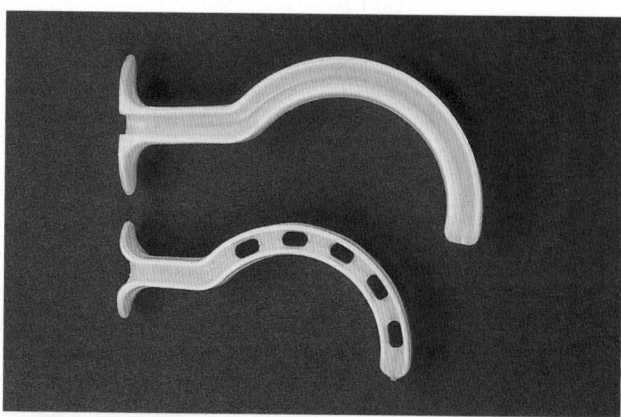

FIGURE 36-9 Examples of oral airways.

NURSING GUIDELINES 36-2

Inserting an Oral Airway

- Gather the following supplies: various sizes of oral airways (most adults can accommodate an 80-mm airway), gloves, a tongue blade, and suction equipment. *Gathering equipment promotes organization and efficient time management.*
- Place the airway on the outside of the client's cheek so that the front portion is parallel with the front teeth. Note whether the back of the airway reaches the angle of the jaw. *Assessment determines the appropriate size to use. (An airway that is too short will be ineffective. An airway that is too long will depress the epiglottis, increasing the risk of airway obstruction.)*
- Wash your hands or use an alcohol-based hand rub (see Chapter 10); put on clean gloves. *These measures reduce the transmission of microorganisms.*
- Explain the procedure to the client. *Instruction provides information that even unconscious clients may comprehend, despite being unable to respond verbally.*
- Perform oral suctioning if necessary. *Doing so clears saliva from the mouth and prevents aspiration.*
- Position the client supine with the neck hyperextended unless contraindicated. *This position opens the airway and facilitates insertion.*

- Open the client's mouth using a gloved finger and thumb or a tongue blade. *Doing so prevents injury to the teeth during insertion.*
- Hold the airway so that the curved tip points upward toward the roof of the mouth (Fig. A) or the side of the cheek. Insert it about halfway. *Such placement prevents pushing the tongue into the pharynx during insertion.*
- Rotate the airway over the top of the tongue and continue inserting it until the front flange is flush with the lips (Fig. B). *This ensures that the artificial airway follows the natural curve of the upper airway.*
- Assess breathing. *Checking breathing validates that the natural airway is patent.*
- Remove the airway every 4 hours, provide oral hygiene, and clean and reinsert the airway. *Hygiene and cleaning remove transient bacteria and promote the integrity of the oral mucosa.*
- As the client's level of consciousness improves, many clients extubate themselves independently.

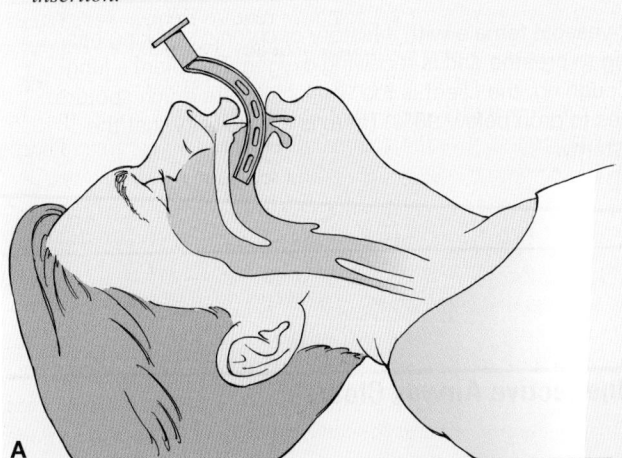

A

The initial insertion position.

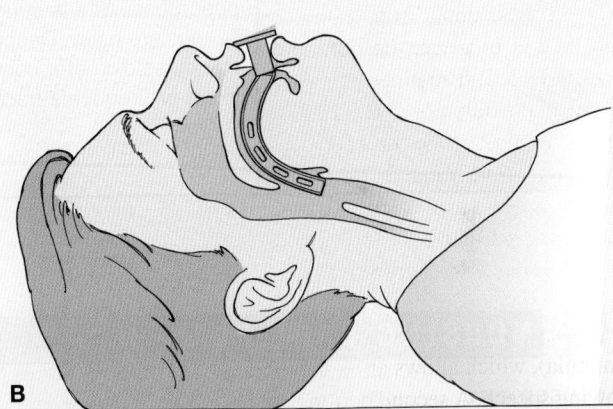

B

The final position after rotation.

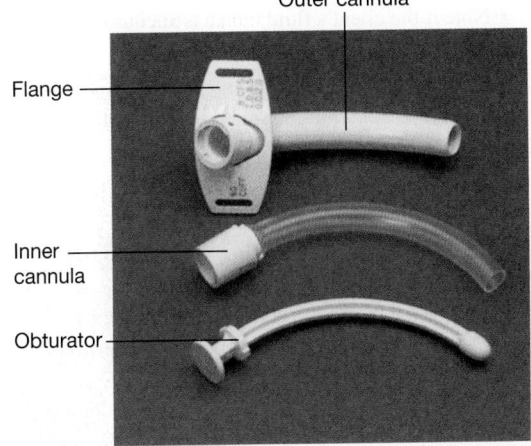
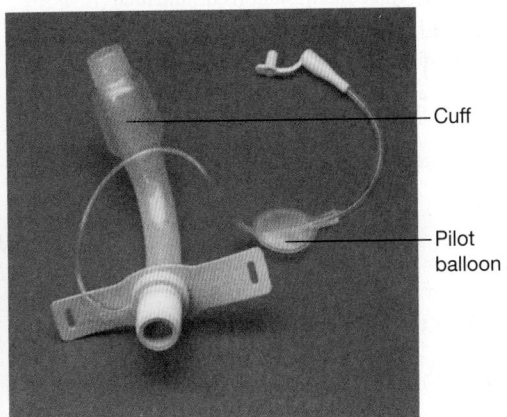

FIGURE 36-10 Examples of uncuffed and cuffed tracheostomy tubes. (From Silbert-Flagg, J. [2022]. *Maternal and child health nursing* [9th ed.]. Lippincott Williams & Wilkins.)

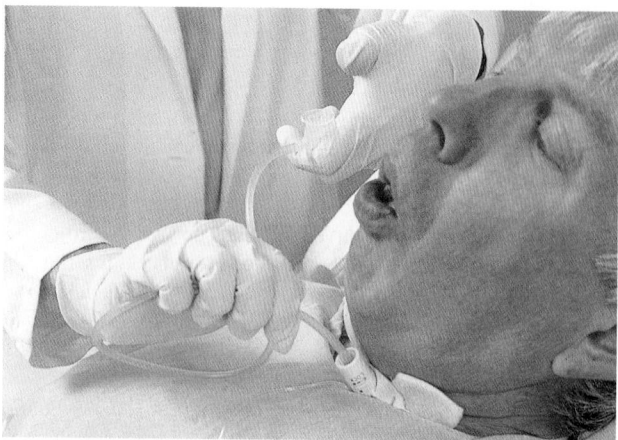

FIGURE 36-11 Suctioning through a tracheostomy tube. (Courtesy of Swedish Hospital Medical Center.)

(Skill 36-2). Nurses perform tracheostomy care at least every 8 hours or as often as clients need to keep the secretions from becoming dried, which may narrow or occlude the airway. They may do tracheal suctioning separately from or at the same time as tracheostomy care.

NURSING IMPLICATIONS

Maintaining an open and patent airway is a priority for nursing care. Lack of oxygen for more than 4 to 6 minutes can result in death or permanent brain damage. Therefore, it is essential to identify nursing diagnoses that apply to respiratory problems and to plan care accordingly for clients at risk. Some possible nursing diagnoses include:

- Ineffective airway clearance
- Impaired gas exchange
- Infection risk
- Acute anxiety
- Knowledge deficiency

Nursing Care Plan 36-1 shows how the nursing process applies to a client with the nursing diagnosis of ineffective airway clearance, defined as the inability to maintain an unobstructed airway.

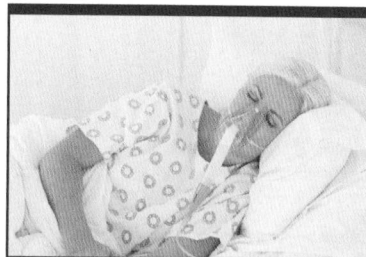

Clinical Scenario A 52-year-old female with a history of chronic smoking has pneumonia. She is struggling to breathe and is receiving oxygen. The client's lung sounds are noisy. Despite coughing, the client is too weak to create much sputum. Her pulse oximeter continues to drop below 90%. There is a possibility that the client will require a tracheostomy.

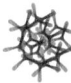

NURSING CARE PLAN 36-1 | Ineffective Airway Clearance

Assessment

- Observe characteristics of the client's breathing and ability to cough forcefully.
- Inspect the sputum for evidence of a viscid consistency.
- Auscultate the lungs to detect adventitious breath sounds suggestive of retained secretions.
- Assess vital signs to detect manifestations of impaired oxygenation.

- Review the client's medical record for conditions that may alter the ability to protect and clear the airway, such as a decreased level of consciousness, unusual weakness or easy fatigability, moderate-to-severe pain, and a surgical incision about the thorax or abdomen.
- Note if the client's fluid intake is adequate.

Nursing Diagnosis. Ineffective airway clearance related to retained secretions as manifested by weak and persistent cough without raising sputum, rapid and shallow respirations, use of accessory muscles, inspiratory gurgles heard in distal right upper lobe both anteriorly and posteriorly, and history of smoking two packs of cigarettes a day

Expected Outcome. The client's airway will be effectively cleared as evidenced by raising sputum sufficiently to keep lung sounds clear by 12/4.

Interventions	Rationales
Auscultate the lungs every shift and before and after coughing or other respiratory therapy.	Auscultation provides data indicating the presence or absence of retained respiratory secretions.
Elevate the head of the bed at all times.	The Fowler position helps provide maximum room for lung expansion.
Maintain 2,000–3,000 mL fluid intake of client's choice (avoid milk) for 24 hours.	Keeping the client well hydrated helps thin respiratory mucus.

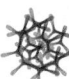

NURSING CARE PLAN 36-1 | **Ineffective Airway Clearance (*continued*)**

Instruct the client to take three deep breaths in through the nose and out the mouth, lean forward, and cough forcefully. Repeat every 1–2 hours while the client is awake.	Deep breathing will help expand the lungs and dilate the airways, subsequently loosening secretions.
Provide a period of rest after forceful coughing.	Repeated coughing creates fatigue that can diminish the effort required for an effective cough.
Administer an expectorant as prescribed by the physician.	Expectorants loosen the adhesive quality of mucus and reduce its gel-like viscosity when it has become attached to cilia.
Perform oral/pharyngeal suctioning if secretions are loose but the client does not expectorate them.	Negative pressure produces a pulling effect, which can remove mucoid secretions that the client cannot clear independently.
Advocate for smoking cessation following recovery from acute illness.	Inhaled smoke increases mucus production; nicotine tends to paralyze the cilia, which decreases the ability to raise pulmonary secretions.

Evaluation of Expected Outcomes

- Client is instructed on deep breathing and the coughing technique.
- Client can raise tenacious, purulent sputum after breathing and coughing.
- Lungs sound less congested.

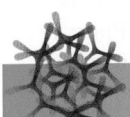

KEY POINTS

- Natural airway management
  - Liquefying secretions
  - Mobilizing secretions: Chest physiotherapy
  - Postural drainage: A positioning technique to assist with draining secretions from the lungs
- Artificial airway management
  - Oral airway
  - Tracheostomy
  - Tracheostomy tube

- Tracheostomy care: Cleaning the skin around the stoma, changing the dressing, and cleaning the inner cannula; performed at least every 8 hours or as often as clients need to keep the secretions from becoming dried, which may narrow or occlude the airway

CRITICAL THINKING EXERCISES

1. What suggestions would you offer an individual to discourage them from continuing to smoke cigarettes?
2. What pulmonary diseases are likely to be diagnosed by examining a sputum specimen, and what nursing actions facilitate an accurate examination of the collected specimen?
3. Explain how body positions that place the head lower than the chest facilitate the expectoration of pulmonary secretions.
4. Discuss ways to relieve the anxiety of a client with a tracheostomy who needs frequent suctioning but fears they will be unable to obtain assistance when needed.

NEXT-GENERATION NCLEX-STYLE REVIEW QUESTIONS

1. Besides describing the characteristics of a client's cough, what other information is most important to document?
   a. The client's family history of respiratory disease
   b. A current assessment of the client's vital signs
   c. The appearance of the respiratory secretions
   d. The types of self-treatments that the client is using
   Test-Taking Strategy: Note the key term and modifier, "most important." Analyze the choices and select the option that correlates with subjective or objective data.
2. Place an "X" on the tracheostomy component that is used only during its insertion but should remain at the bedside in the event that the client accidentally becomes extubated.

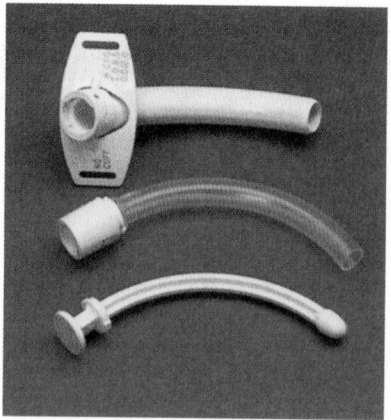

Test-Taking Strategy: Recall the components of a tracheostomy tube and their uses.

3. What time of the day is it best for the nurse to attempt to obtain a sputum specimen?
   a. Before bedtime
   b. After a meal
   c. Between meals
   d. Upon awakening

Test-Taking Strategy: Note the key term, "best." Analyze the choices and select the option that is better than any of the others at identifying a time when the volume of mucus is most abundant.

4. When suctioning a client with a tracheostomy tube, when is the best time to occlude the vent on the suction catheter?
   a. When inserting the catheter
   b. When inside the inner cannula
   c. When withdrawing the catheter
   d. When the client begins coughing

Test-Taking Strategy: Note the key term and modifier, "best time." Select the option that describes the time that is least likely to deplete the client's level of oxygen.

5. When suctioning the airway of a client with a tracheostomy, the nurse applies suction for no longer than how long?
   a. 5 to 7 seconds
   b. 10 to 15 seconds
   c. 15 to 20 seconds
   d. 20 to 30 seconds

Test-Taking Strategy: Analyze the choices and select the option that is within a time range that facilitates safe suctioning.

NEXT-GENERATION NCLEX-STYLE CLINICAL SCENARIO QUESTIONS

Clinical Scenario:

A 52-year-old female with a history of chronic smoking has pneumonia. She is struggling to breathe and is receiving oxygen. The client's lung sounds are noisy. Despite coughing, the client is too weak to create much sputum. Her pulse oximeter continues to drop below 90%. There is a possibility that the client will require a tracheostomy.

1. Select all of the indicators that may suggest a cause for concern regarding the client's inability to clear her airway for adequate ventilation.
   a. Chronic smoking
   b. Diagnosis of pneumonia
   c. Congested lung sounds
   d. Adventitious lung sounds
   e. Inability to cough up sputum
   f. Pulse oximeter at 98%
   g. Pulse oximeter at less than 90%
   h. The client's weakness

2. Place an "x" under "effective" identifying actions that would help the client clear her airway. Place an "x" under "ineffective" identifying actions that may contribute to ineffective airway clearance.

ACTIONS	EFFECTIVE	INEFFECTIVE
Elevate the head of the bed at all times.		
Provide a period of rest after forceful coughing.		
Have the client lie in a supine position.		
Advocate for smoking cessation following recovery from acute illness.		
Decrease fluid intake.		
Perform oral/pharyngeal suctioning if secretions are loose but the client does not expectorate them.		

SKILL 36-1 Suctioning the Airway

Suggested Action	Reason for Action
ASSESSMENT	
Assess the client's lung sounds, respiratory effort, and oxygen saturation level.	Determines the need for suctioning
Determine how much the client understands about suctioning the airway.	Provides an opportunity for health teaching
Inspect the nose to determine which nostril is more patent.	Eases insertion of the catheter
PLANNING	
Consider using a face shield and wearing a cover gown in addition to gloves when suctioning a client.	The nurse can choose to wear a face shield and cover gown as part of standard precautions
Obtain a suction kit. All kits contain a basin and one or two sterile gloves. Some also contain a sterile suction catheter.	Promotes organization and efficient time management
If the kit does not include a catheter, select one that will not occlude the nostril; usually a 12- to 18-F catheter is appropriate for adults.	Promotes comfort and reduces the potential for injury
Obtain a flask of sterile normal saline and a suction machine if a wall outlet is unavailable.	Provides items that are not prepackaged
Attach the suction canister to the wall outlet or plug a portable suction machine into an electrical outlet.	Provides a source for negative pressure
Connect the suction tubing to the canister.	Provides a means for connecting the canister to the suction catheter
Turn on the suction machine, occlude the suction tubing, and adjust the pressure gauge to the desired amount.	Ensures safe pressure during suctioning
Open the container of saline.	Reduces the risk for later contamination
IMPLEMENTATION	
Pull the privacy curtains.	Demonstrates respect for the client
Elevate the head of the bed unless contraindicated.	Aids in ventilation
Wash your hands or use an alcohol-based hand rub (see Chapter 10).	Reduces the transmission of microorganisms
Preoxygenate the client for 1–2 minutes until the SpO$_2$ is maintained at 95%–100%.	Reduces the risk for hypoxemia
Open the suction kit without contaminating the contents.	Follows the principles of asepsis
Put on sterile glove(s). If the kit provides only one, put one clean glove on the nondominant hand and then put the sterile glove on the dominant hand.	Prevents the transmission of microorganisms
Pour sterile normal saline into the basin with your nondominant hand.	Prepares the solution for wetting and rinsing the suction catheter
Consider the nondominant hand contaminated.	Follows principles of asepsis
Pick up the suction catheter with your sterile (dominant) hand and connect it to the suction tubing (Fig. A).	Completes the circuit for applying suction

Connecting the catheter. (Photo by B. Proud.)

(continued)

SKILL 36-1 Suctioning the Airway (*continued*)

Suggested Action	Reason for Action
Place the catheter tip in the saline and occlude the vent (Fig. B).	Wets the outer and inner surfaces of the catheter, which reduces friction and facilitates insertion

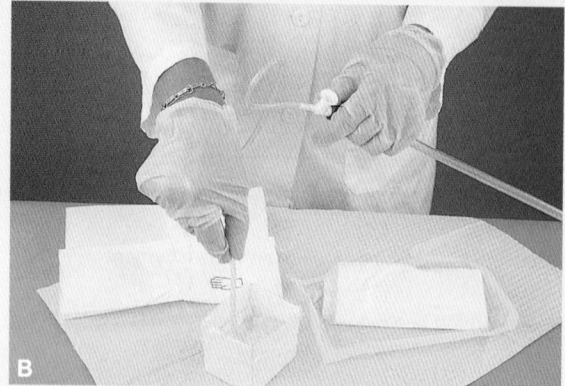

Wetting the catheter. (Photo by B. Proud.)

Suggested Action	Reason for Action
Insert the catheter without applying suction along the floor of the nose or side of the mouth (Fig. C).	Reduces the potential for sneezing or gagging

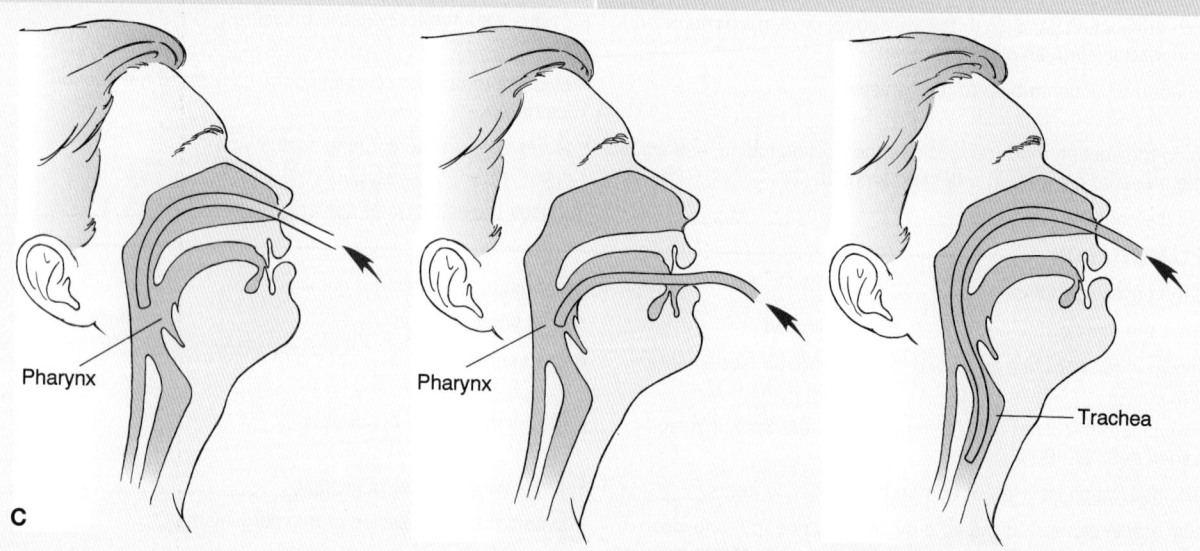

Catheter placement: nasopharyngeal (*left*), oropharyngeal (*center*), and nasotracheal (*right*).

Suggested Action	Reason for Action
Advance the catheter 5–6 in (12.5–15 cm) in the nose or 3–4 in (7.5–10 cm) in the mouth.	Places the distal tip in the pharynx
For tracheal suctioning, wait until the client takes a breath and then advance the tubing 8–10 in (20–25 cm).	Eases insertion below the larynx
Encourage the client to cough if coughing does not occur spontaneously.	Breaks up mucus and raises secretions
Occlude the air vent and rotate the catheter as it is withdrawn (Fig. D).	Maximizes the effectiveness of suctioning

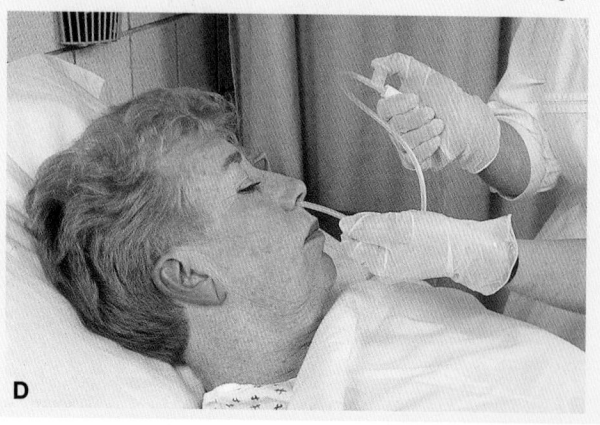

Rotating and withdrawing the catheter. (From Rosdahl, C. B., & Kowalski, M. T. [2012]. *Textbook of basic nursing* [10th ed.]. Lippincott Williams & Wilkins.)

SKILL 36-1 Suctioning the Airway (*continued*)

Suggested Action	Reason for Action
Complete the process in no more than 15 seconds from insertion to removal of the catheter, occluding the vent no longer than 10 seconds.	Prevents hypoxemia
Rinse secretions from the catheter by inserting its tip in the basin of saline and applying suction.	Flushes the mucus from the inner lumen
Provide 2–3 minutes of rest while the client continues to breathe oxygen.	Reoxygenates the blood
Suction again if necessary.	Bases decision on individual assessment data
Remove the gloves to enclose the suction catheter in an inverted glove (Fig. E).	Encloses the soiled catheter, reducing the transmission of microorganisms

Enclosing the catheter. (Photo by B. Proud.)

Discard the suction kit, catheter, and gloves in a lined waste receptacle.	Follows principles of asepsis

EVALUATION

- The airway is cleared of secretions.
- The SpO_2 level remains at 95% or higher.
- The client demonstrates breathing that requires less effort.

DOCUMENT

- Preassessment data
- Type of suctioning performed
- Appearance of secretions
- Client's response

SAMPLE DOCUMENTATION

Date and Time Respirations are moist and noisy. SpO_2 shows a drop from 95% to 90% during the last 15 minutes. Coughing effort is weak and ineffective. Raised to a high Fowler position and oxygenated at 4 L per nasal cannula. Tracheal suctioning performed and reoxygenated. Lungs sound clear at this time. Pulse oximeter indicates SpO_2 at 95% at this time.
———————————————— J. Doe, LPN

SKILL 36-2 Providing Tracheostomy Care

Suggested Action	Reason for Action
ASSESSMENT	
Check the nursing care plan to determine the schedule for providing tracheostomy care.	Provides continuity of care
Review the client's record for documentation concerning previous tracheostomy care.	Provides a database for comparison
Assess the condition of the dressing and the skin around the tracheostomy tube.	Determines the need for a dressing change and skin care
Determine the client's understanding of tracheostomy care.	Provides an opportunity for health teaching

(continued)

SKILL 36-2 Providing Tracheostomy Care (*continued*)

Suggested Action	Reason for Action
PLANNING	
Consult with the client on an appropriate time for tracheostomy care if only routine care is needed.	Demonstrates respect for the client's right to participate in decisions
Consider using a face shield and wearing a cover gown in addition to gloves when suctioning a client.	The nurse can choose to wear a face shield and cover gown as part of standard precautions.
Obtain a container of hydrogen peroxide and a flask of normal saline. Remove the cap from each container.	Provides items that are not prepackaged and prevents the contamination of one gloved hand later in the procedure
IMPLEMENTATION	
Wash your hands or use an alcohol-based hand rub (see Chapter 10).	Removes colonizing microorganisms
Raise the bed to an appropriate height.	Prevents back strain
Place the client in a supine or low Fowler position.	Facilitates access to the tracheostomy tube
Put on a clean glove; remove the soiled stomal dressing and discard it, glove and all, in a lined waste receptacle.	Follows the principles of asepsis
Wash your hands or use an alcohol-based hand rub again.	Reduces the transmission of microorganisms
Open the tracheostomy kit, taking care not to contaminate its contents.	Provides access to and maintains the sterility of supplies
Put on sterile gloves.	Prevents transferring microorganisms to the lower airway
Add equal parts of sterile normal saline and sterile hydrogen peroxide to one basin and sterile normal saline to the other (Fig. A).	The diluted hydrogen peroxide cleans mucoid secretions; the sterile normal saline rinses the peroxide solution from the skin and inner cannula.

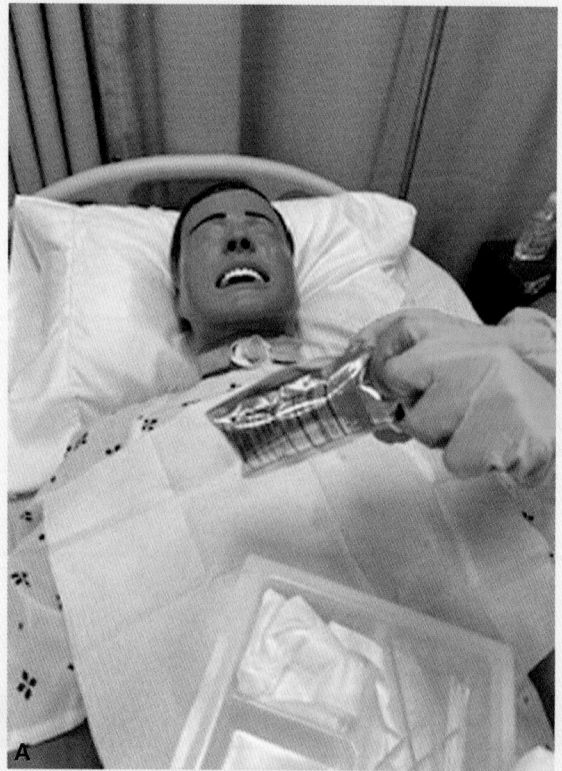

Adding the cleaning solutions. (Photos by L. Moreno.)

Suggested Action	Reason for Action
Unlock the inner cannula (using one hand, which is now considered contaminated) by turning it counterclockwise; deposit it in the basin with the hydrogen peroxide and saline solution (Fig. B).	Loosens protein secretions and reduces colonizing microorganisms

SKILL 36-2 Providing Tracheostomy Care (*continued*)

Suggested Action	Reason for Action
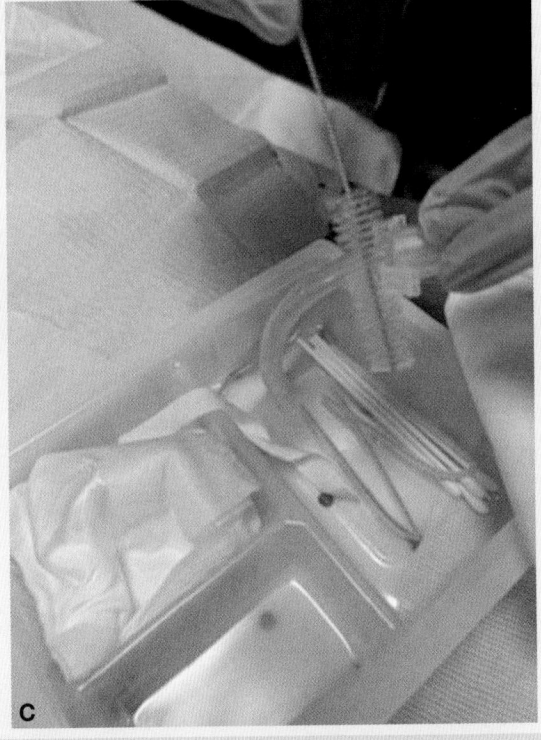 **B**	Removing the inner cannula.(Photos by L. Moreno.)
Clean the inside and outside of the cannula (Fig. C).	Removes gross debris
C	Cleaning the inner cannula. (Photos by L. Moreno.)
Deposit contaminated supplies in a lined or waterproof waste receptacle.	Reduces the potential for contaminating sterile supplies

(continued)

SKILL 36-2 Providing Tracheostomy Care (*continued*)

Suggested Action	Reason for Action
Rinse the cleaned cannula in the basin of normal saline.	Removes remnants of hydrogen peroxide
Tap the rinsed cannula against the edge of the basin and wipe the excess solution with a gauze square.	Removes large droplets of fluid
Replace the inner cannula and turn it clockwise within the outer cannula (Fig. D).	Secures the inner cannula

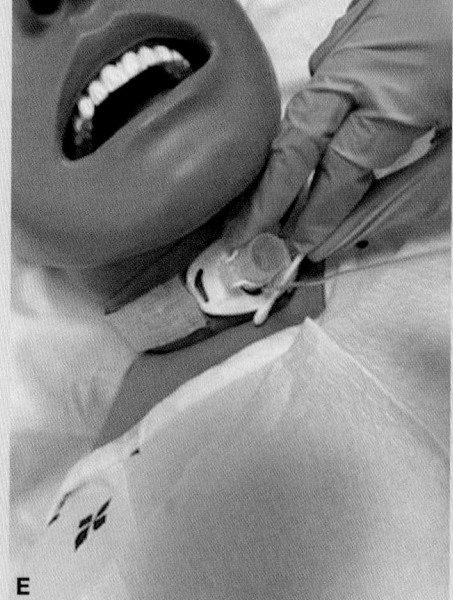

D

Replacing the inner cannula. (Photos by L. Moreno.)

Suggested Action	Reason for Action
Clean around the stoma with an applicator moistened with the diluted peroxide (Fig. E).	Removes secretions and colonizing microorganisms from the tracheal opening

E

Cleaning the stoma. (Photos by L. Moreno.)

Suggested Action	Reason for Action
Never go back over an area once you have cleaned it.	Follows principles of asepsis
Wipe the same area in the same manner with another applicator moistened with saline.	Removes hydrogen peroxide from the skin

SKILL 36-2 Providing Tracheostomy Care (*continued*)

Suggested Action	Reason for Action
Place the sterile stomal dressing beneath the flanges and outer cannula of the tracheostomy tube (Fig. F).	Absorbs secretions and keeps the stomal area clean

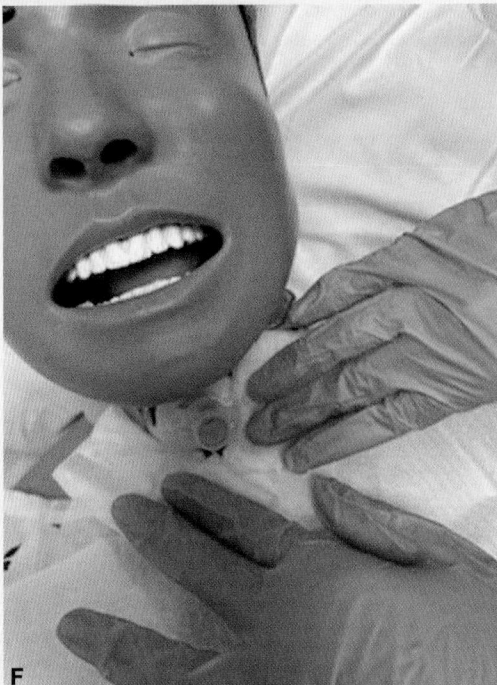

Applying the stomal dressing. (Photos by L. Moreno.)

Suggested Action	Reason for Action
Change the tracheostomy ties by threading them through the slits of each flange of the tracheostomy tube and tying them in place (Fig. G).	Holds the tracheostomy tube in place

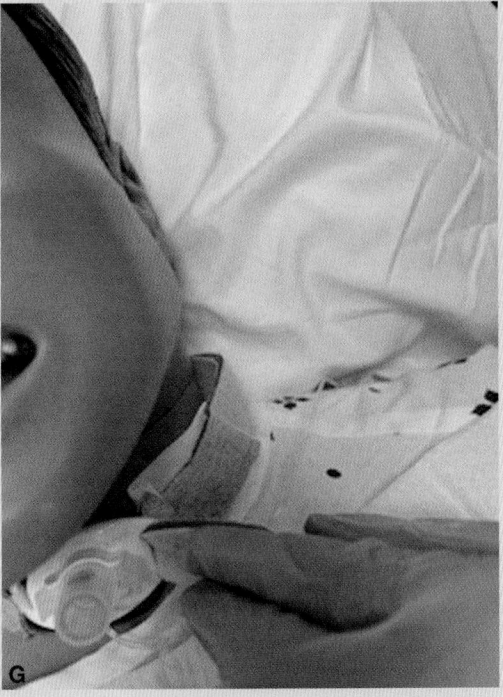

Securing the tracheostomy Velcro strap. (Photos by L. Moreno.)

Suggested Action	Reason for Action
Wait to remove the previous ties until after the new ones are secure, if working alone. Otherwise, have an assistant stabilize the tracheostomy tube while you cut the soiled ties and apply the new ties.	Prevents accidental extubation

(*continued*)

SKILL 36-2 Providing Tracheostomy Care (*continued*)

Suggested Action	Reason for Action
Tie the two ends snugly, but not tightly, at the side of the neck. Make sure there is room to insert your little finger within the ties before securing the ends.	Prevents skin impairment
Discard all soiled supplies, remove your gloves, and wash your hands or use an alcohol-based hand rub.	Follows the principles of asepsis
Return the client to a safe and comfortable position.	Demonstrates concern for the client's well-being
Restore a means that the client can use to signal for assistance (e.g., call button, bell).	Facilitates meeting the client's needs in emergencies and nonemergencies

EVALUATION

- The tracheostomy tube remains patent.
- The stomal opening is clean and without evidence of infection.
- The dressing is clean and dry.
- The skin around the neck is intact.

DOCUMENT

- Preassessment data
- Procedure as it was performed
- Appearance of skin and secretions
- Client's response

SAMPLE DOCUMENTATION

Date and Time   Respirations are quiet and effortless. Routine tracheostomy care provided. Moderate amount of clear mucus removed from inner cannula during cleaning. Stomal skin is pink, but there is no redness, tenderness, swelling, or purulent drainage. Neck skin is intact; skin color is comparable to surrounding areas. _____ J. Doe, LPN

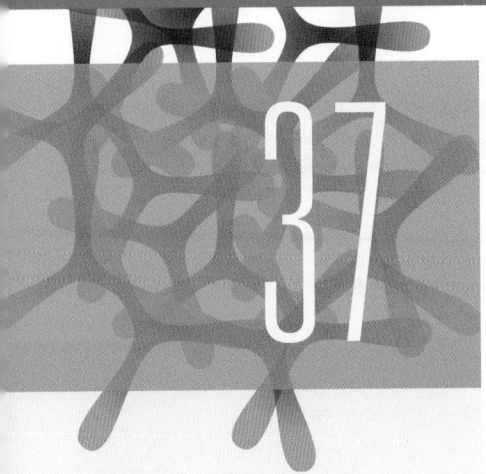

Resuscitation

Words To Know

activation
advanced life support
asystole
automated external defibrillator
cardiac arrest
cardiopulmonary resuscitation
chain of survival
code
complete airway obstruction
defibrillation
head-tilt/chin-lift technique
Heimlich maneuver
jaw-thrust maneuver
partial airway obstruction
recognition
recovery position
rescue breathing
resuscitation team
subdiaphragmatic thrust
ventricular fibrillation

Learning Objectives

On completion of this chapter, the reader should be able to:

1. Identify signs of an airway obstruction and explain why an airway obstruction is life-threatening.
2. Describe appropriate actions if a client has a partial airway obstruction.
3. Explain the purpose of the Heimlich maneuver and describe the circumstances for using subdiaphragmatic and chest thrusts.
4. Identify the recommended action for relieving an airway obstruction in an infant and in an unconscious person.
5. List the five steps in the chain of survival.
6. Explain cardiopulmonary resuscitation (CPR) and the associated steps in **c**irculation, **a**irway, and **b**reathing (CAB).
7. Describe the purpose of chest compression.
8. Name techniques for opening the airway and list ways a trained rescuer administers rescue breathing.
9. Discuss the appropriate use of an automated external defibrillator (AED).
10. Describe criteria used in the decision to discontinue resuscitation efforts.

INTRODUCTION

Nurses are often the first to respond to pulmonary or cardiac emergencies. The information in this chapter reflects the American Heart Association's International Cardiopulmonary Resuscitation (CPR) and Emergency Cardiovascular Care Guidelines of 2020 and 2023 Focused Updates for performing basic life support techniques.

 Gerontologic Considerations

■ In the performance of chest compressions, older adults are at a greater risk for fractured ribs because of the increased likelihood of osteoporosis. Similarly, those with vascular disease may not receive adequate blood perfusion of the brain during CPR, and they may experience brain damage as a result.

■ Older adults who take an anticoagulant are more apt to bleed internally during chest compressions.

■ Older adults may need clear and pertinent descriptions of various treatments and measures for resuscitation addressed in advance directives. An older adult's advance directive should specify the types of medical care they wish. For example, some clients approve the use of emergency drugs but refuse mechanical ventilation.

■ Nurses are responsible for ascertaining whether an older client has an existing advance directive and ensuring that the directions continue to reflect the client's wishes.

■ Some older adults fear that if they specify that they do not wish to be resuscitated, they will receive less than appropriate care and treatment of their illness. The client's record must contain their resuscitation status. If no information is documented, CPR is administered in any life-threatening situation, regardless of the client's age.

■ Family caregivers, particularly those designated as having health care powers of attorney, should be included in discussions about resuscitation efforts. In many situations, it is appropriate to facilitate a referral to a geriatric health care professional with expertise in palliative and hospice care.

AIRWAY OBSTRUCTION

The upper airway can become occluded for various reasons (Box 37-1). Sometimes, the airway swells because of injury; in such cases, the client may need an artificial airway to promote and sustain breathing (see Chapter 36). A bolus of food or some other foreign object may cause a mechanical airway obstruction. Regardless of the cause, airway obstruction compromises air exchange and subsequent oxygenation of cells and tissues. For this reason, an unrelieved airway obstruction will lead to a loss of consciousness and eventually death if it remains unresolved.

>> *Stop, Think, and Respond 37-1*

Discuss circumstances in which a person is at high risk for mechanical airway obstruction.

Identifying Signs of Airway Obstruction

Signs of airway obstruction (Box 37-2) generally occur while the person is eating. The victim may immediately grasp their throat with hands (Fig. 37-1) and make aggressive efforts to cough and breathe. They may make a high-pitched sound while inhaling. The face initially reddens, then becomes pale or blue.

Relieving Airway Obstruction

If the victim can speak or cough, they are exchanging some air, which indicates only a **partial airway obstruction**. Because infants cannot talk or make the universal choking sign, the ability to cry is the best evidence of a partial obstruction in this age group. Other than encouraging and supporting the

BOX 37-1	Common Causes of Airway Obstruction

- Compromised swallowing
- Aspiration of vomitus
- Insufficient chewing
- Consuming large pieces of food
- Laughing or talking while chewing
- Eating when intoxicated
- Inhaling foreign objects from the mouth

BOX 37-2	Signs of a Partial or Complete Airway Obstruction

- Coughing or gagging while eating
- Audibly wheezing
- Persistently attempting to clear throat
- Making hoarse or wet vocal sounds
- Resisting efforts to be fed
- Being unable to speak
- Holding throat
- Being unable to breathe
- Exhibiting cyanosis

victim, a partial airway obstruction requires no additional resuscitation efforts.

If the victim's independent efforts to relieve a partial obstruction are unsuccessful or if the situation worsens, activating the emergency medical system (EMS) is appropriate. In the hospital, staff members do this by calling a **code** (summoning personnel trained in advanced life support techniques). In the community, people can obtain assistance by dialing 911 or another emergency number.

A **complete airway obstruction** (inability to ventilate) requires immediate action to dislodge the obstruction and restore breathing. When the victim is *conscious*, the **Heimlich maneuver** (the method for relieving a mechanical airway obstruction) is appropriate. It involves the use of **subdiaphragmatic thrusts** (pressure to the abdomen) or chest thrusts. Figure 37-2 shows variations for clearing an airway obstruction depending on age and level of consciousness.

Airway Obstructions in Infants

For infants (children younger than 1 year), the rescuer supports the baby over their forearm. Holding the infant prone with the head downward, the rescuer uses the heel of one hand to administer five back slaps between the shoulder blades (Fig. 37-2A). The rescuer turns the infant supine

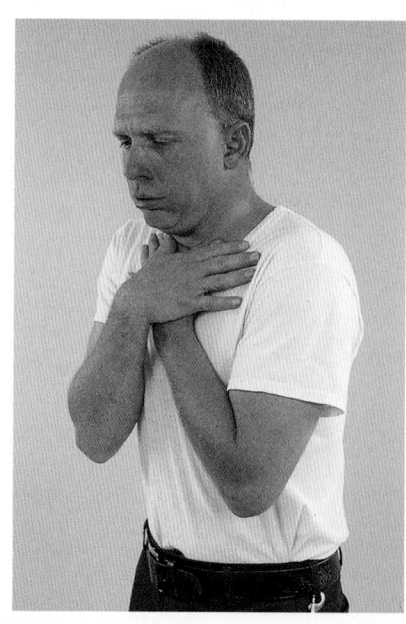

FIGURE 37-1 The universal sign for choking. (Photo by B. Proud.)

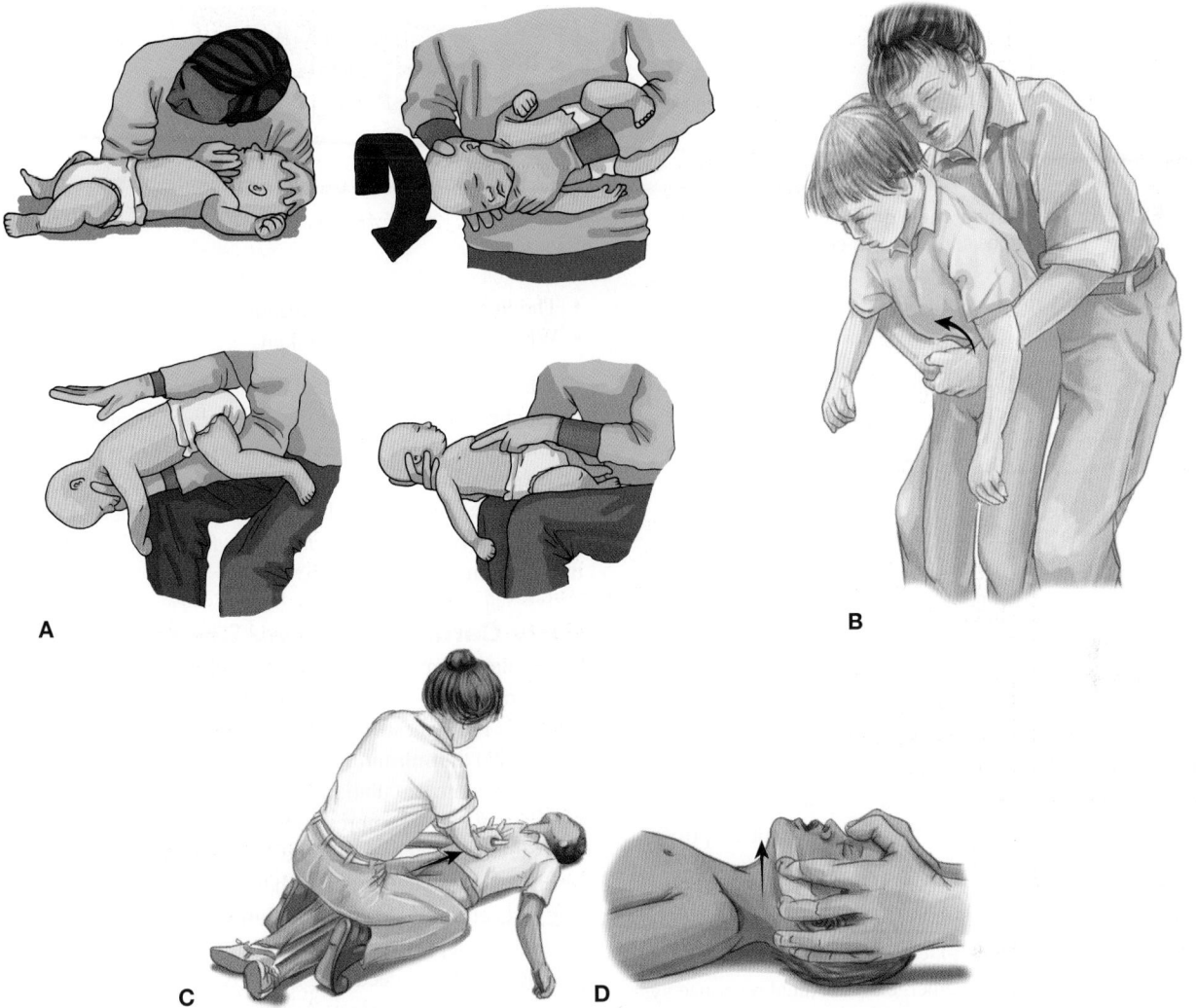

FIGURE 37-2 Relieving an airway obstruction. **A.** Back blows and chest thrust in an infant. **B.** Abdominal thrusts in a conscious child or adult. **C.** Abdominal thrusts in an unconscious child or adult. **D.** Jaw-thrust technique in a child. (**A.** Double Rain/Shutterstock. **B–D.** From Hatfield, N. T. [2021]. *Introductory maternity and pediatric nursing* [5th ed.]. Lippincott Williams & Wilkins.)

and uses two fingers to give five chest thrusts at approximately one per second to the middle of the breastbone, just below the nipple line. They repeatedly alternate five back blows and chest thrusts until the object is dislodged or the infant fails to respond. The rescuer does not use finger sweeps unless they can see the obstructing object. If the infant becomes unconscious, the rescuer performs CPR (described later).

Airway Obstructions in People Older Than 1 Year

For all people older than 1 year, the rescuer gives a series of five quick subdiaphragmatic (abdominal) upward thrusts slightly above the navel to increase intrathoracic pressure equivalent to a cough (Fig. 37-2B). The rescuer opens the victim's airway with the head-tilt/chin-lift maneuver (described later) and continues administering upward thrusts if initial efforts are not successful. They avoid blind finger sweeps unless the object in the airway is visible. If the person becomes unconscious, the rescuer supports the victim to the floor (Fig. 37-2C), activates the emergency response system, and begins performing CPR. The victim's mouth is

checked for any visible object when each attempt at ventilation is made.

When the victim is *unconscious*, increasing the intrathoracic pressure in the airway using chest thrusts can help dislodge the foreign object. When a choking victim becomes unresponsive, the rescuer begins the steps of CPR, starting with compressions. The only difference is that each time the airway is opened, the rescuer looks for the obstructing object before giving each breath. The rescuer removes the object if it is visible.

CHAIN OF SURVIVAL

If a person's unresponsiveness may be the result of **cardiac arrest** (the cessation of heart contraction or a life-sustaining heart rhythm), rescuers implement a six-step intervention process known as the **chain of survival** (Fig. 37-3). Survival rates following cardiac arrest depend greatly on the speed with which rescuers initiate the chain of survival. The faster the steps occur, the better the victim's chances. Outcomes are best when rescuers perform these steps rapidly.

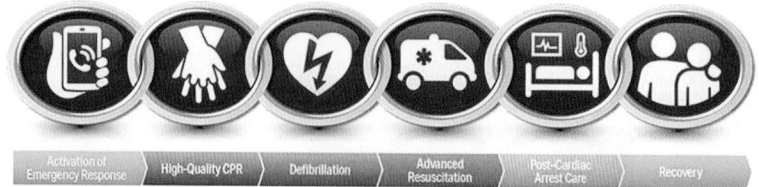

FIGURE 37-3 Out-of-hospital chain of survival. (From American Heart Association. [2023]. *AHA guidelines for CPR and ECC.* https://cpr.heart.org/en/resources/cpr-facts-and-stats/out-of-hospital-chain-of-survival)

The six links in the adult out-of-hospital Chain of Survival are as follows:

- **Recognition** of cardiac arrest and **activation** of the emergency response system
- Early cardiopulmonary resuscitation (CPR) with an emphasis on chest compressions
- Rapid **defibrillation**
- Advanced resuscitation by Emergency Medical Services and other health care providers
- Post–cardiac arrest care
- Recovery (including additional treatment, observation, rehabilitation, and psychological support)

Early Recognition and Access of Emergency Services

Responsiveness is determined initially by shouting and shaking the victim (Fig. 37-4). With the victim in a supine position on a dry, firm surface, a quick assessment taking no more than 10 seconds is performed to determine unresponsiveness and the absence of normal breathing or a pulse (Fig. 37-5).

If the victim appears lifeless or is not breathing normally, it is essential to activate the emergency medical response system, whether outside or within a health care facility. This can be done by a bystander or second rescuer as well. In most locations, emergency medical assistance is obtained by dialing 911 and providing information to a central phone operator. The person making the call gives the following facts:

- The address where assistance is needed
- A description of the situation

- The victim's current condition
- What actions have been taken

Emergency medical technicians or paramedics are then dispatched to the scene. If the emergency involves someone within a health care agency, the **resuscitation team** (a group of people who have been trained and certified in advanced cardiac life support [ACLS] techniques) is alerted by notifying the switchboard operator that assistance is needed and the location of the emergency.

Early Cardiopulmonary Resuscitation

Resuscitation must proceed with circulation, airway, and breathing (CAB) if the rescuer is a trained health care provider or hands-only chest compressions if untrained in defibrillation, or **cardiopulmonary resuscitation** (CPR), a technique used to restore circulation and breathing. Going directly to hands-only chest compressions is recommended for lay rescuers, evidence shows that the risk of harm to a victim who receives chest compressions when not in cardiac arrest is low. Lay rescuers are not able to determine with accuracy whether a victim has a pulse and if the risk of withholding CPR from a pulseless victim exceeds the harm from unneeded chest compressions (American Heart Association, 2020).

Promoting Circulation

Circulation is achieved by performing chest compressions. Chest compression promotes circulation in one of two ways.

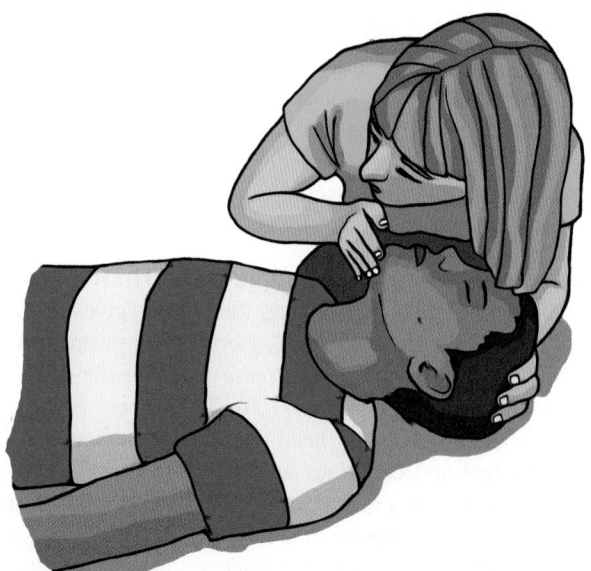

FIGURE 37-4 Determining responsiveness. (SORN340 Studio Images/Shutterstock.)

FIGURE 37-5 Checking for breathing. (Double Rain/Shutterstock.)

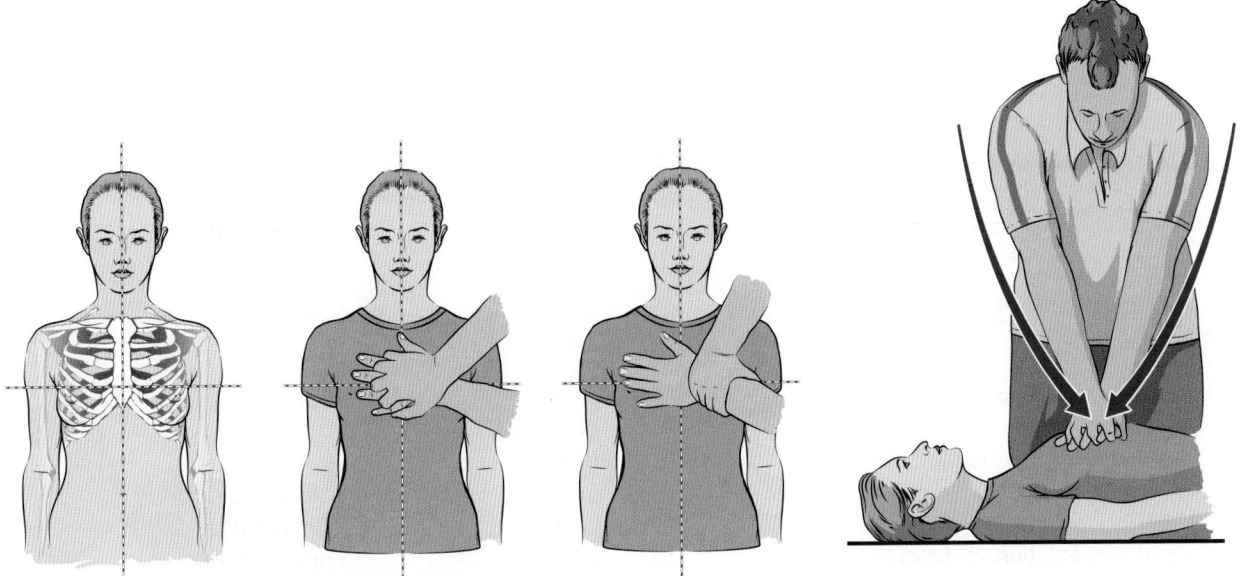

FIGURE 37-6 Hands and back positions for administering chest compressions. (EreborMountain/Shutterstock.)

Squeezing the heart between the sternum and the vertebrae increases pressure in the ventricles, which is thought to push blood into the pulmonary arteries and aorta. Chest compressions are also thought to increase pressure in thoracic blood vessels, promoting systemic blood flow. For chest compressions to be effective, the rescuer must deliver them hard and fast. Administer chest compressions before giving rescue breaths because giving rescue breaths first delays the time for circulating oxygenated blood still within arterial blood. When administering chest compressions, the chest of an adult victim should be depressed to at least 2 to 2.4 in at a rate of 100 to 120 times per minute.

The correct sequence is 30 chest compressions followed by two rescue breaths for rescuers who are able to do so, or a ratio of 30:2 (whether by one or two rescuers) for children older than 1 year of age. If there are two rescuers and the victim is younger than 1 year of age, the ratio is 15 compressions to two breaths (15:2); if the rescuer is alone, a 30:2 ratio is maintained.

Correct placement of the hands and the body is essential during chest compressions. The rescuer puts the heel of one hand over the lower half of the victim's sternum but above the xiphoid process and the other hand on top, then interlocking or extending their fingers. The rescuer positions their body over the hands to deliver a straight downward motion with each compression and to allow the chest wall to recoil afterward. The hands remain in contact with the chest, and the elbows stay locked without leaning on the chest or rocking back and forth over the victim (Fig. 37-6). If two people are available to perform compressions, one should replace the other every 2 minutes to avoid fatigue. Table 37-1 lists variations in rescue breathing and chest compressions

TABLE 37-1 Differences in Cardiopulmonary Resuscitation among Infants, Children, and Adults

TECHNIQUE	INFANT (UP TO 1 YEAR)	CHILD (1–8 YEARS)	ADULT (OVER 8 YEARS)
Compressions			
Location	In the midline, one finger width below the nipples	Center of the chest between the nipples	Center of the chest between the nipples
Hand use	Two thumbs with the hands encircling the chest for two rescuers or two fingers on the breastbone if alone	Heel of one hand with the second hand on top, or heel of one hand only	Two hands; heel of one hand with the other hand on top
Rate	100/minute	100–120/minute	100–120/minute
Depth	At least one third of the depth of the chest, about 1½ in	At least one third of the depth of the chest, about 2 in	2–2.4 in
Rescue Breaths			
Compressions only when the rescuer is untrained or trained but not proficient	One breath every 6 seconds (10/minute)	One breath every 6 seconds (10/minute)	One breath every 6 seconds (10/minute)
Ratio of compressions to ventilation until advanced airway is in place	30:2 (one rescuer)15:2 (two rescuers)	30:2 (one or two rescuers)	30:2 (one or two rescuers)
Duration	1 second with visible rise in chest	1 second with visible rise in chest	1 second with visible rise in chest

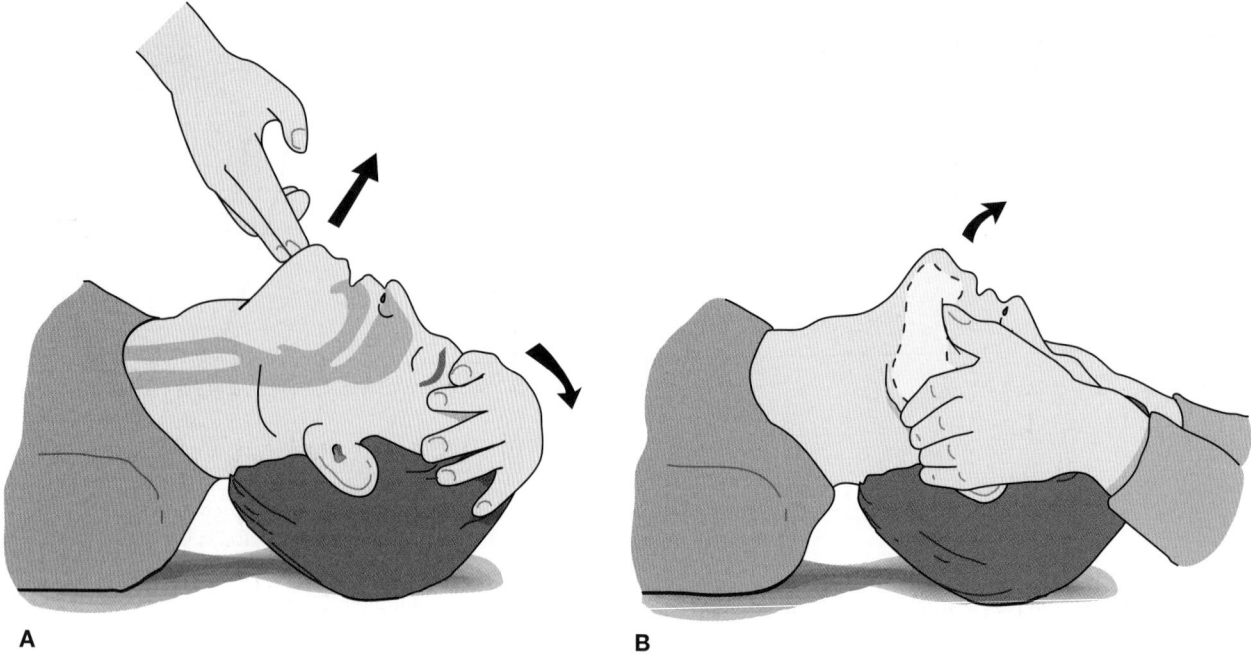

FIGURE 37-7 Techniques to open the airway. **A.** The head-tilt/chin-lift technique. **B.** The jaw-thrust technique. (From LifeART ©2016, Lippincott Williams & Wilkins. All rights reserved.)

to accommodate anatomic differences and the physiologic needs of various age groups.

Basic CPR is not interrupted for more than 10 seconds, except when:

- There is a pulse and the victim resumes breathing.
- The rescuer becomes exhausted.
- The victim's condition deteriorates despite resuscitation efforts.
- There is written evidence that resuscitation is contrary to the victim's wishes.
- ACLS measures such as defibrillation are administered.

Opening the Airway

In the absence of head or neck trauma and taking care not to twist the spine in case there is unidentified trauma, a rescuer can use the **head-tilt/chin-lift technique** (a method of choice for opening the airway; Fig. 37-7A) or the **jaw-thrust maneuver** (an alternative method for opening the airway by grasping the lower jaw and lifting it while tilting the head backward; Fig. 37-7B). The jaw-thrust maneuver is not recommended for lay rescuers because it is difficult to perform safely and may cause injury to the spine. When the airway is opened, rescuers remove any foreign material that is visible within the victim's mouth.

After opening the airway, the presence of spontaneous breathing can be determined, but minimizing hands-off time is essential. Rescuers observe for the rising and falling of the chest and listen and feel for air escaping from the nose or mouth (Fig. 37-8). A breathing victim is placed in the **recovery position** (a side-lying position that helps maintain an open airway and prevent aspiration of fluid; Fig. 37-9). If breathing is not restored within 10 seconds, the victim remains supine and CPR is continued.

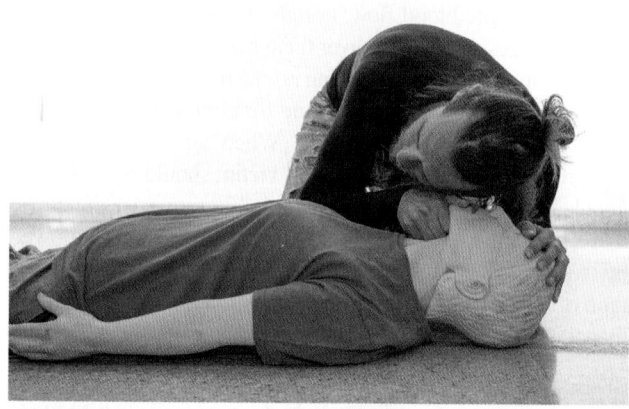

FIGURE 37-8 Listening for breathing. (R.O.M./Shutterstock.)

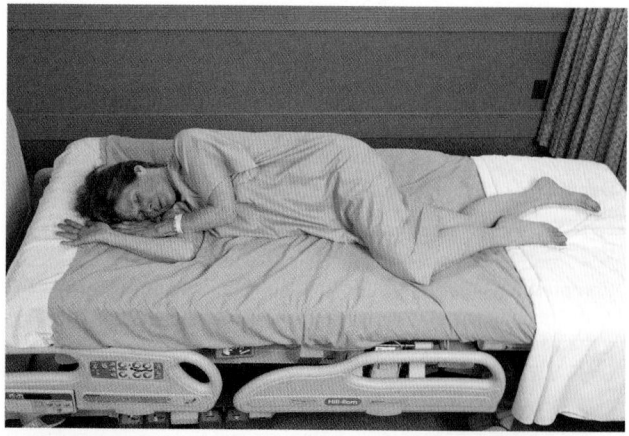

FIGURE 37-9 The recovery position is used when a client has a pulse and is breathing. (From Lynn, P. [2022]. *Taylor's clinical nursing skills* [6th ed.]. Lippincott Williams & Wilkins. Photo by B. Proud.)

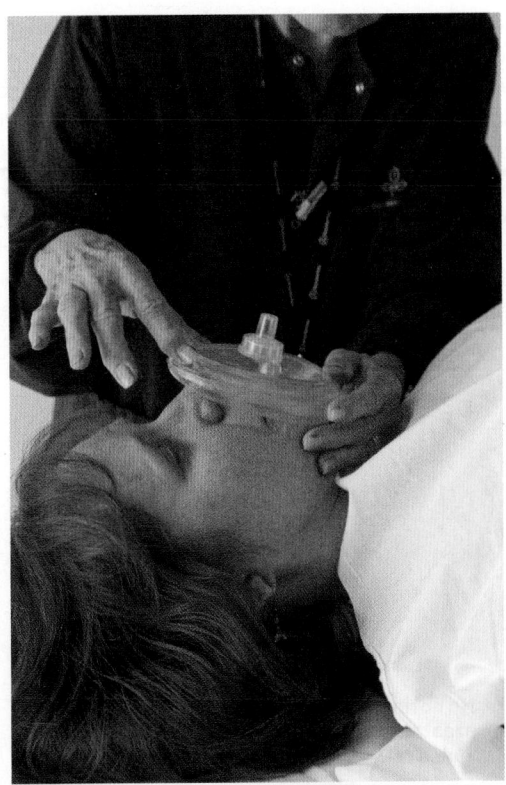

FIGURE 37-10 A mask with a one-way valve can be used in place of mouth-to-mouth rescue breathing. (From Ryan, T. A. [2023]. *Torres' patient care in imaging technology* [10th ed.]. Lippincott Williams & Wilkins.)

Performing Rescue Breathing

Rescuers who are health care providers perform **rescue breathing** (the process of ventilating the lungs) through the victim's mouth, nose, or stoma. They should use a one-way valve mask or other protective face shield if available (Fig. 37-10). These devices theoretically reduce the potential for acquiring infectious diseases; however, the lack of a barrier device should not interfere with attempting rescue breathing.

Because many lay bystanders are unwilling to perform mouth-to-mouth ventilation for fear of disease transmission, continuous chest compressions alone are better than totally avoiding efforts at resuscitation. Continuous chest compressions alone doubled to tripled the survival rates in out-of-hospital resuscitation (Bystander, 2023).

When the rescuer is trained, rescue breathing is administered at a rate of 10 breaths per minute for infants, children, and adults without a pause in chest compression. Each rescue breath should last 1 second and should cause the chest to rise visibly. Rescue breathing continues at the rate of two breaths for every 30 compressions for an adult for one or two rescuers; for children or infants, the rate is two breaths for every 30 compressions for a single trained rescuer or two breaths for every 15 compressions when administered by two trained rescuers.

Mouth-to-Mouth Breathing

In mouth-to-mouth breathing, a rescuer seals the victim's nose, uses their mouth to cover the victim's mouth, and blows air into the victim (Fig. 37-11). Giving a breath that lasts a full second reduces the potential for distending the esophagus and stomach, which may promote regurgitation and aspiration. If

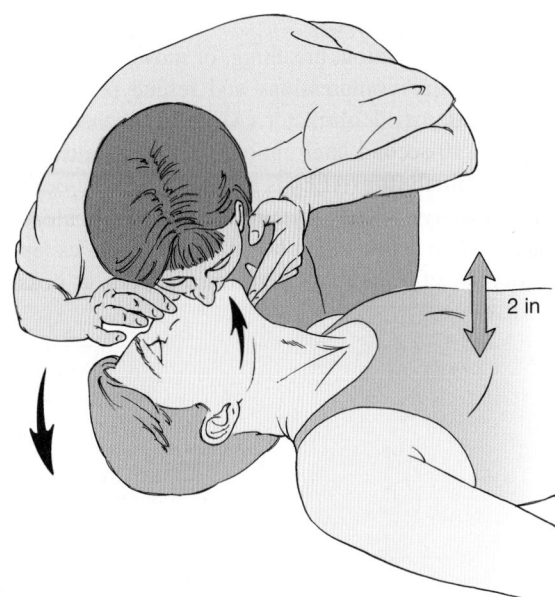

FIGURE 37-11 Mouth-to-mouth rescue breathing.

breathing is not restored, the victim remains supine, an advanced airway is placed, and rescue breathing continues at the rate of one breath every 6 seconds (10 breaths per minute) without interrupting chest compressions.

Mouth-to-Nose Breathing

Mouth-to-nose breathing is necessary when the victim is an infant or a small child or when mouth-to-mouth breathing is impossible or unsuccessful. In mouth-to-nose breathing, the rescuer closes the victim's mouth and blows air into the nose.

 Concept Mastery Alert

Mouth-to-Mouth Breathing

When performing mouth-to-nose breathing, in addition to making sure that the airway is open, be sure that the mouth is closed. Closing the mouth is crucial so that when breaths are given through the nose, the air enters the airway and does not exit through the mouth.

Mouth-to-Stoma Breathing

The rescuer can give rescue breathing to a client with a laryngectomy by sealing their mouth over the victim's stoma. Because the upper airway is essentially a blind pathway, the nose does not require sealing. For clients with a tracheostomy tube, rescue breathing is through the tube with the mouth or a one-way valve mask. If the tracheostomy tube does not have an inflated cuff, the rescuer must seal the victim's nose.

 Pharmacologic Considerations

Opioid overdose can cause a person to stop breathing. In situations where naloxone (Evzio), a single-dose autoinjector opioid antagonist, is available, it should be used. The drug injector provides visual and audio instructions on how to deliver the injection. A family member or caregiver can stimulate breathing before emergency personnel arrive.

Early Defibrillation

If there is no circulation, breathing, or movement after five cycles of cardiac compressions and rescue breathing, an automated external defibrillator (AED) is attached without exceeding a 10-second interruption in CPR. An **automated external defibrillator** (AED) is a portable, battery-operated device that analyzes heart rhythms and delivers an electrical shock to restore a functional heartbeat. With the exception of newborns, defibrillation is performed as soon as possible in victims experiencing **ventricular fibrillation**, an ineffective heart rhythm (Fig. 37-12). In children from 1 to 8 years old or who weigh less than 55 lb, the AED is best when delivering a pediatric shockable dose using pediatric pads and cables that reduce the amount of energy directed at the heart (American Heart Association, 2023).

Ideally, an AED is used as rapidly as possible. **Asystole**, the absence of any heart rhythm, quickly follows ventricular fibrillation. The survival rate of deploying the AED within

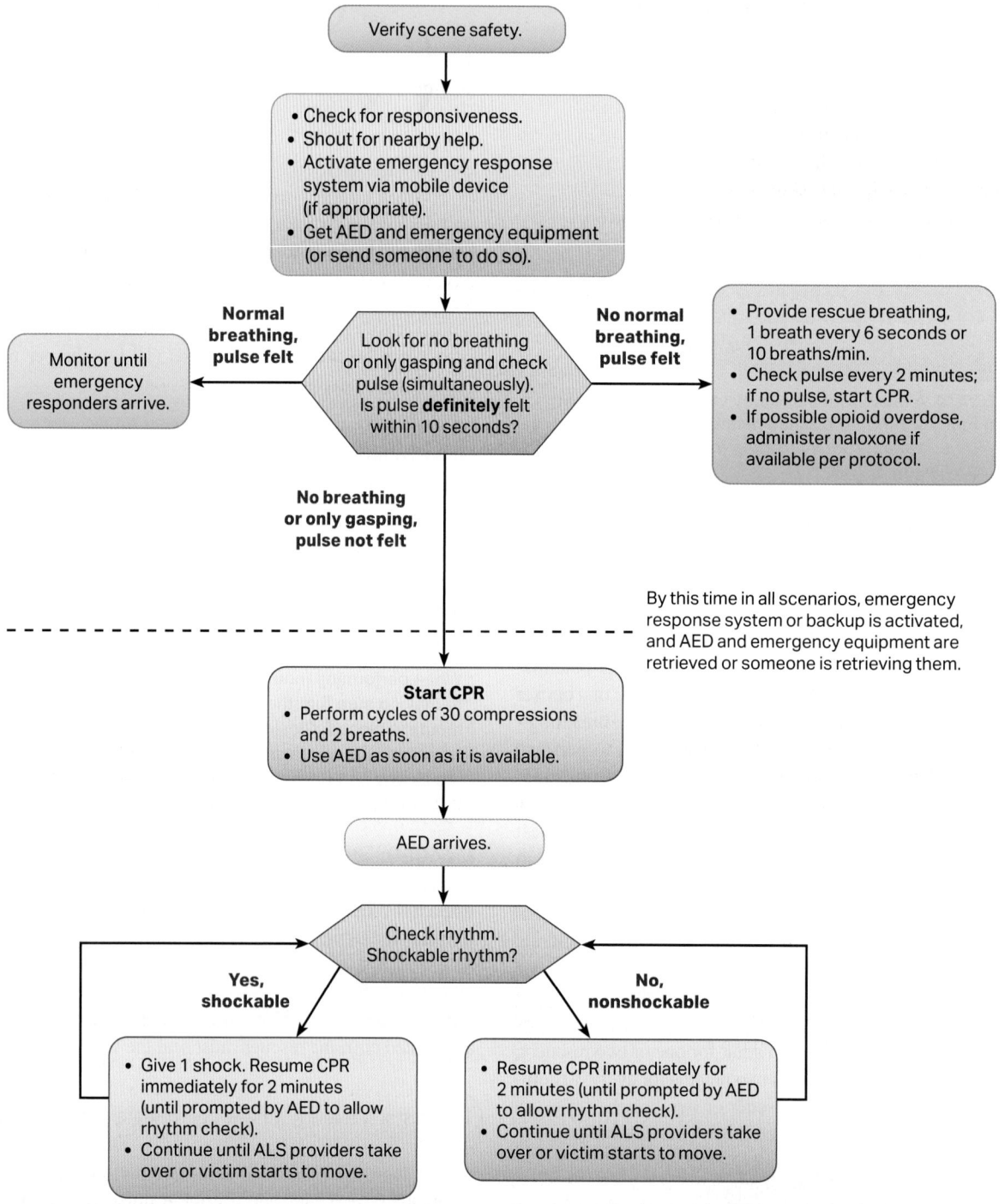

© 2020 American Heart Association

FIGURE 37-12 An algorithm for resuscitation. AED, automated external defibrillator; ALS, advanced life support; CPR, cardiopulmonary resuscitation. © 2020 American Heart Association.

1 minute of collapse is 90% and decreases to 50% if delayed by 5 minutes (AED Facts, 2023). Survival rates after cardiac arrest decrease significantly with every minute that defibrillation is delayed.

AEDs are located in many public access locations, such as schools, airports, and police stations. In addition, many businesses in the private sector have purchased AEDs to be put up throughout the company offices.

Once obtained, the user turns on the AED, so that they can observe its monitor screen. Most AEDs have pictorial instructions and the capacity to provide voice instructions.

Attaching the Electrode Pads

The rescuer attaches the preconnected electrode pads to the victim's skin (Fig. 37-13). If the monitor displays an error message, it may be because the victim's skin is diaphoretic or extremely hairy, which interferes with effective contact. The rescuer can wipe the skin with a towel, shave or clip chest hair, and apply a second set of electrode pads.

Analyzing the Rhythm

When the electrode pads are in place and the victim is motionless, the rescuer presses an analyze button on the AED or the process occurs automatically. After 5 to 15 seconds, the AED provides a message indicating that the victim needs "shock" or "no shock."

Administering a Shock

When the AED indicates "shock," the rescuer looks to make sure that no one is touching the victim. Saying "clear" or "everybody clear" in a loud voice is recommended before pressing the shock button. The AED discharges the shock, which is confirmed by the victim's sudden muscle contraction. CPR resumes immediately after the shock and continues for five cycles (approximately 2 minutes) before analyzing the rhythm again with the AED. The rescuer then facilitates another analysis of the rhythm and waits for the next message to shock or not shock. The rescuer repeats the shock, if indicated, followed by 2 minutes of CPR, and then the analysis steps again and again until the AED gives a "no shock" message, the victim begins to move, or health care providers with ACLS skills arrive to assist.

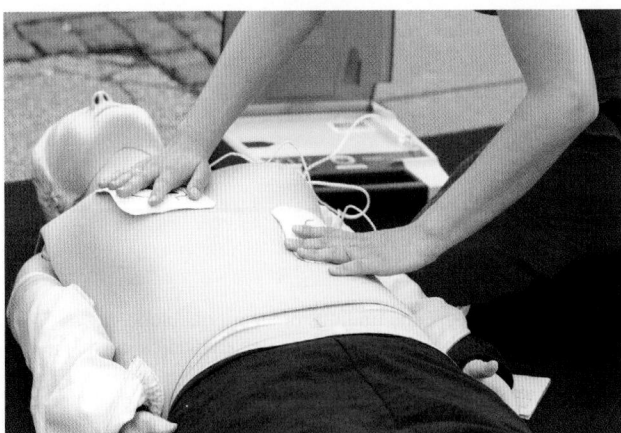

FIGURE 37-13 Applying automated external defibrillator electrodes. (wellphoto/Shutterstock.)

Continuing Cardiopulmonary Resuscitation without Defibrillation

When an AED is not available and the arrival of emergency resuscitation personnel is delayed, those trained and proficient in CPR continue at a rate of 30 compressions to two ventilations. Periodically, rescuers assess the victim to determine whether CPR is effective. They should perform an assessment initially after five cycles (2 minutes) of compressions and ventilations. An assessment for signs of spontaneous breathing can take place only by interrupting chest compressions; such interruptions should last no more than 10 seconds and preferably less. Resuscitation should continue until there are signs of movement or emergency medical personnel arrive and assume care of the victim.

Early Advanced Life Support

Emergency medical support personnel such as paramedics provide early **advanced life support**, procedures such as inserting an endotracheal tube and administering supplemental oxygen. They also carry an AED as part of their resuscitative equipment and can administer defibrillation if a public access defibrillator is unavailable. Paramedics administer emergency medications that can improve the potential for resuscitation before and during the transport of the victim to a hospital's emergency department.

Recovery from Resuscitation

When there is evidence of circulation and breathing, rescuers place the victim in a recovery position (refer to Fig. 37-9). If an AED has been used, the electrodes remain in place. Rescuers continue to monitor the victim and stand prepared to reactivate the defibrillator if the victim's condition worsens again. Once the victim is stable, rescuers evaluate their interventions and operation of the AED for quality assurance. Internal self-evaluation provides a means to improve similar resuscitation efforts in the future.

Following resuscitation, the highest available oxygen concentration is administered with a goal of reaching and maintaining a partial pressure of arterial oxygen (PaO_2) at 94% to 99% and normocarbia ($PaCO_2$) of 35 to 45 mm Hg. The resuscitated client's blood pressure is corrected to keep the systolic pressure above 90 mm Hg. Induced hypothermia may be used to reduce the client's body temperature to within a range of 89.6° to 96.8°F for at least 24 hours.

DISCONTINUING RESUSCITATION

Not every resuscitation attempt is successful. Severe neurologic deficits often result even when a victim's life is saved. Success is measured more appropriately by the victim's quality of life rather than its quantity. There often comes a time, in the absence of a "do not resuscitate" (DNR) order or advance directive, when a team must decide to discontinue both basic and advanced life support efforts. Efforts to terminate resuscitation may be supported using end-tidal carbon dioxide ($ETCO_2$), the concentration of carbon dioxide at the end of an exhaled breath. Maintaining the $ETCO_2$ measurement between 10 and 22 mm Hg during CPR signifies that compressions are being done correctly and are of high quality (Clinical Correlations, 2018). Clients who had an $ETCO_2$ of less than 10 mm Hg before, during, and after CPR were not successfully resuscitated (Clinical Correlations, 2018).

Because no clear-cut guidelines for suspending resuscitation have been established, efforts may extend for long periods. The decision in a health care facility to stop resuscitation is a medical judgment made by the physician or leader of the code. The decision to stop resuscitation efforts is often based on the time that elapsed before resuscitation was begun, the length of time that resuscitation has continued without any change in the victim's condition, the age and diagnosis of the victim, and objective data such as arterial blood gas results and electrolyte studies. Regardless of the basis for the decision, it is not made lightly, and those involved in an unsuccessful code need support from their colleagues. It has been noted that family presence during resuscitation has positive psychological value, regardless of the outcome. It is also important that a staff member supports the observers throughout the experience as well as afterward.

NURSING IMPLICATIONS

Nurses have several responsibilities associated with resuscitation. They must learn to perform basic cardiac life support measures, which include the correct use of an AED, and they must maintain their certification to do so. If nurses do not use or refresh these skills at least every 2 years, their abilities may be less than adequate. They may also support and participate in efforts to teach laypeople, both adults and children, how to perform CPR and carry out the chain of survival. Nurses must discuss advance directives (see Chapter 3) with all clients, regardless of the reason for admission to a health care agency. Honoring the client's right to participate in the decision-making process is important.

The following nursing diagnoses may be relevant in a resuscitation situation:

- Ineffective airway clearance
- Altered breathing pattern
- Impaired gas exchange
- Altered tissue perfusion

Nursing Care Plan 37-1 shows how nurses can use the steps in the nursing process for a client with altered breathing pattern, defined as having an abnormal respiratory rate and rhythm that is labored.

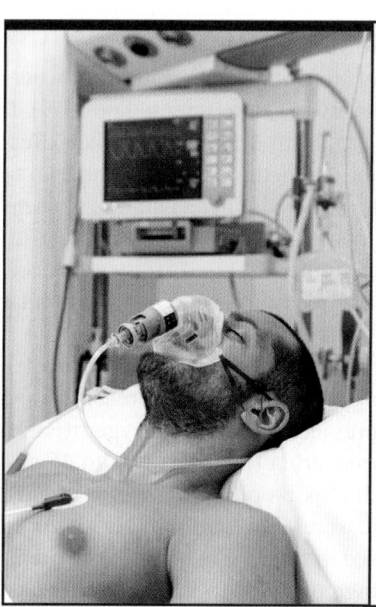

Clinical Scenario A 39-year-old male has been transferred from the emergency department to the intensive care unit (ICU) following impaired breathing that worsened at home. The client and his advance directive indicate that emergency measures are to be used in the event that his condition becomes life-threatening. He is currently receiving oxygen by mask, but the nurse anticipates that the client may require mechanical ventilation.

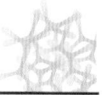

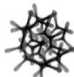

NURSING CARE PLAN 37-1   Altered Breathing Pattern

Assessment

- Monitor respiratory rate and breathing pattern.
- Observe for tachypnea, bradypnea, and periods of apnea.
- Note signs of respiratory distress such as the use of accessory muscles, sitting upright, nasal flaring, restlessness, and cyanosis.
- Ask the client if they are choking or look for the universal sign of the hand to the throat.
- Check for tachycardia.
- Apply a pulse oximeter and note the SpO_2 level.

- Obtain and analyze the findings of an arterial blood gas.
- Determine whether the client has received medication that causes respiratory depression.
- Check the cause for high—or low-pressure alarms on a mechanical ventilator; it could be malfunctioning.
- Assess the client's level of consciousness and responsiveness.
- Determine whether there is an absence of breathing, coughing, and movement.

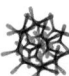

NURSING CARE PLAN 37-1 — Altered Breathing Pattern (*continued*)

Nursing Diagnosis. Risk for **altered breathing pattern**, related to progressive respiratory muscle weakness secondary to amyotrophic lateral sclerosis (Lou Gehrig disease) as manifested by shallow respirations of 32 per minute; SpO_2 of 85% with oxygen at 6 L per mask; difficulty talking and swallowing; and statement, "It has been more and more difficult for me to breathe. My doctor told me that's the usual outcome from this disease."

Expected Outcome. The client will breathe spontaneously at a ventilation rate to sustain life.

Interventions	Rationales
Maintain the client in a Fowler position.	Fowler position facilitates chest expansion by lowering abdominal organs away from the diaphragm, thus increasing the potential for a greater volume of inspired air.
Administer oxygen at 45% using a Venturi mask if a simple mask does not improve oxygenation.	A Venturi mask delivers the exact amount of prescribed oxygen; 45% oxygen is slightly double the amount of oxygen in room air; supplemental oxygen helps to relieve hypoxemia.

Interventions	Rationales
Replace the Venturi mask with a nonrebreather mask if SpO_2 falls below 80%.	A nonrebreather mask can deliver 90%–100% oxygen until the client can receive ventilation assistance.
Obtain arterial blood gas when SpO_2 is sustained below 80% for more than 10 minutes.	An arterial blood gas identifies several important measurements, such as pH of the blood, PaO_2, $PaCO_2$, and HCO_3. Findings will facilitate the subsequent medical management of the client.
Follow the chain of survival if respiratory or cardiac arrest occurs.	The chain of survival has the greatest potential for resuscitating a lifeless person.

Evaluation of Expected Outcomes

- Client continues to breathe spontaneously.
- The client's SpO_2 is 90% with 45% oxygen via a Venturi mask.

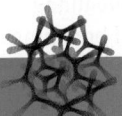

KEY POINTS

- Airway obstruction
  - Partial airway obstruction: Can speak or cough; air is being exchanged
  - Complete airway obstruction: Inability to ventilate
- Heimlich maneuver: The method for relieving a mechanical airway obstruction
  - Subdiaphragmatic thrusts: Pressure to the abdomen
  - Chest thrusts
  - Infants younger than 1 year: Administer back slaps between the shoulder blades and then chest thrusts to the middle of the breastbone, just below the nipple line.
- Chain of survival
  - Activation of emergency response
  - High-quality CPR
  - Defibrillation
  - Advanced resuscitation
  - Post–cardiac arrest care
  - Recovery
- Opening the airway
  - Head-tilt/chin-lift technique: Tilt the head and lift jaw; method of choice if feasible
  - Jaw-thrust maneuver: Grasp the lower jaw and lift it while tilting the head backward; used with suspected head or neck injuries.
- Resuscitation
  - CPR: Airway ventilation and chest compression
  - Rescue breathing: Mouth to mouth, mouth to nose
  - Compressions only (out of hospital)
- AED: A portable, battery-operated device that analyzes heart rhythms and delivers an electrical shock to restore a functional heartbeat
- Discontinuing resuscitation efforts
  - DNR order
  - A medical judgment made by the physician or leader of the code in a health care facility

CRITICAL THINKING EXERCISES

1. Arrange the following adult resuscitation steps in the correct sequence.
1. Combine compressions with ventilations at a rate of 30:2.
2. Check for breathing.
3. Activate the EMS.
4. Provide CPR for 2 minutes, reanalyze heart rhythm, and check for a pulse.
5. Open the airway.
6. Check for breathing.
7. Administer chest compressions at a rate of 100 to 120 per minute.
8. Assess responsiveness.
9. Attach an AED, and follow instructions.

2. Explain the reason that chest compressions are now initially preferable before administering rescue breathing upon finding someone who is unresponsive and not breathing normally.
3. Give a reason for the deemphasis on checking a pulse as a method for determining heart contractions on individuals who are unresponsive.
4. What criteria are used to determine whether rescue breathing is being delivered effectively?

NEXT-GENERATION NCLEX-STYLE REVIEW QUESTIONS

1. A nurse is managing care for all the following clients. For whom would the nurse most anticipate an airway obstruction?
   a. Client A, who has had a cerebral vascular accident (stroke)
   b. Client B, who has had a full mouth extraction of teeth
   c. Client C, who has had a biopsy of a tongue lesion
   d. Client D, who has had facial cosmetic surgery
   Test-Taking Strategy: Note the key word and modifier, "most anticipate." Use the process of elimination and select the option that describes a client at the highest risk for impaired swallowing.
2. Which should the nurse instruct the parents of a 6-month-old child to avoid purchasing because of the risk of accidental choking?
   a. A teething ring with gel filling
   b. A stuffed animal with button eyes
   c. A mobile with suspended objects
   d. A ball measuring 5 in in diameter
   Test-Taking Strategy: Analyze the options and select the option that is most likely to be inhaled by an infant.
3. Which is the best evidence that the nurse should implement the Heimlich maneuver to relieve an airway obstruction in a conscious person?
   a. Forceful coughing
   b. Attempts to clear throat
   c. Inability to speak
   d. Audible wheezing
   Test-Taking Strategy: Note the key word and modifier, "best evidence." Eliminate options that are characteristic of a partial airway obstruction.
4. When a person is in cardiac arrest, what is the first step the nurse takes in the chain of survival?
   a. Early CPR
   b. Early cardiac defibrillation
   c. Early activation of emergency services
   d. Early advanced life support

Test-Taking Strategy: Note the key word and modifier, "first step." Review the choices and select the option that represents the initial action when finding a person who is unresponsive.

5. Before administering the shock from an AED, what action should the nurse take first?
   a. Implement the recovery position.
   b. Loosen the victim's belt.
   c. Shout, "Everybody clear."
   d. Give three rescue breaths.
   Test-Taking Strategy: Note the key word, "before." Analyze the choices and select the option that precedes the administration of an electrical shock to the client.

NEXT-GENERATION NCLEX-STYLE CLINICAL SCENARIO QUESTIONS

Clinical Scenario:
A 39-year-old male has been transferred from the emergency department to the ICU following impaired breathing that worsened at home. The client and his advance directive indicate that emergency measures are to be used in the event that his condition becomes life-threatening. He is currently receiving oxygen by mask, but the nurse anticipates that the client may require mechanical ventilation.

1. From the following list, select the circumstances that are contributing to the client's worsening breathing.
   a. Recent ICU hospitalization for impaired breathing
   b. Oxygen use
   c. O_2 saturation at 82% room air
   d. O_2 saturation at 94% room air
   e. Advanced directives
   f. Impaired breathing at home
2. Choose the most likely option for the information missing from the following statement by selecting from the list of options provided.
   The client may not be maintain his _____1_____ on room air and may need the use of oxygen by _____2_____, or by _____3_____ if his impaired breathing symptoms worsen.

OPTION 1	OPTION 2	OPTION 3
blood pressure	nasal cannula	Venturi mask
international normalized ratio (INR)	mask	ventilator
O_2 saturation	T-piece	oxygen concentrator

UNIT 11 | Caring for the Terminally Ill

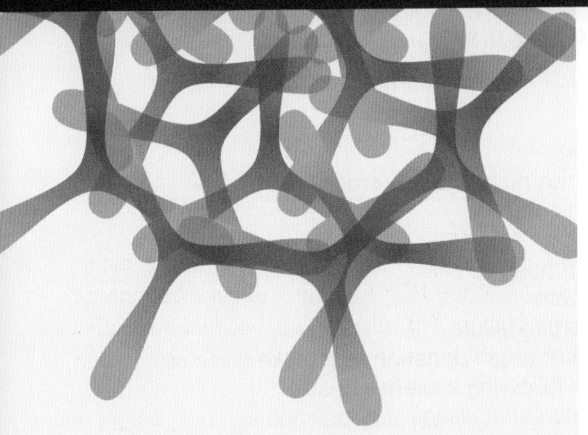

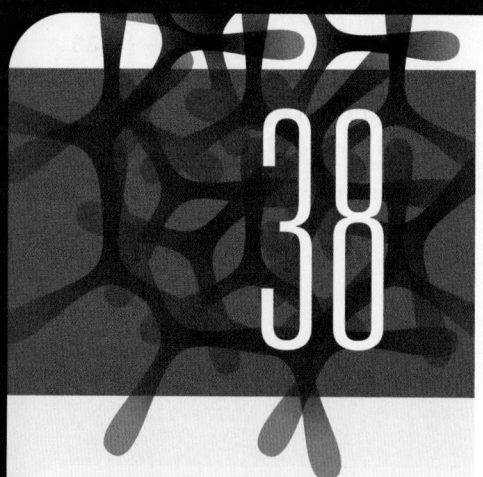

38

End-of-Life Care

Learning Objectives

On completion of this chapter, the reader should be able to:

1. Define terminal illness.
2. Name the stages of dying.
3. Describe methods by which nurses can promote the acceptance of death in dying clients.
4. Define respite care.
5. Discuss the philosophy of hospice care.
6. List aspects of terminal care.
7. Name signs of multiple organ failure.
8. Explain why a discussion of organ donation must take place as expeditiously as possible following a client's death.
9. Explain the difference between a clinical autopsy and a forensic autopsy and the manner in which postmortem care is implemented.
10. Name components of postmortem care.
11. Discuss the benefit of grieving and signs that grief is being resolved.

INTRODUCTION

There was a decrease in life expectancy, 77.0 to 76.1, in the year 2020 to 2021 in the United States, according to the Centers for Disease Control and Prevention (CDC) National Center for Health Statistics (NCHS, 2022). The United States has not seen a decline in life expectancy to this degree since 1996 (Centers for Disease Control and Prevention, 2016) (Fig. 38-1).

Nurses and other health care providers are probably more involved than any other group with people who experience impending death. This chapter deals with aspects of caring for terminally ill clients and the grieving experience for all those involved in the dying process.

 Gerontologic Considerations

■ Older adults may read obituaries and death notices in the newspaper daily in an effort to keep up with acquaintances. Although this activity may seem depressing to some, it may be an effective coping mechanism in helping develop a peaceful and accepting attitude toward death.

■ Include all older adults in as many aspects of care and decision-making as possible. The emphasis is on maintaining self-esteem and personal dignity.

■ Clients of all ages may feel that the use of machines and equipment designed to maintain life support threatens their dignity.

■ Death is an individualized experience that is highly influenced by many factors, including prior experiences, cultural practices, religious beliefs, and level of personal development. Many older adults are realistically aware of pending and inevitable death. Often, they are relieved when health care providers are comfortable discussing death with them. Older adults may benefit from counseling regarding end-of-life concerns, especially if they have a history of accepting help in coping with challenging issues.

■ Hospice services should be considered for older adults with chronic life-limiting conditions, such as dementia or heart failure.

■ Often, families and older adults are relieved when providers discuss hospice care so they can be involved in choices about the type of care they receive.

■ Nurses can encourage older adults and their families to explore these resources because they may benefit from the hospice approach to care, which includes a wide range of support services.

■ Nurses have important roles in teaching older adults about advance directives concerning their health care and identifying a person with a durable power of health care at the same time they prepare a will (see Chapter 3). These advance directives must be reviewed and updated periodically and should be accessible to all those involved in care.

■ It is not uncommon for people to develop life-threatening illnesses and die within 6 months of the death of a spouse. Encouraging older adults who have experienced the death of a close friend or family member to express feelings associated with grieving is important. Referrals for individual counseling or grief support groups are appropriate.

TERMINAL ILLNESS AND CARE

A **terminal illness** means a condition from which recovery is beyond a reasonable expectation. Such a diagnosis is devastating news. Upon learning that death is imminent, clients tend to experience several stages as they process the information.

Stages of Grief

Dr. Elisabeth Kübler-Ross (1969), a psychiatrist and authority on death and dying, established the five stages of grief (the Kübler-Ross model). These are denial, anger, bargaining, depression, and acceptance (Table 38-1). These stages, which represent a pattern of adjustment, may occur in a progressive manner, or a person can move back and forth among the stages. There is no specific time period for the rate of progression, duration, or completion of the stages.

Denial

Denial, the psychological defense mechanism by which a person refuses to believe certain information, helps people to cope initially with the reality of death. Terminally ill clients may first refuse to believe that their diagnosis is accurate. They may speculate that test results are wrong or that their reports have been confused with those of others.

Anger

Anger (the emotional response to feeling victimized) occurs because there is no way to retaliate against fate. Clients often displace their anger onto nurses, physicians, family

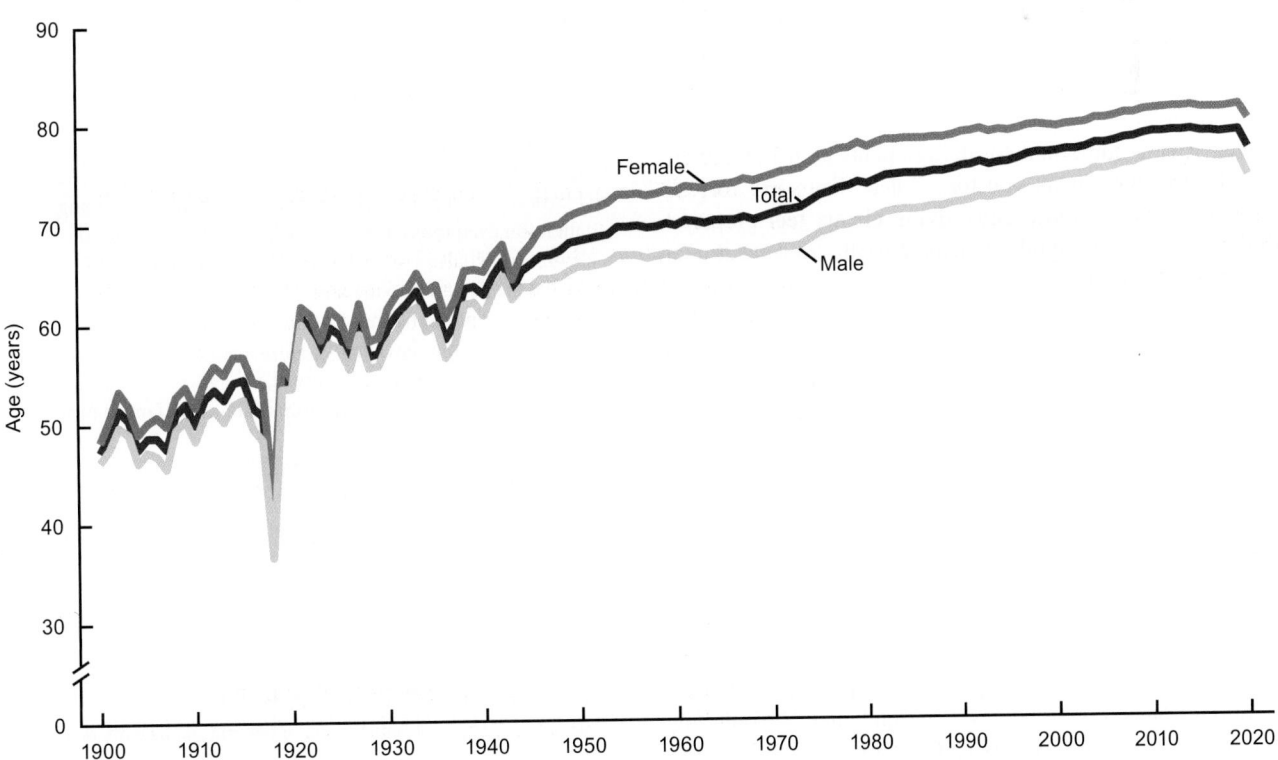

SOURCE: National Center for Health Statistics, National Vital Statistics System, Mortality.

FIGURE 38-1 U.S. life expectancy. (Arias, E., & Xu, J. Q. [2022]. United States life tables, 2020. *National Vital Statistics Reports*, *71*[1]. National Center for Health Statistics. https://doi.org/10.15620/cdc:118055.)

TABLE 38-1 Stages of Grief

STAGE	TYPICAL EMOTIONAL RESPONSE	TYPICAL COMMENT
First stage	Denial	"No, not me."
Second stage	Anger	"Why me?"
Third stage	Bargaining	"Yes, me, but if only...."
Fourth stage	Depression	"Yes, me."
Fifth stage	Acceptance	"I am ready."

members, or even a higher power. They may express anger in less than obvious ways, for example, by complaining about care or overreacting to even the slightest annoyances.

Bargaining

Bargaining, a psychological mechanism for delaying the inevitable, involves a process of negotiation, usually with God or some other higher power. Usually, dying clients have come to terms with their death but want to extend their lives temporarily until some significant event takes place (e.g., a child's wedding).

Depression

Depression (a prolonged deeply sad mood) indicates the realization that death will come sooner rather than later. The sad mood is a result of confronting potential losses.

Acceptance

Acceptance (an attitude of complacency) occurs after clients have dealt with their losses and completed unfinished business. Kübler-Ross describes unfinished business in two ways. Literally, it refers to completing legal and financial matters to provide the best security for survivors. It also refers to addressing social and spiritual matters, such as saying goodbye to loved ones and making peace with a higher power. It is as important for dying clients as it is for their families to say, "Thank you for..." and "I'm sorry for...." After tying up all loose ends, dying clients feel prepared to die. Some even happily anticipate death, viewing it as a bridge to a better dimension.

Promoting Acceptance

Nurses can help clients pass from one stage to another by providing emotional support and by supporting the client's choices concerning terminal care. Facilitating the client's directives helps maintain the client's personal dignity and locus of control.

Emotional Support

Emotional support is always part of nursing care; however, it may be more necessary for dying clients than for some other clients. Sometimes, a dying client simply wants an opportunity to express their feelings and verbally work through emotions. Nurses can act as a nonjudgmental sounding board in such instances (Nursing Guidelines 38-1).

In addition to being available for conversation, nurses provide emotional support to dying clients by acknowledging them as unique and worthwhile. **Dying with dignity**

 NURSING GUIDELINES 38-1

Helping Dying Clients Cope

- Accept the client's behavior, no matter what it is. *Doing so demonstrates respect for individuality.*
- Provide opportunities for the client to express feelings freely. *Giving such opportunities demonstrates attention to meeting individual needs.*
- Try to understand the client's feelings. *Understanding reinforces the client's uniqueness.*
- Use statements with broad openings, such as "It must be difficult for you" and "Do you want to talk about it?" *Such language encourages communication and allows the client to choose the topic or manner of response.*

means the process by which the nurse cares for dying clients with respect, no matter what their emotional, physical, or cognitive state. This process reflects the concepts stated in the Dying Patient's Bill of Rights (Box 38-1).

Arrangements for Care

Respecting the rights of dying clients includes helping them choose how and where they want to receive terminal care.

BOX 38-1 | **The Dying Person's Bill of Rights**

- I have the right to be treated as a living human being until I die.
- I have the right to maintain a sense of hopefulness, however changing its focus may be.
- I have the right to be cared for by those who can maintain a sense of hopefulness, however changing their focus might be.
- I have the right to express my feelings and emotions about my approaching death in my own way.
- I have the right to participate in decisions concerning my care.
- I have the right to expect continuing medical and nursing attention even though "cure" goals must be changed to "comfort" goals.
- I have the right not to die alone.
- I have the right to be free from pain.
- I have the right to have my questions answered honestly.
- I have the right not to be deceived.
- I have the right to have help from and for my family in accepting my death.
- I have the right to die in peace and dignity.
- I have the right to retain my individuality and not be judged for my decisions, which may be contrary to beliefs of others.
- I have the right to discuss and enlarge my religious and/or spiritual experiences, whatever these may mean to others.
- I have the right to expect that the sanctity of the human body will be respected after death.
- I have the right to be cared for by caring, sensitive, knowledgeable people who will attempt to understand my needs and will be able to gain some satisfaction in helping me face my death.

From Barbus, A. J. (1975). The dying person's bill of rights. © 1975, American Journal of Nursing Company. Reprinted with permission from the *American Journal of Nursing*, 75(1), 99. http://hdl.handle.net/10822/770449

Clients may find it comforting to prepare an advance directive (see Chapter 3). Many also appreciate learning about available settings for care. In general, clients have four choices: home care, hospice care (which may be the same as home care), residential care, and acute care.

Home Care

Many clients with terminal illnesses remain at home (Fig. 38-2). They may travel to and from a hospital or clinic for brief treatments, tests, and medical evaluations. Nurses may help coordinate community services, secure home equipment, and arrange for home nursing visits.

Because the major burden of home care often falls on a spouse, family member, or significant other, nurses who care for homebound clients periodically assess the toll this burden takes on the primary caregiver. The focus of support may shift back and forth from the client to the caregiver. **Respite care** (relief for the caregiver by a surrogate) is important because it gives the caregiver an opportunity to enjoy brief periods away from home. Nurses can encourage the caregiver to identify relatives or friends who will volunteer relief time with the client. If no one is available, short-term respite care can be arranged in an inpatient facility, hospital, or nursing home for up to 5 days each time; inpatient respite care pays 95% of the Medicare-approved amount (Medicare. gov, 2023).

Hospice and Palliative Care

The term **hospice** is used to indicate both a facility for providing the care of terminally ill clients and the concept of such care itself. The word originally derives from a place of refuge for travelers. Today's hospice movement is modeled after facilities established by Dr. Cicely Saunders in England in the late 1960s; the movement spread to the United States in the 1970s. Hospice care involves helping clients live their final days in comfort with dignity in a caring environment (Fig. 38-3, Box 38-2). In 1983, the U.S. Congress adopted the Medicare Hospice Benefits program to provide funds for hospice care (Centers for Medicare & Medicaid Services, 2023).

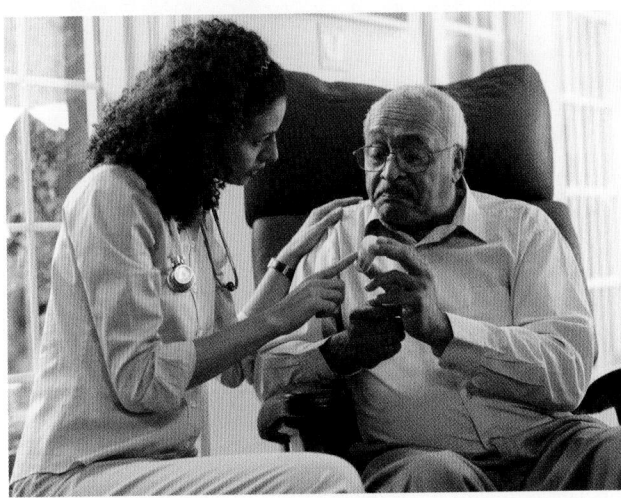

FIGURE 38-2 Home care.

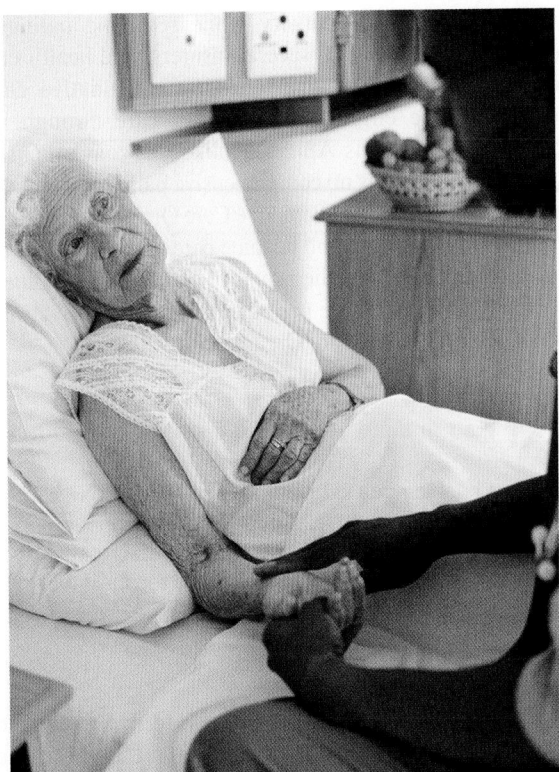

FIGURE 38-3 A hospice client and nurse.

The National Hospice Organization, now known as the *National Hospice and Palliative Care Organization*, was formed in 1978. **Palliative care** is a resource for anyone living with a serious medical illness. Patients can continue to receive curative and therapeutic care such as chemotherapy,

BOX 38-2	Medicare Home Hospice Benefits

- Hospice nurse and physician on call 24 hours a day, 7 days a week
- Hospice aide and homemaker services
- Medications for symptom control or pain relief[a]
- Medical supplies and equipment
- Physical therapy, occupational therapy, and speech-language pathology services
- Social work and counseling services for the client and caregivers
- Dietary counseling services
- Short-term respite care[a]
- Short-term inpatient care for pain and symptom management
- Grief and loss counseling for client and family
- Any other Medicare-covered services needed to manage pain and other symptoms as recommended by the hospice team

Medicare will pay for hospice care if all the following requirements are met: (1) the terminal illness is certified by a physician; (2) the client elects the hospice benefit; and (3) the hospice program is Medicare-certified.

Medicare.gov. (2023). *Hospice care.* https://www.medicare.gov/coverage/hospice-care.
[a]There may be a small copayment.

radiation, dialysis, and surgery while receiving palliative care. Medicare, Medicaid, several insurers, and health care plans will cover the medical portions of palliative care. Veterans may be eligible for palliative care through the Department of Veterans Affairs. Unlike the comprehensive hospice benefit, there is no comprehensive palliative care benefit (National Hospice and Palliative Care Organization, 2023)

Both palliative care and hospice care are focused on the needs of the patient and their quality of life, but hospice is specifically focused on the period closest to death (National Hospice and Palliative Care Organization, 2023).

 Pharmacologic Considerations

To support hospice goals, health care providers may suggest simplifying drug administration by the compounding of drugs. A drug given by the oral or parenteral route may be mixed with an agent and administered topically with the intent of systemic absorption.

Eligibility for Hospice Care

In general, clients with 6 months or less to live as certified by a physician are accepted for hospice care in the United States. If a client survives beyond 6 months, they continue to receive care as long as the physician certifies that the client continues to meet hospice criteria. While receiving hospice care, the client must accept palliative comfort care instead of care to cure the terminal illness.

 Pharmacologic Considerations

Palliative care uses medications to manage many of the symptoms experienced during the dying process. Pharmacologic symptom management treats pain, breathlessness, fatigue, anorexia, nausea, vomiting, constipation, anxiety, depression, dry mouth, and sleep disturbances.

Hospice Services

Most hospice clients receive care in their own homes. A multidisciplinary team of hospice professionals and volunteers supports care provided by the family (see Box 38-2). Hospice organizations also provide support programs for family members and significant others. They offer individual and group counseling both during and after the client's death to help survivors cope with grief.

Terminating Hospice Care

Hospice services can be terminated when (1) a client's health improves, (2) the client's illness goes into remission, or (3) the client withdraws for any reason. Once hospice care is terminated, care can be provided under the client's original Medicare coverage. However, the client can reapply for hospice care at any time if circumstances change.

Residential Care

Residential care is a form of intermediate care. Nursing homes or long-term care facilities are the usual settings for long-term subacute care. These facilities provide round-the-clock nursing care for clients who cannot live independently (Fig. 38-4). Family members have peace of mind knowing that the loved one is receiving care, and they enjoy the opportunity to visit as much as possible. Such care, however, is costly. Some purchase long-term care insurance while still healthy. Long-term care insurance helps people with chronic illnesses, disabilities, or other conditions with daily needs such as simple activities to skilled care over an extended period of time when the need becomes necessary. However, there are many variations in policies among different insurers; clients should carefully review policies pertaining to long-term care insurance.

Acute Care

A client needs **acute care** with its sophisticated technology and labor-intensive treatment if their condition is unstable (Fig. 38-5). This form of care is the most expensive. Expenses for acute care provided in the hours, days, or weeks before a client's death can be significant. Although most clients prefer to die at home, as of 2019, approximately 30% actually do so (Edwards, 2019). Many in terminal stages of a life-threatening illness die in settings where the focus is on curing and prolonging life.

Providing Terminal Care

Throughout **terminal care** and immediately before a client's death, nurses meet the client's basic physical needs for hydration, nourishment, elimination, hygiene, positioning, and comfort. Nurses implement many of the skills described throughout this text to meet the multiple problems that dying clients experience.

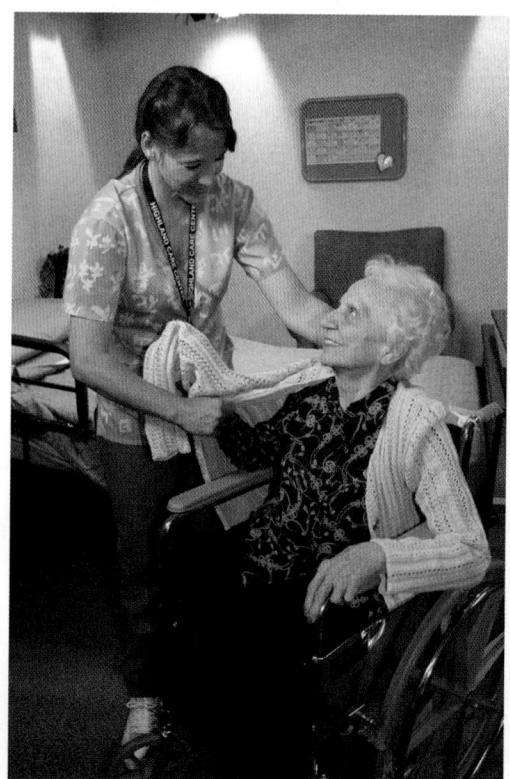

FIGURE 38-4 Residential care.

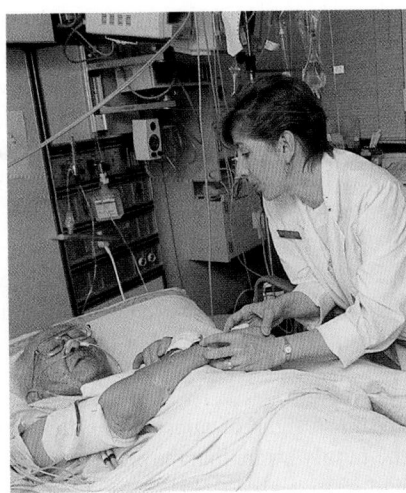

FIGURE 38-5 Acute care.

Hydration

Hydration involves the maintenance of an adequate fluid volume. If the client's swallowing reflex remains intact, the nurse offers water and other beverages frequently. As swallowing becomes impaired, the client is at risk for aspiration, followed by pneumonia. Sucking is one of the last reflexes to disappear as death approaches. Therefore, the nurse can provide a moist cloth or wrapped ice cubes for the client to suck. Some are of the opinion that avoiding parenteral fluids and allowing dehydration for someone who is actively dying may be beneficial. It may relieve choking, lessen chest congestion, decrease urine output, and reduce vomiting and diarrhea.

Nourishment

Some terminally ill clients have little interest in eating. The effort may be too exhausting, or nausea and vomiting may result. Poor nutrition can lead to weakness, infection, and other complications, such as pressure sores. A full-liquid diet may be an alternative approach to solid foods. Nausea may be controlled with rectal medications like prochlorperazine (Compazine) or ondansetron (Zofran) administered subcutaneously.

 Nutrition Notes

■ There is strong clinical, ethical, and legal support both for and against artificial nutrition and hydration when it is not clear what the individual wants or what is clinically warranted (Schwartz et al., 2021).

■ Although nutrition and hydration can maintain life, by themselves, they cannot prevent imminent death.

■ The decision to provide, withdraw, or withhold artificial nutrition and hydration includes consideration for protecting a client's right to life, not unnecessarily prolonging suffering, and the individual's and family's preferences.

Schwartz, D. B., Barrocas, A., Annetta, M. G., Stratton, K., McGinnis, C., Hardy, G., Wong, T., Arenas, D., Turon-Findley, M. P., Kliger, R. G., Corkins, K. G., Mirtallo, J., Amagai, T., Guenter, P., & ASPEN International Clinical Ethics Position Paper Update Workgroup. (2021). Ethical aspects of artificially administered nutrition and hydration: An ASPEN position paper. *Nutrition in Clinical Practice, 36*(2), 254–267. https://pubmed.ncbi.nlm.nih.gov/33616284/

Elimination

Some terminally ill clients are incontinent of urine and stool; others experience urinary retention and constipation. All these conditions are uncomfortable. A physician may order cleansing enemas or suppositories. Catheterization may also be necessary. Skin care becomes particularly important for incontinent clients because urine and stool left in contact with the skin contribute to skin breakdown and produce foul odors. If urinary or bowel incontinence is minimal, it can be managed with absorbent pads.

Hygiene

The dignity of clients is related largely to personal appearance. Therefore, nurses strive to keep dying clients clean, well groomed, and free of unpleasant odors. Frequent mouth care may be necessary. Oral suctioning helps remove mucus and saliva that the client cannot swallow or expectorate. A lateral position keeps the mouth and throat free of accumulating secretions. The lips may need periodic lubrication because they may become dried from mouth breathing or the administration of oxygen. A scopolamine transdermal patch when ordered by the physician may be applied and changed every 72 hours, or subcutaneous administration of glycopyrrolate (Robinul) may reduce oral secretions when the client is disturbed by coughing spells that interfere with sleep or worsen dyspnea.

Positioning

The lateral position helps prevent choking and aspiration. Nevertheless, the nurse may raise the client's head to improve breathing and change the client's position at least every 2 hours (as for any other client) to promote comfort and circulation.

Breathlessness

For clients who experience shortness of breath, the nurse can place the client in a high Fowler position and keep activity to a minimum. Oxygen via a nasal cannula rather than a face mask is preferable so as to avoid interfering with communication, taking oral food and fluids, or causing distress. At home, a window may be opened and/or a fan may be used.

Comfort

Relieving pain may be the most challenging problem when caring for dying clients. The goal is to keep clients free from pain, but not to dull consciousness, suppress respiration, or inhibit the ability to communicate. Most clients initially receive nonopioids for pain; later, the physician may change the drug order to a combination of a nonopioid and opioid analgesic or, eventually, a potent opioid. The physician may also change the route from oral to parenteral or transdermal (refer Chapter 20).

Analgesia may be more effective when the client receives the drug on a routine schedule. Giving pain medication regularly, such as every 4 hours or by continuous release through a transdermal patch rather than on an as-needed (prn) basis, maintains a consistent level of pain relief. The dosage will probably need to be increased because of drug tolerance (see Chapter 20).

Fear of addiction should not interfere with efforts to relieve pain. Unfortunately, nurses and physicians often misinterpret increased requests for pain medication as evidence of addiction. In reality, an increased desire for pain medication may be the result of the development of drug tolerance or an increase in pain related to disease progression.

Clients develop tolerance to the pain-relieving property of analgesic drugs; however, clients who are tolerant to opioids concomitantly develop resistance to respiratory depression, a common side effect of narcotic analgesics. Sedation generally precedes respiratory depression. Therefore, as long as the client is alert, the potential for respiratory depression is minimized. Opioid antagonists can be given for severe respiratory depression, should it develop, but the dosage must be reduced to avoid producing withdrawal symptoms and eliminating the desired analgesic state. Constipation may be a more common consequence of continuous opioid analgesia. Drugs such as naloxegol, lubiprostone, methylnaltrexone, and others are used to manage opioid-induced constipation.

 P h a r m a c o l o g i c   C o n s i d e r a t i o n s

Constipation that leads to the potential for obstruction is an uncomfortable side effect of opioid treatment in the severely ill. Typically, laxatives are used to prevent this condition. Methylnaltrexone is the first drug of its kind that blocks the opioid binding specifically on gastrointestinal tract receptors. Clients need to be monitored for opioid withdrawal symptoms when taking this drug.

Family Involvement

Family members may appreciate involvement in the client's care because they often feel helpless. Involvement tends to maintain family bonds and helps survivors cope with future grief. Many welcome the opportunity to assist. Nevertheless, nurses should not burden family members with major responsibilities.

Some terminally ill clients forestall dying when they feel that their loved ones are not yet prepared to deal with their death. This has been described as the **waiting for permission phenomenon**, because death often occurs shortly after a significant family member communicates that they are strong enough and ready to "let go." Nurses must support family members at this time because family members may feel as though they have given up and let down the loved one.

Approaching Death

As death nears, the client exhibits signs indicating a decrease and ultimately a cessation of function. As these signs appear, the nurse informs the client's family that death is approaching.

Multiple Organ Failure

The signs of approaching death are the result of **multiple organ failure** (a condition in which two or more organ systems gradually cease to function), which directly relates to the quality of cellular oxygenation. When the supply of oxygen begins to fall below the levels required to sustain life, cells, followed by tissues and organs, begin to deteriorate. The cardiovascular, pulmonary, hepatic, and renal systems are most vulnerable to failure.

As they cease to function, cells release their intracellular chemicals. Preexisting hypoxia is first complicated by a localized rather than a generalized inflammatory response (see Chapter 28) that causes the signs of multiple organ failure, heralding approaching death (Table 38-2). This process may take place gradually over hours or days.

Family Notification

As the client shows signs of approaching death, the nurse must make the family aware that the end is near. If the client is in a hospital or extended care facility, the nurse informs the physician first (Nursing Guidelines 38-2).

The physician is responsible for contacting the family and releasing that information. Sometimes, the physician delays the news until they can talk with the family in person to avoid precipitating acts such as suicide or contributing to a traffic accident.

Meeting Relatives

To promote a smooth transition, relatives of the dying client are met by the nurse who informed them. If that is not possible, another support person is designated.

Upon arrival, the nurse shows family members to a private room or area or takes them directly to the client's bedside, depending on their wishes. Privacy allows people the freedom to express feelings without social inhibitions. People have different ways of expressing grief. Some weep and sob uncontrollably; others do not. Nurses remember that those with less outward signs of grief may be feeling sorrow that is just as strong as those who cry and grieve openly.

It is important that nurses remain objective and supportive when there are cultural differences surrounding a death.

TABLE 38-2 Signs of Multiple Organ Failure	
ORGAN	**SIGNS**
Heart	Hypotension
	Irregular, weak, and rapid pulse
	Cold, clammy, and mottled skin
Liver	Internal bleeding
	Edema
	Jaundice
	Impaired digestion, distention, anorexia, nausea, and vomiting
Lungs	Dyspnea
	Accumulation of fluid ("death rattle")
Kidneys	Oliguria
	Anuria
	Pruritus (itching skin)
Brain	Fever
	Confusion and disorientation
	Hypoesthesia (reduced sensation)
	Hyporeflexia (reduced reflexes)
	Stupor
	Coma

NURSING GUIDELINES 38-2

Summoning the Family of a Dying Client

- Plan to notify the family in a timely manner. *Prompt attention allows the family to be with the client at death.*
- Check the client's medical record for the next of kin or a responsible party. *Doing so ensures that the nurse notifies someone significantly involved in the client's well-being.*
- Identify yourself by name, title, and location. *Identification provides more personal communication.*
- Ask for the family member by name. *Doing so ensures you communicate information to the appropriate person.*
- Speak in a calm and controlled voice. *Doing so conveys a serious, competent demeanor.*
- Use short sentences to provide small bits of information. *This technique helps the listener to process and comprehend the news.*
- Explain that the client's condition is deteriorating. *This explanation clarifies the purpose for the call.*
- Pause after giving the most important information. *A pause allows the family member to respond.*
- Give brief answers to questions. Emphasize the level of care that the client is receiving. *Such responses reinforce that the client is receiving appropriate care.*
- Urge family members to come as soon as possible. *This ensures the people most important to the client are there at death.*
- Document the time, the person to whom you communicated the information, and the message. *Appropriate documentation provides a permanent record.*

For example, Native American Lakota Sioux females wail loudly while the males sing mourning songs at the bedside. In some Hindu-Indian cultures, family members chant holy songs, and afterward, the body is cremated. Cremation is considered the only way a spirit can be freed (Hindu, 2023). Similarly, people from Bali, whose religion is a combination of Hinduism, Buddhism, and Islamic concepts mixed with ancient beliefs and customs, control the demonstration of emotions in the belief that their gods will not hear prayers that are offered hysterically.

Discussing Organ and Tissue Donation

Virtually anyone, from the very young to older adults, may be an organ donor. If the donor is younger than 18 years, they must sign a donor card, along with the parents or legal guardian. Age requirements and organ acceptance are determined on an individual basis at the time of death and organ procurement. Some people communicate ahead of time whether they are interested in organ donation; others do not. In either case, if the dying or dead client meets the donation criteria, the possibility of harvesting organs is considered.

Organ donation may or may not be discussed with the next of kin based on guidelines in the 2009 revision of the Uniform Anatomical Gift Act (UAGA):

1. If a dying or deceased person has a document identifying an intention to donate organs or has expressly refused organ donation, the next of kin or someone with a power of attorney for health care need not be involved.

2. If no documentation of intent is available, consent for organ donation on behalf of the client can be sought.
3. Finally, without a signed refusal, life support may not be withdrawn until the potential for organ donation is determined even if doing so contradicts a person's advance directives because life support that has the potential to save lives overrides the desire to withhold or withdraw life support (Smith, 2022).

Involving the next of kin or the person with a power of attorney for health care concerning organ donation is generally a courtesy even when it is not absolutely required. This is done delicately by an organ procurement officer. This person is trained in techniques for sensitively requesting organ donations from family members grieving the death of a loved one. The health care agency selects the person who will solicit organ donations. Typically, the facility's transplant coordinator is the organ procurement officer.

Solicitation for organ donation cannot be delayed; some organs, such as the heart and lungs, must be harvested within a few hours to ensure a successful transplant. In some cases, the client is kept on life support before removing organs. To protect the health care facility from any legal consequences, permission may be obtained in writing (Fig. 38-6).

Confirming Death

Death is generally determined on the basis that breathing and circulation have ceased. In most cases, when these criteria are met, there is no question that the person is dead. Legally, a physician, physician's assistant, medical examiner, or coroner is responsible for pronouncing a client dead; in 20 states, nurses are authorized to do so (RegisteredNursing.org, 2024).

Brain Death

In some situations involving irreversible brain damage, a mechanical ventilator can sustain breathing and circulation that continues reflexively.

Brain death is considered to have occurred when all functions of the entire brain, including the brainstem, have irreversibly ceased (Nair-Collins, 2023). Subsequently, the irreversible cessation of circulatory and respiratory functions or a cessation of all brain functions is considered the most incontestable criterion for establishing whether a person is dead or alive. Based on guidelines set by the American Academy of Neurology (2023), irreversible brain death is considered to be present if, in the absence of hypothermia, central nervous system depressants, or conditions that may simulate brain death, there is:

- A lack of all evidence of responsiveness
- Absence of brainstem reflexes such as pupillary response in both eyes, ocular movements, corneal reflex, facial muscle movement to a noxious stimulus, and pharyngeal and tracheal reflexes
- Absence of breathing drive after disconnection from the ventilator, no respiratory movements for 8 to 10 minutes, and repeated again for 10 to 15 minutes after being adequately preoxygenated

Organ Procurement Agency of Michigan

Subsidiary Of
TRANSPLANTATION SOCIETY OF MICHIGAN
2203 Platt Road, Ann Arbor, Michigan 48104

1-800-482-4881   (313) 973-1577   Detroit—464-7988

ANATOMICAL GIFT DONATION STATEMENT

I understand that in the present state of medical practice, several organs and tissues are being removed from persons who have died unexpectedly, and are being used for transplantation to living persons or for medical or scientific research. I understand that organs are removed after my relative has died, and before the organs suffer any damage, (usually within eight [8] hours) and that this gift authorizes all examinations of the body which are necessary to assure the medical acceptability of the gift.

I appreciate the benefits that come from organ donation and also understand the criteria used in determining death in the case of decedent. I am the surviving:

(1) _____ Spouse
(2) _____ Adult son or daughter
(3) _____ Mother or Father
(4) _____ Adult brother or sister
(5) _____ Guardian of the patient at the time of death
(6) _____ Other person authorized or obligated to
            dispose of the body

_____
                    Relationship

Relatives or persons in a class before my class are not available to sign this form (or have already signed such a form). I have no knowledge that during his or her lifetime the decedent, _____, was opposed to or said things against making an anatomical gift or organ donation such as the one described below. I do not know of any relative or person in a class before mine who is opposed to this gift, nor do I know of any person in the same class as myself who is opposed to this gift.

I hereby make the following anatomical gift from the body of
_____:
( ) Any needed organs or parts, or
( ) Only the following organs or parts:

_____
     (Please specify the organ(s) or part(s))
The specified organ(s) and/or part(s) may be used for any of the purposes allowed by law, i.e. transplantation, therapy, medical research and education.

WITNESSES:

_____   _____
                                            Name

_____   _____
                                          Relation

                                 _____
                                            Date

FIGURE 38-6 An organ procurement form.

Following the determination of brain death, an organ procurement organization is contacted. If the deceased has not provided evidence of a desire for organ donation or the next of kin refuses, the physician issues a death certificate and obtains written permission for an autopsy if one is desirable.

Death Certificate

A **death certificate** (a legal document attesting that the person named on the form has been found dead) also indicates the presumptive cause of the person's death. Death certificates are sent to local health departments that use the information to compile mortality statistics. The statistics are important in identifying trends, needs, and problems in the fields of health and medicine.

The **mortician** (the person who prepares the body for burial or cremation) is responsible for filing the death certificate with the proper authorities. The death certificate also carries the mortician's signature and, in some states, their license number.

Permission for Autopsy

A **clinical autopsy** is an examination of the organs and tissues of a human body after death. It is not necessary after all deaths, but it is useful for determining more conclusively the cause of death. The findings may affect the medical care of blood relatives who may be at risk for a similar disorder, or the results may contribute to medical science. It is usually the physician's responsibility to obtain permission for an autopsy.

Deaths that are seemingly unnatural or suspicious may fall under the jurisdiction of a **medical examiner**, a physician who has specialized training in forensic pathology. Instead of a medical examiner, there may be a **coroner**, a public official who does not necessarily have a medical background. Both have legal authority to investigate deaths that may not be the result of natural causes (Box 38-3) and order a forensic autopsy to investigate a death. A **forensic autopsy** is a medico-legal examination to determine whether a crime has been committed. A forensic autopsy does not require permission from the next of kin.

Performing Postmortem Care

Postmortem care (care of the body after death) involves cleaning and preparing the body to enhance its appearance during viewing at the funeral home, ensuring proper identification, and releasing the body to mortuary personnel (Skill 38-1).

> ### ≫ *Stop, Think, and Respond 38-1*
> *Discuss nursing activities that demonstrate dignity and respect for the dead person's body.*

Deaths that are seemingly unnatural or suspicious generally involve an examination of the external and internal components of the body. Consequently, intravenous needles and lines, endotracheal and gastrointestinal tubes, drains, and airways must remain with the body. They should be firmly taped or secured to avoid the risk of leaking or injuring the examiner. The body is not washed—even if soiled or bloody—to avoid removing evidence.

GRIEVING

Grieving means the process of feeling acute sorrow over a loss. It is a painful experience, but it helps survivors resolve the loss. Some people experience **anticipatory grieving**, or grieving that begins before the loss occurs. The longer people have to anticipate a loss, the sooner they eventually resolve it. **Grief work** (activities involved in grieving) includes participating in the burial rituals common to a culture. Although such rituals differ, the **grief response** (the psychological and physical phenomena experienced by those grieving) is universal. Psychological reactions are commonly identified as the stages of grief:

- Shock and disbelief: the refusal to accept that a loved one is about to die or has died
- Developing awareness: the physical and emotional responses such as feeling sick, sad, empty, or angry
- Restitution period: a recognition of the loss
- Idealization: an exaggeration of the good qualities of the deceased

Some survivors may say they have **paranormal experiences** (experiences outside scientific explanation), such as seeing, hearing, or feeling the continued presence of the deceased. The nurse needs to be supportive and nonjudgmental of the survivor, validating the individual's beliefs.

Survivors feel physical symptoms more acutely immediately after the death of a loved one. Some grieving people report symptoms such as anorexia, tightness in the chest and throat, difficulty breathing, lack of strength, and sleep disturbances. No identifiable pathologic state other than grief can explain these symptoms.

Pathologic Grief

With **pathologic grief**, also called *dysfunctional grief*, a person cannot accept someone's death. Sometimes, people manifest pathologic grief by unusual or morbid behaviors. For example, survivors may keep the possessions of a deceased loved one exactly as they were at the time of death for a prolonged period. Others may attempt to contact the deceased supernaturally. In rare instances, survivors may keep a corpse in the home for an extended period after death.

Resolution of Grief

Mourning takes longer for some than for others; there is no standard length of time for "normal" grieving. One sign that a person is resolving their grief is an ability to talk about the dead person without becoming emotionally overwhelmed. Another sign is that the grieving person describes the good and bad qualities of the deceased.

BOX 38-3	Examples of Deaths Reportable to Medical Examiner

- Sudden while in apparent good health
- Criminally violent such as a homicide
- Suicide suspicious or in unusual circumstances
- While in police custody
- While in prison
- Criminal abortion
- Potential threat to public health

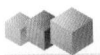 **Concept Mastery Alert**

Grieving Time Frames

People often ask about what is considered the normal time frame for someone to resolve their grief. They are seeking information, not advice. The answer is that there is no specific time frame for what is considered normal. If a person is still unable to talk about the deceased person without becoming overly emotional even after a year, then that is considered normal for this person.

NURSING IMPLICATIONS

Nurses who care for dying clients, their family members, and their friends may identify many different nursing diagnoses:

- Acute (or chronic) pain
- Impaired comfort
- Fear
- Psychosocial/spiritual needs
- Coping impairment

- Grief
- Caregiver fatigue
- Death anxiety

Nursing Care Plan 38-1 applies the nursing process to the care of a client with a nursing diagnosis of death anxiety, defined as fear of death or terminal illness, fear of the unknown of what occurs after death, and fear of the pain and suffering that can accompany death.

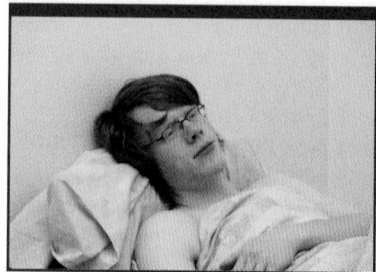

Clinical Scenario A 29-year-old male with acquired immunodeficiency syndrome (AIDS) has been hospitalized with respiratory symptoms. He has been treated for pneumocystis pneumonia several times in the past but has developed it again. Other than his partner, he has neither family nor friends for support. He is torn between treating his current respiratory illness and choosing palliative care. He feels he will eventually die an early death with or without treatment.

 NURSING CARE PLAN 38-1 **Death Anxiety**

Assessment

- Monitor the client's physical manifestations such as loss of appetite, weight loss, fatigue, and sleep disturbances.
- Observe behavioral manifestations such as reduced motivation, passivity, neglect of hygiene, withdrawal, reduced verbal interaction, and disinterest in the future.
- Observe emotional manifestations such as feelings of helplessness, apathy, sadness, defeat, and abandonment.

- Observe cognitive manifestations such as suicidal ideation, decreased attention and concentration, illogical thinking, decreased ability to process or integrate information, and fixation on loss(es).
- Listen for verbal cues that suggest despair, resignation, and surrender.

Nursing Diagnosis. Death anxiety related to psychological distress over the development of AIDS-related complication (*Pneumocystis carinii* pneumonia) as manifested by little eye contact during interaction, staring out of window, and the statement, "It doesn't matter what's done or not done anymore. One of these days you won't be able to stop the infections," and partner's statement, "I'm afraid he'll just stop eating and taking his medications."

Expected Outcome. The client and partner will identify emotions and fears regarding death and will use effective coping mechanisms and sources of support.

Interventions	Rationales
Reinforce at appropriate times that drug therapy can cure the pneumonia and control the primary illness indefinitely.	Remaining compliant with drug therapy reduces the potential for drug resistance and extends survival.
Share normal as well as abnormal findings after periodic physical examinations or laboratory tests.	Sharing positive information may encourage the client to believe in the likelihood for an improved health status.
Provide active listening and answer questions honestly.	Practicing active listening skills creates a safe space for the client to express themselves openly.
Assess the client and significant other for the stage of grief currently being experienced.	Knowledge about the grieving process reinforces the normality of feelings and or reactions being experienced and can help the client deal more effectively with them.

Evaluation of Expected Outcomes

- The client identifies effective coping mechanisms evidence, to encourage support for him and his partner.
- Client verbalizes understanding of the stages of grief and loss and discusses conflicts and feelings related to illness and death.

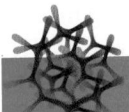

KEY POINTS

- Terminal illness: A condition from which recovery is beyond reasonable expectations
- Kübler-Ross's stages of dying:
  - Denial
  - Anger
  - Bargaining
  - Depression
  - Acceptance
- Dying with dignity: The process that includes the nurse caring for dying clients with respect, no matter what their emotional, physical, or cognitive state
- Arrangements for care
  - Home care: Terminally ill client remains at home with care from family and outside services
  - Respite care: Relief for the caregiver by a surrogate if a terminally ill client remains at home
  - Hospice: Providing care for terminally ill clients either at home or in a facility
  - Palliative care: Providing relief from distressing symptoms, easing pain, and enhancing quality of life
- Multiple organ failure: A sign of approaching death in which two or more organ systems gradually cease to function
- Brain death: A condition in which there is an irreversible loss of function of the whole brain, including the brainstem
- Deaths reportable to medical examiner
  - Sudden while in apparent good health

- Criminally violent such as a homicide
- Suicide suspicious or in unusual circumstances
- While in police custody
- While in prison
- Criminal abortion
- Potential threat to public health
- Postmortem care: Care of the body after death, involves cleaning and preparing the body to enhance its appearance during viewing at the funeral home, ensuring proper identification, and releasing the body to mortuary personnel
- Grieving: The process of feeling acute sorrow over a loss
  - Anticipatory grieving: Begins before the loss occurs; the longer people have to anticipate a loss, the sooner they eventually resolve it
  - Grief work: Activities involved in grieving; includes participating in the burial rituals common to a culture
  - Grief response: The psychological and physical phenomena experienced by those grieving
  - Pathologic grief: Dysfunctional grief; a person cannot accept someone's death
  - Stages of grief
    - Shock and disbelief
    - Developing awareness
    - Restitution period
    - Idealization

CRITICAL THINKING EXERCISES

1. Does being maintained on life support equipment contradict the right to die in peace and dignity (see section "The Dying Person's Bill of Rights")?
2. Select a right from the Dying Person's Bill of Rights and explain how it might be violated. How can nurses protect this right?
3. What qualities would be helpful for someone who is an organ procurement officer?
4. How is grieving over an unexpected death different than grieving the death of a person suffering from a prolonged illness or disorder?

NEXT-GENERATION NCLEX-STYLE REVIEW QUESTIONS

1. When the nurse cares for a client with no hope of recovery, which is the most conclusive criterion for declaring the person brain dead?
   a. A lack of response to verbal stimulation
   b. Urine output less than 100 mL/24 hours
   c. No spontaneous respiratory efforts
   d. Unequal pupils in response to light

Test-Taking Strategy: Note the key word and modifier, "most conclusive." Select the option that corresponds with evidence-based criteria for establishing brain death.

2. Place the stages of grief in order as identified by Dr. Elisabeth Kübler-Ross.
   a. Depression
   b. Anger
   c. Acceptance
   d. Denial
   e. Bargaining

Test-Taking Strategy: Recall the common sequence of behaviors that dying clients experience initially until the final terminal stage.

3. Which statement by a terminally ill client indicates the client is in the bargaining stage?
   a. "There must be some mistake in the pathology report."
   b. "If I can just live until my son graduates, I won't ask for anything else."
   c. "I don't know why I would deserve to die at such a young age."
   d. "I hope my death comes quickly; I'm ready to go."

Test-Taking Strategy: Note the key word and modifier, "best evidence." Use the process of elimination to select the one that corresponds with bargaining.

4. When a terminally ill client refuses to eat or drink, what nursing measures can be independently implemented? Select all that apply.

    a. Inserting a nasogastric feeding tube

    b. Providing frequent oral hygiene measures

    c. Humidifying the room air

    d. Offering hard candies periodically

    e. Administering intravenous fluids

Test-Taking Strategy: Note the key word, "independently." Use the process of elimination to exclude options that require collaboration with a physician.

5. When a client has died, under what circumstance can health care providers proceed with the protocol for harvesting organs for transplantation?

    a. The deceased client has a document indicating their desire to be an organ donor.

    b. The nursing supervisor believes the deceased has suitable organs for transplantation.

    c. The deceased client has died of homicide or suicide rather than natural causes.

    d. The physician has declared and documented the client's time of death.

Test-Taking Strategy: Eliminate any statements that contradict the criteria for donation of organs and tissue.

NEXT-GENERATION NCLEX-STYLE CLINICAL SCENARIO QUESTIONS

Clinical Scenario:

A 29-year-old male with AIDS has been hospitalized with respiratory symptoms. He has been treated for pneumocystis pneumonia several times in the past but has developed it again. Other than his partner, he has neither family nor friends for support. He is torn between treating his current respiratory illness and choosing palliative care. He feels he will eventually die an early death with or without treatment.

1. Select all of the indicators that may be a cause for concern regarding the client's nursing diagnosis of death anxiety.

    a. Medical diagnosis of AIDS

    b. Current hospitalization for pneumocystis pneumonia

    c. No support of friends and family

    d. Choosing to be placed on palliative care

    e. Treating his respiratory illness

    f. Normal physical examination

    g. Normal blood tests

2. Place an X under "effective" identifying interventions that would help the client cope with his anxiety of dying. Place an X under "ineffective" identifying interventions that would be ineffective in helping him cope.

INTERVENTIONS	EFFECTIVE	INEFFECTIVE
Promote reduction of stress through relaxation techniques.		
Encourage the asking of questions to prevent misconceptions or assumptions.		
Promote the identification and use of positive and effective coping mechanisms.		
Give client pamphlets on AIDS and human immunodeficiency virus (HIV).		
Collaborate with social services for palliative care as appropriate.		

SKILL 38-1 Performing Postmortem Care

Suggested Action	Reason for Action
ASSESSMENT	
Determine that the client is dead by assessing breathing and circulation.	Confirms that the client is lifeless in all but cases in which life support equipment is used
Determine whether the physician and family have been notified.	Establishes the chain of communication
Ensure that a person of authority has pronounced the death.	Authority to pronounce a death may vary among states
Notify the nursing supervisor and switchboard of the client's death.	Makes others aware of a change in the client's status
Check the medical record for the name of the mortuary where the body will be taken.	Facilitates collaboration
PLANNING	
Inform mortuary personnel that the family has chosen them to manage the burial.	Communicates a need for services
Ask when to expect mortuary personnel.	Facilitates efficient time management
Contact any individuals involved in organ procurement.	Promotes the timely harvesting of organs
Obtain a postmortem kit or supplies for cleaning, wrapping, and identifying the body if there will be a delay in transport to a mortuary.	Promotes organization when preparing a body that will be temporarily held in the **morgue** (an area where bodies of dead persons are temporarily held or examined)
IMPLEMENTATION	
Pull the curtains around the bed and close the room door.	Ensures privacy
Put on gloves and personal protective garments as deemed necessary.	Follows standard precautions
Place the body supine with the arms extended at the sides or folded over the abdomen.	Prevents skin discoloration in areas that will be visible in a casket
Remove all medical equipment[a] such as intravenous catheters, urinary catheters, and dressings unless this is a case for the medical examiner or coroner.	Eliminates unnecessary equipment, except what may be required for a forensic autopsy
Remove hairpins or clips.	Prevents accidental trauma to the face
Close the eyelids.	Ensures that eyes will close when the body is prepared
Replace or keep dentures in the mouth.	Maintains the natural contour of the face
Place a small rolled towel beneath the chin to close the mouth.	Promotes a natural appearance
Cleanse secretions and drainage from the skin unless a forensic autopsy will be performed.	Ensures the delivery of a hygienic body or protects evidence
Apply one or more disposable pads between the legs and under the buttocks.	Absorbs urine or stool should they escape
Attach an identification tag to the ankle or wrist; pad the wrist first if it is used.	Facilitates the accurate identification of the body; prevents damage to tissue that will be visible
Wrap the body in a paper **shroud** (a covering for the body); cover the body with a sheet.	Demonstrates respect for the dignity of the deceased person
Tidy the bedside area; dispose of soiled equipment.	Follows the principles of medical asepsis
Remove gloves and wash your hands.	Removes colonizing microorganisms
Leave the room and close the door, or transport the body to the morgue (see figure).	Provides a temporary location for the body until mortuary personnel arrive

A morgue cart. (Photo by B. Proud.)

(continued)

SKILL 38-1 Performing Postmortem Care (*continued*)

Suggested Action	Reason for Action
Make an inventory of valuables and send them to an administrative office for placement in a safe.	Ensures the safekeeping and accountability for valuables until a family member can claim them
Notify housekeeping after the body is removed from the room.	Facilitates cleaning and the preparation for another admission

EVALUATION

- The body is cleaned and prepared appropriately for family viewing or left undisturbed for a forensic autopsy.
- The body is transferred to the morgue or mortuary personnel.

DOCUMENT

- Assessments that indicate the client is dead
- Time of death
- People notified of death
- Care of the body
- Time body is transported to the morgue or transferred to mortuary personnel

SAMPLE DOCUMENTATION

Date and Time No breathing noted and no pulse at 1400. Dr. Williams notified at 1415. Dr. Williams pronounced death and called client's wife. Foster's Funeral Home notified. Mortuary personnel unavailable until 1800. Postmortem care provided. Body transported to morgue after wife and children departed. _____ J. Doe, LPN

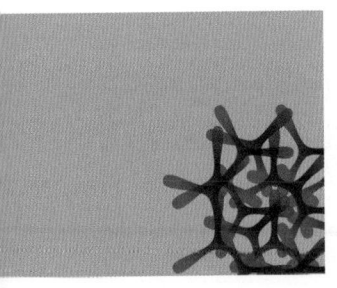

References and Suggested Readings

CHAPTER 1

AACN Fact Sheet-Nursing. (2022). www.aacnnursing.org

American Association of Colleges of Nursing. (2023). *AACN finds slow enrollment growth at schools of nursing.* From https://www.aacnnursing.org/news-data/all-news/new-data-show-enrollment-declines-in-schools-of-nursing-raising-concerns-about-the-nations-nursing-workforce

American Association of Colleges of Nursing. (2024). *Scholarships and Financial Aid.* From https://www.aacnnursing.org/students/scholarships-financial-aid

American Association of Colleges of Nursing. (2022). *Nursing shortage.* From https://www.aacnnursing.org/Portals/0/PDFs/Fact-Sheets/Nursing-Shortage-Factsheet.pdf

American Nurses Association. (2010). *Nursing: A social policy statement* (3rd ed.). Author.

American Nurses Association, & National Council of State Boards of Nursing. (2019). *Joint statement on delegation.* From https://www.nursingworld.org/practice-policy/nursing-excellence/official-position-statements/id/joint-statement-on-delegation-by-ANA-and-NCSBN/

ATrain Education. (n.d.). *The history of nurse practice acts.* Retrieved February 19, 2015, from https://www.atrainceu.com/course-module/2011915-110_florida-laws-and-rules-module-01

Barrow, J. M., & Sharma, S. (2023). *Five Rights of Nursing Delegation.* https://www.ncbi.nlm.nih.gov/books/NBK519519/

Biennial Survey of Schools of Nursing. (2018). *Percentage of enrolled students by program type, 2018.* From https://www.nln.org/news/research-statistics/newsroomnursing-education-statistics/biennial-survey-of-schools-of-nursing-academic-year-2017-2018-a1ac-c95c-7836-6c70-9642-ff00005f0421

Bureau of Labor Statistics, & U.S. Department of Labor. (2013). *Occupational outlook handbook, 2014–2015 edition, occupational employment and wages, May 2013.* Retrieved February 17, 2015, from http://www.bls.gov/oes/current/oes292061.htm

Bureau of Labor Statistics, & U.S. Department of Labor. (2014). *Occupational outlook handbook, 2014–2015 edition, licensed practical and licensed vocational nurses.* Retrieved February 17, 2015, from http://www.bls.gov/ooh/healthcare/licensed-practical-and-licensed-vocational-nurses.htm

Council of Economic Advisors. (2014). *The fifth anniversary of the American Recovery and Reinvestment Act.* Retrieved February 22, 2015, from https://www.whitehouse.gov/blog/2014/02/17/fifth-anniversary-american-recovery-and-reinvestment-act

Donahue, M. P. (1985). *Nursing: The finest art.* Mosby.

Egenes, K. J. (2009). *Nursing during the U.S. civil war: A movement toward the professionalization of nursing.* Retrieved February 17, 2015, from https://hekint.org/2017/02/24/nursing-during-the-us-civil-war-a-movement-toward-the-professionalization-of-nursing-2/#:~:text=Nursing%20during%20the%20US%20Civil%20War%3A%20a,toward%20the%20professionalization%20of%20nursing&text=At%20the%20outbreak%20of%20the,a%20typical%20feminine%20role%20assignment.&text=Another%20group%20interested%20in%20the,the%20Army%20physicians%20and%20surgeons

Egenes, K. J. (n.d.). *History of nursing.* Retrieved February 17, 2015, from http://www.jblearning.com/samples/0763752258/52258_CH01_roux.pdf

Exam Statistics & Publications. https://www.ncsbn.org/exams/exam-statistics-and-publications.page

Harrington, N., & Terry, D. L. (2013). *LPN to RN transitions, achieving success in your new role.* Lippincott Williams & Wilkins.

Health Resources and Services Administration. (2020). *HRSA requests information on the Nurse Faculty Loan Program.* aacnnursing.org

Hill, S. S., & Howlett, H. S. (2012). *Success in practical/vocational nursing: From student to leader* (7th ed.). Saunders.

Johnston, D. F. (1966). *History and trends of practical nursing.* Mosby.

Kaiser Family Foundation. (n.d.). *Breaking a 10-year streak, the number of uninsured Americans rises.* https://khn.org/news/number-of-americans-without-insurance-rises-in-2018/

Kaufman KA. Findings from the Annual Survey of Schools of Nursing academic year 2010-2011: NLN survey finds unremitting demand for entry into programs while student demographics continue to shift. *Nursing Education Perspectives.* July-August 2012;33(4):281-2. PMID: 22916636.

Lindell, A. (2015). *The graying of nurse educators, how to revive a declining field.* Retrieved March 1, 2015, from http://nursing.advanceweb.com/Archives/Article/The-Graying-of-Nurse-Educators.aspx

Masters, K. (2011). *Nursing theories: A framework for professional practice.* Saunders.

NAPNES. https://napnes.org/drupal-7.4/index.php

National Council of State Boards of Nursing. (2015). *Exam statistics & publications.* Retrieved February 18, 2015, from http://www.ncsbn.org/exam-statistics-and-publications.htm

National Council of State Boards of Nursing. (2018). *2018 NCLEX examination statistics.* Retrieved from https://www.ncsbn.org/publications/2018-NCLEX-Examination-Statistics

National League for Nursing. (2013b). *Recognizing the vital contributions of the licensed practical/vocational nurse.* From https://www.nln.org/detail-pages/resource/Reflection-Dialogue-8-Recognizing-the-Vital-Contributions-of-the-Licensed-Practical-Vocational-Nurse-September-2011

National League for Nursing. (2014). *Percentage of qualified applications that were rejected by program type, 2014.* From https://www.nln.org/news/research-statistics/newsroomnursing-education-statistics/nursing-shortage-7a36b25c-7836-6c70-9642-ff00005-f0421pdf)c664bd5c78366c709642ff00005f0421.pdf?sfvrsn=0

National League for Nursing. (n.d.). *Nursing education statistics.* From https://www.nln.org/nlnNews/newsroom/nursing-education-statistics

Penn Nursing Science. (n.d.). *American nursing: An introduction to the Past.* Pennsylvania School of Nursing. Retrieved February 17, 2015, from http://www.nursing.upenn.edu/nhhc/Welcome%20Page%20Content/American%20Nursing.pdf

Population Reference Bureau. (2019). *Fact sheet aging in the United States.* https://www.prb.org/aging-unitedstates-fact-sheet/

Schaefer, N. (2007). *LPN trends.* Retrieved February 17, 2015, from http://nursing.advanceweb.com/Article/LPN-Trends-2.aspx

Smith, J. C., & Medalia, C. (2014). Health insurance coverage in the United States: 2013. Washington, DC: US Department of Commerce, Economics and Statistics Administration, Bureau of the Census.

Smithsonian. (2011). *The diary of a Civil War nurse.* Retrieved February 18, 2015, from http://americanhistory.si.edu/documentsgallery/exhibitions/nursing_2.html

Tavernise, S. (2014). *Number of Americans without health insurance falls, survey shows.* Retrieved July 19, 2015, from http://www.nytimes.com/2014/09/16/us/number-of-americans-without-health-insurance-falls-survey-shows.html?_r=2

Terry, A. J. (2012). *The LPN-to-RN bridge: Transitions to advance your career.* Jones & Bartlett.

The 2020 National Nursing Workforce Survey. From https://www.ncsbn.org/public-files//2020_NNW_Executive_Summary.pdf

The origins of nursing (The nature of nursing) Part 2. (n.d.). From https://www.elitelearning.com/resource-center/nursing/a-history-of-nursing-part-2-a-nursing-revolution/

CHAPTER 2

Abbott, S. (Ed.). (2014). Hidden curriculum. In *The glossary of education reform.* Retrieved February 26, 2015, from http://edglossary.org/hidden-curriculum

American Nurses Association. (2021). *Nursing: Scope and standards of practice* (4th ed.). Author.

American Sentinel. (2012). *Critical thinking can make or break a nursing career.* Retrieved July 21, 2016, from http://www.nursetogether.com/critical-thinking-can-make-or-break-nursing-career

Austin Community College. (n.d.). *Critical thinking strategies: Concept mapping.* Retrieved February 24, 2015, from http://www.austincc.edu/adnfac/collaborative/onsite_conceptmap.htm

Carpenito-Moyet, L. J. (2012). *Nursing diagnosis: Application to clinical practice* (14th ed.). Lippincott Williams & Wilkins.

Deringer, S. O., Filburn, M. J., Lum, G. D., & Maneval, R. E. (2011). Concept mapping: Does it improve critical thinking ability in practical nursing students? *Nursing Education Perspectives, 32*(4), 229–233.

Foundation for Critical Thinking. (2013). *Our concept and definition of critical thinking.* Retrieved February 26, 2015, from http://www.criticalthinking.org/pages/our-concept-of-critical-thinking/411

Garwood, J. K., Ahmed, A. H., & McComb, S. A. (2018). The effect of concept maps on undergraduate nursing students' critical thinking. *Nursing Education Perspectives, 39*(4), 208–214. https://doi.org/10.1097/01.NEP.0000000000000307

Gibbons, C. (2013). Nursing student perceptions of concept maps: From theory to practice. *Nursing Education Perspectives, 34*(6), 395–399.

Harris, C., & Zha, S. (2013). Concept mapping: A critical thinking technique. *Education, 134*(2), 207–211.

National Council of State Boards of Nursing. (2022). *Practical nurse scope of practice white paper.* https://www.ncsbn.org/papers/practical-nurse-scope-of-practice-white-paper

Roberts, C. (n.d.). *What are the four types of nursing diagnosis statements?* Retrieved February 25, 2015, from http://www.ehow.com/info_8240403_four-types-nursing-diagnosis-statements.html

Schuster, P. M. (2012). *Concept care mapping: A critical-thinking approach to care planning* (3rd ed.). F. A. Davis.

Veo, P. (2010). Concept mapping for applying theory to nursing practice. *Journal for Nurses in Professional Development, 26*(1), 17–22.

Zepure, S., Miller, T., & Haras, M. S. (2014). Using high-fidelity simulation and concept mapping to cultivate self-confidence in nursing students. *Nursing Education Perspectives, 35*(6), 408–409.

CHAPTER 3

American Nurses Association. (2015a). *Code of ethics with interpretive statements.*

American Nurses Association. (2015b). *Code of ethics with interpretive statements (view only for members and non-members).* Retrieved March 3, 2015, from http://www.nursingworld.org/codeofethics

American Nurses Association. (2015). *Code of ethics with interpretive statements.* From https://www.nursingworld.org/practice-policy/nursing-excellence/ethics/code-of-ethics-for-nurses/

Cambell, A., & Gormley-Fleming, L. (2011). Factors involved in young people's decisions about their health care. *Nursing Children and Young People, 23*(9), 19–22.

Cornock, M. (2011). Confidentiality: The legal issues. *Nursing Children and Young People, 23*(7), 18–19.

Current NLC States and Status. *Nurse license compact states.* https://www.ncsbn.org/nurse-licensure-compact.htm

DeWitt, A. (2014). Ethical pitfalls in nursing home litigation. *Trial, 50*(9), 16–21.

National Council of State Boards of Nursing. (2020a). *National Practitioner Database (NPDB).* http://www.ncsbn.org/418.htm

National Council of State Boards of Nursing. (2020b). *Nurse licensure compact.* http://www.ncsbn.org/nurse-licensure-compact.htm

Nursing Practice Act, Nursing Peer Review, & Nurse Licensure Compact Texas Occupations code. From https://www.bon.texas.gov/pdfs/law_rules_pdfs/nursing_practice_act_pdfs/NPA2023.pdf

Prideaux, A. (2010). Male nurses and the protection of female dignity. *Nursing Standard, 25*(13), 42–49.

Reynolds, L. (n.d.). *What is the patient bill of rights?* http://www.ehow.com/facts_4868817_what-patient-bill-rights.html?ref=Tract2utm_source=ask

Rock, M. J., & Hoebeke, R. (2014). Informed consent: Whose duty to inform? *MedSurg Nursing, 23*(3), 189–191.

State by State Guide to Assisted Suicide. (2018). *But some believe it is ethical.* https://euthanasia.procon.org/view.resource.php?resourceID=000132

United States Department of Health and Human Services. (2017). *Health information privacy.* From https://www.hhs.gov/hipaa/index.html

CHAPTER 4

American Hospital Association. (2022). *Fact sheet: Strengthening the health care workforce.* https://www.aha.org/fact-sheets/2021-05-26-fact-sheet-strengthening-health-care-workforce

Berg, J. G., & Dickow, M. (2014). Nurse role exploration project: The Affordable Care Act and new nursing roles. *Nurse Leader, 12*(5), 40–44. https://doi.org/10.1016/J.MNL.2014.07.001

Clarke, S. P. (2013). Healthcare reform in 2013: Enduring and universal challenges. *Nursing Management, 44*(3), 45–47. https://doi.org/10.1097/01.NUMA.0000427185.42306.14

Cohen, R. A., & Martinez, M. E. (2014). *Health insurance coverage: Early release of estimates from the National Health Interview Survey, January–March 2014*. Retrieved March 10, 2015, from http://www.cdc.gov/nchs/data/nhis/earlyrelease/insur201409.pdf

HealthyPeople.gov. (n.d.). *Healthy People 2030 framework*. https://health.gov/healthypeople/about/healthy-people-2030-framework

Jeffers, B. R., & Astroth, K. S. (2013). The clinical nurse leader: Prepared for an era of healthcare reform. *Nursing Forum, 48*(3), 223–239. https://doi.org/10.1111/nuf.12032

Kaiser Family Foundation. (2015). *Explaining health care reform: Questions about health insurance subsidies*. Retrieved March 10, 2015, from http://kff.org/health-reform-issue-brief/explaining-health-care-reform-questions-about-health/

Maslow, A. H. (1997). *Motivation and personality* (3rd ed.). Pearson.

McComb, S., & Hebdon, M. (2013). Enhancing patient outcomes in healthcare systems through multidisciplinary teamwork. *Clinical Journal of Oncology Nursing, 17*(6), 669–672. https://doi.org/10.1188/13.CJON.669-670

MedicalNewsToday. (n.d.). *What are the leading causes of death in the US?* https://www.medicalnewstoday.com/articles/282929.php

Medicaid Eligibility. (n.d). From https://www.medicaid.gov/medicaid/eligibility/index.html

Miller, C. (2014). *Nursing for wellness in older adults* (7th ed.). Lippincott Williams & Wilkins.

Needleman, J., Buerhaus, P., Pankratz, V. S., Leibson, C. L., Stevens, S. R., & Harris, M. (2011). Nurse staffing and inpatient hospital mortality. *New England Journal of Medicine, 364*(11), 1037–1045. https://doi.org/10.1056/NEJMsa1001025

Sommerfeldt, S. C. (2013). Articulating nursing in an interprofessional world. *Nurse Education in Practice, 13*(6), 519–523. https://doi.org/10.1016/j.nepr.2013.02.014

Terlizzi, E. P., Cohen, R. A., & Martinez, M. E. (2019). *Health insurance coverage: Early release of estimates from the National Health Interview Survey, January–September 2018*. https://www.cdc.gov/nchs/data/nhis/earlyrelease/insur201902.pdf

Tessler, C. (2014). *Medicare part C (Medicare Advantage)*. Retrieved March 11, 2015, from http://medicare.com/medicare-advantage-part-c/about-medicre-advantage-part-c/medicare-part-c

U.S. Department of Health and Human Services. (2022). *New HHS report shows national uninsured rate reached all-time low in 2022*. https://www.hhs.gov/about/news/2022/08/02/new-hhs-report-shows-national-uninsured-rate-reached-all-time-low-in-2022.html

Volland, J. (2014). Creating a new healthcare landscape. *Nursing Management, 45*(4), 22–28. https://doi.org/10.1097/01.NUMA.0000444871.32074.36

WebMD. (2021). *What to Know About Medicare Premiums*. https://www.webmd.com/health-insurance/what-to-know-about-medicare-premiums

CHAPTER 5

Cherry, K. (2021). *How prolonged stress impacts your health*. http://www.verywellmind.com/prolonged-stress-symptoms-causes-impact-and-coping-5092113

Cleveland Clinic. (2024). *Endorphins*. From https://my.clevelandclinic.org/health/body/23040-endorphins

Holmes, T. H., & Rahe, R. H. (1967). The social readjustment rating scale. *Journal of Psychosomatic Research, 11*(2), 213–218. https://doi.org/10.1016/0022-3999(67)90010-4

Jankovic, J. (2022). Neuropeptides, neurotransmitters, and neurohormones. (8th ed.). In *Bradley and Daroff's neurology in clinical practice*. Elsevier.

Porth, C. (2014). *Essentials of pathophysiology: Concepts of altered health states* (4th ed.). Lippincott Williams & Wilkins.

Randall, M. (2011). *The physiology of stress: Cortisol and the hypothalamic-pituitary-adrenal-axis*. From https://sites.dartmouth.edu/dujs/2011/02/03/the-physiology-of-stress-cortisol-and-the-hypothalamic-pituitary-adrenal-axis/

CHAPTER 6

ACL. (2024). *Fact Sheet: Aging in the United States*. From https://www.prb.org/resources/fact-sheet-aging-in-the-united-states/#:~:text=The%20number%20of%20Americans%20ages,from%2017%25%20to%202023%25.&text=The%20U.S%20population%20is%20older%20today%20than%20it%20has%20ever%20been

Acutrans. (2022). *Top 10 most spoken languages*. https://acutrans.com/top-10-most-spoken-languages/

AFS. (2023). *What are generalizations & stereotypes*. https://www.afsusa.org/study-abroad/culture-trek/culture-points/what-are-generalizations-and-stereotypes/

American Addiction Centers. (2022). *Risks of alcoholism among Native Americans*. https://americanaddictioncenters.org/alcoholism-treatment/native-americans

American Psychological Associatione (2024). *Race and Ethnicity*. From https://www.apa.org/topics/race-ethnicity

Andrews, J. D., Boyle, J. S., Collins, J.W. (2019). *Transcultural concepts in nursing care* (8th ed.). Philadelphia, PA: Lippincott Williams & Wilkins.

Britannica. (2024). *Minority*. In *Encyclopedia Britannica*. Retrieved January 18, 2024, from https://www.britannica.com/topic/minority

Center for Immigration Studies. (2019). *67.3 million in the United States spoke a foreign language at home in 2018*. https://cis.org/Report/673_million-united-states-spoke-foreign-language-home-2018

Centers for Disease Control and Prevention. (2013). *The Tuskegee timeline*. Retrieved April 1, 2015, from http://www.cdc.gov/tuskegee/timeline.htm

Cleveland Clinic. (2023). *Pharmacogenomics*. https://my.clevelandclinic.org/health/articles/pharmacogenomics

Clockify. (2021). *The perception of time in different cultures*. https://clockify.me/blog/managing-time/time-perception

Cullum, S. (2013). *Theory of transcultural nursing*. Retrieved March 31, 2015, from http://www.slideshare.net/ShelleyCullum/transcultural-nursing-powerpoint-presentationdr-madeleine-leininger

Cyracom. (n.d.). *Joint commission standards for qualified interpretation*. http://blog.cyracom.com/joint-commission-standards-for-qualified-interpretation

Department of the Interior, Bureau of Indian Affairs. (2015). *What we do*. From https://www.bia.gov/bia#:~:text=Our%20mission%20is%20to%20enhance,%2C%20grants%2C%20or%20compact%20agreements

Diamond, L., Wison-Stronks, A., & Jacobs, E. (2010). Do hospitals measure up to the culturally and linguistically appropriate services standards. *Medical Care, 48*(12), 1080–1087. https://doi.org/10.1097/MLR.0b013e3181f380bc

Dudek, S. G. (2021). *Nutrition essentials for nursing practice* (9th ed.). Lippincott Williams & Wilkins.

Eliopoulos, C. (2013). *Gerontological nursing* (8th ed.). Philadelphia, PA: Lippincott Williams & Wilkins.

Evanson, N. (2024). *Saudi Arabian culture: Communication. Cultural Atlas.* https://culturalatlas.sbs.com.au/saudi-arabian-culture/saudi-arabian-culture-communication

Giger, J. N. (2013). *Transcultural nursing* (6th ed.). St. Louis, MO: Elsevier.

Helal, M. (2017). *The language of eyes in Arab culture.* Arab America. https://www.arabamerica.com/language-eyes-arab-cultures/

Hinkle, J. L., & Cheever, K. H. (2021). *Brunner & Suddarth's textbook of medical-surgical nursing* (14th ed.). Lippincott Williams & Wilkins.

Islamic-laws.com. (n.d.). *Eating etiquettes in Islam.* http://islamic-laws.com/eatinghabbit.htm

Judaism 101. (n.d.). *Kashrut: Jewish dietary law.* http://www.jewfaq.org/kashrut.htm

Koithan, M., & Farrell, C. (2010). Indigenous native American healing traditions. *Journal for Nurse Practitioners, 6*(6), 477–476. https://doi.org/10.1016/j.nurpra.2010.03.016

Larson, K., Mathews, H. F., Torres, E., & Lea, C. S. (2017). Responding to health and social needs of aging Latinos in new-growth communities: A qualitative study. *BMC Health Services Research, 17,* 601. https://doi.org/10.1186/s12913-017-2551-2

Learn Religions. (2022). *Native American spirituality.* (2022). https://www.learnreligions.com/native-american-spirituality-2562540

Leininger, M. (2008). *Overview of Leininger's theory of culture care diversity and universality.* Retrieved March 31, 2015, from http://www.madeleine-leininger.com/cc/overview.pdf

Lipson, J. G., & Dibble, S. L. (2012). *Culture and clinical care* (2nd ed.). UCSF Nursing Press.

MegaEssays.com. (n.d.). Culturally sensitive nursing care essays. www.megaessays.com/viewpaper/88079.html

Merschel, M. (2023). *New report details how to fine-tune Asian diets for better heart health.* American Heart Association. https://www.heart.org/en/news/2023/05/08/new-report-details-how-to-fine-tune-asian-diets-for-better-heart-health

Migration Policy Institute. (n.d.). *Language diversity and English proficiency in the United States.* https://www.migrationpolicy.org/article/language-diversity-and-english-proficiency-united-states

National Congress of American Indians. (2022). Tribal nations and the United States: An introduction. https://ncai.org/about-tribes

Native Hope. (2023). *Native connection to Unci Maka-Mother Earth.* https://blog.nativehope.org/we-are-the-land

Ndugga, N., & Artiga, S. (2023). *Disparities in health and health care: 5 key questions and answers.* KFF. https://www.kff.org/racial-equity-and-health-policy/issue-brief/disparities-in-health-and-health-care-5-key-question-and-answers/

New Cultural Frontiers. (2022). *The definition of culture.* https://www.newculturalfrontiers.org/the-definition-of-culture

Olafuyi, O., Prekh, N., Wright, J., & Koenig, J. (2021). Inter-ethnic differences in pharmacokinetics—Is there more that unites than divides? *Pharmacology Research & Perspectives, 9*(6), e00890. https://doi.org/10.1002/prp2.890

Patak, L., Wilson-Stronks, A., Costello, J., Kleinpell, R. M., Henneman, E. A., Person, C., & Happ, M. B. (2009). Improving patient-provider communication: A call to action. *Journal of Nursing Administration, 39*(9), 372–376. https://doi.org/10.1097/NNA.0b013e3181b414ca

Pew Research Center. (2011). *A demographic portrait of Muslim Americans.* Retrieved March 23, 2015, from http://www.people-press.org/2011/08/30/section-1-a-demographic-portrait-of-muslim-americans/

Roberio, R. (2012). *AT&T goes multilingual, launches outsourced interpreter services and translator app.* Retrieved March 31, 2015, from http://www.biztechmagazine.com/article/2012/07/att-goes-multilingual-launches-outsourced-interpreter-services-and-translator-app

Ruiz, N. G., Shao, S., & Shah, S. (2022). *What it means to be Asian in America.* Pew Research Center. https://www.pewresearch.org/race-ethnicity/2022/08/02/what-it-means-to-be-asian-in-america/

Satter, D. E., Randall, L. L., & Solomon, T. G. A. (2014). *Conducting health research with native American communities.* American Public Health Association.

Saumure, C., Plouffe-Demers, M. P., Fiset, D., Cormier, S., Zhang, Y., Sun, D., Feng, M., Luo, F., Kunz, M., & Blais, C. (2023). Differences between East Asians and Westerners in the mental representations and visual information extraction involved in the decoding of pain facial expression intensity. *Affective Science, 4,* 332–349. https://link.springer.com/article/10.1007/s42761-023-00186-1

The Joint Commission. (2010). *Advancing effective communication, cultural competence, and patient- and-family centered care.* From https://www.jointcommission.org/-/media/tjc/documents/resources/patient-safety-topics/health-equity/aroadmapforhospitalsfinalversion727pdf.pdf

U.S. Census Bureau. (2010). *Languages used in the United States in 2011.* https://www.census.gov/library/publications/2013/acs/acs-22.html

U.S. Census Bureau. (2022a) *Projections of the size and composition of the U.S. Population: 2014 to 2060.* https://www.census.gov/content/dam/Census/library/publications/2015/demo/p25-1143.pdf

U.S. Census Bureau. (2022b). Facts for features: American Indians and Alaska native heritage month: November 2022. https://www.census.gov/newsroom/facts-for-features/2022/aian-month.html

U.S. Census Bureau. (2022c). *2020 census redistricting data (Public Law 94-171) summary file.* http://www.census.gov/prod/cen2020/doc/pl94-171.pdf

Van Wicklin, S. A. (2020). Ageism in nursing. *Plastic Surgical Nursing, 40*(1), 20–24. https://pubmed.ncbi.nlm.nih.gov/32102075/

Vidal, G. (2023). Vodou and Voodoo as alternative religion. *Nova Religio, 26*(4), 1–7. https://doi.org/10.1525/nr.2023.26.4.1

Weil, A. (2012). *What is integrative medicine?* Retrieved March 21, 2012, from http://www.drweil.com/drw/u/ART02054/Andrew-Weil-Integrative-Medicine.html

Wilson-Stronks, A. L. (2008). The role of nursing in meeting the healthcare needs of diverse populations. *Journal of Nursing Care Quality, 23*(4), 289–291. https://doi.org/10.1097/01.NCQ.0000336669.79853.38

Wilson-Stronks, A., & Mutha, A. (2010). From the perspective of CEOs: What motivates hospitals to embrace cultural competence? *Journal of Healthcare Management, 55*(5), 339–351. https://doi.org/10.1097/00115514-201009000-00009

Wilson-Stronks, A., Lee, K. K., Cordero, C. L., Kopp, A. L., & Galvez, E. (2008). *One size does not fit all: Meeting the healthcare needs of diverse populations.* From https://www.issuelab.org/resources/10463/10463.pdf

Yale, S., Tekiner, H., & Yale, E. S. (2021). Reimagining the terms Mongolian Spot and sign. *Cureus, 13*(12), e20396. https://doi.org/10.7759/cureus.20396

Zborowski, M. (1952). Cultural components in response to pain. *Journal of Social Issues, 8*(4), 16–30. https://doi.org/10.1111/j.1540-4560.1952.tb01860.x

Zborowski, M. (1969). *People in pain.* Jossey-Bass/Wiley.

CHAPTER 7

American Stroke Association. (2024). *Technology for people with aphasia.* American Heart Association. https://www.stroke.org/en/about-stroke/effects-of-stroke/communication-and-aphasia/stroke-and-aphasia/technology-for-people-with-aphasia

Belcher, A. (2014). Express yourself. *Nursing Standard, 28*(50), 63. https://doi.org/10.7748/ns.28.50.63.s49

Boscart, V., Fox, M., McGilton, K., Sorin-Peters, R., Sidani, S., & Rochon, E. (2011). Focus on communication: Increasing the opportunity for successful staff-patient interactions. *International Journal of Older People Nursing, 6*(1), 13–24. https://doi.org/10.1111/j.1748-3743.2010.00210.x

Chillot, R. (2013). *The power of touch.* Retrieved April 6, 2015, from https://psychologytoday.com/articles/201303/the-power-touch

Douglas KS (2012). Through the eyes of gratitude. *Nursing Economics.* January–February 2012;30(1):42-4, 49. PMID: 22479964.

Fogle, C., & Reams, P. (2014). Taking a uniform approach to nursing attire. *Nursing, 44*(6), 50–54. https://doi.org/10.1097/01.NURSE.0000444535.96822.3b

Green, C. (2013). Philosophic reflections on the meaning of touch in nurse-patient interactions. *Nursing Philosophy, 14*(4), 242–253. https://doi.org/10.1111/nup.12006

Hall, E. T. (1959). *The silent language.* Faucett.

Hall, E. T. (1963). A system for the notation of proxemic behavior. *American Anthropologist, 63*(3), 1003–1006. https://doi.org/10.1525/aa.1963.65.5.02a00020

Hall, E. T. (1966). *The hidden dimension.* Anchor Books.

Haugan, G. (2014). The relationship between nurse-patient interaction and meaning-in-life in cognitively intact nursing home patients. *Journal of Advanced Nursing, 70*(1), 107–120. https://doi.org/10.1111/jan.12173

Lattavo, Kathleen, MSN, RN, CNS-MS,C.M.S.R.N., R.N.-B.C.,. (2014). The Importance of Words. *Medsurg Nursing, 23*(4), 209-10. http://hallmarkuniversity.idm.oclc.org/login?url=https://www.proquest.com/scholarly-journals/importance-words/docview/1558468862/se-2.

Short, C. (2010). Time is no barrier to forming a close nurse-patient relationship. *Nursing Standard, 24*(26), 29. https://doi.org/10.7748/ns.24.26.29.s33

The University of Texas Permian Basin. (2022). *How much of communication is nonverbal?* https://online.utpb.edu/about-us/articles/communication/how-much-of-communication-is-nonverbal/

The Joint Commission. (n.d.). *National patient safety goals.* https://www.jointcommission.org/standards/national-patient-safety-goals/

Van der Cingel, M. (2014). Compassion: The missing link in quality of care. *Nursing Education Today, 34*(9), 1253–1257. https://doi.org/10.1016/j.nedt.2014.04.003

Waters, A. (2010). The human touch: Nurses are being reminded to value their senses over electronic equipment when they assess patients. *Nursing Standard, 25*(1), 16. https://doi.org/10.7748/ns.25.1.16.s25

CHAPTER 8

Anderson, L. W., & Krathwohl, D. R. (Eds.) (2001). *A taxonomy for learning, teaching, and assessing: A revision of Bloom's taxonomy of educational objectives.* Pearson Allyn & Bacon.

Bloom, B. S., Engelhart, M. D., Furst, E. J., Hill, W. H., & Krathwohl, D. R. (1956). *Taxonomy of educational objectives: The classification of educational goals. Handbook I: Cognitive domain.* David McKay Company.

Buppert, C. (2014). *What does a nurse's signature mean on discharge papers.* Retrieved April 16, 2015, from http://www.medscape.com/viewarticle/824924

Centre for Disease Control and Prevention. (2022). What is Health Literacy? 2023. From https://www.cdc.gov/healthliteracy/learn/index.html

Centers for Disease Control and Prevention. (2023). *Health literacy.* http://www.cdc.gov/healthliteracy/learn/

Elmore, T. (2014). *Contrasting generation Y and Z.* Retrieved April 19, 2015, from http://www.huffingtonpost.com/tim-elmore/contrasting-generation-y_b_5679434.html

Generational Differences in the Workplace. (2024). From https://www.purdueglobal.edu/education-partnerships/generational-workforce-differences-infographic/

Giang, V. (2013). *Here are the strengths and weaknesses of millennials, gen X, and boomers.* Retrieved April 19, 2015, from http://www.businessinsider.in/Here-Are-The-Strengths-And-Weaknesses-Of-Millennials-Gen-X-And-Boomers/articleshow/25666991.cms

Harrow, A. (1972). *A taxonomy of psychomotor domain: A guide for developing behavioral objectives.* David McKay Company.

Health Literacy Universal. (2015) From Phttps://www.ahrq.gov/health-literacy/improve/precautions/tool5.html

Institute for Healthcare Improvement. (2015). *Always use teach back!* Retrieved April 19, 2015, from http://www.ihi.org/resources/Pages/Tools/AlwaysUseTeachBack!.aspx

Krathwohl, D. R., Bloom, B. S., & Masia, B. B. (1973). *Taxonomy of educational objectives, the classification of educational goals. Handbook II: Affective domain.* David McKay Company.

Literacy Statistics. (2024-2025). (Where are we now). 2024. From https://www.thenationalliteracyinstitute.com/literacy-statistics

LPN Scope of Practice for the Licensed Practical Nurse in College Health. (2023). From https://www.acha.org/documents/resources/guidelines/ACHA_Scope_of_Practice_for_College_Health_LPNs_Feb2023.pdf

LUCIDWAY. (2022). *The psychomotor domain-get physical.* https://www.lucidway.com/the-psychomotor-domain-get-physical/

Patient Education & Information Overload. (2023). From https://www.clinicaladvisor.com/home/topics/practice-management-information-center/patient-education-information/#:~:text=Research%20has%20consistently%20found%20that,to%20them%20by%20their%20physicians.&text=Patients%20can%20immediately%20forget%2040,it%20is%20typically%20recalled%20correctly.

Psychomotor learning. (2022). https://www.britannica.com/science/psychomotor-learning

The Adult Learning Theory-Andragogy- Malcom Knowles. (2013). From https://elearningindustry.com/the-adult-learning-theory-andragogy-of-malcolm-knowles

The Joint Commission on Accreditation of Healthcare Organizations. (2010). *Comprehensive accreditation for hospitals: The official handbook.* Author.

Ward, J. (2012). *Patient care: The nurse's role in discharge planning.* Retrieved April 16, 2015, from http://www.nursetogether.com/patient-care-the-nurses-role-in-discharge

Wilson, L. O. (2016). *Anderson and Krathwohl—Bloom's taxonomy revised.* 2016. From https://quincycollege.edu/wp-content/uploads/Anderson-and-Krathwohl_Revised-Blooms-Taxonomy.pdf

Wylie Communications. (2021). *What's the latest U.S. literacy rate?* https://www.wyliecomm.com/2021/08/whats-the-latest-u-s-literacy-rate/

CHAPTER 9

Abramson, E. L., McGinnis, S., Moore, J., Kaushal, R., & HITEC investigators. (2014). A statewide assessment of electronic health record adoption and health information exchange among nursing homes. *Health Services Research, 49*(1), 361–372. https://doi.org/10.1111/1475-6773.12137

Blair, W., & Smith, B. (2012). Nursing documentation: Frameworks and barriers. *Contemporary Nurse*, *41*(2), 160–168. https://doi.org/10.5172/conu.2012.41.2.160

Brandon, D. H., Docherty, S. L., & Kelley, T. F. (2011). Electronic nursing documentation as a strategy to improve quality patient care. *Journal of Nursing Scholarship*, *43*(2), 154–162. https://doi.org/10.1111/j.1547-5069.2011.01397.x

Campos, N. K. (2010). The legalities of nursing documentation. *Men in Nursing*, 40(1), 7–9. DOI: 10.1097/01.NUMA.0000359202.59952.d2.

Charles, D., Gabriel, M., & Searcy, T. (2015). *Adoption of electronic health record systems among U.S. non-federal acute care hospitals: 2008-2014.* Retrieved September 14, 2015, from http://www.healthit.gov/sites/default/files/data-brief/2014HospitalAdoptionDataBrief.pdf

Cipriano PF. The future of nursing and health IT: The quality elixir. *Nursing Economics*. September-October 2011;29(5):286-9, 282. PMID: 22372088.

Documentation by the Nurse. (n.d.) From https://www.hhs.texas.gov/sites/default/files/documents/doing-business-with-hhs/provider-portal/QMP/NurseDocumentationPPT.pdf.

Electronic Medical Records/Electronic Health Records (EMRs/EHRs). (2022). From https://www.cdc.gov/nchs/fastats/electronic-medical-records.htm

Evaluation of a Problem-Specific SBAR Tool to Improve After-Hours Nurse-Physician Phone Communication: A Randomized Trial. From https://doi.org/10.1016/S1553-7250(13)39065-5

Fields, W., McCullough, S., & Jacoby, J. (2011). The effect of computerized provider order entry on nurses and nurses' work. *Journal of Healthcare Information Management*, *25*, 48–53.

Forman, Tracia M.; Armor, David A.; Miller, Ava S. A Review of Clinical Informatics Competencies in Nursing to Inform Best Practices in Education and Nurse Faculty Development. *Nursing Education Perspectives* 41(1):p E3-E7, 1/2 2020. DOI: 10.1097/01.NEP.0000000000000588

Heisey-Grove, D., & Patel, V. (2014). *Physician motivations for adoption of electronic health records.* Retrieved September 14, 2015, from http://www.healthit.gov/sites/default/files/oncdatabrief-physician-ehr-adoption-motivators-2014.pdf

HHS.gov. (2017). *Guidance on HIPAA & cloud computing.* https://www.hhs.gov/hipaa/for-professionals/special-topics/cloud-computing/index.html

HIPAA Journal. (2022). *Recent HIPAA changes.* Retrieved from https://www.hipaajournal.com/recent-hipaa-changes/

How nurses drive rapid electronic records implementation. (2013). From https://www.myamericannurse.com/how-nurses-drive-rapid-electronic-records-implementation/

Howie, W. O., & McMullen, P. C. (2010). Can checklists minimize legal liability and improve the quality of patient care? *Journal for Nurse Practitioners*, *6*(9), 694–697. https://doi.org/10.1016/j.nurpra.2010.07.006

Jeffries, D. (2012). Communicate with clarity: Correct use of abbreviations and phrases in nursing records is vital for care efficiency and safety. *Nursing Standard*, *26*, 62–63. doi: 10.7748/ns2012.06.26.40.62.p8509

Kohle-Ersher, A., Chatterjee, P., Osmanbeyoglu, H. U., Hochheiser, H., & Bartos, C. (2012). Evaluating the barriers to point-of-care documentation for nursing staff. *Computers Informatics Nursing*, *30*, 126–133. https://doi.org/10.1097/NCN.0b013e3182343f14

Morales, K. (2013). *17 tips to improve your nursing documentation.* Retrieved April 22, 2015, from http://www.nursetogether.com/nurse-documentation-helpful-tips-every-nurs

Murphy J. The journey to meaningful use of electronic health records. *Nursing Economics*. July-August 2010;28(4):283-6. PMID: 21761616.

Murphy J. Nursing and technology: A love/hate relationship. *Nursing Economics*. November-December 2010;28(6):405-8. PMID: 21291063.

Murphy J. Nursing informatics: The intersection of nursing, computer, and information sciences. *Nursing Economics*. May-June 2010;28(3):204-7. PMID: 20672545.

Murphy, J. (2013). Progress report: Electronic health records and hit in the United States. *American Nurse Today*, *8*(11), SR10.

Nurses Hate EHRs Too. From https://www.healthitoutcomes.com/doc/nurses-hate-ehrs-too-0001

Progress report: Electronic health records and HIT in the United States. (2013). https://www.myamericannurse.com/progress-report-electronic-health-records-and-hit-in-the-united-states/

Springhouse. (2007). *Lippincott manual of nursing practice series: Documentation.* Lippincott Williams & Wilkins.

Stokowski, L. A. (2013). *Electronic nursing documentation: Charting new territory.* Retrieved April 22, 2015, from http://www.medscape.com/viewarticle/810573

Struck, R. (2013). Telling the patient's story with electronic health records. *Nursing Management*, *44*, 13–15. https://doi.org/10.1097/01.NUMA.0000431433.46631.cc

Technology, transformation, and the nursing workforce. (2013). From https://www.myamericannurse.com/technology-transformation-and-the-nursing-workforce/

Thede, L. (2012). Informatics: Where is it? *The Online Journal of Issues in Nursing*, *17*(1). https://doi.org/10.3912/OJIN.Vol17No1InfoCol01

U.S. Department of Health and Human Services. (2022). *Right to access medical records.* http://www.hhs.gov/hipaa/for-professionals/faq/right-to-access-medical-records

U.S. Department of Health & Human Services. (n.d.). *Guidance on HIPPA and cloud computing.* https://www.hhs.gov/hipaa/for-professionals/special-topics/cloud-computing/index.html

Yee, T., Needleman, J., Pearson, M., Parkerton, P., Parkerton, M., & Wolstein, J. (2012). The influence of integrated electronic medical records and computerized nursing notes on nurses' time spent in documentation. *Computers Informatics Nursing*, *30*, 287–292. https://doi.org/10.1097/NXN.0b013e31824af835

CHAPTER 10

Boyce, J. M., & Pittet, D. (2002). Guideline for hand hygiene in health-care settings: Recommendations of the Healthcare Infection Control Practices Advisory Committee and the HICPAC/SHEA/APIC/IDSA Hand Hygiene Task Force. *Morbidity & Mortality Weekly Report*, *51*(RR16), 1–44. Retrieved May 4, 2015, from http://www.cdc.gov/mmwr/preview/mmwrhtml/rr5116a1.htm

Centers for Disease Control and Prevention. (2014). *Respiratory protection in health-care settings.* Retrieved May 7, 2015, from https://www.cdc.gov/tb/publications/factsheets/prevention/rphcs.htm

Centers for Disease Control and Prevention. (2020). *Reported tuberculosis in the United States, 2022.* From https://www.cdc.gov/tb/

Centers for Disease Control and Prevention. (2022a). *Nail hygiene.* https://www.cdc.gov/hygiene/personal-hygiene/nails.html

Centers for Disease Control and Prevention. (2022b). *When and how to wash your hands.* https://www.cdc.gov/features/handwashing/

Ethics, Accountability Must Drive Healthcare Workers' Handwashing Behavior. (2013) https://www.infectioncontroltoday.com/view/ethics-accountability-must-drive-healthcare-workers-handwashing-behavior

Fox, M. (2015). *Lyme disease is spreading, government research finds.* Retrieved October 18, 2015, from http://www.nbcnews

.com/health/health-news/lyme-disease-spreads-government-report-finds-n392626

Hand Hygiene. (2024). From https://www.who.int/teams/integrated-health-services/infection-prevention-control/hand-hygiene

Hand washing stops infections, so why do health care workers skip it?. (2016). From https://ihpi.umich.edu/news/hand-washing-stops-infections-so-why-do-health-care-workers-skip-it

Infection Control Today & Informa Life Sciences Exhibitions Announce Nursing Conference at 2017 FIME. (2027). From https://www.infectioncontroltoday.com/view/ict-and-informa-life-sciences-exhibitions-announce-nursing-conference-2017

National Institute for Occupational Safety and Health. (2013). *Respirator awareness: Your health may depend on it.* Retrieved May 7, 2015, from http://www.cdc.gov/niosh/docs/2013-138/pdfs/2013-138.pdf

National Institute of Allergy and Infectious Diseases. (2014). *NIAID's antibacterial resistance program: Current status and future directions.* From https://www.niaid.nih.gov/sites/default/files/arstrategicplan2014.

National Institute of Allergy and Infectious Diseases. (2018). *Recent NIAID research initiatives on antimicrobial resistance.* https://www.niaid.nih.gov/search/niaidsite

National Institute of Allergy and Infectious Diseases. (2020). *Basic research on antimicrobial (drug) resistance.* https://www.niaid.nih.gov/research/antimicrobial-resistance-basic-research-support

Nursing's Role in Hand Hygiene Compliance. (2019). From https://www.elitelearning.com/resource-center/nursing/nursings-role-in-hand-hygiene-compliance/

QIAGEN. (2022). *Tuberculosis prevention in long-term care.* https://www.qiagen.com/us/applications/tbmanagement/risk-groups/long-term-care

Rowe, T. A., & Juthani-Mehta, M. (2013). Urinary tract infection in older adults. *Aging Health, 9*(5). Retrieved October 18, 2015, from http://www.ncbi.nlm.nih.gov/pmc/articles/PMC3878051/

Tuberculosis prevention in long-term care. (2022). From https://www.qiagen.com/us/applications/tb-management/risk-groups/long-term-care

Unsplash. (n.d.). *N95 mask.* https://unsplash.com/s/photos/n95-mask

World Health Organization. (2022). *WHO guidelines on hand hygiene in healthcare.* Author.

Widmer, A. F. (2013). Surgical hand hygiene: Scrub or rub? *Journal of Hospital Infection, 83*(Suppl. 1), S35–S39. https://doi.org/10.1016/S0195-6701(13)60008-0

CHAPTER 11

Centers for Medicare and Medicaid Services. (2017). *Medicare coverage of skilled nursing facility (SNF) care.* https://www.medicare.gov/coverage/skilled-nursing-facility-care.html

CTLawHelp. (2013). *Transfers/discharges from a nursing home and your rights.* Retrieved May 18, 2015, from http://ctlawhelp.org/self-help-guides/elder-law/transfers-discharges-From-nursing-home

Davis, C. P. (2015). *Hospital admissions.* Retrieved May 18, 2015, from http://www.emedicinehealth.com/hospital_admissions/article_em.htm

Hallstrom, L. (2023). *Total and percentage of elderly in nursing homes: 2023 data.* https://www.aplaceformom.com/senior-living-data/articles/elderly-nursing-home-population

Levy, F., Mareiniss, D. P., & Iacovelli, C. (2012). *The importance of a proper against-medical-advice (AMA) discharge.* Retrieved May 18, 2015, from http://www.medscape.com/viewarticle/770719

Malzone, L. (2023). *Does Medicare cover nursing homes.* https://www.medigap.com/faqs/does-medicare-pay-for-nursing-homes/

Markowitz, A. (2022). *Finding the right long-term care for your loved one.* https://www.aarp.org/caregiving/basics/info-2020/long-term-care.html

McGillis Hall, L., Wodchis, W. P., Ma, X., & Johnson, S. (2013). Changes in patient health outcomes from admission to discharge in acute care. *Journal of Nursing Care Quality, 28*(1), 8–16. https://doi.org/10.1097/NCQ.0b013e3182665dab

National Institute of Aging. (2023). *Long-term care facilities: Assisted living, nursing homes, and other residential care.* https://www.nia.nih.gov/health/assisted-living-and-nursing-homes/long-term-care-facilities-assisted-living-nursing-homes

Ortega, B., Salazar, A., Jovell, A., Escarrabill, J., Marca, G., & Corbella, X. (2012). Standardizing admission and discharge processes to improve patient flow: A cross sectional study. *BMC Health Services Research, 12*, 180. Retrieved May 18, 2015, from http://www.biomedcentral.com/1472-6963/12/180

Pearson, K. (2013). *Emergency transfers of the elderly from nursing facilities to critical access hospitals: Opportunities for improving patient safety and quality.* https://www.flexmonitoring.org/sites/flexmonitoring.umn.edu/files/media/policybrief32-transfer-protocols-with-appendix.pdf

Spiva, L., & Johnson, D. (2012). Improving nursing satisfaction and quality through the creation of admission and discharge nurse team. *Journal of Nursing Care Quality, 27*(1), 89–93. https://doi.org/10.1097/NCQ.0b013e318227d645

Sturdy, D., & Heath, H. (2010). Support for discharge planning. *Nursing Standard, 24*(28), 15. https://doi.org/10.7748/ns.24.28.15.s15

The Joint Commission. (2023). *National Patient Safety Goals® Effective January 2024 for the Ambulatory Health Care Program.* https://www.jointcommission.org/-/media/tjc/documents/standards/national-patient-safety-goals/2024/npsg_chapter_ahc_jan2024.pdf

U.S. Department of Health and Human Services. (2012). *A profile of older Americans.* https://acl.gov/sites/default/files/Aging%20and%20Disability%20in%20America/2012profile.pdf

U.S. Department of Health and Human Services. (2020). *Your guide to choosing a nursing home or other long-term services & supports.* https://www.hhs.gov/guidance/document/your-guide-choosing-nursing-home-or-other-long-term-services-supports

CHAPTER 12

Alexander, L. (2022). *Have a fever over 100? Here's what to do about fever in adults.* https://www.healthpages.org/health-a-z/fever-adults/

American Heart Association. (n.d.). *High blood pressure normal BP.* https://newsroom.heart.org/search?ct=releases&q=HBP

American Heart Association. (2020). *The facts about high blood pressure.* https://www.heart.org/en/health-topics/high-blood-pressure

American Heart Association. (2024). *Understanding blood pressure readings.* https://www.heart.org/en/health-topics/high-blood-pressure

American Heart Association. (2024). *High blood pressure.* https://www.heart.org/en/health-topics/high-blood-pressure

Appel, L., Moore, T., Obarzanek, E., Vollmer, W. M., Svetkey, L. P., Sacks, F. M., Bray, G. A., Vogt, T. M., Cutler, J. A., Windhauser, M. M., Lin, P. H., & Karanja, N. (1997). A clinical trial of the effects of dietary patterns on blood pressure. DASH Collaborative Research Group. *The New England Journal of Medicine, 336*(16), 1117–1124. https://doi.org/10.1056/NEJM199704173361601

Brose, R. D., Shin, G., McGuinness, M. C., Schneidereith, T., Purvis, S., Dong, G. X., Keefer, J., Spencer, F., & Smith, K. D. (2012). Activation of the stress proteome as a mechanism for small molecule therapeutics. *Human Molecular Genetics, 21*(19), 4237–4252. https://doi.org/10.1093/hmg/dds247

Cleveland Clinic. (2020). *Hypothermia (low body temperature)*. https://my.clevelandclinic.org/health/diseases/21164-hypothermia-low-body-temperature

Freeman, R. (2008). Clinical practice. Neurogenic orthostatic hypotension. *The New England Journal of Medicine, 358*(6), 615–624. https://doi.org/10.1056/NEJMcp074189

Grimes, A. C. (2022). *The lowest temperature a human can actually survive*. https://www.grunge.com/164461

Holland, K. (2013). *What is thermoregulation?* Retrieved May 25, 2015, from http://www.healthline.com/health/thermoregulation

James, P. A., Oparil, S., Carter, B. L., Cushman, W. C., Dennison-Himmelfarb, C., Handler, J., Lackland, D. T., LeFevre, M. L., MacKenzie, T. D., Ogedegbe, O., Smith, S. C., Jr., Svetkey, L. P., Taler, S. J., Townsend, R. R., Wright, J. T., Jr., Narva, A. S., & Ortiz, E. (2014). 2014 Evidence-based guideline for the management of high blood pressure in adults: Report from the panel members appointed to the Eighth Joint National Committee (JNC 8). *JAMA, 311*(5), 507–520. Retrieved June 3, 2015, from http://jama.jamanetwork.com/article.aspx?articleid=1791497

Jastroch, M., Oelkrug, R., & Keipert, S. (2018). Insights into brown adipose tissue evolution and function from non-model organisms. *The Journal of Experimental Biology, 221*(Pt Suppl 1), jeb169425. https://doi.org/10.1242/jeb.169425

Krakoff, L. R., Gillespie, R. L., Ferdinand, K. C., Fergus, I. V., Akinboboye, O., Williams, K. A., Walsh, M. N., Bairey Merz, C. N., & Pepine, C. J. (2014). 2014 Hypertension recommendations from the eighth Joint National Committee panel members raise concerns for elderly black and female populations. *Journal of the American College of Cardiology, 64*(4), 394–402. https://doi.org/10.1016/j.jacc.2014.06.014

Lanier, J. B., Mote, M. B., & Clay, E. C. (2011). Evaluation and management of orthostatic hypotension. *American Family Physician, 84*(5), 527–536. Retrieved June 5, 2015, from http://www.aafp.org/afp/2011/0901/p527.html

LeWine, H. E. (2024). *Reading the new blood pressure guidelines*. https://www.health.harvard.edu/heart-health/reading-the-new-blood-pressure-guidelines

LogicalScience. (2022). *Increase BA tissue & boost weight loss by 7 times—Science or scam*. https://logicalscience.com/2022/05/increase-ba-tissue-boost-weight-loss-by-7-times-science-or-scam/

McCallum, L., & Higgins, D. (2012). Measuring body temperature. *Nursing Times, 108*(45), 20–22.

Moser, M. (2014). *Hypertension in the elderly—Deserves more attention*. Retrieved June 3, 2015, from http://www.medicinenet.com/script/main/art.asp?articlekey=18397

Naccarato, M., Leviner, S., Proehl, C. J., Cen, C. P. E. N., Barnason, F. S., Brim, C., & Crowley, M. (2011). *Clinical practice guideline: Orthostatic vital signs*. Emergency Nurses Association.

National Heart, Lung, and Blood Institute. (2012). *What is high blood pressure?* Retrieved June 3, 2015, from http://nhlbi.nih.gov/health/health-topics/topics/hbp

Page, M. R. (2014). The JNC 8 hypertension guidelines: An in-depth guide. *The American Journal of Managed Care, 20*(1 Spec No.), E8. Retrieved June 3, 2015, from http://www.ajmc.com/journals/evidence-based-diabetes-management/2014/January-2014/The-JNC-8-Hypertension-Guidelines-An-In-Depth-Guide

RegisteredNurseRN.com. (n.d.). *How to take a temperature 6 different ways*. https://www.registerednursern.com/take-temperature-6-different-ways/

Sisson, M. (2016). *The new primal blueprint: Reprogram your genes for effortless weight loss, vibrant health and boundless energy*. Bradventures LLC.

Torgan, C. (2014). *Cool temperature alters human fat and metabolism*. Retrieved May 25, 2015, from https://www.nih.gov/news-events/nih-research-matters/cool-temperature-alters-human-fat-metabolism

Tousseau, J. (2013). *What is the most accurate way to take a temperature?* Retrieved May 29, 2015, from http://saidsupport.org/what-is-the-most-accurate-way-to-take-a-temperature-is-oral-temporal-ear-or-rectal-best/

CHAPTER 13

American Cancer Society. (n.d.). *American Cancer Society recommendations for the early detection of breast cancer*. https://www.cancer.org/cancer/breast-cancer/screening-tests-and-early-detection/american-cancer-society-recommendations-for-the-early-detection-of-breast-cancer.html

American Cancer Society. (2022). *American Cancer Society screening recommendations for women at average breast cancer risk*. https://www.cancer.org/cancer/breast-cancer/screening-tests-and-early-detection/american-cancer-society-recommendations-for-the-early-detection-of-breast-cancer.html

Anderson, B., Nix, E., Norman, B., & McPike, H. D. (2014). An evidence based approach to undergraduate physical assessment practicum course development. *Nurse Education in Practice, 14*(3), 242–246. https://doi.org/10.1016/j.nepr.2013.08.007

Bickley, L. S. (2012). *Bates' guide to physical examination and history taking* (11th ed.). Lippincott Williams & Wilkins.

Bornais, J. A. K., Raiger, J. E., Krahn, R. E., & El-Masri, M. M. (2012). Evaluating undergraduate nursing students' learning using standardized patients. *Journal of Professional Nursing, 28*(5), 291–296. https://doi.org/10.1016/j.profnurs.2012.02.001

Chircop, A., Edgecombe, N., Hayward, K., Ducey-Gilbert, C., & Sheppard-Lemoine, D. (2013). Evaluating the integration of cultural competence skills into health and physical assessment tools: A survey of Canadian schools of nursing. *Journal of Transcultural Nursing, 24*(2), 195–203. https://doi.org/10.1177/1043659612472202

Craven, R. F., Hirnle, C. J., & Jensen, S. (2012). *Fundamentals of nursing*. Lippincott Williams & Wilkins.

Dugdale, D. C. (2015). *Capillary nail refill test*. Retrieved June 15, 2015, from http://www.nlm.nih.gov/medlineplus/ency/article/003394.htm

Jensen, S. (2014). *Nursing health assessment*. Lippincott Williams & Wilkins.

Larocque, M., Luctkar-Flude, M., & Wilson-Keates, B. (2012). Evaluating high-fidelity human simulators and standardized patients in an undergraduate nursing health assessment course. *Nursing Education Today, 32*(4), 448–452. https://doi.org/10.1016/j.nedt.2011.04.011

Lippincott Advisor. (2022). https://advisor-edu.lww.com/lna/document.do?bid43&did=1119938

Lippincott Williams & Wilkins. (2012). *Assessment made incredibly easy*.

McCaughey, C. S., & Traynor, M. K. (2010). The role of simulation in nurse education. *Nurse Education Today, 30*(8), 827–832. https://doi.org/10.1016/j.nedt.2010.03.005

National Center for Cultural Competence. (n.d.). https://nccc.georgetown.edu/

Norman, K., Haß, U., & Pirlich, M. (2021). Malnutrition in older adults-recent advances and remaining challenges. *Nutrients, 13*(8): 2764. https://doi.org/10.3390/nu13082764

Pellico, L. H. (2012). *Focus on adult health*. Lippincott Williams & Wilkins.

Roberts, D. (2011). Grading the performance of clinical skills: Lessons to be learned from the performing arts. *Nursing Education Today, 31*(6), 607–610. https://doi.org/10.1016/j.nedt.2010.10.017

Study.com. (2022). *Cultural competence in health care policy & law.* https://study.com/academy/lesson/cultural-competence-in-heath-care-policy-law.html

Taylor, C., Lillis, C., & Lynn, P. (2014). *Fundamentals of nursing* (8th ed.). Lippincott Williams & Wilkins.

U. S. Preventive Services Task Force. (2016). *Breast cancer: Screening.* https://www.uspreventiveservicestaskforce.org/uspstf/recommendation/breast-cancer-screening

Weber, J. R., & Kelley, J. H. (2014). *Health assessment in nursing.* Lippincott Williams & Wilkins.

CHAPTER 14

American Cancer Society. (2023). *Colorectal cancer facts & figures 2023-2025.* https://www.cancer.org/content/dam/cancer-org/research/cancer-facts-and-statistics/colorectal-cancer-facts-and-figures/colorectal-cancer-facts-and-figures-2023.pdf

American College of Obstetricians and Gynecologists. (2024). *Cervical cancer screening.* https://www.acog.org/womens-health/faqs/cervical-cancer-screening#:~:text=Women%20who%20are%2021%20to,%2Dtesting)%20every%205%20years

American College of Obstetricians and Gynecologists. (2022). *Cervical cancer screening.* https://www.acog.org/womens-health/infographics/cervical-cancer-screening

American Diabetes Association. (2022). *Insulin pumps: Relief and choice.* https://diabetes.org/healthy-living/medication-treatments/insulin-other-injectables/insulin-pumps-relief-and-choice

American Diabetes Association. (2024). *The big picture: Checking your blood glucose.* https://diabetes.org/living-with-diabetes/treatment-care/checking-your-blood-sugar#:~:text=People%20with%20diabetes%20check%20their,by%20talking%20to%20your%20doctor

American Psychiatric Association. (2024). *What are anxiety disorders?* https://www.psychiatry.org/patients-families/anxiety-disorders/what-are-anxiety-disorders

Fischbach, F., Fischbach, M., & Stout, K. (2021). *A manual of laboratory and diagnostic tests* (11th ed.). Lippincott Williams & Wilkins.

Mayo Clinic. (n.d.). *New protocols allow for MRI in selected pacemaker patients.* http://www.mayoclinic.org/medical-professionals/clinical-updates/cardiovascular/new-protocols-allow-mri-selected-pacemaker-patients

Mayo Clinic. (2021). *'Intelligently aggressive' approach to MRI for people with implanted devices.* https://www.mayoclinic.org/medical-professionals/neurology-neurosurgery/news/intelligently-aggressive-approach-to-mri-for-people-with-implanted-devices/mac-20524720

National Cancer Institute. (2022). HPV and pap test results: Next steps after an abnormal cervical cancer screening test. https://www.cancer.gov/types/cervical/screening/abnormal-hpv-pap-test-results

RadiologyInfo.org. (2024). *MRI safety.* https://www.radiologyinfo.org/en/info/safety-mr

CHAPTER 15

Beltrán-Sánchez, H., Harhay, M. O., Harhay, M. M., & McElligott, S. (2013). Prevalence and trends of metabolic syndrome in the adult U.S. population, 1999–2010. *Journal of the American College of Cardiology, 62*(8), 697–703. https://doi.org/10.1016/j.jacc.2013.05.064

Cleveland Clinic. (2024). *Subcutaneous fat.* https://my.cleveland-clinic.org/health/diseases/23968-subcutaneous-fat

Dalleck, L. C. (2021). *Client-centered Assessments: Past, Present and Future.* https://www.acefitness.org/continuing-education/certified/september-2021/7940/client-centered-assessments-past-present-and-future/

Harvard Health Publishing. (2015). *Vegetarian diet linked to lower colon cancer risk.* https://health.harvard.edu/blog/vegetarian-diet-linked-to-lower-colon-cancer-risk-201503117785

Healthline Media. (2021). *The recommended cholesterol levels by age.* https://www.healthline.com/health/high-cholesterol/levels-by-age

Healthy People 2030. (2020). *Environmental health.* https://health.gov/healthypeople/objectives-and-data/browse-objectives/environmental-health

Mayo Clinic. (2022). *Mayo Clinic BMI and waist circumference calculator.* https://mayoclinic.org/diseases-conditions/obesity/in-depth/bmi-calculator/itt-20084938

Mayo Clinic Staff. (2013). *Statin side effects: Weigh the benefits and risks.* Retrieved October 19, 2015, from http://www.mayoclinic.org/diseases-conditions/high-blood-cholesterol/in-depth/statin-side-effects/art-20046013

Mechanick, J. I., Farkouh, M. E., Newman, J. D., & Garvey, W. T. (2020). Cardiometabolic-based chronic disease, addressing knowledge and clinical practice gaps: JACC state-of-the-art review. *Journal of the American College of Cardiology, 75*(5), 539–555. https://doi.org/10.1016/j.jacc.2019.11.046

Medical News Today. (2022). *What are the health benefits of dark chocolate?* https://www.medicalnewstoday.com/articles/dark-chocolate#anti-inflammatory-effects

Mellardo, A. (2022). This one cause of abdominal fat will shock you, new study reveals. https://www.eatthis.com/news-insufficient-sleep-abdominal-fat/

Narla, R., Peck, S. B., & Qiu, K. M. (2014). Fish oil for treatment of dyslipidemia. *American Family Physician, 89*(4), 288–290. Retrieved October 19, 2015, from http://www.aafp.org/afp/2014/0215/p288.html

National Heart, Lung, and Blood Institute. (n.d.). *Body mass index table.* https://www.nhlbi.nih.gov/health/educational/lose_wt/BMI/bmi_tbl.pdf

National Heart, Lung, and Blood Institute. (2024). *Assessing your weight and health risk.* https://www.nhlbi.nih.gov/health/educational/lose_wt/risk.htm

National Institute of Medicine. (2005). *Clinical guidelines on the identification, evaluation, and treatment of overweight and obesity in adults.* https://www.nhlbi.nih.gov/files/docs/guidelines/ob_gdlns.pdf

Office of Disease Prevention and Health Promotion. (n.d.). *Healthy people 2030 framework.* https://www.healthypeople.gov/2020/About-Healthy-People/Development-Healthy-People-2030/Framework

Tucker, M. E. (2013). *Endocrinology group rejects new AHA/ACC CVD guidelines.* Retrieved July 17, 2015, from http://www.medscape.com/viewarticle/817810

Umay, E., Eyigor, S., Bahat, G., Halil, M., Giray, E., Unsal, P., Unlu, Z., Tikiz, C., Vural, M., Cincin, A. T., Bengisu, S., Gurcay, E., Keseroglu, K., Aydeniz, B., Karaca, E. C., Karaca, B., Yalcin, A., Ozsurekci, C., Seyidoglu, D., Yilmaz, O., …, Ozturk, E. A. (2022). Best practice recommendations for geriatric dysphagia management with 5 Ws and 1H. *Annals of Geriatric Medicine and Research, 26*(2), 94–124. https://doi.org/10.4235/agmr.21.0145

U. S. Department of Agriculture. (2016). *MyPlate daily checklist.* https://chsciowa.org/sites/chsciowa.org/files/resource/files/myplate_dailychecklist_age14plus.pdf

U. S. Department of Agriculture. (2024a). *Learn how to eat healthy with MyPlate.* https://www.myplate.gov/

U. S. Department of Agriculture. (2024b). *Dietary guidelines for Americans 2020-2025.* https://www.dietaryguidelines.gov/sites/default/files/2020-12/Dietary_Guidelines_for_Americans_2020-2025.pdf

U.S. Department of Health and Human Services. (2015). *Healthy people, 2020.* Retrieved July 17, 2015, from http://www.healthypeople.gov

U.S. Department of Health and Human Services & U.S. Department of Agriculture. (2011). *Dietary guidelines for Americans, 2010.* Retrieved July 16, 2015, from http://www.health.gov/dietaryguidelines/dga2010/DietaryGuidelines2010.pdf

U.S. Department of Health and Human Services. (2019). *Physical activities, guidelines for Americans* (2nd ed.). https://health.gov/sites/default/files/2019-09/Physical_Activity_Guidelines_2nd_edition.pdf

U.S. Food and Drug Administration. (2013). *Guidance for industry: Food labeling guide.* https://www.fda.gov/regulatory-information/search-fda-guidance-documents/guidance-industry-food-labeling-guide

U.S. Food and Drug Administration. (2022). *Final determination regarding partially hydrogenated oils (removing trans fat).* https://www.fda.gov/food/food-additives-petitions/final-determination-regarding-partially-hydrogenated-oils-removing-trans-fat

U. S. Food and Drug Administration. (2024). *Label claims for conventional foods and dietary supplements.* https://www.fda.gov/food/food-labeling-nutrition/label-claims-conventional-foods-and-dietary-supplements

CHAPTER 16

American National Red Cross. (n.d.). *Eligibility criteria: Alphabetical.* https://www.redcrossblood.org/donate-blood/how-to-donate/eligibility-requirements/eligibility-criteria-alphabetical.html

American Nurses Association. (2015). *Sharps injury prevention.* Retrieved July 27, 2015, from http://www.nursingworld.org/safeneedles

American Red Cross. (2020). *Infectious disease, HLA and ABO donor qualification testing.* https://www.redcrossblood.org/biomedical-services/blood-diagnostic-testing/blood-testing.html

Association for the Advancement of Blood & Biotherapies. (n.d.). *Donor safety, screening and testing.* http://www.aabb.org/advocacy/regulatorygovernment/donoreligibility/Pages/default.aspx

Business Wire. (2014). *Oxygen Biotherapeutics announces halt of Oxycyte phase IIb traumatic brain injury trial.* Retrieved July 27, 2015, from http://www.businesswire.com/news/home/20140911006403/en/Oxygen-Biotheraptics-Annouces-Halt-Oxycyte-Phase-IIb#.VbZex31RGM8

Bouya, S., Balouchi, A., Rafiemanesh, H., Amirshahi, M., Dastres, M., Moghadam, M. P., Behnamfar, N., Shyeback, M., Badakhsh, M., Allahyari, J., Al Mawali, A., Ebadi, A., Dezhkam, A., & Daley, K. A. (2020). Global prevalence and device related causes of needle stick injuries among health care workers: A systematic review and meta-analysis. *Annals of Global Health, 86*(1), 35. https://doi.org/10.5334/aogh.2698

Cardinale, M., Owusu, K., & Malm, T. (2017). Chapter 29—Blood, blood components, plasma, and plasma products. *Side Effects of Drugs Annual, 39,* 331–343. https://doi.org/10.1016/bs.seda.2017.06.011

Centers for Disease Control and Prevention. (2017). *Guidelines for the prevention of intravascular catheter-related infections.* http://www.cdc.gov/hicpac/pdf/guidelines/bsi-guidelines-2011.pdf

Dudek, S. G. (2021). *Nutrition essentials for nursing practice* (9th ed.). Lippincott Williams & Wilkins.

Fischbach, F., Fischbach, M., & Stout, K. (2021). *A manual of laboratory and diagnostic tests* (11th ed.). Lippincott Williams & Wilkins.

Food and Drug Administration. (2017). *Recommendations for assessment of blood donor eligibility, donor deferral and blood product management in response to Ebola virus.* https://www.fda.gov/media/94902/download

Hinkle, J. L., & Cheever, K. H. (2021). *Brunner & Suddarth's textbook of medical-surgical nursing* (15th ed.). Lippincott Williams & Wilkins.

Infusion Nurse Blog. (n.d.). *Poll results: Gloves vs no gloves during vein palpation.* Retrieved July 28, 2015, from https://infusionnurse.org/2012/06/09/poll-results-gloves-vs-no-gloves-during-vein-palpation/

Kakaei, N., Amirian, R., Azadi, M., Mohammadi, G., & Izadi, Z. (2023). Perfluorocarbons: A perspective of theranostic applications and challenges. *Frontiers in Bioengineering and Biotechnology, 11,* 1115254. https://doi.org/10.3389/fbioe.2023.1115254

Moore, E. E., Moore, F. A., Fabian, T. C., Bernard, A. C., Fulda, G. J., Hoyt, D. B., Duane, T. M., Weireter, L. J., Jr., Gomez, G. A., Cipolle, M. D., Rodman, G. H., Jr., Malangoni, M. A., Hides, G. A., Omert, L. A., Gould, S. A., & PolyHeme Study Group. (2009). Human polymerized hemoglobin for the treatment of hemorrhagic shock when blood is unavailable: The USA multicenter trial. *Journal of the American College of Surgeons, 208*(1), 1–13. https://doi.org/10.1016/j.jamcollsurg.2008.09.023

Moosmosis. (2020). *Glucose transporters GLUT and SGLT: Biochemistry, MCAT, and USMLE.* https://moosmosis.org/2020/07/21/glucose-transporters-glut-and-sglt-biochemistry/

Patrician, P. A., Pryor, E., Fridman, M., & Loan, L. (2011). Needlestick injuries among nursing staff: Association with shift-level staffing. *American Journal of Infection Control, 39*(6), 477–482. https://doi.org/10.1016/j.ajic.2010.10.017

Ray, S. D. (Ed.). (2017). *A worldwide yearly survey of new data in adverse drug reactions* (Vol. 44). Elsevier. https://www.sciencedirect.com/topics/medicine-and-dentistry/haemoglobin-based-oxygen-carriers

CHAPTER 17

Ashkenazi, M., Yaish, Y., Yitzhak, M., Sarnat, H., & Rakocz, M. (2013). The relationship between nurses' oral hygiene and the mouth care of their patients. *Special Care in Dentistry, 33*(6), 280–285. https://doi.org/10.1111/j.1754-4505.2012.00306.x

Coker, E., Ploeg, J., Kaasalainen, S., & Fisher, A. (2013). A concept analysis of oral hygiene care in dependent older adults. *Journal of Advanced Nursing, 69*(10), 2360–2371. https://doi.org/10.1111/jan.12107

Cowdell, F., & Radley, K. (2014). What do we know about skin-hygiene care for patients with bariatric needs? Implications for nursing practice. *Journal of Advanced Nursing, 70*(3), 543–552. https://doi.org/10.1111/jan.12208

Dupont, R. (2022). Dementia care: Bathing without a battle. https://www.aplaceformom.com/caregiver-resources/articles/bathing-and-dementia

El-Solh, A. A. (2011). Association between pneumonia and oral care in nursing home residents. *Lung, 189*(3), 173–180. https://doi.org/10.1007/s00408-011-9297-0

Lindqvist, L., Seleskog, B., Wardh, I., & von Bültzingslöwen, I. (2013). Oral care perspectives of professionals in nursing homes for the elderly. *International Journal of Dental Hygiene, 11*(4), 298–305. https://doi.org/10.1111/idh.12016

Lippincott. (2011). *Lippincott's visual nursing* (2nd ed.). Lippincott Williams & Wilkins.

Özden, D., Türk, G., Düger, C., Güler, E. K., Tok, F., & Gülsoy, Z. (2014). Effects of oral care solutions on mucous membrane integrity and bacterial colonization. *Nursing in Critical Care, 19*(2), 78–86. https://doi.org/10.1111/nicc.12057

Poor Hygiene: Hygiene in the Nursing Home. (2024). https://www.nursinghomeabusecenter.com/nursing-home-neglect/poor-hygiene/

Sonnenberg, A. (2015). *Electric vs. manual toothbrushes: Which should you choose?* Retrieved August 4, 2015, from http://www.besthealthmag.ca/best-you/oral-health/electric-vs-manual-toothbrushes-which-should-you-choose/#Iv2tasC1WTpL7G36.97

Stolt, M., Suhonen, R., Puulla, P., Viitanen, M., Voutilainen, P., & Leino-Kilpi, H. (2013). Nurses' foot care activities in home health care. *Geriatric Nursing, 34*(6), 491–497.

Willumsen, T., Karlsen, L., Naess, R., & Bjørntvedt, S. (2012). Are the barriers to good oral hygiene in nursing homes within the nurses or the patients? *Gerondontology, 29*(2), e748–e755. https://doi.org/10.1111/j.1741-2358.2011.00554.x

CHAPTER 18

American Psychiatric Association. (2013). *Diagnostic and statistical manual of mental disorders* (5th ed.). American Psychiatric Publishing.

American Sleep Apnea Association. (2015). *The state of sleep health in America.* https://www.sleephealth.org/sleep-health/the-state-of-sleephealth-in-america/

American Sleep Association. (n.d.). *Insomnia: Symptoms, causes & treatment.* https://www.sleepassociation.org/sleep-disorders/insomnia

Armon, C. (2014). *Polysomnography.* Retrieved August 9, 2015, from http://emedicine.medscape.com/article/1188764-overview

ASA.org. (2020). *Sleep apnea, testing and diagnostics.* https://www.sleepapnea.org/treat/getting-sleep-apnea-diagnosis/

Centers for Medicare & Medicaid Services. (2020). *Polysomnography and sleep testing.* https://www.cms.gov/medicare-coverage-database/view/lcd.aspx?lcdId=33405&ver=25

Cherry, K. (2022). *The 4 stages of sleep. What happens in the brain and body during NREM and REM sleep.* https://verywellhealth.com/the-four-stages-of-sleep-2795920

Division of Sleep and Medicine Harvard Medical School. (2024). *Genetics, aging and sleep: Sleep and aging.* https://sleep.hms.harvard.edu/education-training/public-education/sleep-and-health-education-program/sleep-health-education-79

Harvard Medical School. (2007). *Healthy sleep.* Retrieved August 11, 2015, from http://healthysleep.med.harvard.edu/healthy/science/what/sleep-patterns-rem-nrem

Herdman, H. T., & Kamitsuru, S. (2018). *NANDA international nursing diagnoses: Definitions & classification 2018–2020* (11th ed.). Thieme.

Institute of Medicine (US) Committee on Sleep Medicine and Research. (2006). *Sleep disorders and sleep deprivation: An unmet public health problem.* National Academies Press.

Khullar, A. (2012). *The role of melatonin in the circadian rhythm sleep-wake cycle.* Retrieved August 8, 2015, from https://www.psychiatrictimes.com/view/role-melatonin-circadian-rhythm-sleep-wake-cycle

Kirsch, D. (2015). *Stages and architecture of normal sleep.* Retrieved August 8, 2015, from http://www.uptodate.com/contents/stages-and-architecture-of-normal-sleep

Markwalk, R. R., Melanson, E. L., Smith, M. R., Higgins, J., Perreault, L., Eckel, R. H., & Wright, K. P., Jr. (2013). Impact of insufficient sleep on total daily energy expenditure, food intake, and weight gain. *Proceedings of the National Academy of Sciences of the United States of America, 110*(4), 5695–5700. https://doi.org/10.1073/pnas.1216951110

National Institute of Neurological Disorders and Stroke. (2014). *Brain basics: Understanding sleep.* Retrieved August 10, 2015, from https://www.ninds.nih.gov/health-information/public-education/brain-basics/brain-basics-understanding-sleep

National Sleep Foundation. (2023a). 2009 Health and safety. *Sleep Health Journal, 4*(2), 83–140.

National Sleep Foundation. (2023b). *Shift work disorder symptoms.* https://www.sleepfoundation.org/shift-work-disorder/symptoms#:~:text=The%20average%20person%20with%20shift,least%20once%20during%20their%20shift

National Sleep Foundation. (2022) *How much sleep do we really need.* Retrieved June 26, 2023, https://www.sleepfoundation.org/articles/how-much-sleep-do-we-really-need

SleepFoundation.org. (2023a). *Obesity and sleep.* https://www.sleepfoundation.org/physical-health/obesity-and-sleep

SleepFoundation.org. (2023b). *Insomnia: Symptoms, causes, and treatments. What it is, how it affects you, and how to help you get back your restful nights.* https://www.sleepfoundation.org/insomnia

Sleephealth.org. (2020). *The state of sleep health in America.* https://www.sleephealth.org/sleep-health/the-state-of-sleephealth-in-america/

CHAPTER 19

American Nurse Today. (n.d.). *When and how to use restraints.* www.AmericanNurseToday.com

American Psychiatric Nurses Association. (2014). *APNA position on the use of seclusion & restraint.* Retrieved August 15, 2015, from http://www.apna.org/i4a/pages/index.cfm?pageid=3730

Bush, E. (2015). *Smoke inhalation is the most common cause of death in house fires.* Retrieved August 14, 2015, from http://msue.anr.msu.edu/news/smoke_inhalation_is_the_most_common_cause_of_death_in_house_fires

Center for Patient Safety. (2024). *Hospital: 2024 national patient safety goals.* https://www.jointcommission.org/standards/national-patient-safety-goals/hospital-national-patient-safety-goals/.

Centers for Disease Control and Prevention. (2023a). *Older adult fall prevention.* https://www.cdc.gov/falls/index.html

Centers for Disease Control and Prevention. (2023b). *Older adult fall prevention facts about falls.* https://www.cdc.gov/falls/facts.html

Healthwise Staff. (2012). *Carbon monoxide poisoning.* Retrieved August 14, 2015, from http://www.webmd.com/first-aid/tc/carbon-monoxide-poisoning-topic-overview

Hendrich, A. (2013). *Fall risk assessment for older adults: The Hendrich II fall risk model™.* Retrieved August 15, 2015, from http://uprightfallprevention.com

Holstege, C. P. (2015). *Smoke inhalation.* Retrieved August 14, 2015, from http://www.emedicinehealth.com/smoke_inhalation/article_em.htm

The Joint Commission. (2022). *Restraint or seclusion—Role of residents enrolled in graduate medical education programs.* https://www.jointcommission.org/standards/standard-faqs/critical-access-hospital/provision-of-care-treatment-and-services-pc/000001359/

The Joint Commission. (2024). *Hospital: 2024 National Patient Safety Goals.* https://www.jointcommission.org/standards/national-patient-safety-goals/hospital-national-patient-safety-goals/

Rodziewicz, T. L., Houseman, B., & Hipskind, J. E. (2024). Medical error reduction and prevention. *StatPearls*. Treasure Island (FL): StatPearls Publishing; https://www.ncbi.nlm.nih.gov/books/NBK499956/

Mercola, J. (2013). *What is the leading cause of death in U.S.?* Retrieved August 12, 2015, from http://blog.world-mysteries.com/science/what-is-the-leading-cause-of-death-in-u-s/

Mercurio, J. (2011). Creating a latex-safe perioperative environment. *OR Nurse, 5*(6), 18–25.

National Conference of State Legislatures. (2020). *Medicare nonpayment for hospital-acquired conditions.* https://www.ncsl.org/research/health/medicare-nonpayment-for-hospital-acquired.aspx

National Fire Protection Association. (2024). *Fire extinguisher information.* https://www.nfpa.org/education-and-research/home-fire-safety/fire-extinguishers

National Fire Protection Association. (2023). *Fire loss in the United States.* https://www.nfpa.org/education-and-research/research/nfpa-research/fire-statistical-reports/fire-loss-in-the-united-states

National Poison Control. (2023). *National poison control call statistics, 2021.* https://www.poison.org/poison-statistics-national

Quigley, P. A., & White, S. V. (2013). *Hospital-based fall program measurement and improvement in high reliability organizations.* Retrieved August 15, 2015, from http://www.medscape.com/viewarticle/813259

Shochat, G. N. (2015). *Carbon monoxide toxicity.* Retrieved August 14, 2015, from http://emedicine.medscape.com/article/819987-overview

Sorensen, A., Jarrett, N., Tant, E., Bernard, S., & McCall, N. (2014). *HAC-POA policy effects on hospitals, other payers, and patients.* Retrieved August 15, 2015, from https://www.cms.gov/mmrr/Downloads/MMRR2014_004_03_a07.pdf

Starfield, B. (2000). Is US health really the best in the world? *Journal of the American Medical Association, 284*(4), 483–485.

CHAPTER 20

Alexander, B. K., & Wong, L. S. (2010). *Demon drug myths: The myth of drug-induced addiction.* Retrieved August 24, 2015, from http://www.brucekalexander.com/articles-speeches/demon-drug-myths

ANA Position Statement. (2018). *The ethical responsibility to manage pain and the suffering it causes.* https://www.nursingworld.org/~495e9b/globalassets/docs/ana/ethics/theethicalresponsibilitytomanagepainandthesufferingitcauses2018.pdf

Arnstein, P., Broglio, K., Wuhrman, E., & Kean, M. B. (2011). Use of placebos in pain management. *Pain Management Nursing, 12*(4), 225–229.

Bernhofer, E. (2011). Ethics and pain management in hospitalized patients. *The Online Journal of Issues in Nursing, 17*(1). Retrieved August 22, 2015, from http://www.nursingworld.org/MainMenuCategories/ANAMarketplace/ANAPeriodicals/OJIN/TableofContents/Vol-17-2012/No1-Jan-2012/Ethics-and-Pain-Management.html

Centers for Disease Control and Prevention. (2023). *Treat opioid use disorder.* https://www.cdc.gov/opioids/overdoseprevention/treatment.html

Centers for Disease Control and Prevention, National Center for Health Statistics, Office of Communication. (2022). *Drug & alcohol deaths on the rise among older Americans.* https://www.cdc.gov/nchs/pressroom/nchs_press_releases/2022/20221130.htm#:~:text=Death%20rates%20from%20drug%20overdoses,women%20in%20the%20recent%20period

Copstead, L. E., & Banasik, J. L. (2012). *Pathophysiology, biological and behavioral perspectives* (5th ed.). Saunders.

Davids, H. R. (2024). *Botulinum toxin in pain management.* https://emedicine.medscape.com/article/325574-overview?form=fpf

Di Maio, G., Villano, I., Ilardi, C. R., Messina, A., Monda, V., Iodice, A. C., Porro, C., Panaro, M. A., Chieffi, S., Messina, G., Monda, M., & La Marra, M. (2023). Mechanisms of transmission and processing of pain: A narrative review. *International Journal of Environmental Research and Public Health, 20*(4), 3064. https://doi.org/10.3390/ijerph20043064

Drugs.com. (2020). *NSAIDs: Do they increase my risk of heart attack and stroke?* https://www.drugs.com/mcf/nsaids-do-they-increase-my-risk-of-heart-attack-and-stroke

Fein, A. (2012). *Nociceptors and the perception of pain.* Retrieved August 20, 2015, from http://cell.uchc.edu/pdf/fein/nociceptors_fein_2012.pdf

Freudenrich, C. (2007). *How pain works.* Retrieved August 20, 2015, from http://science.howstuffworks.com/life/inside-the mind/human-brain/pain4.htm

Kendroud, S., Fitzgerald, L. A., Murray, I. V., & Hanna, A. (2024). *Physiology, nociceptive pathways.* StatPearls Publishing. https://www.ncbi.nlm.nih.gov/books/NBK470255/

Lohman, D., Schleifer, R., & Amon, J. J. (2010). *Access to pain treatment as a human right. BMC Medicine, 8,* 8. https://doi.org/10.1186/1741-7015-8-8

Maxwell, K. (2012). *The challenges of cancer pain assessment and management.* Retrieved August 22, 2015, from http://www.ncbi.nlm.gov/pmc/articles/PMC3605546/

McCaffery, M., & Ferrell, B. (1999). Opioids and pain management: What do nurses know? *Nursing, 29*(3), 48–52.

MD Anderson Cancer Center. (2009). *Botulinum toxin for the treatment of chronic pain syndromes.* Retrieved August 22, 2015, from http://www.mdanderson.org/transcripts/botulinum-toxin-transcript.html

Medscape. (2016). *Botulinum toxin in pain management.* https://emedicine.medscape.com/article/325574-overview#showall

Melzack, R. (1999). From the gate to the neuromatrix. *Pain, 82*(Suppl. 6), S121–S126.

Melzack, R., & Wall, P. D. (1965). Pain mechanisms: A new theory. *Science, 150*(3699), 971–979.

National Institute of Drug Abuse. (2022). *Opioid overdose crisis.* https://www.drugabuse.gov/drugs-abuse/opioids/opioid-overdose-crisis

National Institute of Neurological Disorders. (2009). Pain: Hope through research. *Journal of Pain & Palliative Care Pharmacotherapy, 23*(3), 307–322.

NCCIH.NIH.gov. (2023). *Glucosamine and chondroitin used for osteoarthritis.* http://nccih.nih.gov/health/glucosaminechondroitin

Physiotherapy-treatment.com. (n.d.). *Gate control theory of pain.* https://www.physiotherapy-treatment.com/gate-control-theory-of-pain.html

Preidt, R. (2014). *Knee pain may not be helped by glucosamine.* Retrieved August 22, 2015, from http://www.webmd.com/pain-management/knee-pain/news/20140311/knee-pain-may-not-be-helped-by-glucosamine

Salmedo, D. (2015). *Fibromyalgia and neuropathic pain have both differences and similarities in sensory profiles.* Retrieved August 21, 2015, from http://fibromyalgianewstoday.com/2015/01/15/fibromyalgia-neuropathic-pain-differences-similarities-sensory-profiles/

Stallard, J. (2013). *Will I become addicted to the pain medications I may need during my cancer treatment?* Retrieved August 24, 2015, from https://www.makcc.org/blog/will-i-become-addicted-pain-medications-i-may-need-during-my-treatment/

Sutherland, S. (2013). *Multiple studies, one conclusion: Some fibromyalgia patients show peripheral nerve pathologies.* Retrieved August 21, 2015, from http://www.painresearchforum

.org/news/33529-multiple-studies-one-conclusion-some-fibromyalgia-patients-show-peripheral-nerve-pathologies

Pasquale, M., Murphy, N. (2022). *The emotional impact of the pain experience.* https://www.hss.edu/conditions_emotional-impact-pain-experience.asp

Upendarrao, G. (2013). *Pain control theories.* Retrieved August 20, 2015, from http://www.slideshare.net/gollaupendarrao/theories-of-pain

What are the key concepts organizations need to understand regarding pain management requirements in the Leadership (LD) and provision of Care, Treatment, and Services (PC) chapters? (2022). https://www.jointcommission.org/standards/standard-faqs/hospital-and-hospital-clinics/provision-of-care-treatment-and-services-pc/000002161/

WebMD. (n.d.). *Neuropathic pain management.* https://www.webmd.com/pain-management/guide/neuropathic-pain#1

World Health Organization. (2022a). *WHO's pain ladder.* who.int.cancer/palliative/painladder/en/

World Health Organization. (2022b). *WHO analgesic ladder.* http://www.ncbi.nlm.nih.gov/books/NBK554435/figure/article-31358.image.f1/

Yang, J., Bauer, B. A., Wahner-Roedler, D. L., Chon, T. Y., & Xiao, L. (2020). The modified WHO analgesic ladder: Is it appropriate for chronic non-cancer pain? *Journal of Pain Research, 13*, 411–417. https://doi.org/10.2147/JPR.S244173

CHAPTER 21

Allen, D. (2007). Oxygen therapy: How much do you really know about oxygen therapy and respiratory diseases. *Nursing Older People, 19*(1), 36. https://doi.org/10.7748/nop2007.02.19.1.36.c4364

American Association for Respiratory Care. (2007). *Oxygen therapy in the home or alternate site health care facility—2007 revision & update AARC clinical practice guideline.* https://www.aarc.org/wp-content/uploads/2014/08/08.07.1063.pdf

American Association of Respiratory Care. (n.d.). *A guide to portable oxygen concentrators.* https://www.aarc.org/wp-content/uploads/2014/08/portable_oxygen_concentrators_guide.pdf

American Lung Association. (2015). *Supplemental oxygen.* Retrieved September 8, 2015, from http://www.lung.org/lung-disease/copd/treating-copd/supplemental-oxygen.html

Anderson, M. A., Hill, P. D., & Johnson, C. L. (2012). Comparison of pulse oximetry measures in a health population. *MedSurg Nursing, 21*(2), 70–75; quiz 76.

Bauman, M. (2011). *Chest-tube care: The more you know, the easier it gets.* Retrieved September 11, 2015, from http://americannursetoday.com/chest-tube-care-the-more-you-know-the-easier-it-gets/

Booker, R. (2008). Pulse oximetry. *Nursing Standard, 22*(30), 39–41. https://doi.org/10.7748/ns2008.04.22.30.39.c6441

Henderson, Y. (2008). Delivering oxygen therapy to acute breathless adults. *Nursing Standard, 22*(35), 46–48. https://doi.org/10.7748/ns2008.05.22.35.46.c6535

Malhatra, A., Schwartz, D. R., & Schwartzstein, R. M. (2015). *Oxygen toxicity.* Retrieved September 8, 2015, from http://www.uptodate.com/contents/oxygen-toxicity

McGloin, S. (2008). Administration of oxygen therapy. *Nursing Standard, 22*(21), 46–48. https://doi.org/10.7748/ns2008.01.22.21.46.c6416

Merritt, S. (2014). *Nursing: Chest tube maintenance and troubleshooting.* Retrieved September 11, 2015, from https://www.youtube.com/watch?v=pFuGwSOEtUk

National Heart Lung Blood Institute. (2022). *Oxygen therapy.* https://www.nhlbi.nih.gov/health/lung-treatments

Peters, B. (2014). *What is the difference between CPAP and BiPAP?* Retrieved September 8, 2015, from http://sleepdisorders.about.com/od/sleepdisorderstreatment/fl/What-Is-the-Difference-Between-CPAP-and-BiPAP.htm

Phillips, K. (2014). *(2023). BiPAP vs. CPAP machines: Breaking down the differences.* https://www.sleepfoundation.org/cpap/cpap-vs-bipap

Sharma, S., Danckers, M., Sanghavi, D.,& Chakraborty, R. K. (2022). High-flow nasal cannula. In *StatPearls* [Internet]. National Center for Biotechnology Information. https://www.ncbi.nlm.nih.gov/books/NBK526071/

Stitch, J. C., & Cassella, D. M. (2009). Oxygen delivery devices. *Nursing, 39*(9), 51–54. https://doi.org/10.1097/01.NURSE.0000360249.26070.d3

Stubblefield, H. (2014). *Oxygen therapy.* Retrieved September 8, 2015, from http://www.healthline.com/health/oxygen-therapy#Overview/

WebMD. (2023). *What is an oxygen concentrator?* https://www.webmd.com/lung/oxygen-concentrator-what-is

Woodrow, P. (2007). Caring for patients receiving oxygen therapy. *Nursing Older People, 19*(1), 31–51. https://doi.org/10.7748/nop2007.02.19.1.31.c4363

CHAPTER 22

Association for Professionals in Infection Control and Epidemiology. (2024). *Follow all posted precaution signs.* https://infectionpreventionandyou.org/protect-your-patients/follow-the-rules-for-isolation-precautions/

Brown, L., Munro, J., & Rogers, S. (2019). Use of personal protective equipment in nursing practice. *Nursing Standard, 34*(5), 59–66. https://doi.org/10.7748/ns.2019.e11260

Beam, E., Gibbs, S. G., Boulter, K. C., Beckerdite, M. E., & Smith, P. W. (2011). A method for evaluating health care workers' personal protective equipment technique. *American Journal of Infection Control, 39*(5), 415–420. https://doi.org/10.1016/j.ajic.2010.07.009

Beam, E., Gibbs, S. G., Hewlett, A. L., Iwen, P. C., Nuss, S. L., & Smith, P. W. (2014). Method for investigating nursing behaviors related to isolation care. *American Journal of Infection Control, 42*(11), 1152–1156. https://doi.org/10.1016/j.ajic.2014.08.001

Beam, E., Gibbs, S. G., Hewlett, A. L., Iwen, P. C., Nuss, S. L., & Smith, P. W. (2015). Clinical challenges in isolation care. *American Journal of Nursing, 115*(4), 44–49. https://doi.org/10.1097/01.NAJ.0000463027.27141.32

Benson, S., & Powers, J. (2011). *Your role in infection prevention.* Retrieved September 17, 2015, from http://www.nursingcenter.com/cearticle?tid=1157225

Carpenito, L. J. (2012). *Nursing diagnosis: Application to clinical practice* (4th ed.). Lippincott Williams & Wilkins.

Centers for Disease Control and Prevention. (2015). *Guidance on personal protective equipment (PPE) in U.S. Healthcare Settings during management of patients confirmed to have selected viral hemorrhagic fevers or patients suspected to have selected viral hemorrhagic fevers who are clinically unstable or have bleeding, vomiting, or diarrhea.* Retrieved September 19, 2015, from http://www.cdc.gov/vhf/ebola/healthcare-us/ppe/guidance.html

Centers for Disease Control and Prevention. (2021). *2019 National and State Healthcare-Associated Infections Progress Report.* https://archive.cdc.gov/www_cdc_gov/hai/data/archive/2019-HAI-progress-report.html

Commiskey, D. (2009). *Contact precautions: You should know them forwards and backwards.* http://allnurses.com/nclex-disscussion-forum/contact-precautions-you-409406.html

HIV.gov. (n.d.). *How do you get or transmit HIV?* https://www.hiv.gov/hiv-basics/overview/about-hiv-and-aids/how-is-hiv-transmitted

About HIV. (2024). From https://www.cdc.gov/hiv/about/

McDonald, M., & Ness, S. M. (2015). *Infection control*. Retrieved September 17, 2015, from http://www.nursingceu.com/courses/485/index_nceu.html

Monsalve, M. N., Pemmaraju, S. V., Thomas, G. W., Herman, T., Segre, A. M., & Polgreen, P. M. (2014). Do peer effects improve hand hygiene adherence among healthcare workers? *Infection Control and Hospital Epidemiology, 35*(10), 1277–1285. https://doi.org/10.1086/678068

Scott, C., Kirking, H. L., Jeffries, C., Price, S. F., & Pratt, R. (2015).Tuberculosis trends—United States, 2014. *Morbidity and Mortality Weekly Report, 64*(10);265-269. https://www.cdc.gov/mmwr/preview/mmwrhtml/mm6410a2.htm#:~:text=In%202014%2C%20a%20total%20of,%25%20from%202013%20(1)

Siegel, J. D., Rhinehart, E., Jackson, M., Chiarello, L., & Health Care Infection Control Practices Advisory Committee (2007). 2007 Guideline for Isolation Precautions: Preventing Transmission of Infectious Agents in Health Care Settings. *American Journal of Infection Control, 35*(10 Suppl 2), S65–S164. https://doi.org/10.1016/j.ajic.2007.10.007

Vyas, J. M. (2014). *Isolation precautions*. Retrieved September 20, 2015, from http://www.ncbi.nlm.nih.gov/books/NBK214342/

Zastrow, R. L. (2011). Emerging infections: The contact precautions controversy. *American Journal of Nursing, 111*(3), 47–53. https://doi.org/10.1097/10.1097/01.NAJ.0000395242.14347.37

CHAPTER 23

American Academy of Pediatrics. (2016). *SIDS and other sleep-related infant deaths: Evidence base for 2016 updated recommendations for a safe infant sleeping environment*. https://pediatrics.aappublications.org/content/pediatrics/138/5/e20162940.full.pdf

American Nurses Association. (2015). *Safe patient handling & mobility*. Retrieved September 24, 2015, from http://www.nursingworld.org/MainMenuCategories/Policy-Advocacy/State/Legislative-Agenda-Reports/State-SafePatientHandling

American Nurses Association. (2024). *Sharps injury prevention*. https://www.nursingworld.org/practice-policy/work-environment/health-safety/safe-needles/

American Nurse Today. (2014). *Current topics in safe patient handling and mobility*. Retrieved September 29, 2015, from http://www.americannursetoday.com/wp-content/uploads/2014/07/ant9-Patient-Handling-Supplement-821a_LOW.pdf

Association of Occupational Health. (2011). *Beyond getting started: A resource guide for implementing a safe patient handling program in the acute care setting*. Retrieved September 24, 2015, from https://www.aohp.org/aohp/Portals/0/Documents/AboutAOHP/BGS_Summer2011.pdf

Centers for Disease Control and Prevention. (2014). *Ergonomics and musculoskeletal disorders*. Retrieved September 23, 2015, from http://www.cdc.gov/niosh/topics/ergonomics

Centers for Disease Control and Prevention. (2015a). *Occupational traumatic injuries among workers in health care facilities—United States, 2012–2014*. Retrieved September 24, 2015, from http://www.cdc.gov/mmwr/preview/mmwrhtml/mm6415a2.htm

Centers for Disease Control and Prevention. (2015b). *Safe patient handling and Mobility (SPHM)*. Retrieved September 24, 2015, from http://www.cdc.gov/niosh/topics/safepatient/

Centers for Disease Control and Prevention. (2022). *Enviromechanical hazards*. https://www.cdc.gov/niosh/learning/safetyculturehc/module-2/6.html

Craven, R. F., Hirnle, C. J., & Jensen, S. (2017). *Fundamentals of nursing* (8th ed.). Lippincott Williams & Wilkins.

deCastro, A. B. (2004). *Handle with care®: The American Nurses Association's campaign to address work-related musculoskeletal disorders*. Retrieved September 24, 2015, from http://www.nursingworld.org/MainMenuCategories/ANAMarketplace/ANAPeriodicals/OJIN/TableofContents/Volume92004/No3Sept04/HandleWithCare.html

GovTrack.us. (2020). *H.R. 4266(114th): Nurse and Health Care Worker Protection Act of 2015*. https://www.govtrack.us/congress/bills/114/hr4266

National Occupational Research Agenda. (2018). *National occupational research agenda for musculoskeletal health*. https://www.cdc.gov/nora/councils/mus/pdfs/National-Occupational-Research-Agenda-for-Musculoskeletal-Health-October-2018.pdf

Obesity Action Coalition. (2015). *What is severe obesity?* Retrieved September 28, 2015, from http://www.obesityaction.org/understanding-obesity/severe-obesity

Occupational Safety and Health Administration. (2009). *Guidelines for nursing homes: Ergonomics for the prevention of musculoskeletal disorders*. Retrieved September 29, 2015, from http://www.osha.gov/ergonomics/guidelines/nursinghome/final_nh_guidelines.html

Occupational Safety and Health Administration. (2024). *Worker safety in hospitals, caring for our caregivers*. https://www.osha.gov/hospitals

Occupational Safety and Health Administration. (2014a). *Safe patient handling—Preventing musculoskeletal disorders in nursing homes*. Retrieved September 24, 2015, from https://www.osha.gov/Publications/OSHA3708.pdf

Occupational Safety and Health Administration. (2014b). *Worker safety in hospitals: Caring for our caregivers*. Retrieved September 24, 2015, from https://www.osha.gov/dsg/hospitals/patient_handling.html

The Joint Commission. (2012). *Improving patient and worker safety: Opportunities for synergy, collaboration and innovation*. Retrieved September 25, 2015, from http://www.jointcommision.org/assets/1/18/TJC-ImprovingPatientAndWorkerSafety-Monograph.pdf

United States House. (2013). *H.R.2480—Nurse and health care worker protection act of 2013*. Retrieved September 24, 2015, from https://www.congress.gov/bill/113th-congress/house-bill/2480

Venus, K., Munshi, L., & Fralick, M. (2020, November 23). Prone positioning for patients with hypoxic respiratory failure related to COVID-19. *Canadian Medical Association Journal, 192*(47), E1532–E1537. https://doi.org/10.1503/cmaj.201201

VISN 8 Patient Safety Center. (2005). *Safe patient handling and movement algorithms*. https://www.lmcins.com/uploads/3/2/0/7/3207324/safe_patient_handling.pdf

CHAPTER 24

10,000 Steps. (2020). *Counting your steps*. https://www.10000steps.org.au/articles/counting-steps/

American College of Sports Medicine. (2011). *(2024) Physical activity guidelines*. https://www.acsm.org/education-resources/trending-topics-resources/physical-activity-guidelines

Centers for Disease Control and Prevention. (2015). *Measuring physical activity intensity*. Retrieved October 2, 2015, from http://www.cdc.gov/physicalactivity/basics/measuring/heartrate.htm

Centers for Disease Control and Prevention. (2020). *Physical activity*. https://www.cdc.gov/physicalactivity/basics/measuring/heartrate.htm

Douglas, P. S. (2014). *Exercise and fitness in the prevention of atherosclerotic cardiovascular disease.* Retrieved October 6, 2015, from http://www.uptodate.com/contents/exercise-and-fitness-in-the-prevention-of-cardiovascular-disease

Flack, K. D., Stults-Kolehmainen, M. A., Creasy, S. A., Khullar, S., Boullosa, D., Catenacci, V. A., & King, N. (2023). Altered motivation states for physical activity and 'appetite' for movement as compensatory mechanisms limiting the efficacy of exercise training for weight loss. *Frontiers in Psychology, 14.* https://doi.org/10.3389/fpsyg.2023.1098394

Foster, H. (2014). *The 3 I's: Isotonic, isometric and isokinetic exercises.* Retrieved October 5, 2015, from http://www.livestrong.com/article/434761-isotonic-isometric-and-isokinetic-exercises

Jackson, B. (2015). *Sobering statistics on physical inactivity in the U.S.* Retrieved October 5, 2015, from http://www.sciencedaily.com/releases/2015/08/150826093015.htm

Lund University. (2015). *Exercise is good for everyone, but some struggle more than others.* Retrieved October 5, 2015, from http://www.sciencedaily.com/releases/2015/10/151002103353.htm

National Institute on Aging. (2015). *Exercise and physical activity.* Retrieved October 5, 2015, from http://www.nia.nih.gov/health/publication/exercise-physical-activity/introduction

Topend Sports Network. (2020). *Harvard step test.* https://www.topendsports.com/testing/tests/step-harvard.htm

Weil, R. (2015a). *Aerobic exercise.* Retrieved October 5, 2015, from http://www.medicinenet.com/aerobic_exercise/article.htm

Weil, R. (2015b). *Pedometers.* http://www.medicinenet.com/pedometers/article.htm

Zelman, K. (2015). *Get motivated to exercise.* Retrieved October 5, 2015, from http://www.medicinenet.com/benefits_of_exercise/article.htm

CHAPTER 25

Brown, J. L. (2014). *Cast care.* Retrieved October 14, 2015, from http://www.emedicinehealth.com/cast_care/article_em.htm

Cincinnati Children's Hospital Medical Center. (2024). What is the care for a hip spica cast?. https://www.cincinnatichildrens.org/health/h/hip-spica

Cone, J., & Inaba, K. (2017). Lower extremity compartment syndrome. *Trauma Surgery & Acute Care Open, 2*(1), e000094. https://doi.org/10.1136/tsaco-2017-000094

Davis, P. (2012). *Skeletal pin traction: Guidelines on postoperative care and support.* Retrieved October 14, 2015, from http://www.nursingtimes.net/Journals/2012/11/09/z/y/a/030527Skeletal-pin-traction-guidelines-on-postoperative-care-and-support.pdf

Drugs.com. (2024). Walking boot. https://www.drugs.com/cg/walking-boot.html#:~:text=The%20boot%20can%20be%20used,mid%2Dway%20up%20your%20calf

Ma, C. B. (2014). *Compartment syndrome.* Retrieved October 13, 2015, from http://www.nlm.nih.gov/medlineplus/ency/article/001224.htm

Nadar, M. S., Alotaibi, N., & Manee, F. (2023). Efficacy of splinting the wrist and metacarpophalangeal joints for the treatment of Carpal tunnel syndrome: an assessor-blinded randomised controlled trial. *BMJ Open, 13*(11), e076961. https://doi.org/10.1136/bmjopen-2023-076961

Nursingfile.com. (2010). *Nursing interventions: Post cast application and cast removal.* https://nursingfile.com/nursing-care-plan/nursing-interventions/nursing-interventions-post-cast-application-and-cast-removal.html

Rasul, T. T. (2015). *Acute compartment syndrome.* Retrieved October 14, 2015, from http://emedicine.medscape.com/article/307668-overview

Roberts, L. (2022). *Orthopedic nursing 101.* https://www.studypool.com/documents/17001115/orthopaedic-nursing-101

Satryb, S. A., Wilson, T. J., & Patterson, M. M. (2011). *Casting: All wrapped up.* Retrieved October 14, 2015, from http://www.nursingcenter.com/cearticle?tid=1125451

Stang, D. (2012). *Traction: Types, risks, & aftercare.* Retrieved October 14, 2015, from http://www.healthline.com/health/traction#Overview1

University of Pittsburg Schools of Health Sciences. (2022). *Pin care.* https://medlineplus.gov/ency/patientinstructions/000481.htm

Wedro, B. (2015). *Compartment syndrome.* Retrieved October 13, 2015, from http://www.medicinenet.com/compartment_syndrome/page3.htm

CHAPTER 26

American Academy of Orthopedic Surgeons. (2015). *How to use crutches, canes, and walkers.* Retrieved October 26, 2015, from http://orthoinfo.aaos.org/topic.cfm?topic=a00181

Antipuesto, D. J. (2011). *Crutch maneuvering techniques.* Retrieved October 26, 2015, from http://nursingcrib.com/demo-checklist/crutch-maneuvering-techniques

Arm Dynamics. (2024). *Prosthetic options.* https://www.armdynamics.com/our-care/prosthetic-options

Drugs.com. (2015). *Crutch instructions.* Retrieved October 26, 2015, from http://www.drugs.com/cg/crutch-instructions-discharge-care.html

Eustice, C. (2022). *How to use a walker correctly.* https://www.verywellhealth.com/tips-for-walker-use-2552074

Inverarty, L. (2024). *How to safely walk with a cane.* https://www.verywellhealth.com/walking-with-a-cane-2696294

Luz, C., Bush, T., & Shen, X. (2017). Do canes or walkers make any difference? Nonuse and fall injuries. *The Gerontologist, 57*(2), 211–218. https://doi.org/10.1093/geront/gnv096

Pullen, R. (2010). Caring for a patient after amputation. *Nursing, 40*(1), 15. https://doi.org/10.1097/01.NURSE.0000365908.40394.4e

Sears, B. (2013). *How to walk with a walker.* Retrieved October 26, 2015, from http://physicaltherapy.about.com/od/Physical-Therapy-For-Seniors/ss/How-To-Walk-With-A-Standard-Walker.htm

Tinoco-Varela, D., Ferrer-Varela, J. A., Cruz-Morales, R. D., & Padilla-García, E. A. (2022). Design and implementation of a prosthesis system controlled by electromyographic signals means, characterized with artificial neural networks. *Micromachines (Basel), 13*(10), 1681. https://doi.org/10.3390/mi13101681

CHAPTER 27

American National Red Cross. (2015). *Autologous and directed donations.* https://www.redcrossblood.org/donate-blood/how-to-donate/types-of-blood-donations/autologous-and-directed-donations.html

American Society of Anesthesiologists. (2011). Practice guidelines for preoperative fasting and the use of pharmacologic agents to reduce the risk of pulmonary aspiration: Application to health patients undergoing elective procedures. *Anesthesiology, 224*(3), 495–511. https://doi.org/10.1097/ALN.0b013e3181fcbfd9

American Society of Anesthesiologists. (2023). Practice guidelines for preoperative fasting and the use of pharmacologic agents to reduce the risk of pulmonary aspiration: Application to healthy patients undergoing elective procedures: An updated report by the American Society of Anesthesiologists Task Force on Preoperative Fasting and the use of pharmacologic agents to reduce the risk of pulmonary aspiration. *Anesthesiology, 126*(3), 376–393. https://doi.org/10.1097/ALN.0000000000001452

Association of periOperative Registered Nurses. (n.d.). *Guidelines for perioperative practice.* https://www.aorn.org/guidelines/about-aorn-guidelines

Association of periOperative Registered Nurses. (2014). *Guidelines for perioperative standards and recommended practices.* Author. Retrieved July 21, 2016, from http://www.aornstandards.org

Campbell, C. M., & Edwards, R. R. (2012). Ethnic differences in pain and pain management. *Pain Management, 2*(3), 219–230. https://doi.org/10.2217/pmt.12.7

Canadian Centre for Occupational Health and Safety. (2014). *Laser plumes—Health care facilities.* Retrieved November 1, 2015, from http://www.ccohs.ca/oshanswers/phys_agents/laser_plume.html

Centers for Disease Control and Prevention. (2014). *Control of smoke from laser/electric surgical procedures.* Retrieved November 1, 2015, from http://www.cdc.gov/niosh/docs/hazardcontrol/hc11.html

Edmiston, C. E., Okoli, O., Graham, M. B., Sinski, S., & Seabrook, G. R. (2010). Evidence for using chlorhexidine gluconate preoperative cleansing to reduce the risk of surgical site infection. *Association of periOperative Registered Nurses Journal, 92*(5), 509–518. https://doi.org/10.1016/j.aorn.2010.01.020

Hinkle, J. L., & Cheever, K. H. (2013). *Brunner & Suddarth's textbook of medical-surgical nursing.* Lippincott Williams & Wilkins.

Johns Hopkins Medicine. (2012). *Informed consent guidance.* Retrieved November 1, 2015, from http://www.hopkinsmedicine.org/institutional_review_board/guidelines_policies/guidelines/informed_consent_i.html

Kumar, D. T. (2013). *Respiratory protection to prevent potential transmission of human papillomavirus during surgical procedures that generate smoke.* https://cdn.ymaws.com/www.cste.org/resource/dynamic/forums/20131112_151658_22377.pdf

McCall, M. (2023). *Understanding informed consent and your rights as a patient.* https://www.findlaw.com/healthcare/patient-rights/understanding-informed-consent-a-primer.html

Peng, L., & Norris, E. J. (2014). *Outpatient surgery instructions, types of anesthesia, risks, and complications.* Retrieved November 1, 2015, from http://www.emedicinehealth.com/outpatient_surgery/article_em.htm

Smith, M. A., Dahlen, N. R., Davis, S., & Heishman, C. (2013). *Clinical practice guideline surgical site infection prevention.* Retrieved November 3, 2015, from http://www.nursingcenter.com/ceaarticle?an=00006416-201309000-00004

Stamenkovic, D. M., Rancic, N. K., Latas, M. B., Neskovic, V., Rondovic, G. M., Wu, J. D., & Cattano, D. (2018). Preoperative anxiety and implications on postoperative recovery: What can we do to change our history. *Minerva Anestesiologica, 84*(11), 1307–1317. https://doi.org/10.23736/S0375-9393.18.12520-X

Tadman, M., Roberts, D., & Foulkes, M. (Eds). (2019). Oxford handbook of cancer nursing (2 ed.). Oxford: Oxford Academic. https://doi.org/10.1093/med/9780198701101.001.0001

The Joint Commission. (2024). *Hospital: 2024 National Patient Safety Goals.* https://www.jointcommission.org/standards/national-patient-safety-goals/hospital-national-patient-safety-goals/

The Joint Commission. (2024). *Universal protocol poster.* https://www.jointcommission.org/standards/universal-protocol/

The University of Texas Medical Branch. (2018). *The medical record and health information management services handbook.* https://www.utmb.edu/him/him-home

CHAPTER 28

Alberts, B., Johnson, A., Lewis, J., Morgan, D., Raff, M., Roberts, K., & Walter, P. (2014). *Molecular biology of the cell* (6th ed.). Garland Science.

Alhajj, M., & Goyal, A. (2022, January). Physiology, granulation tissue. *StatPearls.* https://www.ncbi.nlm.nih.gov/books/NBK554402/

Bryant, J. (2011). *Changing a wound VAC dressing.* Retrieved November 12, 2015, from https://www.youtube.com/watch?v=skLm5D3KY-4

Daley, B. J. (2015). *Wound care treatment & management.* Retrieved November 10, 2015, from http://emedicine.medscape.com/article/194018-treatment

Gestring, M., Berman, R. S., & Cochran, A. (2023). Negative pressure wound therapy. *UpToDate.* https://www.uptodate.com/contents/negative-pressure-wound-therapy

Hakakian, D., & Suzuki, K. (2014). *What you should know about emerging wound care dressings.* Retrieved November 16, 2015, from http://www.podiatrytoday.com/what-you-should-know-about-emerging-wound-care-dressings

Healthline. (2021). *Bedsores: What you should know about decubitus ulcers.* https://www.healthline.com/health/pressure-ulcer

Kirman, C. N. (2024). Pressure injuries (pressure ulcers) and wound care guidelines. *eMedicine.* https://emedicine.medscape.com/article/190115-guidelines

Manley, S., & Mitchell, A. (2022). The impact of nutrition on pressure ulcer healing. *British Journal of Nursing, 31*(12), S26–S30. https://www.britishjournalofnursing.com/content/nutrition/the-impact-of-nutrition-on-pressure-ulcer-healing

Mercandetti, M., & Molnar, J. A. (2021). *Wound healing and repair.* https://emedicine.medscape.com/article/1298129-overview

Miller, J., Hayes, D. D., & Carey, K. W. (2015). Evidence-based practice or sacred cow? *Nursing, 45*(8), 46–55. https://doi.org/10.1097/01.NURSE.0000469234.84277.95

Ranaweera, A. (2014). *Negative pressure wound therapy.* Retrieved November 12, 2015, from http://www.dermnetnz.org/procedures/negative-pressure.html

Rivera, N. S., & Wu, S. C. (2011). *Keys to effective wound dressing selection.* Retrieved November 10, 2015, from http://www.podiatrytoday.com/keys-effective-wound-dressing-selection

Wake Forest Baptist Health. (2015). *Vacuum-assisted closure device (V.A.C.).* Retrieved November 11, 2015, from http://www.wakehealth.edu/Plastic-Surgery/Wound-Care/Vacuum-Assisted-Closure.htm

WebMD. *Stitches, staples, glue: Which do you need?* https://www.webmd.com/first-aid/stitches-staples-glue#2

Woodash, A. J. (2012). Wet-to-dry dressings do not provide moist wound healing. *Journal of the American College of Clinical Wound Specialists, 4*(3), 63–66. Retrieved November 16, 2015, from http://www.ncbi.nlm.nih.gov/pmc/articles/PMC4511549

CHAPTER 29

American Association of Critical-Care Nurses. (2020). *Initial and ongoing verification of feeding tube placement in adults.* https://www.aacn.org/clinical-resources/practice-alerts/initial-and-ongoing-verification-of-feeding-tube-placement-in-adults

American Meteorological Society. (2016). Initial and ongoing verification of feeding tube placement in adults (applies to blind insertions and placements with an electromagnetic device). *Critical Care Nurse, 36*(2), e8–e13. https://doi.org/10.4037/ccn2016141

American Nurses Association. (2017). *Nutrition and hydration at the end of life.* https://www.nursingworld.org/~4af0ed/globalassets/docs/ana/ethics/ps_nutrition-and-hydration-at-the-end-of-life_2017june7.pdf

Bankhead, R., Boullata, J., Brantley, S., Corkins, M., Guenter, P., Krenitsky, J., Lyman, B., Metheny, N. A., Mueller, C., Robbins, S., Wessel, J., & A.S.P.E.N. Board of Directors. (2009). Enteral nutrition practice recommendations. *Journal of Parenteral Enteral Nutrition, 33*(2), 122–167. https://doi.org/10.1177/0148607108330314

Bionex. (2022). *Patients with enteral feeding tubes.* https://bionix.com/articles/enteral-feeding-tube-decloggers-patients-with-enteral-feeding-tubes

Dudek, S. G. (2021). *Nutrition essentials for nursing practice* (9th ed.). Lippincott, Williams & Wilkins.

Eveleigh, M., Pullyblank, A., & Bennett, J. (2011). Nasogastric feeding tube placement: Changing culture. *Nursing Times, 107*(41), 14–16.

Fessler, T. A. (2010). *Gastric residuals—Understand their significance to optimize care.* Retrieved December 4, 2015, from http://www.todaysdietitian.com/newarchives/060210p8.shtml

Gerritsen, A., Rooij, T., Dijkgraaf, M. G., Busch, O. R., Bergman, J. J., Ubbink, D. T., van Duijvendijk, P., Erkelens, G. W., Molenaar, I. Q., Monkelbaan, J. F., Rosman, C., Tan, A. C., Kruyt, P. M., Bac, D. J., Mathus-Vliegen, E. M., & Besselink, M. G. (2015). *Electromagnetic guided bedside or endoscopic placement of nasoenteral feeding tubes in surgical patients (CORE trial): Study protocol for a randomized controlled trial.* Retrieved December 1, 2015, from http://www.ncbi.nlm.nih.gov/pmc/articles/PMC4390000/

Gok, F., Kilicasian, A., & Yosunkaya, A. (2015). Ultrasound-guided nasogastric feeding tube placement in critical care patients. *Nutrition in Clinical Practice, 30*(2), 257–260. https://doi.org/10.1177/0884533614567714

Humphries, L. (2011–2012). *NG tubes policy and guidelines ICU adult.* Retrieved December 1, 2015, from http://www.slideshare.net/lianne463/ng-tubes-policy-and-guidelines-icu-adult

Kim, H. M., So, B. H., Jeong, W. J., Choi, S. M., & Park, K. N. (2012). *The effectiveness of ultrasonography in verifying the placement of a nasogastric tube in patients with low consciousness at an emergency center.* Retrieved December 2, 2012, from http://www.ncbi.nlm.nih.gov/pmc/articles/PMC3477076

Mathus-Vliegen, E. M., Duflou, A., Spanier, M. B., & Fockens, P. (2010). Nasoenteral feeding tube placement by nurses using an electromagnetic guidance system (with video). *Gastrointestinal Endoscopy, 71*(4), 728–736. https://doi.org/10.1016/j.gie.2009.10.046

Miller, J., Hayes, D. D., & Carey, K. W. (2015). 20 questions: Evidence-based practice or sacred cow? *Nursing, 45*(8), 46–55. https://doi.org/10.1097/01.NURSE.0000469234.84277.95

Nickson, C. (2014). *Gastric residual volume.* https://litfl.com/gastric-residual-volume/

Nurseslabs. (2022). *Aspiration risk & aspiration pneumonia nursing care plan & management.* https://nurseslabs.com/risk-for-aspiration/

Nutrient Component. (n.d.). *Nutrient composition of adult commercial enteral formulas and modular formulas available at UCSF.* https://nutrition.ucsfmedicalcenter.org/internalsite/inpatient/Adult_Enteral_Formulary.pdf

Pennsylvania Patient Safety Authority. (2006). Confirming feeding tube placement: Old habits die hard. *Patient Safety Advisory, 3*(4), 23–30. https://patientsafety.pa.gov/ADVISORIES/documents/200612_23.pdf

Simons, S. R., & Abdallah, L. M. (2012). Bedside assessment of enteral tube placement: Aligning practice with evidence. *American Journal of Nursing, 112*(2), 40–46. https://doi.org/10.1097/01.NAJ.0000411178.07179.68

CHAPTER 30

ACI Urology Network. (2012). *Collection of urine midstream.* Retrieved December 9, 2015, from http://www.aci.health.nsw.gov.au/__data/assets/pdf_file/0005/165920/Collection-of-Urine-Midstream-Toolikit.pdf

Agency for Healthcare Research and Quality. (2015). *Toolkit for reducing CAUTI in hospitals.* Retrieved December 11, 2015, from http://www.ahrq.gov/professionals/quality-patient-safety/hais/tools/cauti-hospitals/index.html

Amalaradjou, M. A. R., & Venkitanarayanan, K. (2013). *Role of bacterial biofilms in catheter-associated urinary tract infections (CAUTI) and strategies for their control.* Retrieved December 13, 2015, from http://www.intechopen.com/books/recent-advances-in-the-field-of-urinary-tract-infections/role-of-bacterial-biofilms-in-catheter-associated-urinary-tract-infections-cauti-and-strategies-for-

American Nurses Association. (2014). *Streamlined evidence-based RN tool: Catheter Associated Urinary Tract Infection (CAUTI) prevention.* https://www.nursingworld.org/~4aede8/globalassets/practiceandpolicy/innovation--evidence/clinical-practice-material/cauti-prevention-tool/anacautipreventiontool-final-19dec2014.pdf

American Nurses Association. (2020). *CAUTI prevention and urinary catheter maintenance.* https://www.myamericannurse.com/cauti-prevention-and-urinary-catheter-maintenance/

American Urological Association. (2019). Diagnosis and treatment of overactive bladder (non-neurogenic) in adults: AUA/SUFU guideline amendment 2019. *The Journal of Urology, 202*(3), 558–563. https://www.auajournals.org/doi/10.1097/JU.0000000000000309

Carpenito, L. J. (2013). *Nursing care plans: Transitional patient & family centered care* (6th ed.). Lippincott Williams & Wilkins.

Centers for Disease Control and Prevention. (2015). *Catheter-associated urinary tract infections (CAUTI).* Retrieved December 11, 2015, from http://www.cdc.gov/HAI/ca_uti/uti.html

Delanghe, J. R., Speeckaert, M. M. (2016). Preanalytics in urinalysis. *Clinical Biochemistry, 49*(18), 1346–1350. https://doi.org/10.1016/j.clinbiochem.2016.10.016

Elist, J. (2022). *What is double voiding and why should you consider it?* https://www.drelist.com/blog/double-voiding-consider/#:~:text=Double%20voiding%20is%20a%20bladder%20emptying%20technique%20and,hands%20must%20be%20placed%20on%20thighs%20or%20knees

Gerard, L., & Sueppel, C. (1997). Lubrication technique for male catheterization. *Urologic Nursing, 17*(4), 156–157.

Hynes, J. (2009). Skill building: Collecting a urine specimen. *LPN, 5*(1), 19. https://www.nursingcenter.com/journalarticle?Article_ID=841490&Journal_ID=522928&Issue_ID=841483

Lachance, C. C., & Grobelna, A. (2019). *Management of patients with long-term indwelling urinary catheters: A review of guidelines.* Canadian Agency for Drugs and Technologies in Health. https://pubmed.ncbi.nlm.nih.gov/31449368/

Lo, E., Nicolle, L. E., Coffin, S. E., Gould, C., Maragakis, L. L., Meddings, J., Pegues, D. A., Pettis, A. M., Saint, S., & Yokoe, D. S. (2014). Strategies to prevent catheter-associated urinary tract infections in acute care hospitals: 2014 update. *Infection Control and Hospital Epidemiology, 35*(5), 464–479. https://doi.org/10.1086/675718

Society of Urologic Nurses and Associates. (2021). Urinary catheterization of the adult male. *Urologic Nursing, 41*(2). https://www.suna.org/sites/default/files/download/resources/SUNA_catheterizationMaleCCP.pdf

Soto, S. M. (2014). *Importance of biofilms in urinary tract infections: New therapeutic approaches.* Retrieved December 13, 2015, from http://www.hindawi.com/journals/ab/2014/543974

WebMD. (2023). *Cranberry—uses, side effects, and more.* https://www.webmd.com/vitamins/ai/ingredientmono-958/cranberry

CHAPTER 31

American Cancer Society. (2023). *Key statistics for colorectal cancer.* https://www.cancer.org/cancer/colon-rectal-cancer/about/key-statistics.html

Centers for Disease Control and Prevention. (2023). *Screening for colorectal cancer.* https://www.cdc.gov/colorectal-cancer/screening/index.html#:~:text=The%20fecal%20immunochemical%20test%20(FIT,lower%20third%20of%20the%20colon

Centers for Disease Control and Prevention. (2024). *Family health history and colorectal (colon) cancer.* https://www.cdc.gov/colorectal-cancer-hereditary/risk-factors/index.html#:~:text=Colonoscopy%20starting%20at%20age%2040,In%20some%20cases%2C%20genetic%20counseling

Dugdale, D. C. (2013). *Fecal immunochemical test (FIT).* Retrieved December 24, 2015, from https://www.nlm.nih.gov/medlineplus/ency/patientinstructions/000704.htm

Imperiale, T. F., Ransohoff, D. F., Itzkowitz, S. H., Levin, T. R., Lavin, P., Lidgard, G. P., Ahlquist, D. A., & Berger, B. M. (2014). Multitarget stool DNA testing for colorectal-cancer screening. *New England Journal of Medicine, 370*(4), 1987–1997. https://doi.org/10.1056/NEJMoa1311194

Johnson, D. A. (2012). *Colorectal cancer screening: Guidelines for best practice.* Retrieved December 25, 2015, from http://www.medscape.com/viewarticle/760214

MedlinePlus. (2023). *Fecal immunochemical test (FIT).* https://medlineplus.gov/ency/patientinstructions/000704.htm

Simon, S. (2024). *Stool DNA test.* https://www.mayoclinic.org/tests-procedures/stool-dna-test/about/pac-20385153#:~:text=Stool%20DNA%20testing%20is%20used,colon%20cancer%20or%20colon%20polyps

The Life Today. (2023). *16 fast facts colon cancer warning signs and symptoms you should not ignore!* https://thelifetoday.com/colon-cancer-symptoms/8/

CHAPTER 32

Carlo, D. (2011). *ER versus SR? What's the difference?* Retrieved January 4, 2016, from http://www.drugs.com/answers/er-versus-sr-486490.html

GoodRx Health. (2023). *Sustained release vs. Extended release (vs. Other modified-release dosage forms).* https://www.goodrx.com/healthcare-access/medication-education/meaning-medication-suffixes-er-sr

Institute for Safe Medication Practices. (2015a). *ISMP's list of confused drug names.* Retrieved January 4, 2016, from http://www.ismp.org/Tools/confuseddrugnames.pdf

Institute for Safe Medication Practices. (2015b). *ISMP's list of error prone abbreviations, symbols, and dose designations.* Retrieved January 6, 2016, from http://www.ismp.org/tools/errorproneabbreviations.pdf

Institute for Safe Medication Practices. (2019). *List of confused drug names.* https://www.ismp.org/recommendations/confused-drug-names-list

Patient Safety Solutions. (2012). *Verbal orders.* Retrieved January 6, 2016, from http://www.patientsafetysolutions.com/docs/January_10_2012_Verbal_Orders.htm

U.S. Food and Drug Administration. (2015). *Computerized prescriber order entry medication safety (CPOEMS).* Retrieved January 7, 2016, from http://www.fda.gov/downloads/Drugs/DrugSafety/MedicationErrors/UCM477419.pdf

CHAPTER 33

Bhandari, S. (2022). *Can you be addicted to nasal spray?* https://www.webmd.com/mental-health/addiction/addicted-nasal-spray

Case-Lo, C. (2013). *Administration of medication.* Retrieved January 17, 2016, from http://www.healthline.com/health/administration-of-medication

Gor, H. B. (2015). *Vaginitis treatment & management.* Retrieved January 17, 2016, from http://emedicine.medscape.com/article/257141-treatment#d8

Graham, L. (2014). *Tips on instilling eyedrops properly.* Retrieved January 16, 2016, from http://www.emedicinehealth.com/how_to_instill_your_eyedrops_properly/article_em.htm

Mortuaire, G., deGabory, L., & Francois, M. (2013). *Rebound congestion and rhinitis medicamentosa: Nasal decongestants in clinical practice. Critical review of the literature by a medical panel.* Retrieved January 16, 2016, from http://www.sciencedirect.com/science/article/pii/S1879729612001378

Nyawira, M., & Kenan, L. (2023). How to use your eye medication. *Community Eye Health, 36*(118), 8. https://www.ncbi.nlm.nih.gov/pmc/articles/PMC10236409/

Seltman, W. (2022). *Tips on instilling your eye drops properly.* https://www.webmd.com/eye-health/how-to-instill-your-eyedrops-treatment

CHAPTER 34

American Diabetes Association. (2024). *Insulin routines.* https://diabetes.org/health-wellness/medication/insulin-routines

Centers for Disease Control and Prevention. (2001). *Occupational exposure to bloodborne pathogens; needlestick and other sharps injuries.* https://www.osha.gov/laws-regs/federalregister/2001-01-18#:~:text=The%20Needlestick%20Safety%20and%20Prevention%20Act%20requires%20employers%2C%20who%20have,control%20plan%20must%20also%20%22document

Centers for Disease Control and Prevention. (2002). *State-by-state provisions of state needle safety legislation.* https://www.ospedalesicuro.eu/storia/materiali/doc/ndl-law-1.html

Centers for Disease Control and Prevention. (2019). *Stop sticks campaign.* https://www.cdc.gov/nora/councils/hcsa/stopsticks/default.html#:~:text=The%20Stop%20Sticks%20campaign%20is,and%20other%20sharps%20related%20injuriesb

Cocoman, A., & Murray, J. (2010). Recognizing the evidence and changing practice on injection sites. *British Journal of Nursing, 19*(18), 1170–1174. https://doi.org/10.12968/bjon.2010.19.18.79050

Drugs.com. (2023). *How to give a subcutaneous injection.* Retrieved January 21, 2016, from https://www.drugs.com/cg/how-to-give-a-subcutaneous-injection.html

Hettinger, F., & Jurkovich, P. (2015). *Evidence-based injection practice: To aspirate or not.* Retrieved January 23, 2015, from http://thenursepath.com/20`15/09/03/intramuscular-injections-should-you-aspirate/

Howard, A., Mercer, P., Nataraj, H. C., & Kang, B. C. (1997). Bevel-down superior to bevel-up in intradermal skin testing. *Annals of Allergy, Asthma, & Immunology, 78*(6), 594–596. https://doi.org/10.1016/S1081-1206(10)63222-X

H.R.5178—Needlestick Safety and Prevention Act. Retrieved January 23, 2016, from https://www.congress.gov/bill/106th-congress/house-bill/5178

Joslin Diabetes Center. (2016a). *How to improve the insulin injection experience*. Retrieved January 22, 2016, from http://www.joslin.org/info/how_to_improve_the_insulin_injection_experience.html

Joslin Diabetes Center. (2016b). *Tips for injecting insulin*. Retrieved January 22, 2016, from http://www.joslin.org/info/tips_for_injecting_insulin.html

McCulloch, D. (2014). *Choosing the best body site for an insulin shot*. Retrieved January 22, 2016, from http://www.ghc.org/healthAndWellness/?item=/common/healthAndWellness/conditions/diabetes/ insu-linShot.html

Miller, I. (2014). *The ventrogluteal injection site*. Retrieved January 23, 2016, from http://thenursepath.com/2014/04/23/the-ventrogluteal-im-injection-site/

Occupational Safety and Health Administration. (2023). *Bloodborne pathogens and needlestick prevention*. Retrieved January 22, 2016, from https://www.osha.gov/bloodborne-pathogens/standards

CHAPTER 35

Alexandrou, E., Ramjan, L. M., Spencer, T., Frost, S. A., Salamonson, Y., Davidson, P. M., & Hillman, K. M. (2011). The use of midline catheters in the adult acute care setting—Clinical implications and recommendations for practice. *Journal of the Association for Vascular Access, 16*(1), 35–41. https://doi.org/10.2309/java.16-1-5

Catudal, J. P., & Sharpe, E. L. (2014). The wandering ways of a PICC line: Case report of a malpositioned peripherally inserted central catheter (PICC) and correction. *Journal of the Association for Vascular Access, 16*(4), 218–220. https://doi.org/10.2309/java.16-4-3

Craven, R. F., Hirnle, C. J., & Jensen, S. (2013). *Fundamentals of nursing. Breaking the ampule* (7th ed.). Lippincott Williams & Wilkins.

Hadaway, L. (2011). Needleless connectors: Improving practice, reducing risks. *Journal of the Association for Vascular Access, 16*(1), 20–30. https://doi.org/10.2309/java.16-1-4

Infusion Therapy Institute. (2013). *IV therapy hands-on training programs for novices and advanced learners*. Retrieved February 2, 2016, from http://infusioninstitute.com

Mathers, D. (2011). Evidence-based practice: Improving outcomes for patients with a central venous access device. *Journal of the Association for Vascular Access, 16*(2), 64–72. https://doi.org/10.2309/java.16-2-3

Meyer, B. M. (2011). Managing peripherally inserted central catheter thrombosis risk. A guide for clinical best practice. *Journal of the Association for Vascular Access, 16*(3), 144–147. https://doi.org/10.2309/java.16-3-3

New York State Education Department, & Office of the Professions. (2021). *The practice of IV therapy by licensed practical nurses in long term care settings*. https://www.coursehero.com/file/77568550/IV-LPNs-Long-Term-Caredoc/

Rutkoff, G. S. (2014). The influence of an antimicrobial peripherally inserted central catheter on central line-associated bloodstream infections in a hospital environment. *Journal of the Association for Vascular Access, 19*(3), 172–179. https://doi.org/10.1016/j.java.2014.06.002

Smith, J. S., Irwin, G., Viney, M., Watkins, L., Pinno Morris, S., Kirksey, K. M., & Brown, A. (2012). Optimal disinfection times for needleless intravenous connectors. *Journal of the Association for Vascular Access, 17*(3), 137–143. https://doi.org/10.1016/j.java.2012.07.008

Villalba-Nicolau, M., Chover-Sierra, E., Saus-Ortega, C., Ballestar-Tarín, M. L., Chover-Sierra, P., & Martínez-Sabater, A. (2022). Usefulness of midline catheters versus peripheral venous catheters in an inpatient unit: A pilot randomized clinical trial. *Nursing Reports, 12*(4), 814–823. https://doi.org/10.3390/nursrep12040079

Whitlock, J. (2015). *What is a PICC line?* Retrieved February 2, 2016, from http://surgery.about.com/od/questionsanswers/fl/PICC-Line-Information.htm

CHAPTER 36

Carpenito, L. J. (2013). *Nursing care plans, transitional patient & family centered care*. Lippincott Williams & Wilkins.

Cleveland Clinic. (2024). *Tracheostomy suctioning*. https://my.clevelandclinic.org/health/procedures/tracheostomy-suctioning

Hess, D. R., & Altobelli, N. R. (2014). *Tracheostomy tubes. Respiratory Care, 59*(6), 956–973. https://doi.org/10.4187/respcare.02920

Johns Hopkins Medicine. (2024). *Tracheostomy*. https://www.hopkinsmedicine.org/health/treatment-tests-and-therapies/tracheostomy

Johnson, W. A. (2015). *Tracheostomy tube change*. Retrieved February 16, 2016, from http://emedicine.medscape.com/article/1580576-overview

Nance-Floyd, B. (2011). *Tracheostomy care: An evidence-based guide*. Retrieved February 15, 2016, from http://www.american-nursetoday.com/tracheostomy-care-an-evidence-based-guide-to-suctioning-and-dressing-changes

Ohio State University Wexner Medical Center. (n.d.). *EMERGENCY REPLACEMENT OF TRACHEOSTOMY TUBE for a ventilator dependent patient*. https://www.myshepherdconnection.org/docs/EMERGENCY_REPLACEMENT.pdf

Ohio State University Wexner Medical Center. (2023). *What is a fenestrated tracheostomy tube?* https://www.healthline.com/health/fenestrated-tracheostomy-tube

Tracheostomy Education. (2021). *Tracheostomy tubes*. https://tracheostomyeducation.com/tracheostomy-tubes/

Varga-Huettner, V. E. (2014). *Dislodged tracheostomy positioning technique*. Retrieved February 16, 2016, from http://emedicine.medscape.com/article/2051313-technique

CHAPTER 37

ACLS Training Center. (2016). *BLS CPR algorithm*. Retrieved February 18, 2016, from https://www.acls.net/bls-cpr-algorithm.htm

AED Facts. (2023). *AED facts | Things to know*. Retrieved February 18, 2016, from https://www.aedstoday.com/AED-Facts_ep_52.html

AHA/ASA Journals. (2000). *Part 4: The automated external defibrillator: Key link in the chain of survival*. Retrieved February 18, 2016, from https://www.ahajournals.org/doi/10.1161/circ.102.suppl_1.I-60

American Heart Association. (n.d.). *Hands-only CPR vs. CPR with breaths*. https://www.heart.org/-/media/Files/Affiliates/WSA/Oregon/Hands-Only-CPR-vs-CPR-with-Breaths.pdf

American Heart Association. (2024). *Automated external defibrillator Q&A*. https://www.uiltexas.org/health/info/automated-external-defibrillator-qa

American Heart Association. (2018). *AED programs Q&A*. Retrieved February 20, 2016, from https://cpr.heart.org/-/media/cpr-files/training-programs/aed-implementation/aed-programs-qa-ucm501519.pdf?la=en&hash=534EDE12A71933EAED3630FEEAE5E7D884E6609C

American Heart Association. (2020). *Highlights of the 2020 American Heart Association guidelines for CPR and ECC*. Retrieved February 20, 2016, from https://cpr.heart.org/-/media/CPR-Files/

CPR-Guidelines-Files/Highlights/Hghlghts_2020_ECC_Guide-lines_English.pdf

American Heart Association. (2023). *CPR & ECC*. Retrieved February 20, 2016, from https://cpr.heart.org/

Bystander. (2023). *Bystander CPR improves survival*. Retrieved February 20, 2016, from https://cpr.heart.org/en/resources/cpr-facts-and-stats

Clinical Correlations. (2018). *End tidal CO₂—How has it changed CPR?* Retrieved February 20, 2016, from https://www.clinicalcorrelations.org/2018/11/15/end-tidal-co2-how-has-it-changed-cpr/

Dumas, F., Rea, T. D., Fahrenbruch, C., Rosenqvist, M., Faxén, J., Svensson, L., Eisenberg, M. S., & Bohm, K. (2013). *Chest compression alone cardiopulmonary resuscitation is associated with better long-term survival compared with standard cardiopulmonary resuscitation*. Retrieved February 19, 2016, from http://circ.ahajournals.org/content/127/4/435.full

Handley, A. (2011). *Emergency medicine—Treating airway obstruction*. Retrieved February 18, 2016, from http://www.gponline.com/emergency-medicine-treating-airway-obstruction/emergency-medicine/article/1057177

Hands-Only CPR vs. CPR with Breaths. (n.d.). from https://www.heart.org/-/media/Files/Affiliates/WSA/Oregon/Hands-Only-CPR-vs-CPR-with-Breaths.pdf

Haskell, S. E., & Atkins, D. L. (2010). Defibrillation in children. *Journal of Emergencies, Trauma, and Shock, 3*(3), 261–266. https://doi.org/10.4103/0974-2700.66526

Hess, D. R., Macintyre, N. R., & Galvin, W. F. (2015). *Respiratory care: Principles and practice*. Jones & Bartlett.

Hughes, S. (2012). *Chest-compression-only CPR shows long-term survival benefit*. Retrieved February 19, 2016, from http://www.medscape.com/viewarticle/776173

Leary, M. (2015). *The science of saving a life*. Retrieved February 18, 2018, from http://www.huffingtonpost.com/marion-leary/the-science-of-saving-a-life_b_8373946.html

National Center for Early Defibrillation. (n.d.). *National Center for Early Defibrillation, fast facts for sudden cardiac arrest*. Retrieved February 18, 2018, from http://www.early-defib.org/

Nichol, G., Leroux, B., Wang, H., Callaway, C. W., Sopko, G., Weisfeldt, M., Stiell, I., Morrison, L. J., Aufderheide, T. P., Cheskes, S., Christenson, J., Kudenchuk, P., Vaillancourt, C., Rea, T. D., Idris, A. H., Colella, R., Isaacs, M., Straight, R., Stephens, S., ... the ROC Investigators. (2015). *Trial of continuous or interrupted chest compressions during CPR*. Retrieved February 19, 2016, from http://www.nejm.org/doi/full/10.1056/NEJMoa1509139

Rapp, A. (2015). *Key changes to the 2015 AHA guidelines update*. Retrieved February 18, 2016, from http://emedcert.com/blog/changes-to-2015-aha-guidelines-update

Science News Daily. (2015). *CPR by medics: Keep pumping or stop for rescue breathing?* Retrieved February 18, 2016, from http://www.sciencedaily.com/releases/2015/11/151109181911.htm

Shaw, R. (2013). *Can I use adult AED pads on a child or infant?* Retrieved February 20, 2016, from http://www.royonrescue.com/2013/07/can-i-use-adult-aed-pads-on-a-child-or-infant

CHAPTER 38

Alexander, B. K., & Wong, L. S. (2010). *Demon drug myths: The myth of drug-induced addiction*. Retrieved March 2, 2016, from http://www.brucekalexander.com/articles-speeches/demon-drug-myths/164-myth-of-drug-induced

American Academy of Neurology. (2023). *Pediatric and adult brain death/death by neurologic criteria consensus guideline*. https://www.neurology.org/doi/10.1212/WNL.0000000000207740

American Association of Retired Persons. (2012). *Understanding long-term care insurance*. Retrieved March 6, 2016, from http://www.aarp.org/health/health-insurance/info-06-2012/understanding-long-term-care-insurance.html

Centers for Disease Control and Prevention. (2016). *QuickStats: Age-adjusted death rates, by sex—United States, 1979–2014*. Retrieved March 6, 2016, from http://www.cdc.gov/mmwr/volumes/65/wr/mm6508a6.htm

Centers for Medicare & Medicaid Services. (2023). *Medicare hospice benefits*. https://www.medicare.gov/Pubs/pdf/02154-Medicare-Hospice-Benefits.PDF

Clarke, G., Harrison, K., Holland, A., Kuhn, I., & Barclay, S. (2013). How are treatment decisions made about artificial nutrition for individuals at risk of lacking capacity? A systematic literature review. *PLoS One, 8*(4), e61475. https://doi.org/10.1371/journal.pone.0061475

Dignity Memorial. (2023). *Hindu funeral traditions: Hindu cremation and Hindu mourning period*. https://www.dignitymemorial.com/support-friends-and-family/hindu-funeral-traditions

Edwards, E. (2019). *More people are choosing to die at home, instead of in a hospital*. https://www.nbcnews.com/health/aging/more-people-are-choosing-die-home-instead-hospital-n1099571

Healy, S., Israel, F., Charles, M. A., & Reymond, L. (2023). An educational package that supports laycarers to safely manage breakthrough subcutaneous injections for home-based palliative care patients: Development and evaluation of a service quality improvement. *Palliative Medicine, 27*(6), 562–570. https://doi.org/10.1177/0269216312464262

Hindu. (2023). *Hindu cremation and Hindu mourning period*. https://www.dignitymemorial.com/support-friends-and-family/hindu-funeral-traditions

Johnson, M. (2009). *Pros and cons of long-term-care insurance*. Retrieved March 6, 2016, from http://health.usnews.com/health-news-managing-your-healthcare/healthcare/articles/2009/12/21/pros-and-cons-of-long-term-care-insurance

Kübler-Ross, E. (1969). *On death and dying*. Macmillan.

Medicare.gov. (2023). *Hospice care*. https://www.medicare.gov/coverage/hospice-care

Nair-Collins, M. (2023). Must hypothalamic neurosecretory function cease for brain death determination? Yes. *Neurology, 101*(3), 134–136. https://www.neurology.org/doi/10.1212/WNL.0000000000207340#:~:text=The%20Uniform%20Determination%20of%20Death,is%20to%20deny%20logic%20itself

National Center for Health Statistics. (2022). *Life expectancy in the U.S. dropped for the second year in a row in 2021*. https://www.cdc.gov/nchs/pressroom/nchs_press_releases/2022/20220831.htm

National Hospice and Palliative Care Organization. (2015). *Palliative care overview*. https://www.nhpco.org/palliativecare/

National Hospice and Palliative Care Organization. (2023a). *What is palliative care?* https://www.caringinfo.org/types-of-care/palliative-care/

National Hospice and Palliative Care Organization. (2023b). *Who pays for palliative care?* https://www.caringinfo.org/types-of-care/palliative-care/

National Institute on Aging. (2021). *Depression and older adults*. https://www.nia.nih.gov/health/mental-and-emotional-health/depression-and-older-adults

RegisteredNursing.org. (2024). *Can RN pronounce death?* https://www.hashtagnursing.com/question/can-rn-pronounce-death/

Schwartz, D. B., Barrocas, A., Annetta, M. G., Stratton, K., McGinnis, C., Hardy, G., Wong, T., Arenas, D., Turon-Findley, M. P., Kliger, R. G., Corkins, K. G., Mirtallo, J., Amagai, T., Guenter, P., & ASPEN International Clinical Ethics Position Paper Update

Workgroup. (2021). Ethical aspects of artificially administered nutrition and hydration: An ASPEN position paper. *Nutrition in Clinical Practice, 36*(2), 254–267. https://pubmed.ncbi.nlm.nih .gov/33616284/

Smith, T. (2022). *When life support is withdrawn, commitment to care must not end.* https://www.ama-assn.org/delivering-carc/ethics/ when-life-support-withdrawn-commitment-care-must-not-end

Stollard, J. (2013). *Will I become addicted to the pain medications I may need during my cancer treatment?* Retrieved August 24, 2015, from http://mskcc.org/blog/will-i-become-addicted-pain- medications-i-may-need-during-my-treatment/

United Nations. (2019). *World population prospects.* https://population. un.org/wpp/Publications/Files/WPP2019_Volume-I_Comprehensive- Tables.pdf

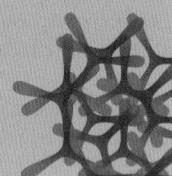

Commonly Used Abbreviations and Acronyms

Symbols

$<$	less than
$\leq$	less than or equal to
$>$	more than
$\geq$	more than or equal to
$\pm$	plus or minus
®	registered name; brand or trade name
™	trade mark
°	degree

Words

ABG	arterial blood gas
ACA	Affordable Care Act
ACIP	Advisory Committee for Immunization Practices
ACS	American Cancer Society
ACTH	adrenocorticotropic hormone
ADA	American Dietetic Association
ADLs	activities of daily living
AED	automated external defibrillator
AHA	American Heart Association
AHCPR	Agency for Health Care Policy and Research
AIDS	acquired immune deficiency syndrome
AK	above the knee
AMA	against medical advice; or American Medical Association
ANA	American Nurses Association
ANS	autonomic nervous system
ASL	American sign language
AX	axillary
b.i.d.	twice a day
BiPAP	bilevel positive air pressure
BK	below the knee
BMI	body mass index
BP	blood pressure
bpm	beats per minute
BSE	breast self-examination
C	Centigrade
cal	calorie
CAM	complementary and alternative medicine; *now integrative medicine*
CAUTI	catheter-associated urinary tract infection
CBC	complete blood count

CDC	Centers for Disease Control and Prevention
CHO	carbohydrate
cm	centimeter
CNS	central nervous system
CO	carbon monoxide
CO_2	carbon dioxide
COA	Council on Aging; also called Commission on Aging
COW	computer on wheels
CPAP	continuous positive air pressure
CPM	continuous passive motion
CPOE	computerized provider order entry
CPR	cardiopulmonary resuscitation
CQI	continuous quality improvement
CR	continuous release
CRF	corticotropin-releasing factor
CT	computed tomography (also CAT)
CVC	central venous catheter
D_5W	dextrose 5% in water
dc	discontinue
DHHS	Department of Health and Human Services
dL	deciliter (100 mL)
DNR	do not resuscitate
DRG	diagnostic-related group
ECG	electrocardiogram (also EKG)
EEG	electroencephalogram
EMG	electromyography
EMLA	eutectic mixture of local anesthetic
EOMs	extraocular movements
ER	extended release; also XR
ESL	English as a second language
$ETCO_2$	end-tidal carbon dioxide at end of exhaled breath
F	Fahrenheit
FDA	Food and Drug Administration
FIO_2	portion of oxygen in relation to total inspired gas
FIT	fecal immunochemical test
FOBT	fecal occult blood test
g	gram
GABA	gamma-aminobutyric acid
GAS	general adaptation syndrome
GI	gastrointestinal
GRV	gastric residual volume
gtt/min	drops per minute

Hb	hemoglobin
HBOT	hyperbaric oxygen therapy
HBV	hepatitis B virus
HCAI	health care–associated infection
Hct	hematocrit
HCV	hepatitis C virus
HDL	high-density lipoprotein
HIPAA	Health Insurance Portability and Accountability Act
HIV	human immunodeficiency virus
HMO	health maintenance organization
HPA	hypothalamus–pituitary–adrenal (axis)
hs	hours of sleep
I & O	intake and output
ICN	International Council of Nurses
ID	intradermal
IM	intramuscular
IPOP	immediate postoperative prosthesis
ISMP	Institute for Safe Medication Practices
IV	intravenous
IVP	IV push
IVPB	IV piggyback
JC	The Joint Commission
kcal	kilocalorie
kg	kilogram (1,000 g)
L	liter
LDL	low-density lipoprotein
LEP	limited English proficiency
LMWH	low-molecular-weight heparin
LPN	licensed practical nurse (also LVN, licensed vocational nurse)
MAR	medication administration record
MASH	military army surgical hospital
MDS	minimum data set
mEq	milliequivalent
MET	metabolic energy equivalent
mg	milligram (one-thousandth g)
mL	milliliter (one-thousandth L)
mm Hg	millimeters of mercury
mph	miles per hour
MRI	magnetic resonance imaging
NAPNES	National Association for Practical Nurse Education and Service
NCCIH	National Center for Complementary and Integrative Health
NCLEX-PN	National Council Licensure Examination for Practical Nurses
NCLEX-RN	National Council Licensure Examination for Registered Nurses
NCSBN	National Council of State Boards of Nursing
NEX	nose-to-earlobe-to-the-xiphoid
NFLPN	National Federation of Licensed Practice Nurses
NFPA	National Fire Protection Association

NG	nasogastric
NHLBI	National Heart, Lung, and Blood Institute
NI	nasointestinal
NIOSH	National Institute for Occupational Safety and Health
NKA	no known allergies
NLC	nurse licensure compact
NLN	National League for Nursing
NPDB	National Practitioner Data Bank
NPO	nil per os (Latin), nothing by mouth
NPSG	National Patient Safety Goals
NPWT	negative-pressure wound therapy; also called vacuum-assisted closure
NREM	non–rapid eye movement (sleep phase)
NSAID	nonsteroidal antiinflammatory drug
NSPA	Needlestick Safety and Prevention Act
NSS	normal saline solution
NWB	non–weight bearing
O	oral
O_2	oxygen
OBRA	Omnibus Budget Reconciliation Act
OTC	over the counter (e.g., nonprescription)
$PaCO_2$	partial pressure of carbon dioxide; that which is dissolved in plasma
PACU	postanesthesia care unit
PaO_2	partial pressure of oxygen; that which is dissolved in plasma
Pap	Papanicolaou
PAPR	powered air-purifying respirator
PAR	postanesthesia reacting
PCA	patient-controlled analgesia
PCT	patient care tech
PEG	percutaneous endoscopic gastrostomy
PEJ	percutaneous endoscopic jejunostomy
PENS	percutaneous electrical nerve stimulation
PERRLA	pupils equally round and respond to light and accommodation
PES	problem etiology, signs, and symptoms
PET	positron emission tomography
pH	measure of hydrogen ion concentration
PHO	partially hydrogenated oil
PICC	peripherally inserted central catheter
PO	per os (Latin), by mouth
POC	point of care
PPE	personal protective equipment
PPN	peripheral parenteral nutrition
PPO	preferred provider organization
PWB	partial weight bearing
q	quaque (Latin), every
q2h	every 2 hours
QA	quality assurance
qhs	every hour of sleep
q.i.d.	four times a day

q.o.d.	every other day	TA	temporal artery
R	rectal	TED	thromboembolic disorder
RAS	reticular activating system	TENS	transcutaneous electrical nerve stimulation
RBC	red blood cell	t.i.d.	three times a day
RC	risk for complication	TM	tympanic membrane
REM	rapid eye movement (sleep phase)	TO	telephone order
RN	registered nurse	TPN	total parenteral nutrition
R/O	rule out; either confirm or eliminate	TPR	temperature, pulse, and respirations
ROM	range of motion	TQI	total quality improvement
SAD	seasonal affective disorder	UAP	unlicensed assistive personnel
SaO$_2$	oxygen saturation of blood obtained in arterial blood	UAGA	Uniform Anatomical Gift Act
SBAR	situation, background, assessment, recommendation	VAC	vacuum-assisted closure; also called negative-pressure wound therapy
SC	subcutaneous		
SNF	skilled nursing facility	VLDL	very-low-density lipoprotein
SpO$_2$	oxygen saturation in blood obtained by pulse oximetry	VO	verbal order
SR	sustained release	WBC	white blood cell
SSE	soapsuds enema	WHO	World Health Organization
STI	sexually transmitted infection		

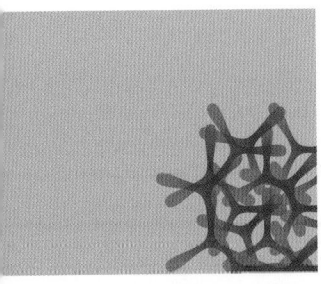

Glossary

A

Abdominal circumference indirect measurement of fatty (adipose) tissue that is distributed in and about the viscera of the abdomen

ABO system method by which blood is identified as one of four blood types: A, B, AB, or O

Acceptance attitude of complacency; last stage of dying, according to Dr. Kübler-Ross

Accommodation pupil constriction when looking at an object close by and dilation when looking at an object in the distance

Active exercise therapeutic activity performed independently

Active listening demonstrating full attention to what is being said; hearing both the content being communicated and the unspoken message

Active transport process of chemical distribution that requires an energy source

Activities of daily living acts that people normally do every day

Acultural nursing care care that lacks concern for cultural differences

Acupressure technique that involves tissue compression to reduce pain

Acupuncture pain management technique in which long, thin needles are inserted into the skin

Acute hypersensitivity an instantaneous or fairly prompt systemic allergic reaction

Acute illness one that comes on suddenly and lasts a short time

Acute pain discomfort of short duration

Adaptation manner in which an organism responds to change

Adapting making minor changes in the performance of the skill when adjustments are necessary

Adjuvants drugs that assist in accomplishing the desired effect of a primary drug

Administrative laws legal provisions through which federal, state, and local agencies maintain self-regulation

Admission entering a health care agency for nursing care and medical or surgical treatment

Advance directive written statement identifying a competent person's wishes concerning terminal care

Advanced life support procedures such as inserting an endotracheal tube and administering supplemental oxygen

Advanced practice specialized areas of nursing expertise, such as nurse practitioner and nurse midwifery

Aerobic bacteria microorganisms that require oxygen to live

Aerobic exercise rhythmically moving all parts of the body at a moderate to slow speed without hindering the ability to breathe

Aerosol mist

Afebrile absence of a fever

Affective domain learning by appealing to a person's feelings, beliefs, or values

Affective touch touching that demonstrates concern or affection

African Americans those whose ancestral origin is Africa

Afterload force against which the heart pumps when ejecting blood

Ageism form of negative stereotypical thinking about older adults

Air embolism bubble of air in the vascular system

Airborne precautions infection control measures that reduce the risk for transmitting pathogens that remain infectious over long distances when suspended in the air

Airway collective system of tubes in the upper and lower respiratory tract

Airway management skills that maintain the patency of natural or artificial airways

Alarm stage the immediate physiologic response to a stressor

Alignment proper relation of one part to another

Allocation of scarce resources process of deciding how to distribute limited life-saving equipment or procedures

Alternative behavioral techniques actions that modify stress in order to take control rather than become immobilized

Alternative lifestyle techniques activities in which people who are prone to stress make a conscious effort to change their patterns of living

Alternative medical therapy treatment outside the mainstream of traditional medicine

Alternative thinking techniques those that facilitate a change in a person's perceptions from negative to positive

Ambulatory electrocardiogram continuous recording of heart rate and rhythm during normal activity

American Sign Language (ASL) communication technique used by deaf persons using signs made by hand movements and finger spelling, an alphabetical substitute for words that have no sign

Ampule sealed glass container for a drug

Anaerobic bacteria microorganisms that exist without oxygen

Anal sphincters ring-shaped bands of muscles in the anus

Analgesic pain-relieving drug

Analyzing a cognitive level that requires using abstract and logical thought processes

Anatomic position standing with arms at the sides and palms forward

Andragogy principles of teaching adult learners

Anecdotal record personal, handwritten account of an incident

Anesthesiologist physician who administers chemical agents that temporarily eliminate sensation and pain

Anesthetist nurse specialist who administers anesthesia under the direction of a physician

Anger emotional response to feeling victimized

Anglo-Americans people who trace their ancestry to the United Kingdom or Western Europe

Anions electrolytes with a negative charge

Ankylosis permanent loss of joint movement

Anorexia loss of appetite

Anthropometric data measurements of body size and composition

Anticipatory grieving grieving that begins before a loss actually occurs

Antiembolism stockings elastic stockings

Antimicrobial agents chemicals that limit the number of infectious microorganisms by destroying them or suppressing their growth

Antineoplastic drugs medications used to destroy or slow the growth of malignant cells

Antipyretics drugs that reduce fever

Antiseptics chemicals such as alcohol that inhibit the growth of, but do not kill, microorganisms

Anuria absence of urine, or up to a 100-mL volume in 24 hours

Apical heart rate number of ventricular contractions per minute

Apical–radial rate number of sounds heard at the apex of the heart and the rate of the radial pulse during the same period

Apnea absence of breathing

Appliance collection bag over a stoma

Applying a cognitive level that requires using principles to solve or interpret information

Aquathermia pad electrical heating or cooling device

Arrhythmia irregular pattern of heartbeats

Art ability to perform an act skillfully

Arterial blood gas laboratory test using blood from an artery

Artifacts distortions on images that interfere with an accurate interpretation of the test results

Asepsis practices that decrease or eliminate infectious agents, their reservoirs, and vehicles for transmission

Aseptic techniques measures that reduce or eliminate microorganisms

Asian Americans people who come from China, Japan, Korea, the Philippines, Thailand, Indochina, and Vietnam

Asphyxiation inability to breathe

Assault act in which there is a threat or attempt to do bodily harm

Assessment systematic collection of information

Assessment skills acts that involve collecting data

Assistive listening systems devices that increase volume and sound to a level that is comparable to that of people with normal hearing

Assumption of risk when a client is forewarned of a potential safety hazard and chooses to ignore the warning

Asystole absence of heart rhythm

Atelectasis airless, collapsed lung areas

Audiometry measurement of hearing acuity at various sound frequencies

Auditors inspectors who examine client records

Auscultation listening to body sounds

Auscultatory gap period during which sound disappears and then reappears when taking a blood pressure measurement

Autologous transfusion self-donated blood

Automated external defibrillator device that delivers an electrical charge to the heart

Automated medication dispensing system on-unit device used to store and release frequently used medications, controlled and emergency drugs

Automated monitoring devices equipment that allows the simultaneous collection of multiple vital sign data

Autonomy a competent person's right to make his or her own choices without intimidation or influence

Axillary crutches standard type of crutches

B

Bag bath technique for bathing that involves the use of eight to 10 premoistened, warmed, disposable cloths contained in a plastic bag

Balance steady position

Bandage strip or roll of cloth

Barcode medication administration system point-of-care software that verifies that the name of the medication, administration time, dosage, drug form, and client for whom the drug is prescribed are accurate by scanning a barcode on the drug and identification band on the client

Bargaining psychological mechanism for delaying the inevitable

Bariatric client person who is severely overweight with a body mass index (BMI) of 30 to 39.9 or morbidly obese with a BMI over 40

Baroreceptors sensory nerves in the walls of large arteries whose function is to maintain arterial pressure

Barrel part of a syringe that holds the medication

Base of support area on which an object rests

Basic care facility agency that provides extended custodial care

Battery unauthorized physical contact

Bed bath washing with a basin of water at the bedside

Bed board rigid structure placed under a mattress

Bedpan seat-like container for elimination

Beliefs concepts that a person holds to be true

Beneficence "doing good" or acting for another's benefit

Beneficial disclosure an exemption whereby an agency can release private health information without a client's prior authorization

Bilingual able to speak a second language

Binder cloth covering applied to a body part such as the abdomen or breast

Biofeedback technique in which the client learns to control or alter a physiologic phenomenon

Biohazard container device usually mounted on the wall within the client's room for used sharp items

Biologic defense mechanisms methods that prevent microorganisms from causing an infectious disorder

BiPAP mask face or nasal mask that provides two different levels of airway pressure; *inspiratory positive airway pressure* that is higher during inhalation and *expiratory positive airway pressure* that is lower during expiration

Bivalved cast cast that is cut into two lengthwise pieces

Blood pressure force exerted by blood in the arteries

Blood substitutes fluids that when transfused carry and distribute oxygen to cells, tissues, and organs; also known as oxygen therapeutics

Board of Nursing regulatory agency that manages the provisions of a state's nurse practice act

Body cast form of a cylinder cast that encircles the trunk of the body instead of an extremity

Body composition amount of body tissue that is lean versus fat

Body mass index numeric data used to compare a person's size in relation to norms for the adult population

Body mechanics efficient use of the musculoskeletal system

Body systems approach collection of data according to the functional systems of the body

Bolus larger dose of a drug administered initially or when pain is intense

Bolus administration undiluted or diluted medication given into a vein in one or more minutes

Bolus feeding instillation of liquid nourishment four to six times a day in less than 30 minutes

Braces custom-made or custom-fitted devices designed to support weakened structures

Bradycardia a pulse rate less than 60 beats per minute (bpm) in an adult

Bradypnea slower-than-normal respiratory rate at rest

Brain death condition in which there is an irreversible loss of function of the whole brain, including the brainstem

Breakthrough pain acute pain that occasionally develops in those who have chronic pain

Bridge dental device that replaces one or several teeth

Broad-spectrum antibiotics drugs prescribed to eliminate a wide range of bacteria

Brown adipose tissue fat cells filled with mitochondria that raise body temperature by increasing metabolism

Bruxism grinding of the teeth

Buccal application drug placement against the mucous membranes of the inner cheek

C

Cachexia general wasting of body tissue

Calorie amount of heat that raises the temperature of 1 g of water by 1°C

Cane handheld ambulatory device made of wood or aluminum with a rubber tip

Capacity to learn intellectual ability to receive, remember, analyze, and apply new information

Capillary action movement of a liquid at the point of contact with a solid

Capillary refill time time duration for blood to resume flowing in the base of the nail beds

Capitation strategy for controlling health care costs by paying a fixed amount per member

Carbohydrates nutrients that contain molecules of carbon, hydrogen, and oxygen

Carboxyhemoglobin compound of carbon monoxide and hemoglobin in the blood

Cardiac arrest cessation of heart contraction or life-sustaining heart rhythm

Cardiac ischemia impaired blood flow to the heart

Cardiac output volume of blood ejected from the left ventricle per minute

Cardiometabolic syndrome cluster of modifiable risk factors that can potentially lead to cardiovascular diseases and type 2 diabetes mellitus if uncontrolled

Cardiopulmonary resuscitation techniques used to restore circulation and breathing for lifeless victims

Caregiver one who performs health-related activities that a sick person cannot perform independently

Caries dental cavities

Caring skills nursing interventions that restore or maintain a person's health

Carriers asymptomatic clients or animals who harbor pathogens but do not show evidence of an infectious disease

Case method pattern in which one nurse manages a client's care for a designated period

Cast rigid mold around a body part

Cataplexy sudden loss of muscle tone, triggered by an emotional change such as laughing or anger

Catastrophize choosing to focus on all the potentially negative outcomes that may result from stressors

Catheter-associated urinary tract infections (CAUTIs) infections acquired by those with indwelling urinary catheters, especially with those that are in place for a prolonged period of time

Catheter care hygiene measures used to keep the meatus and adjacent area of the catheter clean

Catheter irrigation flushing the lumen of a catheter

Catheterization act of applying or inserting a hollow tube

Cations electrolytes with a positive charge

Cellulose undigestible fiber in the stems, skin, and leaves of fruits and vegetables

Center of gravity point at which the mass of an object is centered

Centigrade scale scale that uses 0°C as the temperature at which water freezes and 100°C as the point at which it boils

Central venous catheter venous access device that extends to the superior vena cava

Certified interpreter translator who is certified by a professional organization through rigorous testing based on appropriate and consistent criteria

Cerumen ear wax

Cervical collar foam or rigid splint around the neck

Chain of infection sequence that enables the spread of disease-producing microorganisms

Chain of survival intervention and rescue process including (1) immediate recognition and access of emergency services; (2) early CPR with a focus on compressions; (3) rapid defibrillation, if appropriate; (4) effective advanced life support; and (5) integrated postcardiac arrest care

Change-of-shift report discussion between a nurse from the shift that is ending and personnel coming on duty

Characterization evidence that a learner continues to practice and act upon acquired information

Chart binder or folder that enables the orderly collection, storage, and safekeeping of a client's medical records

Charting process of entering information

Charting by exception documentation method in which only abnormal assessment findings or care that deviates from the standard is charted

Checklist form of documentation in which the nurse indicates with a check mark or initials that routine care has been performed

Chemical restraint sedative medication that is not a standard treatment or dosage for the client's condition that is used to manage a violent or self-destructive client's behavior or freedom of movement

Chest physiotherapy techniques for mobilizing pulmonary secretions

Chronic illness one that comes on slowly and lasts a long time

Chronic pain discomfort that lasts longer than 6 months

Circadian rhythm phenomena that cycle on a 24-hour basis

Circulatory overload severely compromised heart function

Civil laws statutes that protect the personal freedoms and rights of individuals

Clean-catch specimen voided sample of urine that is considered sterile

Climate control mechanisms for maintaining temperature, humidity, and ventilation

Clinical autopsy postmortem examination to determine cause of death

Clinical pathways standardized multidisciplinary plans for a specific diagnosis or procedure that identifies specific aspects of care to be performed during a designated length of stay

Clinical resume summary of previous care

Clinical thermometers instruments used to measure body temperature

Closed drainage system device used to collect urine from a catheter

Closed wound one in which there is no opening in the skin or mucous membrane

Code summoning personnel to administer advanced life support techniques

Code of ethics statements describing ideal behavior

Code status manner in which nurses or health care personnel must manage the care of a client during cardiac or respiratory arrest

Cognitive domain style of processing information by listening or reading facts and descriptions

Cold spot area with little or no radionuclide concentration

Collaborative problem physiologic complication whose treatment requires both nurse- and physician-prescribed interventions

Collaborator one who works with others to achieve a common goal

Collagen protein substance that is tough and inelastic

Colloid solutions water and molecules of suspended substances, such as blood cells, and blood products such as albumin

Colloidal osmotic pressure force for attracting water

Colloids undissolved protein substances

Colonization condition in which microorganisms are present but the host manifests no signs or symptoms of infection

Colonography inspection of the colon using a CT scan instead of a colonoscope

Colonoscopy visual inspection of the entire interior colon using a flexible lighted endoscope

Colostomy opening to some portion of the colon

Comfort state in which a person is relieved of distress

Comforting skills interventions that provide stability and security during a health crisis

Commode portable chair used for elimination

Common law decisions based on prior cases of a similar nature

Communicable diseases infectious diseases that are transmitted from one source to another

Communication exchange of information

Community-acquired infections infections that are not present or incubating prior to care provided by health care

Compartment syndrome complication following the application of a cast caused by pressure due to swelling within inelastic fascia that surrounds muscles

Complementary and alternative medicine combination of conventional medical practice with nontraditional physical and nonphysical approaches for which there is some scientific evidence of safety and effectiveness; now called integrative medicine

Complete airway obstruction inability to ventilate

Complete proteins those that contain all of the essential amino acids

Compresses moist cloths that may be warm or cool

Computed tomography form of roentgenography that shows planes of tissue

Computerized provider order system method in which physicians can provide medical orders using a computer when unable to provide them verbally

Concept mapping organizing information in a graphic or pictorial form

Concurrent disinfection measures that keep the client environment clean on a daily basis

Conductor substance that facilitates the flow of electrical current

Confidentiality safeguarding a client's health information from public disclosure

Congenital disorder disorder present at birth that results from faulty embryonic development

Conscious sedation state in which clients are sedated, relaxed, and emotionally comfortable, but not unconscious

Consensual response brisk, equal, and simultaneous constriction of both pupils when one eye and then the other are stimulated with light

Constipation condition in which dry, hard stool is difficult to pass

Contact dermatitis delayed localized skin reaction

Contact precautions infection control measures used to block the transmission of pathogens by skin-to-skin contact with an infected or colonized person or touching a contaminated intermediate object in the client's environment

Contagious diseases diseases that can spread rapidly among individuals in close proximity to each other

Continence training process of restoring control of urination

Continent ostomy surgically created opening in which liquid stool or urine is removed by siphoning

Continuity of care uninterrupted client care despite the change in caregivers

Continuous feeding instillation of liquid nutrition without interruption

Continuous infusion parenteral instillation over several hours

Continuous irrigation ongoing instillation of solution

Continuous passive motion machine electrical device that exercises joints

Continuous quality improvement process of promoting care that reflects established agency standards

Continuous release form of drug designed to dissolve slowly and be released over time; also called extended release

Contractures permanently shortened muscles that resist stretching

Contrast medium substance that adds density to a body organ or cavity, such as barium sulfate or iodine

Controlled substances drugs whose prescription and dispensing are regulated by federal law because they have the potential for abuse

Coping mechanisms unconscious tactics used to protect the psyche

Coping strategies stress-reduction activities selected on a conscious level

Cordotomy surgical interruption of pain pathways in the spinal cord

Core temperature warmth at the center of the body

Coroner person legally designated to investigate deaths that may not be the result of natural causes

Cortisol a stress hormone, from the adrenal cortex

Counseling skills interventions that include communicating with clients, actively listening to the exchange of information, offering pertinent health teaching, and providing emotional support

CPAP mask device that maintains positive pressure in the airway throughout the respiratory cycle

Creating cognitive level that involves inventing, modifying, substituting, and reorganizing information to fashion new ideas

Credé maneuver act of bending forward and applying hand pressure over the bladder to stimulate urination

Criminal laws penal codes that protect citizens from persons who are a threat to the public good

Critical thinking process of objective reasoning; analyzing facts to reach a valid conclusion

Cross-trained ability to assume a nonnursing job position, depending on the census or levels of client acuity on any given day

Crutch palsy weakening of forearm, wrist, and hand muscles because of nerve impairment in the axilla caused by incorrectly fitted crutches or poor posture

Crutches ambulatory aid, generally in pairs, constructed of wood or aluminum

Crystalloid solution water and other uniformly dissolved crystals, such as salt and sugar

Cultural shock bewilderment over behavior that is culturally atypical

Culturally sensitive nursing care care that is respectful of and is compatible with each client's culture

Culture (1) values, beliefs, and practices of a particular group; (2) incubation of microorganisms

Cutaneous pain discomfort that originates at the skin level

Cutaneous triggering the act of lightly massaging or tapping the skin above the pubic area to stimulate urination

Cuticles thin edge of skin at the base of the nail

Cyclic feeding continuous instillation of liquid nourishment for 8 to 12 hours

Cylinder cast rigid mold that encircles an arm or leg

D

Dangling sitting on the edge of a bed

Database assessment initial information about the client's physical, emotional, social, and spiritual health

Deaf unable to hear well enough to process information

Death certificate legal document confirming a person's death

Debridement removal of dead tissue

Decompression removal of gas and secretions from the stomach or bowel

Defamation act in which untrue information harms a person's reputation

Defecation bowel elimination

Defendant person charged with violating the law

Dehiscence the separation of wound edges

Dehydration fluid deficit in both extracellular and intracellular compartments

Delegator one who assigns a task to someone

Deltoid site injection area in the lateral upper arm

Dementia impairment of intellectual functioning

Denial psychological defense mechanism in which a person refuses to believe that certain information is true

Dentures artificial teeth

Deontology ethical study based on duty or moral obligations

Depilatory agent chemical that removes hair

Depression sad mood

Developmental level physical, cognitive, social/emotional, and language characteristics that are norms at particular stages in life from infancy through adulthood

Diagnosis identification of health-related problems

Diagnostic examination procedure that involves physical inspection of body structures and evidence of their function

Diagnostic-related group classification system used to group clients with similar diagnoses

Diaphragmatic breathing breathing that promotes the use of the diaphragm rather than upper chest muscles

Diarrhea urgent passage of watery stools

Diastolic pressure pressure in the arterial system when the heart relaxes and fills with blood

Diet history assessment technique used to obtain facts about a person's eating habits and factors that affect nutrition

Directed donors relatives and friends who donate blood for a client

Discharge termination of care from a health care agency

Discharge instructions directions for managing self-care and medical follow-up

Discharge planning predetermining a client's postdischarge needs and coordinating the use of appropriate community resources to provide a continuum of care

Disinfectants chemicals that destroy active microorganisms but not spores

Distraction intentional diversion of attention

Disuse syndrome signs and symptoms that result from inactivity

Diversity differences among groups of people

Documentation record keeping

Documenting process of entering information

Doppler stethoscope device that helps detect sounds created by the velocity of blood moving through a blood vessel

Dorsal recumbent position reclining posture with the knees bent, hips rotated outward, and feet flat

Dorsogluteal site injection area in the upper outer quadrant of the buttocks

Dose amount of drug

Double-bagging infection control measure in which one bag of contaminated items, such as trash or laundry, is placed within another, keeping the outer surface of the second bag clean

Double charting repetitious entry of the same information in the medical record

Douche procedure for cleansing the vaginal canal

Drains tubes that provide a means for removing blood and drainage from a wound

Drape sheet of soft cloth or paper

Drawdown effect cooling of the ear when it comes in contact with a thermometer probe

Dressing cover over a wound

Drop factor number of drops per milliliter in intravenous tubing

Droplet precautions measures that block transmission of infectious pathogens within moist droplets larger than 5 microns that are present in respiratory secretions or mucous membranes

Drowning situation in which fluid occupies the airway and interferes with ventilation

Drug diversion obtaining a drug through illicit methods such as theft from a person for whom the drug has been prescribed, "doctor shopping," purchase from illegal internet pharmacies, prescription forgery, or unnecessary prescriptions from less than ethical physicians

Drug tolerance diminished effect of a drug at its usual dosage range

Dry powder inhaler device containing a reservoir of pulverized drug and a carrier substance that relies on the client's inspiratory effort to deliver the drug into the lungs

Dumping syndrome cluster of symptoms resulting from the rapid deposition of calorie-dense nourishment into the small intestine

Durable power of attorney for health care proxy for making medical decisions when a client becomes incompetent or incapacitated and cannot make decisions independently

Duty obligation to provide care for a person claiming injury or harm

Dying with dignity treating a terminally ill person with respect regardless of his or her emotional, physical, or cognitive state

Dysphagia difficult swallowing

Dyspnea difficult or labored breathing

Dysrhythmia irregular pattern of heartbeats

Dysuria difficult or uncomfortable voiding

E

Echography soft tissue examination that uses sound waves in ranges beyond human hearing

Edema excessive fluid in tissue

Educator one who provides information

Electrical shock discharge of electricity through the body

Electrocardiography examination of the electrical activity in the heart

Electrochemical neutrality balance of cations with anions

Electroencephalography examination of the energy emitted by the brain

Electrolytes chemical compounds, such as sodium and chloride, that are dissolved, absorbed, and distributed in body fluid and possess an electrical charge

Electromyography examination of the energy produced by stimulated muscles

Electronic charting documenting client information with a computer

Emaciation excessive leanness

Emancipated minor adolescent living independent of parents or guardians and supporting him or herself

Emboli moving clots

Emesis substance that is vomited

Emotional health when one feels safe and copes effectively with the stressors of life

Empathy intuitive awareness of what the client is experiencing

Emulsion mixture of two liquids, one of which is insoluble in the other

Endocrine system a group of glands found throughout the body that produce hormones

Endogenous opioids naturally produced morphine-like chemicals

Endorphins natural body chemicals that produce effects similar to those of opiate drugs such as morphine

Endoscopy visual examination of internal structures

Enema introduction of a solution into the rectum

Energy capacity to do work

English as a second language (ESL) other than primary spoken language

Enteral nutrition nourishment provided via the stomach or small intestine rather than via the oral route

Enteric-coated tablet tablet covered with a substance that does not dissolve until it is past the stomach

Enterostomal therapist a nurse certified in caring for ostomies and related skin problems

Environmental hazards potentially dangerous conditions in the physical surroundings

Environmental psychologist specialist who studies how the environment affects behavior

Equianalgesic dose oral dose that provides the same level of pain relief as a parenteral dose

Ergonomics field of engineering science devoted to promoting comfort, performance, and health in the workplace

Eructation belching

Essential amino acids protein components that must be obtained from food because they cannot be synthesized by the body

Ethical dilemma choice between two undesirable alternatives

Ethics moral or philosophical principles

Ethnicity bond or kinship a person feels with his or her country of birth or place of ancestral origin

Ethnocentrism belief that one's own ethnicity is superior to all others

Evaluating cognitive level that involves an ability to appraise a situation or information and to defend or support a selected action

Evaluation process of determining whether a goal has been reached

Evidence-based practice scientific knowledge used to predict nursing interventions most likely to produce a desired outcome

Evisceration wound separation with the protrusion of organs

Exacerbation reactivation of a disorder, or one that reverts from a chronic to an acute state

Excoriation chemical skin injury

Exercise purposeful physical activity

Exit route means by which microorganisms escape from their original reservoir

Expiration exhalation; breathing out

Expressive aphasia inability to use verbal language skills

Extended care services that meet the health needs of clients who no longer require acute hospital care

Extended care facility health care agency that provides long-term care

Extended release form of drug designed to dissolve slowly and be released over time; also called continuous release

External catheter device applied to the skin that collects urine

External fixator metal device inserted into and through one or more bones

Extracellular fluid fluid outside cells

Extraocular movements eye movements controlled by several pairs of eye muscles

F

Face tent device that provides oxygen in an area around the nose and mouth

Facilitated diffusion process in which certain dissolved substances require the assistance of a carrier molecule to pass from one side of a semipermeable membrane to the other

Fahrenheit scale scale that uses 32°F as the temperature at which water freezes and 212°F as the point at which it boils

False imprisonment interference with a person's freedom to move about at will without legal authority to do so

Fat nutrient that contains molecules composed of glycerol and fatty acids called glycerides

Fat-soluble vitamins those carried and stored in fat; vitamins A, D, E, and K

Febrile elevated body temperature

Fecal immunologic test self-collected stool test for colorectal disorders that uses antibodies to detect globin, a protein removed from heme, that is present exclusively in the lower intestine

Fecal impaction condition in which it is impossible to pass feces voluntarily

Fecal incontinence inability to control the elimination of stool

Fecal occult blood test self-collected screening test for colorectal disorders to detect heme, an iron compound in blood within stool

Feces stool

Feedback loop mechanism that turns hormone production off and on

Felony serious criminal offense

Fenestrated drape one with an open circle at its center

Fenestrated tracheostomy tube one with holes in the outer cannula that allows air to pass through the vocal cords allowing speech

Fever body temperature that exceeds 99.3°F (37.4°C)

Fidelity being faithful to work-related commitments and obligations

Fifth vital sign client's pain assessment that is checked and documented, in addition to his or her temperature, pulse, respirations, and blood pressure

Fight-or-flight response physiologic process used to attack a stressor in an effort to overcome the danger it represents, or flee from the stressor to escape its threat

Filtration process that regulates the movement of water and substances from a compartment where the pressure is high to one where the pressure is lower

Fire plan procedure followed if there is a fire

First-intention healing reparative process when wound edges are directly next to one another

Fitness capacity to exercise

Fitness exercise physical activity performed by healthy adults

Flatulence accumulation of intestinal gas

Flatus gas formed in the intestine and released from the rectum

Flora microorganisms

Flow sheet form of documentation that contains sections for recording frequently repeated assessment data

Flowmeter gauge used to regulate the number of liters of oxygen delivered to the client

Fluid imbalance condition in which the body's water is not in proper volume or location in the body

Fluoroscopy form of radiography that displays an image in real time

Focus assessment information that provides more details about specific problems

Focus charting modified form of SOAP charting

Folk medicine health practices unique to a particular group of people

Fomites nonliving reservoirs of pathogens

Foot drop permanent dysfunctional position caused by shortening of the calf muscles and lengthening of the opposing muscles on the anterior leg

Forced coughing coughing that is purposely produced

Forearm crutches crutches with an arm cuff but no axillary bar

Forensic autopsy medicolegal examination to determine if a crime has been committed

Formal teaching instruction that requires a plan

Fowler position upright seated position

Fraction of inspired oxygen portion of oxygen in relation to total inspired gas

Freeze response a stress response that simulates the appearance of death by slowing down physiologic responses

Frenulum structure that attaches the undersurface of the tongue to the fleshy portion of the mouth

Frequency need to urinate often

Functional assessment determining a person's ability to perform self-care task

Functional braces braces that provide stability for a joint

Functional mobility alignment that maintains the potential for movement and ambulation

Functional nursing pattern in which each nurse on a unit is assigned specific tasks

Functional position position that promotes continued use and mobility

Functionally illiterate possessing minimal literacy skills

G

Gastric reflux reverse flow of gastric contents

Gastric residual volume of liquid remaining in the stomach

Gastrocolic reflex increased peristaltic activity

Gastrostomy tube; G-tube transabdominal tube located in the stomach

Gauge diameter

Gavage provision of nourishment

General adaptation syndrome collective physiologic processes that occur in response to a stressor

Generalization supposition that a person shares cultural characteristics with others of a similar background

Generic name chemical drug name that is not protected by a manufacturer's trademark

Gerogogy techniques that enhance learning among older adults

Gingivitis inflammation of the gums

Globin protein removed from heme that is present exclusively in the lower intestine

Glucometer instrument that measures the amount of glucose in capillary blood

Gluteal setting contraction and relaxation of the gluteus muscles to strengthen and tone them

Goal expected or desired outcome

Good Samaritan laws legal immunity for passersby who provide emergency first aid to accident victims

Gram staining process of adding dye to a microscopic specimen

Granulation tissue combination of new blood vessels, fibroblasts, and epithelial cells

Gravity force that pulls objects toward the center of the earth

Grief response psychological and physical phenomena experienced by those who grieve

Grief work activities involved in grieving

Grieving process of feeling acute sorrow over a loss

Gross negligence total disregard for another's safety

Ground diverts leaking electrical energy to the earth

H

Hand antisepsis removal and destruction of transient microorganisms from the hands

Hand hygiene methods for removing surface contaminants on the skin

Handwashing aseptic practice that involves scrubbing the hands with plain soap or detergent, water, and friction

Hard of hearing state of having limited hearing, in which communication is nonetheless possible

Head tilt/chin lift technique preferred method for opening the airway

Head-to-toe approach gathering data from the top of the body to the feet

Health state of complete physical, mental, and social well-being; not merely the absence of disease or infirmity

Health care–associated infections infections acquired while a person is receiving care in a health care agency

Health care system network of available health services

Health insurance marketplaces state organizations that provide a means for individuals or employers with small numbers of employees to purchase affordable private health insurance

Health Insurance Portability and Accountability Act legislation that sets national standards for the security of health information, ensures that an individual's electronic, paper, or oral health information is protected

Health literacy degree to which individuals have the capacity to obtain, process, and understand basic health information and services needed to make appropriate health decisions

Health maintenance organizations corporations that charge members preset, fixed, yearly fees in exchange for providing health care

Health promotion diagnosis a concern with which a healthy person desires nursing assistance to maintain or achieve a higher level of wellness

Hearing acuity ability to hear and to discriminate sound

Heimlich maneuver method for removing a mechanical airway obstruction

Heme iron compound in blood

Hereditary condition disorder acquired from the genetic codes of one or both parents

Holism philosophical concept of interrelatedness

Home health care in-home health care provided by an employee of a home health agency

Homeostasis relatively stable state of physiologic equilibrium

Hospice facility for or concept addressing the care of terminally ill clients

Hospital-acquired condition complication of hospitalization that is reasonably preventable

Hot spot area where radionuclide is intensely concentrated

Human needs factors that motivate behavior

Humidifier device that produces small water droplets

Humidity amount of moisture in the air

Hydrostatic pressure pressure exerted against a membrane

Hydrotherapy therapeutic use of water

Hygiene personal cleanliness practices that promote health

Hyperbaric oxygen therapy delivery of 100% oxygen at three times the normal atmospheric pressure in an airtight chamber

Hypercarbia excessive levels of carbon dioxide in the blood

Hyperendemic infections infections that are considered highly dangerous in all age groups

Hypersomnia sleep disorder characterized by feeling sleepy despite getting a normal amount of sleep

Hypersomnolence excessive sleeping

Hypertension high blood pressure

Hyperthermia excessively high core temperature

Hypertonic solution solution that is more concentrated than body fluid

Hyperventilation rapid or deep breathing, or both

Hypervolemia higher-than-normal volume of water in the intravascular fluid compartment

Hypnogogic hallucinations dream-like auditory or visual experiences while dozing or falling asleep

Hypnogogic jerks muscle twitches that occur during the onset of sleep

Hypnosis therapeutic technique in which a person enters a trancelike state

Hypnotic agent that produces sleep

Hypoalbuminemia deficit of albumin in the blood

Hypopnea hypoventilation

Hypotension low blood pressure

Hypothalamus temperature-regulating structure in the brain

Hypothalamus–pituitary–adrenal (HPA) axis pathway of physiologic communication among the central nervous, endocrine, and immune systems

Hypothermia core body temperature less than 95°F (35°C)

Hypotonic solution one that contains fewer dissolved substances than normally found in plasma

Hypoventilation diminished breathing

Hypovolemia low volume in the extracellular fluid compartments

Hypoxemia insufficient oxygen in arterial blood

Hypoxia inadequate oxygen at the cellular level

I

Idiopathic illness one in which the cause is unexplained

Ileostomy surgically created opening to the ileum

Illiterate unable to read or write

Illness state of being unwell

Imagery using the mind to visualize an experience

Imitating attempt to duplicate what has been observed

Immobilizers commercial splints made from cloth and foam

Implementation carrying out a plan of care

Incentive spirometry technique for deep breathing using a calibrated device

Incident report written account of an unusual event involving a client, employee, or visitor that has the potential for being injurious

Incomplete proteins those that contain some, but not all, of the essential amino acids

Incontinence inability to control either urinary or bowel elimination

Individual supply single container of drugs with several days' worth of doses

Induration area of hardness

Infection condition that results when microorganisms cause injury to a host

Infection control precautions physical measures designed to curtail the spread of infectious diseases

Infectious diseases diseases that spread from one person to another

Infiltration escape of intravenous fluid into the tissue

Inflammation physiologic defense that occurs immediately after tissue injury

Inflatable splints immobilizing devices that become rigid when filled with air; also called pneumatic splints

Informal teaching instruction that is unplanned and occurs spontaneously

Informatics collection, storage, retrieval, and sharing of recorded data

Informed consent permission that a person gives after having the risks, benefits, and alternatives explained

Infusion device electric or battery-operated machine that regulates and monitors the administration of IV solutions

Infusion pump device that uses pressure to infuse solutions

Inhalant route drug administration into the lower airways

Inhalation therapy respiratory treatments that provide a mixture of oxygen, humidification, and aerosolized medication

Inhalers handheld devices for delivering medication to the respiratory passages

Inner cannula component of a tracheostomy tube that can be temporarily removed and cleaned

Inpatient surgery operative procedures performed on persons admitted to a hospital and expected to remain for a period of time

Insomnia sleep disorder involving early awakening or difficulty falling asleep or staying asleep

Inspection purposeful observation

Inspiration inhalation; breathing in

Insulator substance that contains electrical current so it does not scatter

Insulin pen hard plastic cylinder that contains a prefilled reservoir of insulin

Insulin pump programmable computerized device that contains rapid-acting insulin released through a catheter attached to a needle in the skin

Insulin syringe syringe that is calibrated in units and holds a volume of 0.5 to 1 mL of medication

Intake and output record of a client's fluid intake and fluid loss over a 24-hour period

Integrated delivery system network that provides a full range of health care services in a highly coordinated, cost-effective manner

Integument covering, the skin

Integumentary system includes the skin, mucous membranes, hair, and nails

Intentional tort lawsuit in which a plaintiff charges that a defendant committed a deliberately aggressive act

Intermediate care facility agency that provides health-related care and services to people who, because of their mental or physical condition, require institutional care but not 24-hour nursing care

Intermittent feeding gradual instillation of liquid nourishment four to six times a day

Intermittent infusion parenteral administration of medication over a relatively short period

Intermittent venous access device sealed chamber that provides a means for administering intravenous medications or solutions on a periodic basis

Interstitial fluid fluid in tissue space between and around cells

Intestinal decompression removal of gas and intestinal contents

Intimate space distance within 6 in of a person

Intracellular fluid fluid inside cells

Intractable pain pain unresponsive to methods of pain management

Intradermal injection parenteral drug administration between the layers of the skin

Intramuscular injection parenteral drug administration into the muscle

Intraoperative period time when a client undergoes surgery

Intraspinal analgesia method of relieving pain by instilling a narcotic or local anesthetic via a catheter into the subarachnoid or epidural space of the spinal cord

Intravascular fluid watery plasma, or serum, portion of blood

Intravenous fluids solutions infused into a client's vein

Intravenous injection parenteral drug administration into a vein

Intravenous route drug administration via peripheral and central veins

Introductory phase period of getting acquainted

Intubation placement of a tube into a structure of the body

Invasion of privacy failure to leave people and their property alone

Ions substances that carry either a positive or a negative electrical charge

Irrigation technique for flushing debris

Isokinetic exercise movement that combines constant speed with a form of resistance

Isometric exercise stationary exercises that are generally performed against a resistive force

Isotonic exercise activity that involves movement and work

Isotonic solution solution that contains the same concentration of dissolved substances as normally found in plasma

J

Jaeger chart visual assessment tool with small print

Jaw-thrust maneuver alternative method for opening the airway

Jejunostomy tube; J-tube transabdominal tube that leads to the jejunum of the small intestine

Jet lag emotional and physical changes experienced when arriving in a different time zone

Justice principle for treating impartially without discrimination according to age, gender, race, religion, socioeconomic status, weight, marital status, or sexual orientation

K

Kardex quick reference for current information about the client and the client's care

Kilocalories 1,000 calories, or the amount of heat that raises the temperature of 1 kg of water by 1°C

Kinesics body language

Knee–chest position position in which the client rests on the knees and chest

Korotkoff sounds sounds that result from the vibrations of blood in the arterial wall or changes in blood flow

L

Laboratory test procedure that involves the examination of body fluids or specimens

Lateral oblique position variation of a side-lying position

Lateral position side-lying position

Latex-safe environment room stocked with latex-free equipment and wiped clean of glove powder

Latex sensitivity allergic response to the proteins in latex

Latinos people who trace their ethnic origin to South America

Lavage wash out; remove poisonous substances

Laws rules of conduct established and enforced by the government of a society

Learning need gap between what a person knows and has yet to learn

Learning readiness capacity to learn because of physical and psychological well-being

Learning style how a person prefers to acquire knowledge

Leukocytes white blood cells

Leukocytosis increased production of white blood cells

Liability insurance contract between a person or corporation and a company that is willing to provide legal services and financial assistance when a policyholder is involved in a malpractice lawsuit

Libel damaging statement that is written and read by others

Limited English proficiency (LEP) inability to speak, read, write, or understand English at a level that permits effective interaction

Line of gravity imaginary vertical line that passes through the center of gravity

Lipoatrophy breakdown of subcutaneous fat at the site of repeated insulin injections

Lipohypertrophy thickening of subcutaneous fat at insulin injection sites

Lipoproteins combinations of fats and proteins

Liquid oxygen unit device that converts cooled liquid oxygen to a gas by passing it through heated coils

Literacy ability to read and write

Lithotomy position reclining posture with the feet in metal supports called stirrups

Living will a person's advance, written directive identifying medical interventions to use or not to use in cases of terminal condition, irreversible coma, or vegetative state with no hope of recovery

Loading dose larger dose of a drug administered initially or when pain is intense

Lockout period of time during which a client cannot self-administer intravenous pain medication

Long-term goals desirable outcomes that take weeks or months to accomplish

Lumbar puncture procedure that involves insertion of a needle between lumbar vertebrae in the spine but below the spinal cord itself

Lumen channel

Lysosomes enzymatic sacs inside phagocytes that digest engulfed matter

M

Macrophages white blood cells that consume cellular debris

Macroshock harmless distribution of low-amperage electricity over a large area of the body

Maggot therapy use of larvae of a species of blow flies that secrete an enzyme that dissolves dead tissue

Magnetic resonance imaging diagnostic tool used to identify disorders that affect structures in the body without performing surgery; a magnetic field excites hydrogen atoms within the body creating a radio signal that is converted into an image on a computer monitor

Malingerer someone who pretends to be sick or in pain

Malnutrition condition resulting from a lack of proper nutrients in the diet

Malpractice professional negligence

Managed care organizations private insurers who carefully plan and closely supervise distribution of their clients' health care services

Managed care practices cost-containment strategies used to plan and coordinate a client's care to avoid delays, unnecessary services, or overuse of expensive resources

Manual traction pulling on the body using a person's hands and muscular strength

Massage stroking the skin

Mattress overlay layer of foam or other devices placed on top of the mattress

Maximum heart rate highest limit for heart rate during exercise

Means of transmission how infectious microorganisms move to another location

Medicaid state-administered program designed to meet the needs of low-income residents

Medical asepsis practices that confine or reduce the numbers of microorganisms

Medical examiner physician who has specialized training in forensic pathology

Medical records written collection of information about a person's health problems, the care provided by health practitioners, and the progress of the client

Medicare federal program that finances health care costs of persons who are 65 years and older, permanently disabled workers and their dependents, and people with end-stage renal disease

Medication administration record agency form used to document drug administration

Medication order directions for administering a drug

Medication reconciliation act of obtaining and verifying medications a client is currently taking

Medications chemical substances that change body function

Meditation concentrating on a word or idea that promotes tranquility

Megadoses amounts exceeding those considered adequate for health

Melatonin hormone that induces drowsiness and sleep

Melena blood in stool

Mental status assessment technique for determining the level of a client's cognitive functioning

Metabolic energy equivalent measure of energy and oxygen consumption during exercise

Metabolic rate use of calories for sustaining body functions

Metered-dose inhaler canister that contains medication under pressure

Microabrasions tiny cuts in the skin that provide an entrance for microorganisms

Microorganisms living animals or plants visible only with a microscope

Microshock low-voltage but high-amperage electricity

Microsleep unintentional sleep lasting 20 to 30 seconds

Midarm circumference measurement used to assess skeletal muscle mass

Military time time based on a 24-hour clock

Minerals noncaloric substances in food that are essential to all cells

Minimum disclosure portions or isolated pieces of information necessary for an immediate purpose

Minority people who differ from the majority in cultural characteristics like language, physical characteristics such as skin color, or both

Misdemeanor minor criminal offense

Modified standing position position in which the upper half of the body leans forward

Modulation last phase of pain impulse transmission when the brain interacts downward with spinal nerves to alter a pain experience

Molded splints orthotic devices made of rigid material

Monocytes type of white blood cells called macrophages that migrate to the site of an injury

Montgomery straps strips of tape with eyelets

Morbidity incidence of a specific disease, disorder, or injury

Morgue area where dead bodies are temporarily held or examined

Mortality incidence of deaths

Mortician person who prepares the body for burial or cremation

Motivation desire to acquire new information or skill

Mucus substance that keeps mucous membranes moist

Multicultural diversity unique characteristics of ethnic groups

Multiple organ failure condition in which two or more organ systems gradually cease to function

Multiple sleep latency test assessment of daytime sleepiness

Muscle spasms sudden, forceful, involuntary muscle contractions

N

N95 respirator device that is individually fitted to each caregiver and can filter particles 1 micron in size, with a filter efficiency of 95% or more, provided it fits the face snugly

NANDA International the authoritative organization for developing and approving nursing diagnoses

Narcolepsy sleep disorder characterized by the sudden onset of daytime sleep, a short NREM period before the first REM phase, and pathologic manifestations of REM sleep

Narrative charting style of documentation generally used in source-oriented records

Nasal cannula hollow tube with prongs that are placed into the client's nostrils for delivering oxygen

Nasal catheter tube for delivering oxygen that is inserted through the nose into the posterior nasal pharynx

Nasogastric intubation insertion of a tube through the nose into the stomach

Nasogastric tube tube that is placed in the nose and advanced to the stomach

Nasointestinal intubation insertion of a tube through the nose to the intestine

Nasointestinal tube tube inserted through the nose for distal placement below the stomach

Nasopharyngeal suctioning removal of secretions from the throat through a nasally inserted catheter

Nasotracheal suctioning removal of secretions from the trachea through a nasally inserted catheter

National Patient Safety Goals objectives designed to reduce the incidence of injuries to those being cared for in health agencies

National Practitioner Data Bank serves as a tracking system designed to protect the public from unfit health care practitioners

Native Americans Indian nations found in North America, including the Eskimos and Aleuts

Nausea feeling that usually precedes vomiting

Nebulizer device that converts liquid inhalant medication to an aerosol using compressed air

Necrotic tissue nonliving tissue

Needleless systems equipment that eliminates the need for needles

Negative pressure wound therapy method of promoting more rapid wound healing by using suction to pull fluid and debris from a wound bed through a foam filler into a collection canister; also called vacuum-assisted closure

Negligence harm that results because a person did not act reasonably

Neuropathic pain pain with atypical characteristics

Neuropeptides chemicals that stimulate nociceptors

Neurotransmitters chemical messengers synthesized in neurons

Neutral position limb that is turned neither toward nor away from the body's midline

Neutrophils white blood cells that migrate to the site of injury

Nociceptors nerve receptors that transmit pain impulses

Nocturia nighttime urination

Nocturnal enuresis bedwetting

Nocturnal polysomnography technique used to obtain physiologic data during nighttime sleep

Noncoring needle one that does not remove a plug from the septum of an implanted port, commonly called a Huber needle

Nonelectrolytes chemical compounds that remain bound together when dissolved in solution

Nonessential amino acids protein components manufactured in the body

Nonmaleficence "doing no harm" or avoiding an action that deliberately harms a person

Nonopioids nonnarcotic drugs

Nonpathogens harmless and beneficial microorganisms

Non-rebreather mask oxygen delivery device in which all the exhaled air leaves the mask rather than partially entering the reservoir bag

Nonverbal communication exchange of information without using spoken or written words

Normal flora microorganisms that reside in and on humans

Nose-to-earlobe-to-the-xiphoid (NEX) measurement method to determine the projected depth of a tube to reach the oropharynx and stomach

Nuclear medicine department unit responsible for radionuclide imaging

Nurse licensure compacts agreements between states in which a nurse licensed in one state can practice in another without obtaining an additional license

Nurse-managed care pattern in which a nurse manager plans the nursing care of clients based on their illness or medical diagnosis

Nurse practice act statute that legally defines the unique role of the nurse and differentiates it from that of other health care practitioners, such as physicians

Nursing care plans written assignments on a standardized worksheet that contains a column for nursing diagnoses, outcome criteria, nursing interventions, and their rationale for each assigned client

Nursing diagnosis health problem that can be prevented, reduced, or resolved through independent nursing measures

Nursing Home Reform Act sets the federal quality standards for nursing homes

Nursing orders directions for a client's nursing care

Nursing process organized sequence of problem-solving steps: assessment, diagnosis, planning, implementation, and evaluation

Nursing skills activities unique to the practice of nursing

Nursing team personnel who care for clients directly

Nursing theory proposal of what is involved in the process of nursing

Nutrition process by which the body uses food

O

Obesity condition in which a person's body mass index exceeds 30 or the triceps skinfold measurement exceeds 15 mm

Objective data facts that are observable and measurable

Observing learning by watching an experienced person

Obturator component of a tracheostomy tube used at the time of tube insertion to protect the edge of the cannula from traumatizing tracheal tissue

Occupied bed changing linen while the client remains in bed

Offsets predictive mathematical conversions

Oliguria urine output of less than 400 mL per 24 hours

Open wound wound in which the surface of the skin or mucous membrane is no longer intact

Ophthalmic application method of applying drugs onto the mucous membrane of one or both eyes

Ophthalmologist medical doctor who treats eye disorders

Ophthalmoscope instrument used to examine structures within the eye

Opioids narcotic drugs; synthetic narcotics

Opportunistic infections disorders caused by nonpathogens that occur in people with compromised health

Optometrist person who prescribes corrective vision lenses

Oral airway curved device that keeps the tongue positioned forward within the mouth

Oral hygiene practices used to clean the mouth, especially the teeth

Oral route drug administration by swallowing or instillation through an enteral tube

Oral suctioning removal of secretions from the mouth

Organization evidence that a learner integrates new information by changing behavior

Orientation helping a person to become familiar with a new environment

Orogastric intubation insertion of a tube through the mouth into the stomach

Orogastric tube tube that is inserted from the mouth into the stomach

Oropharyngeal suctioning removal of secretions from the throat through a catheter inserted through the mouth

Orthopnea breathing that is facilitated by sitting up or standing

Orthopneic position seated position with the arms supported on pillows or the armrests of a chair

Orthoses orthopedic devices that support or align a body part and prevent or correct deformities

Orthostatic hypotension sudden but temporary drop in blood pressure when rising from a reclining or seated position

Osmosis process that regulates the distribution of water

Ostomy surgically created opening

Otic application drug instillation in the outer ear

Otoscope instrument used to examine the tympanic membrane of the ear

Outcome criteria specific evidence for each nursing diagnosis that a client's problem is trending toward resolution or has been resolved

Outer cannula component of a tracheostomy tube that remains in place until the entire tube is replaced or removed

Outpatient surgery operative procedures from which clients recover and return home on the same day

Over-the-counter medication nonprescription drug

Oxygen analyzer device that measures the percentage of oxygen a client is receiving

Oxygen concentrator machine that collects and concentrates oxygen from room air and stores it for client use

Oxygen tent clear plastic enclosure that provides cooled, humidified oxygen

Oxygen therapeutics fluids that when transfused carry and distribute oxygen to cells, tissues, and organs; also known as blood substitutes

Oxygen therapy therapeutic intervention for administering more oxygen than exists in the atmosphere

Oxygen toxicity lung damage that develops when oxygen concentrations of more than 50% are administered for longer than 48 to 72 hours

P

Pack commercial device for applying moist heat

Pain unpleasant sensation usually associated with disease or injury

Pain management techniques for preventing, reducing, or relieving pain

Pain threshold point at which sufficient pain-transmitting neurochemicals reach the brain to cause awareness of discomfort

Pain tolerance amount of pain a person endures once the pain threshold is surpassed

Palliative care providing relief from distressing symptoms, easing pain, and enhancing quality of life

Palpation lightly touching the body or applying pressure

Palpitation awareness of one's own heart contraction without having to feel the pulse

Pap test screening test that detects abnormal cervical cells, the status of reproductive hormone activity, or the presence of normal or infectious microorganisms in the uterus or vagina

Paracentesis procedure for withdrawing fluid from the abdominal cavity

Paralanguage vocal sounds that are not actually words

Parallel bars double row of stationary bars

Paranormal experiences those outside scientific explanation

Parasomnia condition associated with activities that cause arousal or partial arousal, usually during transitions in NREM periods of sleep

Parenteral nutrition nutrients, such as proteins, carbohydrate, fat, vitamins, minerals, and trace elements, which are administered intravenously

Parenteral route route of drug administration other than oral or through the gastrointestinal tract; administration by injection

Partial airway obstruction condition in which some air is being exchanged and person can speak or cough

Partial bath washing only the areas of the body that are subject to the greatest soiling or that are sources of body odor

Partial rebreather mask oxygen delivery device through which a client inhales a mixture of atmospheric air, oxygen from its source, and oxygen contained in a reservoir bag

Passive diffusion physiologic process in which dissolved substances, such as electrolytes and gases, move from an area of higher concentration to one of lower concentration through a semipermeable membrane

Passive exercise therapeutic activity performed with assistance

Paste vehicle that contains a drug in a viscous base

Pathogens microorganisms that cause illness

Pathologic grief condition in which a person cannot accept someone's death

Patient-controlled analgesia intervention that allows clients to self-administer pain medication

Patient Protection and Affordable Care Act a health reform law enabling many uninsured people to acquire health insurance

Pedagogy the science of teaching children or those with cognitive ability comparable to children

Pedometer self-monitoring motion-sensing device that tracks total steps and distance walked

Pelvic examination physical inspection of the vagina and cervix, with palpation of the uterus and ovaries

Pelvic floor muscle exercises (Kegel exercises) isometric exercises to improve the ability to retain urine within the bladder

Perception conscious experience of discomfort

Percussion (1) striking or tapping a part of the body; (2) type of chest physiotherapy performed by rhythmically striking the chest wall

Percutaneous applications drugs rubbed into or placed in contact with the skin

Percutaneous electrical nerve stimulation pain management technique involving a combination of acupuncture needles and transcutaneous electrical nerve stimulation

Percutaneous endoscopic gastrostomy (PEG) tube transabdominal tube inserted into the stomach under endoscopic guidance

Percutaneous endoscopic jejunostomy (PEJ) tube tube that is passed through a PEG tube into the jejunum

Perineal care techniques used for cleansing the perineum

Periodontal disease condition that results in destruction of the tooth-supporting structures and jawbone

Perioperative care care that clients receive before, during, and after surgery

Peripheral parenteral nutrition isotonic or hypotonic intravenous nutrient solution instilled in a vein distant from the heart

Peristalsis rhythmic contractions of gastrointestinal smooth muscle

Peristomal skin skin around a stoma

PERRLA abbreviation that means *p*upils *e*qually *r*ound and *r*eact to *l*ight and *a*ccommodation

Personal protective equipment garments that block the transfer of pathogens from one person, place, or object to oneself or others

Personal space distance of 6 in to 4 ft

Petals strips of adhesive tape or moleskin applied to the rough edges of a cast for the purpose of reducing skin irritation

Phagocytosis process in which white blood cells consume cellular debris

Phlebitis inflammation of a vein

Photoperiod number of daylight hours

Phototherapy technique for suppressing melatonin by stimulating light receptors in the eye

Physical assessment systematic examination of body structures

Physical health when body organs function normally

Physical restraint method of immobilization that reduces the ability of a client to freely move his or her arms, legs, body, or head

PIE charting method of recording the client's progress under the headings of problem, intervention, and evaluation

Piloerection contraction of arrector pili muscles in skin follicles

Pin site location where pins, wires, or tongs enter or exit the skin

Placebo inactive substance or treatment measure that charades as one that is legitimate

Plaintiff person who claims injury

Planning process of prioritizing nursing diagnoses and collaborative problems, identifying measurable goals or outcomes, selecting appropriate interventions, and documenting the plan for care

Plaque substance composed of mucin and other gritty substances that deposits on teeth

Platform crutches crutches that support the forearm

Plume vaporized tissue, carbon, and water released during laser surgery

Plunger part of a syringe inside the barrel that moves back and forth to withdraw and instill medication

Pneumatic compression device machine that promotes circulation of venous blood and the movement of excess fluid into the lymphatic vessels

Pneumatic splints immobilizing devices that become rigid when filled with air; also called inflatable splints

Pneumonia lung infection

Podiatrist person with special training in caring for feet

Poisoning injury caused by the ingestion, inhalation, or absorption of a toxic substance

Polymorphonuclear leukocytes type of white blood cells called neutrophils that migrate to the area of tissue injury

Polypharmacy administration of multiple drugs to the same person

Polyuria larger-than-normal urinary volume

Port sealed opening

Portal of entry site where microorganisms find their way onto or into a host

Positive airway pressure machines devices that help to relieve impaired oxygen levels caused by apnea or hypopnea during sleep

Positron emission tomography radionuclide scanning with the layered analysis of tomography

Postanesthesia care unit area in the surgical department where clients are intensively monitored

Postmortem care care of the body after death

Postoperative care nursing care after surgery

Postoperative period interval that begins after surgery is completed

Postural drainage positioning technique that facilitates drainage of secretions from the lungs

Postural hypotension sudden but temporary drop in blood pressure when rising from a reclining or seated position

Posture position of the body, or the way in which it is held

Powered air-purifying respirator alternative device for a caregiver who has not been fitted with an N95 respirator; works by blowing atmospheric air through belt-mounted, air-purifying canisters to the facepiece via a flexible tube

Practicing performing an action repeatedly

Precipitate solid particles originally dissolved in liquid

Preferred provider organizations agents for health insurance companies that control health care costs on the basis of competition

Prefilled cartridge sealed glass cylinder of parenteral medication with a preattached needle

Preload volume of blood that fills the heart and stretches the heart muscle fibers during its resting phase

Preoperative checklist form that identifies the status of essential presurgical activities

Preoperative period time that starts when the client is informed that surgery is necessary and ends when he or she is transported to the operating room

Pressure ulcer wound caused by prolonged capillary compression sufficient to impair circulation to the skin and underlying tissue

Primary illness one that develops independently of any other disease

Primary nursing pattern in which the admitting nurse assumes responsibility for planning client care and evaluating the progress of the client

Primary prevention actions used to eliminate the potential for illness before it occurs

Problem-focused diagnosis a problem that currently exists

Problem-oriented records records organized according to the client's health problems

Progressive care units units for clients who were once in critical condition but have recovered sufficiently to require less-intensive nursing care

Progressive relaxation therapeutic exercise whereby a person actively contracts and then relaxes muscle groups

Projectile vomiting vomiting that occurs with great force

Proliferation period during which new cells fill and seal a wound

Prone position position in which the client lies on the abdomen

Prophylactic braces braces used to prevent or reduce the severity of a joint injury

Prospective payment system one that uses financial incentives to decrease total health care charges by reimbursing hospitals on a fixed rate basis

Prosthetic limb substitute for an arm or leg

Prosthetist person who constructs prosthetic limbs

Protein nutrient composed of amino acids; chemical compounds made up of nitrogen, carbon, hydrogen, and oxygen

Protein complementation combining plant sources of protein

Protocol plan or set of steps to follow when implementing an intervention

Proxemics relation of space to communication

Pseudoconfirmatory gurgling sound made when air enters the esophagus or small intestine causing a misinterpretation of a gastric location of a tube's tip

Psychomotor domain learning by doing

Public space distance of 12 ft or more

Pulmonary embolus blood clot that travels to the lung

Pulse wave-like sensation that can be palpated in a peripheral artery

Pulse deficit difference between the apical and radial pulse rates

Pulse oximetry noninvasive, transcutaneous technique for periodically or continuously monitoring the oxygen saturation of blood

Pulse pressure difference between systolic and diastolic blood pressure measurements

Pulse rate number of peripheral arterial pulsations palpated in a minute

Pulse rhythm pattern of the pulsations and pauses between them

Pulse volume quality of the pulsations that are felt

Pursed-lip breathing form of controlled ventilation in which the expiration phase of breathing is consciously prolonged

Purulent drainage white- or green-tinged fluid

Pyrexia fever

Q

Quadriceps setting isometric exercise in which a client alternately tenses and relaxes the quadriceps muscles

Quality assurance process of promoting care that reflects established agency standards

R

Race biologic variations

Radiography diagnostic procedures that use X-rays

Radionuclides elements whose molecular structures are altered to produce radiation

Range-of-motion exercises therapeutic activity in which joints are moved

Rebound effect swelling of the nasal mucosa within a short time of inhaled decongestant drug administration

Receiving evidence that a learner is attending to instruction

Receiving room presurgical holding area

Reciprocity licensure based on evidence of having met licensing criteria in another state

Reconstitution process of adding liquid to a powdered substance

Recording process of writing information

Recovery index guide for determining a person's fitness level

Recovery position side-lying position that helps to maintain an open airway and prevent aspiration of liquids

Rectus femoris site injection area in the anterior thigh

Referral process of sending someone to another person or agency for special services

Referred pain discomfort perceived in an area of the body away from the site of origin

Reframing an alternative thinking behavior that helps a person analyze a stressful situation from various perspectives and ultimately conclude that the situation is not as bad as it once seemed

Regeneration cell duplication

Regurgitation bringing stomach contents to the throat and mouth without the effort of vomiting

Rehabilitative braces braces that allow protected motion of an injured joint that has been treated surgically

Relationship association between two people

Relative humidity ratio between the amount of moisture in the air and the greatest amount of water vapor the air can hold at a given temperature

Relaxation technique for releasing muscle tension and quieting the mind

REM rebound sleep deviation of normal sleep cycle when REM is interrupted characterized by returning to REM earlier than usual and staying in REM longer

Remembering recalling information from prior learning

Remission disappearance of signs and symptoms associated with a particular disease

Remodeling period during which a wound undergoes changes and maturation

Repetitive strain injuries disorders that result from cumulative trauma to musculoskeletal structures

Rescue breathing process of ventilating a nonbreathing victim's lungs

Reservoir place where microbes grow and reproduce, providing a haven for sustaining microbial survival

Resident microorganisms generally nonpathogens that are constantly present on the skin

Residual urine urine that remains in the bladder after voiding

Resolution process by which damaged cells recover and reestablish their normal function

Respiration exchange of oxygen and carbon dioxide

Respiratory hygiene/cough etiquette infection control measures used when there are signs of illness suggesting an undiagnosed transmissible respiratory infection

Respiratory rate number of ventilations per minute

Respite care relief for a caregiver

Responding willingness to participate in learning

Rest waking state characterized by reduced activity and reduced mental stimulation

Restless legs syndrome movement, typically in the legs, but occasionally in the arms or other body parts, to relieve disturbing skin sensations

Restraint alternatives protective or adaptive devices that promote client safety and postural support, but which the client can release independently

Restraints devices or chemicals that restrict movement or access to one's body

Resuscitation team group of people trained and certified in advanced cardiac life support (ACLS) techniques

Retching act of vomiting without producing vomitus

Retention catheter urinary tube that is left in place for a period of time

Retention enema solution held temporarily in the large intestine

Reticular activating system area of the brain through which a network of nerves pass linking the body and the mind

Reversal drugs medications that counteract the effects of those used for conscious sedation

Rhizotomy surgical sectioning of a nerve root close to the spinal cord

Rinne test assessment technique for comparing air versus bone conduction of sound

Risk diagnosis a problem the client is uniquely at risk for developing

Risk management process of identifying and reducing the costs of anticipated losses

Roentgenography general term for procedures that use X-rays

Rounds visits to clients on an individual basis or as a group

Route of administration oral, topical, inhalant, or parenteral route where a drug is administered

S

Safe injection practices infection control measures that prevent the transmission of blood-borne pathogens through the use of aseptic techniques involving the preparation and administration of parenteral medications

Safety measures that prevent accidents or unintentional injuries

Saturated fats lipids that contain as much hydrogen as their molecular structure can hold

SBAR format model for effective communication identifying *s*ituation, *b*ackground, *a*ssessment, and *r*ecommendation

Scar formation replacement of damaged cells with fibrous tissue

Science body of knowledge unique to a particular subject

Scoop method technique for threading the needle of a syringe into the cap without touching the cap itself

Scored tablet tablet with a groove in its center

Second-intention healing reparative process when wound edges are widely separated

Secondary care health services to which primary caregivers refer clients for consultation and additional testing

Secondary illness disorder that develops from a preexisting condition

Secondary infusion administration of a diluted intravenous drug at the same time a solution is infusing, or intermittently with an infusing solution

Secondary prevention actions used to screen for risk factors that provide a means for early diagnosis of disease

Sedative drug that produces a relaxing and calming effect

Sensory manipulation using sensory stimuli to alter moods, feelings, and physiologic responses

Sepsis potentially fatal systemic infection

Sequelae consequences of a disease or its treatment

Serous drainage leaking plasma

Set point optimal body temperature

Shaft long portion of a needle

Shearing force exerted against the surface and layers of the skin as tissues slide in opposite but parallel directions

Shearing force effect that moves layers of tissue in opposite directions

Shell temperature warmth at the skin surface

Short-term goals outcomes that can be met in a few days to a week

Shroud covering for a dead body

Sigmoidoscopy visual endoscopic inspection limited to the sigmoid portion of the large intestine

Signs objective data; information that is observable and measurable

Silence intentionally withholding verbal comments

Simple mask device for administering oxygen that fits over the nose and mouth

Sims position lying on the left side with the chest leaning forward, the right knee bent toward the head, the right arm forward, and the left arm extended behind the body

Sitz bath soak of the perianal area

Skeletal traction pull exerted directly on the skeletal system by attaching wires, pins, or tongs into or through a bone

Skilled nursing facility nursing home that provides 24-hour nursing care under the direction of a registered nurse

Skin patches drugs that are bonded to an adhesive bandage

Skin tear shallow break in the skin

Skin traction pulling effect on the skeletal system by applying devices to the skin

Slander character attack uttered in the presence of others

Sleep state of arousable unconsciousness

Sleep apnea/hypopnea syndrome sleep disorder in which the sleeper stops breathing or the breathing slows for 10 seconds or longer, five or more times per hour

Sleep diary daily account of sleeping and waking activities

Sleep inertia feeling of incomplete awakening or grogginess as though still in a sleep state when a sleep cycle is interrupted

Sleep paralysis inability to move for a few minutes just before falling asleep or awakening

Sleep rituals habitual activities performed before retiring

Sleep–wake cycle disturbance condition that results from a sleep schedule that involves daytime sleeping

Sling cloth device used to elevate, cradle, and support parts of the body

Slough dead tissue on a wound surface that is moist, stringy, yellow tan, gray, or green

Smelling acuity ability to smell and identify odors

Snellen eye chart tool for assessing far vision

Soak procedure in which a part of the body is submerged in fluid

SOAP charting documentation style more likely to be used in a problem-oriented record

Social health feeling accepted and useful

Social space distance of 4 to 12 ft

Somatic pain discomfort generated from deeper connective tissue

Somnambulism sleepwalking

Sordes dried crusts around the mouth containing mucus, microorganisms, and epithelial cells shed from the oral mucous membrane

Source-oriented records records organized according to the source of information

Spacer chamber that is attached to an inhaler

Speaking valve device inserted into a tracheostomy tube that directs exhaled air through the upper airway allowing speech

Specimens samples of tissue or body fluids

Speculum metal or plastic instrument for widening the vagina or other body cavity

Sphygmomanometer device for measuring blood pressure

Spica cast rigid mold that encircles one or both arms or legs and the chest or trunk

Spinal tap procedure that involves insertion of a needle between lumbar vertebrae in the spine but below the spinal cord itself

Spiritual health the result of believing that one's life has purpose

Splint device that immobilizes and protects an injured part of the body

Spore temporarily inactive microbial life form

Sputum mucus raised to the level of the upper airways

Stage of exhaustion the last phase in the general adaptation syndrome that develops when one or more adaptive or resistive mechanisms can no longer protect a person experiencing a stressor

Stage of resistance second phase in the general adaptation syndrome characterized by physiologic changes designed to restore homeostasis

Standard precautions infection control measures for reducing the risk of transmission among all clients, regardless of suspected or confirmed infection status

Standards for care policies that ensure quality client care

Staples wide metal clips

Stasis lack of movement

Statute of limitations designated amount of time within which a person can file a lawsuit

Statutory laws laws enacted by federal, state, or local legislatures

Stent tube that keeps a channel open

Step test submaximal fitness test involving a timed stepping activity

Stepdown units units for clients who were once in critical condition but have recovered sufficiently to require less-intensive nursing care

Stereotypes fixed attitudes about all people who share a common characteristic

Sterile field work area free of microorganisms

Sterile technique practices that avoid contaminating microbe-free items

Sterilization physical and chemical techniques that destroy all microorganisms, including spores

Stertorous breathing noisy ventilation

Stethoscope instrument that carries sound to the ears

Stimulants drugs that excite structures in the brain

Stock supply drugs kept in a nursing unit for use in an emergency

Stoma entrance to a surgically created opening

Straight catheter urine drainage tube that is inserted but not left in place

Strength power to perform

Stress physiologic and behavioral reactions that occur in response to disequilibrium

Stress electrocardiogram test of electrical conduction through the heart during maximal activity

Stress management techniques therapeutic activities used to re-establish balance between the sympathetic and parasympathetic nervous systems

Stress-reduction techniques methods that promote physiologic comfort and emotional well-being

Stress-related disorders diseases that result from prolonged stimulation of the autonomic nervous and endocrine systems

Stressors changes that have the potential for disturbing equilibrium

Stridor harsh, high-pitched sound heard on inspiration when there is laryngeal obstruction

Stylet metal guidewire

Subcultures unique cultural groups that coexist among the dominant culture

Subcutaneous injection parenteral drug administration beneath the skin but above the muscle

Subdiaphragmatic thrust pressure to the abdomen

Subjective data information that only the client feels and can describe

Sublingual application placement of a drug under the tongue

Submaximal fitness test exercise test that does not stress a person to exhaustion

Substituted judgment court belief that a client would issue consent if he or she had the capacity to do so

Suctioning technique for removing liquid secretions with a catheter

Suffering emotional component of pain

Sump tubes tubes that contain a double lumen

Sundown syndrome onset of disorientation as the sun sets

Sunrise syndrome early morning confusion

Supine position position in which the person lies on the back

Suppository medicated oval- or cone-shaped mass

Surfactant lipoprotein produced by cells in the alveoli that promotes elasticity of the lungs and enhances gas diffusion

Surgical asepsis measures that render supplies and equipment totally free of microorganisms

Surgical hand antisepsis medically aseptic hand hygiene procedure that is performed prior to the nurse donning sterile gloves and garments in an operative or obstetric procedure

Surgical waiting area room where family and friends await information about the surgical client

Susceptible host one whose biologic defense mechanisms are weakened in some way

Sustained release drug that dissolves at timed intervals

Sutures knotted ties that hold an incision together

Sympathy feeling as emotionally distraught as the client

Symptoms subjective data; that which only the client can identify

Syndrome diagnosis cluster of problems that is present due to an event or situation

Systolic pressure pressure in the arterial system when the heart contracts

T

Tachycardia heart rate between 100 and 150 beats per minute (bpm) at rest

Tachypnea rapid respiratory rate

Tamponade controlling gastric bleeding with internal pressure via a tube

Target heart rate goal for heart rate during exercise

Tartar hardened plaque

Task-oriented touch personal contact that is required when performing nursing procedures

Teach-back method technique for confirming that a person has understood what has been taught by asking the person to repeat the information in his or her own words

Team nursing pattern in which nursing personnel divide the clients into groups and complete their care together

Telehealth services technology that facilitates the transmission of health assessment and monitoring data with audio, video, and internet-based devices

Telehome care visiting clients electronically in their homes for the purpose of seeing and communicating in real time

Telenursing health triage, or information through electronic or telephonic access

Teleology ethical theory based on final outcomes

Telephonic interpreting language translation via telephone

Temperature translation conversion of tympanic temperature into an oral, rectal, or core temperature

Temporal artery thermometer noninvasive device that scans body temperature in the temporal artery at the skin surface

Tension pneumothorax extreme air pressure in the lung when there is no avenue for its escape

Terminal disinfection measures used to clean the client environment after discharge

Terminal illness illness with no potential for cure

Terminating phase ending of a nurse–client relationship when there is mutual agreement that the client's immediate health problems have improved

Tertiary care health services provided at hospitals or medical centers that offer specialist and complex technology

Tertiary prevention actions that minimize the consequences of a disorder through aggressive rehabilitation or appropriate management of the disease

The Joint Commission a not-for-profit organization that accredits health care organizations in the United States

Theory opinion, belief, or view that explains a process

Therapeutic baths baths performed for other than hygiene purposes

Therapeutic exercise activity performed by people with health risks or those being treated for a health problem

Therapeutic relationship association between people whose objective is to achieve a higher state of health

Therapeutic verbal communication using words and gestures to accomplish a particular objective

Thermal burn skin injury caused by flames, hot liquids, or steam

Thermistor temperature sensor

Thermistor catheter heat-sensing device at the tip of an internally placed tube

Thermogenesis heat production

Thermoregulation ability to maintain stable body temperature

Third-intention healing reparative process when a wound is widely separated and later brought together with some type of closure material

Third-spacing movement of intravascular fluid to nonvascular fluid compartments, where it becomes trapped and useless

Thrombophlebitis inflammation of a vein caused by a thrombus

Thrombus stationary blood clot

Thrombus formation development of a stationary blood clot

Tidaling rhythmic rise and fall of water in a chest tube drainage system

Tilt table device that raises client from a supine to a standing position

Tip part of a syringe to which the needle is attached

Tone ability of muscles to respond when stimulated

Topical route drug administration to the skin or mucous membranes

Tort litigation in which one person asserts that an injury, which may be physical, emotional, or financial, occurred as a consequence of another's actions or failure to act

Total parenteral nutrition hypertonic solution of nutrients designed to meet almost all the caloric and nutritional needs of clients

Total quality improvement process of promoting care that reflects established agency standards

Touch tactile stimulus produced by making personal contact with another person or an object

Towel bath technique for bathing in which a single large towel is used to cover and wash a client

T-piece device that fits securely onto a tracheostomy tube or endotracheal tube

Tracheostomy surgically created opening into the trachea

Tracheostomy care hygiene and maintenance of a tracheostomy and tracheostomy tube

Tracheostomy collar device that delivers oxygen near an artificial opening in the neck

Tracheostomy tube curved, hollow plastic tube in the trachea

Traction pulling on a part of the skeletal system

Traction splints metal devices that immobilize and pull on muscles that are in a state of contraction

Trade name name by which a pharmaceutical company identifies its drug

Traditional time time based on two 12-hour revolutions on a clock

Training effect heart rate and consequently pulse rate become consistently lower than average with regular exercise

Tragus Skin-covered cartilage at the opening of the external ear

Tranquilizer drug that produce a relaxing and calming effect

Trans fats unsaturated, hydrogenated fats

Transabdominal tubes tubes placed through the abdominal wall

Transcultural nursing providing nursing care in the context of another's culture

Transcutaneous electrical nerve stimulation medically prescribed pain management technique that delivers bursts of electricity to the skin and underlying nerves

Transdermal application method of applying a drug on the skin and allowing it to become passively absorbed

Transducer instrument that receives and transmits biophysical energy

Transduction conversion of chemical information at the cellular level into electrical impulses that move toward the spinal cord

Transfer (1) discharging a client from one unit or agency and immediately admitting him or her to another; (2) moving a client from place to place

Transfer summary written review of the client's previous care

Transient microorganisms pathogens picked up during brief contact with contaminated reservoirs

Transitional care unit area for clients initially in a critical or unstable condition, but sufficiently recovered to require less intensive nursing care

Transmission phase during which stimuli move from the peripheral nervous system toward the brain

Transmission-based precautions measures for controlling the spread of highly transmissible or epidemiologically important infectious agents from clients when the known or suspected route(s) of transmission is (are) not completely interrupted using standard precautions alone

Transtracheal catheter hollow tube inserted into the trachea to deliver oxygen

Trauma injury

Triceps skinfold measurement data for estimating the amount of subcutaneous fat deposits

Tripod position seated position with the arms supported on pillows or the armrests of a chair

Truth telling ethical principle proposing that all clients have the right to receive complete and accurate information

Tuberculin syringe syringe that holds 1 mL of fluid and is calibrated in 0.01-mL increments

Turgor resiliency of the skin

Twenty-four-hour specimen collection of all the urine produced in a full 24-hour period

U

Ultrasonography soft tissue examination that uses sound waves in ranges beyond human hearing

Undermining erosion of tissue from underneath intact skin at a wound edge

Understanding evidence of learning that requires explaining ideas or concepts

Unintentional tort situation that results in an injury, although the person responsible did not mean to cause harm

Unit dose self-contained packet that holds one tablet or capsule

Universal protocol preoperative process to prevent surgery on wrong site, wrong procedure, wrong person

Unlicensed assistive personnel (UAP) perform tasks and duties assigned by RNs and/or LPN/LVNs for clients

Unoccupied bed changing the linen when the bed is empty

Unsaturated fats lipids that are missing some hydrogen

Urgency strong feeling that urine must be eliminated quickly

Urinal cylindrical container for collecting urine

Urinary diversion procedure in which one or both ureters are surgically implanted elsewhere

Urinary elimination process of releasing excess fluid and metabolic wastes

Urinary retention condition in which urine is produced but is not released from the bladder

Urine fluid in the bladder

Urostomy urinary diversion that discharges urine from an opening on the abdomen

V

Vacuum-assisted closure use of negative pressure to promote more rapid wound healing by using suction to pull fluid and debris from a wound bed through a foam filler into a collection canister; also known as negative pressure wound therapy

Valsalva maneuver act of closing the glottis and contracting the pelvic and abdominal muscles to increase abdominal pressure

Values ideals that a person believes are important

Valuing evidence that a learner accepts or is committed to acquired information

Vapotherm oxygen delivery system that uses a nasal cannula to deliver high-flow oxygen

Vasovagal response reflex that occurs when circulating blood is diverted to the legs rather than the head resulting in dizziness and fainting

Vastus lateralis site injection area in the outer thigh

Vegan person who relies exclusively on plant sources for protein

Vegetarian person who restricts consumption of animal food sources

Venipuncture accessing the venous system by piercing a vein with a needle

Ventilation (1) movement of air in and out of the lungs; (2) movement of air in the environment

Ventricular fibrillation life-threatening dysrhythmia in which the heart muscle quivers and cannot contract sufficiently to circulate blood

Ventrogluteal site injection area in the hip

Venturi mask oxygen delivery device that mixes a precise amount of oxygen and atmospheric air

Veracity the duty to be honest and avoid deceiving or misleading a client

Verbal communication communication that uses words

Vial glass or plastic container of parenteral medication with a self-sealing rubber stopper

Vibration type of chest physiotherapy used to loosen retained secretions

Viral load number of viral copies

Viral replication multiplication or copying of viruses

Virulence the ability to overcome the immune system and the person's state of health

Visceral pain discomfort arising from internal organs

Visual acuity ability to see both far and near

Visual field examination assessment of peripheral vision and continuity in the visual field

Vital signs body temperature, pulse rate, respiratory rate, and blood pressure

Vitamins chemical substances that are necessary in minute amounts for normal growth, maintenance of health, and functioning of the body

Voided specimen freshly urinated sample of urine

Voiding reflex spontaneous relaxation of the urinary sphincter in response to physical stimulation

Volumetric controller electronic infusion device that instills intravenous solutions by gravity

Vomiting loss of stomach contents through the mouth

Vomitus substance that is vomited

W

Waiting-for-permission phenomenon a terminally ill client's forestalling of death when he or she feels that loved ones are not yet prepared to deal with the client's death

Walk-a-mile test fitness test that measures the time it takes a person to walk a mile

Walker ambulatory aid constructed of curved aluminum bars that form a three-sided enclosure, with four legs for support

Walking belt safety device applied around the client's waist used to provide ambulatory support and assistance

Water-seal chest-tube drainage technique for evacuating air or blood from the pleural cavity

Water-soluble vitamins vitamins present and carried in body water; B complex and vitamin C

Weber test assessment technique for determining equality or disparity of bone-conducted sound

Wellness full and balanced integration of all aspects of health

Wellness diagnosis situation in which a healthy person obtains nursing assistance to maintain his or her health or perform at a higher level

Wheal elevated circle on the skin

Whistle-blowing reporting incompetent or unethical practices

White adipose tissue fat cells that provide heat insulation and cushioning of internal structures

White coat hypertension condition in which the blood pressure is elevated when taken by a health care worker but is normal at other times

Window square of plaster removed from a cast that provides an area for inspecting or treating underlying tissue

Working phase period during which the nurse and the client plan the client's care and put the plan into action

Wound damaged skin or soft tissue

X

Xerostomia dry mouth

Z

Z-track technique injection method that prevents medication from leaking outside the muscle

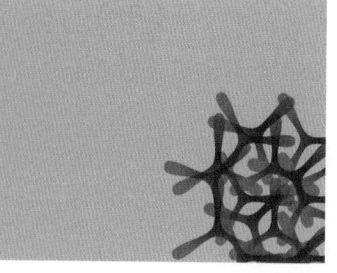

Index

Note: Page numbers followed by *f* indicate figures; those followed by *t* indicate tables; those followed by *b* indicate box and display text.

A

Abbreviations, in documentation, 114–115, 115*t*
Abdominal assessment, 233–235, 234*b*, 234*f*
Abdominal circumference, 279, 281*f*
Abdominal girth, 235, 235*f*
Abdominal quadrants, 233, 234*f*
Abnormal blood pressure measurement, 198–201, 198–199*t*, 199*f*, 201*b*
Abrasion, 226
Acceptance, in terminal illness, 826
Accommodation, 222, 223*b*
Accreditation, documentation in, 109
Acculturation, 74*b*
Acne, 336*t*
Active exercise, 514–515
Active listening, 90
  use of, 11
Active transport, 298, 298*f*
Activities of daily living (ADL), 11, 172*f*, 517–518*b*
Activity intolerance, 562–563*b*
Activity monitoring, 512, 512*t*
Acupressure, 423–424, 424*f*
Acupuncture, 423–424, 424*f*
Acute anxiety, 257*b*
Acute care, 828, 829*f*
Acute hypersensitivity, 392, 392*f*
Acute illness, 45
Acute pain, 414, 415*t*
  nursing care plan for, 426*b*
Adaptation
  physiologic, 55–58, 55*f*, 56*f*, 57*f* (*See also* Homeostasis)
  to stress, 58–62, 59*f*, 60*t*, 61*t*, 62*t*
Adaptation theory, 5*t*
Adenosine triphosphate (ATP), 298
Adipocytes, 181
Adjustable bed, 488, 488*f*
Adjuvant drugs, 420–421
Administrative laws. *See under* Law(s)
Admission, 158–164
  admitting department, 159, 159*f*
  client orientation in, 160
  client's personal items in, 160, 160*f*
  client undress, helping, 161
  client welcome in, 159–160, 160*f*
  defined, 158
  medical admission responsibilities, 161, 162*b*
  medical authorization, 159
  medications, reconciling, 161
  nursing admission activities, 159–161
  nursing data base, 161, 161*f*, 174–175*b*
  nursing plan for care, 161
  responses to
    altered health maintenance, 164
    anxiety, 162, 162–163*b*
    fear, 164
    self-esteem, 164
  room preparation in, 159, 159*b*
  types of, 158*t*
Admission assessment form, 17*f*
Adolescents, safety concerns for, 391
Adults, safety concerns for, 391, 393*t*
Advanced cardiac life-support (ACLS), 814
Advance directives, 38, 40*b*

Adventitious sounds, 230
Aerobic bacteria, 127
Aerobic exercise, 513, 514*f*
Aerosol, 744, 793, 795*f*
Afebrile, 188
Affective domain, in learning, 99
Affective touch, 92, 92*f*
African Americans, 70, 73
Afterload, 193
Against Medical advice (AMA), 164
Ageism, 68
Airborne precautions, 466*t*, 467, 467*f*
Air bubbles in IV tubing, 307, 312*b*
Air embolism, 309
Air-fluidized bed, 492*t*, 493, 493*f*
Air pressure mattress, static, 491
Airway
  anatomy of, 793, 794*f*
  definition of, 792
  occlusion, postoperative, 590*t*
  oral, 797, 798*b*, 798*f*
Airway management, 792–810
  anatomic aspects of, 793, 794*f*
  artificial, 796–800
  cardiopulmonary resuscitation in, 814–817, 815–817*f*, 815*t*
  chest physiotherapy in, 793
  client teaching, 795
Airway obstruction
  causes of, 812, 812*b*
  in infants, 812, 813*f*
  in people older than one year, 812–813, 813*f*
  relieving, 812 -813, 813*f*
  in resuscitation, 812*b*, 812–813, 812*f*
  signs of, 812, 812*b*, 812*f*
Airway opening, 816, 816*f*
Alarm stage of stress response, 59–60, 60*t*
Alcohol
  rubs, 133
  sleep and, 372
Alcohol dehydrogenase (ADH) deficiency, 78
Alginate dressings, 606–607
α-tocopherol, 276*t*
Altered breathing pattern, 745*b*
Altered health maintenance, 164
Altered tissue perfusion, 538*b*
Alternating air mattress, 492, 492*f*
Alternative activities in stress management, 64
Alternative medical therapy, 80*b*
Aluminum canes, 556, 557*b*
Alzheimer disease, 93
Ambulation, 556–560. *See also* Crutches
  assistive devices for, 555–556, 555*f*
    parallel bars, 555, 555*f*
    walking belt, 555, 555*f*
  lower limb prosthesis, 561, 562*f*
  nursing implications, 561, 562–563*b*
  preparation for
    dangling, 554, 554*b*, 554*f*
    exercises for, isometric, 553, 553*b*
    tilt table, 554, 555*f*
    upper arm strengthening, 553–554, 554*f*
  prosthetic limbs for, 560–561, 560–561*f*, 572–573*b*
  walkers, 556–558, 558*f*, 565–567*b*

Ambulatory aids
  canes, 556, 556*f*, 567*b*
  crutches, 558–559, 558*f*
  crutch-walking gaits, 559, 559–560*t*, 568–571*b*
Ambulatory electrocardiogram, 510–511, 511*f*
Ambulatory surgery, 577
American College of Cardiology, 270
American Congress of Obstetricians and Gynecologists (ACOG), 247
American Heart Association (AHA), 273
American Nurses Association (ANA), 6, 14, 486
American Pain Society, 415
American Red Cross, 312
American Sign Language (ASL), 93
American Society for Pain Management Nursing, 425
American Society of Anesthesiology's guidelines (2017), 584
Amino acids, 272
Ampules, 756, 757*b*
Amputation, 560
Anaerobic bacteria, 127
Anal sphincters, 693
Anecdotal record, 34–35
Aneroid manometer, 195, 195*f*, 196*t*
Anesthesia, 587–588
  for surgery, 579*t*, 587–588, 587*f*
  for test, 250
Anesthesiologist, 577
Anesthetist, 577
Anger, in terminal illness, 825–826
Anions, 297
Ankylosis, 515
Anorexia, 283, 284*b*
Anthropometric data, 279–281, 279*f*, 281*t*
Antianxiety drugs, 372, 585
Antibiotic drug resistance, causes of, 129*b*
Antibiotics, 585*b*
Anticholinergics, 585*b*
Anticipatory grieving, 833
Anticonvulsants, 420
Antidepressants, 420
Antiembolism stockings, 583, 595–597*b*
Anti-infective drugs, 132
Antimicrobial agents, 131–132, 132*t*
Antineoplastic drugs, 783, 783*f*
Antipyretics, 188
Antiseptics, 131
Anuria, 663
Anus, assessment of, 236, 236*f*
Anxiety, 162
  nursing care plan for, 162–163*b*
Apical heart rate, 191, 191*f*
Apical-radial rate, 191–192, 192*f*
Apnea, 193
Appliance, 702
Aquathermia pad, 615, 615*f*
Arm sling, 531, 532*f*, 540–542*b*
Arm strengthening exercises, 553–554, 554*f*
Arrhythmia, 190
Arterial blood gases (ABG), 436, 436*t*, 437*b*
Artifacts, 511
Artificial airway, 796–800
Ascorbic acid, 275*t*
Asepsis, 131–139. *See also* Microorganisms